The 5-Minute Neurology Consult

D. JOANNE LYNN, MD

ASSOCIATE PROFESSOR

DEPARTMENT OF NEUROLOGY

THE OHIO STATE UNIVERSITY COLLEGE OF

MEDICINE AND PUBLIC HEALTH

CO-DIRECTOR, MULTIPLE SCLEROSIS CENTER

THE OHIO STATE MEDICAL CENTER

COLUMBUS, OHIO

HERBERT B. NEWTON, MD, FAAN

ASSOCIATE PROFESSOR

DEPARTMENTS OF NEUROLOGY AND PEDIATRICS

THE OHIO STATE UNIVERSITY COLLEGE OF

MEDICINE AND PUBLIC HEALTH

DIRECTOR, DIVISION OF NEURO-ONCOLOGY

DEPARTMENT OF NEUROLOGY

THE OHIO STATE MEDICAL CENTER

DIRECTOR, DARDINGER NEURO-ONCOLOGY CENTER

JAMES CANCER HOSPITAL AND SOLOVE RESEARCH INSTITUTE

COLUMBUS, OHIO

ALEXANDER D. RAE-GRANT, MD, FRCP(C)

PRESIDENT, MEDICAL STAFF

DIVISION OF NEUROLOGY

DEPARTMENT OF MEDICINE

LEHIGH VALLEY HOSPITAL AND HEALTH NETWORK

ALLENTOWN, PENNSYLVANIA

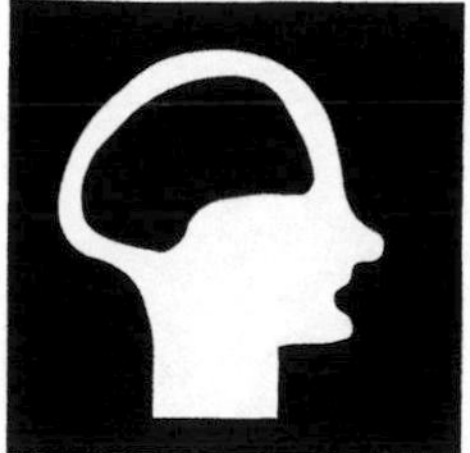
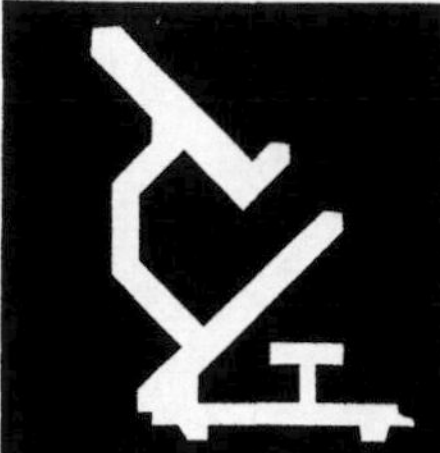
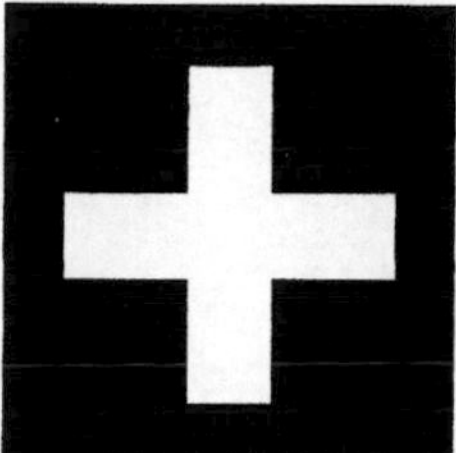
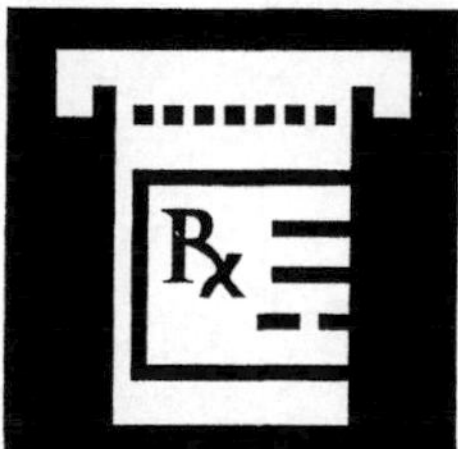

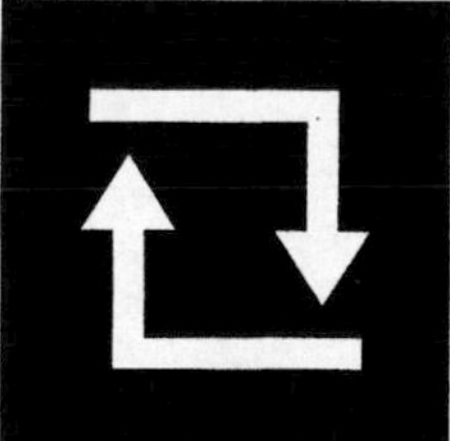
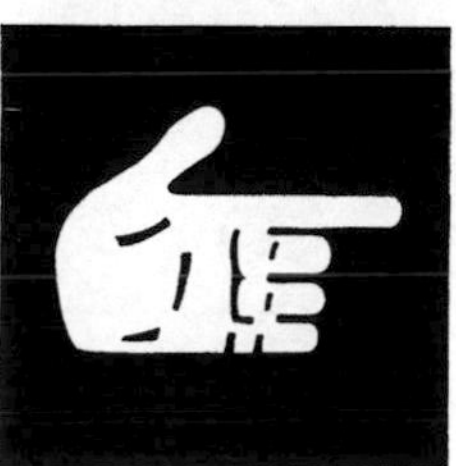

The 5-Minute Neurology Consult

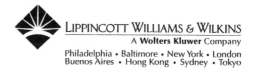
LIPPINCOTT WILLIAMS & WILKINS
A Wolters Kluwer Company
Philadelphia • Baltimore • New York • London
Buenos Aires • Hong Kong • Sydney • Tokyo

Acquisitions Editor: Charley Michell
Developmental Editor: Keith Donnellan
Production Manager: Toni Ann Scaramuzzo
Production Editor: Michael Mallard
Manufacturing Manager: Colin Warnock
Cover Designer: Christine Jenny
Compositor: TechBooks
Printer: Maple-Press

530 Walnut Street
Philadelphia, PA 19106 USA
LWW.com

ISBN-13: 978-0-683-30723-8
ISBN-10: 0-683-30723-1

Note: The contributions of Drs. Barner, Brugge, Campbell, Ferri, and Wicklund were performed outside the scope of their employment as U.S. government employees. Their work represents their personal and professional views and not necessarily those of the U.S. government.

Printed in the USA

10 9 8 7 6 5 4 3

To all of my patients, students and others who bring inspiration and grace into my life (including Drs. Kottil Rammohan, John Stang, Ralph Józefowicz, John Kissel, Miriam Freimer, Sheryl Pfeil, and Jerry Mendell) and, most of all, to my daughters Kate and Patty who are not always patient, but who never fail to bring the blessing of love to each of my days.

D. J. L.

To my wife, Cheryl, and my children, Alex and Ashley, for their love, support, and patience. In addition, I'd like to thank all of my neuro-oncology patients for the inspiration they have given me.

H.B.N

To my wife, Mary Bruce, and my four children Michael, Tucker, George and Sasha, for being patient with their father. Thanks to Dr. Lawrence Levitt for encouraging my interest in neurological education.

A.D.R-G.

Contents

SECTION IV: SHORT TOPICS / 445

Contributors

MOHAMMED I. AKHTAR, MD
Consultant Neurologist
Southern Ohio Medical Center
Portsmouth, Ohio

JAMES W. ALBERS, MD, PHD
Professor
Department of Neurology
University of Michigan
Director, EMG Laboratory
University of Michigan Health System
Ann Arbor, Michigan

ROULA AL-DAHHAK, MD
Fellow, Department of Neurology
The Ohio State University
College of Medicine and Public Health
Columbus, Ohio

MONIQUE A. ANAWIS, MD, JD
Clinical Instructor
Department of Ophthalmology
The Chicago Medical School
Director of Ophthalmology Teaching
Department of Medicine
Weiss Memorial Hospital/University of Chicago Hospital
Chicago, Illinois

RUSSELL J. ANDREWS, MD
Ames Associate
NASA Ames Research Center
Moffett Field, California

MIRIAM ANIXTER, MD
Department of Anesthesiology
The University of Pittsburgh School of Medicine
Pittsburgh, Pennsylvania

RAJU S.V. BALABHADRA, MD
Department of Neurosurgery
Stanford School of Medicine
Stanford, California

PETER J. BARBOUR, MD
Clinical Associate Professor of Medicine
Department of Medicine
College of Medicine of Pennsylvania State University
Hershey, Pennsylvania
Medical Director, Parkinson's Disease
Movement Disorder Program
Good Shepard Outpatient Rehabilitation
Division of Neurology
Lehigh Valley Hospital
Allentown, Pennsylvania

KRISTEN C. BARNER, MD
MAJ, MC, USA
Department of Neurology
Walter Reed Army Medical Center
Washington, D.C.

RONNIE BERGEN, MD
Assistant Professor of Clinical Neurology
Department of Neurology
Arizona Health Sciences Center and
University Medical Center
Tucson, Arizona

XABIER BERISTAIN, MD
Assistant Professor of Neurology
Department of Neurology
School of Medicine
Indiana University-Purdue University Indianapolis
Indianapolis, Indiana

FRANCOIS BETHOUX, MD
Associate Staff
Department of Neurology
Department of Physical Medicine and Rehabilitation
The Cleveland Clinic
Cleveland, Ohio

DAVID BEVERSDORF, MD
Assistant Professor of Cognitive Neurology
Department of Neurology
The Ohio State University College of Medicine and Public Health
Columbus, Ohio

MARK BORSODY, MD, PHD
Department of Neurology
Northwestern Memorial Hospital
Chicago, Illinois

ERIC C. BOUREKAS, MD
Associate Professor of Radiology
Section of Diagnostic and Interventional Neuroradiology
The Ohio State University College of Medicine and Public Health
Columbus, Ohio

BARBARA BRANDOM, MD
Professor, Department of Anesthesiology
The University of Pittsburgh School of Medicine
Department of Anesthesiology
Children's Hospital
Pittsburgh, Pennsylvania

DANIEL BROWN, MD
Vice Chairperson, Department of Pathology
Lehigh Valley Hospital
Allentown, Pennsylvania

KAREN L. BRUGGE, MD
Medical Officer
Psychiatric Drug Products Group
Division of Neuropharmacological Drug Products
Center for Drug Evaluation and Research
Food and Drug Administration
Rockville, Maryland

RICHARD E. BURGESS, MD, PHD
Department of Neurology
Barnes-Jewish Hospital/Washington University
St. Louis, Missouri

PETER A. CALABRESI, MD
Associate Professor
Department of Neurology
Director, Neuroimmunology and Multiple Sclerosis Center
Johns Hopkins Hospital
Baltimore, Maryland

WILLIAM W. CAMPBELL, MD, MSHA
LTC, MC, USAR
Department of Neurology
Walter Reed Army Medical Center
Washington, D.C.

JOHN CASTALDO, MD
Professor of Clinical Medicine
Lehigh Valley Hospital and Health Network
Allentown, Pennsylvania

ROBERT CAVALIERE, MD
Instructor, Department of Neurology
Staff Physician
Neurology Services
University of Virginia Health System
Charlottesville, Virginia

THOMAS C. CHELIMSKY, MD
Assistant Professor
Department of Neurology
Case Western Reserve University
Director, University Pain Center and Autonomic Laboratory
University Hospitals of Cleveland
Cleveland, Ohio

GREGORY CHRISTOFORIDES, MD
Associate Professor of Radiology
Section of Diagnostic and Interventional Neuroradiology
The Ohio State University College of Medicine and Public Health
Columbus, Ohio

JAMES C. CLELAND, MBCHB
Fellow, Neuromuscular Diseases
Department of Neurology
University of Rochester
Rochester, New York

BRADLEY COLE, MD
Staff Neurologist
Beaver Medical Group, Redlands Community Hospital
Loma Linda University
Loma Linda, California

DOROTHEE COLE, MD
Assistant Professor
Department of Neurology
Loma Linda University
Loma Linda, California

TODD CZARTOSKI, MD
Fellow, Department of Neurology
University of Washington Medical Center
Seattle, Washington

KAY E. DAVIES, MA, DPHIL, CBE
Professor, Department of Human Anatomy and Genetics
University of Oxford
Oxford, United Kingdom

DR. PETER PAUL DEDEYN
A.Z. Middelheim Hospital
Antwerp, Belgium

ROBERT L. DODD, MD, PHD
Department of Neurosurgery
Stanford University
Department of Neurosurgery
Stanford University Medical Center
Stanford, California

SAMUEL DZODZOMENYO, MD
Medical Staff
Neurology Section
Columbus Children's Hospital
Columbus, Ohio

LAWRENCE W. ELMER, MD, PHD
Assistant Professor of Neurology
Director, Parkinson's Disease and Movement Disorders Program
Movement Disorders Clinic
Department of Neuroscience
Medical College of Ohio
Toledo, Ohio

SAID ELSHIHABI, MD
Department of Neurosurgery
University of Arkansas for Medical Sciences
Little Rock, Arkansas

SCOTT ELTON, MD
Surgical Staff
Division of Neurosurgery
The Ohio State University Medical Center
Columbus, Ohio

SEVIM ERDEM, MD
Assistant Professor
Department of Neurology
Hacettepe University
Ankara, Turkey

DORUK ERKAN, MD
Assistant Attending Physician
Division of Rheumatology
Hospital for Special Surgery, Weill Medical College of Cornell University
New York, New York

RANDOLPH W. EVANS, MD
Chief, Neurology Section
Park Plaza Hospital
Houston, Texas

ROBERT G. FELDMAN, MD (*DECEASED*)
Professor

Department of Neurology
Boston University School of Medicine
Boston, Massachusetts

MAGALI FERNANDEZ, MD
Assistant Professor of Medicine
Deptartment of Medicine
Division of Human Genetics
The Ohio State University College of Medicine and Public Health
Columbus, Ohio

RAYMOND FERRI, MD
National Institues of Health
Bethesda, Maryland

ROBERT J. FOX, MD
Department of Neurology
Cleveland Clinic Foundation
Cleveland, Ohio

MIRIAM L. FREIMER, MD
Assistant Professor
Director, Electromyography Laboratory
Department of Neurology
The Ohio State University College of Medicine and Public Health
Columbus, Ohio

ELLIOT M. FROHMAN, MD, PHD
Director, Mutiple Sclerosis Program
Assistant Professor,
Department of Neurology and Opthamology
University of Texas Southwestern Medical Center
Dallas, Texas

DAVID H. GARABRANT, MD, MPH
Professor of Occupational Medicine
Department of Environmental Health Sciences
School of Public Health
University of Michigan
Associate Professor of Occupational Medicine
Department of Internal Medicine
University of Michigan Health System
Ann Arbor, Michigan

JOSEPH GASTALDO, MD
Department of Infectious Diseases
Riverside Methodist Hosptial
Columbus, Ohio

DANIEL W. GIANG, MD
Associate Professor
Chief, Neurology Service
Neurology Department
Loma Linda University
Loma Linda, California

MARK R. GIBSON, MD
Department of Neurology
Mayo Clinic
Rochester, Minnesota

BARBARA S. GIESSER, MD
Associate Professor of Clinical Neurology
Department of Neurology
UCLA School of Medicine
Reed Neurological Research Center
Los Angeles, California

STEPHEN J. GOMEZ, MD
Resident Neurologist
Department of Neurology
Vanderbilt University Medical Center
Nashville, Tennessee

PATRICK M. GROGAN, MD
Department of Neurology
Stanford University
Palo Alto, California

KEVIN V. HACKSHAW, MD
Associate Professor of Internal Medicine
Division of Immunology/Rheumatology and Allergy
The Ohio State University College of
Medicine and Public Health
Columbus, Ohio

JULIE E. HAMMACK, MD
Department of Neurology
Mayo Clinic
Rochester, Minnesota

SUSAN L. HICKENBOTTOM, MD
Clinical Assistant Professor
Director, Stroke Program
Department of Neurology
University of Michigan
Ann Arbor, Michigan

DONALD HIGGINS JR., MD
Associate Professor
The Neuroscience Institute
Albany Medical College
Albany, New York

BRIAN E. HIGGINS, DO
Medical Director, Interventional Spine Pain
Physical Medicine and Rehabilitation Spine,
Sports and Industrial Rehabilitation
Lancaster, Ohio

HOLLI HORAK, MD
Assistant Professor of Neurology
University Hospital
Department of Neurology
Indiana University School of Medicine
Indianapolis, Indiana

YIQUN HU, MD
Assistant Professor
Department of Neurology
The Ohio State University College of
Medicine and Public Health
Columbus, Ohio

SAFWAN S. JARADEH, MD
Chairman and Professor
Department of Neurology
Medical College of Wisconsin
Milwaukee, Wisconsin

ROBERT WALTER JENSEN, MD, JD, FCLM
Assistant Professor of Neurology, Otoneurology,
and Neuro-Ophthalmology
Department of Neurology
The Ohio State University College of Medicine and Public Health
Columbus, Ohio

H. A. JINNAH, MD, PHD
Assistant Professor of Neurology
Department of Neurology
The Johns Hopkins Hospital
Baltimore, Maryland

S. ANNE JOSEPH, MD
Assistant Clinical Professor of Neurology
Division of Pediatric Neurology
Department of Neurology
Medical College of Wisconsin
Milwaukee, Wisconsin

VERN JUEL, MD
Associate Professor of Neurology
Student Clerkship Director
Department of Neurology
University of Virginia Health System
Charlottesville, Virginia

STEPHEN E. KATZ, MD
Associate Professor of Ophthalmology
William H. Havener Eye Center
The Ohio State University College of Medicine and Public Health
Columbus, Ohio

JONATHAN S. KATZ, MD
Assistant Professor
Department of Neurology and Neurological Sciences
Stanford University
Palo Alto, California

THOMAS C. KEELING, MD
Department of Infectious Diseases
Grant Medical Center
Columbus, Ohio

ANDREW KIRK, MD, FRCP(C)
Division of Neurology
University of Saskatchewan
Royal University Hospital
Saskatoon, Saskatchewan, Canada

JAWAD F. KIRMANI, MD
Department of Neurology
The Ohio State University College of Medicine and Public Health
Columbus, Ohio

JOHN KISSEL, MD
Professor of Neurology
Department of Neurology
The Ohio State University College of Medicine and Public Health
Columbus, Ohio

EMILY KLATTE, MD
Department of Neurology
The Ohio State University College of Medicine and Public Health
Columbus, Ohio

JENNIFER L. KLAUS, MD
Division of Infectious Diseases
Department of Internal Medicine
The Ohio State University College of Medicine and Public Health
Columbus, Ohio

BOYD M. KOFFMAN, MD, PHD
Assistant Professor of Neurology
Department of Neurology
Medical College of Ohio
Toledo, Ohio

SUSAN L. KOLETAR, MD
Professor of Clinical Internal Medicine
Fellowship Program Director
Division of Infectious Diseases
Department of Internal Medicine
The Ohio State University College of Medicine and Public Health
Columbus, Ohio

GORDON J. KORBY, DC, DO
Private Practice - Physical Medicine and Rehabilitation
Spine, Sports and Industrial Rehabilitation
Medical Director, Musculoskeletal and Integrative Pain Medicine
Columbus, Ohio

SANDRA K. KOSTYK, MD, PHD
Assistant Professor of Neurology
Department of Neurology
The Ohio State University College of Medicine and Public Health
Columbus, Ohio

GARY KRAUS, MD
Neurosurgeon
Kettering Medical Center
Kettering, Ohio

LAURA KRIETMEYER, MD
Department of Neurology
The Ohio State University College of Medicine and Public Health
Columbus, Ohio

ALI F. KRISHT, MD
Associate Professor of Neurosurgery
Director of Neuroendocrine Clinic
University of Arkansas for Medical Sciences
Neuroendocrine Clinic
Little Rock, Arkansas

ROGER KURLAN, MD
Professor of Neurology
Unit Chief, Cognitive and Behavioral Neurology
Department of Neurology
University of Rochester Medical Center
Rochester, New York

JEFFREY S. KUTCHER, MD, MPH
Resident Physician
Department of Neurology
University of Michigan
Ann Arbor, Michigan

THOMAS D. LAMARRE JR., MD
Division of Infectious Diseases
Department of Internal Medicine
Cincinnati, Ohio

JAMES LAMB, MD
Associate Professor
Department of General Internal Medicine
The Ohio State University College of Medicine and Public Health
Department of Internal Medicine
The Ohio State University Medical Center
Columbus, Ohio

MANFRED LANGE, MD
Vice-Chief, Department of Neurosurgery
Academic Hospital of the University of Freiburg
Vice-Chief, Department of Neurosurgery
Klinikum VS-Schwenningen
VS-Schwenningen, Germany

BETH LEEMAN, MD, PHD
Department of Neurology
School of Medicine
Washington University in St. Louis
St. Louis, Missouri

LAWRENCE P. LEVITT, MD
Professor of Clinical Medicine
Lehigh Valley Hospital and Health Network
Allentown, Pennsylvania

JUN LI, MD, PHD
Assistant Professor of Neurology
Department of Neurology
Wayne State University
Detroit,Michigan

P. MARK LI, MD, PHD
Chief, Division of Neurological Surgery
Neurosurgical Associates of Lehigh Valley Physician Group
Allentown, Pennsylvania

YELENA LINDENBAUM, MD
Assistant Professor of Clinical Neurology
Division of Neuromuscular Diseases
Columbia University
New York, New York

BRIAN W. LITTLE, MD, PHD
Assistant Professor
Department of Pathology
Thomas Jefferson University
Philadelphia, Pennsylvania
Vice President, Academic Affairs and Research
Christiana Care Health Services
Wilmington, Delaware

ERIC L. LOGIGIAN, MD
Professor of Neurology
Department of Neurology
University of Rochester Medical Center
Director, EMG Laboratory
Department of Neurology
Strong Memorial Hospital
Rochester, New York

D. JOANNE LYNN, MD
Associate Professor
Department of Neurology
The Ohio State University College of Medicine and Public Health
Co-Director, Multiple Sclerosis Center
The Ohio State Medical Center
Columbus, Ohio

DAUNE L. MACGREGOR, MD, FRCPC
Fellow, Department of Paediatrics
Division of Neurology
The Hospital for Sick Children
University of Toronto
Toronto, Ontario, Canada

GLENN A. MACKIN, MD
Department of Neurology
Lehigh Valley Hospital and Health Network
Allentown, Pennsylvania

KAZI IMRAN MAJEED, MD
Consulting Staff
Neurology Consultants P.C.
Genesis Medical Center of Davenport
Davenport, Iowa

JULIE E. MANGINO, MD
Associate Professor of Clinical Internal Medicine
Division of Infectious Diseases
Department of Internal Medicine
The Ohio State University Medical Center
Columbus, Ohio

BERNARD L. MARIA, MD, MBA
Professor and Chairman
Department of Child Health
Pediatrician-in-Chief of Children's Hospital
University of Missouri Health Sciences Center
Columbia, Missouri

CHRISTINA M. MARRA, MD
Professor
Neurology and Medicine
Division of Allergy and Infectious Diseases
Department of Neurology
University of Washington Medical Center
Seattle, Washington

ALEXANDER M. MASON, MD
Appointed Assistant Professor
Departments of Neurology and Pediatrics
University of Pennsylvania School of Medicine
Philadelphia, Pennsylvania

CHARLES C. MATOUK, MD
Resident, Division of Neurosurgery
University of Toronto
Toronto, Ontario, Canada

PATRICK MCDONALD MD, FRCSC
Assistant Professor, Section of Neurosurgery
University of Manitoba
Pediatric Neurosurgeon, Winnipeg Children's Hospital
Winnipeg, Manitoba, Canada

JOHN MCGREGOR, MD
Assistant Professor of Surgery
Division of Neurological Surgery
The Ohio State University College of Medicine and Public Health
Columbus, Ohio

JAMES A. MCHALE, MD
William H. Havener Eye Center
The Ohio State University College of
Medicine and Public Health
Columbus, Ohio

THOMAS J. MEHELAS, MD
Associate Professor
Chief, Division of Opthamology
Department of Surgery
Medical College of Ohio
Toledo, Ohio

CHRIS MELTON, MD
Assistant Professor
Department of Emergency Medicine
University of Arkansas for Medical Sciences
Little Rock, Arkansas

LAWRENCE MERVIS, MD (*DECEASED*)
Department of Neurology
The Ohio State University College of Medicine and Public Health
Columbus, Ohio

MICHAEL MINER, MD, PHD
Director, Division of Neurosurgery (Retired)
The Ohio State University College of Medicine and Public Health
Columbus, Ohio

YOUSEF MOHAMMAD, MD, MSC
Assistant Professor of Neurology
Department of Neurology
The Ohio State University College of Medicine and Public Health
Columbus, Ohio

J. LAYNE MOORE, MD
Assistant Professor of Clinical Neurology
Co-director, Comprehensive Epilepsy Program
Department of Neurology
The Ohio State University College of Medicine and Public Health
Columbus, Ohio

PAUL L. MOOTS, MD
Associate Professor of Neurology
Department of Neurology
Vanderbilt University Medical Center
Nashville, Tennessee

RUTH MULLOWNEY-AGRA, MD
Fellow, Division of Infectious Disease
The Ohio State University College of Medicine and Public Health
Fellow, Department of Infectious Disease
The Ohio State University Medical Center
Columbus, Ohio

MARIE A. NAMEY, RN, MSN
The Mellon Center for Multiple Sclerosis Treatment and Research
Cleveland Clinic Foundation
Cleveland, Ohio

STEVEN NASH, MD
Assistant Professor of Clinical Neurology
Department of Neurology
The Ohio State University College of Medicine and Public Health
Columbus, Ohio

HERBERT B. NEWTON, MD, FAAN
Associate Professor
Departments of Neurology and Pediatrics
The Ohio State University College of Medicine and Public Health
Director, Division of Neuro-Oncology
Department of Neurology
The Ohio State Medical Center
Director, Dardinger Neuro-Oncology Center
James Cancer Hospital and Solove Research Institute
Columbus, Ohio

VERA NOVAK, MD, PHD
Assistant Professor
Department of Neurology
Harvard Medical School
Cambridge, Massachusetts

W. JERRY OAKES, MD
Professor and Chief
Division of Pediatric Neurosurgery
Children's Hospital of Alabama
Birmingham, Alabama

RUSSELL C. PACKARD, MD, FACP
Professor of Neurology and Neuropsychiatry
Department of Neuropsychiatry and Behavioral Science, Texas Tech University
Health Sciences Center
Lubbock, Texas

STEVEN A. PAGET, MD
Physician-in-Chief and Chairman of the Division of Rheumatology
Hospital for Special Surgery
New York, New York

DONNA PALUMBO, PHD
Associate Professor of Neurology and Pediatrics
Department of Neurology
University of Rochester Medical Center
Rochester, New York

JULIANN M. PAOLICCHI, MD
Director, Comprehensive Epilepsy Center
Department of Neurology
Columbus Children's Hospital
Columbus, Ohio

STEVEN G. PAVLAKIS, MD
Clinical Associate Professor
Developmental Medicine and Child Neurology
Maimonides Medical Center
Brooklyn, New York

ISABEL PERIQUET, MD
Department of Neurology
The Ohio State University College of Medicine and Public Health
Columbus, Ohio

NOOR A. PIRZADA, MD
Assistant Professor
Department of Neurology
Medical College of Ohio
Medical College Hospital
Toledo, Ohio

CHARLES P. POLLAK, MD
Associate Professor, Sleep Disorders
Department of Neurology
Weill Cornell Medical College
Cornell University
Ithaca, New York

J. NED PRUITT II, MD
Assistant Professor of Neurology
Department of Neurology
Medical College of Georgia
Augusta, Georgia

NIALL P. QUINN
Professor of Clinical Neurology
Sobell Department of Motor Neuroscience and Movement Disorders
Institute of Neurology
Honorary Consultant Neurologist

National Hospital for Neurology and Neurosurgery
London, United Kingdom

ALEXANDER D. RAE-GRANT, MD, FRCP(C)
President, Medical Staff
Division of Neurology
Department of Medicine
Lehigh Valley Hospital and Health Network
Allentown, Pennsylvania

SUBHA V. RAMAN, MD
Division of Cardiology
The Ohio State University College of Medicine and Public Health
Columbus, Ohio

KOTTIL W. RAMMOHAN, MD
Professor of Neurology
Department of Neurology
The Ohio State University College of Medicine and Public Health
Columbus, Ohio

MARCIA H. RATNER, PHD
Departments of Neurology, and Pharmacology and Experimental Therapeutics
Boston University School of Medicine
Boston, Massachusetts

GARY L. REA, MD, PHD
Neurosurgeon
Division of Neurosurgery
The Ohio State University College of Medicine and Public Health
Columbus, Ohio

BERND F. REMLER, MD
Associate Professor of Neurology and Ophthalmology
Departments of Neurology and Ophthalmology
Medical College of Wisconsin, Milwaukee
Froedtert Memorial Lutheran Hospital, Milwaukee
Milwaukee, Wisconsin

DEBORAH L. RENAUD, MD
Mayo Clinic
Department of Pediatric and Adolescent Medicine
Rochester, Minnesota

SARAH M. RODDY, MD
Associate Professor
Department of Pediatrics and Neurology
Loma Linda University
Department of Pediatrics
Loma Linda University Children's Hospital
Loma Linda, California

STEPHEN I. RYU, MD
Departments of Neurosurgery
Stanford University and Stanford University Medical Center
Stanford, California

RICHARD L. SABINA, PHD
Associate Professor
Department of Biochemistry
Medical College of Wisconsin
Milwaukee, Wisconsin

ZARIFE SAHENK, MD, PHD
Professor of Neurology
Department of Neurology
The Ohio State University College of Medicine and Public Health
Columbus, Ohio

RADU V. SAVEANU, MD
Chair, Department of Psychiatry
Neuropsychiatric Facility
The Ohio State University College of Medicine and Public Health
Columbus, Ohio

STEPHEN F. SCHAAL, MD
Division of Cardiology
The Ohio State University College of Medicine and Public Health
Columbus, Ohio

DOUGLAS W. SCHARRE, MD
Assistant Clinical Professor
Departments of Neurology and Psychiatry
The Ohio State University College of Medicine and Public Health
Director, Division of Cognitive Neurology
Department of Neurology
The Ohio State University Medical Center
Columbus, Ohio

CARMEN SERRANO-MUNUERA, MD
Visiting Scholar
Fellow in Neuromuscular Diseases
Department of Neurology
The Ohio State University College of Medicine and Public Health
Columbus, Ohio

JAMES SHARPE, MD
Senior Scientist
Division of Applied and Interventional Research
Toronto Western Research Institute
University of Toronto
Toronto, Ontario, Canada

LORI SHUTTER, MD
Director of Neurorehabilitation
Department of Neurology
Loma Linda University
Loma Linda, California

JOSEPH I. SIRVEN, MD
Department of Neurology
Mayo Clinic
Scottsdale, Arizona

ANDREW SLIVKA, MD
Associate Professor
Department of Neurology
The Ohio State University College of Medicine and Public Health
Department of Neurology
The Ohio State University Medical Center
Columbus, Ohio

H. WAYNE SLONE, MD
Associate Professor
Department of Radiology
The Ohio State University College of Medicine and Public Health
Columbus, Ohio

TERESA L. SMITH, MD
Department of Neurology
University of Virginia
Charlottesville, Virginia

LORRAINE SPIKOL, MD
Assistant Professor
Department of Medicine
Milton S. Hershey Medical Center
Hershey, Pennsylvania
Associate Chief
Department of Neurology
Lehigh Valley Hospital
Allentown, Pennsylvania

STACY STATLER, PA-C
Lehigh Neurology
Lehigh Valley Hospital
Allentown, Pennsylvania

GARY K. STEINBERG, MD, PHD
Chair, Neurosurgery
Lacroute-Hearst Professor
Stanford University Medical Center
Palo Alto, California

LAEL STONE, MD
Staff Neurologist, Mellen Center
Mellen Center for Multiple Sclerosis Treatment and Research
Department of Neurology
The Cleveland Clinic Foundation
Cleveland, Ohio

KEVIN TALBOT, MD, DPHIL
Honorary Consultant Neurologist
University Department of Clinical Neurology
MRC/GlaxoSmithKline Clinician Scientist
Honorary Consultant Neurologist
Radcliffe Infirmary
Oxford, United Kingdom

ERSIN TAN, MD
Associate Professor
Department of Neurology
Hacettepe University and Haceteepe University Hospitals
Ankara, Turkey

RABI TAWIL, MD
Associate Professor of Neurology
Director, Muscle and Nerve Pathology Lab
Co-Director, Neuromuscular Disease Clinic
Neuromuscular Disease Center Unit
Department of Neurology
University of Rochester Medical Center
Rochester, New York

ROBERT M. TAYLOR, MD
Mount Carmel Hospice
Columbus, Ohio

KAREN M. THOMAS, DO
Madden/National Parkinson Foundation Center of Excellence
The Ohio State University Medical Center
Columbus, Ohio

GRETCHEN TIETJEN, MD
Associate Professor
Chair, Department of Neurosciences
Medical College of Ohio
Toledo, Ohio

EVELINE C. TRAEGER, MD
Assistant Professor
Department of Pediatrics
Robert Wood Johnson Medical School
New Brunswick, New Jersey

CHANG-YONG TSAO, MD, FAAN, FAAP
Clinical Professor
Department of Pediatrics
The Ohio State University College of Medicine and Public Health
Child Neurologist
Department of Pediatrics
Columbus Children's Hospital
Columbus, Ohio

R. SHANE TUBBS, MS, PA-C, PHD
Assistant Professor of Neurosurgery
Pediatric Neurosurgery
Children's Hospital Birmingham
Birmingham, Alabama

TARVEZ TUCKER, MD
Associate Professor
University Hospitals of Cleveland
Cleveland, Ohio

ALLAN TUNKEL, MD
Pathway Director and Site Coordinator:
Department of Medicine
Drexel University College of Medicine
Philadelphia, Pennsylvania

ROXANNE VALENTINO MD
Senior Resident Physician
Department of Neurology
Cleveland Clinic Foundation
Cleveland, Ohio

AKILA VENKATARAMAN, MD
Department of Developmental Medicine and Child Neurology
Maimondes Medical Center
Brooklyn, New York

AMIR VOKSHOOR, MD
Staff, Department of Neurosurgery
Woodland Hills Medical Center
Woodland Hills, California

PAUL G. WASIELEWSKI, MD
Senior Staff Neurologist
Division of Movement Disorders
Department of Neurology
Henry Ford Hospital
Detroit, Michigan

MATTHEW WICKLUND, MD, LT COL, USAF, MC
Chairman and Program Director
Department of Neurology
San Antonio Uniformed Services Health Education Consortium
Neurology Flight Commander
Department of Neurology
Wilford Hall Medical Center
Lackland AFB, Texas

ADRIAN J. WILLS, MD
Consultant Neurologist

Department of Neurology
Queens Medical Centre
Nottingham, United Kingdom

JOANNE M. WOJCIESZEK, MD
Associate Professor of Neurology
Movement Disorders Program
Department of Neurology
Indiana University School of Medicine
Indianapolis, Indiana

R. THEODORE WOODRUFF
Department of Neurology
The Ohio State University College of Medicine and Public Health
Columbus, Ohio

BRADFORD BURKE WORRALL, MD, MSC
Department of Neurology
The Stroke Center
University of Virginia
Charlottesville, Virginia

ABUTAHER M. YAHIA, MD
Associate Professor
Neurocritical Care Stroke Unit Director
Department of Neurosciences
New Jersey Medical School
Newark, New Jersey

G. BRYAN YOUNG, MD, FRCPC
Professor of Neurology
Department of Clinical Neurological Sciences
University of Western Ontario
Consultant Neurologist
Department of Clinical Neurological Sciences
London Health Sciences Center
London, Ontario, Canada

DAVID YOUNGER, MD
Clinical Associate Professor
Department of Neurology
New York Unviersity School of Medicine
New York, New York

KHALED ZAMEL, MD
Assistant Professor of Clinical Pediatrics
Columbus Children's Hospital
Columbus, Ohio

DOUGLAS W. ZOCHODNE, MD
University of Calgary
Department of Clinical Neurosciences
Calgary, Alberta, Canada

Preface

We are pleased to bring a Neurology volume to the 5-Minute Consult series. This book is intended to present current clinical information to several groups:

- Busy clinical practitioners in neurology, general practice, emergency rooms, and nonneurologic specialties who need rapid access to basic data about diagnosis and treatment for various neurologic conditions
- Residents and students seeking a reference where they can quickly refresh their knowledge about the basics of a neurologic condition
- Patients and their families who want quick information about their diagnoses and referrals to patient information and support organizations

Neurology is an area of medicine that incites anxiety and discomfort for many students, nurses, and physicians who have not trained in the specialty. In this decade following the *Decade of the Brain,* therapeutic interventions for neurologic disease are flourishing; every practitioner must understand the diagnosis and treatment of basic neurologic conditions. We hope that this rapid information source will help all to approach patients suffering from neurologic disorders with more confidence.

Information is provided in a structured format that allows easy access and rapid assimilation. We have attempted to offer relevant and current references. The information is readily adaptable to handheld devices and will be available from the publisher in that format shortly following publication of the book.

It has been a great honor and pleasure to work with the many chapter authors who have shared their expertise in and enthusiasm for clinical neurology. Some are young stars while others are accomplished masters in neurology, but all have attempted to provide the best distillation of relevant information for each condition. The staff at Lippincott Williams & Wilkins, including Keith Donnellan and Charley Mitchell, kept us on track in this effort with advice, encouragement, and humor.

Practice is science touched with emotion.

–Stephen Paget, *Confessio Medici,* 1909

D.J.L.
H.B.N.
A.D.R-G.

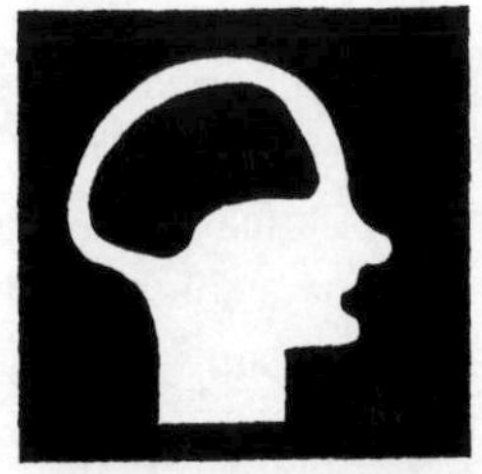
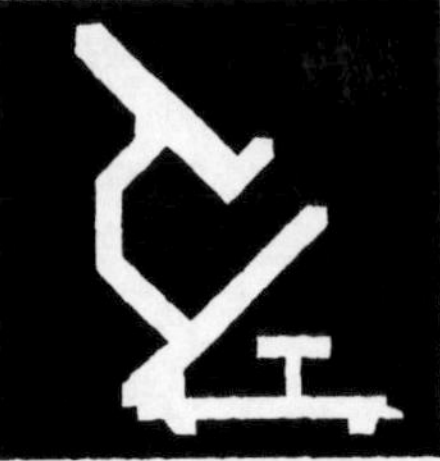
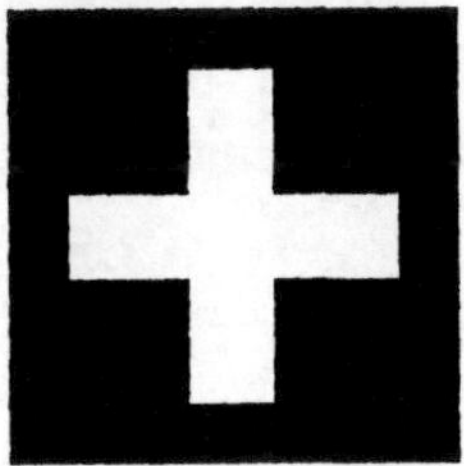
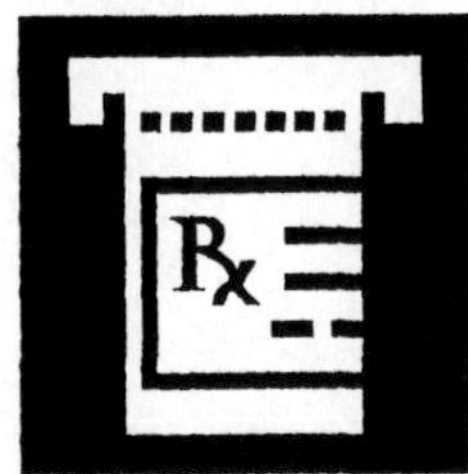

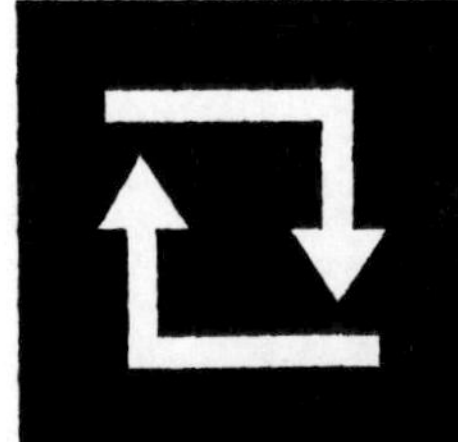
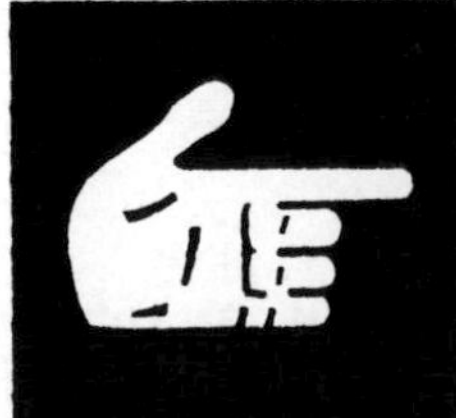

The 5-Minute Neurology Consult

The 5-Minute Neurology Consult

D. JOANNE LYNN, MD

ASSOCIATE PROFESSOR

DEPARTMENT OF NEUROLOGY

THE OHIO STATE UNIVERSITY COLLEGE OF

MEDICINE AND PUBLIC HEALTH

CO-DIRECTOR, MULTIPLE SCLEROSIS CENTER

THE OHIO STATE MEDICAL CENTER

COLUMBUS, OHIO

HERBERT B. NEWTON, MD, FAAN

ASSOCIATE PROFESSOR

DEPARTMENTS OF NEUROLOGY AND PEDIATRICS

THE OHIO STATE UNIVERSITY COLLEGE OF

MEDICINE AND PUBLIC HEALTH

DIRECTOR, DIVISION OF NEURO-ONCOLOGY

DEPARTMENT OF NEUROLOGY

THE OHIO STATE MEDICAL CENTER

DIRECTOR, DARDINGER NEURO-ONCOLOGY CENTER

JAMES CANCER HOSPITAL AND SOLOVE RESEARCH INSTITUTE

COLUMBUS, OHIO

ALEXANDER D. RAE-GRANT, MD, FRCP(C)

PRESIDENT, MEDICAL STAFF

DIVISION OF NEUROLOGY

DEPARTMENT OF MEDICINE

LEHIGH VALLEY HOSPITAL AND HEALTH NETWORK

ALLENTOWN, PENNSYLVANIA

SECTION I

Neurologic Symptoms and Signs

Aphasia

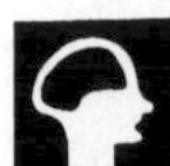

Basics

DESCRIPTION

Aphasia is an acquired impairment of language characterized by word-finding difficulty and paraphasias with a variable disturbance of comprehension. In right-handed people and most left-handers, aphasia results from a lesion in the left cerebral hemisphere. Occasionally a right-hander is seen with aphasia due to a right hemisphere lesion, a phenomenon known as "crossed aphasia." The term *aphasia* refers to spoken language, but aphasics almost always have impaired reading (alexia) and writing (agraphia).

DEFINITIONS

Paraphasias are errors in word production. They may be *phonemic,* with substitution of a wrong sound ("bup" for "cup"); *semantic,* with substitution of a wrong word that is often related in meaning ("dinner" for "cup"); or *neologisms,* with production of a meaningless nonword ("bitko" for "cup").

Fluency refers to the flow of speech and may be thought of as number of words per unit time or length of longest utterance. Nonfluent speech is halting, with long pauses and phrases shorter than four words. Fluent speech retains long phrases and normal melody of speech. Nonfluent aphasics can often make themselves understood in a few words produced with great effort, while fluent aphasics often make very little sense despite lengthy output.

CLINICAL CHARACTERISTICS

Aphasia is usually readily apparent during history-taking. The patient exhibits word-finding difficulty resulting in paraphasias, circumlocutory descriptions ("that thing you write with" for "pen"), or obvious searching for words with pauses and filler phrases ("oh, um, you know"). Aphasia, a disorder of language, must be distinguished from disorders of speech. *Dysarthria* is a disturbance of articulation usually due to lesions lower in the nervous system. Although aphasia and dysarthria may coexist, a patient with only dysarthria should be able to read and write normally. *Dysphonia,* a disturbance of voice, may be due to problems with the larynx or its innervation.

Aphasia must also be distinguished from more diffuse disturbances of cerebral function such as delirium or dementia where disturbances of attention or other cognitive functions are also found.

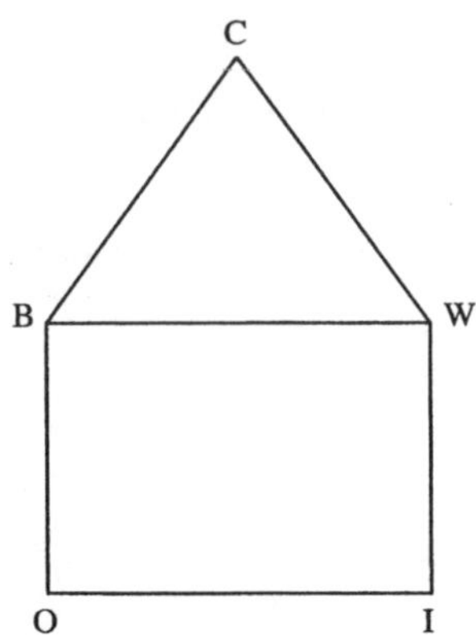

Figure 1. Lichtheim's house.

PATHOPHYSIOLOGY

Language centers surround the left sylvian fissure within territory supplied by the middle cerebral artery (MCA). The diagram of "Lichtheim's house" (Fig. 1) presents a schematic of language processing based on the work of Lichtheim. While obviously a gross oversimplification of a complex process, it nonetheless serves as a useful mnemonic for bedside assessment of aphasia. Auditory input (I) is presented to Wernicke's area (W) in the posterior third of the superior temporal gyrus where sounds heard are linked to representations of words that Lichtheim called "auditory word engrams." Broca's area (B) in the inferior frontal gyrus programs lower centers to articulate a word, producing speech output (O) and may be thought of as containing Lichtheim's "motor word engrams." Broca's area is also important in producing correct word order so that sentences make grammatical sense. Wernicke's and Broca's areas are strongly connected by white matter tracts such as the arcuate fasciculus (the line W–B). Lichtheim visualized an extra-sylvian area of concepts (C) where engrams were linked to actual meanings of words and, while there is no one brain area corresponding to this, C may be thought of as the rest of the cerebrum, beyond left MCA territory.

Lesions disrupting the line C–B–O impair fluency. Lesions along I–W–C impair comprehension. Repetition is impaired by lesions along I–W–B–O.

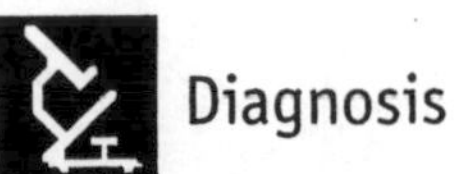

Diagnosis

DIFFERENTIAL DIAGNOSIS

Aphasia is most often due to ischemic or hemorrhagic stroke within or adjacent to the territory of the left MCA but may result from trauma, tumor, infection, or other lesions in this location. Aphasia is uncommon in a white matter disease like multiple sclerosis and is also distinctly uncommon with compressive lesions such as subdural hematomas. A hemiparetic patient with aphasia is thus likely to have an intraparenchymal rather than an extraparenchymal lesion. Language disturbance is often present in cortical dementias such as Alzheimer's disease and is often prominent in frontotemporal dementia.

SIGNS AND SYMPTOMS

Patients' spontaneous speech reveals paraphasias and word-finding difficulty and is also used to judge whether they are fluent or nonfluent. Naming is tested by showing patients objects to name. Patients with mild aphasia may name common objects well but have more difficulty producing less common words such as parts of objects. Thus, aphasics tend to have more difficulty naming a watch strap than a watch. Comprehension is tested by asking the patient to carry out commands of varying levels of difficulty. One can begin with simple one-step commands and progress to complex three-stage commands. Repetition is tested beginning with single words and progressing to complex phrases such as "no ifs, ands, or buts."

Peri-sylvian aphasias (Broca's, Wernicke's, conduction, and global) are typically due to infarcts in left MCA territory and since all disrupt I–W–B–O, they have in common a disturbance of repetition.

Broca's Aphasia

A lesion in Broca's area (B) causes nonfluent speech with poor repetition but relatively preserved comprehension, particularly for nouns and verbs. Since Broca's area is adjacent to the precentral gyrus, this is usually accompanied by right hemiparesis.

Wernicke's Aphasia

A lesion in Wernicke's area (W) results in fluent speech with impaired comprehension and repetition. Although it may be accompanied by a right superior homonymous quadrantanopia due to involvement of temporal fibers of the optic radiations, Wernicke's aphasia is generally not accompanied by hemiparesis. Due to the paucity of other findings on examination it is not unusual to see a patient referred with "confusion" who actually has Wernicke's aphasia.

Conduction Aphasia

A lesion between Wernicke's and Broca's areas in the arcuate fasciculus/insular area (W–B) results in fluent speech with good comprehension and poor repetition.

Global Aphasia

A large middle cerebral territory infarct causes nonfluent speech with poor comprehension and repetition and is typically accompanied by severe hemiparesis. Global aphasia unaccompanied by hemiparesis suggests multiple lesions sparing motor cortex, often of cardioembolic or metastatic origin.

Transcortical Aphasias

These result from lesions in the watersheds between middle, anterior and posterior cerebral arteries (ACA and PCA) or within ACA or PCA territory, disconnecting peri-sylvian language centers from the rest of the cerebrum. Watershed infarcts may result from hypotension, a shower of small emboli, or carotid occlusion. During cardiac surgery, either of the first two of these may occur and this is a typical clinical setting for transcortical aphasia. Because peri-sylvian language centers are spared, repetition is intact.

Transcortical Motor Aphasia

A frontal lesion outside of Broca's area (C–B) results in a language deficit similar to Broca's aphasia except that repetition is preserved.

Transcortical Sensory Aphasia

Temporo-occipital lesions (W–C) may result in a deficit similar to Wernicke's aphasia except that repetition is preserved.

Mixed Transcortical Aphasia

An aphasia similar to global aphasia but with preserved repetition may result from a large MCA/PCA/ACA watershed infarcts (C–B and W–C).

Anomic Aphasia

Impairment of naming with good comprehension, repetition, and fluency is a common but poorly localizing aphasia type. Lesions in many left cerebral areas may cause this mild aphasia.

Subcortical Aphasias

Lesions in thalamus or subcortical white matter can cause aphasia syndromes rather similar to the cortical aphasia types described above. Associated deficits may be atypical (e.g., Wernicke's like aphasia with dense hemiparesis). These patients are often quite dysarthric and repetition is often relatively preserved. Particularly with thalamic lesions, patients may fluctuate dramatically between near-normal output and mumbled jargon.

LABORATORY PROCEDURES

N/A

IMAGING STUDIES

CT or MRI scanning confirms the localization and nature of the causative lesion.

SPECIAL TESTS

Bedside examination is generally sufficient to determine aphasia type and severity, but numerous standardized aphasia test batteries provide more detailed assessment. These range from 3- to 10-minute screening tests, such as the Frenchay Aphasia Screening Test, to the Boston Diagnostic Aphasia Examination, which may take several hours. In 45 minutes the Western Aphasia Battery determines the type and severity of aphasia.

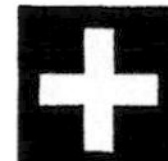

Management

GENERAL MEASURES

The underlying lesion type determines overall management.

SURGICAL MEASURES

Determined by underlying lesion.

SYMPTOMATIC TREATMENT

Determined by underlying lesion. Patients with poor comprehension often benefit from being told information repeatedly and in different words.

ADJUNCTIVE TREATMENT

Large trials suggest that speech therapy by speech pathologists improves recovery.

ADMISSION/DISCHARGE CRITERIA

Usually determined by underlying condition.

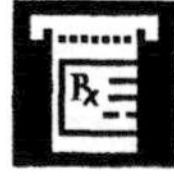

Medications

DRUG(S) OF CHOICE

Although some reports suggest that bromocriptine or stimulant drugs may improve speech output, pharmacotherapy of aphasia has been disappointing and is not generally used.

ALTERNATIVE DRUGS

N/A

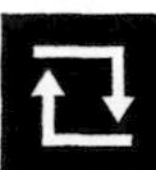

Follow-Up

PATIENT MONITORING

Usually determined by the underlying cause.

EXPECTED COURSE AND PROGNOSIS

Aphasia following stroke generally improves the most in the first 3 months but may continue at a slower rate for 1 to 2 years. Global aphasia may evolve into Broca's, while Wernicke's may become conduction or anomic aphasia during recovery.

PATIENT EDUCATION

Family members benefit from an explanation of language impairment. They often do not understand that patients' answers may not reflect true understanding of questions asked. National Aphasia Association, 156 5th Avenue, Suite 707, New York, NY 10010, (800)922-4622, *www.aphasia.org*.

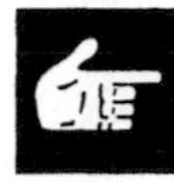

Miscellaneous

SYNONYMS

Dysphasia.

ICD-9-CM: 784.3 Aphasia

SEE ALSO: CEREBROVASCULAR DISEASE

REFERENCES

- Kirk A, Kertesz A. Cortical and subcortical aphasias compared. Aphasiology 1994;8:65–84.
- Kirshner HS. Aphasia. In: Bradley WG, et al., eds. Neurology in clinical practice, vol 1. Boston, Butterworth-Heinemann, 2000:141.
- Lichtheim L. On aphasia. Brain 1885;7:433–484.
- Mesulam M-M. Aphasias and other focal cerebral disorders. In: Fauci AS, et al., eds. Harrison's principles of internal medicine. New York: McGraw-Hill, 1998:134.
- Robey RR. A meta-analysis of clinical outcomes in the treatment of aphasia. J Speech Lang Hearing Res 1993;41: 172–187.

Author(s): Andrew Kirk, MD, FRCP(C)

Ataxia

Basics

DESCRIPTION

Ataxia is defined as incoordination of movements, especially voluntary movements. Gait, limb movements, balance, speech, eye movements, and tone can be involved. Movements appear clumsy or irregular. Velocity and force may not be normally regulated, leading to overshoot of movements.

DEFINITIONS

N/A

CLINICAL CHARACTERISTICS

Ataxia may be of sudden or insidious onset. Disorderly and irregular movements are observed. These are especially prominent with directed movements of the limbs and become more pronounced closer to the target (hypermetria, intention tremor). Gait may appear similar to the gait observed with alcohol intoxication—wide based and unsteady. Speech may be hesitant or explosive. Nystagmus and irregular eye movements may be seen. Association with acute headache, nausea, vomiting, and/or diplopia may be a sign of acute cerebellar infarct or hemorrhage and should be treated as potentially life threatening.

Hereditary ataxias progress slowly and are divided by pattern of inheritance and genotype. In autosomal-dominant ataxias risk to offspring is 50%. In autosomal-recessive forms risk to siblings is a 25% chance of being affected, 50% of being an unaffected carrier, and 25% chance of being unaffected and not a carrier. Offspring of an affected individual are obligate carriers. In X-linked recessive inheritance, all daughters of an affected male are carriers; sons are not affected. For siblings, if the mother of the affected individual is a carrier, brothers are at 50% risk of being affected; sisters have a 50% chance to be carriers and unaffected.

PATHOPHYSIOLOGY

Varies depending on the specific cause of ataxia. Ataxia is most commonly related to disruption of cerebellar pathways. However, coordinated movements require synchronization of multiple sensory and motor pathways and injury to the spinal cord, brainstem, cortex or peripheral nervous system can also cause ataxia.

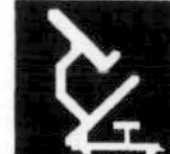

Diagnosis

DIFFERENTIAL DIAGNOSIS

- Vascular: infarcts (cerebellum, brainstem, anterior thalamus, frontal cortex, or parietal lobe), hemorrhage, basilar migraine
- Structural: tumors, abscess, arteriovenous malformations, Chiari malformations, Dandy-Walker malformation, and hydrocephalus
- Multiple sclerosis
- Infectious: postinfectious cerebellitis, Gerstmann-Sträussler syndrome, Creutzfeldt-Jakob disease
- Toxins: alcohol, anticonvulsants, heavy metals (thallium, lead, mercury, lithium), toluene, cytarabine (Ara-C), cyclosporine
- Endocrine: hypothyroidism
- Nutritional: vitamin E deficiency, vitamin B_{12} deficiency, Wernicke-Korsakoff disease
- Immune: gluten sensitivity and glutamic acid decarboxylase antibodies, Miller-Fisher variant of Guillain-Barré syndrome
- Paraneoplastic cerebellar degeneration, opsoclonus-myoclonus
- Sporadic neurodegenerative diseases: olivopontocerebellar atrophy, cerebellar cortical atrophy, multiple system atrophy
- Hereditary:
  - —Autosomal dominant: SCA1-21, DRPLA, episodic ataxia type 1 (EA1), episodic ataxia type 2 (EA2).
  - —Autosomal recessive: Friedreich ataxia, ataxia telangiectasia, ataxia with vitamin E deficiency (AVED), infantile-onset spinocerebellar ataxia (IOSCA), ataxia with oculomotor apraxia, Marinesco-Sjögren, spastic ataxia (ARSACS), myoclonus-ataxia syndromes, ataxia with hypogonadism.
  - —X-linked: X-linked ataxia with spasticity, X-linked ataxia with sideroblastic anemia, X-linked ataxia with deafness and blindness and other reported families
  - —Mitochondrial: NARP (neuropathy, ataxia, and retinitis pigmentosa) and MERRF (myoclonic epilepsy with ragged red fibers)
  - —Metabolic: abetalipoproteinemia, hexosaminidase deficiency, Refsum disease, cerebrotendinous xanthomatosis, metachromatic leukodystrophy, adrenoleukomyeloneuropathy, urea cycle disorders, intermittent branched-chain ketoaciduria, Hartnup disease, pyruvate dehydrogenase deficiency

SIGNS AND SYMPTOMS

Ataxic disorders cause static or progressive generalized incoordination affecting gait, limb coordination, speech, and/or extraocular movements. The brainstem, basal ganglia, spinal cord, retina, or peripheral nervous system are often involved. Other signs of neurologic dysfunction may be seen in vascular disease or multiple sclerosis. Parkinsonian features and autonomic failure may be seen in multisystem atrophy and SCA3.

There is great overlap in the phenotype of the hereditary spinocerebellar ataxias. Most are caused by trinucleotide repeat expansions. There are a few distinguishing features for some types. Molecular diagnosis is needed for definitive classification.

- Distinguishing features of some of the autosomal-dominant hereditary ataxias:
  - —SCA2: Slow saccadic eye movements, hyporeflexia or areflexia
  - —SCA4: Sensory axonal neuropathy
  - —SCA6: Sometimes episodic ataxia is present
  - —SCA7: Visual loss with retinopathy
  - —SCA10: May be associated with seizures
  - —SCA12: Early tremor, late dementia
  - —SCA13: Mild mental retardation and short stature
  - —SCA14: Early axial myoclonus
  - —SCA16: Head and hand tremor
  - —DRPLA: Chorea, seizures, and myoclonus
  - —EA1: Episodic ataxia lasting seconds/minutes, myokymia
  - —EA2: Episodic ataxia lasting minutes to hours, nystagmus
- Distinguishing features of the autosomal-recessive disorders:
  - —Friedreich ataxia (FA): hyporeflexia or areflexia, extensor plantars, depressed vibratory/proprioceptive sense, cardiac involvement
  - —Ataxia with vitamin E deficiency: similar to FA, plus head titubation and dystonia
  - —Ataxia telangiectasia: telangiectasia, immunodeficiency, cancer and endocrine abnormalities
  - —Ataxia with oculomotor apraxia: oculomotor apraxia, choreoathetosis and mental retardation
  - —Spastic ataxia (ARSACS): pyramidal signs, peripheral neuropathy, and retinal striations

LABORATORY PROCEDURES

Serum levels of vitamin B_{12}, thyroid-stimulating hormone (TSH), and vitamin E should be checked. Heavy metal screening in cases of suspected exposure. Plasma amino acids and urine organic acids are helpful when an inherited metabolic cause is suspected. If the Miller-Fisher variant of Guillain-Barré syndrome is suspected (ataxia with areflexia and ophthalmoplegia), lumbar puncture for cell count and protein level and nerve conduction studies should be considered.

IMAGING STUDIES

Cranial MRI may identify structural abnormalities including infarcts, hemorrhage, tumors, and demyelination. Atrophy of involved structures in the brain or spinal cord can be found in some neurodegenerative disorders.

SPECIAL TESTS

Antigliadin antibodies and glutamic acid decarboxylase antibodies (GAD-Abs) should be searched in all patients with cerebellar ataxia of unknown etiology. Paraneoplastic cerebellar syndrome is associated with anti-Yo, -Hu -Ri, -Ta, -Ma, or -CV2. Paraneoplastic symptoms may be the first sign of an occult cancer. In cases where a hereditary disorder is suspected, DNA testing is commercially available for SCA1, SCA2, SCA3, SCA6, SCA7, SCA8, SCA10, DRPLA, Friedreich ataxia, and ataxia-telangiectasia. These tests are expensive. Genetic counseling prior to testing is advised. In ataxia-telangiectasia serum electrophoresis shows decreased concentrations of immunoglobulin A (IgA) and IgG, while serum α-fetoprotein levels are elevated. Cultured cells show cytogenetic abnormalities and increased sensitivity to ionizing radiation. Muscle biopsy may confirm a mitochondrial disorder.

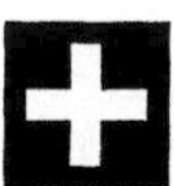

Management

GENERAL MEASURES

Protect from fall risks. Acute-onset ataxia needs to be treated as a possible neurosurgical emergency. Cerebellar hemorrhages and large infarcts are associated with a high risk of swelling and may compromise brainstem respiratory centers leading to death. CT scan or MRI should be obtained immediately.

SURGICAL MEASURES

Decompression of hematomas or infarcts associated with edema compressing the cerebellum, brainstem, and fourth ventricle. Surgical removal of tumors.

SYMPTOMATIC TREATMENT

Antiemetics for nausea and vomiting; eye patching for diplopia. Antispastic medications for those with spasticity.

ADJUNCTIVE TREATMENTS

Physical, occupational, and speech therapy. Patients with antigliadin antibodies may respond to a gluten-free diet. Patients with GAD-Abs and the Miller-Fisher variant of Guillain-Barré syndrome may respond to IV immunoglobulin.

ADMISSION/DISCHARGE CRITERIA

Acute ataxia associated with inability to walk generally requires admission and evaluation. Ataxia of insidious onset can be evaluated as an outpatient after radiologic studies rule out mass lesions. Individuals with ataxia secondary to intoxication with alcohol or phenytoin may need admission until levels decrease. Discharge criteria include assurance of safety from falls.

Medications

DRUG(S) OF CHOICE

In most cases, no effective medications are available.

- Adults with vitamin E deficiency: replace with 60 to 75 IU PO or IM. Adjust dosage to normal plasma levels.
- Thiamine deficiency in chronic alcoholics and malnourished patients: thiamine 50 mg PO daily. In Wernicke encephalopathy, thiamine 50 to 100 mg IV and IM immediately, 50 mg/day IM for 3 days, and then 50 mg PO daily.
- Vitamin B_{12} deficiency: cyanocobalamin 1,000 μg IM daily for 5 to 7 days, then weekly for a month and then monthly for life.
- For episodic ataxia: acetazolamide.
- Stroke prevention, multiple sclerosis, or cancer treatment as indicated.

Contraindications

Limit medications with cerebellar toxicity (anticonvulsants).

Precautions

Alcohol and benzodiazepines may worsen symptoms.

ALTERNATIVE DRUGS

N/A

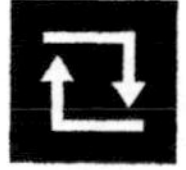

Follow-Up

PATIENT MONITORING

In ataxia secondary to acute cerebellar stroke or hemorrhage, patients are followed closely (often in the ICU) for cerebral edema and brainstem compromise. Offer genetic counseling to those with hereditary ataxias.

EXPECTED COURSE AND PROGNOSIS

Prognosis depends on the underlying etiology. Recovery after cerebellar insult is possible. Ataxia secondary to tumors, multiple sclerosis, or other areas of infarction may improve. Recovery from alcohol or toxin exposure depends on degree of exposure. Idiopathic and hereditary cerebellar ataxias have a progressive course, and life span may be decreased.

PATIENT EDUCATION

- National Ataxia Foundation, 2600 Fernbrook Lane, Suite 119, Minneapolis, MN 55447. Phone: 763-553-0020, Web: www.ataxia.org
- WE MOVE (Worldwide Education and Awareness for Movement Disorders), 204 East 84th St., New York, NY 10024. Phone: 212-875-8312, Web: www.wemove.org
- International Network of Ataxia Friends (INTERNAF), Web: www.internaf.org

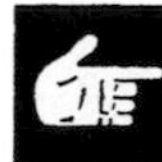

Miscellaneous

SYNONYMS

Cerebellar ataxia
Spinocerebellar ataxia

ICD-9-CM: 334.2 Primary cerebellar degeneration (familial); 334.3 Cerebellar ataxia; 334.8 Ataxia telangiectasia; 334.9 Spinocerebellar degeneration; 331.9 Cerebral ataxia; 781.3 Ataxia NOS; 781.2 Ataxic gait; 303.9 Alcohol associated

SEE ALSO: FRIEDREICH'S ATAXIA, SPINOCEREBELLAR ATAXIAS

REFERENCES

- Abele M, Weller M, Mescheriakov S, et al. Cerebellar ataxia with glutamic acid decarboxylase autoantibodies. Neurology 1999;52:857–859.
- Bird TD. Ataxia overview. In: GeneClinics: clinical genetic information resource [database online]. Copyright, University of Washington, Seattle. Available at *http://www.geneclinics.org/profiles/ataxias.*
- Conner KE, Rosenberg RN. The genetic basis of ataxia. In: Rosenberg RN, Prusiner SB, DiMauro S, et al., eds. The molecular and genetic basis of neurological disease, 2nd ed. Boston: Butterworth-Heinemann 1997:503–544.
- Evidente VG, Gwinn-Hardy KA, Caviness JN, et al. Hereditary ataxias. Mayo Clin Proc 2000;75:475–490.
- Jankovic JJ, Deirkiran M. Classification of paroxysmal dyskinesias and ataxia. Adv Neurol 2002;89:387–400.
- Pellecchia MT, Scala R, Perreti A, et al. Cerebellar ataxia associated with subclinical celiac disease responding to gluten-free diet. Neurology 1999;53:1606–1608.

Author(s): Magali Fernandez, MD; Sandra K. Kostyk, MD, PhD

Back Pain

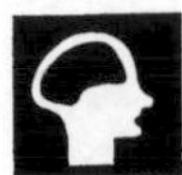

Basics

DESCRIPTION

Back pain is a constellation of signs of symptoms that can be of mechanical, neurologic (nonmechanical), or visceral origin. The clinical presentation can be categorized into central and peripheral components. The neurologic complaints may not always match the clinical and neurologic findings. Fifty-six percent of adults have back pain and 3% have pain lasting greater than 3 months.

DEFINITIONS

- *Axial pain*: pain centralized to the midline structures of the back to include pain from the facet joints, intervertebral disc, vertebral body, sacroiliac joint, and spinal ligaments and muscles.
- *Dermatomal pain*: pain in a specified area of skin in the distribution of a single nerve root with or without neurologic changes.
- *Discogenic pain*: pain emanating from the intervertebral disc with or without neurologic symptoms or findings (such as annular tears, protrusions, and degenerative disc disease).
- *Myofascial pain*: pain in the musculoligamentous structures with discrete and defined tender or trigger points with reproducible referred pain patterns.
- *Myotomal pain*: pain in a muscle group innervated by a single nerve root with or without neurologic change.
- *Peripheral pain*: spinal pain referred to an extremity with or without neurologic findings.
- *Radicular pain*: pain sensation in the distribution of a single nerve root without neurologic deficits.
- *Radiculopathy*: pain associated with neurologic deficits in the distribution of a single nerve root.
- *Referred pain*: pain referred from a remote structure or organ without neurologic deficit. The pain patterns depend on the dermatomal, myotomal, and sclerotomal of the inciting structure or organ.
- *Sclerotomal (somatic) pain*: pain in bone and fascia in distribution of a single nerve root.

CLINICAL CHARACTERISTICS

Back pain can be associated with acute trauma, single mechanical injury, cumulative trauma, degenerative changes, and no identifiable events. It can be associated with remote internal organ disease processes with local or metastatic pathology. Back pain with peripheral symptoms may not have classic neurologic deficits and clinical findings even though identifiable pathology is present, such as discogenic pain that may have radicular pain but not true radiculopathy. Back pain may be axial, unilateral, or bilateral with or without radiation to the gluteal region, iliac crest, or extremities. It may be associated with decreased range of motion, muscle spasm, trigger point tenderness and referral pain patterns, antalgic trunk deviation and gait abnormalities, body posture and altered function.

PATHOPHYSIOLOGY

Degenerative and cumulative trauma may lead to alteration of the weight distribution between the anterior elements, disc and vertebral body, and the posterior elements, facet joints and capsule, ligaments and muscles. This trauma leads to annular tears, loss of disc height, osteophyte formation, facet synovial reaction and menisci tear, cartilage destruction, and facet capsular laxity and subluxation. This trauma also leads to spinal canal and neural foraminal stenosis with resulting neural element encroachment and compromise. Before mechanical compromise occurs, chemical substances producing inflammation from various structures in the back can produce symptoms and physical findings with minimal neural compromise. Some of the known mediators are phospholipase A_2, leukotrienes, prostaglandins, platelet-activating factors, bradykinins, cytokines, interleukins, nitric oxide, tumor necrosis factor, macrophages, and other inflammatory cells. The dorsal root ganglion is sensitive to mechanical compression and chemical or inflammatory mediators and it will increase nerve fiber firing and alter neural pathways and increases pain perception. Neural sensitivity increases as the biomechanical deterioration occurs.

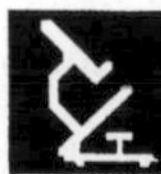

Diagnosis

DIFFERENTIAL DIAGNOSIS

- Axial pain: lumbosacral sprain and strain, internal disc disruption and annular tears, facet joint pathology, (arthropathy, capsulitis, and synovitis), sacroiliac joint dysfunction, myofascial dysfunction, spondylolisthesis and pars defects, vertebral compression fracture, and vertebral somatic and segmental dysfunctions.
- Radicular pain: discogenic pain with chemical radiculopathy, disc herniation, spinal and foraminal stenosis, spondylolisthesis with nerve root compromise, degenerative disc disease, tumors (primary and metastatic), arachnoiditis, diabetic neuropathies, piriformis syndrome, hypertrophic facet joint changes with foraminal stenosis, and vertebral trauma with cord or nerve root compromise.
- Visceral pain: gynecologic, urologic, renal, stomach and duodenal ulcers, pancreatic pathology, and retroperitoneal pathology.
- Miscellaneous: rheumatic diseases, spinal infections, vascular pathology, abdominal aortic aneurysm.
- Nonorganic/psychogenic: depression, anxiety, somatization, and malingering.

SIGNS AND SYMPTOMS

Axial

- *Lumbosacral sprain and strain:* caused by unaccustomed eccentric contraction, trauma, muscle strain, back pain with 24- to 28-hour delay, tenderness in lumbar paraspinal muscles.
- *Internal disc disruption/annular tear/discogenic pain:* caused by high-speed accidents, extreme axial loads, trauma, twisting, and degenerative changes. Deep "axial ache" and can progress to radicular symptoms. Pain decreased with unloading axial spine; flexion increases pain; usually neurologic findings are absent unless significant disc degeneration occurs.
- *Facet arthropathy/capsulitis:* can be caused by trauma, degeneration, arthritis, lifting, extension and torsional injury; 15% to 30% of back pain. Pain increases with extension and rotation and may radiate to buttock and leg. Neurologic exam is normal.
- *Sacroiliac (SI) dysfunction:* can be caused by a fall, step off a curb, or heavy lifting. Pain and tenderness at SI joint, Patrick's test (also called the FABERE test: flexion, abduction, external rotation, and extension) and pelvic rock are positive on involved side, asymmetric pelvis, no neurologic findings.

- *Myofascial pain:* can be caused by sprain, whiplash, and industrial and cumulative trauma. Pain is localized with discrete trigger points and has nondermatomal radiation pattern. Palpation of muscle reproduces the pain and a localized muscle twitch may be present. No neurologic findings are present.
- *Spondylolisthesis:* can be caused by congenital or acute or chronic trauma. Low back pain is present, possibly radiates to leg, and increases with activity. Decreased range of motion may be present.
- *Vertebral compression fracture:* may be secondary to osteoporosis, major trauma; pain is localized to back and is worse with movement, especially flexion. Neurologic symptoms are usually absent unless bone fragment is in spinal or neural foraminal canal. If greater than 50% loss of vertebral body height, consider the fracture unstable.
- *Vertebral somatic/segmental dysfunction:* caused by major or minor trauma, overuse, and lifting. Altered segmental motion is present, decreased tissue compliance; radicular symptoms may be present without neurologic findings.

Radicular

- *Patterns of radicular findings*
  —L2-3: Motor—hip flexion; sensory—groin
  —L3-4: Motor—knee extension; sensory—medial ankle
  —L4-5: Motor—extensor hallucis longus (EHL) and ankle dorsiflexion; sensory—dorsal foot
  —L5-S1: Motor—plantar flexion and ankle eversion; sensory—lateral foot
- *Discogenic pain with radicular symptoms:* causes as above but with radicular symptoms and findings secondary to chemical radiculopathy or mechanical nerve root compromise.
- *Disc herniation:* can be caused by flexion, extension, or rotational injury with or without axial load. Prominent in 30- to 40-year-olds. Low back and radicular pain with or radicular findings. Straight leg test positive, deep tendon reflexes may be absent, dermatomal sensory loss may be present, and muscular weakness specific to a nerve root injury may be present.
- *Spinal stenosis/foraminal stenosis:* commonly degenerative, but may be traumatic with leg pain with activity/walking; may be relieved by forward flexed posture, and nighttime pain relieved by walking. Paresthesia and weakness may be present. In foraminal stenosis, extension may produce radicular symptoms from nerve root compromise. Must differentiate neurogenic from vascular claudication.
- *Degenerative disc disease:* degenerative process with progressive symptoms. Symptoms and findings are similar to those of discogenic pain and spinal stenosis.
- *Spinal tumors:* pain and symptoms may progress as tumor grows. Pain may be constant and worse at night, associated with red flags (unexplained fever, chills, weight loss, anorexia) change in bowel and bladder function, and neurologic symptoms and findings may be present. Tumor may be in spinal canal or extension from bone and associated with pathologic fracture. Evaluate for primary tumor with bone metastasis (lung, breast, prostate, and renal are most common).
- *Arachnoiditis:* cause is from adhesions and scar formation from previous back surgery, disc space infection, myelography, intrathecal drugs, and radiation therapy. Radicular pain is present but neurologic findings may or may not be present. Flexion of spine may increase radicular symptoms.
- *Diabetic neuropathy:* sensory and motor symptoms are present, pain is constant, worse at night, and may be associated with weight loss. May be confused with herniated disc.
- *Piriformis syndrome:* cause may be from acute or chronic trauma, hip fracture or surgery, and extended driving. Pain is in buttocks but may have radicular symptoms. Internal rotation of hip will increase pain. Tenderness along piriformis muscle. (Muscle courses from sacrum to greater trochanter.)
- *Hypertrophic facet joint pain with foraminal stenosis:* see Spinal stenosis/foraminal stenosis, above.
- *Vertebral trauma:* cause may be fall, motor vehicle accident, or other trauma. Symptoms vary according to degree of nerve root or cord compromise from disc herniation or vertebral fracture.
- *Visceral/miscellaneous/nonorganic/psychogenic:* a detailed history, physical examination, and diagnostic workup help to differentiate these causes and proper referral.

LABORATORY PROCEDURES

If symptoms warrant or clinical red flags are present, consider the following diagnostic laboratory procedures: ESR, ANA, rheumatoid factor, CBC with differential, CPK, thyroid panel, comprehensive metabolic panel, SPEP, or urine analysis.

IMAGING PROCEDURES

- MRI is helpful to identify soft tissue pathology, such as tumors and disc. CAT scan is best to evaluate bone pathology. CT-myelogram helps to evaluate both bone and nerve or cord compression. Bone scan is useful for metabolic and metastatic pathology and stress fractures. Provocative discography is helpful for internal disc disruption and annular tears. Plain films are good for fractures, degenerative changes, postural analysis, to evaluate pars defects, and spondylolisthesis. Flexion and extension views are important to evaluate segmental instability. Oblique views are best to evaluate pars defects.
- Significance of imaging studies, in particular disc changes on MRI, need to be viewed and interpreted based on clinical examination and findings. Diagnostic ultrasound has not proven to be effective for evaluation of low back pain.

SPECIAL TESTS

EMG/NCV studies are of benefit to evaluate degree of nerve root damage or compromise and to differentiate peripheral neuropathy from radiculopathy and myopathic diseases. Medial branch blocks and intraarticular facet injections can evaluate facet joints as a pain generator. Three-phase bone scan of the legs is helpful if reflex sympathetic dystrophy (RSD) is suspected.
Selective nerve root blocks are helpful to determine the level of nerve root compromise.

Back Pain

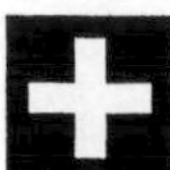

Management

GENERAL MEASURES

Limited rest may be of benefit with initial injury. Cold packs for acute pain and inflammation. Heat after acute episode. Home exercise for strengthening, flexibility, and stretching. Analgesics are of benefit. Start with nonsteroidal antiinflammatory drugs (NSAIDs) and opioids for intense pain.

SURGICAL MEASURES

After conservative treatment has been exhausted, referral to a neurosurgeon or orthopedic spine surgeon is appropriate. Cauda equina syndrome is a surgical emergency. Spinal tumors require a surgical evaluation. Surgical considerations may include open and percutaneous and microdiscectomy, laminectomy, fusion with and without instrumentation.

SYMPTOMATIC TREATMENT

- NSAIDs and opiates for acute pain. If radicular symptoms are present, oral or IM steroids.
- Muscle relaxants for spasm. Antiepileptic medications for neurogenic and nociceptive pain. Antidepressants for chronic pain and improved sleep. Lumbar supports and bracing may help with pain and posturing. Transcutaneous electrical nerve stimulation (TENS) unit for pain.

ADJUNCTIVE TREATMENTS

- Physical therapy to include modalities, aquatic therapy, active therapy, aerobic reconditioning, proprioceptive and dynamic lumbar stabilization exercises. Chiropractic and osteopathic spinal manipulation and massage.
- For radicular symptoms: lumbar epidural steroid injection, selective nerve root blocks, spinal endoscopy for delivery of steroids and adenolysis. Discogenic pain: intradiscal electrothermal therapy (IDET), nucleoplasty (coblation), laser decompression, percutaneous disc decompressor.
- Facet pain: intraarticular facet joint injections with steroids, medial branch blocks, radiofrequency lesioning of the medial branch nerve.
- Myofascial pain: trigger point injections, botulinum toxin injections, prolotherapy/regenerative injection therapy.
- Sacroiliac dysfunction: SI joint injection with steroids, radiofrequency lesioning, prolotherapy.
- Pain: acupuncture, spinal cord stimulator, intrathecal opiates via pump. Alternative and complementary pain management.

ADMISSION/DISCHARGE CRITERIA

Cauda equina syndrome for surgical intervention. Acute and progressive neurologic compromise and urgent surgical evaluation.

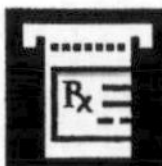

Medications

DRUG(S) OF CHOICE

Acute/Subacute Medications

The primary goal at this stage is symptom control with analgesics, muscle relaxants, and antiinflammatory drugs, both steroidal and nonsteroidal.

Persistent/Chronic Medications

The goal is to control the pain and discomfort and to improve function with scheduled medications and reducing the frequency of dosage. Use a long-acting scheduled preparation with a short-acting one for breakthrough pain.

Analgesics

- Acute/breakthrough pain
  - —Mild pain
    - -Tramadol 50–100 mg q6–8h PRN (Ultram)
    - -Tramadol 37.5 mg/APAP 1–2 q6–8h PRN (Ultracet)
    - -Propoxyphene 100 mg/APAP q4–6h PRN (Darvocet)

  ibuprofen/naproxen/rofecoxib/celecoxib (See NSAIDs below.)
  - —Moderate pain
    - -Hydrocodone 5–10 mg/APAP q4–6h PRN (Vicodin, Lortab)
    - -Hydrocodone 7.5 mg/ibuprofen q4–6h PRN (Vicoprofen)
    - -Oxycodone 5–7.5–10 mg/APAP q4–6h (Percocet, Endocet)
    - -Oxycodone 5 mg q4–6h PRN (OxyIR)
  - —Severe pain
    - -Hydrocodone 10 mg/APAP q4–6h PRN (Percocet)
    - -Oxycodone 15–30 mg q4–6h PRN (Roxicodone)
    - -Hydromorphone 2–4 mg q4–6h (Dilaudid)
  - —Persistent/chronic pain
    - -Oxycodone 10–160 mg q12h (scheduled and not PRN) (OxyContin)
    - -Fentanyl transdermal 25–100 μg q3d (Duragesic patch)
    - -Morphine sustained release
    - -MS Contin 15–200 mg q12h
    - -Kadian 30–100 mg q12–24h
    - -Avinza 30–120 mg q24h

NSAIDs

There is an abundance of these medications. We are listing a limited few and you must determine those that are effective for your use.

- Ibuprofen 400–800 mg q6–8h
- Naproxen 250–500 mg q12h
- Rofecoxib 25–50 mg q24h (Vioxx)
- Celecoxib 200–400 mg q24h (Celebrex)
- Valdecoxib 10–20 mg q24h (Bextra)

Steroidal Antiinflammatory

These medications are used to reduce the inflammation of disc herniation on the nerve root (chemical and compressive radiculitis) and for the inflammatory diseases of the spine (ankylosing spondylitis). Dosages and protocols vary. Below are options.

- Methylprednisolone 2 mg, prepackaged dosing (Medrol)
- Prednisone 20 mg: 3 PO qd for 3 days; 2 PO qd for 3 days; 1 PO qd for 3 days

Muscle Relaxants

- Cyclobenzaprine 5–10 mg q8h PRN (Flexeril)
- Tizanidine 1–4 mg hs to qid (Zanaflex)
- Baclofen 5–20 mg hs to qid (Lioresal)
- Carisoprodol 350 mg q6–8h
- Diazepam 5–10 mg qhs to qid (Valium)

Anticonvulsants

These are used for acute radicular symptoms and chronic pain (neurogenic and nociceptive pain). The list below is abbreviated. Many are available.

- Gabapentin 100–3,600 mg per day in divided doses (Neurontin)
- Topiramate 25–400 mg q24h (Topamax)
- Tiagabine 4–32 mg qd to qid in divided dosages (Gabitril)

Antidepressants

These are initially used for acute and chronic pain. In the chronic state, depression may accompany the chronic back pain. Many antidepressants are available and used for pain. A partial list of commonly used medications is listed below.

- Amitriptyline 10–100 mg qhs (Elavil)
- Nortriptyline 10–100 mg qhs (Pamelor)
- Fluoxetine 10–80 mg daily (Prozac)
- Paroxetine 10–40 mg daily (Paxil)
- Venlafaxine 37.5–200 mg qd to bid (Effexor)

Contraindications

NSAIDs can cause peptic ulcer disease (PUD), and some are contraindicated with anticoagulants. Renal and hepatic side effects are possible. Opioid medications need to be titrated for pain relief and side effects. Tolerance and dependence can develop, especially in long-term use, and must be differentiated from addiction. In general most of the medications used can cause anticholinergic side effects, fatigue and drowsiness, and impaired mental functions.

Precautions

Polypharmacy is possible and drug interactions and physical and mental functional status should be monitored. Alcohol and recreational drugs may be used by the patient, especially in chronic pain. Caution must be used, and consideration may be given to compliance drug screening.

ALTERNATIVE DRUGS

Lidoderm patch, capsaicin cream, acetaminophen, and herbal and nutritional supplements.

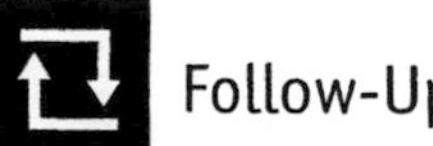

Follow-Up

PATIENT MONITORING

Patients should be monitored for their pain, neurologic symptoms and findings, and their functional status and medications.

EXPECTED COURSE AND PROGNOSIS

Prognosis is usually good, with 3% becoming chronic back pain sufferers. Concomitant diseases, and psychosocial, employment, and financial issues may complicate and impede recovery.

PATIENT EDUCATION

Patient education has proven to be effective in the treatment of back pain. There are many preprinted materials, supportive organizations, and Web sites available.

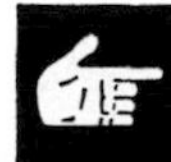

Miscellaneous

SYNONYMS

- Sciatica
- Radiculopathy
- Pinched nerve
- Muscle strain
- Ruptured disc
- Slipped disc
- Back arthritis
- Back and disc degeneration

ICD-9-CM: 846.0 Lumbosacral sprain and strain; 847.2 Lumbar sprain and strain; 846.1 Sacroiliac sprain and strain; 724.2 Lumbar back pain syndrome; 724.5 Mechanical back pain; 729.1 Myofascial pain and fibromyalgia; 721.3 Facet arthropathy/spondylosis without myelopathy; 724.02 Lumbar spinal stenosis; 738.4 Spondylolisthesis, acquired and degenerative; 733.13 Pathologic fracture of vertebra; 805.4 Closed fracture of lumbar spine; 724.2 Lumbar radiculopathy; 729.1 Neuralgia/neuritis; 724.2 Sciatica; 720.2 Sacroiliitis; 722.83 Postlaminectomy syndrome; 722.52 Lumbar disc degeneration; 722.10 Lumbar disc displacement without myelopathy; 722.73 Lumbar disc displacement with myelopathy; 355.0 Sciatic nerve lesion; 728.85 Muscle spasm; Piriformis syndrome is coded as a combination code (355.0 and 728.85)

SEE ALSO: N/A

REFERENCES

- Cailliett R. Low back disorders, a medical enigma. Philadelphia: Lippincott Williams & Wilkins, 2003.
- Cole AJ, Herring SA. The low back pain handbook, 1st ed. Philadelphia: Hanley and Belfus, 1997.
- Omberregt L, Bisschop P, ter Veer H, eds. A system of orthopedic medicine, 2nd ed. Philadelphia: Churchill-Livingston 2003:3–131, 699–983.

Author(s): Gordon J. Korby, DO, DC; Brian E. Higgins, DO

Brain Herniation Syndromes

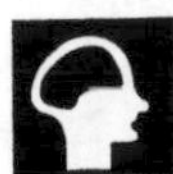

Basics

DESCRIPTION

The intracranial space is filled with brain, CSF, and blood. Since this is a nonexpandable space, any increase in one of the constituents of the compartment must be balanced by a reduction of another constituent, or must cause an increase in the intracranial pressure. Mass lesions of various types, and brain swelling of various etiologies, can cause increase in the intracranial pressure. Above a threshold of pressure, the contents of the intracranial compartment begin to move through into spaces of lower pressure, causing brain herniation. There are well-defined major types of brain herniation that occur under these circumstances.

DEFINITIONS

Herniation: a shift of brain tissue from its proper location to another location due to an imbalance of pressure between the two locations.

CLINICAL CHARACTERISTICS

Brain swelling occurs under a variety of conditions: infarction, hemorrhage, infection (including abscess), neoplasia, toxic injury, and ischemia. When there is enough difference in pressure between contiguous spaces intracranially, the brain may herniate to the space of lower pressure. The location of herniation determines the general characteristic of the herniation syndrome.

Lateral Herniation

Laterally placed mass lesions of the brain, usually extracerebral or in the temporal lobe, cause a side-to-side shift of the brain contents. Such mass lesions displace the brain medially, both pushing the medial temporal lobe inward, and distorting the midbrain. Clinical characteristics include alterations of consciousness (confusion, stupor, coma). Pupillary dilatation, which traditionally is ipsilateral to the mass lesions, may occur on either side. A contralateral hemiparesis may occur, but on occasion pressure of the midbrain against the rigid dural edge contralaterally may cause an ipsilateral hemiparesis, a "false" localizing sign (Kernohan's phenomenon).

Central Herniation

Downward pressure from supratentorial mass lesions may cause central herniation syndromes. These are due to downward pressure on the diencephalon and midbrain. Clinically this causes an altered consciousness early in the syndrome, followed by progressively worsened consciousness, posturing, and respiratory dysfunction. Such "rostrocaudal" deterioration does not necessarily occur in a stepwise pattern, but may occur suddenly.

Subfalcine Herniation

Laterally placed supratentorial lesions may cause herniation of the cingulate gyrus under the falx cerebri. Such herniation may compromise blood flow in the anterior cerebral arteries, ultimately leading to leg weakness due to infarction in the territory of the anterior cerebral arteries.

Infratentorial Herniation

Less commonly recognized, this syndrome develops when lesions in the infratentorial compartment cause upward herniation of the brainstem and cerebellum through the tentorium. This may result in midbrain dysfunction (pupillary dysfunction, loss of up and down gaze), decerebrate posturing, abnormal respirations, and coma.

Cerebellar Herniation

Herniation of the cerebellar tonsils into the foramen magnum may occur. This may cause compression of the medulla, with altered respiration, meningismus, altered autonomic function, vertigo, skew deviation, vomiting, coma, and death.

PATHOPHYSIOLOGY

Herniation of brain material causes injury to the brain in various manners:

- Direct pressure on brain tissue may cause ischemic change with a loss of neural function.
- Compression of arteries may cause infarction in the territory of that artery. Most commonly the artery affected is the posterior cerebral artery compressed over the edge of the tentorium in a lateral herniation syndrome, causing hemorrhagic infarction of the occipital lobe. The anterior cerebral artery may be compressed by a subfalcine herniation syndrome, causing infarction in one or both anterior cerebral artery territories.
- Torting of neural structures. Elegant work by Ropper et al. has shown that torting (twisting) of the midbrain may underlie the symptoms of the lateral herniation syndrome, rather than direct tissue compression. Thus, while it is clinically taught that the ipsilateral third nerve becomes compressed in the lateral herniation syndrome, in fact either third nerve may become dysfunctional, and both pupillary constriction and dilatation may occur.
- Occasionally lateral lesions will cause secondary hydrocephalus due to compression of cerebrospinal outflow, increasing intracranial fluid and further compromising the situation. Lesions in the posterior fossa commonly block CSF flow at the level of the aqueduct of Sylvius, again causing obstructive hydrocephalus.

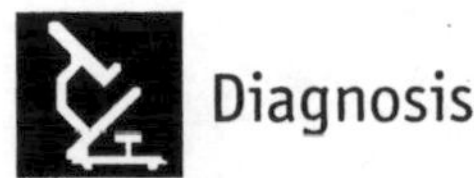

Diagnosis

DIFFERENTIAL DIAGNOSIS

Any pathology that causes increased intracranial pressure can cause cerebral herniation syndromes. Diffuse processes are less likely to cause herniation due to the general distribution of the pressure. Focal lesions, particularly laterally placed lesions and infratentorial lesions, are most likely to cause herniation, particularly if they are rapidly progressive. Various pathologic processes may cause the common pathway of brain herniation to occur.

SIGNS AND SYMPTOMS

Key to the diagnosis of cerebral herniation syndrome is the recognition of the possibility that they might occur. Patients with any intracranial mass lesion should be observed for signs of herniation. New or progressive neurologic symptoms, altered consciousness, or progressive headache are all signs of impending herniation. Uncontrolled vomiting may presage more severe herniation. Signs of cerebral herniation depend on the type of herniation as detailed above, but key in the diagnosis is recognizing changing signs indicating ongoing alteration of neurologic activity.

LABORATORY PROCEDURES

N/A

IMAGING STUDIES

Neuroimaging is key to the diagnosis and management of cerebral herniation syndromes. Frequently patients are known to have an underlying lesion, and the role of neuroimaging is to rapidly diagnose the type and extent of herniation, presence of secondary pathologies, and presence of specific treatable components of the herniation syndrome. Either CT or MRI may be used. CT scanning may be preferred since scanning times tend to be shorter, depending on the scan sequences used for MRI. Newer scan methodologies may allow for more rapid MRI evaluation. Key features to note on scanning are the location of the primary lesions (tumor, abscess, etc.), location of the herniation syndrome, secondary infarctions, and the presence of obstructive hydrocephalus. Such imaging is key to planning of surgical approaches to treating cerebral herniation.

SPECIAL TESTS

N/A

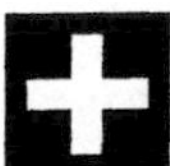

Management

GENERAL MEASURES

Patient should be kept well oxygenated to avoid secondary injury due to hypoxia. The head of the bed should be kept upright to avoid increasing intracranial pressure due to positioning. Similarly keeping the neck in a neutral position may reduce pressure on the jugular veins with secondary increases in back flow pressure. Patients should be kept NPO until the situation is stabilized in case they require emergency surgery.

SURGICAL MEASURES

Neurosurgical consultation is key in the management of cerebral herniation syndromes. Definitive treatment may depend on removal or debulking of the primary mass lesion; ventricular drainage for secondary hydrocephalus; removal of infarcted brain tissue causing herniation; and occasionally hemicraniectomy for massive unilateral brain swelling with cerebral infarction. The placement of a ventricular pressure measurement device may aid in the treatment of increased intracranial pressure, reducing the likelihood of secondary herniation syndromes.

SYMPTOMATIC TREATMENT

While cerebral herniation syndrome is a medical emergency, some attention to pain management in patients with headache is appropriate. It is best to avoid oral dosing of medications. Treatment of intracranial pressure (ICP) elevation is a crucial component of care, and ICP monitoring devices may aid in the rational provision of care. Cerebral blood flow needs to be maintained with a cerebral perfusion pressure of 70 mm Hg or more being optimal.

ADJUNCTIVE TREATMENT

- IV fluids should be kept isotonic and at a low rate, to avoid the risk of overhydration. Mechanical hyperventilation may be used to rapidly reduce ICP, by achieving pco_2 of 20 to 25 mm Hg. This maneuver is only effective for a few minutes. Achievement of lower pco_2 values risks secondary arterial constriction, which is counterproductive.
- In patients with brain neoplasms, radiation therapy may be used to reduced the mass size, depending on the tumor and the clinical situation.

ADMISSION/DISCHARGE CRITERIA

Patients with increased ICP or with signs of cerebral herniation syndromes should be admitted to the hospital, and remain there until the situation is definitively stabilized.

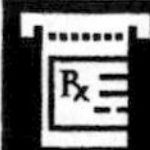

Medications

DRUG(S) OF CHOICE

- Mannitol is the most commonly used medication for increased ICP (see Increased Intracranial Pressure). Recently hypertonic saline has been used with some benefit in patients with raised ICP. Once herniation syndromes are apparent, attention to surgical approaches may be more important than medical management.
- In patients with known intracerebral brain tumors, dexamethasone given either orally or IV may reduce mass effect. For patients with impending herniation syndrome, higher doses may be used (e.g., 10 mg IV q6h), though no precise data exist on dosing regimens in this situation. Again, medical therapy tends to be a temporizing strategy, not the definitive therapy.

Contraindications

Mannitol may be contraindicated in patients with congestive heart failure or specific allergy to mannitol.

Precautions

Hyperventilation may cause a reflex vasoconstriction of the pco_2 is dropped below 25 mm Hg. Hyperosmotic agents such as mannitol may cause a rebound in intracranial pressure when stopped. Careful attention to fluid and electrolyte management is imperative during the management of brain herniation syndromes. Excessive hypernatremia or dehydration may be counterproductive.

ALTERNATIVE DRUGS

N/A

Follow-Up

PATIENT MONITORING

The ICU is necessary for patients with impending herniation syndromes. Cardiac monitoring, ICP pressure, respiratory monitoring, and fluid status monitoring are all important.

EXPECTED COURSE AND PROGNOSIS

Course and prognosis depends on the extent of the herniation, its potential for treatment, secondary injury, and the primary pathology underlying the herniation syndrome.

PATIENT EDUCATION

N/A

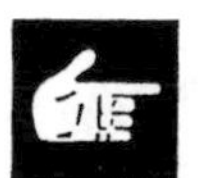

Miscellaneous

SYNONYMS

Cerebral herniation

ICD-9-CM: 348.4 Herniation, cerebral or brainstem

SEE ALSO: INCREASED INTRACRANIAL PRESSURE, HYDROCEPHALUS

REFERENCES

- Fisher CM. Brain herniation: a revision of classical concepts. Can J Neurol Sci 1995;22(2):83–91.
- Ropper AH. Lateral displacement of the brain and level of consciousness in patients with acute hemispheral mass. N Engl J Med 1986;314:953–958.
- Wijdicks EF, Miller GM. MR imaging of progressive downward herniation of the diencephalon. Neurology 1997;48(5):1456–1459.

Author(s): Alexander D. Rae-Grant, MD, FRCP(C)

Choreoathetosis

Basics

DESCRIPTION

Choreoathetosis is a combination of the term *chorea* and the term *athetosis*. These are two abnormal types of movement that are often combined in the same disorder. Chorea refers to rapid, involuntary, brief, irregular, and unpredictable jerks of muscles and can occur in the limbs, face, or trunk muscles. Athetosis is characterized by slow, writhing, uncoordinated involuntary movements usually involving the limbs, though similar movements may affect the face and trunk muscles as well.

DEFINITIONS

Chorea: rapid, involuntary, brief, irregular movements

Athetosis: writhing, involuntary, slow, uncoordinated movements

Parakinesia: a choreic movement camouflaged by a superimposed purposeful act

CLINICAL CHARACTERISTICS

Choreoathetosis may occur acutely or on a chronic basis, be transient, or be a persistent, lifelong phenomenon. It may interfere with the ability to speak, use the limbs, walk, or stand still. The movements may be unilateral (hemichorea), and at times are flinging (merging into hemiballismus, a separate but related disorder). Tone is usually reduced, but strength is unaffected. Patients may be unable to sustain a tight hand grip (milkmaid's hand). The tongue may dart in and out irregularly while attempting to protrude it.

PATHOPHYSIOLOGY

Choreoathetosis is caused by a degeneration or fixed injuries to the striatum (putamen, globus pallidus, caudate), or to a biochemical imbalance affecting these parts of the brain. The basal ganglia are critical in modulating motor activity from the corticospinal tract, and help maintain the posture, tone, and amplitude of motor activity both at rest and in action.

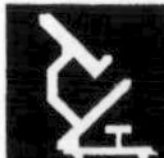

Diagnosis

DIFFERENTIAL DIAGNOSIS

- *Huntington disease* (HD): autosomal dominant, onset in 20s and 30s, with a combination of progressive chorea, a personality disorder and dementia. HD gene *(IT15)* on short arm of chromosome 4 (4p16.3).
- *Sydenham chorea*: (rheumatic chorea) in childhood and adolescence, often hemichorea, occurring after rheumatic fever, now rare. Self-limited disease.
- *Senile chorea*: late onset, generalized chorea, no family history, no dementia. Mild, slowly progressive. Various causes.
- *Chorea gravidarum*: chorea occurring with pregnancy. May also be seen with use of oral contraceptives.
- *Choreoathetosis with medications*: may occur with dopaminergic medications (L-dopa, bromocriptine, newer dopaminergic medications). Occasionally with famciclovir (in dialysis patients), digoxin, oral contraceptives, and gabapentin. Case reports with cocaine use.
- *Choreoathetosis with systemic diseases*: may occur with lupus erythematosus, thyrotoxicosis, polycythemia vera, and hyperosmolar, nonketotic hyperglycemia, antiphospholipid antibody syndrome, Creutzfeldt-Jakob disease. Rarely postpump choreoathetosis after cardiac surgery.
- *Neuroacanthocytosis*: familial multisystem progressive disorder with chorea, cognitive impairment, neuropathy, reduced reflexes, abnormal red cells (acanthocytes).
- *Developmental disorders*: a variety of prenatal and perinatal insults including kernicterus may cause choreoathetosis, which is nonprogressive and present from infancy or early childhood.
- *Rarer associations with choreoathetosis*: neuro-Behçet's disease, stroke, tumors, vascular malformations, moyamoya, tuberculous meningitis, multiple sclerosis, Wilson disease.
- *Hereditary nonprogressive chorea*: rare autosomal-dominant disorder, with chorea, no dementia or progression, no other neurologic signs.
- *Paroxysmal kinesigenic choreoathetosis*: choreoathetotic movements brought on by volitional movements. May be familial.
- *Dentatorubral-pallidoluysian atrophy*: rare autosomal-dominant disorder sometimes confused with Huntington disease. Patients show chorea, myoclonus, ataxia, seizures, and dementia.

SIGNS AND SYMPTOMS

In a patient presenting with choreoathetosis, symptoms suggesting cognitive dysfunction (memory loss, altered judgment, impulsivity, altered sexuality) may suggest Huntington disease. The clinical setting suggests Sydenham chorea, chorea gravidarum, and chorea related to systemic disease or medications. Choreoathetosis related to prenatal and perinatal insults is usually self-evident. Signs to seek include presence of associated neurologic findings (hyporeflexia, sensory loss suggesting neuropathy; cognitive dysfunction; presence of focal signs suggesting stroke).

LABORATORY PROCEDURES

Directed by clinical circumstances. In suspected cases of systemic causes of choreoathetosis, with blood smear (polycythemia vera, neuroacanthocytosis), glucose (hyperosmolar nonketotic hyperglycemia), thyroid indices (thyrotoxicosis), liver function studies (Wilson disease, kernicterus), antiphospholipid antibodies (antiphospholipid antibody syndrome). Genetic testing is available in Huntington disease but should be linked with counseling.

IMAGING STUDIES

CT scanning and MRI may both show focal basal ganglia lesions causing choreoathetosis. In situations such as acute chorea, imaging to assess for infarction, hemorrhage, tumor, or vascular malformation may be useful. Carbon monoxide poisoning may show hypodensities in the globus pallidus bilaterally. In Huntington disease, MRI later in disease may show atrophy of both caudate nuclei.

SPECIAL TESTS

For specific diseases special tests may be applicable. Tuberculous meningitis requires lumbar puncture, moyamoya may require angiography, multiple sclerosis may require evoked potentials and lumbar puncture. Positron emission tomography (PET) scanning may show caudate nucleus hypometabolism early in Huntington disease.

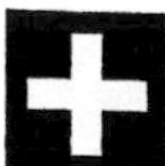

Management

GENERAL MEASURES

There are no specific measures to treat choreoathetosis. Treatment is directed at symptomatic management of the movements of chorea and athetosis, if necessary. If choreoathetosis is the result of a specific disease, that disease management should be used.

SURGICAL MEASURES

N/A

SYMPTOMATIC TREATMENT

Using neuroleptic medications can control choreic movements. These include dopamine receptor blocking agents (such as haloperidol and perphenazine). Other medications that deplete presynaptic dopamine, such as reserpine or tetrabenazine, can be used. Newer atypical antipsychotic agents (e.g., quetiapine or olanzapine) may be tried.

ADJUNCTIVE TREATMENT

N/A

ADMISSION/DISCHARGE CRITERIA

Patients with acute onset of chorea may require hospitalization for diagnosis and stabilization. Patients with Huntington disease may require admission if at risk of harming themselves or others based on their psychiatric state.

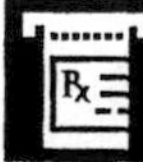

Medications

DRUG(S) OF CHOICE

See individual diseases for drug information.

Follow-Up

PATIENT MONITORING

See individual disease chapters.

EXPECTED COURSE AND PROGNOSIS

See individual disease chapters.

PATIENT EDUCATION

See Huntington disease section for patient education.

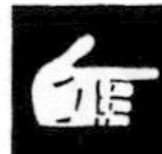

Miscellaneous

SYNONYMS

- St. Vitus dance, chorea minor, acute chorea, rheumatic chorea (Sydenham chorea)
- Chorea-acanthocytosis (neuroacanthocytosis)
- Benign hereditary chorea (hereditary nonprogressive chorea)

ICD-9-CM: 333.4 Chorea, Huntington's; 333.5 Choreathetosis (paroxysmal); 333.5 Chorea, senile; 392.9 Chorea, Synderhams; 780.3 Chorea, gravidarum

SEE ALSO: CEREBROVASCULAR DISEASE, ANTIPHOSPHOLIPID ANTIBODY SYNDROME, HUNTINGTON'S DISEASE, SYDENHAM'S CHOREA, PARKINSON'S DISEASE, SYSTEMIC LUPUS ERYTHEMATOSUS

REFERENCES

- Alarcon F, Duenas G, Cevallos N, et al. Movement disorders in 30 patients with tuberculous meningitis. Mov Disord 2000;15(3):561–569.
- Fernandez M, Raskind W, Matsushita M, et al. Hereditary benign chorea: clinical and genetic features of a distinct disease. Neurology 2001;57(1):106–110.
- Rinne JO, Daniel SE, Scaravilli F, et al. The neuropathological features of neuroacanthocytosis. Mov Disord 1994;9:297–304.
- Ross CA, Margolis RL, Rosenblatt A, et al. Huntington disease and the related disorder, dentatorubral-pallidoluysian atrophy. Medicine 1997;76:305–338.

Author(s): Alexander D. Rae-Grant, MD, FRCP (C)

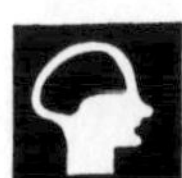

Basics

DESCRIPTION

Coma is the most severe form of unresponsiveness. The subject is unarousable. Either there is severe diffuse cerebral dysfunction or significant brainstem impairment. Structural, metabolic, and infectious causes are typical. Clinical presentation, neurologic assessment, neuroimaging, and laboratory evaluations determine the specific cause and guide treatment options.

DEFINITION

Coma is a state of unconsciousness with complete absence of awareness of the environment even when externally stimulated. A persistent vegetative state usually emerges in about 2 weeks and refers to unresponsiveness despite wakefulness with return of sleep-wake cycles. Related terms include stupor, where subjects can be aroused with noxious stimuli, and lethargy, referring to someone arousable with verbal stimuli. Acute confusional states represent levels of attentional deficits between full responsiveness and lethargy. A locked-in state subject is mute and quadriplegic but conscious and can blink or vertically move the eyes on command. Brain death is declared when there is irreversible cessation of all brain and brainstem function from a known and explainable cause.

CLINICAL CHARACTERISTICS

The subject lies with eyes closed and cannot be aroused verbally or with noxious painful stimuli. There is no spontaneous eye opening, facial movements, utterances, or body movements. Painful stimuli may produce nondirected reflexive movements related to spinal cord or lower brainstem pathways, but will not result in any conscious responsiveness.

PATHOPHYSIOLOGY

Coma results only from conditions that disrupt both cerebral hemispheres or the brainstem ascending reticular activating system. Conscious behavior requires both arousal and cognitive processing. The brainstem reticular activating system extending from the midpons to the hypothalamus is responsible for arousal. The cerebral hemispheres are responsible for cognitive abilities. The locked-in syndrome results from conditions affecting the nervous system below the midpons, which preserves that portion of the reticular activating system responsible for arousal and consciousness.

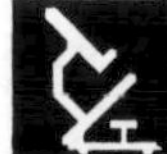

Diagnosis

DIFFERENTIAL DIAGNOSIS

Diffuse Encephalopathies

- Cerebral anoxia/ischemia
- Encephalitis/meningitis
- Subarachnoid hemorrhage
- Vasculitis
- Metabolic encephalopathy (eg. uremia)
- Hyponatremia
- Diabetes (ketoacidosis, hypoglycemia, nonketotic hyperosmolar coma)
- Nutritional deficiency (thiamine)
- Alcohol/narcotic abuse
- Drug overdose/intoxication
- Hepatic encephalopathy
- Hypothyroidism
- Multiorgan failure
- Sepsis
- Seizures (complex partial status epilepticus, nonconvulsive status)
- Hypothermia/hyperthermia
- Hypertensive encephalopathy

Structural Lesions

- Brain herniation syndromes
- Brain tumor
- Brain abscess
- Epidural/subdural hematoma
- Subdural empyema
- Intracerebral infarction or hemorrhage
- Brainstem infarction or hemorrhage
- Cerebellar infarction or hemorrhage
- Basilar artery thrombosis
- Head trauma (cerebral contusion)

SIGNS AND SYMPTOMS

History

- Ask about onset and time course. Sudden onset with rapid progression suggests stroke or hemorrhage, whereas subacute course may indicate tumor or abscess. Coma preceded by acute confusional states without focal neurologic complaints suggests diffuse encephalopathies.
- Ask about recent head trauma, progressive neurologic deficits (brain tumor), fever, infection, severe headache, stroke risk factors, seizures, current medications, drug or alcohol abuse, nutritional deficiencies, depression, diabetes, and organ failure.

General Exam

- Observe for signs of head trauma.
- Evaluate for stiff neck common with meningitis or subarachnoid hemorrhage.
- Check vital signs and temperature. Elevated blood pressure is common with hemorrhage, stroke, or hypertensive encephalopathy. Hypothermia is seen with certain drug intoxications, hepatic encephalopathy, hypothyroidism, and hypoglycemia. Hyperthermia is seen with anticholinergic drug intoxications, heat stroke, status epilepticus, and certain hypothalamic lesions.

Fundi

- Papilledema and retinal hemorrhages suggest increased intracranial pressure.

Pupils

- Normal to smaller and reactive: diffuse encephalopathies or hypothalamic compression.
- Bilateral dilated and fixed: midbrain lesion, anoxia, or drug intoxications usually anticholinergic, sympathomimetic, barbiturates, or glutethimide.
- Unilateral dilated and fixed: third nerve palsy.
- Pinpoint and reactive: pontine lesion, narcotic intoxications, organophosphate poisoning, or miotic eye drops.

Extraocular Movements

- Check primary gaze for skews or deviations, look for roving eye movements, test oculocephalic reflexes (doll's-head reflex), and/or oculovestibular reflexes (calorics).
- Normal primary gaze with intact oculocephalics and oculovestibulars showing slow lateral deviation without nystagmus: diffuse encephalopathies.
- Normal primary gaze with impaired oculocephalics and oculovestibulars: occasionally seen with certain drug intoxications (barbiturates, benzodiazepines, tricyclics, succinylcholine, phenytoin, or antibiotics) or preexisting vestibular dysfunction.
- Dysconjugate gaze: structural lesions.
- Deviated eyes at rest (to side of lesion) with intact oculocephalics and oculovestibulars showing slow lateral deviation without nystagmus: supratentorial structural lesion.
- Single deviated eye at rest that fails to adduct with either oculocephalics or oculovestibulars: third nerve palsy lesion.
- Skewed, deviated at rest (away from lesion) or normal primary gaze with absent oculocephalics and absent oculovestibulars: pontine lesion.

Brainstem Reflexes

- Corneal reflexes: normal direct and consensual responses suggest an intact midbrain and pons.
- Gag responses: if present, suggest an intact medulla.

Motor Exam

- Look for spontaneous movements, check posture (laterally rotated legs, facial droop), tone, reflexes, and response to noxious stimuli applied to an extremity or face to help detect hemiparesis, facial weakness, and other focal neurologic deficits.
- Repetitive movements of a limb or face: think of seizures or status.
- Tremors, myoclonus, or asterixis: diffuse encephalopathies.
- Flaccid tone: diffuse encephalopathies, pontine lesions, or medulla lesions.
- Decorticate posturing (arm flexion, leg extension) to noxious stimuli: diffuse encephalopathies, supratentorial lesions, or thalamic lesions.

- Decerebrate posturing (arm and leg extension) to noxious stimuli: subtentorial or brainstem lesions.

Transtentorial Brain Herniation

- Results from progressive downward pressure on thalamus and brainstem due to supratentorial structural lesions and/or edema.
- Pupils: initially, small, reactive to light and progressing to midsized and nonreactive as the upper brainstem is compressed.
- Extraocular movements: eyes may be deviated or have dysconjugate gaze, and oculocephalic and oculovestibular reflexes become impaired as brainstem is compressed.
- Motor exam: initially usually asymmetric but responsive to pain, progressing to decorticate posturing as the thalamus and hypothalamus are compressed, then to decerebrate posturing as the midbrain is compressed, and finally progressing to a flaccid state.

Uncal Brain Herniation

- Results from progressive lateral pressure on the thalamus and upper brainstem due to temporal lobe structural lesions and/or edema.
- Pupils: dilated and fixed ipsilateral to lesion.
- Extraocular movements: eye ipsilateral to lesion may be deviated laterally and fails to adduct with either oculocephalics or oculovestibulars.
- Motor exam: hemiplegia may occur ipsilateral to lesion due to the opposite cerebral peduncle being compressed against the incisura of the tentorium (Kernohan's notch).

Respiratory Breathing Patterns

- Cheyne-Stokes: periodic episodes of apnea alternating with hyperpnea, seen with either diffuse encephalopathies or structural lesions.
- Central neurogenic hyperventilation: sustained, rapid hyperpnea often associated with midbrain/upper pons damage, but can be seen with diffuse encephalopathies or structural lesions.
- Apneustic: pausing at full inspiration seen with pontine damage and, occasionally, anoxia, meningitis, or hypoglycemia.
- Ataxic: irregular pattern of shallow, deep breaths seen with medullary damage.

LABORATORY PROCEDURES

- Lab tests should include arterial blood gas, electrolytes, BUN, creatinine, glucose, calcium, magnesium, liver function tests, ammonia, CBC, PT, PTT, sedimentation rate, thyroid function tests, and toxicology screen.
- Cervical spine films if trauma suspected.
- Lumbar puncture: cerebrospinal fluid may identify meningitis or encephalitis. Should be avoided with mass lesions as herniation can occur.
- Electrocardiogram to evaluate the heart.
- Electroencephalogram if seizures suspected.

IMAGING STUDIES

- CT and MRI scans will show structural lesions. MRI is better for visualizing the brainstem.

SPECIAL TESTS

N/A

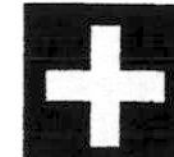

Management

GENERAL MEASURES

- Airway, breathing, and circulation.
- Check for and stabilize cervical spine fractures before examination.
- Every comatose patient should be given thiamine 100 mg IV for possible Wernicke's encephalopathy, 50% dextrose 50 mL IV for possible hypoglycemic coma, and naloxone 0.4–1.2 mg IV for possible opiate overdose.
- Treat seizures.
- Perform laboratory and imaging studies to determine cause of the coma.
- Wean off any sedative medications.

SURGICAL MEASURES

- Neurosurgical evaluation is helpful in the management and treatment of patients with subarachnoid hemorrhage, intracerebral hemorrhage, hematoma, tumor, abscess, and brain herniation.

SYMPTOMATIC TREATMENT

- Stabilize vital signs.
- Correct metabolic and other treatable causes.
- Meningitis, encephalitis, and brain abscess are treated with antibiotics.
- Decreasing protein intake and reducing ammonia levels with lactulose and neomycin can treat hepatic encephalopathy.

Treatment of Herniation Syndromes and Cerebral Edema

- Ischemic stroke causing cerebral edema and transtentorial herniation is not helped by osmotic diuretics or corticosteroids.
- Elevate head.
- Intubate and hyperventilate to reduce P_{CO_2} to 25 mm Hg.
- Administer mannitol 20% 1.5–2.0 g/kg IV over 30 to 60 minutes.
- Give normal saline two-thirds maintenance.
- For those with tumor, abscess, and possibly intracerebral hemorrhage, give dexamethasone 10 mg IV then 4 mg PO or IV every 6 hours with an H_2 blocker and monitor blood sugar.

ADJUNCTIVE TREATMENT

Supportive care is critical.

ADMISSION/DISCHARGE CRITERIA

- Admit to the intensive care unit for initial evaluation and treatment.
- Discharges to convalescent or rehabilitation units occur if recovery is not complete.

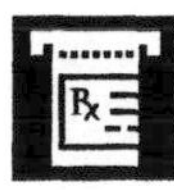

Medications

DRUG(S) OF CHOICE

- See general measures and symptomatic treatment sections above.

Contraindications

N/A

Precautions

N/A

ALTERNATIVE DRUGS

N/A

Follow-Up

PATIENT MONITORING

Neurologic checks required frequently for detecting changes in neurologic function.

EXPECTED COURSE AND PROGNOSIS

- If the underlying cause of the coma can be treated, prognosis depends on how much irreversible brain damage has occurred.
- Given the severe nature of many of the underlying causes of coma, mortality is high.

PATIENT EDUCATION

Provide strategies to reduce reoccurrence of preventable metabolic or other forms of coma.

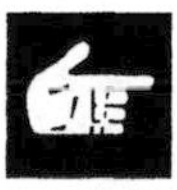

Miscellaneous

SYNONYMS

N/A

ICD-9-CM: 780.01 Coma

SEE ALSO: N/A

REFERENCES

- Levy DE, Caronna JJ, Singer BH, et al. Predicting outcome from hypoxic-ischemic coma. JAMA 1985;253:1420–1426.
- Plum F, Posner JB. The diagnosis of stupor and coma, 3rd ed. Vol. 19 of Contemporary Neurology Series. Philadelphia: F. A. Davis, 1980.
- Simon RP. Coma. In: Joynt RJ, Griggs RC, eds. Clinical neurology. Philadelphia: Lippincott-Raven, 1997.

Author(s): Douglas W. Scharre, MD

Delirium/Encephalopathy

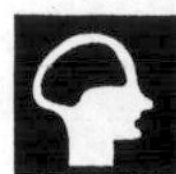

Basics

DESCRIPTION

Delirium describes a state where the patient is confused, with an agitated, inattentive behavior. Delirious patients frequently hallucinate or have delusional thoughts. This syndrome develops over a brief period of time, usually hours or days. Patients often have an autonomic disorder with sweating, tachycardia, and excessive movement. Encephalopathy is a more nonspecific term that describes a state of altered consciousness that is usually acute, caused by metabolic or systemic disorders, and often is reversible (see specific chapters on encephalopathies).

DEFINITIONS

- Delirium: acute confusional state in patients with agitation and hallucinations.
- Dementia: chronic, progressive cognitive impairment in alert patients.
- Encephalopathy: nonspecific term for altered mental state, usually of acute onset.

CLINICAL CHARACTERISTICS

Delirium and acute encephalopathy are common in the inpatient setting. The prevalence of delirium has been estimated at 10% to 30% of inpatient medical populations. Up to 50% of patients with hip fractures experience delirium at some time, and delirium is common in patients with severe burns. Clinical characteristics of delirium include an acute onset of mental status changes, usually over hours or a few days. The mental state is marked by inattention, in which the patient cannot focus on specific stimuli for any period of time. Patients are either drowsy or hypervigilant, and show an altered response to their environment. Patients have difficulty interacting for mental status testing, and tend to either not interact appropriately with the examiner or make errors in orientation, repetition, and memory testing related to their inattention and clouded sensorium. Characteristic of delirium is agitation, frequently with hallucinations, which may be visual, and at times formed (e.g., insects crawling). Patients may make perceptual errors, misidentifying objects in the room. Patients may also have signs of autonomic hyperactivity, including tachycardia, diaphoresis, flushed facies, and hyperventilation.

PATHOPHYSIOLOGY

Delirium is caused by a variety of toxic, metabolic, infectious, and medication-related disorders. Thus the specific pathophysiology of neurologic dysfunction depends on the etiology. Different delirious states have in common dysfunction of CNS neurons, due to reduced/altered substrates, acid-base disorders, hypoxemia, toxins or medications that affect neuronal function, secondary immunologic effects, or inflammatory activity in the CNS. Each of these causes an alteration function of CNS neurons, leading to the clinical state.

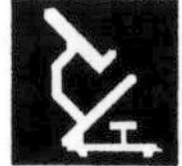

Diagnosis

DIFFERENTIAL DIAGNOSIS

A variety of disorders may cause delirium or encephalopathy during their course. Patients with underlying brain disorders are more likely to show delirium or encephalopathy as a result of disease. Thus patients with senile dementia who have new infections commonly become delirious. Patients who are either very old or very young are at more risk of responding to disease with delirium or encephalopathy. Other risk factors include a history of alcohol abuse, multiple medical problems, visual or hearing impairment, and sleep deprivation.

- Medical/surgical diseases: sepsis, focal infections, postoperative states, endocrine disorders (e.g., thyrotoxicosis, Cushing's disease), metabolic disorders (e.g., hyponatremia, hyperglycemia, hypoglycemia, etc.), hepatic or renal failure, hypoxia or hypercarbia.
- Neurologic diseases: meningitis, encephalitis, subarachnoid hemorrhage, traumatic brain injury, vascular, neoplastic, inflammatory, or other disorders. May occur after seizures.
- Drug or medication use or withdrawal states: street drugs, alcohol withdrawal or intoxication, sedative/hypnotic agents, opiates, anticholinergics, atropine, amphetamines, drug overdoses, steroids.
- Toxins: organophosphates, heavy metals, organic solvents, etc.

SIGNS AND SYMPTOMS

Patients with delirium show inattention, with difficulty doing tasks such as counting backward by 7 from 100, listing the months backward, etc. They drift off in conversation, and are unable to give a history. More complex tasks of mental status are clouded by inattention. Patients are often restless, but usually show no focal neurologic signs. Reflexes and cranial nerves are unaffected. The toes are usually downgoing unless there is neurologic disease causing delirium. Patients may show signs of hallucinating. They may be drowsy or frankly stuporous. Patients may have asterixis, particularly with hepatic encephalopathy.

LABORATORY PROCEDURES

Depending on the history, laboratory studies may assist in diagnosis. CBC (for increased WBC); electrolytes (for hypo- or hypernatremia, low bicarbonate associated with metabolic acidosis); glucose (for hypo- or hyperglycemia); liver function tests; BUN and creatinine; drug screen; levels of therapeutic medications for intoxication. Arterial blood gases. Consider vitamin B_{12}, autoimmune studies, sedimentation rate in selected cases.

IMAGING STUDIES

Imaging of the brain may be important to exclude focal disorders causing encephalopathy. Depending on the clinical circumstance, CT scanning or MRI may be used.

SPECIAL TESTS

Lumbar puncture should be used once an intracranial mass lesion is excluded in those patients considered to have an intracranial infection (encephalitis or meningitis). If CT scanning is negative and subarachnoid hemorrhage is suspected, lumbar puncture may be diagnostic. EEG may be useful in showing triphasic waves, characteristic of metabolic encephalopathy, as well as excluding nonconvulsive status epilepticus.

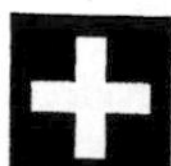

Management

GENERAL MEASURES

Careful attention must be given to the maintenance or establishment or an airway, breathing, and circulation. Any evidence of cardiovascular instability must be treated immediately. IV access is important to allow medication to be provided, as well as electrolyte solutions. Consider providing IV thiamine (patients suspected of having Wernicke syndrome), glucose (suspected hypoglycemia), and naloxone (opioid intoxication). Measures should be taken to protect patients from harming themselves; a bed check may help prevent falls, or if necessary, restraints or provision of 1:1 nursing may be helpful. Consider a secure environment if the patient is a potential threat to others.

SURGICAL MEASURES

N/A

SYMPTOMATIC TREATMENT

Once an etiology or delirium or encephalopathy is determined, treating the cause of this state is required. Treatment guidelines pertinent to the etiology should be followed.

ADJUNCTIVE TREATMENT

Ensure that all drugs or toxins that may be causing the delirium are withdrawn. Make sure that fluid requirements, particularly in patients with autonomic overactivity, are met.

ADMISSION/DISCHARGE CRITERIA

Patients with delirium or encephalopathy require admission for their diagnosis and safety. Such patients are at risk of falls and injuries in the home setting. Patients should be fully alert and oriented if possible before discharge. They should usually be discharged into the care of a responsible party if possible.

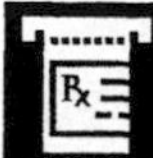

Medications

DRUG(S) OF CHOICE

The primary treatments for delirium or encephalopathy are to treat the underlying disorder. At times patients may require treatment to reduce their symptoms of agitation or restlessness. Care should be taken to avoid respiratory suppression by medications in such patients. If necessary, medication such as haloperidol in low doses may be useful without significant risk of respiratory compromise. Haloperidol 0.5–2 mg IM or IV repeated q4–6h as needed, depending on age, weight, degree of agitation. Switch to oral when possible. For alcohol withdrawal use benzodiazepines.

Contraindications

Avoid with significant hypotension or sensitivity to similar medications.

Precautions

Watch for dystonic reactions and hypotension.

ALTERNATIVE DRUGS

Risperidone may be used.

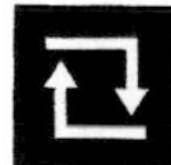

Follow-Up

PATIENT MONITORING

Patients with delirium or encephalopathy should be closely monitored until stabilization occurs.

EXPECTED COURSE AND PROGNOSIS

Delirium and encephalopathy are self-limited conditions that should resolve with improvement of the medical condition. Prognosis is related to the underlying medical conditions.

PATIENT EDUCATION

Since this is a self-limited disorder, patient education is limited to reassurance, reorientation, and explanation of the clinical condition after the patient has returned to a more normal mental status.

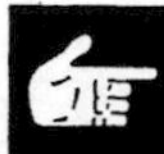

Miscellaneous

SYNONYMS

Acute confusional state

ICD-9-CM: 291.0 Acute alcohol delirium; 293.0 Acute psychotic delirium; 293.1 Subacute delirium; 292.81 Drug-induced delirium; 349.82 Toxic encephalopathy; 348.3 Encephalopathy NOS

SEE ALSO: DEMENTIA; ENCEPHALOPATHY, HEPATIC; ENCEPHALOPATHY, SEPTIC; ENCEPHALOPATHY, RENAL

REFERENCES

- Francis J, Martin D, Kapoor WN. A prospective study of delirium in hospitalized elderly. JAMA 1990;265: 1097–1101.
- Levkoff SE, Evans DA, Liptzin B, et al. Delirium. Arch Intern Med 1992;152: 334–340.
- Schor JD, Levkoff SE, Lipsitz LA, et al. Risk factors for delirium in hospitalized elderly. JAMA 1992;267:827–831.

Author(s): Alexander D. Rae-Grant, MD, FRCP (C)

Dizziness

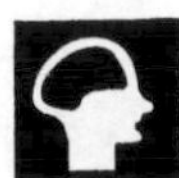

Basics

DESCRIPTION

Dizziness is a common, nonspecific symptom that affects approximately 15% to 30% of the population at some point during one's lifetime. It describes an altered sense of position of patients in relation to their surroundings. The etiology can be central or peripheral with a broad differential ranging from benign to life-threatening conditions.

DEFINITIONS

Dizziness can be defined as central or peripheral in origin. Peripheral etiologies refer to lesions of the temporal bone, middle ear, labyrinth, and cranial nerve VIII before it enters the brainstem. Central etiologies include lesions of the vestibular nuclei, brainstem, cerebellum, or cerebrum.

CLINICAL CHARACTERISTICS

Dizziness can affect patients of all ages; however, it is more common in elderly patients. There is a slight female preponderance. All races are affected equally. Risk factors to develop dizziness include older age, infections, inner ear problems, vision problems, trauma, hypertension, dehydration, orthostatic hypotension, atherosclerotic vascular disease, anemia, menopause, and familial factors.

PATHOPHYSIOLOGY

The two most common causes of dizziness are vestibular disorders (35%–55%) and psychiatric illnesses (10%–25%). The most common CNS cause is cerebrovascular ischemia or infarction (2%–10%). Neoplasms are an infrequent cause of dizziness, noted in less than 1% of patients. Dizziness can be secondary to inflammation, infections, metabolic abnormalities, autoimmune disorders, medications (e.g., ototoxins), developmental anomalies, autonomic nervous system dysfunction, neurodegenerative diseases, trauma, and other systemic disorders. The cause of dizziness is often multifactorial, especially in elderly patients. In 15% to 25% of patients the etiology remains unknown. Familial causes of vertiginous dizziness have been reported.

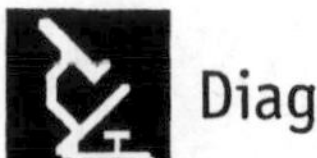

Diagnosis

DIFFERENTIAL DIAGNOSIS

- Benign paroxysmal positional vertigo
- Vestibular neuronitis
- Ramsay Hunt syndrome
- Meniere's disease
- Meniere's syndrome
- Multiple sclerosis
- Vertebrobasilar migraine
- Autonomic dysfunction
- Orthostatic hypotension
- Hypoglycemia
- Infectious (otitis media, syphilitic, delayed-onset Meniere's disease, meningitis, AIDS, viral encephalitis)
- CNS vasculitis
- Cerebellar lesion (infarct, vascular malformation, hemorrhage, neoplasm)
- Lateral medullary syndrome
- Pontine syndrome
- Posterior fossa neoplasm (e.g., vestibular schwannoma, brainstem glioma)
- Neurofibromatosis type 2
- Paraneoplastic syndrome
- Posterior fossa structural lesion (e.g., Chiari malformation)
- Postconcussion syndrome
- Alcoholic cerebellar degeneration
- Vitamin E deficiency
- Vitamin B_{12} or folate deficiency

SIGNS AND SYMPTOMS

Dizziness can be divided into four major categories: vertigo, presyncope, dysequilibrium, and light-headedness. The symptoms can range from mild light-headedness, the sensation of losing one's balance when standing or walking (dysequilibrium), spinning movements relative to the surroundings (vertigo), to an impending loss of consciousness (presyncope). The onset of dizziness can be spontaneous or provoked by certain movements or head position, and be episodic or persistent. Dizziness is commonly associated with varying degrees of nausea, vomiting, pallor, and perspiration. It also can be associated with tinnitus, hearing loss, aural fullness, ataxia, headache, vision disturbances, memory difficulties, seizures, and focal neurologic deficits. Focal neurologic findings such as cranial neuropathies, hemiparesis, dysarthria, dysphagia, diplopia, ataxia, and dysmetria suggest a central etiology.

LABORATORY PROCEDURES

Blood tests have a low yield in identifying a specific cause of dizziness. Lumbar puncture is important in evaluating CNS infection and idiopathic intracranial hypo- or hypertension. Spinal fluid can also be tested for cytology, VDRL, ACE level, oligoclonal bands, and IgG synthesis index.

IMAGING STUDIES

MRI with and without contrast is important to exclude structural lesions or malformations, infarction, demyelinating disorders, or upper cervical spine dysfunction. Imaging studies are strongly indicated for patients with focal neurologic findings and persistent vertigo or imbalance for longer than 6 months. MR and cerebral angiography are used to identify vertebrobasilar insufficiency or atherosclerosis.

SPECIAL TESTS

The Dix-Hallpike test can be helpful to distinguish peripheral from central causes of dizziness. Tests of vestibular function may be of benefit, including audiometry, electronystagmography, and rotational testing. Cardiac evaluation may be indicated in some patients. Neurologic studies may include autonomic function testing, EEG, brainstem auditory evoked responses, and EMG.

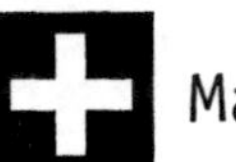

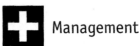

Management

GENERAL MEASURES

Specific therapies are directed to the underlying etiology of the dizziness. Antibiotics, antiviral, or antifungal agents may be used for infection. Antiepileptic drugs are effective in treating paroxysmal vestibular disorders. Beta-blockers are effective for basilar or vestibular migraine attacks. Corticosteroids can be used in inflammatory processes such as vestibular neuritis or Cogan's disease. Antiplatelet and anticoagulation therapies are indicated for infarction and dizziness associated with vascular etiologies. Vestibular exercises and rehabilitation programs are designed to readjust perceptual, vestibulo-ocular, and vestibulospinal reflexes by fostering central compensation of vestibular tone imbalance.

SURGICAL MEASURES

Surgery is the treatment of choice for posterior fossa tumors and cysts. It is also appropriate for rotational vertebral artery syndrome or upper cervical spine dysfunction. In patients with refractory Meniere's disease, surgical intervention such as endolymphatic shunt placement and selective vestibular nerve section can be performed. Surgical patching may be necessary for refractory cases of perilymphatic fistula.

SYMPTOMATIC TREATMENT

Most causes of dizziness are benign and self-limiting disorders, and antivertiginous drugs and antiemetics can provide symptomatic relief in the acute phase. Symptomatic therapy for hypertension, hypoglycemia, anemia, arrhythmia, seizures, headache, muscle spasm, and thyroid and other systemic disorders may be indicated for specific etiologies. For psychogenic dizziness, reassurance, short-term benzodiazepines, selective serotonin reuptake inhibitors (SSRIs), or psychiatric consultation may be needed.

ADJUNCTIVE TREATMENTS

In the acute phase, bed rest, mental relaxation, and visual fixation are helpful. Vestibular habituation and balance retraining exercises are beneficial for chronic persistent dizziness secondary to multiple sensory deficits. Physical and occupational therapies involving eye, head, and body movements are also beneficial for dizziness due to upper cervical dysfunction and CVA, and should be begun as soon as the acute stage of nausea and vomiting has ended.

ADMISSION/DISCHARGE CRITERIA

Patient with profound disequilibrium or intractable vomiting may require hospitalization and IV rehydration. Patients with acute onset and severe dizziness of central origin (e.g., cerebellar or brainstem stroke) are admitted for evaluation and close monitoring through the acute phase.

Medications

DRUG(S) OF CHOICE

Vestibular Suppressants

- Antihistamines: meclizine (Antivert 25–50 mg q6h PRN) is most commonly used; dimenhydrinate (Dramamine 50 mg q4–6h PO or IM), diphenhydramine, and cyclizine are also used as vestibular sedative medications. Central anticholinergic activity may be the underlying mechanism.
- Benzodiazepines: diazepam (Valium 2.5–5 mg PO, IM, or IV tid or PRN) or clonazepam (Klonopin 0.5 mg PO tid) can be helpful in alleviating severe vertigo and anxiety.
- Anticholinergics: scopolamine (0.6 mg q4–6h or transdermal patch 1 q3d, no longer than 10 days) is effective for motion sickness and posttraumatic vertigo.

Antiemetics

Promethazine (Phenergan, 25 mg q6h PO, IM, supp, IV, PRN) and prochlorperazine (Compazine 5–10 mg PO im q6h or 25 mg supp q12h) are useful in relieving the severe nausea associated with vertigo. Ondansetron (4 mg q8h PRN) and prochlorperazine are used for severe nausea from central vertigo.

For *Meniere's disease,* low-sodium diet and diuretics (acetazolamide 250–500 mg bid) for 3 months to 1 year have been recommended. Also, a trial course of prednisone at 1 mg/kg for 10 days given orally or intramuscular injection of methylprednisolone 60–80 mg followed by oral prednisone taper are recommended for Meniere's disease, vestibular neuritis, or inner ear autoimmune process.

Contraindications

Prior history of hypersensitivity or allergic reaction. Transtympanic aminoglycoside treatment of Meniere's disease is associated with risk of profound hearing loss; bilateral involvement of Meniere's disease is a relative contraindication for ototoxic treatment.

Precautions

Drowsiness is commonly associated with antihistamines and antiemetics. Steroid therapy for vestibular neuritis or autoimmune inner ear disease can be associated with hypertension, hyperglycemia, gastric ulcers, osteoporosis, and cataract.

ALTERNATIVE DRUGS

Sympathomimetic agents such as amphetamine and ephedrine may be useful in specific situations. Baclofen (20 mg tid PO) has been used for downbeat or upbeat nystagmus. SSRIs such as paroxetine (Paxil 10–20 mg qd) are used for chronic anxiety. Glycopyrrolate (Robinul, 2 mg bid or tid PO) can be tried in cases of antihistamine failure in patients without glaucoma, congestive heart failure, hyperthyroidism, or gastroesophageal reflux.

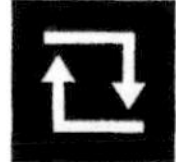

Follow-Up

PATIENT MONITORING

Patients are followed to monitor progression and recurrence of symptoms and efficacy of pharmacologic and rehabilitation therapy. This can be done with serial physical exams and specific outcome measures as the Dizziness Handicap Inventory, Activities Specific Balance Confidence Scale, Computerized Dynamic Posturography, and gait measures.

EXPECTED COURSE AND PROGNOSIS

Clinical course and prognosis varies with etiology. Most cases of dizziness are benign and self-limited, and recover spontaneously over several weeks to months. Symptomatic recovery is due to vestibular compensation (central reorganization of vestibular circuits). Prognosis is better if the symptoms are due to vestibular dysfunction. In dizziness of central origin or from systemic illness, success depends on treating the underlying disorder.

PATIENT EDUCATION

- Vestibular Disorders Association, P.O. Box 4467, Portland, OR 97208-4467. Website *www.vestibular.org.*
- Balance and Dizziness Disorders Society in Canada, or 5525 West Boulevard, #325, Vancouver, BC, Canada V6M 3W6. Website *www.BalanceAndDizziness.org.*
- Meniere's Society, 98 Maybury Rd., Working Surrey, GU21 5HX, UK.

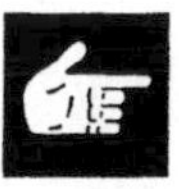

Miscellaneous

SYNONYMS

Vertigo, disequilibrium, presyncope

ICD-9-CM: 386 Vertiginous syndromes; 386.01 Meniere's disease (active); 386.10 Peripheral vertigo, unspecified; 386.11 Benign paroxysmal positional vertigo; 386.12 Vestibular neuronitis; 386.2 Vertigo of central origin; 386.3 Labyrinthitis; 780.2 Presyncope; 780.4 Dizziness and giddiness; 306.9 Unspecified psychophysiological malfunction (including psychogenic dizziness)

SEE ALSO: MENIERE'S SYNDROME

REFERENCES

- Baloh RW. Vertigo. Lancet 1998;352: 1841.
- Derebery MJ. The diagnosis and treatment of dizziness. Med Clin North Am 1999;83: 163.
- El-Kashlan HK, Telian SA. Diagnosis and initiating treatment for peripheral system disorders: imbalance and dizziness with normal hearing. Otolaryngol Clin North Am 2000;33:563.
- Hoffman RM, Einstadter D, Kroenke K. Evaluating dizziness. Am J Med 1999; 107:468.
- Koelliker P, Summers RL, Hawkins B. Benign paroxysmal positional vertigo: diagnosis and treatment in the emergency department—a review of the literature and discussion of canalith-repositioning maneuvers. Ann Emerg Med 2001;37: 392.
- Rubin AM, Zafar SS. The assessment and management of the dizzy patient. Otolaryngol Clin North Am 2002;35:255.
- Sajjadi H. Medical management of Meniere's disease. Otolaryngol Clin North Am 2002;35:581.
- Solomon D. Distinguishing and treating causes of central vertigo. Otolaryngol Clin North Am 2000;33:579.

Author(s): Yiqun Hu, MD, PhD

Dysarthria

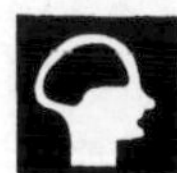

Basics

DESCRIPTION

Dysarthria is defined as a defect in the production of speech affecting the volume, rate, tone, or quality of spoken language. Abnormalities in a number of neurologic structures can lead to dysarthria by altering the function of the muscles of phonation and articulation. Dysarthria must be discriminated from aphasia, in which there is a disorder of the production of language with or without an articulation disorder.

DEFINITIONS

Phonation: the production of vocal sounds.
Articulation: contractions of the pharynx, palate, tongue, and lips that alter the vocal sound to form components of speech.
Anarthria: inability to produce speech with sparing of comprehension of speech and ability to read and write.

CLINICAL CHARACTERISTICS

The origin of dysarthria is neurologic, associated with damage to either the central or peripheral nervous system. It is a disorder of movement and abnormal speech execution, disrupting the range, timing, speed, or accuracy of the movement producing speech. It does not therefore disrupt the structure of speech, or its linguistic or cognitive components. Disorders affecting the physical structures of the speech apparatus, such as a cleft lip or palate, are not referred to as dysarthrias.
Dysarthria can be characterized by the major neurologic abnormality causing it. Each level of the neuraxis causes a different quality of dysarthric speech.
Lower motor neuron dysarthria (bulbar palsy): speech slurred, nasal, drooling, raspy quality, monotonous, indistinct. Tongue atrophy, flaccid palate, reduced gag.
Spastic dysarthria (pseudobulbar palsy): speech explosive, forced, effortful. No tongue atrophy, brisk jaw jerk, brisk gag. Slow tongue movements.
Extrapyramidal dysarthria: rapid, slurred speech, low pitched, trailing off at the end of sentences. May be whispering.
Ataxic dysarthria: arrhythmic, slurred, syllables of words broken up (scanning speech). Variable force, rate, rhythm of speech.
Choreiform dysarthria: prolonged sentences interspersed with silences, improper stresses in words. Speech may come in outbursts.

PATHOPHYSIOLOGY

Speaking depends on the coordinated movement of the respiratory muscles, the pharynx and larynx, the lips, palate, tongue, and jaw. These structures are innervated by cranial nerve nuclei (facial, trigeminal, vagal, hypoglossal, and phrenic). They are controlled by corticobulbar connections and ultimately by the motor cortex. There are influences from cerebellar and extrapyramidal inputs, which modify the rate, range, volume, and force of speech. By varying the amount of expelled air, the physical qualities of the sound passage, and the tension of the vocal cords, various sounds and words can be developed. Thus disorders at multiple levels of the nervous system may lead to dysarthria.

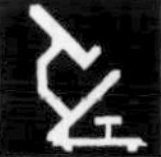

Diagnosis

DIFFERENTIAL DIAGNOSIS

- Muscular disorders: muscular dystrophies may occasionally cause slurred speech of the bulbar type.
- Neuromuscular disorders: myasthenia gravis may cause bulbar muscles; involvement with characteristics of a fluctuating, bulbar dysarthria.
- Cranial nerve diseases: combinations of disorders of vagal, hypoglossal, and facial nerves may cause dysarthria, whose characteristics are those of the specific cranial nerve involvement. Chronic meningitis, leptomeningeal disorders, skull base tumors, inflammatory disorders.
- Brainstem diseases: bulbar or pseudobulbar speech, depending on the level in the brainstem. Stroke, demyelination, tumor, vascular malformations, etc.
- Cerebellar and cerebellar connection disorders: ataxic dysarthria associated with gait ataxia, nystagmus, and incoordination. Various causes.
- Extrapyramidal disorders: Parkinson's and related disorders, Huntington's and other choreoathetotic disorders.
- Corticobulbar disorders: strokes, cerebral palsy, anoxic encephalopathy, etc. Motor neuron disease may give a mixture of upper and lower motor neuron signs, i.e., wasted tongue, brisk gag, pseudobulbar affect, etc.

SIGNS AND SYMPTOMS

Ask about difficulty swallowing liquids and solids, other cranial nerve symptoms (diplopia, facial numbness, vertigo), parkinsonian symptoms, muscular weakness, toxin or chemical ingestion, medical problems. Evaluate oropharynx for mass lesions. Listen to the quality of speech and reading. Have patient repeat linguals (sounds l and t), labials (b, p), and gutterals (nk, ng). Have the patient hold a vowel to assess the stability of phonation.

LABORATORY PROCEDURES

Depends on underlying disorders.

IMAGING STUDIES

Depends on level of neuraxis affected.

SPECIAL TESTS

Patients with unexplained dysarthria should be considered for a Tensilon test for myasthenia gravis and other neuromuscular disorders. EMG-NCS may be helpful in muscular disorders and neuromuscular disorders.

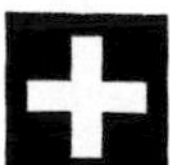

Management

GENERAL MEASURES

Speech therapy to retrain speech precision, or if necessary training in alternative communication strategies may be useful. For severe dysarthria, alternative or augmentative communication strategies may be useful. These include communicators or computer systems that may incorporate computer-synthesized voice. Speech therapy should be aimed at the particular aspect of speech that is most affected to improve comprehensibility and speech output.

SURGICAL MEASURES

For patients with certain kinds of dysarthria, there may be surgical options. A pharyngeal flap may be considered for patients with hypernasal speech. Procedures aimed at improving vocal cord apposition may help speech in disorders of vocal cord paralysis.

SYMPTOMATIC TREATMENT

Depends on specific diagnosis.

ADJUNCTIVE TREATMENT

Depends on specific diagnosis.

ADMISSION/DISCHARGE CRITERIA

Dysarthria does not usually require hospital admission. But associated neurologic problems such as aspiration due to dysphagia, respiratory disorders, and weakness may require admission.

Medications

DRUG(S) OF CHOICE

This depends on the clinical basis of dysarthria. For example, for myasthenia gravis, use of pyridostigmine (Mestinon), steroids, or other immunomodulating therapy may improve speech. Treatment of Parkinson's disease with L-dopa or dopaminergic agents may modulate speech disorders.

CONTRAINDICATIONS

N/A

PRECAUTIONS

N/A

ALTERNATIVE DRUGS

N/A

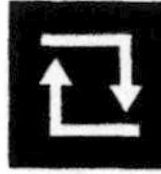

Follow-Up

PATIENT MONITORING

Depends on specific diagnosis.

EXPECTED COURSE AND PROGNOSIS

Depends on specific diagnosis.

PATIENT EDUCATION

Depends on specific diagnosis.

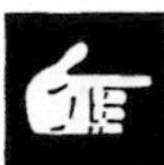

Miscellaneous

SYNONYMS

None

ICD-9-CM: 784.5 Dysarthria

SEE ALSO: MYASTHENIA GRAVIS, AMYOTROPHIC LATERAL SCLEROSIS AND OTHER MOTOR NEURON, PARKINSON'S DISEASE

REFERENCES

- Darley FL, Aronson AE, Brown JR. Differential diagnostic patterns of dysarthria. J Speech Hear Res 1969;12: 246–269.
- Duffy JR. Motor speech disorders: substrates, differential diagnosis, and management. St. Louis: Mosby, 1995.

Author(s): Alexander D. Rae-Grant, MD

Basics

DESCRIPTION

Falls are a common and serious problem encountered by older persons associated with significant morbidity and mortality, reduced functioning, and an increased chance of nursing home admission. A complex interaction among host factors, activities (situational), and environmental factors is usually required to predispose an individual to falling. Evaluating fall risk and instituting preventive measures has been shown to be effective in reducing falls in the older population.

DEFINITION

A fall is an unintentional coming to rest on the ground, floor, or other lower level. A drop attack is a sudden loss of postural tone leading to a fall without warning.

CLINICAL CHARACTERISTICS

- Most falls are multifactorial. Causes of falls include (in descending order of frequency): environmental hazards, gait and balance disorders, weakness, dizziness and vertigo, drop attacks, confusion, postural hypotension, visual disorders, syncope, and miscellaneous (arthritis, acute illness, drugs, alcohol, pain, epilepsy, falling from bed). Environmental hazards interact with individual susceptibilities (due to age and disease) to encompass the largest cause of falls. Age-related changes (stiffer gait, decreased muscle strength and step height), specific diseases (parkinsonism, stroke, arthritis), and deconditioning contribute to gait disorders and weakness. Dizziness can be due to a variety of disorders (vertigo, near-syncope, gait dysfunction). Drop attacks occur without associated dizziness, loss of consciousness, or postictal symptoms. They are often provoked by a sudden change in head position. Confusion as a cause of falls may be due to an acute medical illness causing delirium or a chronic dementia that impairs judgment or perception. Orthostatic hypotension is common in normal older persons (5–25%); in those with autonomic dysfunction, hypovolemia, and parkinsonism; and in those taking certain medications (sedative-hypnotics, vasodilators, tricyclic antidepressants). Defined as a drop of at least 20 mm Hg in systolic blood pressure, it can cause falls, although many individuals can compensate without falling. Syncope is underrepresented as a cause of falls because many studies have excluded this cause, and some patients have difficulty remembering the exact circumstances of their fall. Up to 30% of older persons with carotid sinus syndrome present with falls. Medications most strongly linked to falls are neuroleptics, benzodiazepines, tricyclic antidepressants, selective serotonin reuptake inhibitors, class I antiarrhythmics, and anticonvulsants. Less common causes include anemia, osteoporosis with spontaneous fracture, and foot problems.
- Risk factors for falls include a history of falls, gait impairments, balance disorders, use of an assistive device, lower extremity weakness, visual deficits, cognitive impairment, age over 80, arthritis, and use of four or more medications. Of these, lower extremity weakness is the most significant. The risk of falling increases as the number of risk factors increases. Using three risk factors (balance deficit, four or more prescription medications, and hip weakness), the risk of falling within 1 year is 12% with zero risk factors to 100% with all three.
- Thirty-five percent to 40% of community-dwelling persons older than 65 and roughly half of those 80 years and older fall annually. Annual incidence rates are 0.2 to 1.6 falls per person per; 16% to 75% of nursing home patients fall each year. Annual incidence of falls in long-term care facilities is 0.2 to 3.6 per bed. Hospital-based annual incidence rates range from 0.5 to 2.7 falls per bed. Accidents are the fifth leading cause of death in older adults; 5% to 10% of falls in older persons in the community result in serious injury; 10% to 25% of institutional falls result in fracture, laceration, or hospitalization.

PATHOPHYSIOLOGY

- Maintenance of locomotion, balance, and adaptive responses requires integration of sensory, central nervous, and musculoskeletal systems. Disturbances in any of these predispose to falls. The aging process itself increases postural sway, reduces postural reflexes and vision, and affects gait. Superimposed upon the predisposing factors of aging and disease are threats (acute illnesses, new medications, environmental hazards) to maintenance of postural stability. Hypotension due to age-related declines in baroreflex sensitivity may lead to decreased cerebral perfusion.
- Drop attacks are thought to result from sudden loss of muscular strength due to corticospinal tract dysfunction at the medulla/high cervical cord level. Once thought to result from vertebrobasilar ischemia, the pathophysiology may involve other mechanisms such as transient compression by excessive odontoid movement (due to unstable atlantoaxial articulation from rheumatoid arthritis or trauma) or knee instability.
- Medications contribute to falls by impairing central processing, cerebral perfusion, or alertness or causing extrapyramidal effects.

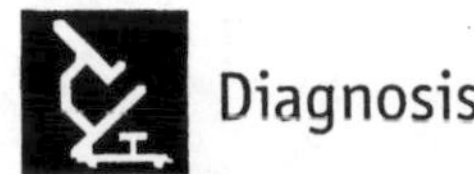

Diagnosis

DIFFERENTIAL DIAGNOSIS

Symptoms of falls and syncope overlap. Persons with preexisting gait instability may develop imbalance secondary to a hypotensive episode. Patients may be unaware of loss of consciousness; syncope should be considered in patients who are "found down." Older persons with carotid sinus hypersensitivity can present with falls. Atonic seizures characterized by sudden loss of muscle tone (more frequent in children) can cause falls.

SIGNS AND SYMPTOMS

- All persons older than 70 years or their caregivers should be assessed annually about balance or gait difficulties and falls. High-risk groups (nursing home residents, injurious falls, recurrent fallers, acute presentation after a fall) require a more comprehensive assessment. History should include circumstances of the fall(s) including activity during the fall, warning/associated symptoms, how the patient felt immediately after the fall, loss of consciousness. Falls that occur immediately after arising from a lying or sitting position could be due to orthostatic hypotension. If the person tripped, environmental hazards should be assessed, as well as the possibilities of weak ankle dorsiflexors, spasticity, or parkinsonism. Collapse at the knees could indicate a syncopal episode, seizure, or knee instability. Falling backward could indicate an extrapyramidal disorder. A fall after a meal could be secondary to postprandial hypotension. Vertigo, vision changes, urinary incontinence (normal pressure hydrocephalus), clumsiness, and impaired judgment should be sought. Medication history should explore use of benzodiazepines, neuroleptics, sedative-hypnotics, alcohol, and vasodilators. Medical comorbidities, functional status, and environmental risks should be assessed.
- Physical examination should include orthostatic blood pressures, strength, sensation (especially proprioception), feet, and gait. A good screening gait exam is the "Get Up and Go" test, which asks a patient to arise from a chair without using arms, walk 10 feet, turn around, and return to sit in the chair. Stride length, steppage, start hesitation, freezing, postural stability, and sway can all be evaluated.

LABORATORY PROCEDURES

Testing based on history and physical examination.

IMAGING STUDIES

MRI/CT scan may be indicated based on symptoms and signs.

SPECIAL TESTS

The following studies may be necessary depending on the history and physical exam:

- Echocardiogram
- EEG
- Nerve conduction studies/EMG
- Holter/event monitor
- Electronystagmogram
- CSF—large volume (30–50 mL) spinal tap for NPH

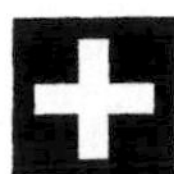

Management

GENERAL MEASURES

- If fall related to syncope, exclude cardiac or neurologic cause.
- If nonsyncopal fall, best results are achieved with multicomponent interventions.
  - —Medication modification—reduce or discontinue psychotropics and other offending meds if possible.
  - —Postural hypotension treatment.
  - —Environmental hazard modification (occupational therapy consult to evaluate home safety and need for raised toilet seat, grab bars, handrails, adequate lighting, removal of loose cords or slip rugs).
  - —Exercise programs with balance (e.g., tai chi) and gait training.
  - —Treatment of cardiovascular disorders (e.g., arrhythmias).
  - —Vision and hearing aids if needed.
- Osteoporosis evaluation (bone densitometry) for age over 65 years (and 60–65 years if risk factors present—thin body habitus, smoker, family history of maternal hip fracture).

SURGICAL MEASURES

May be necessary if injury from the fall.

SYMPTOMATIC TREATMENT

Determined by underlying etiology.

ADJUNCTIVE TREATMENT

- Physical therapy/occupational therapy.
- Treat osteoporosis if present.
- Hip protectors do not affect falling risk, and use for prevention of hip fractures is controversial—recent study showed no benefit.
- No evidence to support restraint use (or removal of restraints) for fall prevention.
- No specific footwear to reduce falls. Gait and balance improved more with walking shoes than barefoot. Balance is better in low-heeled rather than high-heeled shoes. Stability in men is improved with high mid-sole hardness and low mid-sole thickness.

ADMISSION/DISCHARGE CRITERIA

Determined by severity of associated injuries and by underlying cause(s) of fall.

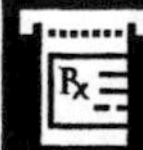

Medications

DRUG(S) OF CHOICE

- No medications indicated for fall prevention or treatment other than in some cases of orthostatic hypotension.
- Minimize medications that affect postural stability.

Contraindications

None

Precautions

None

ALTERNATIVE DRUGS

- Fludrocortisone or midodrine may be necessary for orthostatic hypotension.
- Calcium 1,500 mg/day, vitamin D 800 units/day, and bisphosphonates (alendronate 70 mg orally once a week or risedronate 35 mg orally once a week) or raloxifene 60 mg orally once a day if osteoporosis.

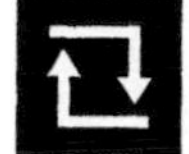

Follow-Up

PATIENT MONITORING

- Determined by underlying cause.
- Ask about falls at each visit in patient with history of fall(s) or gait/balance disorder.

EXPECTED COURSE AND PROGNOSIS

- Fifty percent of fallers have multiple falls.
- Determined by underlying cause and interventions to reduce/prevent falls.

PATIENT EDUCATION

- Does not reduce falls when used as an isolated intervention.
- Benefit is demonstrated when education is included as part of a multifactorial intervention.
- Home safety modifications.
- Strategies for what to do if person falls and cannot get up (accessible telephone; emergency-response system).
- Calcium and vitamin D for bone protection.
- Review risk factors for falling.

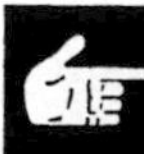

Miscellaneous

SYNONYMS

N/A

ICD-9-CM: E885.9 Fall from other slipping, tripping, or stumbling

SEE ALSO: N/A

REFERENCES

- Ishiyama G, Ishiyama A, Jacobson K, et al. Drop attacks in older patients secondary to an otologic cause. Neurology 2001;57(6):1103–1106.
- Kenny RA, Richardson DA, Steen N. Carotid sinus syndrome: a modifiable risk factor for nonaccidental falls in older adults. J Am Coll Cardiol 2001;38: 1491–1496.
- Rubenstein LZ, Josephson KR. The epidemiology of falls and syncope. Clin Geriatr Med 2002;18(2):141–158.
- Rubenstein TC, Alexander NB, Hausdorff JM. Evaluating fall risk in older adults. Clin Geriatr 2003;11(1):52–60.
- Tinetti ME. Preventing falls in elderly persons. N Engl J Med 2003;348(1):42–49.

Author(s): James F. Lamb, MD

Gait Disorders

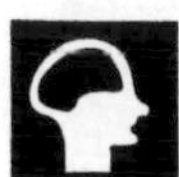

Basics

DESCRIPTION

Walking is a complex, fundamental human skill that is often taken for granted. Many neurologic systems are required for effective walking and balance. Disorders of many types involving these systems may cause disorders of gait. Disorders of gait may be characterized by the level in the nervous system, the particular nervous system structure, or the underlying disease that causes them. Gait disorders are common in the elderly. In a cohort of the elderly from Sweden, one in four patients age 79 used mechanical aids for walking. All of those studied had slower gait than normal for the overall Swedish population. Falls are common in the elderly and contribute to the estimated 200,000 hip fractures per year in the United States; 40% to 50% of nursing home patients have difficulty with walking.

DEFINITIONS

Gait disorder: a problem with the initiation or maintenance of walking.

CLINICAL CHARACTERISTICS

Patients with gait disorders present with a variety of symptoms. Often they present with falling repeatedly, not noticing that they have an altered gait. They may complain of wooziness or imbalance, a vague sense of instability when walking. Their family may notice an altered pattern of walking or posture, or may be worried that they may fall. The patients may limit their activities in an attempt to avoid dangerous areas for walking (outside, slippery surfaces, on an incline, etc.). They may have associated leg weakness, numbness, back pain, or other symptoms depending on the specific cause of gait dysfunction. Often gait disorders are progressive depending again on the underlying cause or causes.

PATHOPHYSIOLOGY

Walking depends on the effective interaction of a number of neurologic systems to integrate the gait into a smooth, balanced activity. Disorders of neurologic systems that underlie gait, or musculoskeletal systems that participate in gait are key to gait disorders. Often patients have more than one neurologic or musculoskeletal system involved (multifactorial gait disorder). The normal gait is complex, though it seldom attracts attention. It consists of a stance phase, in which the foot is in contact with the ground, and a swing phase, which begins when the foot leaves the ground. Normal gait requires antigravity support of the body, stepping, the maintenance of equilibrium, and propulsion. Antigravity support requires input from vestibular, proprioceptive, and visual responses integrated at multiple levels. Stepping is a basic motor pattern present at birth and depends on spinal cord, midbrain, and diencephalic interactions. Locomotor pattern generators permit rhythmic motion. Equilibrium depends on highly tuned interactions between reflex arcs and input from visual, vestibular, and proprioceptive systems. Propulsion depends on muscles generating appropriate timed force, as well as the appropriate inhibition of antagonistic muscle groups. All of the above can be overridden by conscious cortical centers so one can go where one wants to. Neurologic systems that are involved in walking include the frontal lobes, basal ganglia, diencephalon and midbrain, spinal cord, peripheral nervous system, vestibular system, and cerebellum.

Diagnosis

DIFFERENTIAL DIAGNOSIS

The analysis of the gait and categorization of the type of gait disorder helps in directing the diagnostic process. Certain kinds of gait are relatively distinctive, while others are harder to characterize.

- *Apraxic gait:* wide based, short steps, uncertain, shuffling. Patient appears unsure how to proceed. Able to do complex movements while lying down (bicycling movements with legs). No ataxia or weakness of individual limb movements. Seen in frontal lobe disorders, multiple infarction syndromes, normal pressure hydrocephalus.
- *Cerebellar gait:* wide based, unsteady, consisting of steps that vary in rate, rhythm, and force. May be described as reeling or drunken. Marked difficulty in walking heel to toe. May be associated with nystagmus or overshoot dysmetria, rebound, intention tremor, hypotonia. Seen in patients with cerebellar disease, and frequently in multiple sclerosis.
- *Choreiform gait:* jerky, irregular, erratic gait, sometimes appears dancing, incorporating choreiform movements. Seen in Huntington's disease and other choreiform disorders.
- *Equine gait:* excessive raising of legs, feet fall limply due to weakness of anterior shin muscles, slapping when foot falls. Seen in neuropathies, spinal muscular atrophies, distal muscular dystrophies.
- *Festinating gait:* shuffling, hastening, with forward flexed posture, associated with difficulty initiating gait and turning. Associated with parkinsonism.
- *Senile gait:* cautious, short steps, unsteady without specific character, stooped posture, slightly widened stance. Seen in patients with multimodal sensory loss, orthopedic disorders, and patients with prior falls.
- *Sensory gait:* Feet placed wide apart, stamping gait, legs flung outward, very positive Romberg sign. Seen in disorders of dorsal column system (classically tabes dorsalis, seen in sensory ganglioneuropathies).
- *Spastic gait:* stiff legged, with tendency for the toes to turn in and scrape, leg circumducts, legs may scissor. Seen with upper motor neuron disorders.
- *Toppling gait:* Patient suddenly, precipitously falls, often without warning. May fall backward. Gait is hesitant, uncertain, but not specifically ataxic. Seen in progressive supranuclear palsy, midbrain strokes.
- *Waddling gait:* Alternating waddle due to weakness of hip girdle muscles, pelvis falls due to weakness of supporting muscles. Seen in proximal myopathies.

SIGNS AND SYMPTOMS

The gait should be assessed by watching the person arise from a chair, walk, stand, turn, and balance. Note whether the patient is unsteady, whether the steps are short or shuffling, and whether there is evidence of a hemiparesis, spasticity, or a foot drop. Signs of a neuropathy (decreased reflexes, distal sensory loss, distal muscle weakness), spinal cord disease (spasticity, brisk reflexes, sensory level, Babinski sign), brainstem disease (diplopia, dysarthria, nystagmus, cranial nerve palsies, long tract signs), and dementia (abnormal cognition, memory, affect, or judgment) should be sought. The Romberg sign (swaying or falling with eyes closed, not with eyes open) is an indication of a proprioceptive deficit. The presence of ataxia and other cerebellar signs should be evaluated (rebound, intention tremor, truncal instability). Hearing and vision should be measured.

LABORATORY PROCEDURES

There are no specific laboratory procedures for this problem. Laboratory studies are directed at specific diseases once the type of gait disorder is ascertained, i.e., cerebellar ataxia, anti-Purkinje cell antibodies.

IMAGING STUDIES

MRI or CT scanning may be useful in excluding intracranial disorders causing gait difficulty (i.e., mass lesions, normal pressure hydrocephalus, stroke). MRI scanning of the spine may be useful in assessing for myelopathic gait disorders.

SPECIAL TESTS

EMG-NCS may document the presence of peripheral neuropathies or polyradiculopathies underlying gait disorders. Computerized gait analysis may be most useful in developing rehabilitative programs for gait disorders.

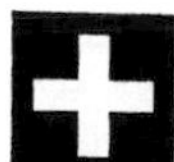

Management

GENERAL MEASURES

The initial measure is to assess for reversible factors contributing to gait dysfunction. Medications contributing to gait disorders include sedative-hypnotics, anxiolytics, anticholinergics, narcotics; drugs and alcohol should be avoided. Visual disorders should be corrected if possible. An assessment of home factors contributing to gait disorders (uneven flooring, lack of a shower mat, lack of banisters for stairs, etc.) may be useful. Stabilizing walking aids such as canes, walkers, rolling rollators, and other supports may be necessary. Specific training is necessary for any walking aid. Physical therapy aimed at strengthening leg muscles may be helpful. If available, a program of computerized evaluation for gait and gait rehabilitation may be used.

SURGICAL MEASURES

Not applicable, unless related to the underlying etiology of gait disorder.

SYMPTOMATIC TREATMENT

Therapies such as antiparkinsonian medication may be useful and are directed at the underlying etiology of gait disorder.

ADJUNCTIVE TREATMENT

Grab bars particularly in the bathroom and shower are worthwhile safety measures. Consider stair glide if stairs are a problem.

ADMISSION/DISCHARGE CRITERIA

Most gait disorders are treated on an outpatient basis. If patients are at risk of falling and cannot ambulate to care for themselves, and do not have support in the home environment, admission may be necessary, with early transfer to a rehabilitative or skilled nursing facility setting. Discharge to rehabilitation or home is based on safe ambulation or a secure environment.

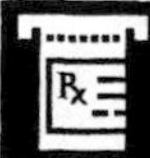

Medications

DRUG(S) OF CHOICE

See specific diseases.

ALTERNATIVE DRUGS

See specific diseases.

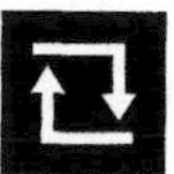

Follow-Up

PATIENT MONITORING

Patients should be followed for changes in gait as a result of therapy.

EXPECTED COURSE AND PROGNOSIS

If a specific disease is identified, the course and prognosis is that of the underlying disease. Patients with multifactorial gait disorders may respond to therapy and changes in walking aids.

PATIENT EDUCATION

Patients should be educated about the multifactorial nature of gait disorders, and on the effect of medication, drugs, and alcohol on gait. They should be taught about home safety and appropriate walking aids. What to do in case of falls should be reviewed with the patient and family.

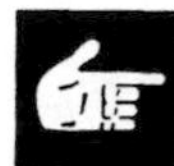

Miscellaneous

SYNONYMS

Ambulation disorders
Balance disorders

ICD-9-CM: 719.79 Multiple gait disorder; 781.2 Ataxia

SEE ALSO: ATAXIA, PARKINSON'S DISEASE

REFERENCES

- Hindmarsh JJ, Estes EH. Falls in older persons. Arch Intern Med 1989;149: 2217–2222.
- Nutt JG, Marsden CD, Thompson PD. Human walking and higher-level gait disorders, particularly in the elderly. Neurology 1993;43:268–279.
- Sudarsky L. Geriatrics: gait disorders in the elderly. N Engl J Med 1990;322: 1441–1446.

Author(s): Alexander D. Rae-Grant, MD

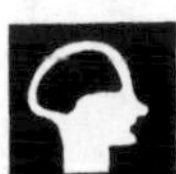

Basics

DESCRIPTION

- Headache is one of the most common medical complaints of modern society, affecting virtually every person during his or her lifetime. Each year, >5% of the US population will seek medical attention for headache. More than 1% of primary care and emergency room visits are because of headache. Most recurrent headaches are symptomatic of a chronic primary headache disorder.

DEFINITIONS

- Primary headaches occur without an underlying cause and include migraine, tension type, cluster, and miscellaneous headaches (such as benign exertional headache). Secondary headaches always have a direct underlying cause (e.g., subarachnoid hemorrhage [SAH], brain tumor, meningitis, carotid dissection, sinusitis), some of which can be life threatening.

CLINICAL CHARACTERISTICS

- Headache history is essential to establish the proper diagnosis. Several key issues should be discussed.
  —*Age of onset:* Migraines usually begin before age 40 years. Temporal arteritis typically begins after age 50.
  —*Time to maximum intensity:* Thunderclap headaches are severe, with maximum intensity within 1 minute, and can be caused by SAH, carotid artery dissection, and migraine. Severe headaches also can have a gradual onset, such as migraine or viral meningitis.
  —*Frequency:* Primary headaches are variable in frequency, ranging from a few migraines in a lifetime to cluster headaches occurring up to eight times daily.
  —*Time of day:* Cluster headaches often occur during certain times of the day and may awaken the sufferer from sleep about the same time. Headaches that awaken the patient from sleep usually are benign (e.g., migraine, cluster); however, they also can occur with brain tumors, meningitis, and SAH. Tension-type headaches often occur in the afternoon.
  —*Duration:* Migraine typically lasts 4–72 hours without treatment. Cluster headaches typically last 15–180 minutes. Tension-type headaches typically last 30 minutes to days. Trigeminal neuralgia is characterized by volleys of pain lasting a few seconds to <2 minutes.
  —*Triggers:* Most migraineurs have one or more triggers that can induce a headache. During periods of cluster headaches, alcohol can be a trigger. Tension-type headaches can be triggered by stress. Stimulation of certain areas of the face may trigger trigeminal neuralgia.

PATHOPHYSIOLOGY

- The pain of headache can be caused by several different mechanisms, including elevated intracranial pressure, inflammation or irritation of pain-sensitive intracranial structures (e.g., vessels, meninges), and inflammation or damage to structures in the head and neck region (e.g., muscles). Migraine pain is incompletely understood but involves dysfunction of brainstem control over the trigeminovascular system, with dilation and inflammation of innervated vessels and release of vasoactive neuropeptides. Cluster headaches may involve abnormal interactions between the trigeminovascular system and the posterior hypothalamic circadian cycling mechanism. Tension headache involves inflammation and tenderness of the pericranial and upper cervical musculature. Central mechanisms also may be involved, including oversensitization to peripheral activation of muscle nociceptive afferent input.

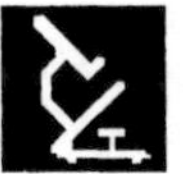

Diagnosis

DIFFERENTIAL DIAGNOSIS

- In addition to the common benign headache syndromes (e.g., migraine, tension, cluster), other secondary headaches to consider include the following. For head and neck trauma, consider subdural or epidural hematoma; headaches during pregnancy and the postpartum period, consider preeclampsia and cortical vein thrombosis; in obese young women, consider pseudotumor cerebri; pheochromocytoma should be considered in patients with paroxysmal hypertension accompanied by headache; new-onset headache in an HIV-positive patient could be due to mass lesion (e.g., lymphoma) or infection (e.g., meningitis); headaches in patients with a cancer diagnosis should be screened for brain metastasis; SAH should be considered in a patient with acute onset of the worst headache of his or her life; frequent use of prescription and over-the-counter drugs (including analgesics) may lead to rebound headaches; oral contraceptives can cause a vascular-type headache in some women; headaches associated with fever, stiff neck, nausea and vomiting, and altered sensorium may be related to CNS infection.

SIGNS AND SYMPTOMS

- About 60% of migraineurs have a prodrome before the headache. Complaints may involve the mental state (irritability, depression, euphoria) and neurologic function (decreased concentration; light, noise, and smell hypersensitivity), as well as more general function (diarrhea or constipation, thirst, sluggish feeling, food cravings, neck stiffness). About 20% of migraines have an aura that generally develop over 5–20 minutes and last <60 minutes. The headache can begin before, during, or after the aura. The most common auras in descending frequency are visual, sensory, motor, and speech and language abnormalities. Prodromal low-grade fever and upper respiratory symptoms or diarrhea frequently are present in viral meningitis.
- Migraine is accompanied by nausea in 90% of patients, vomiting in 30%, and light/noise sensitivity in 80%. These same symptoms often are present in headaches due to SAH or meningitis. Ipsilateral conjunctival injection, tearing, and nasal congestion or drainage typically occur during cluster headaches. Ipsilateral ptosis and miosis are present in 30% of cases.
- An important feature of the headache is the location of the pain. Cluster headaches are always unilateral, whereas about 40%–60% of migraines are unilateral. Trigeminal neuralgia typically is unilateral, occurring more often in the second or third trigeminal distributions than in the first. Headaches from brain tumors or subdural hematomas can be bilateral or unilateral.
- Quality of pain is another important aspect. In about 85% of cases, migraine pain is throbbing, pounding, or pulsatile. Tension-type headaches present as a pressure, aching, tight, or squeezing sensation. Cluster headaches are described as boring or burning. Trigeminal neuralgia is usually an electrical or stabbing pain. Headaches due to brain tumors can produce a variety of pains, ranging from a dull steady ache to throbbing.
- Severity of pain can help differentiate headache syndromes. Migraine pain can vary from mild to severe in general, and from attack to attack. Severity of pain does not equate with the presence of life-threatening causes. The vast majority of severe headaches are due to migraine or cluster types. However, a patient complaining of acute onset of the worst headache of his or her life should be evaluated for SAH.
- After the headache resolves, many migraineurs report feeling tired and drained, with decreased mental acuity. Depression or euphoria sometimes is reported. In some systemic disorders, high fever and headache may be followed by other symptoms or signs.

LABORATORY PROCEDURES

- Erythrocyte sedimentation rate (ESR) is necessary when temporal arteritis is under consideration. A vasculitis screen (e.g., ESR, antinuclear antibody, rheumatoid factor, extractable nuclear antigen) is helpful in patients with headache and arthralgias. Endocrine and metabolic testing may be necessary to rule out other systemic disorders that can cause secondary headache.

IMAGING STUDIES

- CT scan of the head will detect most pathology able to cause headaches and is the preferred study for acute head trauma and SAH. MRI scan of the brain (with and without gadolinium) is more sensitive than CT and is superior for the evaluation of all other causes. MR angiography may detect intracranial aneurysms and carotid dissection. The yield of a CT or MRI scan in a patient with headache and a normal neurologic examination is about 2%.

SPECIAL TESTS

- Lumbar puncture, usually after CT/MRI, may be helpful to exclude SAH, infection (e.g., meningitis, encephalitis, HIV), or low or high CSF pressure.

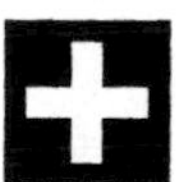

Management

GENERAL MEASURES

- Will vary with the specific form of primary or secondary headache disorder

SURGICAL MEASURES

- Surgery is not indicated for primary headache disorders but may be appropriate for specific secondary headache disorders (e.g., brain tumor, SAH, abscess).

SYMPTOMATIC TREATMENT

- Will vary significantly depending on the type of headache disorder; see specific form of headache

ADJUNCTIVE TREATMENT

- Nonpharmacologic methods of treatment may be helpful. Migraine headaches may resolve with sleep or improve with lying down in a dark quiet room. Application of ice to the forehead may help. Tension-type headaches may improve with relaxation techniques in some patients and an exercise regimen in others.

ADMISSION/DISCHARGE CRITERIA

- Admission is not indicated for most patients with primary headache disorders, except for treatment of status migrainosus. Admission often is appropriate for workup and treatment of patients with secondary headache syndromes (e.g., SAH, brain tumor, meningitis).

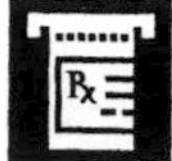

Medications

DRUG(S) OF CHOICE

- For abortive treatment of migraine, the triptan medications are preferred. For prophylactic treatment, choices include β-blockers, valproate, and amitriptyline. Cluster headaches respond best to oxygen and subcutaneous sumatriptan; corticosteroids also may be of benefit.

Contraindications

- Hypersensitivity to medication

Precautions

N/A

ALTERNATIVE DRUGS

- Other drugs to consider for migraine or cluster headaches include ergot derivatives, serotonin antagonists, calcium channel blockers, gabapentin, nonsteroidal antiinflammatory drugs, topiramate, and selective serotonin reuptake inhibitors.

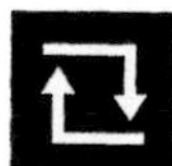

Follow-Up

PATIENT MONITORING

- Patients with primary and secondary headaches will need intermittent follow-up to assess response to treatment and, in some cases, to follow neurologic status.

EXPECTED COURSE AND PROGNOSIS

- The course and prognosis for most patients with primary headache disorders are good, with adequate control of headache pain after appropriate diagnosis and treatment. For secondary headache disorders, the course and prognosis are quite variable and depend on the specific cause.

PATIENT EDUCATION

- Patients with primary headache disorders should be thoroughly educated about the specifics of their form of headache and instructed about behavioral and lifestyle changes that might improve control (e.g., avoidance of triggers).

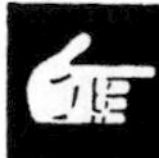

Miscellaneous

SYNONYMS

- Migraine
- Cluster headache
- Tension headache
- Exertional headache

ICD-9-CM: 784.0 Headache; 346.2 Cluster headache; 346.9 Migraine headache; 307.81 Tension headache; 349.0 Post LP headache

SEE ALSO: HEADACHE, MIGRAINE; CEREBROVASCULAR DISEASE, INTRACRANIAL ANEURYSMS AND SUBARACHNOID HEMORRHAGE; BRAIN TUMOR; MENINGITIS; ENCEPHALITIS

REFERENCES

- Evans RW, Mathew NT. Handbook of headache. Philadelphia: Lippincott Williams & Wilkins, 2000.
- Evans RW, ed. Saunders manual of neurologic practice. Philadelphia: WB Saunders, 2003.
- Silberstein SD, Lipton RB, Dalessio SJ. Wolff's headache and other head pain, 7th ed. New York: Oxford University Press, 2001.

Author(s): Randolph W. Evans, MD; Herbert B. Newton, MD

Muscle Cramps and Pain

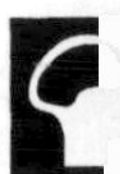

Basics

DESCRIPTION

- Myalgia or muscle pain may be of varying intensity and character and may involve any muscle. Muscle cramps are associated with severe pain of acute onset and short duration.

DEFINITIONS

- Muscle pain is a sensation. A cramp or spasm is an involuntary contraction of muscle.

CLINICAL CHARACTERISTICS

- Patients use subjective terms, such as "charley horse," "spasm," "seizing up," and "lameness," to describe muscle pain. Cramps are associated with a hard muscular contraction and are relieved by stretching the muscle.

PATHOPHYSIOLOGY

- Muscle pain during exercise may result from ischemia, claudication, tearing of muscle fibers, rupture of muscle tendons, muscle cramping, or exhaustion of fuel supply with resultant contracture in patients with metabolic defects.

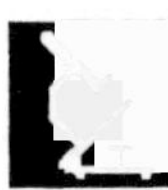

Diagnosis

DIFFERENTIAL DIAGNOSIS

- Muscle disorders
  —Inflammatory myopathy: dermatomyositis, polymyositis with collagen vascular disease, viral, bacterial, and parasitic myositis
  —Substrate utilization defects: glycogenolysis, glycolysis, fatty acid oxidation, purine nucleotide cycle
  —Toxic myopathy: alcohol, narcotics, clofibrate, zidovudine
  —Endocrinopathies: hypothyroidism, hyperthyroidism, hypoparathyroidism, hyperparathyroidism
  —Metabolic disorders: lowered sodium, potassium, calcium, magnesium, phosphate; elevated sodium, calcium
  —Metabolic myopathies, such as McArdle's disease
  —Myotonia (occasionally may cause cramps)
  —Local muscle injury, such as neoplasm, hematoma, ruptured tendon
- Nonmuscle disease
  —Joint disease, such as lumbar stenosis
  —Peripheral neuropathies of many different causes can cause both muscle pains and cramps
  —Circulatory insufficiency
  —Anterior horn cell disease, such as amyotrophic lateral sclerosis (ALS)
  —"Growing pains"
  —Fasciitis
  —Restless leg syndrome
  —Fibromyalgia: generalized pain at rest without weakness, tender spots, normal CK level with no objective laboratory or clinical abnormalities
  —Polymyalgia rheumatica: pain at rest without weakness; in patients >50 years, pain is proximal with stiffness, often accompanied by weight loss and low-grade fever; no muscle tenderness; ESR nearly always elevated
  —Stiff person syndrome: cramps and spasms
  —Bone diseases: pain and myopathic weakness but normal CK. Bones hurt during movement and are tender to pressure or percussion.
  —Cramps may occur in normal individuals (during swimming and at night). The cramps are of explosive onset, visible contraction, painful, may leave soreness, tend to be confined to one muscle or parts of a muscle, start and end with twitching, and occur after forceful contraction, especially when muscle shortens. Usually can be terminated by passive stretching of the muscle.

SIGNS AND SYMPTOMS

- In taking a medical history, it is useful to inquire whether the pain occurs at rest or only during exercise. Severe pain and cramps are associated with other symptoms that vary depending on the etiology:
  —Muscle pain and severe cramps that occur after exertion and are associated with ecchymosis and local swelling are due to tearing of muscle fibers or rupturing of the tendon.
  —In metabolic myopathies, associated features include a "second-wind" phenomenon (i.e., improvement of the cramps after resting for a short time). Cramps are induced with exercise, never spontaneously at rest. They are electrically silent on EMG.
  —Joint pain and swelling
  —Skin rash in dermatomyositis
  —Contractures: active muscle contraction that is not dependent on excitation of the outer muscle membrane; EMG electrically silent.
  —Stiffness induced by certain condition (by cold in certain myotonias)
  —Dark urine if myoglobinuria occurs
  —Muscle atrophy in cases of anterior horn cell diseases
  —Hypertrophic calves muscles in some dystrophies
  —Pathologic reflexes and spasticity in patients with ALS
  —Tender points, fatigue, disturbed sleep pattern, and morning stiffness in patients with fibromyalgia

LABORATORY PROCEDURES

Blood Tests

- Creatine kinase may be elevated, indicating muscle damage. If CK levels are >10,000, then myoglobinuria is expected. Normal CK excludes necrotizing myopathy.
- Electrolytes, thyroid function tests, creatine (will be below normal in patients with severe muscle wasting from any cause)
- ESR, ANA if autoimmune disease is suspected
- Specific enzymes such as myophosphorylase in metabolic myopathies
- Forearm ischemic exercise test is indicated in patients with suspected metabolic myopathies due to defect in glycogenolysis. It should be performed under careful monitoring to prevent ischemia. Lactate and ammonia levels are evaluated. In the normal condition, both levels are increased after the test; in metabolic defects, lactate level does not increase after exercise.

IMAGING STUDIES

- Plain x-ray views of the joint or bones if injury is suspected.
- Plain roentgenography of muscle is helpful in evaluation of mass lesions for calcium, fat, or tumor.
- CT scan and MRI of the muscle show distinctive and diagnostically helpful abnormalities in many muscle diseases. They are particularly helpful in differentiating fat from muscle, thus helping to distinguish true hypertrophy from pseudohypertrophy of muscle. They also may aid in differentiating inflammatory myopathy from muscular dystrophy.
- Radionuclide scanning with gallium can detect muscle abscesses in patients with pyomyositis.
- NMR spectroscopy to evaluate muscle metabolism. Phosphocreatine, inorganic phosphate, intracellular pH, APT, and lactate level are monitored continuously during exercise.

SPECIAL TESTS

- Electromyography/nerve conduction velocity (EMG/NCV) studies
  —EMG/NCV studies are useful to confirm a clinical diagnosis of myopathic or neuropathic muscle weakness. These electrophysiologic studies also are helpful in the diagnosis of myotonia, motor neuron disease, or neuromuscular junction disease as a cause for the pain and cramps.
  —Cramps are characterized on EMG by repetitive firing of normal motor unit potentials. The EMG shows a full recruitment pattern on the oscilloscope screen.
  —Cramps may be electrically silent on EMG in some conditions, as mentioned earlier.
- Muscle biopsy
  —Useful in evaluating for storage diseases, focal myopathy, inflammatory myopathy, and necrosis

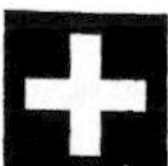

Management

GENERAL MEASURES

- Patient assurance is very important.
- Prevent the pain and cramps by limiting the triggering activity.
- It is advisable to limit activity at the onset of symptoms in patients with second-wind phenomenon.
- Genetic evaluation of the patient and family members if indicated (in cases of motor neuron diseases, muscular dystrophies).

SURGICAL MEASURES

- Surgical treatment is considered for
  —Tendon rupture with severe pain that did not respond to conservative management
  —Localized abscess that did not respond to a full course of antibiotics
  —Inserting devices for pain control in certain conditions

SYMPTOMATIC TREATMENT

- Local massage to relieve the contractions; passive stretching of the contracted muscle may be helpful.
- Fluid replacement is indicated in certain conditions.
- Analgesics can be given in severe cases.

ADJUNCTIVE TREATMENT

- Physical and occupational therapy
- Hypnotics provide short-term benefit for sleep disturbances, but long-term value not established
- Aerobic exercise program, physical conditioning

ADMISSION/DISCHARGE CRITERIA

- Patients are admitted for the severity of symptoms and deficits in cases of acute crisis with myoglobinuria. They need close monitoring for pain control and for aggressive hydration to prevent renal insufficiency. Cardiac monitoring is also indicated in these conditions, as cardiomyopathy may be another manifestation of the disease.
- In patients with inflammatory myopathy, intravenous steroids, plasma exchange, or immunoglobulin therapy in sometimes indicated. Respiratory function, as well as renal and cardiac function, should be monitored to prevent complications.
- Patients may need subacute inpatient rehabilitation care, depending on the condition.

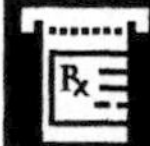

Medications

DRUG(S) OF CHOICE

- Nonsteroidal antiinflammatory drugs (NSAIDs) are helpful in reducing pain and inflammation. In patients who previously experienced less than optimal relief with NSAIDs, it is important for psychological reasons to start a new and as yet untried drug.
- Antidepressants
  —Tricyclic antidepressants, such as amitriptyline and nortriptyline, increase serotonin, thus lowering the perception of pain. They also cause drowsiness, which may help with sleep in cases of chronic pain and fibromyalgia.
  —Selective serotonin reuptake inhibitors (SSRIs), such as sertraline and venlafaxine, may lower perception of pain by their effects on serotoninergic pain systems.
- Anticonvulsants, such as gabapentin, carbamazepine, phenytoin, and clonazepam, are very helpful for muscle cramps and control of neuropathic pain.
- Muscle relaxants, such as the benzodiazepines, baclofen, and dantrolene.
- Quinine sulfate 325 mg given at night will provide some relief from the cramps. It is especially helpful for cramps induced by anterior horn cell disease.

Contraindications

- Quinine sulfate is contraindicated in pregnancy because of its potential teratogenicity (particularly the development of deafness).
- Dantrolene is used less often than baclofen. Its serious side effects include fulminant liver failure.

Precautions

- Side effects of NSAIDs include, but are not limited to, GI discomfort, anaphylactic reaction, interstitial nephritis, and renal toxicity. Serious hepatic reactions may occur.
- Major side effects of SSRIs include serotonin syndrome, GI upset, and sleep disturbances.
- Side effects of anticonvulsants include fatal aplastic anemia and serious liver toxicity in the case of carbamazepine. Skin rash and cardiac arrhythmias can occur with dilantin. Dependency with tolerance can develop with benzodiazepines.
- Side effects of antidepressants include sedation and anticholinergic effects (tachycardia, orthostatic hypotension, urinary retention).

ALTERNATIVE DRUGS

- Dantrolene

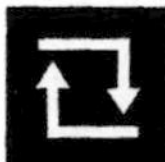

Follow-Up

PATIENT MONITORING

- Frequent clinical evaluation with adjustment of medications according to the response and tolerance.
- Periodic blood tests (CBC, hepatic and kidney function) may be indicated in patients who are taking anticonvulsants.

EXPECTED COURSE AND PROGNOSIS

- Most conditions that cause muscle pain and cramps are benign and self-limited. Prognosis in general is good, except in certain conditions such as anterior horn cell disease where the symptoms of weakness continue to progress with association of dysphagia and respiratory insufficiency.

PATIENT EDUCATION

- Patient assurance is recommended. It is very important to educate patients about their condition and how to avoid activities and vigorous exercise that trigger their muscle pain.

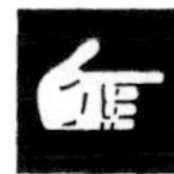

Miscellaneous

SYNONYMS

- Myalgias
- Cramps

ICD-9-CM: 728.85 Spasm of muscle; 729.1 Myalgia and myositis, unspecified, fibromyositis NOS; 729.82 Cramps

SEE ALSO: N/A

REFERENCES

- Griggs RC, Mendell JR, Miller RG. Evaluation and treatment of myopathies. Philadelphia: FA Davis, 1995:389–399.
- Pestronk A. Muscle pain and cramps. In: Bradley W, Fenichel G, Daroff R, eds. Neurology in clinical practice, vol. 1. Boston: Butterworth Heinemann, 2000: 397–402.

Author(s): Roula al-Dahhak, MD

Syncope

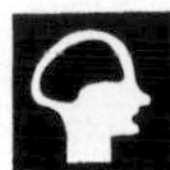

Basics

DESCRIPTION

Transient loss of consciousness and postural tone with spontaneous recovery.

DEFINITIONS

N/A

CLINICAL CHARACTERISTICS

The onset of syncope may either be abrupt or subacute with or without prodromal symptoms. The patient may only recall "passing out," while someone who observed the event may provide more detailed information. Thus, a thorough history involves both the patient and any observers the patient wishes to include in the interview.

PATHOPHYSIOLOGY

Syncope occurs as a result of global reduction in cerebral blood flow. In cardiac disorders such as hypertrophic cardiomyopathy or severe aortic stenosis, syncope results from obstruction to cardiac output. Any mechanical obstruction to cerebral blood flow may produce syncope in a similar mechanism; less frequent causes include ascending aortic dissection flap or occlusion of the left ventricular outflow tract by a dislodged left atrial myxoma. In neurocardiogenic syncope, reflective changes in heart rate or blood pressure fail to appropriately maintain cardiac output; this may include an abnormal fall in heart rate or blood pressure or simply a failure to adequately augment these parameters. Faulty signals from baroreceptor feedback to CNS centers may impair the execution of appropriate compensatory changes that would otherwise stabilize the patient. Cardiac arrhythmias may produce syncope; bradyarrhythmias in particular should be considered in elderly patients with resting bradycardia or atrioventricular conduction disease.

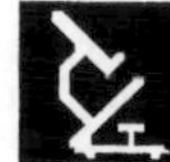

Diagnosis

DIFFERENTIAL DIAGNOSIS

Establishing that syncope occurred is usually straightforward; the patient will say, "I passed out." Distinguishing near-syncope from vertigo or nonspecific neurologic syndromes may be more challenging. The history from the patient or an observer will allow the clinician to distinguish vestibular phenomena from true syncope. In eliciting a history of tonic-clonic movements or incontinence, keep in mind that seizure-like activity may ensue from syncope of any etiology, but focal neurologic signs should prompt consideration of a primary neurologic disorder. Identifying other autonomic disturbances raises the possibility of diseases such as Shy-Drager syndrome, Parkinson's disease, and diabetic neuropathy. Volume depletion due to any cause may predispose a susceptible patient to syncopal episodes.

SIGNS AND SYMPTOMS

In the majority of cases the clue to the etiology of syncope results from a careful history. The history begins with characterizing the onset of syncope; for example, focal dysesthesias may suggest that the syncope is related to a seizure disorder. If syncope is preceded by lightheadedness upon standing, consider postural hypotension or vasodepressor syncope. Prodromal nausea and warmth often signal vasodepressor syncope. Certain maneuvers such as micturition, defecation, cough, and sneezing may trigger neurally mediated syncope. Identifying a history of coronary artery disease or cardiovascular risk factors as well as an abnormal cardiac examination should flag patients in whom structural heart disease is suspected. A family history of sudden death or drowning may help identify arrhythmic causes of syncope. History related by a witness often yields pertinent information; for example, a spouse may observe tonic-clonic movements in a patient with seizure-induced syncope or pallor and diaphoresis in vasodepressor syncope.

LABORATORY PROCEDURES

Most patients with syncope warrant surface electrocardiography (ECG). Review of the baseline ECG permits identification of intrinsic conduction system disease such as bradycardic rhythms, high-grade A-V block, or significant His-Purkinje system abnormalities. Measurement of the baseline QT interval may identify patients at risk for torsade de pointes. ECG performed at the time of the event, if feasible, may capture tachycardia or bradycardia.

IMAGING STUDIES

Assessment for structural heart disease is mandated in elderly patients with syncope or any patient with risk factors or physical findings of cardiovascular disease. In general, this is performed with surface echocardiography. If the history suggests exertional syncope or angina, stress testing should be considered. Caution should be exerted in the patient suspected of having aortic stenosis or any mechanical obstruction to cardiac output prior to treadmill exercise testing; a significant fall in peripheral vascular resistance without the ability to augment cardiac output adequately may produce syncope or cardiac arrest.

SPECIAL TESTS

- A history of syncope only after prolonged standing coupled with orthostatic vital sign measurement at the bedside concludes the diagnostic workup in an otherwise healthy patient. Tilt testing can be useful given the same history when bedside measures are nondiagnostic.
- Appropriate use of initially expensive diagnostic tests may prevent the greater cost to patient and society of an erroneous diagnosis. One such test is the electrophysiologic study (EPS), which is indicated if an arrhythmic event has occurred or is suspected based on other findings. In the CAD population, EPS has been shown to identify high-risk patients. Syncope that occurs in the setting of known CAD or remote myocardial infarction merits EPS, particularly in those patients with reduced LV function. EPS should also be performed for patients with symptomatic hypertrophic cardiomyopathy.
- Capturing an arrhythmic cause of syncope may be difficult, especially with infrequent episodes; 24- or 48-hour ambulatory ECG monitoring may be useful, but longer periods of monitoring may be required. This can be done with external 30-day event monitors or implantable electrocardiographic event monitors; the latter can capture an arrhythmic diagnosis several months after implantation.

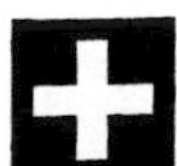

Management

GENERAL MEASURES

The key to selecting an appropriate management strategy for the patient with syncope is risk stratification. The clinician must determine the likelihood of a recurrent syncopal event, and estimate the risk to the patient in the event of recurrent syncope.

SURGICAL MEASURES

- Bradycardia that results in syncope may be treated with pacemaker implantation. Permanent pacing may also be indicated in vasodepressor syncope when profound chronotropic incompetence is part of the pathophysiology producing syncope.
- Surgical measures are reserved for treating mechanical causes of syncope such as aortic stenosis (AS) and hypertrophic obstructive cardiomyopathy. The vast majority of sudden deaths in AS occur only in patients who had previously been symptomatic, further underscoring the need for surgical evaluation in the patient with syncope due to AS.
- Altering the sequence of myocardial activation with permanent pacemaker implantation in hypertrophic obstructive cardiomyopathy has shown mixed results in preventing syncope, but may be an option for the patient who does not respond to medical therapy and is not a candidate for surgery. Surgical myectomy or percutaneous alcohol septal ablation effectively removes the myocardium obstructing the left ventricular outflow tract; these therapies may be considered depending on the availability of experienced operators.

SYMPTOMATIC TREATMENT

N/A

ADJUNCTIVE TREATMENT

- Since vasodepressor syncope is the most common cause of syncope, such patients should be instructed on the use of self-therapy measures that can be highly effective. These include avoidance of abrupt standing, liberalization of water and sodium intake, and avoidance of prolonged standing. Use of compression stockings meets with occasional patient acceptance and symptomatic improvement.
- In patients with ventricular tachycardia or ventricular fibrillation as the cause of syncope, implantation of a cardiac defibrillator (ICD) may prove lifesaving. All current-generation defibrillators also provide antitachycardia pacing routines. These can terminate sustained tachycardias often without administration of a shock. Note that the substrate for syncope is not altered; thus, to avoid frequent firings of the ICD, the underlying substrate should be altered if possible. An example of this is the patient with sustained VT and CAD; identifying reversible ischemia should prompt revascularization if possible or concomitant use of antiarrhythmic drug therapy.

ADMISSION/DISCHARGE CRITERIA

Any episode of syncope resulting in significant harm to the patient mandates inpatient evaluation. Furthermore, patients with structural heart disease and syncope probably should be admitted to a telemetry ward given the risk of sudden death. On the other hand, a young person with a clearly identified reversible precipitant such as dehydration or presumed vasodepressor (neurocardiogenic) syncope could be managed as an outpatient in the absence of high-risk features.

Medications

DRUG(S) OF CHOICE

In general, drug therapy for syncope is reserved for the patient with vasodepressor syncope whom adjunctive measures have failed. Useful drugs include midodrine, which stimulates α_1-adrenergic receptors, and fludrocortisone, which augments renal retention of water and sodium.

- In the absence of contraindications, patients with orthostatic hypotension requiring drug therapy may be treated with midodrine 2.5–5 mg tid as tolerated. Fludrocortisone 0.1 mg can be given once daily. Careful patient selection and follow-up minimizes the risk of supine hypertension with these drugs.
- Theophylline (300 mg once daily or in divided doses) may help some patients with its propensity to produce tachycardia, though patients should be queried as to possible sleep disturbances, tremor, or palpitations that may ensue.
- Selective serotonin reuptake inhibitors (SSRIs) such as fluoxetine and sertraline may also be useful.

Contraindications

Midodrine should not be used in patients with hypertension, significant cardiovascular disease, acute renal disease, pheochromocytoma, or thyrotoxicosis.

Precautions

N/A

ALTERNATIVE DRUGS

N/A

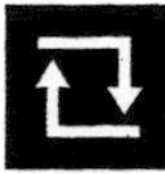

Follow-Up

PATIENT MONITORING

Patient monitoring is indicated particularly if an arrhythmic cause is suspected but a diagnosis has not been made.

EXPECTED COURSE AND PROGNOSIS

Prognosis in syncope is intimately related to etiology and management. Patients with cardiovascular disease likely have a worse prognosis because of the underlying disorders (e.g., CAD, hypertension, AS) compared with patients with vasodepressor syncope. Primary arrhythmic disorders such as the congenital long QT syndromes have varying long-term survival rates; further studies of risks associated with various genetic polymorphisms may help define prognosis for these patients.

PATIENT EDUCATION

Symptoms of noncardiac syncope are briefly outlined at this NIH Web site: http://www.ninds.nih.gov/health_and_*medical/disorders/syncope_*doc.htm.

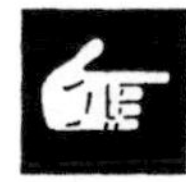

Miscellaneous

SYNONYMS

Fainting, spells, loss of consciousness.

ICD-9-CM: 780.2 Syncope and collapse

SEE ALSO: AUTONOMIC REFLEX TESTING, ORTHOSTATIC HYPOTENION, EPILEPSY

REFERENCES

- Fenton AM, Hammill SC, Rea RF, et al. Vasovagal syncope. Ann Intern Med 2000;133(9):714–725.
- Kapoor WN. Syncope N Engl J Med 2000;343(25):1856–1862.
- Schnipper JL, Kapoor WN. Diagnostic evaluation and management of patients with syncope. Med Clin North Am 2001; 85(2):423–456.

Author(s): Subha V. Raman, MD; Stephen F. Schaal, MD

Tremor

Basics

DESCRIPTION

Tremor is involuntary repetitive contraction of agonist and antagonist muscles producing rhythmic oscillation about a joint at a regular frequency.

DEFINITION

Rest Tremor

Exhibited with complete relaxation.

- Parkinsonian tremor
  - —Idiopathic Parkinson's disease (PD)
  - —Parkinsonian syndromes: Parkinson's plus
  - —Drug-induced parkinsonism
  - —Heredodegenerative disease
- Nonparkinsonian rest tremor
  - —Drug-induced tremor
  - —Metabolic abnormalities
  - —Heredodegenerative disease

Action Tremor

Exhibited with muscle activity

- Postural tremor—during held posture
  - —Enhanced physiologic tremor
  - —Essential tremor (ET)
  - —Drug-induced, dystonic, and neuropathic tremor
- Kinetic tremor—during volitional movement
  - —Midbrain tremor
  - —Cerebellar tremor
  - —Task-specific tremor

If mixed pattern present, observe for associated findings; or consider psychogenic origin.

CLINICAL CHARACTERISTICS

The clinical spectrum of tremor disorders is of diverse phenomenology and etiology. Most tremors are worsened by anxiety and improved during sleep.

PATHOPHYSIOLOGY

General

- Central—nests of oscillatory CNS neurons generate tremor
- Peripheral—tissue properties, rhythmicity of respiration and cardiac movements create resonating frequency

Rest Tremor

- Idiopathic PD and Parkinson's plus syndromes—degeneration of dopaminergic neurons; likely multifactorial cause, including genetic and environmental
- Drug-induced parkinsonism—dopamine blockers, other agents
- Cerebrovascular disease, toxins, trauma, endocrine abnormalities, infectious/ postinfectious, normal pressure hydrocephalus, and heredodegenerative diseases
- Nonparkinsonian rest tremor—caused by tremorogenic drugs, heredodegenerative diseases
- Essential tremor may be severe enough to appear at rest
- Palatal tremor and myorhythmia—slow rest tremors, secondary to brainstem pathology, infectious (Whipple's disease) or idiopathic (essential palatal tremor)

Action tremor

- Postural
  - —Enhanced physiologic tremor—natural resonance may increase with certain metabolic conditions (e.g., hyperthyroidism), medications (e.g., stimulants), toxins or alcohol withdrawal
  - —Essential tremor (ET)
    - -Most common
    - -Familial tendency—likely autosomal-dominant inheritance
    - -Loci at 3q13 and 2p22-25 have been noted
    - -Likely a heterogeneous condition
  - —Secondary postural tremor—medications, trauma, cerebrovascular disease, toxins, and heredodegenerative disorders (e.g., Wilson's disease, Hallervorden-Spatz syndrome)
  - —Task-specific—limited to the performance of a certain task (e.g., handwriting, shaving); idiopathic, may be dystonic
  - —Dystonic tremor—involuntary muscle contraction causes abnormal posture, movement opposing direction of posture causes rhythmic movements
  - —Isometric tremor—during sustained isometric contraction: idiopathic, trauma, neuropathic
  - —Orthostatic tremor
  - —Neuropathic tremor—impaired neuromuscular feedback
- Kinetic tremor
  - —Often brainstem abnormalities or lesions of the olivocerebellorubro-thalamic pathway
  - —Common etiologies—stroke, demyelination, trauma, Infectious processes and drug intoxication

Diagnosis

DIFFERENTIAL DIAGNOSIS

Rest Tremor

PD, Parkinson's syndromes, drug-induced tremor, normal pressure hydrocephalus, conditions of calcium or iron abnormalities, cerebrovascular disease, psychogenic.

- Tremor-like movements—tics, myoclonus, chorea

Action Tremor

- Postural—ET, physiologic tremor, drug-induced tremor, dystonia, neuropathy, cerebellar lesion (titubation), psychogenic
- Kinetic—midbrain (stroke, multiple sclerosis, neoplasm) cerebellar lesion, psychogenic
- Tremor-like movements—myoclonus, asterixis, tics, chorea

SIGNS AND SYMPTOMS

- Rhythmic oscillation about a joint.
- Note enhancing positions, and activity during distraction.
- Note associated neurologic findings—rigidity, bradykinesia, gait disturbance, dystonia, neuropathy.
- Note pattern and location of onset, work, social, medication and health history, psychiatric history.
- Rest tremor—observed with relaxation of involved part, attenuates during voluntary movement.
  - —Parkinsonian tremor
    - -4- to 7-Hz frequency
    - -Commonly involving upper extremity, jaw, or lower extremity
    - -Unilateral onset in typical PD (bilateral onset indicating atypical parkinsonian syndrome, secondary parkinsonism)
    - -Accompanied by bradykinesia and/or rigidity
  - —Faster rest tremor and no other parkinsonian signs: toxin exposure, heredodegenerative disease, or tremorogenic drugs
  - —Myorhythmia: 1- to 3-Hz frequency; usually face or proximal upper extremities
  - —Palatal tremor: 2-Hz frequency; rhythmic elevation of soft palate often producing subjective "clicking" sound in ear
- Postural tremor—during held posture (arms outstretched or winged position)
  - —Resting the part decreases tremor
  - —ET
    - -Onset insidious
    - -Fine motor tasks impaired
    - -No bradykinesia or rigidity
    - -4- to 12-Hz frequency
  - —Distal extremities with flexion/extension movements
    - May be whole head or voice tremor
    - -Handwriting, drawing Archimedes spiral, or water pouring enhances tremor
    - -Alcohol intake reduces ET in 50%
    - -Worsens with stress, fatigue, excitement, or stimulants (common to many tremors)
  - —Enhanced physiologic tremor
    - -Similar to ET, finer amplitude, faster frequency (8–12 Hz)
    - -Usually symmetrical
  - —Orthostatic tremor
    - -Standing in one position, relieved by movement
    - -Subjective discomfort or pain in legs immediately relieved with movement
    - -Best observed by electrophysiologic studies due to 10- to 18-Hz frequency and extremely fine amplitude

- Kinetic tremor—during volitional movement
  - —High amplitude, chaotic, rhythmic movements, enhanced with target-directed actions
  - —Chaotic appearance from proximal musculature involvement
  - —Findings of brainstem or cerebellar dysfunction usually present
- Psychogenic tremor—variable presentation
  - —Often present in all actions
  - —Lessens as patient fatigues or is distracted
  - —Embellished with focus
  - —Variable amplitude, frequency, and direction
  - —May "travel" from one body part to another
  - —Careful history may uncover psychosocial pathology

LABORATORY PROCEDURES

- PD, ET, and drug-induced tremor—no extensive laboratory workup
- Uncertainty—test for metabolic causes (e.g., hyperthyroidism, hypoparathyroidism)
- Unusual presentations, suspicious family history—serum ceruloplasmin, urine copper, peripheral blood smear to detect Wilson's disease or acanthocytic disorders

IMAGING STUDIES

CT or MRI brain scanning may demonstrate focal lesion, diffuse white matter disease, hydrocephalus, or basal ganglia deposition of calcium or iron in atypical presentations.

SPECIAL TESTS

- Genetic studies for Huntington's disease considered with positive family history
- If normal pressure hydrocephalus is suspected (may produce Parkinsonism), cerebrospinal fluid cisternography

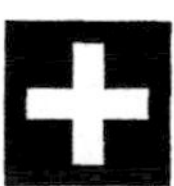

Management

GENERAL MEASURES

Depends on the tremor type and severity. Medications may ameliorate many types of tremor. Severe tremors may prompt consideration of neurosurgical approaches.

SURGICAL MEASURES

- Ablative
  - —Permanent lesion produced in the involved pathway—commonly the ventral thalamus
- Nonablative
  - —Deep brain stimulation with reversible implantation of electrodes into specific nuclei. Ventral thalamus stimulation effective for many tremors, subthalamic or pallidal stimulation for PD

SYMPTOMATIC TREATMENT

N/A

ADJUNCTIVE THERAPY

Stress management, proper sleep, and medication caution helpful.

ADMISSION/DISCHARGE CRITERIA

Admission is rarely required for tremor.

Medications

DRUG(S) OF CHOICE

- Parkinson's disease
  - —Carbidopa/levodopa, benserazide/levodopa
  - —Ropinirole, pramipexole, pergolide
  - —Amantadine
  - —Trihexyphenidyl, benztropine, biperiden
- Essential tremor: Propranolol, nadolol, primidone, gabapentin, topiramate, alprazolam, clonazepam
- Dystonic tremor: Trihexyphenidyl, benztropine
- Task-specific tremor: Clonazepam, botulinum toxin injections
- Kinetic tremor: Clonazepam, trihexyphenidyl, benztropine, carbidopa/levodopa, propranolol, carbamazepine
- Isometric/orthostatic tremor: Clonazepam, gabapentin

Contraindications

Beta-blockers in reactive airway disease, congestive heart failure.

Precautions

- Primidone: flu-like symptoms, drowsiness.
- Anticholinergic effects in trihexyphenidyl and benztropine.
- Benzodiazepines have addiction potential.

ALTERNATIVE DRUGS

- ET—acetazolamide, clozapine
- PD and ET—Mirtazapine

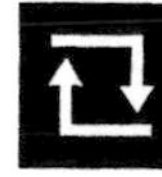

Follow-Up

PATIENT MONITORING

- Monitor effectiveness of therapy and untoward effects.
- Some medications require lab monitoring (e.g., weekly WBC counts with Clozaril).

EXPECTED COURSE AND PROGNOSIS

- PD
  - —Progressive neurodegenerative disease
  - —As rigidity and bradykinesia worsen, tremor lessens
- ET—Benign
  - —Subtle for years, increasing with age
- Dystonic tremor; dystonia often progresses over 3 to 5 years, then plateaus
- Task-specific tremor
  - —Worsens with repetition of specific task
  - —Avoidance of or changing performance may alleviate symptoms

PATIENT EDUCATION

- Community support groups for ET, PD, and dystonia
- National organizations:
  - —International Tremor Foundation (ITF), 7046 West 105th Street, Overland Park, KS 66212-1803; Tel: 913-341-3880, *www.essentialtremor.org*.
  - —WE MOVE, 204 West 84th Street, New York, NY 10024; Tel: (U.S.): 800-437-MOV2; (outside U.S.): 212-875-8312, *www.wemove.org*.

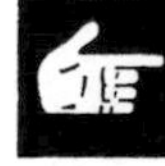

Miscellaneous

SYNONYMS

- *Parkinson's disease*: paralysis agitans, shaking palsy
- *Essential tremor*: benign essential tremor, familial tremor
- *Cervical dystonia*: spasmodic torticollis
- *Midbrain kinetic tremor*: rubral tremor
- *Cerebellar tremor*: intention tremor, titubation

ICD-9-CM: 332.0 PD; 333.1 ET; 781.0 Tremor (NOS); 333.83 Cervical dystonia

SEE ALSO: TREMOR, ESSENTIAL; PARKINSON'S DISEASE

REFERENCES

- Deuschl G, Koster B, Lucking C. Diagnostic and pathophysiological aspects of psychogenic tremors. Mov Disord 1998;13:294–302.
- Deuschl G, Toro C, Hallet M. Symptomatic and essential palatal tremor: differences of palatal movements. Mov Disord 1994;9(6):676–678.
- Elble R. The pathophysiology of tremor. In: Watts R, Koller W, eds. Movement disorders: principles and practice. New York: McGraw-Hill, 1997:405–417.
- Jankovic J. Essential tremor: clinical characteristics. Neurology 2000;S4,54(11):21–25.
- Lou J, Jankovic J. Essential tremor: clinical correlates in 350 patients. Neurology 1991;41:234–238.

Author(s): Karen M. Thomas, DO

Weakness

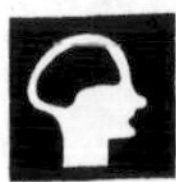

Basics

DESCRIPTION

- Weakness can be defined as a deficit in the motor system, with decreased strength in one or more muscles or limbs, or generalized weakness. Patients may use the term weakness to refer to other problems, such as fatigue, muscle and joint pain, and incoordination. Therefore, it is important to explore with the patient exactly what is meant when the term weakness is used.

DEFINITIONS

- Upper motor neuron deficit refers to an injury to the central nervous system (brain or spinal cord) causing weakness. A lower motor neuron syndrome refers to weakness caused by injury to any of several levels of the peripheral nervous system (including anterior horn cell, nerve root, plexus, nerve, neuromuscular junction, and, for general purposes, muscle).

CLINICAL CHARACTERISTICS

- The most important factors to ascertain the correct etiology of weakness include rapidity of onset and speed of development of weakness, distribution of weakness, fluctuating versus fixed weakness, and associated findings such as abnormal reflexes, sensory loss, impaired bowel and bladder function, exposure to toxins, and family history of weakness.
  —In developed countries, the most common causes of acute weakness are Guillain-Barré syndrome (GBS), myasthenia gravis, drug effects, botulism, rhabdomyolysis, and hypokalemic weakness.
  —Family history of episodes of acute weakness may suggest porphyria, periodic paralysis, or rhabdomyolysis.
  —In-hospital onset suggests hypermagnesemia, hypokalemia, myasthenia gravis, GBS, antibiotic-induced weakness, botulism, critical illness polyneuropathy, or myopathy.
  —Travel history suggests fish poisoning, polio, diptheria, botulism, tick paralysis, rabies, or snake or other envenomation.
  —Gastrointestinal symptoms suggest porphyria, botulism, or organophosphate, thallium, or arsenic poisoning.

PATHOPHYSIOLOGY

- Weakness of upper motor neuron etiology is caused by injury to the major descending motor pathway, the corticospinal tract. The corticospinal tract may be injured at multiple levels, including its cortical origin, through the cerebral white matter, internal capsule, caudal brainstem, or within the spinal cord. Lower motor neuron weakness is caused by more diverse sites of injury, including the anterior horn cells of the spinal cord, roots, plexus, nerves, neuromuscular junction, and muscle.

Diagnosis

DIFFERENTIAL DIAGNOSIS

- The differential diagnosis of weakness is extremely broad and only a few major causes are listed here.
  —Cerebrum/brainstem
    -Cerebrovascular accident
    -Multiple sclerosis
    -Mass lesions (tumors, abscess)
    -Trauma
  —Spinal cord
    -Trauma
    -Compressive myelopathy (neoplastic, herniated disc, spondylotic)
    -Transverse myelitis
    -Anterior spinal artery syndrome
  —Motor neuron
    -Amyotrophic lateral sclerosis
    -Acute anterior poliomyelitis
  —Peripheral nerve
    -GBS
    -Porphyria
    -Toxic neuropathies (heavy metals [e.g., arsenic, lead, thallium, gold], hexacarbons, nitrofurantoin, lithium, disulfiram)
    -Diphtheria
    -HIV-associated neuropathies
  —Neuromuscular junction
    -Myasthenia gravis and myasthenic syndromes
    -Organophosphate poisoning
    -Drug-induced neuromuscular blockade
    -Botulism
    -Animal venoms/poisons
    -Electrolyte derangements (hypermagnesemia)
  —Muscle
    -Muscular dystrophies
    -Inflammatory myopathies
    -Rhabdomyolysis
    -Periodic paralysis
    -Electrolyte derangements (hypokalemia, hypophosphatemia)

SIGNS AND SYMPTOMS

- Upper motor neuron weakness typically is associated with hypertonia or spasticity, hyperreflexia, and extensor plantar responses. Myelopathy that develops slowly is generally associated with hyperactive reflexes and Babinski signs. Acute spinal cord injury may present with "spinal shock" and flaccid areflexic paralysis, which can be confused with a lower motor neuron pathology. Differentiation from root, plexus, or peripheral nerve disease usually can be made based on determination of sensory level, urinary symptoms (urinary retention, urgency, frequency, and incontinence), frequent asymmetry of weakness, and eventual development of upper motor neuron signs.
- Lower motor neuron weakness typically is associated with hypotonia or flaccidity if the weakness is severe, with hyporeflexia or areflexia and flexor or absent plantar responses. Fasciculations may be present if the anterior horn cell or motor nerve has been injured with resultant denervation of muscle.
- Patterns of weakness help to localize the site of pathology.
  —Hemiparesis that includes the face suggests cerebral or high brainstem lesions.
  —Hemiparesis without facial and other cranial nerve involvement suggests lower brainstem or spinal cord.
  —Myotomal level suggests spinal cord pathology.
  —Proximal weakness in all limbs suggests myopathy.
  —Distal weakness suggests peripheral neuropathy.
- Weakness of eye movements suggests a differential diagnosis of botulism, myasthenia gravis, hypermagnesemia, diphtheria, antibiotic-induced weakness, tick paralysis, and thallium intoxication.
- Decreased or absent pupillary responses suggest a differential diagnosis of diphtheria, botulism, anticholinergic toxicity, antibiotic-induced weakness, snake venoms, and Lambert-Eaton syndrome.
- Various types of pain may suggest different causes of weakness.
  —Neck and back pain may herald weakness for GBS, porphyria, polio
  —Tender muscles: rhabdomyolysis
  —Proximal myalgias: periodic paralysis, GBS
  —Distal dysesthesias: toxic neuropathies
- Respiratory failure disproportionate to limb weakness: myasthenia gravis, botulism, antibiotic-induced weakness, hypermagnesemia, hypophosphatemia, rabies, amyotrophic lateral sclerosis, high cervical cord lesions, critical care polyneuropathy, rabies, snake envenomations

LABORATORY PROCEDURES

- Electrolytes
- Creatine kinase for question of muscle injury
- Antiacetylcholine receptor antibodies for suspicion of myasthenia gravis
- Cerebrospinal fluid analysis for evaluation of GBS (elevation of protein with normal or near-normal cell count), carcinomatous meningitis (cytology, tumor markers), multiple sclerosis (IgG synthesis rate and index and oligoclonal bands), transverse myelitis
- Serum levels of organophosphates (TEPP, parathion)
- Urine studies for toxins such as arsenic
- Serum, feces, and gastric contents for botulinum toxin assay
- Hair and fingernail analysis for metals such as arsenic and thallium

IMAGING STUDIES

- CT brain to investigate for mass lesion or stroke
- MRI brain to investigate for stroke, mass lesion, or multiple sclerosis
- MRI spine to evaluate for compressive myelopathy (e.g., stenosis, disc herniation, tumor, abscess) or demyelination/inflammation
- MRI cauda equina to evaluate for compressive lesions or thickening of roots that might represent neoplastic infiltration
- MRI plexus occasionally helpful to investigate neoplastic involvement of plexus

SPECIAL TESTS

- Nerve conduction velocity studies/electromyography to investigate pattern and type of radiculopathy, plexopathy, neuropathy, or myopathy
- Repetitive stimulation nerve study to explore neuromuscular junction function in suspected myasthenia gravis, myasthenic syndromes, or botulinum poisoning
- Edrophonium (Tensilon) test for suspected myasthenia gravis

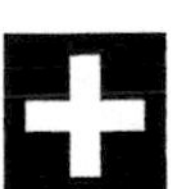

Management

GENERAL MEASURES

- The initial approach to treatment of weakness depends upon the etiology. Separate chapters on causes of weakness will go into greater detail. Patients with progressive generalized weakness with possibility of threatened respiratory insufficiency must be monitored closely for vital capacities and inspiratory pressures to determine the need for intubation and ventilation.

SURGICAL MEASURES

- Potential surgical measures include
  - —Decompression/excision of cord lesions
  - —Stabilization of vertebral fractures or spinal instability
  - —Biopsy of cerebral/cord lesions
  - —Release of nerve entrapments as in carpal tunnel syndrome

SYMPTOMATIC TREATMENT

- Physical therapy, including range of motion and frequent turning for those with severe weakness
- Splinting to prevent contractures
- Occupational therapy
- Measures to prevent deep vein thrombosis if patient is nonambulatory
- Speech therapy if weakness affects the ability to speak

ADJUNCTIVE TREATMENT

N/A

ADMISSION/DISCHARGE CRITERIA

- Admission criteria for this diverse group of causes of weakness vary but include
  - —Rapidly progressive course of generalized weakness
  - —Impending respiratory failure or inability to protect the airway
  - —Need for expedited workup
  - —Inability to perform activities of daily living and transfers

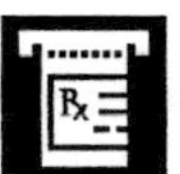

Medications

DRUG(S) OF CHOICE

- The choice of medications for the vast spectrum of disorders that can cause weakness depends on the cause. Treatments for some of the commonly considered causes of weakness include
  - —Patients with weakness from acute cerebral infarction who present within 3 hours and meet inclusion/exclusion criteria should be considered for treatment with thrombolytic therapy.
  - —Treatment with high-dose corticosteroids should be considered for patients with weakness from acute exacerbations of multiple sclerosis, transverse myelitis, spinal cord compression, myasthenia gravis, inflammatory myopathies, and CIDP.
  - —GBS, CIDP, myasthenia gravis, and inflammatory myopathies may respond to intravenous immunoglobulin therapy.
  - —Porphyric neuropathy may respond to infusions of intravenous glucose 10–20 g/hour and hematin 4 mg/kg every 12 hours.
  - —Atropine and pralidoxime (a cholinesterase reactivator) for organophosphate poisoning
  - —Botulinum antitoxin for botulism
  - —IV calcium gluconate for hypermagnesemia

Precautions

- See specific disease chapters for details

Contraindications

- Known hypersensitivity to medications

ALTERNATIVE DRUGS

N/A

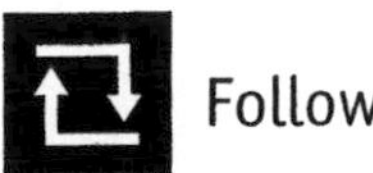

Follow-Up

PATIENT MONITORING

- Patients with acute weakness must be followed closely for development of respiratory failure and, after the etiology of the weakness is discovered, for response to therapy if one is available. After discharge to home or a rehabilitation facility, monitoring should continue to assess continued course.

EXPECTED PROGNOSIS AND COURSE

- Expected course and prognosis are dependent upon the underlying cause of the weakness.

PATIENT EDUCATION

- See separate chapters for sources of information on disorders causing weakness

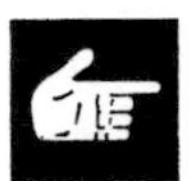

Miscellaneous

SYNONYMS

- Paralysis
- Paresis

ICD-9-CM: 780.7 Weakness (generalized); 728.8 Weakness, muscle; 344.1 Paraplegia; 344.9 Paralysis (with many subheadings)

SEE ALSO: NEUROPATHY, PERIPHERAL; GUILLAIN-BARRÉ SYNDROME; MYASTHENIA GRAVIS; LAMBERT-EATON SYNDROME; TRANSVERSE MYELITIS; POLYMYOSITIS; DERMATOMYOSITIS

REFERENCES

- Knochel JP. Neuromuscular manifestations of electrolyte disorders. Am J Med 1982;72;521–533.
- LoVecchio F, Jacobson S. Approach to generalized weakness and peripheral neuromuscular disease. Emerg Med Clin North Am 1997;15(3):605–623.
- Sliwa JA. Acute weakness syndromes in the critically ill patient. Arch Phys Med Rehabil 2000;81[3 Suppl 1]:845–852.

Author(s): D. Joanne Lynn, MD

SECTION II

Neurologic Diagnostic Tests

Neurologic Examination

Mental Status

- A rough assessment of mental status can be made just by observing the patient during history taking and examination. Patients should be observed for signs of self-neglect, depression, anxiety, inappropriate behavior, emotional lability, thought disorder, and disorders of memory, language, and other cognitive functions.
- Screening tests include
  —Simple questions to test orientation to time, place, and person
  —Digit span to assess attention: Ask patient to repeat presented numbers forward or backward, starting with three or four digits and increasing up to seven digits
  —Assess registration: Ask patient to repeat back three objects
  —Short-term memory: Ask patient to recall these objects at 5 minutes
  —Assess calculations with tasks such as serial subtractions of 7's or 3's or simple addition problems
  —Abstract thoughts, such as proverbs, similarities, estimations
  —Spatial: Ask patient to draw in a clock face, place major cities on a map outline, draw interlocking pentagons
  —Visual and body perception: Ask patient to recognize famous faces, identify his or her own index finger, touch right ear with left index finger, test stereognosis and graphesthesia
  —Test for apraxias

Cranial Nerves

CRANIAL NERVE I (OLFACTORY)

- Cranial nerve I is tested by asking the patient to smell bedside objects, such as food or formally prepared substances. Anosmia may be caused by rhinitis, trauma, degenerative illnesses such as Parkinson's and Alzheimer's disease, medications, and frontal meningiomas. Hyposmia is common with aging.

CRANIAL NERVE II (OPTIC)

- Cranial nerve II is tested by checking pupillary responses, visual acuity, visual fields, and fundi.
  —The pupillary light response is mediated via cranial nerve II as the afferent limb and parasympathetic fibers on both sides as the efferent limb. Note whether the pupils are equal or different in size (anisocoria). Shine a bright light in one pupil and observe the direct pupillary response in that eye and the consensual pupillary response in the other eye while the patient looks into the distance. Then have the patient look from the distance to your finger located a few inches from his or her nose and watch the pupils for the reaction to accommodation.
  —Swinging light test: Swing a bright light from one pupil to the other and assess pupillary constriction, which should be equal in both eyes. If one pupil dilates when the light is swung to it, a relative afferent pupillary defect or Marcus Gunn pupil is present, representing a lesion anterior to the optic nerve chiasm.
  —Assess visual acuity with Snellen chart, near vision chart or card, or ask if the patient can read bedside materials, count fingers, see hand movements, or perceive light.
  —Funduscopic examination: Examine the optic disk, blood vessels, and retinal background.

CRANIAL NERVES III, IV, AND VI (EYE MOVEMENTS)

- Look at position of eyes in primary gaze: Are they conjugate or dysconjugate?
- Test movements to cardinal positions, noting any positions in which the patient develops diplopia. Note any pathologic nystagmus.

CRANIAL NERVE V (TRIGEMINAL)

- Sensory: Test light touch and pinprick for each division of the trigeminal nerve (V1—forehead, V2—cheek, V3—lower lip). If a sensory deficit is found, map out the edges.
- Motor: muscles of mastication
  —Look for wasting of the temporalis muscle.
  —Ask the patient to clench the jaw and palpate the masseter and temporalis muscles. Try to open the jaw.
  —Ask the patient to forcefully open the mouth against the resistance of your hand beneath the jaw. Look for deviation of the jaw to one side.
- Jaw jerk: Ask the patient to let the mouth hang open loosely. Place your finger on his or her chin and percuss it with hammer. Observe jaw movement.

CRANIAL NERVE VII (FACIAL)

- Motor: Examine facial symmetry, nasolabial folds, forehead wrinkles, smiling, eye closure. Ask patient to show teeth, close eyes tightly, look up at the ceiling, whistle.
- Upper motor neuron lesions spare forehead compared with lower face. Lower motor neuron or nuclear lesions involve upper and lower face equally. Taste may be altered because the facial nerve carries taste fibers for the anterior two thirds of the tongue.

CRANIAL NERVE VIII (AUDITORY)

- Assess hearing acuity with whispered speech or a ticking watch, or rub fingers in each ear. If there is a decrease in acuity in one ear, perform the Rinne and Weber tests.
  —Rinne: Hold a 516-Hz tuning fork on the mastoid process and then in front of the ear and ask the patient which is louder.
  —Weber: Position the end of the tuning fork on the vertex of the head and ask if the sound is louder in the good ear or the deaf ear.
  —In conductive hearing loss, bone conduction via the mastoid is better than air conduction, and the sound is heard loudest in the affected ear on Weber testing. In sensorineural hearing loss, air is better than bone conduction, and the sound is heard loudest in the good ear.
  —Vestibular nerve dysfunction is associated with unilateral horizontal nystagmus that is associated with vertigo. Gait may be unsteady, veering toward the side of the lesion. In the Hallpike test, the patient is brought quickly from a sitting to a supine position, with head tilted below the horizontal and turned 45 degrees to the right or left. Fatigable rotary nystagmus with delay indicates a peripheral vertigo syndrome.

CRANIAL NERVES IX (GLOSSOPHARYNGEAL) AND X (VAGUS)

- Watch resting position and then movement of the uvula when the patient says "ahh." Touch the pharyngeal wall behind the pillars to elicit a "gag reflex" and observe the uvula: Does it lift, and is the movement symmetric or deviated to one side: Also ask about sensation in the pharynx. Movement of the uvula to one side suggests upper or lower motor neuron lesion of the vagus on the other side. If the uvula does not move at all, bilateral palatal muscle paresis may be suggested.

CRANIAL NERVE XI (ACCESSORY)

- This nerve arises from the medulla with contributions from C2–4. The ipsilateral cerebral hemisphere innervates the ipsilateral sternocleidomastoid and the contralateral trapezius. Examine for wasting or fasciculation of the sternocleidomastoid muscle. Have the patient turn the head to either side against your resistance and to shrug shoulders, noting any asymmetry of the trapezii muscles.

CRANIAL NERVE XII (HYPOGLOSSAL)

- Examine the tongue for size and fasciculations (when the tongue is at rest in the mouth), and ask the patient to protrude the tongue, noting any deviation. Test power by asking the patient to push the tongue into each cheek. Deviation to one side suggests weakness on the side to which the tongue moves. This can be upper motor neuron weakness if associated with hemiparesis. Lower motor neuron weakness is associated with atrophy and fasciculations.

Motor/Reflexes

- Motor examination assesses not only the strength of various muscle groups but also bulk, tone, and abnormal spontaneous movements of the muscles. Judgment should be made as to whether muscle tone is decreased, normal, or increased. Hypertonicity may be due to spasticity, rigidity, or paratonia. Patients with weakness should be assessed for atrophy and fasciculations.
- Power should be graded and reported on a scale such as the Medical Research Council scale:
  —5 = Full strength
  —4 = Movement against some resistance
  —3 = Movement against gravity
  —2 = Movement with gravity eliminated
  —1 = Trace movement
  —0 = No movement
- Muscle stretch reflexes are tested at the
  —Biceps C5
  —Brachioradialis C6
  —Triceps C7
  —Finger flexors C8
  —Knees L2–4
  —Ankles S1
- Reflexes are recorded on a scale of 0 = absent, 1 = normal or mildly pathologically reduced depending on the context, 2 = normal, 3 = hyperreflexic, and 4 = hyperreflexic with clonus. The examiner should note asymmetries and spread to adjacent segments of the body.

Sensory

- The primary sensory modalities, that is, light touch, vibration, proprioception, pinprick (pain), and temperature sense, should be assessed in each limb starting distally and moving proximally as a quick screen. More extensive testing, such as touching upon each dermatome and major nerve distribution, is required if there are sensory complaints. A 128-Hz tuning fork is needed for testing of vibration.
- Higher integrative sensory modalities may be checked if the primary modalities are found to be intact. These include two-point discrimination and sensory inattention. A blunted pair of compasses or two pins can be used to test two-point discrimination; normal values include index finger <5mm, little finger <7 mm, great toe <10 mm. In parietal lobe injury, primary modalities may be intact, but the patient may localize these inputs poorly with decreased two-point discrimination, astereognosis, and sensory inattention.

Cerebellar

- Several different tests assess cerebellar function.
  —Finger-to-nose testing and heel-to-shin testing to look for ipsilateral limb ataxia, which may be manifest as intention tremor, dysmetria, and dysdiadochokinesia (incoordination or disorganization in tests of repeated movements or rapid alternating movements).
  —Rebound: Ask the patient to hold arms out and close eyes. Then push the arms up or down suddenly and see if the patient has an exaggerated correction.
  —Observation of gait may show evidence of midline cerebellar dysfunction with truncal ataxia with broad base and/or titubation. If there is very severe truncal ataxia, the patient may not be able to sit without falling to one side.
  —Dysarthria, cerebellar type

Stance and Gait

- Patients who can stand should be asked to do so normally, with feet touching and eyes closed for Romberg testing. Heel-to-toe walking stresses normal balance mechanisms. Patients should be assessed for narrow versus broad base, shuffling, ataxia, circumduction, footdrop, and apractic gait.

Author(s): D. Joanne Lynn, MD

Autonomic Reflex Testing (ART)

Description of Procedure

Noninvasive ART techniques are designed to detect and quantitate autonomic failure by evaluation of sudomotor, cardiovagal, and adrenergic autonomic functions.

QUANTITATIVE SUDOMOTOR AXON REFLEX TEST (QSART)

Evaluates postganglionic sudomotor function. Acetylcholine (10% sterile saline solution) is iontophoresed into the skin, where it activates the axon terminal of the nearest sweat gland. This impulse propagates antidromically to the branching point and then travels orthodromically to the nearby sweat gland where sweat is released.

Recording Sites

Dorsum of the foot (sural nerve), distal leg (saphenous), proximal leg (peroneal), and medial forearm (ulnar).

Normal Response

Similar volume on all sites; men > women; declines with age.

Abnormal Response

Reduced, excessive, persistent sweating.

SILASTIC IMPRINTS

Measures direct sweat gland response to iontophoresis of 1% pilocarpine or acetylcholine. Silastic material is spread onto skin and sweat droplets are imprinted into it.

SYMPATHETIC SKIN RESPONSES (SSR)

The sympathetic skin response measures change in skin resistance using EMG electrodes using electrical or other stimulation (deep breathing, noise).

Recordings Sites

Palm/dorsum of hand, sole/dorsum of foot.

Normal Response

Readily elicitable, amplitude in hands > foot.

Abnormal Response

Absent or <50%.

THERMOREGULATORY SWEAT TEST (TST)

TST evaluates the *entire* efferent sympathetic cholinergic pathway. Body is covered by a mixture of alizarin red/corn starch/sodium carbonate (50:100:50 g) which turns red with sweating. Sweating is induced by rising oral temperature by at least 1.0°C in a heated cabinet. Anhidrosis (white areas) is measured as percent of total sweat area (red areas).

Normal Response

Homogeneous sweating.

Abnormal Response

Distal, segmental, regional, focal, mixed, and global sweat loss patterns.

DEEP BREATHING TEST (DB)

Cardiovagal and adrenergic functions are evaluated using deep breathing, Valsalva maneuver, and head-up tilt with beat-to-beat heart rate and blood pressure monitoring. Heart rate variation to DB is measured at maximum inspiration and expiration at breathing frequency 6/cycles/min.

Normal Response

Age 20–39 (14–41 bpm), 40–59 (10–33 bpm), ≥60 (7–27 bpm).

Abnormal Response

Reduced heart rate variation is an early sign of autonomic neuropathy and is associated with increased cardiovascular risks.

VALSALVA MANEUVER (VM)

The subject performs a forced expiration for 15 seconds, against a fixed resistance, maintaining an expiratory pressure of 40 mm Hg. Valsalva ratio evaluates parasympathetic; beat-to-beat blood pressure profile evaluates peripheral adrenergic function.

- Phase I: Respiration.
- Phase II–early (II_E): Progressive fall of blood pressure, venous return and cardiac output compensated with baroreflex-mediated tachycardia.
- Phase II–late (II_L): Restoration blood pressure to the resting level occurs due to increasing peripheral resistance.
- Phase III: Inspiration.
- Phase IV: Blood pressure overshoots baseline, as venous return and cardiac output have returned to normal but peripheral vasoconstriction persists. Baroreflex-mediated bradycardia is present.

Valsalva ratio: an index of baroreflex integrity is calculated ratio between tachycardia during phase II and bradycardia during phase IV.

Abnormal Response

Adrenergic overactivity—reduced pulse pressure, increased phase IV
Adrenergic failure—increased fall of blood pressure, reduced or absent late phase II, reduced phase IV
Cholinergic failure—flat heart rate response

HEAD-UP TILT (HUT)

Blood pressure and heart rate are continuously recorded for 5 to 45 minutes during a head-up tilt to 60 to 80 degrees. Prolonged HUT is recommended for evaluation of syncope.

Normal Response

Heart rate increment >10 and <30 bpm, stable blood pressure and cerebral blood flow.

Abnormal Response

- Orthostatic intolerance: heart rate increment >30 bpm and <120 bpm, pulse pressure reduced <50% of baseline.
- Postural tachycardia syndrome (POTS): heart rate >120 bpm, pulse pressure falls >50% of baseline, >10% reduction of cerebral blood flow
- Syncope: rapid fall of blood pressure with brady- or tachycardia and cerebral hypoperfusion
- Orthostatic hypotension: sustained fall of blood pressure >30/10 mm Hg for 3 minutes with or without orthostatic symptoms

Time-Frequency Analysis

Power spectrum of R-R intervals, beat-to-beat variation, etc., are sensitive methods for evaluation of heart rate variability

Indications

Unexplained loss of consciousness (seizures vs. syncope), dizziness, light-headedness, orthostatic and postprandial hypotension, Parkinson's disease, multiple system atrophy, peripheral neuropathies (diabetes), small fiber neuropathy, hypo- or hyperhidrosis, chronic pain.

Strengths

Noninvasive and reproducible.

Limitations

Interpretation may be limited in older people with medications (anticholinergic, sympatholytics, and sympathomimetics). Withdrawal of these medications for 24 hours may be indicated. Heart rate variation is reduced by aging, tachycardia, hypocapnia, anticholinergic medications.

Risks

HUT may induce orthostatic hypotension, syncope with tachy-, bradycardia, or rarely sinus arrest. Risks of stopping cardioactive medications, e.g., beta-blockers.

Contraindications

Caution needed for tilt testing of older people with cardiac disease and pacemakers.

Preparation/Special Instructions for Patients

No caffeine or cigarettes for 8 hours and 1 hour after meal.

Miscellaneous

None

Author(s): Vera Novak, MD

Description of Procedure

Cerebral angiography provides images depicting contrast material as it flows through the vasculature of the CNS, head, and neck. A catheter is entered into the peripheral vasculature (typically via the common femoral artery), and access is gained into the head and neck vasculature. An iodine-based contrast is injected through the catheter and into the vessels as sequential x-ray images are taken over 5 to 20 seconds in order to record the contrast flowing through the head and neck arteries, capillaries, and veins.

Indications

Because of its invasive nature and potential risks, angiography should be considered in situations where diagnostic information regarding the CNS vasculature is not adequately evaluated by other imaging modalities such as MRI, MRA, CTA, or SPECT. Cerebral angiography, therefore, can be considered under the following circumstances:

- Suspicion for asymptomatic cerebrovascular disease based on physical findings such as a bruit, ophthalmoscopic findings, or neurologic findings suggesting potential disease involving the carotid or vertebrobasilar systems.
- Screening for cerebrovascular source of disease following a transient ischemic attack or stroke involving the carotid or vertebrobasilar territories.
- Fixed or worsening focal neurologic deficit, occurring for less than 6 hours, suspected to be due to acute cerebrovascular occlusion.
- Suspicion for nonatherosclerotic occlusive cerebrovascular disease such as vasculitis, vasculopathy, vasospasm, or venous occlusive disease.
- Unexplained or suspected subarachnoid hemorrhage.
- Unexplained intraparenchymal hemorrhage.
- Penetrating injury to the head and neck.
- Unexplained neurologic findings following blunt trauma.
- Head and neck trauma with suspicion for dissection, traumatic aneurysms, traumatic arteriovenous fistulas, traumatic venous thrombosis.
- Vascular malformations or arteriovenous fistulas.
- Functional testing for speech and memory prior to epilepsy surgery (Wada test).
- Presurgical investigation and embolization of hypervascular tumors.
- Vertebrospinal angiography.

Strengths

Relative to other angiographic modalities, conventional angiography provides greater spatial resolution. As a result, it is the most precise and accurate imaging method in assessing intracranial and extracranial carotid and vertebral territory cerebrovascular disease allowing for the detection of smaller vascular lesions and disease in smaller vessels. Furthermore, due to its temporal fashion of acquisition, angiography is able to depict collateral blood flow and delayed cerebrovascular blood flow. Transcatheter interventions can be performed during angiography if needed.

Limitations

Although it is possible to deduce the approximate anatomic location based on the identification of the intracranial cerebrovascular structures, cross-sectional imaging can identify structural CNS abnormalities in a more precise and accurate fashion than conventional angiography.

Risks

The incidence of cerebrovascular ischemic events within 24 hours of cerebral angiography (<1%) varies according to the angiographer's experience, the length of the procedure, and the degree of carotid artery disease. Anaphylactoid reactions to contrast medium can result in hives or pruritus; however, 1 in 40,000 patients undergoing diagnostic examinations using nonionic iodinated contrast medium suffer anaphylactic shock and death. Significant hematoma formation at the puncture site is common (6.9–10.7%). Other complications may include death, myocardial infarction, angina pectoris, retroperitoneal hematoma, pseudoaneurysm at the puncture site, abscess at the puncture site, nausea, vomiting, benign bradycardia, transient leg paresthesia due to local anesthesia, aneurysm rupture during angiography, transient global amnesia, and cortical blindness.

Contraindications

Relative contraindications to angiography include:

- Renal failure
- Prior contrast reaction
- Pregnancy
- Bleeding diathesis

Preparation/Special Instructions for Patients

Patients are asked not to eat or drink anything with the exception of oral medications beginning 4 hours prior to the exam. Premedication with steroid and Benadryl reduces the risk for contrast reaction in patients with prior history of contrast reaction. Patients with poor renal function who are not being dialyzed are hydrated before and after the procedure. Glucophage (metformin) should be withheld temporarily (48 hours) prior to myelography due to potential risk for renal failure and reinstated only after renal function has been reevaluated and found to be normal. Correction of any bleeding diathesis prior to the procedure may reduce the risk of hemorrhagic complications. Consideration should be given to the administration of anxiolytics or conscious sedation during the examination.

Miscellaneous

At the end of the procedure the catheter is removed and pressure is applied over the arteriotomy to achieve hemostasis. In the setting of bleeding diathesis, an arteriotomy closure device may be deployed for hemostasis. Following the procedure the patient is placed on strict bed rest while keeping the puncture sight immobilized, and oral fluids are encouraged. The patient is asked not to drive or operate heavy machinery for 24 hours and avoid activities during the next 2 to 3 days that may stress the incision site, such as lifting heavy objects or repeated movements that flex the joint around the incision site.

Author(s): Gregory Christoforides, MD

Biopsy, Brain

Description of Procedure

Brain biopsy can be obtained by open craniotomy or via computer-assisted stereotactic procedures (i.e., needle biopsies using a stereotactic frame, under local anesthesia). Several considerations are important in deciding between the two techniques and whether or not to pursue surgery. The most important issues relate to the lesion or process in the brain: Is it too deep or too small to be accessible? Is it located in an eloquent region of brain? Are the lesions solitary or multiple? Is the process too diffuse to define an adequate target? Other considerations focus on the patients, such as, Are they too old or too ill to undergo biopsy? Do they have a specific preference? Lesions that are generally considered most appropriate for stereotactic biopsy include those that are small and deep, located in eloquent cortex, diffuse within deep portions of the brain, and multifocal. Biopsy by open craniotomy requires general anesthesia and is most appropriate for lesions of non-eloquent cortical and adjacent subcortical tissues, and the meninges. A wedge of tissue that includes the cortex, meninges, and underlying white matter is usually optimal.

Indications

Diseases that require biopsy may be infectious, neoplastic, degenerative, vascular, metabolic, or developmental. The differential diagnosis of diseases where biopsy may be helpful is broad and includes enhancing lesions (infarct, abscess, glioma, metastasis, necrosis), tumors (primary versus metastasis), degenerative or dementing illnesses (prion diseases, Pick's disease, Lewy body disease), skull and soft tissue disorders (histiocytosis X), inflammatory conditions (vasculitis, tumefactive multiple sclerosis, neurosarcoidosis), infectious processes (abscess, progressive multifocal leukoencephalopathy), and AIDS patients (lymphoma, toxoplasmosis).

Strengths

Diagnostic accuracy based on neuroimaging criteria alone is limited. Clinically significant alterations of the preoperative diagnosis occur in 12% to 25% of cases after tissue is obtained and analyzed. In many patients, this allows for the administration of more specific and appropriate therapy.

Limitations

The major limitation of brain biopsy involves the decision of which region of the mass lesion or abnormal area of brain to access. If there is not a well-defined target, it is possible to miss the target and obtain normal or nondiagnostic tissue. This can also occur with a mass lesion, if the needle removes tissue only from the edge or transition zone. Biopsy of the center of a mass may also be nondiagnostic, by obtaining only necrotic tissue. There is an 8% to 9% failure rate associated with brain biopsy, in which the obtained tissue does not result in a definitive histologic or microbiologic diagnosis. The problem of sampling error is improved by taking multiple samples of the lesion, as well as samples of the region of interface between the lesion and normal brain. Intraoperative pathologic assessment by frozen section is also useful to ensure diagnostic adequacy of samples.

Risks

- The risks involved in brain biopsy include those to the patient, in the form of surgical complications during or after the brain biopsy, as well as potential risks to the surgical team and pathologist. In most series of brain biopsy, surgical mortality is less than 1%, while surgical morbidity ranges between 1% and 6%. The most significant risks during the procedure are intracranial hemorrhage, brain swelling and edema, and new focal neurologic deficits. Other potential risks include cerebral infarction, infection, and scarring with formation of an epileptic focus.
- The surgical team and pathology staff must handle specimens with care, since they may be at risk for infection from agents such as HIV, hepatitis, and Creutzfeldt-Jakob disease.

Contraindications

Include patients at high risk of hemorrhage due to excessive anticoagulation, liver abnormalities, thrombocytopenia, and related conditions. Patients who are medically unstable or too ill may not be suitable for anesthesia and brain biopsy.

Preparation/Special Instructions for Patients

The pathologist should be aware of the differential diagnosis before surgery to ensure proper tissue handling and to improve diagnostic yield at the time of frozen section review. For a frozen section, biopsy tissue is snap frozen in liquid nitrogen and then prepped onto slides for microscopic interpretation. Based on this preliminary diagnosis (which takes 15 to 20 minutes), the pathologist advises the neurosurgeon about the need for further samples. The definitive diagnosis will be made after review of the permanent (i.e., paraffin embedded) tissue slides.

Miscellaneous

- Special stains may be helpful to improve diagnostic accuracy. Immunohistochemical analyses of specific protein antigens on the cell surface or in the nucleus are particularly useful for differentiating between categories of disease (e.g., lymphoma versus an inflammatory condition). Genetic studies may also be of benefit for diagnosis (e.g., immunoglobulin gene rearrangement studies of lymphoma) or prognosis (e.g., chromosome 1p and 19q deletion status of oligodendroglial neoplasms).
- A postoperative CT scan is necessary to screen for hemorrhage and to evaluate the accuracy of the biopsy in relation to the target lesion.

Author(s): Dan Brown, MD; Herbert B. Newton, MD

Description of Procedure

- Muscle may be biopsied using either a needle or open surgical technique. Open muscle biopsy is generally preferred to needle biopsy in most cases because of the larger samples obtained. The muscles often biopsied are the biceps, quadriceps (usually vastus lateralis), and deltoid. It is usually best to biopsy a muscle with moderate weakness in a chronic situation, as a severely weak muscle may yield pathology of end-stage scarring and fibrosis that obscures the underlying disorder. It is best to avoid muscles that were the site of EMG investigation, injections, etc., because of traumatic pathologic changes. Sometimes the peroneus brevis muscle is biopsied at the same time as the superficial peroneal nerve when vasculitis is suspected to increase diagnostic yield.
- A skin incision is made after local anesthesia. The muscle fascia is then anesthetized and opened. Sections of muscle are excised, and samples are sent for frozen section (for histochemistry and light microscopy), fixation in glutaraldehyde, embedding in plastic (for ultrastructural analysis), and embedding in paraffin (for examination for inflammation).
- Needle biopsy may be used for sampling of multiple sites and provides samples sufficient for biochemical and DNA studies. However, the samples obtained by needle biopsy are smaller and less satisfactory for electron microscopy.

Indications

A muscle biopsy is indicated for investigation of etiology when a patient presents with clinical and laboratory evidence of myopathy such as weakness, myopathic EMG findings, elevated serum creatine kinase, and/or chronic or intermittent muscle pain. A muscle biopsy may also be useful for diagnosis of systemic conditions that may have relatively silent muscle manifestations such as vasculitis or sarcoidosis.

Strengths

Many muscle disorders such as dystrophies and inflammatory myopathies have distinct cytoarchitectural characteristics that readily allow diagnosis. Patterns and distribution of inflammatory cells may help distinguish polymyositis, dermatomyositis, vasculitis, fasciitis, and other inflammatory disorders. Special histochemical analysis may identify disorders such as lipid-storage myopathy, inclusion body myositis, or mitochondrial myopathies (ragged-red fibers). Immunochemistry for dystrophin may confirm Duchenne dystrophy when DNA studies are uninformative. Histologic features of individual muscle fibers may suggest a neuropathic cause (fiber type grouping, atrophic and angular fibers, and target fibers) but muscle biopsy is rarely diagnostic for neurogenic etiologies.

Limitations

Unfortunately, many types of muscle disease may share common pathologic features on biopsy, such as increased connective tissue, changes in fiber size and shape, and fiber necrosis. In recent years, expanding knowledge of the genetic defects that cause many myopathies has supplemented routine muscle histology to increase definitive diagnosis. Muscle biopsy cannot differentiate between various neuropathic causes for weakness. In addition, there is the risk of sampling error in multifocal disease such as polymyositis. Needle biopsies are even more prone to miss patchy (as in inflammatory myopathies) or endomysial pathology.

Risks

Risks include hemorrhage, hematoma, infection, and pain.

Contraindications

Contraindications include uncorrected coagulopathy and thrombocytopenia.

Preparation/Special Instructions for Patients

Patients should limit heavy use of the biopsied limb for several days after biopsy, and monitor for signs of infection such as excessive drainage, swelling, or erythema. No submersion in water for bathing or showering until the sutures have been removed. Sutures are generally removed in 7 to 10 days.

REFERENCES

- Griggs RC, Mendell JR, Miller RG. Evaluation and treatment of myopathies. Philadelphia: F. A. Davis, 1995:54–70.
- Younger DS, Gordon PH. Diagnosis in neuromuscular diseases. Neurol Clin 1996;14(1):135–168.

Author(s): D. Joanne Lynn, MD

Biopsy, Nerve

Description of Procedure

Nerve biopsy for diagnosis of the cause of peripheral neuropathy is most commonly performed on the sural nerve, but also on the superficial peroneal and occasionally the superficial radial nerve. For sural nerve biopsy, an incision is made, after local anesthesia, approximately 25 cm above the plantar surface of the heel, 1 cm lateral to the midline, and the nerve is dissected out. One segment is frozen for identification of immune deposits; immunocytochemistry studies are useful to stain for immunoglobulin and complement deposition. A second segment is placed in buffered formalin to be processed for paraffin sections, most useful for demonstration of vasculitis, inflammation, and granulomas. Another section is fixed in glutaraldehyde for preparation for light microscopy. Nerve fascicles are separated for single nerve fiber teasing, which allows detailed determination of nerve pathology, e.g., axonal vs. demyelinating.

Indications

Peripheral nerve biopsy is indicated to evaluate for a specific cause of neuropathy, which may be diagnosed with certainty only by pathologic examination.
Conditions for which peripheral nerve biopsy is most helpful for diagnosis include:

- Vasculitis
- Sarcoidosis
- Amyloidosis
- Tumor infiltration
- Leprosy
- Fabry disease
- Storage diseases (Niemann-Pick disease, metachromatic leukodystrophy, sialidosis, Farber disease)
- Hereditary neuropathy with liability to pressure palsies
- Neuropathy associated with antibody to MAG (myelin-associated glycoprotein)

Strengths

The nerve biopsy is especially useful to identify changes in blood vessels and connecting tissue elements of the nerve. This makes it most useful to identify inflammatory changes in vasculitis, granulomatous disease such as sarcoidosis, neoplastic infiltration, and infection such as leprosy.
If there is clinical evidence of peripheral nerve involvement in suspected multisystem vasculitis, peripheral nerve may be the least invasive site for biopsy. The yield of biopsy is usually greater if a nerve is biopsied that is abnormal on electrophysiologic studies.

Limitations

Peripheral nerves respond to the myriad diseases that affect them with a narrow spectrum of pathologic responses. This limits the diagnostic utility of nerve biopsy in most patients presenting with common types of neuropathy. It should be emphasized that the diagnosis of peripheral neuropathy is generally based on neurologic examination and electrophysiologic study findings. In addition, sampling error may be an issue with nerve biopsy; sampling of a single segment of a single nerve may miss multifocal pathology such as vasculitic lesions that may occur in the nerve proximal or distal to the site of biopsy. In addition, nerve biopsy may fail to demonstrate significant pathology in small-fiber neuropathies. In that situation, skin biopsy to examine intraepidermal small nerve fibers may be a more powerful technique.

Risks

Nerve biopsy is a surgical procedure and is associated with the typical risks of hemorrhage, hematoma, wound infection, and wound dehiscence. It can also be painful, both during the procedure and in the postoperative period.

Contraindications

Uncorrected coagulopathy or thrombocytopenia. The risk/benefit ratio should be evaluated appropriately in patients with diabetes mellitus, peripheral vascular disease, and significant edema, as complications such as infection are more common in these groups.

Preparation/Special Instructions for Patients

There is no special preoperative preparation required except for temporary discontinuation of anticoagulation if present (after judicious consideration of risk/benefit ratio for doing so). However, patients should be apprised of what to expect after the biopsy. Patients often experience spontaneous paresthesias starting 24 to 48 hours after the biopsy, which may be precipitated by stretching of the proximal nerve stump by certain movements or positions of the involved limb. Pain usual wanes by 2 to 3 weeks, but lesser discomfort may persist for much longer. Electric dysesthesias or hypersensitivity to touch may persist for more than a year in a minority of patients. For sural nerve biopsies, there is a sensory deficit along the lateral aspect of the foot, which generally recedes or even resolves by 18 months.

Miscellaneous

N/A

REFERENCES

- Mendell JR, Erdem S, Agamanolis DP. The role of peripheral nerve and skin biopsies. In: Mendell JR, Kissel JT, Cornblath DR, eds. Diagnosis and management of peripheral nerve disorders. New York: Oxford University Press, 2001:90–123.

Author(s): D. Joanne Lynn, MD

Computed Tomography of the Brain and Spine

Description

Computed tomography (CT), or computed axial tomography, is an imaging technique that uses x-rays to obtain cross-sectional images. The appearance of x-ray imaged structures depends on their density. Water is arbitrarily assigned the value of zero, with denser structures like bone having positive values and less dense tissues such as fat and air having negative values. Most CT scanners today are third generation (spiral) or fourth generation (multislice, volumetric acquisition). Multislice detectors allow faster imaging, acquisition of thinner slices, faster reconstruction, and improved image quality.

TECHNIQUES AND APPLICATIONS

- Conventional CT
  - —Axial images only, except for the head—direct coronal images can be obtained if the patient is able to lay prone with head extended.
- Reconstructions—computer generated: sagittal, coronal, 3D
- Cisternography and myelography—after the intrathecal administration of contrast
- CT angiography (CTA)—requires contrast with 3D reconstructions
  - —Circle of Willis
  - —Carotid arteries
- Functional CT
  - —CT perfusion—requires contrast, cerebral blood flow imaging
  - —Xenon CT—cerebral blood flow imaging
- Interventional
  - —CT fluoroscopy—real-time imaging
- Intraoperative CT, portable CT

Indications

INDICATIONS FOR HEAD CT

Examination of choice for evaluation of acute intracranial hemorrhage, calcifications, and cortical bone:

- Acute intracranial hemorrhage—subdural, epidural, subarachnoid, intraparenchymal, intraventricular
- Mental status/neurological change—rule out (R/O) hemorrhage
- Headache—for "worst headache of my life"; R/O subarachnoid hemorrhage. For chronic headaches MR is preferable, although imaging is generally not indicated.
- Stroke—R/O hemorrhage; early CT findings of acute ischemic stroke:
  - —Hyperdense artery sign: thrombus seen in 35% to 50% with clinical signs of acute middle cerebral artery (MCA) stroke; poor prognostic sign
  - —Obscuration of lentiform nucleus
  - —Insular ribbon sign
  - —Sulcal effacement
  - —Parenchymal hypodensity
- Trauma—R/O hemorrhage, edema, herniation, pneumocephalus, fracture.
  - —Any patient with loss of consciousness, neurologic deficit, anisocoria, fixed or dilated pupils, bleeding diathesis, or anticoagulation, and all penetrating head injuries.
- Hydrocephalus
- New-onset seizure
- Postoperative craniotomy—R/O hemorrhage, herniation
- In patients where MR is contraindicated (e.g., pacemaker) for:
  - —Tumor
  - —Infection—abscess, empyema, AIDS
  - —Seizures
  - —Multiple sclerosis
  - —Neurodegenerative disorders
  - —Granulomatous disease

INDICATIONS FOR SPINE CT

- Trauma—R/O fracture
- Postoperative fusion—metal will cause some artifacts limiting the exam
- Spondylolysis
- Arthritis
- Spinal stenosis (MR is examination of choice)
- Disc disease (MR is examination of choice)
- Cord compression—only postmyelography with injection of intrathecal contrast
- Characterization of an isolated indeterminate bone lesion noted on MR or nuclear medicine scan (e.g., hemangioma).
- In patients where MR is contraindicated (e.g., pacemaker) for:
  - —Tumor—ideally after intrathecal contrast
  - —Infection—epidural abscess, discitis, osteomyelitis, although CT even with contrast is relatively insensitive.

INDICATIONS FOR CONTRAST WITH HEAD CT

- Tumor—(MR is exam of choice)
- Infection—abscess, empyema, AIDS, (MR is exam of choice)
- Seizure—R/O tumor (MR is exam of choice)
- Arteriovenous malformations
- CT angiography/venography
- CT perfusion

INDICATIONS FOR INTRAVENOUS CONTRAST WITH SPINE CT

- Tumor—if MR contraindicated
- Infection—if MR contraindicated
- Disc disease—to enhance the epidural space/veins and better define the margins of the discs, although MR still best

INDICATIONS FOR INTRATHECAL CONTRAST WITH SPINE CT (POSTMYELOGRAM CT)

- Cord compression—when MR is contraindicated
- Disc disease, spinal stenosis, radiculopathy—if MR is contraindicated or if MR findings do not correlate with clinical findings

Strengths

- Readily available 24/7 even at small hospitals
- Noninvasive
- Fast—ideal for uncooperative and critically ill patients
- Extremely sensitive for acute intracranial hemorrhage
- Ideal for evaluation of calcifications and cortical bone

Limitations

- Beam-hardening artifacts limit posterior fossa evaluation
- Insensitive to acute ischemia
- Limited spinal cord evaluation
- Axial plane only
- Limited soft tissue contrast
- Metal streak artifacts

Contraindications

- If giving contrast: contrast allergy, renal insufficiency, multiple myeloma are relative contraindications.
- Pregnancy—relative contraindication especially first trimester; contrast contraindicated.

Preparation/Special Instructions for Patients

Patients who are scheduled for a CT with contrast are instructed to be NPO 2 hours prior to the exam. At the time of the exam they are asked to remove earrings, hair clips, hearing aids, glasses, and removable dental work.

Miscellaneous

Approximately 1% of patients are claustrophobic and require some sedation. Diazepam 5 to 10 mg PO is adequate for most.

REFERENCES

- Tanenbaum LN, ed. CT in neuroimaging revisited. Neuroimag Clin North Am 8(3).1998;

Author(s): Eric C. Bourekas, MD; H. Wayne Slone, MD

Magnetic Resonance Imaging of the Brain and Spine

Description Of Procedure

- Magnetic resonance imaging (MRI) uses a powerful magnetic field and radiofrequency waves to produce images. No ionizing radiation is involved. Most MRI units in clinical use are 1.5 tesla.
- Depending on imaging parameters, different pulse sequences can be obtained producing images yielding different information. Traditional imaging involves T1-weighted (T1W) and T2-weighted (T2W) spin echo imaging. Gradient echo imaging allows for faster imaging. T1W images are obtained after intravenous contrast, which does not affect T2W images very much. Fat suppression images help identify lesions obscured by fat. Proton density and FLAIR images are useful in evaluation of white matter disease. Functional imaging such as diffusion and perfusion imaging is invaluable in evaluation of stroke. MR angiography (MRA) and venography (MRV) are noninvasive means of evaluation of the vasculature of the head and neck.

Indications

INDICATIONS FOR BRAIN MRI

- Stroke—diffusion imaging very sensitive to acute ischemia
- Tumor
- Infection—encephalitis, abscess, empyema
- Demyelinating disorders—MS
- Seizures
- Neurodegenerative disorders—Alzheimer's, parkinsonism
- Granulomatous disease—sarcoid
- Negative CT with continuing neurologic deficits

INDICATIONS FOR BRAIN MRI WITH CONTRAST

- Tumor
- Infection
- Demyelinating disorders—helpful to monitor disease activity
- Seizures—new onset to R/O tumor

INDICATIONS FOR SPINE MRI

- Tumor—primary spinal cord, metastatic to bone, R/O cord compression, leptomeningeal carcinomatosis, R/O drop metastases
- Infection—osteomyelitis, discitis, epidural abscess
- Trauma—cord or ligamentous injury
- Degenerative disc disease—R/O disc herniation, spinal or foraminal stenosis
- Cord abnormalities—tumor, demyelination, extremity weakness, incontinence, paralysis

INDICATIONS FOR CONTRAST FOR SPINE MRI

- Tumor
  —NOT necessary for vertebral metastases
  —Primary spinal cord or nerve root tumors, leptomeningeal carcinomatosis
- Infection—osteomyelitis, discitis, epidural abscess
- Demyelination
- Granulomatous disease
- Any cord lesion
- Prior lumbar spine surgery—R/O epidural scar

Strengths

- Superior soft tissue contrast/resolution
- Direct multiplanar imaging
- No ionizing radiation
- No beam hardening artifacts related to bone

Limitations

- Length of exam—at least 20 minutes
- Sensitivity to motion
- Cost
- Difficulty in monitoring critically ill patients—ECGs don't work during scanning; only pulse oximeter monitoring available; MR compatible ventilator required.
- Difficulty in obtaining STAT off hours—technologist availability limited
- Metal artifacts
- Cortical bone, although MR is excellent for evaluation of bone marrow

Contraindications

Many contraindications are relative; it is best to consult MR facility for local policy. Electrically, magnetically, or mechanically activated implants are generally contraindicated.

ABSOLUTE CONTRAINDICATIONS

- Pacemakers
- Defibrillators
- Neurostimulators
- Bone growth stimulators
- Cochlear implants
- Ocular metallic foreign bodies
- Swan-Ganz catheters
- Allergy to IV gadolinium (MR) contrast for contrast study

RELATIVE CONTRAINDICATIONS

- Aneurysm clips—most used today are MR compatible; however, safety concerns exist and many facilities consider them absolute contraindications
- Heart valves—current valves are not contraindicated; old Starr Edwards (pre-6000 series) contraindicated
- IVC filters—current filters mostly MR compatible, although recommendations are to wait 2 to 6 weeks after insertion prior to imaging
- Inner ear implants—cochlear implants contraindicated, some stapes implants
- Drug infusion pumps—generally not contraindicated, although MR may stop infusion and necessitate pump reprogramming
- Bullets, pellets, shrapnel—must use judgment; duration, proximity to vessel? Most bullets are not contraindicated.

NOT CONTRAINDICATED

Hemostatic clips, wire sutures, plates, pins, screws, nails, dental devices (e.g., braces, bridges despite artifacts), orthopedic implants (joint replacements, spinal rods), ocular implants, ventricular shunts.

Preparations/Special Instructions for Patients

Patients must remove all jewelry and metal items from their body and clothing, including glasses, dentures and all other removable dental work, wigs, and hairpins. An extensive history and screening form designed to ensure that there are no contraindications and safety of the exam is filled out.

Miscellaneous

Claustrophobia is a problem in 5% to 10% of patients. Often this is transient and eliminated by reassurance from the technologist. Most are able to get through the exam with mild sedation usually 5 mg PO of Valium. Approximately 1% will require heavy sedation in order to complete the exam in a closed MR. Open MRIs accommodate such patients at the cost of reduced image quality.

MR has not been proven safe in pregnancy but is not believed hazardous. It is indicated in pregnancy if it will provide information critical to the patient's well-being or because the patient would otherwise require exposure to ionizing radiation.

REFERENCES

- Atlas SW. Magnetic resonance imaging of the brain and spine, 3rd ed. Philadelphia: Lippincott Williams & Wilkins, 2002.
- Kanal E, Borgstede JP, Barkovich AJ, et al. American College of Radiology White Paper on MR safety. AJR 2002;178:1335–1347.
- Shellock FG, Crues JV III. MR safety and the American College of Radiology White Paper. AJR 2002;178:1349–1352.

Author(s): Eric C. Bourekas, MD; H. Wayne Slone, MD

Description of Procedure

Myelography is an invasive imaging test that allows for the radiographic depiction of the spinal cord and associated nerve roots within the thecal sac via the intrathecal injection of water-soluble nonionic iodinated contrast agents. Changes in the contour of the thecal sac and its contents allows for the indirect diagnosis of extradural compression of spinal nerve roots and spinal cord as well as the inference of intradural neoplasms, arachnoiditis, and arachnoid cysts. Plain myelography does not accurately depict nerve root structures after exiting the thecal sac; however, the adjunct use of CT immediately following myelography (CT myelography) allows for a more accurate delineation of the anatomic relationship between discogenic and osseous structures in relation to the nerve roots and its contents. As a result, CT is almost always performed immediately following myelography.

Indications

MRI has replaced myelography as a screening tool for spinal disease. There are, however, circumstances where myelography can provide useful information. In general myelography provides higher spatial resolution than MRI and depicts osseous structures more consistently than MRI. This information is often useful for surgical planning especially in the cervical spine. If MRI is contraindicated or not possible, myelography can provide diagnostic information screening for spinal cord or nerve root compression. Keeping this in mind, myelography and CT myelography can be considered under the following circumstances:

- Suspected nerve root or spinal cord compression based on clinical symptoms such as radiculopathy or lower extremity weakness or incontinence
- Suspected spinal AVM
- Suspected tumor affecting the spinal canal
- Suspected arachnoiditis
- Suspected meningeal cyst (arachnoid cyst, meningocele, perineural cyst)

Strengths

Myelography with CT myelography provide high-resolution images depicting the relationship of osseous structures to the thecal sac and its contents in a more precise manner than MRI. Even though the sensitivity of MRI is at least as good, CT myelography is felt to more accurately depict symptomatic pathology in the setting of degenerative spine disease. Certain pathologies are more readily depicted on myelography rather than plain CT or MRI. These include arachnoid cysts, meningoceles, and arachnoiditis. Plain film myelography is less encumbered by surgically placed metallic hardware than other MRI. Furthermore, myelography allows for the collection of spinal fluid for analysis.

Limitations

Myelography can depict spinal cord morphology but cannot identify intrinsic lesions of the spinal cord such as demyelination or transverse myelitis. Infectious processes such as discitis or epidural abscess and spinal canal neoplasms are more readily identified on MRI than on myelography or CT myelography.

Risks

Complications associated with myelography include headache, nausea, vomiting, cerebrospinal fluid leak, seizure, infection, vasovagal reaction, spinal cord injury, and nerve root damage. Improper injection of contrast medium into the epidural or subdural space may confound the examination and transiently exacerbate symptoms.

Contraindications

Relative contraindication to myelography include:

- Raised intracranial pressure (papilledema)
- Bleeding abnormalities (elevated PT, PTT, decreased platelet count or patients on anticoagulation)
- Allergy to iodinated contrast agents
- Medications that lower seizure threshold such as phenothiazines, tricyclic antidepressants, CNS stimulants, MAO inhibitors
- Glucophage (metformin) should be withheld temporarily (48 hours) prior to myelography due to potential risk for renal failure
- Pregnancy
- Bacteremia or sepsis

Preparation/Special Instructions for Patients

Patients are asked not to eat or drink anything with the exception of oral medications beginning 4 hours prior to the exam. In patients with a prior history of contrast reaction, premedication with steroid and Benadryl reduces their risk for contrast reaction. Patients with poor renal function who are not being dialyzed are hydrated prior to the procedure. Glucophage (metformin) should be withheld temporarily (48 hours) prior to myelography due to potential risk for renal failure and reinstated only after renal function has been reevaluated and found to be normal. Additionally, phenothiazines, tricyclic antidepressants, or Tigan is held prior to the examination. Sedation is not typically required; however, consideration should be given to the administration of anxiolytics or conscious sedation during the examination under appropriate circumstances.

Miscellaneous

With regard to nerve root compression due to degenerative disease of the spine, clinical decisions should not be based exclusively on the basis of imaging findings alone. Objective clinical findings should be supported by radiologic findings.
To reduce the risk for cerebrospinal fluid leakage and headache following the procedure, patients are placed on strict bed rest for 4 hours, with the head of bed elevated 30 degrees, and are limited to light activity for 24 to 48 hours following the procedure. Oral fluids are encouraged following the procedure. Additionally, phenothiazines, tricyclic antidepressants, or Tigan is held for 48 hours after the study.

Author(s): Gregory Christoforidis, MD

Nerve Conduction Studies/Electromyography

Description of Procedure

- Series of diagnostic tools that evaluate the integrity and function of nerve and muscle
- *Nerve conduction velocity (NCV)* studies rely on the ability of nerve to conduct electrical potentials.
  - —Usually use surface stimulation, less often near-needle or, rarely, magnetic stimulation.
  - —Usually recorded with surface electrodes, less often with near-needle electrodes.
  - —Small electric shocks are applied over a nerve and the response is recorded.
- *Electromyography (EMG)* studies rely on the electrical activity of the muscle membrane.
  - —Usually performed using a small needle placed into the muscle(s) of interest.
- Electrodiagnostic studies are an extension of the neurologic exam to localize disorders of:
- Peripheral nerve
  - —Sensory and/or motor nerves
  - —Small or large diameter fibers
- Plexus
  - —Brachial
  - —Lumbosacral
- Nerve root
- Motor neuron
- Sensory ganglion
- Muscle
- Neuromuscular junction

Indications

- Useful in answering questions raised by the clinical exam.
- What is the pattern of injury?
  - —Is it distal or proximal?
  - —Is it diffuse?
  - —Is it symmetric or asymmetric?
  - —Is it multifocal?
  - —Is it focal in a named nerve distribution?
  - —Is it focal in a nerve root (or radicular) pattern?
- What is the underlying pathophysiology?
  - —Is it primarily demyelinating?
  - —Is it primarily axonal?
- Is this a nerve and/or a muscle process?
  - —If just muscle, what are the characteristics of the EMG?
  - —Is it a primary neuromuscular junction disorder?
- To confirm a clinical diagnosis
- To aid in differential diagnosis and direct further evaluation if necessary
- To identify subclinical disease
- To characterize the disease
- To quantitate the disease
- Symptoms that might have an etiology elucidated by NCV/EMG:
  - —Numbness
  - —Pain
  - —Weakness
  - —Cramping
- Diseases or disorders that can be diagnosed by NCV/EMG:
  - —Neuropathies
  - —Nerve entrapments
  - —Plexopathies
  - —Radiculopathies
  - —Motor neuron diseases (e.g., amyotrophic lateral sclerosis)
  - —Myopathies (e.g., muscular dystrophies, polymyositis, dermatomyositis)
  - —Neuromuscular junction disorders (e.g., myasthenia gravis, Lambert-Eaton syndrome)

Strengths

- Noninvasive
- Can narrow the differential diagnosis in order to more efficiently direct other forms of testing

Limitations

- Nerve conduction studies are useful in evaluating large fiber neuropathies. Other modalities may be necessary to define small fiber neuropathies:
  - —Quantitative sensory testing (QST)
  - —Autonomic reflex testing
  - —Skin biopsy
- Evaluation of proximal nerves is technically difficult and less reliable.
- Timing of evaluation is important.
  - —In Guillain-Barré syndrome (GBS), findings may be minimal for 7 to 10 days.
  - —In axonal injuries, nerve conduction studies may be normal for 10 to 14 days.
  - —In long-standing and/or severe neuropathies, nerve responses may be unevokable.
- Etiology cannot be determined by electrodiagnostic testing.

Risks

- Equipment must be properly grounded to avoid electrical injury to the patient.
- Patients must be properly grounded.
- Extra care should be taken with patients with indwelling cardiac catheters.
- Care should be taken when performing needle EMG on patients with bleeding diatheses or coagulopathies. Deep muscles where local pressure cannot be applied should be avoided.

Contraindications

- EMG in patients with platelets counts below 20,000 should be avoided or limited as much as possible.
- Needle EMG may interfere with histologic findings in a muscle biopsy. Avoid placing a needle in a muscle that will be biopsied.
- Needle EMG may artificially elevate the serum CK. Obtain blood samples prior to EMG.

Preparation/Special Instructions for Patients

- Inform the physician of any medications that thin blood or increase bleeding times.
- Wear loose fitting clothing.
- Do not apply lotions or creams to skin on day of test.
- If the patient is referred for evaluation of a neuromuscular junction disorder (e.g., myasthenia gravis), hold pyridostigmine (Mestinon) for 12 hours before the test.

Miscellaneous

If patient has excessive anxiety regarding this test, administration of a benzodiazepine (diazepam 10 mg) before the test is acceptable

REFERENCES

- Brown W, Bolton C, eds. Clinical electromyography. Boston: Butterworth-Heinemann, 1993.
- Daube J, eds. Clinical neurophysiology. Philadelphia: F. A. Davis, 1996.
- Kimura J, eds. Electrodiagnosis in diseases of nerve and muscle: principles and practice. Philadelphia: F. A. Davis, 2001.

Author(s): Miriam L. Freimer, MD

Description of Procedure

- Doppler ultrasonography is a noninvasive method of examining the extracranial arteries supplying the brain that relies on the Doppler effect to generate audio signals and frequency spectrum. Three measurements used to diagnose internal carotid artery stenosis are peak systolic velocity, end diastolic velocity, and the ratio of peak systolic velocity in the internal carotid artery to that in the ipsilateral middle to distal common carotid artery. The peak systolic velocity is the most accurate and reproducible Doppler parameter measured and is therefore the most commonly reported. Stenosis results are reported as 0–15%, 16–49%, 50–79%, 80–99%, or occlusion. The frequency spectrum and waveform appearance of the internal, external, and common carotid arteries are different and distinguishable.
- Continuous-wave Doppler systems are instruments with two transducers that continuously emit and receive ultrasound signals. Pulse wave Dopplers are used in duplex systems in combination with B-mode ultrasonography. A single transducer alternatively emits and then receives ultrasound signals. The method allows distance measurements to be made from the transducer probe to the ultrasound-reflecting source.
- Conventional duplex scanning and color Doppler flow imaging are ultrasonographic techniques that use high-resolution B-mode scanning to generate a gray scale picture of soft tissue structures and vessels. Measurements of percent stenosis or cross-sectional area can be made in sagittal or transverse images, respectively. Color Doppler flow imaging adds color-coded blood flow patterns. Using a defined color scale, the direction and average mean velocity of blood cells moving in a sample volume at a given point in time is assigned a color.
- Gel is used to improve ultrasound conductance, and the transducer probe is moved on the neck from above the clavicle to the angle of the jaw. Several longitudinal planes and the transverse plane are routinely scanned allowing evaluation of the proximal, middle, and distal common carotid arteries, carotid bulb, and proximal internal and external carotid arteries.

Indications

Doppler ultrasonography and B-mode imaging is a noninvasive method to evaluate the extracranial carotid and vertebral arteries in patients with carotid or subclavian bruits, transient ischemic attacks, or stroke as a preangiography screening test to detect carotid stenosis in patients who are carotid endarterectomy candidates.

Strengths

As a noninvasive screen for carotid artery stenosis, ultrasonography is less costly than CT or magnetic resonance angiography. The procedure is well tolerated and can be completed in 20 to 40 minutes. Sonography does not involve the use of contrast agents and has no risks or contraindications. Carotid ultrasound results correlate well with angiographic findings. The sensitivity and specificity of Doppler threshold measurements for detecting stenosis of greater than 50% by angiography is in the 85% to 95% range.

Limitations

The quality of ultrasonographic results is dependent on the experience of the examiner and interpreter as well as the equipment used. Some patients image poorly, and those with large, thick necks may be difficult to study. Depending on the level of the carotid bifurcation relative to the mandible, 3 to 4 cm of the proximal internal or external carotid artery can be studied. With high bifurcations these arteries may not be visualized at all. Examination of the vertebral artery is limited by anatomic accessibility to the origin, proximal pretransverse segment, and intertransverse segments between the third and sixth cervical vertebra and the atlas loop. Frequent arterial caliber variations and asymmetries of the vertebral arteries make correct assessment of stenosis or occlusion difficult.

Risks

Although there are two potential physical effects of ultrasonography related to safety, cavitation, which involves ultrasound-induced production and motion of bubbles in a fluid, and thermal effects from heating of the insinuated medium due to conversion of ultrasound energy, no clinical adverse effects from diagnostic ultrasonography have been reported.

Contraindications

None.

Preparation/Special Instructions for Patients

None.

Miscellaneous

Although some practitioners rely solely on carotid duplex results to make decisions about carotid endarterectomy, concern about the extension of the stenosis into the inaccessible distal internal carotid artery, the possible presence of significant stenosis in the cavernous carotid artery, the coincidental existence of unsuspected intracranial aneurysms, and the presence of intraluminal thrombus beyond the stenosis are deterrents to making decisions to proceed with surgery based on ultrasound results alone.

Several large multiinstitutional studies suggest that Doppler and duplex ultrasonography do not have the high specificities and sensitivities reported by selected individual laboratories. Furthermore the risk of stroke and benefit from carotid endarterectomy correlate with the degree of stenosis determined angiographically. Such a correlation has not been demonstrated with percent stenosis measured by ultrasonography. For these reasons most practitioners use ultrasonography as a screening tool to exclude patients with no carotid artery stenosis from further testing and rely on results from conventional angiography before recommending carotid endarterectomy.

Author(s): Andrew Slivka, MD

SECTION III

Neurologic Diseases and Disorders

Acquired Immunodeficiency Syndrome: Neurologic Complications

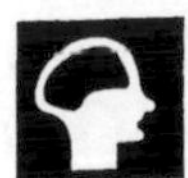

Basics

DESCRIPTION

Neurologic complications are common in patients with HIV infection and AIDS, affecting all levels of the central and peripheral nervous system. The etiology of these disorders is variable and may result from direct effects of HIV infection, damage from inflammatory processes and cytokine production, neoplasms, opportunistic infections, metabolic abnormalities, vascular damage, and toxic effects of HIV therapy.

EPIDEMIOLOGY

Incidence/Prevalence

Exact incidence/prevalence figures are not available. Before highly active antiretroviral therapy (HAART), it was estimated that 10% of AIDS patients presented with a neurologic complaint, while 30% to 50% developed neurologic complications during their disease. The incidence of HIV dementia was estimated to be 7.5% to 20% in retrospective studies. More recently, the incidence of neurologic complications appears to be decreasing, likely due to widespread use of HAART.

Race

All races affected; most common in Caucasians and blacks.

Age

Any age can be affected; most common 20 to 40 years of age.

Sex

Both sexes can be affected; most often diagnosed in males.

ETIOLOGY

- The etiology is variable and depends on the specific process involving the nervous system. In severely immunocompromised patients, opportunistic infections and neoplasms can involve the central or peripheral nervous system, including toxoplasmosis, cryptococcal and tuberculous meningitis, neurosyphilis, progressive multifocal leukoencephalopathy (PML; papovavirus), cytomegalovirus (CMV), herpes simplex virus, and primary CNS lymphoma (PCNSL).
- HIV is neurotropic and can be cultured early from the nervous system. However, productive infection within neural tissues does not appear to be the major cause of HIV dementia, vacuolar myelopathy, myopathy, or peripheral neuropathy. Although HIV does shed toxic substances such as gp 120, viral initiation of inflammation and secretion of toxic cytokines (e.g., tumor necrosis factor-α, interleukins 1β and 6) may be more critical in mediating neural tissue injury.
- Neurologic complications can also develop as a result of treatment with antiretroviral therapy (e.g., zidovudine myopathy).

Genetics

Genetic factors have not been identified.

RISK FACTORS

No specific risk factors have been identified other than diagnosis of HIV infection, low CD4 counts (i.e., less than 100/μL), and lack of antiretroviral therapy.

PREGNANCY

Pregnancy has not been shown to affect the neurologic complications of HIV.

ASSOCIATED CONDITIONS

N/A

Diagnosis

DIFFERENTIAL DIAGNOSIS

The differential diagnosis is extensive and includes any non–HIV-related disease with a similar presentation affecting the nervous system. See Dementia, Focal Brain Lesions, and neuromuscular topics for a more detailed differential diagnosis.

SIGNS AND SYMPTOMS

- HIV dementia (i.e., AIDS dementia complex) usually manifests with progressive impairment of short-term memory, cognition, concentration, and motivation. Associated motor abnormalities include unsteady gait, leg weakness, tremor, and incoordination. Late-stage patients have global dementia with severe psychomotor slowing, confusion, reduced verbal output, weakness, and spasticity.
- Space-occupying lesions include cerebral toxoplasmosis, PCNSL, PML, tuberculous or fungal abscess, focal viral encephalitis, and metastatic tumors (e.g., lymphoma or Kaposi's sarcoma). Symptoms consist of progressive headache, confusion, lethargy, personality changes, memory loss, seizures, nausea/emesis, and focal deficits (e.g., hemiparesis, dysphasia).
- Encephalitis typically develops from toxoplasmosis, CMV, and herpes simplex virus, while meningitis is most frequently caused by cryptococcus and other fungi, tuberculosis, and leptomeningeal lymphoma. HIV can cause an aseptic meningitis syndrome. Encephalitic patients present with acute confusion, lethargy, seizures, fever, headache, and meningismus. Patients with meningitis develop subacute headache, fever, meningismus, lethargy, and nausea.
- Vacuolar myelopathy usually develops as part of HIV dementia, but can occur in isolation. It presents as a progressive myelopathy with spastic paraparesis, hyperactive reflexes, Babinski's signs, gait ataxia, tremor, and urinary incontinence. In some patients, a sensory level may be appreciated.
- Neuromuscular complications present as polyradiculopathy, neuropathy, or myopathy. Polyradiculopathy (usually caused by CMV) is characterized by a painful, subacute, progressive loss of strength and reflexes that ascends from lower to upper extremities. Most of the neuropathies cause a progressive mixture of motor and sensory loss in the extremities, accompanied by reduced or absent distal reflexes. The acute inflammatory demyelinating polyneuropathy type is clinically similar to Guillain-Barré syndrome. Autonomic neuropathy causes orthostatic dizziness, fainting, impotence, diarrhea, and urinary dysfunction. Myopathies all cause slowly progressive, painless, proximal extremity weakness.

LABORATORY PROCEDURES

In general, the most important tests consist of blood counts (including CD4 counts, to determine stage of HIV infection), infectious cultures of appropriate tissues, and serum antibody titers of various infectious agents. Other specific tests may be helpful in certain cases, such as VDRL or vitamin B_{12} levels.

IMAGING STUDIES

Magnetic resonance imaging (MRI), with and without gadolinium, is the most sensitive technique to evaluate HIV patients with cranial or spinal neurologic complaints. HIV dementia may demonstrate atrophy or scattered, nonenhancing, white matter lesions. Similarly, PML presents with patchy, nonenhancing, periventricular white matter lesions that slowly enlarge and coalesce. Cerebral toxoplasmosis usually demonstrates multiple ring enhancing lesions with surrounding edema. PCNSL presents as a solitary or multifocal lesion within the deep periventricular white matter that typically enhances with contrast. Mild edema and/or mass effect may be noted. Tuberculous or fungal abscesses cause ring-enhancing lesions with surrounding edema. Focal viral encephalitis (e.g., CMV, varicella-zoster virus, herpes simplex virus) may produce mass lesions with minimal enhancement. Other potential enhancing mass lesions include metastatic systemic lymphoma and Kaposi's sarcoma.

SPECIAL TESTS

Lumbar puncture is often helpful to differentiate the etiology of brain or spinal processes, and should at least include routine CSF studies, bacterial/fungal antigens, cytology, CSF bacterial/viral/fungal cultures, smear and culture for acid-fast bacilli, and VDRL. Other tests that may be helpful in selected patients include electroencephalography (i.e., seizure activity), electromyography and nerve conduction studies (i.e., neuropathy and myopathy), and neuropsychological testing (i.e., HIV dementia).

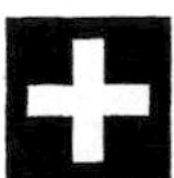

Management

GENERAL MEASURES

Antiretroviral therapy should be maximized, if possible (i.e., HAART). HAART consists of a combination of two nucleoside reverse transcriptase inhibitors (e.g., zidovudine, didanosine, abacavir) and at least one protease inhibitor (e.g., saquinavir, indinavir), and/or one nonnucleoside reverse transcriptase inhibitor (e.g., nevirapine, delavirdine). Nutritional and metabolic deficiencies should be corrected, especially those that might impact on neurologic function. All systemic infections should be diagnosed and treated. Medications should be reviewed for potential central or peripheral neurotoxicity.

SURGICAL MEASURES

Biopsy may be required to differentiate focal intracranial lesions. Less often, biopsy may be helpful to diagnose the cause of neuropathy or myopathy.

SYMPTOMATIC TREATMENT

Patients with HIV dementia may stabilize or improve slightly on antiretroviral therapy (zidovudine or HAART). Cerebral toxoplasmosis usually responds to combination therapy with pyrimethamine (50–75 mg/d), sulfadiazine (100 mg/d), and leucovorin (10 mg/d). Patients with PCNSL should receive whole brain irradiation (4,000–5,000 cGy), although chemotherapy can be beneficial in selected patients with good performance status. Infectious neurologic complications require therapy specific to the agent involved. The acute and chronic forms of demyelinating polyneuropathy may respond to plasmapheresis or IVIG. Inflammatory myopathy secondary to HIV may respond to corticosteroids. Painful neuropathic symptoms often improve with tricyclic antidepressants or anticonvulsants. There are no proven beneficial therapies for PML.

ADJUNCTIVE TREATMENTS

N/A

ADMISSION/DISCHARGE CRITERIA

Patients are generally admitted for acute neurologic changes such as altered level of consciousness, confusion, focal or generalized weakness, seizure activity, headache, and focal neurologic deficits. Patients with persistent neurologic deficits should be considered for rehabilitation.

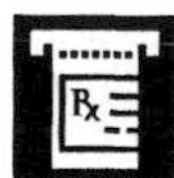

Medications

DRUG(S) OF CHOICE

All patients should be evaluated for HAART, since this may prevent or abrogate the direct effects of HIV on the nervous system. In addition, HAART may prevent or reduce the risk of opportunistic infectious and neoplastic complications. All other drug decisions have to be individualized to the specific neurologic complication of each patient.

ALTERNATIVE DRUGS

N/A

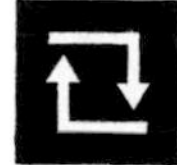

Follow-Up

PATIENT MONITORING

Follow-up of neurologic status is required. This is particularly true for some of the infectious complications that need long-term therapy (e.g., toxoplasmosis, CMV).

EXPECTED COURSE AND PROGNOSIS

The course and prognosis for many of the neurologic complications mentioned above is quite poor, since most occur in patients with low CD4 counts and advanced disease. The 6-month cumulative mortality rate for stage 2 to 4 HIV dementia is 67%. Similar 6-month cumulative mortality rates are noted for PML (85%), PCNSL (70%), and cerebral toxoplasmosis (51%). Some infectious complications caused by specific agents may respond to appropriate therapy, such as CMV encephalitis and neurosyphilis.

PATIENT EDUCATION

AIDS Daily Summary: *www.cdcnpin.org.*
AIDS Education Global Information System: *www.aegis.com.*
AIDS Treatment Data Network: *www.aidsnvc.org.*
Centers for Disease Control (CDC) AIDS Information: *www.cdcnpin.org.*
National Association of People with AIDS: *www.rainbow.net.au/~napwa/.*
National AIDS Treatment Advocacy Project: *www.natap.org.*

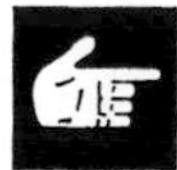

Miscellaneous

SYNONYMS

N/A

ICD-9-CM: 331.9 Cerebral degeneration, unspecified (HIV dementia); 322.9 Meningitis, cause unspecified; 321.0 Cryptococcal meningitis; 323.9 Encephalitis, cause unspecified; 336.9 Myelopathy, unspecified; 046.3 Progressive multifocal leukoencephalopathy; 191.9 Malignant neoplasm of brain, unspecified (PCNSL); 357.9 Polyneuropathy, unspecified; 359.9 Myopathy, unspecified

SEE ALSO: ACQUIRED IMMUNODEFICIENCY SYNDROME: DEMENTIA, HIV; ACQUIRED IMMUNODEFICIENCY SYNDROME: NEUROMUSCULAR COMPLICATIONS; ACQUIRED IMMUNODEFICIENCY SYNDROME: FOCAL BRAIN LESIONS

REFERENCES

- Antinori A, Ammassari A, De Luca A, et al. Diagnosis of AIDS-related focal brain lesions: a decision-making analysis based on clinical and neuroradiologic characteristics combined with polymerase chain reaction assays in CSF. Neurology 197;48: 687–694.
- Atwood WJ, Berger JR, Kaderman R, et al. Human immunodeficiency virus type 1 infection of the brain. Clin Microbiol Rev 1993;6:339–366.
- Clumeck H, De Wit S. Update on highly active antiretroviral therapy: progress and strategies. Biomed Pharmacother 2000; 54:7–12.
- Epstein LG, Gendelman HE. Human immunodeficiency virus type 1 infection of the nervous system: pathogenetic mechanisms. Ann Neurol 1993;33:429–436.
- Lipton SA, Gendelman HE. Dementia associated with the acquired immunodeficiency syndrome. N Engl J Med 1995;332:934–940.
- Newton HB. Common neurologic complications of HIV-1 infection and AIDS. Am Fam Physician 1995;51:387–398.
- Sharer LR. Pathology of HIV-1 infection of the central nervous system. A review. J Neuropathol Exp Neurol 1992;51:3–11.
- Simpson DM, Tagliati M. Neurologic manifestations of HIV infection. Ann Intern Med 1994;121:769–785.

Author(s): Herbert B. Newton, MD

Acquired Immunodeficiency Syndrome: Dementia, HIV

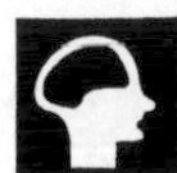

Basics

DESCRIPTION

HIV dementia (i.e., AIDS dementia complex, HIV encephalopathy, HIV-1–associated cognitive/motor complex) is a syndrome of progressive deterioration of memory, cognition, behavior, and motor function in HIV-infected individuals during the late stages of the disease, when immunodeficiency is severe.

EPIDEMIOLOGY

Incidence/Prevalence

Exact incidence and prevalence figures are not available. HIV dementia is the most common neurologic complication of HIV infection and is estimated to have an overall incidence of 7.5% to 20% in retrospective studies. The incidence varies with CD4 counts: 7.3 cases/100 person-years with CD4 counts less than 100, 3.0 cases/100 person-years with CD4 counts between 101 to 200, 1.5 cases/100 person-years with CD4 counts between 201 and 500, and 0.5 cases/100 person-years with CD4 counts above 500. More recently, the incidence appears to be decreasing, most likely due to widespread use of highly active antiretroviral therapy (HAART).

Race

All races affected; most common in Caucasians and blacks.

Age

Any age can be affected; most common 20 to 40 years of age.

Sex

Both sexes can be affected; most often diagnosed in males.

ETIOLOGY

Neuropathologic evaluation of patients with HIV dementia often reveals cortical atrophy and ventricular dilatation, as well as abnormalities of deep structures including the hemispheric white matter, basal ganglia, and thalamus, consistent with a subcortical dementing process. Histologically, there is diffuse white-matter pallor and vacuolation, astrocytic gliosis, and cortical neuronal loss. Regions of HIV encephalitis contain multiple foci of multinucleated giant cells, foamy macrophages, lymphocytes, and microglia. The characteristic histologic findings of vacuolar myelopathy consist of spongiform (vacuolar) changes of the dorsal and lateral columns, in association with lipid-filled macrophages.

HIV is neurotropic and can be cultured early from the nervous system. However, productive infection within neurons or astrocytes does not appear to be the major cause of HIV dementia or vacuolar myelopathy. Brain macrophages (i.e., microglia) can develop productive HIV infection and are the major vehicle for introducing the virus into the nervous system. Recent hypotheses suggest that neural injury and dysfunction may be due to an innocent-bystander effect. HIV does shed toxic substances, such as whole or fragmented gp 120 envelope glycoprotein, which can cause neuronal death *in vitro*. In addition, other neurotoxic substances can be released in areas of productive infection and cause injury to neurons and astrocytes, such as tumor necrosis factor-α, interleukin-1β, interleukin-6, and quinolinic acid. The proposed "final common pathway" of neurotoxicity is excessive stimulation of *N*-methyl-D-aspartate (NMDA) receptors. Overstimulation of NMDA receptors by gp 120, quinolinic acid, and other substances could cause toxic buildup of intracellular calcium, thereby killing neuronal cells.

Genetics

Genetic factors have not been identified.

RISK FACTORS

No specific risk factors have been identified other than diagnosis of HIV infection, low CD4 counts (i.e., less than 200/μL) and an advanced stage of disease, and lack of antiretroviral therapy.

PREGNANCY

Pregnancy has not been shown to affect the course of HIV dementia.

ASSOCIATED CONDITIONS

Vacuolar myelopathy.

Diagnosis

DIFFERENTIAL DIAGNOSIS

The differential diagnosis includes HIV-related and non–HIV-related diseases that can lead to deterioration of memory and cognition. HIV-related diseases to consider include progressive multifocal leukoencephalopathy (PML), cerebral toxoplasmosis, primary CNS lymphoma (PCNSL), bacterial or fungal abscess, and various toxic/metabolic encephalopathies. See chapter on Dementia and AIDS: Focal Brain Lesions.

SIGNS AND SYMPTOMS

Patients with HIV dementia demonstrate progressive dysfunction of memory, cognition, behavior, and motor function. During early stages of disease (stages 0.5, 1, and 2), patients note difficulty with concentration, mild memory impairment, loss of mental agility, behavioral changes, and slowness of thinking. Mild motor dysfunction may occur, affecting strength, gait, balance, and coordination. The neurologic examination often reveals subtle psychomotor slowing, mild memory deficits, reduced concentration, saccadic ocular pursuit movements, and soft motor signs (e.g., mild leg weakness, hyperreflexia, slowed rapid alternating movements, unsteady gait, tremor, frontal lobe release reflexes).

In advanced stages of HIV dementia (stages 3 and 4), patients develop progressively more severe neurologic dysfunction with pronounced psychomotor slowing, reduced verbal output, apathy, confusion, disorientation, disinhibition, and reduced awareness of illness. Smooth-pursuit ocular movements become very saccadic, and frontal lobe release reflexes are common. Motor dysfunction becomes profound and may include ataxia, severe leg weakness and spasticity, hyperreflexia, Babinski's signs, tremor, myoclonus, and bowel and bladder incontinence.

Vacuolar myelopathy usually develops as part of the motor component of HIV dementia, but can occur in isolation. It is clinically similar to subacute combined degeneration (i.e., vitamin B_{12} deficiency) and presents as a progressive myelopathy with spastic paraparesis, hyperactive reflexes, Babinski's signs, gait ataxia, tremor, and urinary incontinence. In some patients, a sensory level may be appreciated.

LABORATORY PROCEDURES

In general, HIV dementia is a diagnosis of exclusion after other infections, space-occupying lesions, and processes are ruled out. The most important tests consist of blood counts (including CD4 counts, to determine stage of HIV infection), infectious cultures of appropriate tissues, and serum antibody titers of various infectious agents. Other specific tests may be helpful in certain cases, such as VDRL or vitamin B_{12} levels.

IMAGING STUDIES

MRI, with and without administration of gadolinium, is the most sensitive technique to evaluate HIV patients with loss of memory and intellectual function. HIV dementia may demonstrate atrophy or scattered, nonenhancing, white matter lesions, as well as ventricular enlargement. Similarly, PML presents with patchy, nonenhancing, periventricular white matter lesions that slowly enlarge and coalesce. Cerebral toxoplasmosis usually demonstrates multiple ring enhancing lesions with surrounding edema. PCNSL presents as a solitary or multifocal lesion within the deep periventricular white matter that typically enhances with contrast. Mild edema and/or mass effect may be noted. Tuberculous or fungal abscesses cause ring-enhancing lesions with surrounding edema.

SPECIAL TESTS

Lumbar puncture is often helpful and should at least include routine CSF studies, bacterial/fungal antigens, cytology, CSF bacterial/viral/fungal cultures, smear and culture for acid-fast bacilli, and VDRL. In addition, surrogate markers of immune activation should be ordered, such as β_2-microglobulin, quinolinic acid, and neopterin. EEG can rule out subclinical seizure activity as a cause for cognitive deterioration. Neuropsychological testing can establish a pattern of memory loss and cognitive dysfunction, and provide a baseline for subsequent follow-up testing.

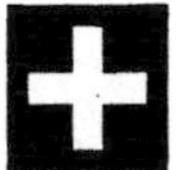

Management

GENERAL MEASURES

Antiretroviral therapy should be maximized, if possible (i.e., zidovudine, HAART). Nutritional and metabolic deficiencies should be corrected, especially those that might impact on neurologic function (e.g., hyponatremia). All systemic infections should be diagnosed and treated.

SURGICAL MEASURES

Biopsy may be required in rare cases to differentiate HIV dementia from other focal intracranial processes.

SYMPTOMATIC TREATMENT

Patients with HIV dementia may stabilize or improve slightly on antiretroviral therapy (zidovudine or HAART). Muscle relaxants such as baclofen may be helpful to reduce spasticity and muscle spasms in patients with advanced motor complications.

ADJUNCTIVE TREATMENT

N/A

ADMISSION/DISCHARGE CRITERIA

Patients are generally admitted for acute neurologic changes such as altered level of consciousness, confusion, focal or generalized weakness, seizure activity, headache, and focal neurologic deficits (e.g., dysphasia, hemianopsia). Patients with persistent neurologic deficits should be considered for rehabilitation.

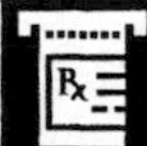

Medications

DRUG(S) OF CHOICE

All patients should be evaluated for zidovudine or HAART, since this may delay the onset or reduce the severity of HIV dementia. HAART usually consists of a combination of two nucleoside reverse transcriptase inhibitors (e.g., zidovudine, didanosine, lamivudine) plus one protease inhibitor (e.g., indinavir, saquinavir). Several randomized, placebo-controlled trials have shown benefit of single-agent zidovudine (1,000 or 2,000 mg/d) for delaying the onset of HIV dementia, or improving neuropsychological test performance in affected patients. More recently, a study by Chang et al. demonstrated that treatment with HAART can induce an improvement in clinical grading of HIV dementia, as well as reduce brain metabolite abnormalities as shown by magnetic resonance spectroscopy. In addition, HAART may prevent or reduce the risk of opportunistic infectious and neoplastic complications.

ALTERNATIVE DRUGS

Nimodipine (calcium channel blocker) was evaluated in a placebo-controlled clinical trial. Although the results did show a trend toward an effect for nimodipine, it was not statistically significant. Similar results have been noted in clinical trials of deprenyl (monoamine oxidase B inhibitor and antiapoptotic agent) and lexipafant (platelet-activating factor inhibitor). A new promising agent is memantine, which blocks ion channels associated with NMDA receptors and inhibits gp 120–associated neuronal injury *in vitro*. Clinical trials using memantine in patients with HIV dementia are currently ongoing.

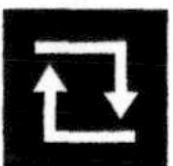

Follow-Up

PATIENT MONITORING

Follow-up of neurologic status is required, especially as patients enter more advanced stages of HIV dementia.

EXPECTED COURSE AND PROGNOSIS

The course and prognosis for HIV dementia is quite poor, since it occurs in patients with low CD4 counts and advanced disease. The 6-month cumulative mortality rate for stages 2 to 4 of HIV dementia is 67%. However, the number of patients developing late-stage HIV dementia appears to be slowing with widespread use of HAART.

PATIENT EDUCATION

AIDS Daily Summary: *www.cdcnpin.org.*
AIDS Education Global Information System: *www.aegis.com.*
AIDS Treatment Data Network: *www.aidsnvc.org.*
Centers for Disease Control (CDC) AIDS Information: *www.cdcnpin.org.*
National Association of People with AIDS: *www.rainbow.net.au/~napwa/.*
National AIDS Treatment Advocacy Project: *www.natap.org.*
International Association of Physicians in AIDS Care: *www.iapac.org.*

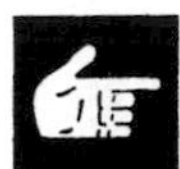

Miscellaneous

SYNONYMS

N/A

ICD-9-CM: 331.9 Cerebral degeneration, unspecified (HIV dementia); 336.9 Myelopathy, unspecified

SEE ALSO: ACQUIRED IMMUNODEFICIENCY SYNDROME: NEUROLOGIC COMPLICATIONS; ACQUIRED IMMUNODEFICIENCY SYNDROME: NEUROMUSCULAR COMPLICATIONS; ACQUIRED IMMUNODEFICIENCY SYNDROME: FOCAL BRAIN LESIONS

REFERENCES

- Atwood WJ, Berger JR, Kaderman R, et al. Human immunodeficiency virus type 1 infection of the brain. Clin Microbiol Rev 1993;6:339–366.
- Chang L, Ernst T, Leonido-Yee M, et al. Highly active antiretroviral therapy reverses brain metabolite abnormalities in mild HIV dementia. Neurology 1999;53:782–789.
- Clifford DB. Human immunodeficiency virus-associated dementia. Arch Neurol 2000;57:321–324.
- Epstein LG, Gendelman HE. Human immunodeficiency virus type 1 infection of the nervous system: pathogenetic mechanisms. Ann Neurol 1993;33:429–436.
- Lipton SA, Gendelman HE. Dementia associated with the acquired immunodeficiency syndrome. N Engl J Med 1995;332:934–940.
- Newton HB. Common neurologic complications of HIV-1 infection and AIDS. Am Fam Physician 1995;51:387–398.
- Sharer LR. Pathology of HIV-1 infection of the central nervous system. A review. J Neuropathol Exp Neurol 1992;51:3–11.
- Simpson DM, Tagliati M. Neurologic manifestations of HIV infection. Ann Intern Med 1994;121:769–785.

Author(s): Herbert B. Newton, MD

Acquired Immunodeficiency Syndrome: Focal Brain Lesions

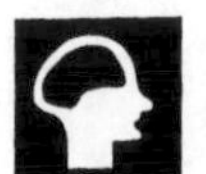

Basics

DESCRIPTION

CNS complications are frequent in patients with HIV infection and often manifest as enhancing or nonenhancing focal lesions of the brain. The most common focal brain lesions in HIV-infected patients are cerebral toxoplasmosis, primary CNS lymphoma (PCNSL), and progressive multifocal leukoencephalopathy (PML). Although the etiology of the focal lesion may vary, the various clinical presentations are often very similar, with signs and symptoms of elevated intracranial pressure, alterations of memory and cognition, and focal neurologic deficits.
If patients don't respond to an empiric trial of antitoxoplasmosis therapy, surgical biopsy is required for a definitive histologic diagnosis.

EPIDEMIOLOGY

Incidence/Prevalence

Exact incidence and prevalence figures are not available. Recent estimates suggest an overall incidence of intracranial mass lesions in roughly 10% of HIV-infected individuals. Cerebral toxoplasmosis occurs in approximately 5% to 12% of all AIDS patients. Primary CNS lymphoma is noted in 3% to 5% of all AIDS patients; the incidence of PCNSL may be increasing.
PML occurs in 2% to 4% of all AIDS patients.
HIV dementia is estimated to have an incidence of 7.5% to 20% in retrospective studies.
The overall incidence of focal brain lesions may be decreasing due to widespread use of highly active antiretroviral therapy (HAART).
Neuroimaging and autopsy studies demonstrate that cerebral toxoplasmosis accounts for 50% to 60% of all intracranial mass lesions, while another 20% to 30% are caused by PCNSL and 10% to 20% arise from PML.

Race

All races affected; most common in Caucasians and blacks.

Age

Any age can be affected; most common 20 to 40 years of age.

Sex

Both sexes can be affected; most often diagnosed in males.

ETIOLOGY

Intracranial mass lesions usually develop in end-stage AIDS patients with CD4 counts below 200/μL. In rare patients, mass lesions can be the presenting manifestation of HIV infection. Cerebral toxoplasmosis is caused by reactivation of an endogenous infection by *Toxoplasma gondii,* an obligate intracellular parasite. The parasite usually reaches the brain by hematogenous spread from infected systemic organs. Pathologically, the abscesses demonstrate regions of necrosis with mild inflammation and *Toxoplasma* cysts, endarteritis, lipid-laden macrophages, extracellular tachyzoites, and encysted bradyzoites.
Primary CNS lymphoma develops from neoplastic lymphocytes (usually B cells). Epstein-Barr virus DNA is present in many of the tumors. Pathologically, the tumors show densely packed neoplastic lymphocytes with diffuse infiltration into surrounding brain, regions of necrosis, and a tendency to spread along perivascular spaces.
PML is caused by reactivation of the JC papovavirus. Once reactivated, the JC virus infects oligodendrocytes, causing progressive demyelination throughout the subcortical and periventricular white matter, cerebellum, and brainstem. Histologically, swelling and degeneration of oligodendrocytes are noted, with minimal inflammation. Viral inclusion bodies may be present within infected cells.
Less common causes of intracranial mass lesions include abscess from other parasites (cysticercosis), fungi (*Cryptococcus neoformans*), and bacteria (*Mycobacterium tuberculosis*); focal viral infections (e.g., cytomegalovirus, herpes simplex virus); gliomas; metastatic brain tumors (e.g., Kaposi's sarcoma, systemic lymphoma); and cerebrovascular disease.
For a detailed discussion of the etiology of AIDS HIV dementia, see that specific chapter.

Genetics

Genetic factors have not been identified.

RISK FACTORS

No specific risk factors have been identified other than diagnosis of HIV infection, low CD4 counts (i.e., less than 200/μL) and advanced stage of disease, and lack of antiretroviral therapy.

PREGNANCY

Pregnancy has not been shown to affect the course of focal brain lesions in HIV patients.

ASSOCIATED CONDITIONS

N/A

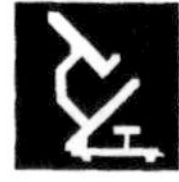

Diagnosis

DIFFERENTIAL DIAGNOSIS

The differential diagnosis is extensive and includes any non-HIV-related diseases that can present as a focal lesion within the brain. See chapters on Brain Tumors, Primary; Brain Tumor, Metastatic; and brain abscess for a more detailed differential diagnosis.

SIGNS AND SYMPTOMS

The temporal profile of cerebral toxoplasmosis is more acute than either PCNSL or PML, with symptoms evolving over several days to a week. The initial symptoms are typically headache and confusion, which develop in over half of all patients. Other frequent symptoms include lethargy, low-grade fever, seizures, and focal neurologic deficits (e.g., hemiparesis, dysphasia, ataxic gait, hemianopsia, sensory loss).
Patients with PCNSL usually develop symptoms that evolve over 1 week to several weeks. The most common symptoms are headache, confusion, lethargy, personality changes, seizures, and memory loss. Focal neurologic signs and symptoms are frequent and similar to that noted above. Fever and other constitutional symptoms are generally absent.
PML is the most indolent of the common focal intracranial lesions and evolves over several weeks or more. Signs and symptoms of elevated intracranial pressure, fever, and constitutional symptoms are absent. Patients complain of slowly progressive deterioration of memory and higher cognitive functions, as well as focal neurologic deficits as listed above.
HIV dementia causes progressive impairment of short-term memory, cognition, concentration, and motivation. Associated motor abnormalities include unsteady gait, leg weakness, tremor, and incoordination.
Less common causes of focal intracranial mass lesions present in a similar fashion.

LABORATORY PROCEDURES

The most important tests consist of blood counts (including CD4 counts, to determine stage of HIV infection), toxoplasmosis serology, and serum antibody titers of other infectious agents.

IMAGING STUDIES

MRI, with contrast, is the most sensitive technique to evaluate for a focal intracranial mass lesion. Cerebral toxoplasmosis usually demonstrates multiple ring-enhancing lesions with surrounding edema, present in the gray matter of the diencephalon and cortex. PCNSL presents as solitary or multifocal lesions within the deep periventricular white matter that enhance diffusely. Mild edema and/or mass effect may be noted. PML presents with patchy, nonenhancing, white matter lesions that slowly enlarge and coalesce. The lesions often begin adjacent to the cortex (i.e., affect subcortical fibers) and do not cause mass effect or edema. HIV dementia may demonstrate atrophy or scattered, nonenhancing, white matter lesions that usually spare the subcortical fibers. Focal viral encephalitis may produce mass lesions with minimal enhancement.
For patients without access to a MRI facility, cerebral CT is still an excellent alternative, especially with double-dose iodinated contrast.
If available, thallium 201 single photon emission computed tomography (SPECT) or fluorodeoxyglucose positron emission tomography (PET) should be obtained.
A positive result is suspicious for PCNSL.

SPECIAL TESTS

Lumbar puncture may be helpful in selected patients (i.e., those who do not undergo immediate surgical biopsy and are not precluded by excessive intracranial pressure and/or mass effect) to differentiate the etiology of focal brain lesions, and should include at least routine CSF studies, bacterial/fungal antigens, cytology, CSF bacterial/viral/fungal cultures, smear and culture for acid-fast bacilli, and VDRL.

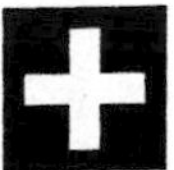

Management

GENERAL MEASURES

Antiretroviral therapy should be maximized, if possible (i.e., HAART). Corticosteroids should be avoided unless brain herniation is suspected.

SURGICAL MEASURES

All large lesions with mass effect and impending herniation require biopsy with decompression. Biopsy is also warranted for patients with positive SPECT or PET studies, those with a single lesion and negative toxoplasma serology, and all patients that have failed an empiric trial of antitoxoplasmosis therapy. Biopsy is accurate for diagnosis in 85% to 90% of cases.

SYMPTOMATIC TREATMENT

All patients, except those listed above, require an empiric trial of antitoxoplasmosis therapy: pyrimethamine (loading dose of 100 to 200 mg, then 25 to 50 mg/d), sulfadiazine (6 to 8 g/d in divided doses), and leucovorin (5 to 10 mg/d). Clinical and radiologic improvement in 10 to 14 days confirms the diagnosis. Patients with PCNSL should receive whole brain irradiation (4,000–5,000 cGy), although chemotherapy (e.g., methotrexate or PCV; procarbazine, CCNU, vincristine) can be beneficial in selected patients with good performance status. Dexamethasone has cytotoxic effects against PCNSL and often reduces tumor size and edema. Although there are no proven beneficial therapies for PML, occasional patients may stabilize or improve with HAART or intravenous cytarabine therapy. HIV dementia may also stabilize or improve slightly on antiretroviral therapy (zidovudine or HAART).

ADJUNCTIVE TREATMENTS

N/A

ADMISSION/DISCHARGE CRITERIA

Patients are admitted for acute neurologic changes related to the focal brain lesion, such as altered level of consciousness, confusion, seizure activity, headache, and focal neurologic deficits. Patients with persistent neurologic deficits should be considered for rehabilitation.

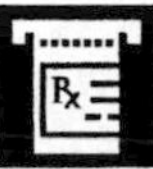

Medications

DRUG(S) OF CHOICE

All patients should be evaluated for HAART, since this may prevent or reduce the risk of opportunistic infectious and neoplastic complications. All other drug decisions have to be individualized to the neurologic complications of each specific focal mass lesion.

ALTERNATIVE DRUGS

N/A

Follow-Up

PATIENT MONITORING

Follow-up of neurologic status is required; particularly for focal lesions that need long-term therapy and serial MRI scans (e.g., PCNSL, toxoplasmosis). Patients with cerebral toxoplasmosis require lifelong maintenance therapy with pyrimethamine (25 to 50 mg/d) and sulfadiazine (2 g/d) to prevent relapses.

EXPECTED COURSE AND PROGNOSIS

The course and prognosis for HIV patients with focal intracranial mass lesions is quite poor, since most occur in patients with advanced disease. However, overall survival may be improving for this group because of the use of HAART. The 6-month cumulative mortality rate for cerebral toxoplasmosis is 51%, although many patients do respond to treatment with improvement of neurologic symptoms and MRI scans. Patients with PCNSL have a median survival of 1 month if untreated and 4 to 6 months following radiation therapy. The median survival for patients with PML is 2 to 4 months. The 6-month cumulative mortality rate for stages 2 to 4 of HIV dementia is 67%. Some focal infectious complications caused by specific agents may respond to appropriate therapy, such as CMV encephalitis.

PATIENT EDUCATION

AIDS Daily Summary: *www.cdcnpin.org.*
AIDS Education Global Information System: *www.aegis.com.*
AIDS Treatment Data Network: *www.aidsnvc.org.*
Centers for Disease Control (CDC) AIDS Information: *www.cdcnpin.org.*
National Association of People with AIDS: *www.rainbow.net.au/~napwa/.*
National AIDS Treatment Advocacy Project: *www.natap.org.*
International Association of Physicians in AIDS Care: *www.iapac.org.*

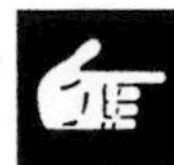

Miscellaneous

SYNONYMS

N/A

ICD-9-CM: 323.9 Encephalitis, cause unspecified; 046.3 Progressive multifocal leukoencephalopathy; 191.9 Malignant neoplasm of brain, unspecified (PCNSL); 331.9 Cerebral degeneration, unspecified (HIV dementia)

SEE ALSO: ACQUIRED IMMUNODEFICIENCY SYNDROME: OVERVIEW OF NEUROLOGIC COMPLICATIONS; ACQUIRED IMMUNODEFICIENCY SYNDROME: DEMENTIA COMPLEX; ACQUIRED IMMUNODEFICIENCY SYNDROME: NEUROMUSCULAR COMPLICATIONS

REFERENCES

- Berger J, Hall C, McArthur J, et al. Evaluation and management of intracranial mass lesions in AIDS. Report of the Quality Standards Subcommittee of the American Academy of Neurology. Neurology 1998;50: 21–26.
- Goldstein JD, Dickson DW, Moser FG, et al. Primary central nervous system lymphoma in acquired immune deficiency syndrome. A clinical and pathologic study with results of treatment with radiation. Cancer 1991;67:2756–2765.
- Holloway RG, Mushlin AI. Intracranial mass lesions in acquired immunodeficiency syndrome: using decision analysis to determine the effectiveness of stereotactic brain biopsy. Neurology 1996;46: 1010–1015.
- Levy RM, Russell E, Yungbluth M, et al. The efficacy of image-guided stereotactic brain biopsy in neurologically symptomatic acquired immunodeficiency syndrome patients. Neurosurgery 1992;30:186–190.
- Porter SB, Sande MA. Toxoplasmosis of the central nervous system in the acquired immunodeficiency syndrome. N Engl J Med 1992;327:1643–1648.
- Whiteman MLH, Post MJD, Berger JR, et al. Progressive multifocal leukoencephalopathy in 47 HIV-seropositive patients: neuroimaging with clinical and pathologic correlation. Radiology 1993;187:233–240.

Author(s): Herbert B. Newton, MD

Acquired Immunodeficiency Syndrome: Neuromuscular Complications

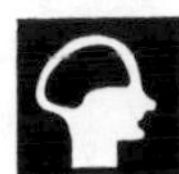

Basics

DESCRIPTION

Neuromuscular complications are common in patients with HIV infection and AIDS, potentially affecting nerve roots, peripheral nerves, and muscles. The etiology of these disorders is variable and may result from direct effects of HIV infection, damage from inflammatory processes and cytokine production, opportunistic infections and neoplasms, metabolic abnormalities, and toxic effects of HIV therapy.

EPIDEMIOLOGY

Incidence/Prevalence

Exact incidence and prevalence figures are not available. Approximately 10% to 40% of patients with HIV-1 and AIDS develop some form of neuromuscular complication. The most common complication is a distal symmetric polyneuropathy (DSP), which is diagnosed in 20% to 30% of patients. Asymptomatic HIV-1–infected patients can also be affected and have an incidence between 2% and 20%, as shown by detailed neurophysiological testing. More recently, the incidence of neuromuscular complications appears to be decreasing, most likely due to widespread use of highly active antiretroviral therapy (HAART).

Race

All races affected; most common in Caucasians and blacks.

Age

Any age can be affected; most common 20 to 40 years of age.

Sex

Both sexes can be affected; most often diagnosed in males.

ETIOLOGY

The etiology is variable and depends on the stage of disease and the specific process involving the peripheral nerves and/or muscles.

In early stages of HIV-1 infection, neuromuscular complications are caused by immune dysregulation. Acute and chronic forms of inflammatory demyelinating polyradiculoneuropathy (AIDP, CIDP) and vasculitic neuropathy are thought to occur by this mechanism. In AIDP and CIDP, an autoimmune process develops that results in damage to peripheral nerve myelin (i.e., myelin antibodies). Vasculitic neuropathy appears to be caused by deposition of HIV-1 antibody/antigen immune complexes into blood vessel walls.

DSP and autonomic neuropathy usually occur in the middle and late stages of HIV-1 infection. Although the etiology of DSP remains unclear, it does not appear to be caused by direct infection of nerves by HIV-1. Instead, nerve damage occurs through indirect means initiated by productive systemic HIV-1 infection. The suspected mediators of this peripheral nerve damage are whole or fragmented gp 120 envelope glycoprotein and cytokines such as tumor necrosis factor-α, interleukin-1β, interleukin-6, transforming growth factor-α, and nitric oxide. Concurrent infections [i.e., cytomegalovirus (CMV)] and malnutrition (e.g., vitamin B_6, vitamin B_{12}) may also contribute to the clinical manifestations of DSP.

During late stages, opportunistic infections and neoplasms can directly involve nerve roots and peripheral nerves. The most common infection is CMV, which can involve the nerve roots (i.e., polyradiculopathy) and/or peripheral nerves (i.e., mononeuropathy multiplex). Other less common infections include herpes zoster ganglionitis, syphilitic radiculopathy, and tuberculous polyradiculopathy. Lymphoma can directly invade nerve roots and cause polyradiculopathy after spreading to the spinal meninges. Infrequently, neuropathies can develop in patients with vitamin B_6 and/or vitamin B_{12} deficiencies.

Toxic neuropathies can arise in a dose-dependent manner from therapy for HIV-1, in particular the antiretroviral dideoxynucleotide analogues didanosine (ddI), zalcitabine (ddC), and stavudine (d4T). The neuropathy may result from damage to cellular mitochondria caused by inhibition of mitochondrial DNA-γ polymerase.

Myopathies can develop as a result of HIV-1 infection or from toxicity of antiretroviral therapy. Productive HIV-1 infection has not been demonstrated in myofibers. Rather, indirect mediators of myofiber damage are suspected, such as gp 120 and inflammatory cytokines. Zidovudine is also implicated as a cause of myopathy and appears to damage myofiber mitochondria, resulting in "ragged-red fibers" and other evidence of dysfunction. The mechanism is through inhibition of mitochondrial DNA-γ polymerase.

Rarely, opportunistic infections can directly involve muscle and present as a myopathy, such as toxoplasmosis or CMV.

Genetics

Genetic factors have not been identified.

RISK FACTORS

No specific risk factors have been identified other than diagnosis of HIV infection, low CD4 counts (i.e., less than 100/μL), and lack of antiretroviral therapy.

PREGNANCY

Pregnancy has not been shown to affect the course of neuromuscular complications of HIV.

ASSOCIATED CONDITIONS

N/A

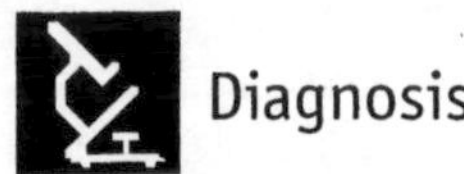

Diagnosis

DIFFERENTIAL DIAGNOSIS

The differential diagnosis is extensive and includes any non–HIV-related disease with a similar presentation affecting the nerve roots, peripheral nerves, or muscles. See chapters on Guillain-Barré Syndrome; Myopathy; and Neuropathy, Peripheral for a more detailed differential diagnosis.

SIGNS AND SYMPTOMS

Patients with DSP usually complain of distal, symmetric numbness, paresthesias, and dysesthesias of the legs and feet that develops over weeks to months; upper extremities can become affected in late stages of disease. Typically, the pain is most severe on the soles of the feet. Light touch and pressure often exacerbate the pain. On examination, most patients have loss of reflexes at the ankles and a distal-to-proximal gradient to pinprick, cold, and vibration; muscle weakness and atrophy is usually mild or absent. Toxic neuropathies from HIV-1 therapy have signs and symptoms similar to DSP.

HIV-1–related AIDP and CIDP have a similar clinical presentation to the idiopathic neuropathies. The patient notes either a rapid (i.e., weeks, for AIDP) or slow (i.e., months, for CIDP) onset of progressive weakness in two or more limbs, generalized areflexia, and mild sensory loss. Muscle atrophy may be noted in patients with long-standing disease.

Patients with autonomic neuropathy complain of fainting, orthostatic dizziness, impotence, diminished sweating, diarrhea, and urinary dysfunction. In addition, cardiac conduction abnormalities may occur.

The various forms of polyradiculopathy present with progressive lower extremity and sacral paresthesias, flaccid paraparesis, areflexia, sensory loss, and urinary dysfunction.

Mononeuropathy multiplex is characterized by multifocal, asymmetric, dysfunction of cutaneous nerves, mixed nerves, and nerve roots that often presents with wrist drop, foot drop, facial palsy, and other focal neuropathic signs. Reflexes are preserved in asymptomatic nerve distributions.

Patients with myopathy complain of slowly progressive, generalized proximal muscle weakness that initially affects activities such as rising from a chair or climbing stairs. Myalgias are noted in 25% to 50% of patients. Reflexes are preserved and sensory function remains intact.

LABORATORY PROCEDURES

The most important tests consist of blood counts (including CD4 counts, to determine stage of HIV infection), infectious cultures of appropriate tissues (e.g., CMV), and serum antibody titers of various infectious agents. Serum creatine kinase levels are moderately elevated (450 to 500 U/L) in patients with myopathy. Other specific tests may be helpful in certain cases, such as VDRL, vitamin B_6, and vitamin B_{12} levels.

IMAGING STUDIES

MRI and CT have limited diagnostic value.

SPECIAL TESTS

Lumbar puncture is often helpful and should at least include routine CSF studies, bacterial/fungal antigens, cytology, CSF bacterial/viral/fungal cultures, smear and culture for acid-fast bacilli, and VDRL. The CSF cell count always demonstrates a pleocytosis (20 to 50 mononuclear cells) in patients with HIV-1-related AIDP and CIDP (usually hypocellular in HIV negative cases). Patients with CMV mononeuropathy multiplex and polyradiculopathy have an elevated CSF protein and mononuclear cell pleocytosis.
Electromyography and nerve conduction testing are helpful for diagnosis. In DSP, the findings are consistent with a distal, symmetrical, sensory more than motor, axonal neuropathy, with evidence for acute and chronic partial denervation and reinnervation of muscles. A similar pattern is seen with toxic neuropathies. AIDP and CIDP demonstrate slowed motor nerve conduction velocities consistent with demyelination, as well as conduction block. Myopathy shows typical myopathic findings of early, polyphasic motor unit potentials, positive sharp waves, and fibrillation potentials.
Autonomic function testing may be helpful to define the presence and extent of autonomic neuropathy.

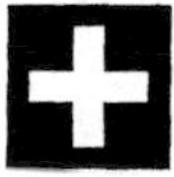

Management

GENERAL MEASURES

Antiretroviral therapy should be maximized, if possible (i.e., HAART). All systemic infections should be diagnosed and treated. Medications that could contribute to a myopathic or neuropathic process (e.g., zidovudine, ddC) should be reviewed and possibly discontinued as a therapeutic trial.

SURGICAL MEASURES

Biopsy of involved nerve roots, peripheral nerves, or muscles may be helpful for definitive diagnosis.

SYMPTOMATIC TREATMENT

Treatment for DSP is symptomatic and consists of a combination of tricyclic antidepressants, selected serotonin reuptake inhibitors, carbamazepine, gabapentin, lamotrigine, and topical agents (i.e., capsaicin).
Toxic neuropathies receive similar treatment to DSP and may improve after cessation of the offending drug. Patients with AIDP and CIDP may respond to plasmapheresis or IVIG, similar to HIV-negative patients. Therapy for autonomic neuropathy consists of fludrocortisone, antiarrhythmic agents, and management of fluids and electrolytes. CMV polyradiculopathy and mononeuropathy multiplex may respond to ganciclovir. HIV myopathy may respond to a course of prednisone (60 mg/d). Zidovudine myopathy should be treated with reduced dosage or cessation of the drug.

ADJUNCTIVE TREATMENTS

N/A

ADMISSION/DISCHARGE CRITERIA

Patients are generally admitted for acute neurologic changes related to the specific neuropathic or myopathic process. The most common causes for admission include focal extremity weakness, generalized weakness, progressive proximal weakness, and exacerbation of extremity pain. Patients with persistent neurologic deficits should be considered for rehabilitation.

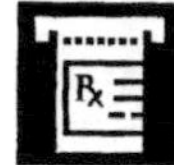

Medications

DRUG(S) OF CHOICE

All patients should be evaluated for HAART, since this may prevent or abrogate the direct and indirect effects of HIV on nerve roots, peripheral nerves, and muscles. In addition, HAART may prevent or reduce the risk of opportunistic infectious and neoplastic neuromuscular complications. All other drug decisions have to be individualized to the specific neuromuscular complication of each patient.

ALTERNATIVE DRUGS

N/A

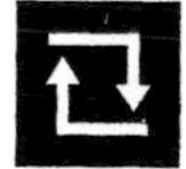

Follow-Up

PATIENT MONITORING

Follow-up of neurologic status is required. This is particularly true for conditions that require long-term therapy, such as distal painful neuropathy or infectious neuromuscular complications (e.g., CMV).

EXPECTED COURSE AND PROGNOSIS

The course and prognosis for many of the neuropathies and myopathies mentioned above is quite poor, since the majority occur in patients with low CD4 counts and advanced disease. However, in some cases treatment may lead to stabilization or improvement. Infectious complications caused by specific agents may respond to appropriate therapy, such as CMV polyradiculopathy or mononeuropathy multiplex, syphilitic radiculopathy, or tuberculous polyradiculopathy. Toxic myopathies and neuropathies may improve if the offending agent is discontinued at an early stage.

PATIENT EDUCATION

AIDS Daily Summary: *www.cdcnpin.org.*
AIDS Education Global Information System: *www.aegis.com.*
AIDS Treatment Data Network: *www.aidsnvc.org.*
Centers for Disease Control (CDC) AIDS Information: *www.cdcnpin.org.*
National Association of People with AIDS: *www.rainbow.net.au/~napwa/.*
National AIDS Treatment Advocacy Project: *www.natap.org.*
International Association of Physicians in AIDS Care: *www.iapac.org.*

Miscellaneous

SYNONYMS

N/A

ICD-9-CM: 357.9 Polyneuropathy, unspecified; 359.9 Myopathy, unspecified

SEE ALSO: ACQUIRED IMMUNODEFICIENCY SYNDROME: OVERVIEW OF NEUROLOGIC COMPLICATIONS; ACQUIRED IMMUNODEFICIENCY SYNDROME: DEMENTIA COMPLICATIONS; ACQUIRED IMMUNODEFICIENCY SYNDROME: FOCAL BRAIN LESIONS

REFERENCES

- Freeman R, Roberts M, Friedman L, et al. Autonomic function and human immunodeficiency virus infection. Neurology 1990; 40:575–580.
- Illa I, Nath A, Dalakas M. Immunocytochemical and virological characteristics of HIV-associated inflammatory myopathies: similarities with seronegative polymyositis. Ann Neurol 1991;29:474–481.
- Mhiri C, Baudrimont M, Bonne G, et al. Zidovudine myopathy: a distinctive disorder associated with mitochondrial dysfunction. Ann Neurol 1991;29:606–614.
- Newton HB. Common neurologic complications of HIV-1 infection and AIDS. Am Fam Physician 1995;51:387–398.
- Simpson DM, Olney RK. Peripheral neuropathies associated with human immunodeficiency virus infection. Neurol Clin 1992;10:685–711.
- Simpson DM, Tagliati M. Neurologic manifestations of HIV infection. Ann Intern Med 1994;121:769–785.
- Verma A, Bradley WG. HIV-1-associated neuropathies. CNS Spectrums 2000;5:66–72.

Author(s): Herbert B. Newton, MD

Alcohol Abuse, Neurologic Complications

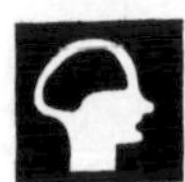

Basics

DESCRIPTION

Alcohol addiction is a major public health problem, accounting for an estimated $117 billion in annual cost in the United States in health expenses and lost productivity. Ethanol-related neurologic complications are diverse and can affect any level of the neuraxis, including brain, spinal cord, cranial and peripheral nerves, and muscle.

EPIDEMIOLOGY

Incidence/Prevalence

In the United States, 7% of adults and 19% of adolescents are considered "problem drinkers"; the estimated prevalence of alcohol abuse and dependence is 7.4% to 12%; ethanol-related deaths exceed 100,000 each year.

Race

All races affected; most common in Caucasians and blacks.

Age

Adults and adolescents can be affected; most commonly diagnosed between 30 to 50 years of age.

Sex

Both sexes can be affected; most often diagnosed in males.

ETIOLOGY

- After ingestion of only 2 oz of 100% ethanol, the blood ethanol level will be 100 mg/dL, requiring 6 hours to be metabolized. Blood ethanol levels of 100 mg/dL and higher result in symptoms of impaired concentration, poor judgment, reduced inhibitions, slurred speech, nystagmus, ataxic gait, and labile mood; levels of 300-400 mg/dL induce stupor and coma.
- Ethanol interacts with nervous system tissues in several ways, including intercalation into cell membranes, increasing membrane fluidity, and perturbing hydrophobic regions of membrane lipids and proteins; ethanol interacts directly with specific neurotransmitter receptors and ion channels in the brain. $GABA_B$ receptors, which regulate potassium and calcium channels, are modulated by ethanol; similarly, it is theorized that ethanol modulates $GABA_A$ receptors by augmenting their response to GABA; excitatory amino acid receptors are also affected by ethanol; ethanol inhibits NMDA-activated Ca^{2+} currents and cellular responses to NMDA receptor activation; chronic ethanol exposure causes increased expression of glutamate receptors, which may contribute to the generation of alcohol withdrawal seizures.
- Chronic alcohol intake leads to poor dietary intake and deficiencies of protein, thiamine, folate, and niacin; in addition, chronic ethanol intake can lead to accumulation of potentially toxic substances (e.g., acetaldehyde).
- Wernicke's encephalopathy results from thiamine deficiency, causing demyelination, necrosis, gliosis, and vascular proliferation in the mammillary bodies, superior vermis, hypothalamic nuclei, and diencephalon. Korsakoff's syndrome is also due to thiamine deficiency, causing lesions of the dorsal medial nuclei of the thalamus. Alcoholic cerebellar degeneration may also be related to thiamine deficiency, in addition to electrolyte derangements and direct neurotoxic effects. Pellagra is caused by niacin deficiency, which induces chromatolysis of neurons in the motor cortex and basal ganglia; alcoholic dementia is multifactorial and can be related to thiamine deficiency, pellagra, hepatocerebral degeneration, Marchiafava-Bignami disease, and direct neurotoxic effects of ethanol; alcoholic polyneuropathy is most likely from nutritional deficiency (thiamine?); alcoholic myopathy is probably due to direct toxic effects of ethanol; the causes of Marchiafava-Bignami disease and central pontine myelinolysis (CPM) remain unknown; CPM usually occurs after overly aggressive correction of hyponatremia, with demyelination of the basis pontis.

Genetics

Alcoholism is seven times more frequent in first-degree relatives of alcoholics than in the general population; 16% to 26% of fathers and 2% to 6% of mothers of alcoholics are alcohol abusers; identical twins have a significantly higher concordance rate for alcoholism than fraternal twins. No consistent genetic locus has been identified.

RISK FACTORS

The risk of developing neurologic complications is related to genetic factors and the duration and severity of the patient's alcoholism.

PREGNANCY

Pregnancy does not affect the course of neurologic complications of alcohol abuse; alcohol abuse during pregnancy may cause the fetal alcohol syndrome (mental retardation, microcephaly, hypotonia, poor coordination, impaired growth, abnormal facies).

ASSOCIATED CONDITIONS

N/A

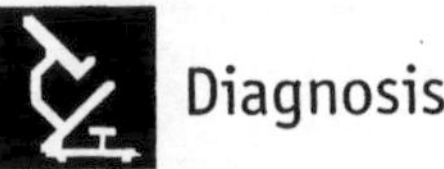

Diagnosis

DIFFERENTIAL DIAGNOSIS

The differential diagnosis is extensive and includes any non-ethanol-related diseases that can have a similar presentation of encephalopathy, seizure activity, dementia, polyneuropathy, myopathy, or cerebellar degeneration.

SIGNS AND SYMPTOMS

- Patients with minor alcohol withdrawal present with tremulousness, insomnia, agitation, flushing, sweating, nausea and emesis, tachypnea, tachycardia, and increased blood pressure. Hallucinations and seizures may also occur; seizures are generally tonic-clonic and occur within 48 hours of abstinence; some patients may progress to delirium tremens, which has similar but more severe symptoms compared to simple withdrawal, as well as fever, delusions, hallucinations, and severe encephalopathy.
- Patients with Wernicke's encephalopathy present with an acute confusional state, ophthalmoplegia, and gait ataxia; ocular findings include nystagmus, unilateral or bilateral lateral rectus palsy, and conjugate gaze palsies; other findings may include hypotension, hypothermia, polyneuropathy, and somnolence; Korsakoff's syndrome often develops after Wernicke's and is characterized by severe anterograde and short-term retrograde amnesia, lack of concern and insight, and confabulation.
- Alcoholic cerebellar degeneration presents with gait ataxia and less severe limb ataxia; symptoms affect the legs more than the arms; dysarthria may occur; usually gradual in onset.
- Alcoholic dementia presents as progressive cognitive decline; in patients without a nutritional or other cause, it is often mild, with anterograde and retrograde memory deficits; on occasion, symptoms can be severe.
- Alcoholic polyneuropathy presents with paresthesias, pain, and weakness of the distal lower extremities; gait may be affected; pain and temperature sensation are reduced; distal atrophy and hyporeflexia are often present.
- Chronic alcoholic myopathy presents with intermittent cramps and painless, progressive proximal weakness of variable severity; atrophy may be present; acute alcoholic myopathy is a necrotizing process, often noted during alcoholic binges, that presents with pain, tenderness, weakness, muscle swelling, myoglobinuria, and cardiac arrhythmias.
- Pellagra presents with an acute confusional state, rigidity, and myoclonus; other signs may include hallucinations, seizures, pyramidal signs, ataxia, and neuropathy.

- Marchiafava-Bignami disease presents with a progressive, subacute confusional state, dementia, seizures, dysarthria, pyramidal signs, and incontinence; stupor and coma may occur.
- CPM presents with acute confusion or coma, spastic paraparesis or quadriparesis, dysarthria, and dysphagia; locked-in syndrome may occur.

LABORATORY PROCEDURES

Patients should be screened for thiamine, niacin, and other vitamin levels, transketolase level, liver panel, ammonia, electrolytes, glucose, renal panel, calcium, and magnesium; ethanol level, toxicology screen, and infectious workup may be of benefit.

IMAGING STUDIES

MRI or CT, with and without contrast, are appropriate in patients with mental status changes, atypical seizures, or focal neurologic findings to rule out intracranial processes.

SPECIAL TESTS

Patients with seizures and/or encephalopathy should undergo lumbar puncture (meningitis?) and an EEG; EMG and nerve conduction testing is helpful for patients with neuropathy and/or myopathy.

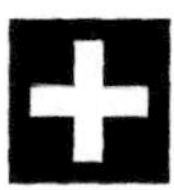

Management

GENERAL MEASURES

Administration of thiamine, niacin, and multivitamins; correction of electrolyte, glucose, and fluid imbalances; hyponatremia should be corrected slowly (i.e., ≤10–12 mmol/L/d); monitoring of heart rhythm; calming environment; seizure precautions; treatment of general medical complications and infections as appropriate.

SURGICAL MEASURES

N/A

SYMPTOMATIC TREATMENT

- Treatment of early alcohol withdrawal consists of oral diazepam (10–40 mg) or chlordiazepoxide (25–100 mg) every 2–4 hours. The addition of atenolol (50 mg qd or bid) or clonidine (0.3 mg bid) may be of benefit. Treatment of delirium tremens consists of intravenous (IV) diazepam (10–40 mg) every 5 to 10 minutes, titrated to clinical effect; maintenance doses of 5–20 mg every 1–4 hours; oral atenolol (50 mg qd or bid) should be considered; hydration, electrolyte replacement, and cooling as needed; withdrawal-related seizures are typically self-limited once treatment has begun; persistent seizures or status epilepticus require IV diazepam or lorazepam and IV phenytoin, similar to non-ethanol-related seizures.
- Wernicke's encephalopathy should be treated with thiamine 100 mg IV, converting to oral therapy at discharge; Korsakoff's syndrome should be treated with thiamine, although it typically does not improve; pellagra responds to multivitamin and niacin (nicotinic acid) replacement; alcoholic polyneuropathy may respond to thiamine and multivitamin replacement.
- There is no specific therapy for alcoholic cerebellar degeneration, it may improve with thiamine and multivitamins; there is no treatment for Marchiafava-Bignami disease or CPM; alcoholic myopathy usually improves with abstinence and supportive care.

ADJUNCTIVE TREATMENT

N/A

ADMISSION/DISCHARGE CRITERIA

Seizure activity, mental status alterations, and focal neurologic deficits are the most common cause for admission; alcohol withdrawal and delirium tremens usually occur after admission and cessation of alcohol intake.
Discharge is appropriate when symptoms of withdrawal, seizures, and other neurologic and medical complications have either stabilized or resolved.

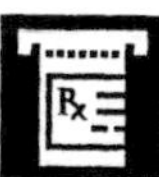

Medications

DRUG(S) OF CHOICE

As above.

ALTERNATIVE DRUGS

N/A

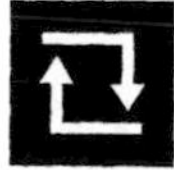

Follow-Up

PATIENT MONITORING

Neurologic follow-up is required; monitoring of abstinence, nutritional status, and compliance with thiamine, multivitamins, and other medications is critical.

EXPECTED COURSE AND PROGNOSIS

The course and prognosis for early alcohol withdrawal is favorable, but becomes more guarded with delirium tremens, due to frequent medical complications. Patients with Wernicke's encephalopathy and Korsakoff's syndrome often have residual neurologic dysfunction (dementia, ataxia). Alcoholic cerebellar degeneration and polyneuropathy usually improve with abstinence and nutritional therapy; recovery from pellagra is excellent with treatment; recovery of myopathy is excellent with abstinence; recovery from Marchiafava-Bignami disease and CPM is poor.

PATIENT EDUCATION

- National Institute on Alcohol Abuse and Alcoholism: *www.niaaa.nih.gov.*
- Medical Council on Alcohol: *www.medicouncilalcol.demon.co.uk.*
- Alcoholism/Treatment: *www.alcoholismtreatment.org.*
- American Council on Alcoholism: *www.nca-usa.org.*
- Alcoholics Anonymous: *www.aa.org.*

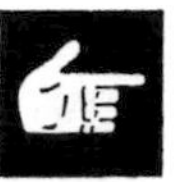

Miscellaneous

SYNONYMS

N/A

ICD-9-CM: 291.0 Alcohol withdrawal delirium; 291.1 Alcohol amnestic syndrome (Korsakoff's, Wernicke-Korsakoff's); 291.2 Other alcoholic dementia; 291.3 Alcohol withdrawal hallucinosis; 303.0; 334.4 Cerebellar ataxia secondary to alcoholism; 357.5 Alcoholic polyneuropathy; 359.9 Myopathy, unspecified

SEE ALSO: ENCEPHALOPATHY, NEUROPATHY, MYOPATHY

REFERENCES

- Brust JCM. Alcoholism. In: Rowland LP, ed. Merritt's neurology, 157:10th ed. Philadelphia: Lippincott Williams & Wilkins, 2000;921–929.
- Charness ME, Simon RP, Greenberg DA. Ethanol and the nervous system. N Engl J Med 1989;321:442–453.
- Greenberg DA. Ethanol and sedatives. Neurol Clin 1993;11:523–534.
- O'Connor PG, Schottenfeld RS. Patients with alcohol problems. N Engl J Med 1998;338:592–602.
- Ragan PW, Singleton CK, Martin PR. Brain injury associated with chronic alcoholism. CNS Spectrums 1999;4:66–87.
- Swift RM. Drug therapy for alcohol dependence. N Engl J Med 1999;340: 1482–1490.

Author(s): Herbert B. Newton, MD

Amnesia, Transient Global

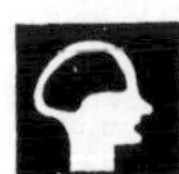

Basics

DESCRIPTION

- Transient global amnesia (TGA), as its name implies, is a self-limited loss of the ability to create new memory. It presents as sudden onset of confusion, best characterized as "bewilderment," on the part of the patient due to the inability to learn new material.

EPIDEMIOLOGY

- Incidence of about 5/100,000 annually
- Usually affects people age >50 years
- No clear sex differences

ETIOLOGY

- No cause of TGA is known. Speculation has revolved around cerebral ischemia, seizure, and migraine; however, it does *not* appear to herald an increased risk for strokes, transient ischemic attacks, or seizures.

RISK FACTORS

- Many TGA patients have a previous history of migraine
- Some studies suggest an increased presence of patent foramen ovale among TGA patients
- Precipitated by Valsalva
  —Exertion
  —Emotional excitement
  —Minor medical procedures (angiography, endoscopy)
  —Cold water

PREGNANCY

N/A

ASSOCIATED CONDITIONS

N/A

Diagnosis

DIFFERENTIAL DIAGNOSIS

- Closed head trauma
  —Concussion
  —Bitemporal cerebral contusions
- Drug effects
  —Benzodiazepines
  —Other sedative/hypnotic agents
  —Alcohol ("blackouts" or delirium tremens)
  —Hallucinogens
- Thiamine deficiency (Wernicke-Korsakoff syndrome) should be considered, especially if there is evidence of ophthalmoparesis or ataxia
  —Thiamine deficiency can occur without alcoholism
- Status epilepticus should be considered in patients with a history of epilepsy
- Encephalitis, especially herpes simplex encephalitis
  —Associated with decreased alertness, headache, or fever
- Psychogenic
  —Psychogenic amnesia produces loss of personal identity ("Who am I?"), but the ability to learn new material is retained. This is in direct contrast to organic amnesia, wherein personal identity is retained, but the patient is unable to learn.

SIGNS AND SYMPTOMS

- Abrupt onset of memory loss, usually including the last few hours, and inability to learn new material
  —Produces bewilderment in the patient who senses something is amiss but cannot recall previous reassurances
  —The patient often will repeatedly ask the same question or perform the same task
- Retained ability to repeat ("immediate memory")
- Retained ability to recall remote memories, including personal identity
- Preserved alertness and other cognitive functions, except for amnesia
- Normal neurologic examination except for amnesia

LABORATORY PROCEDURES

- Consider urine drug screen for benzodiazepines
- There are no laboratory studies for TGA

IMAGING STUDIES

- Consider CT of the head in cases of possible head trauma
- Diffusion-weighted MRI of the brain may show transient abnormalities
- There are no imaging studies for TGA

SPECIAL STUDIES

- Consider EEG for nonconvulsive status epilepticus if the patient has a history of seizures
- There are no special studies for TGA

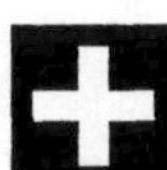

Management

GENERAL MEASURES

- Repeatedly reassure the patient and family of the patient's eventual recovery

SURGICAL MEASURES

N/A

SYMPTOMATIC TREATMENT

N/A

ADJUNCTIVE TREATMENT

N/A

ADMISSION/DISCHARGE CRITERIA

- Patients should be observed until they have sufficient recent memory to return home without undue anxiety

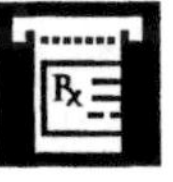

Medications

DRUG OF CHOICE

- Consider thiamine 100 mg IV if any possibility of thiamine deficiency exists
- Benzodiazepines are contraindicated

ALTERNATIVE DRUGS

N/A

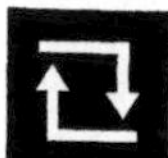

Follow-Up

PATIENT MONITORING

- Check for evidence of altered alertness that would suggest one of the differential diagnoses

EXPECTED COURSE AND PROGNOSIS

- Gradual return of the ability to learn new material, usually within 12 hours
- The patient will not recall events that occur while amnestic
- Recurs in <20% of patients
- Does not convey any increased risk for stroke or seizure

PATIENT EDUCATION

- TGA may recur in a minority of patients
- TGA does not herald an increased risk of stroke or seizures
- TGA is not a psychogenic reaction to stress
- No modification of lifestyle is required by the diagnosis of TGA per se

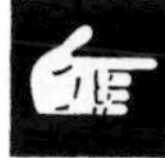

Miscellaneous

SYNONYMS

- TGA

ICD-9-CM: 294.8 Amnestic disorder not otherwise specified

SEE ALSO: WERNICKE-KORSAKOFF SYNDROME

REFERENCES

- Fisher CM, Adams RA. Transient global amnesia. Acta Neurol Scand 1964; 40[Suppl 9]:7–82.
- Hinge HH, Jensen TS, Kjaer M, et al. The prognosis of transient global amnesia. Results of a multicenter study. Arch Neurol 1986;43:673–676.
- Klotzsch C, Sliwka U, Berlit P, et al. An increased frequency of patent foramen ovale in patients with transient global amnesia. Analysis of 53 consecutive patients. Arch Neurol 1996;53:504–508.
- Lauria G, Gentile M, Fassetta G, et al. Incidence of transient global amnesia in the Belluno province, Italy: 1985 through 1995. Results of a community-based study. Acta Neurol Scand 1997;95:303–310.
- Schmidtke K, Ehmsen L. Transient global amnesia and migraine. A case control study. Eur Neurol 1998;40:9–14.

Author(s): Daniel W. Giang, MD

Amyotrophic Lateral Sclerosis and Other Motor Neuron Diseases

Basics

DESCRIPTION

- Amyotrophic lateral sclerosis (ALS) is an idiopathic, progressive CNS disease resulting in death of brain upper motor neurons (UMN), brainstem bulbar motor neurons, and spinal cord lower motor neurons (LMN), and causing weakness of corticobulbar and corticospinal innervated muscles. ALS starts focally in a bulbar or limb muscle and spreads, resulting in death, usually by respiratory failure.

EPIDEMIOLOGY

Incidence

- 2/100,000/year

Age

- All ages, highest between 50 and 70 years, mean 58, uncommon <40

Sex

- Slight male predominance of 1.3:1, especially in younger ages; 1:1 <65

Race

- Fairly uniform geographic and ethnic distribution

Prevalence

- 6/100,000

ETIOLOGY

- Unknown; theories include apoptosis, autoimmunity, excitotoxicity, free-radical formation, mitochondrial dysfunction, paraneoplastic, viral infection

Genetics

- Familial ALS (FALS, 5%–10% of all ALS): younger age onset, mean 45.
- Multiple gene mutations; most are autosomal dominant; 20% of FALS due to mutation in copper zinc superoxide dismutase gene

RISK FACTORS

- Genetic (FALS)
- Lymphoproliferative disease (rare association)
- ? Environmental (e.g., ALS/parkinsonism–dementia complex of Guam)

PREGNANCY

- SOD_1 gene test available for prenatal testing (covers 1% of all ALS)

ASSOCIATED CONDITIONS

- N/A

Diagnosis

DIFFERENTIAL DIAGNOSIS

ALS Phenotype

- Familial ALS
- ALS with lymphoproliferative disease, monoclonal gammopathy, or other malignancy
- ALS-like disease with HIV infection
- ALS/parkinsonism–dementia complex of Guam

LMN Disorders

- Spinal muscular atrophy (SMA): most are autosomal recessive (5q11.2-13.3); onset birth to young adult
- Spinal bulbar muscular atrophy (SBMA, "Kennedy's disease"): X-linked, CAG trinucleotide repeat in androgen receptor gene; adolescence and older; slow, proximal > distal LMN; chin fasciculations; gynecomastia
- Progressive muscular atrophy (PMA): adult onset; minimal bulbar signs; slower than ALS, but "PMA" LMN onset frequently turns out to be ALS
- Viral: poliomyelitis, other enteroviruses

UMN Disorders

- Primary lateral sclerosis (PLS): adult onset; rare, sporadic; UMN limb signs, gait impairment, spastic dysarthria, dysphonia, dysphagia; normal EMG; slower than ALS, but "PLS" UMN onset usually turns out to be ALS
- Hereditary spastic paraplegia (HSP)
- Viral myelopathy: HTLV-1 (tropical spastic paraparesis) and HIV
- Other CNS: Creutzfeldt-Jakob, progressive supranuclear palsy, corticobasal degeneration, diffuse Lewy body disease, multiple systems atrophy, syphilis

Disorders That May Be Confused with ALS

- Cervical myelopathy: spondylotic, Chiari malformation, tumor, syringomyelia
- Lumbosacral spinal stenosis
- Subacute combined degeneration
- Inclusion-body myositis (IBM): older male predominance; slowly progressive distal arm weakness; hip flexor weakness; dysphagia
- Multifocal motor neuropathy (MMN): sporadic LMN syndrome; middle age and older; male predominance; weakness without numbness out of proportion to atrophy, fasciculations; antibody-mediated multifocal demyelinating motor neuropathy; confirm via NCS, motor conduction blocks, high-titer anti-G_{M1} ganglioside antibody (50%)
- Chronic inflammatory demyelinating polyneuropathy
- Amyotrophy (diabetic or monomelic)
- Stroke
- Multiple sclerosis
- Myasthenia gravis
- Heavy metal intoxication
- Hyperthyroidism, hyperparathyroidism
- Benign cramp-fasciculation syndrome

SIGNS AND SYMPTOMS

- UMN signs: spasticity, hyperreflexia, Babinski and Hoffman signs, emotional lability ("pseudobulbar")
- LMN signs: weakness and atrophy, fasciculations, hyporeflexia, flaccidity, muscle cramps; widespread fasciculations are sensitive but not specific, seen especially in tongue, upper chest, proximal limbs
- Bulbar: tongue atrophy and fasciculations, dysarthria (flaccid or spastic), jaw jerk/gag (reduced or hyperactive), dysphagia, laryngospasm, sialorrhea
- Respiratory: exertional dyspnea, orthopnea
  —Chronic ventilatory insufficiency: heralded by fitful sleep, awakenings, emergence, or change in snoring quality, orthopnea, nightmares, morning headache, excessive daytime somnolence
- Cognitive dysfunction (5%–10+% of cases)
- El Escorial Criteria (World Federation of Neurology): requires progressive motor weakness; no alternative explanation; "regions" defined as bulbar, cervical myotomes, thoracic myotomes, and lumbosacral myotomes
- Definite ALS: UMN and LMN signs in 3 regions (bulbar + 2 spinal, or 3 spinal)
- Probable ALS: UMN and LMN signs in 2 regions, some UMN rostral to LMN
- Possible ALS: UMN and LMN signs in 1 region

LABORATORY PROCEDURES

- No serologic confirmatory test
- EMG/nerve conductions: single most useful test
  —Looking for at least 3-limb acute and chronic denervation and reinnervation
  —Helpful in showing widespread LMN involvement if clinically unclear
- Laboratory tests to evaluate differential diagnosis:
  —CBC, ESR
  —CK (in ALS, normal or mild to moderately elevated)
  —T_4, TSH
  —Vitamin B_{12}(methylmalonic acid)
  —SIEP/SIFX, UIEP/UIFX (exclude monoclonal)
  —ANA, rheumatoid factor
  —Lyme, HIV titers (depending on risk), RPR
  —Urine heavy metals (lead, mercury)
  —Acetylcholine receptor antibody
  —GM_1 ganglioside antibody (40%–60% MMN cases with high titers)
  —Hexosaminidase A
  —Gene tests: FALS, SBMA, SMA (SMN, survival motor neuron gene)
  —Hexosaminidase A deficiency

IMAGING STUDIES

- Cervical MRI (to exclude cervical stenosis, especially if both UMN and LMN signs in upper extremities)
- Brain, thoracic, lumbosacral MRI (depending on presentation)

SPECIAL TESTS

- Muscle biopsy (ALS shows nonspecific "neurogenic" changes); exclude inclusion-body myositis, dystrophy
- Cerebrospinal fluid if atypical presentation; exclude meningeal carcinomatosis

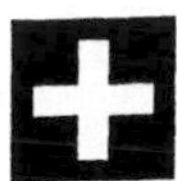

Management

GENERAL MEASURES

- Accurate diagnosis by ALS-experienced neurologist is essential to enable patient and family to come to terms and to rationally choose among options
- Earliest feasible diagnosis helps avert unnecessary operations
- Encourage second diagnostic opinion if uncertain, or to facilitate "closure"
- Choice of ALS center for principal neurologic care requires ALS-specialized neurologist and multidisciplinary care setting
- Compassion in "breaking the news"
- Discuss early and periodically review end-of-life wishes, advance directives, and durable power of attorney (health care); have non-rushed talks *before the need*
- Respite care and psychological support for the spouse or caregiver
- Deep vein thrombosis (DVT) prophylaxis
- Keep vaccinations current

SURGICAL MEASURES

- PEG: elective, most safely performed when forced vital capacity (FVC) >50%
- Tracheostomy: airway protection; enable long-term ventilation (if desired)

SYMPTOMATIC TREATMENT

- Dyspnea
  - —Indications for respiratory support: dyspnea, excessive daytime sleepiness, morning headaches, frequent nocturnal awakenings
  - —Nocturnal bi-PAP is treatment of choice for nocturnal ventilation; nasal O_2 less effective, may cut hypoxemic drive in hypercapnia
  - —Elevate head of bed
  - —Aggressive early treatment of respiratory infections
  - —Establish wishes regarding intubation, short- and long-term ventilation
  - —Terminal care to prevent air hunger for patients declining ventilator
- Speech: as dysarthria progresses, low tech (notepads, letter boards) to high tech (computer voice synthesizers, headset laser pointer)
- Salivation: sialorrhea—glycopyrrolate, hyoscyamine (Levsin), tricyclics, hycosamine, scopolamine patches; suction and quarterly botulinum toxin type A (BOTOX) parotid injections; parotid irradiation causes undesirable dryness
- Thick phlegm: suction, guaifenesin, nebulized acetylcysteine, propranolol; nasal congestion, postnasal drip: loratadine (Claritin)
- Swallowing: swallowing therapy, videofluoroscopy; PEG tube placement
- Pain control
- Spasticity: baclofen, tizanidine, diazepam
- Cramps and myalgias: quinine, calcium/magnesium/zinc, vitamin E, gabapentin
- Jaw clenching: clonazepam, diazepam, botulinum toxin
- Cognitive impairment: consider trial of donepezil
- Depression and anxiety: medications, counseling, psychology/psychiatry liaison, support groups, respite
- Pseudobulbar affect: amitriptyline, carbamazepine, fluoxetine, paroxetine
- Sleep disturbance: consider change in nocturnal breathing, possible nocturnal hypoventilation, sleep apnea; other causes are depression, anxiety, pain
- Constipation: stool softener, bulk, sorbitol, other laxatives

ADJUNCTIVE TREATMENT

- Physical and occupational therapy
- Durable goods: ankle-foot orthoses, cane, walker, wheelchair scooter, head support, hospital beds
- Domestic modifications: wheelchair ramps and vans, grab bars, lift devices
- Meticulous symptom management and palliative care at end of life

ADMISSION/DISCHARGE CRITERIA

- Avoid hospitalizations, "elective" spinal surgery
- PEG placement
- Pneumonia

Medications

DRUG(S) OF CHOICE

- Riluzole: only FDA-approved, disease-modifying ALS drug; 3-month survival advantage in placebo trials. Antiglutamate excitotoxicity mechanism of action. Dosing: 50 mg PO q12h. Expensive. Side effects are fatigue, nausea, vomiting. Rarely discontinue for fivefold elevation in LFTs.

Contraindications

- Caution with impaired hepatic and renal function, hypertension, history of neutropenia, hypersensitivity to drug class

Precautions

- Monitor LFTs monthly for first 3 months, then every 3 months

ALTERNATIVE DRUGS

Unproven But Commonly Prescribed

- β-Carotene
- Coenzyme Q10
- Creatine (1–2.5 g bid) may improve mitochondrial function, GI side effects
- Vitamin C (1,000–2,000 mg daily)
- Vitamin E (800–1,200 IU daily)

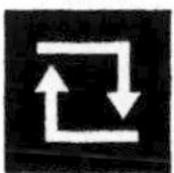

Follow-Up

PATIENT MONITORING

- Clinically: every 3 months, more frequently near diagnosis and end stages.
- FVC: every 3 months

EXPECTED COURSE AND PROGNOSIS

- Mean survival 3- to 4-year range; variable

PATIENT EDUCATION

- ALS Association, 27001 Agoura Road, Suite 150, Calabasas Hills, CA 91301. Phone: 818-880-9007, website: *www.alsa.org*
- Muscular Dystrophy Association–USA, 3300 E. Sunrise Drive, Tucson, AZ 85718. Phone: 1-800-572-1717, website: *www:mdausa.org*

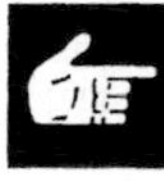

Miscellaneous

SYNONYMS

- Lou Gehrig's disease

ICD-9-CM: 335.20 Amyotrophic lateral sclerosis (including bulbar ALS); 335.29 Motor neuron diseases other

SEE ALSO: N/A

REFERENCES

- Katirji B, Kaminski HJ, Preston DC, et al., eds. Neuromuscular disorders in clinical practice. Boston: Butterworth-Heinemann, 2002.
- Miller RG, Rosenberg JA, Gelinas DF, et al., and the ALS Practice Parameters Task Force. Practice parameter: the care of the patient with amyotrophic lateral sclerosis (an evidence-based review). Neurology 1999;52:1311–1323.
- Pascuzzi RM. ALS, motor neuron disease and related disorders: a personal approach to diagnosis and management. Semin Neurol 2002;22:75–87.
- Rowland LP, Shneider NA. Amyotrophic lateral sclerosis. N Engl J Med 2001;344:1688–1700.

Author(s): Glenn A. Mackin, MD

Antiphospholipid Antibody Syndrome, Neurologic Complications

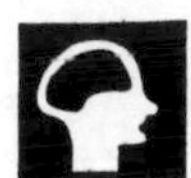

Basics

DESCRIPTION

Antiphospholipid syndrome consists of thrombotic events, thrombocytopenia, and recurrent fetal loss, in the presence of circulating antiphospholipid antibodies (aPLs). Antiphospholipid syndrome (APS) can be primary or secondary to connective tissue disorders such as systemic lupus erythematosus (SLE), infectious diseases, or neoplastic disorders. Neurologic manifestations of APS are variable, and are most often due to recurrent cerebral ischemia.

EPIDEMIOLOGY

Incidence/Prevalence

The incidence of stroke in patients under 50 years of age is 0.05%/year. The prevalence of aPLs in the population is 2% to 5%, with the majority of subjects being asymptomatic.

Race

While APS has not been reported in African-Americans as frequently as in other ethnic groups, IgA and IgM aCL isotypes appear to be more prevalent in this subgroup.

Age

Although the syndrome is more common in younger patients, 27% of patients with APS are over 60. It is estimated that 20% to 30% of young adults with thromboembolic events have positive anticardiolipin antibodies (aCLs) and/or lupus anticoagulant (LA), and 7% to 10% of total patients with stroke are aPL positive if all ages are considered.

Sex

The female to male ratio varies from 1.5-2:1 in primary APS, and up to 9:1 in patients with APS associated with SLE.

ETIOLOGY

APS is linked to the presence of aPLs—acquired antibodies against anionic phospholipid-containing moieties in cell membranes. LA and aCL, especially the IgG isotype, were identified as risk factors for ischemic strokes. Although the mechanism of thrombosis is uncertain, it is believed that aPLs promote platelet aggregation and disruption of coagulation cascade with subsequent inhibition of the production of prostagland E_2—a potent vasodilator.

The binding of aCL phospholipid is dependent on the presence of a β_2-glycoprotein (β_2-GPI), a plasma protein with high affinity to anionic phospholipids, creating an immunologic reaction that may lead to thrombosis.

APL can interfere with protein C activity and decrease protein S levels, leading to inhibition of plasminogen activator protein.

Genetics

Familial aPL positivity has been linked to human leukocyte antigens (HLAs) DR7, DR4, DQw7, and DRw53. Familial coexistence has been linked to factor V Leiden mutation.

RISK FACTORS

SLE

PREGNANCY

Antiphospholipid antibodies can cause spontaneous abortion.

ASSOCIATED CONDITIONS

- SLE
- Sneddon's syndrome (livedo reticularis and stroke)
- Sjögren's syndrome
- Primary inflammatory vasculitis
- Rheumatoid arthritis
- Budd-Chiari syndrome
- Addison's disease
- Degos syndrome (malignant atrophic papulosis)
- Cerebral atrophy

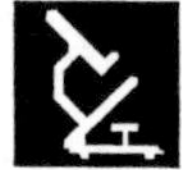

Diagnosis

DIFFERENTIAL DIAGNOSIS

APS should be considered in patients with stroke, especially in the absence of recognized risk factors. Other causes of unexplained arterial or venous thrombosis should be excluded:

- Protein C or S deficiency
- Homocystinuria
- Antithrombin III deficiency
- CNS vasculitis
- Coagulation factors disorders
- Factor V Leiden mutation
- Sickle cell disease
- Underlying malignancy with hypercoagulability
- Conditions associated with transient elevation of aPL, such as AIDS, neuroleptic agents (in particular phenothiazines), recombinant tissue plasminogen activator (rt-PA), aging (50% of patients over 80 are aPL positive), and insulin-dependent diabetes mellitus.

SIGNS AND SYMPTOMS

Neuropsychiatric Manifestations

- Cerebral infarct: arterial infarct (thrombotic, cardioembolic); venous infarct
- TIA
- Transient global amnesia
- Headache: migraine-like headaches or auras; benign intracranial hypertension
- Seizures
- Dementia, including vascular dementia
- Encephalopathy
- Movement disorders: chorea; dystonia; tics, including Tourette's syndrome; ballistic movements; akathisia
- Transverse myelopathy
- Guillain-Barré syndrome
- Reflex sympathetic syndrome
- Psychiatric disorders: unexplained behavioral disorder; attention deficit; memory difficulties; psychomotor delay; lethargy; major depression; schizophrenia

Non-Neurologic Manifestations

- Recurrent miscarriages
- Cutaneous manifestations: livedo reticularis; necrotizing vasculitis; livedoid vasculitis; thrombophlebitis; cutaneous ulceration and necrosis; erythematous macules; purpura; ecchymoses; painful skin nodules; subungual splinter hemorrhages; pyoderma gangrenosum
- Ocular manifestations: retinal vein thrombosis; central retinal artery occlusion; ischemic optic neuropathy
- Cardiac valvular abnormalities
- Pulmonary hypertension/embolism
- Deep venous thrombosis
- Renal vein thrombosis
- Addison's disease
- Adult respiratory distress syndrome
- Multiple organ failure
- Hematologic disorders: hemolytic anemia; autoimmune thrombocytopenic purpura; hemolytic-uremic syndrome

LABORATORY PROCEDURES

The presence of one or both of the circulating aPLs (LA or IgG-aCL) in the blood of patients with signs and symptoms of recurrent venous thrombosis is suggestive of the diagnosis of APS. Hematologic abnormalities that may be associated with APS include:

- Thrombocytopenia (26%–31%)
- Prolonged aPTT (50%)
- Positive Coombs test
- False-positive VDRL
- Neutropenia
- Lymphopenia
- Decreased C_4 levels

IMAGING STUDIES

- CT and MRI findings are nonspecific. At least 50% of patients with APS will show a single lesion on CT, and about half this number will have multiple infarcts. Less common findings include white matter abnormalities, cortical atrophy, and sinus thrombosis
- Conventional cerebral angiography or MRA may show evidence of intracranial stenosis in 40% of patients, half of which are in the MCA branches. Only 22% of patients may show extracranial lesions. Dural sinus thrombosis is a common finding. Rarely, the angiogram picture may be suggestive of vasculitis.

SPECIAL TESTS

None

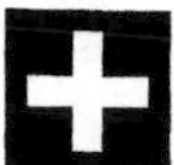

Management

GENERAL MEASURES

There are no good prospective studies to support any particular mode of therapy. Different therapeutic strategies include the use of antiplatelet agents, anticoagulants and immunomodulators individually or in combination. Multicenter collaborative trials are studying the usefulness of aspirin-warfarin in APS.

Control of Risk Factors

- Avoid smoking, excessive alcohol intake, and oral contraceptive pills.
- Management of blood pressure

SURGICAL MEASURES

N/A

SYMPTOMATIC TREATMENT

Varies widely with symptoms.

ADJUNCTIVE TREATMENT

N/A

ADMISSION/DISCHARGE CRITERIA

Admission is required for management of acute stroke or neuropsychiatric symptoms.

Medications

DRUG(S) OF CHOICE

Antiplatelet Agents

- Aspirin: aspirin reduces the risk of stroke recurrence by inhibiting platelet aggregation through inhibition of endothelial prostacyclin synthesis. Although it has been widely used as a prophylactic agent for stroke, the efficacy of aspirin in APS is uncertain. Aspirin can be used in variable doses of 81 to 1,300 mg, in patients with a single thromboembolic event and positive aCLs.
- Other antiplatelet agents: ticlopidine, clopidogrel, and dipyridamole have not been studied in the aCL-positive subgroup of stroke patients.

Anticoagulants

- Warfarin is an effective therapy for recurrent thromboembolic events, with an international normalized ratio (INR) aim of >3. Abrupt discontinuation of the medication may increase the probability of recurrent thrombosis. A combination of aspirin and warfarin has been used for patients who continue to have recurrent events on warfarin alone.
- Heparin: high doses of unfractionated heparin or low molecular weight heparin appear to be efficacious in protecting against recurrent thrombosis.

Thrombolytics

Alteplase rtPA has been successfully used in few patients with APS, and can be used in selective patients with acute stroke.

Plasma Exchange

Plasma exchange may lower the level of circulating antibodies; repeated exchanges may be required to avoid a rapid rise in aPL titers.

Steroids

There is no conclusive evidence for a positive role for steroids in aCL-positive stroke patients. Its use in pregnant women was associated with decrease incidence of fetal loss, especially in patients with SLE.

Immunoglobulin Therapy

The role of intravenous immunoglobulin (IVIG) in APS is not well understood, but is thought to binds to receptors on the endothelial cells prohibiting the interaction of aPL with receptors. Immunoglobulin therapy may cause thrombosis especially in elderly patients and in patients with other risk factors for thrombosis.

Immunosuppressive Agents

Azathioprine, cyclophosphamide, and methotrexate, with or without corticosteroids, have been used in refractory APS, with remarkable decrease of aCL titers and LA activity.

Contraindications

Known hypersensitivity reactions for any of the above drugs. Warfarin is contraindicated in those with active or potential sources of bleeding or frequent falls.

Precautions

N/A

ALTERNATIVE DRUGS

Fish oil derivatives may help in preventing recurrent miscarriage in APS women.

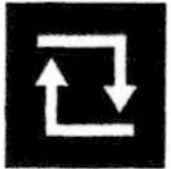

Follow-Up

PATIENT MONITORING

Patients should be reevaluated for new neurologic complaints. Those on warfarin require routine monitoring of coagulation parameters.

EXPECTED COURSE AND PROGNOSIS

The disease duration is thought to be longer in secondary APS, after the initial manifestations or after the detection of circulating aCLs. The rate of recurrence of stroke or TIA in patients with APS is 35% to 50%.

PATIENT EDUCATION

N/A

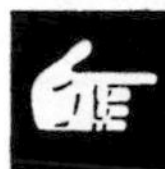

Miscellaneous

SYNONYMS

Hughes' syndrome

ICD-9-CM: 795.79 Anticardiolipin antibody syndrome and antiphospholipid syndrome, with the code given for nonspecific immunologic findings, should be used in conjunction with codes for the specific symptoms/disorders associated with the presence of circulating aPLs; 436 Stroke; 435 TIA; 362.31 Central retinal artery occlusion; 363.5 Central retinal vein occlusion; 362.34 Amaurosis fugax; 695.4 Lupus

SEE ALSO: N/A

REFERENCES

- Antiphospholipid Antibodies in Stroke Study Group (APASS). Anticardiolipin Antibodies are an independent risk factor for first ischemic stroke. Neurology 1993;43:2069–2073.
- Dafer RM, Tietjen GE, Asherson RA. Drug treatment of stroke in patients with antiphospholipid antibodies. CNS Drugs 1997;8:219–226.
- Feldmann E, Levine SR. Cerebrovascular disease with antiphospholipid antibodies: immune mechanisms, significance, and therapeutic options. Ann Neurol 1995; 37 (S1):S114–S130.
- Gelfand YA, Dori D, Miller B, et al. Visual disturbances and pathologic ocular findings in primary antiphospholipid syndrome. Ophthalmology 1999;106:1537–1540.
- Jacobson MW, Rapport LJ, Keenan PA, et al. Neuropsychological deficits associated with antiphospholipid antibodies. Clin Exp Neuropsychol 1999;21: 251–264.
- Khamashta MA, Cuadrado MJ, Mujic F, et al. The management of thrombosis in the antiphospholipid-antibody syndrome. N Engl J Med 1995;332:993–997.
- Tietjen GE, Day M, Norris L, et al. Role of anticardiolipin antibodies in young persons with migraine and transient focal neurologic events: a prospective study. Neurology 1998;50:1433–1440.
- Verro P, Levine SR, Tietjen GE. Cerebrovascular ischemic events with high positive anticardiolipin antibodies. Stroke 1998;29:2245–2253.

Author(s): Rima M. Dafer, MD; Gretchen E. Tietjen, MD

Arachnoiditis

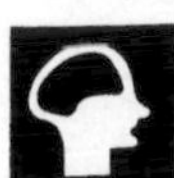

Basics

DESCRIPTION

- Arachnoiditis is a nonspecific inflammatory process of the arachnoid (middle) layer of the meninges, classically the result of an insult to the membrane by an irritant, infection, or other foreign body introduced into the subarachnoid space of the spinal cord. The disease process of lumbosacral arachnoiditis is perhaps best viewed on a continuum, ranging from a mild thickening of the arachnoid membranes that is clinically asymptomatic to the progressive heavy scarring of adhesive arachnoiditis. In the most severe cases, spinal cord roots may be compressed by bands of collagen scar tissue and lead to a clinically debilitating myeloradiculopathy with weakness and paraesthesias of the lower limbs.

EPIDEMIOLOGY

Incidence/Prevalence

- Clinically significant arachnoiditis is much less common than radiographic evidence of the disease. The incidence is 1.6% of patients with a history of an iodophendylate (Pantopaque or Myodil) myelogram, an oil-based intrathecal contrast agent that was used in the United States until the 1980s.

Race

- No demonstrated ethnic predominance

Age

- Adults of all ages are at risk for arachnoiditis; risk is increased for older patients because of the increased frequency of lumbar disc disease; 25- to 65 year-old patients are at highest risk.

Sex

- May affect men more frequently than women.

ETIOLOGY

- Arachnoiditis is classically caused by a local inflammatory reaction of the arachnoid matter covering the nerve roots of the spinal cord in response to the presence of irritants, infections, or foreign bodies. The inflammatory process may be contained to a minimal/self-limited local response without clinical significance, or it can progress to complete obliteration of the subarachnoid space by swollen arachnoid sheaths. A more chronic phase is characterized by the deposition of scar tissue, causing the protective layers and the nerve roots to adhere to one another. In a small percentage of patients, this will calcify. Common causes include local spinal trauma from postsurgical procedures, lumbar puncture, spinal anesthesia, postoperative infection (after spine surgery), and, most commonly in modern western cultures, myelography, especially with oil-based contrast agents. Other known etiologies include herniated spinal disc, primary spinal stenosis, intrathecal blood or subarachnoid hemorrhage, intrathecal steroids, or chemotherapeutic agents. Although arachnoiditis classically involves the lumbosacral roots of the cauda equina, it can involve the arachnoid membrane in any part of the CNS.

Genetics

N/A

RISK FACTORS

- There are several well-known risk factors, including previous myelography, especially with oil-based intrathecal radiographic contrast materials with risk increasing for multiple or traumatic myelograms. A significant span of time may elapse between administration and clinical presentation (as long as decades). Although most commonly associated with intrathecal contrast agents, there are other, less frequently associated risk factors, including postoperative wound infections in the lumbar region after spinal surgery, previous spinal surgery, repeated lumbar procedures (particularly failed back syndrome), primary spinal stenosis, and intrathecal or epidural administration of therapeutic agents, including spinal anesthesia.

PREGNANCY

- There are no well-reported complications with pregnancy.

ASSOCIATED CONDITIONS

- Arachnoiditis can be seen in association with failed back syndrome (11% of patients). Other disease associations include sarcoidosis, spinal stenosis, ankylosing spondylitis, and fibromyalgia.

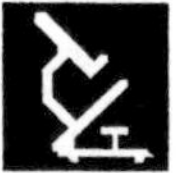

Diagnosis

DIFFERENTIAL DIAGNOSIS

- Herniated disc
- Degenerative joint/disc disease
- Chronic back pain
- Infection
- Muscle or ligament strain
- Metastatic bone disease
- Osteopenic states
- Paget's disease
- Structural/congenital abnormalities
- Referred pain
- Multiple myeloma
- Psychogenic
- Other

SIGNS AND SYMPTOMS

- An alternative diagnosis to arachnoiditis should be considered if there is sudden pain following an intraspinal procedure or if the presentation is acute. Development of arachnoiditis depends on the etiology and can present months after a failed back surgery or as long as decades after myelography. Arachnoiditis represents a nonspecific, sometimes confusing, clinical picture. It can present with burning pain in one or both legs and/or the lower back; back pain made worse with activity; sciatica; positive straight-leg raise; tenderness at the sciatic notch; muscle spasm and leg cramps; limited trunk movement/lumbar stiffness; or motor, sensory, and/or reflex changes that occur bilaterally in as many as two thirds of selected patient groups. Such changes can involve only one root or can be more widespread, involving many roots. This can progress to monoparesis or paraparesis. Urinary frequency, urgency, or incontinence sometimes is seen.

LABORATORY PROCEDURES

- There are no reliable blood or CSF tests to help diagnose arachnoiditis.

IMAGING STUDIES

- MRI is the primary imaging modality for arachnoiditis. Findings include abnormal position and/or morphology of nerve roots, often with adhesion to the surrounding arachnoid membranes. Radiographic evidence of arachnoiditis occurs frequently in asymptomatic patients. Arachnoiditis tends to coexist with additional pathology; this pathology is important in treatment planning because it can represent potential curative aspects of the disease. Myelography often is avoided because of the success of less invasive imaging studies.

SPECIAL TESTS

- Infectious etiologies can be evaluated with CSF analysis.

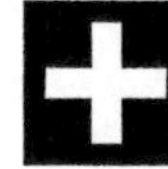

Management

GENERAL MEASURES

- Despite many promising treatment possibilities, arachnoiditis generally responds poorly to treatment and is considered a permanent condition by some clinicians, with therapy related only to symptomatic care. Prevention is an important component of arachnoiditis.
- Specific treatment should be given if any underlying pathology is detected, such as a herniated lumbar disc or focus of infection, such as tuberculosis arachnoiditis.

SURGICAL MEASURES

- Correlation between clinical and radiologic findings may be difficult because of the frequency of asymptomatic radiographic findings on imaging studies. Clinical presentation and a history of classic etiologies with associated MRI findings may provide the most accurate means of evaluation. Surgical intervention is controversial. Exploratory surgery in the absence of progressive neurologic deficit or with well-controlled pain usually is not indicated. Surgical intervention with the presence of potentially curable pathology, including disc disease or other focal abnormality, is reasonable. In selected patients with progressive neurologic deficits, surgical neural micro-decompression with lysis of arachnoid scarring may be considered.
- Initial operative success may be tempered by long-term follow-up, which suggests that long-term symptomatic relief may be reduced to <50%. Inherent risks of surgery include bowel or bladder dysfunction, little or no relief of symptoms, or saddle anesthesia. Unfavorable prognosis is associated with higher-grade cases of arachnoiditis.

SYMPTOMATIC TREATMENT

- Definitive treatment for arachnoiditis is limited to eliminating possible sources of irritants through prevention, medical therapy, or surgical intervention.
- Conservative care includes symptomatic relief with antiinflammatory and pain medications, patient education, and behavioral control.

ADJUNCTIVE TREATMENT

- Several different adjunctive treatments can be considered, including dorsal column stimulators, transcutaneous electrical nerve stimulators for pain control, or intrathecal morphine or baclofen. Use of epidural steroids is controversial, because some investigators have related this treatment to actually causing arachnoiditis. Intrathecal hyaluronidase in spinal arachnoiditis caused by tuberculosis meningitis has been reported as successful, although preservative-free hyaluronidase is not FDA approved for use in the United States. Cordotomies usually are not recommended.

ADMISSION/DISCHARGE CRITERIA

- Patients generally are evaluated and treated as outpatients. Admission may be indicated for patients with intractable pain or with acute changes in neurologic status.

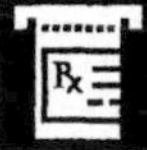

Medications

DRUG(S) OF CHOICE

- For pain control, consider gabapentin (Neurontin), start 300 mg PO qhs, increase by 300 mg/day over several days, maximum dose of 3,600 mg/day; or amitriptyline, start 10–25 mg PO qhs, gradually increase to effective dose of 100 mg/day.

Contraindications

- Amitriptyline should not be used in conjunction with monoamine oxidase inhibitors. Adjunctive pain control medication and referral to a pain management specialist can be considered in patients with intractable pain.

Precautions

- Gabapentin: Decrease dose in renal impairment; not FDA approved for neuropathic pain
- Amitriptyline and nortriptyline: Orthostatic hypotension, arrhythmias, and anticholinergic side effects; not FDA approved for chronic pain

ALTERNATIVE DRUGS

- Muscle relaxants on a short-term basis may provide relief in selected patients.

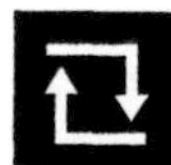

Follow-Up

PATIENT MONITORING

- Arachnoiditis is a chronic disease with the usual associated patient and caretaker issues. Regular scheduled follow-up is important. Although serial imaging studies are not customarily needed, any changes in neurologic or pain status should prompt a more complete workup. No regular patient monitoring of laboratory tests or imaging studies are required once a firm diagnosis is made. However, proper attention to changes in neurologic or pain status should prompt workup to rule out additional pathology.

EXPECTED COURSE AND PROGNOSIS

- There is no cure for arachnoiditis. There is a wide spectrum of clinical disease ranging from mild to very severe. In one study with long-range follow-up, pain and functional disability tended to remain the same as they were at the time of diagnosis. Although most patients were able to walk and drive a car, their ability to return to full-time work was limited. This study also noted that a majority of subjects depended on daily narcotic analgesics.

PATIENT EDUCATION

- National Organization for Rare Disorders, Inc.(NORD), P.O. Box 8923, New Fairfield, CT 06812-8923. Website: *www.nord-rdb.com*
- NIH/National Institute of Neurological Disorders and Stroke, 31 Center Drive, MSC 2540, Building 31, Room 8A16, Bethesda, MD 20892. Website: *www.ninds.nih.gov*

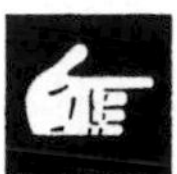

Miscellaneous

SYNONYMS

- Lumbosacral adhesive arachnoiditis
- Chronic adhesive arachnoiditis
- Serous circumscribed meningitis
- Spinal arachnoiditis

ICD-9-CM: 322.9 Arachnoiditis; 036.0 Meningococcal arachnoiditis; 013.0 Tuberculous arachnoiditis; 724.1 Pain in thoracic spine; 724.2 Low back pain/syndrome; 724.3 Sciatica; 724.5 Backache not otherwise specified; 724.9 Other unspecified back disorder

SEE ALSO: N/A

REFERENCES

- Burton CV. Lumbosacral arachnoiditis. In: Youman JR, ed. Youmans neurological surgery, vol. III, part IX, 4th ed. Philadelphia: WB Saunders, 1996: 2483–2491.
- Delamarter RB. Diagnosis of lumbar arachnoiditis by magnetic resonance imaging. Spine 1990;15:304–310.
- Dolan RA. Spinal adhesive arachnoiditis. Surg Neurol 1993;39:479–484.
- Guyer DW. The long-range prognosis of arachnoiditis. Spine 1989;14:1332–1337.
- Hoffman GS. Spinal arachnoiditis: what is the clinical spectrum? Spine 1983;8: 538–551.
- Roca J. The results of surgical treatment of lumbar arachnoiditis. Int Orthop 1993;17:77–81.

Author(s): L. Mervis, MD; Alexander M. Mason, MD

Arsenic Poisoning

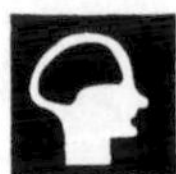

Basics

DESCRIPTION

- Arsenic neuropathy is part of a systemic illness due to excessive exposure to this toxic metalloid. Arsenic is easily obtained because it is commonly used as a rodenticide, herbicide, and insecticide. It has a long history of medicinal applications, but it is also a notorious homicidal or suicidal agent. The neurologic consequences of recurrent or chronic intoxication are similar to those of acute intoxication.

EPIDEMIOLOGY

Incidence

- Little information exists, but its presence undoubtedly exceeds its recognition. There is no known predilection for individuals of any race, age, or sex.

ETIOLOGY

- Homicidal and suicidal applications account for most cases of acute intoxication. Other considerations include iatrogenic medicinal exposures (usually folk medicines) and inadvertent exposure to contaminated foods, beverages, water, or combustion fumes. Arsenic is a general protoplasmic poison that interferes with cellular energy metabolism.

Risk Factors

- The primary risk factor is excessive arsenic exposure from any source.

PREGNANCY

- There is no known relationship with pregnancy. Arsenic is not known to present any particular danger to the fetus at typical environmental concentrations.

ASSOCIATED CONDITIONS

- In addition to neuropathy, associated conditions are toxic encephalopathy, chemical hepatitis, pancytopenia, renal tubular necrosis, dermatitis with hyperkeratosis, pancreatitis, and cardiomyopathy. Inorganic arsenic compounds are human carcinogens associated with hepatic angiosarcoma and skin cancer.

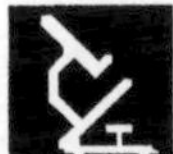

Diagnosis

DIFFERENTIAL DIAGNOSIS

- Guillain-Barré syndrome (GBS), acute porphyric neuropathy, HIV-associated neuropathy, confluent vasculitic mononeuritis multiplex, chronic inflammatory demyelinating polyneuropathy, other dysimmune neuropathies associated with plasma cell dyscrasias (Waldenström's macroglobulinemia, γ heavy-chain disease, cryoglobulinemia, systemic lupus erythematosus, Castleman's disease), lymphoma or occult malignancy, other toxic neuropathies (amiodarone, carbon disulfide, cytosine arabinoside, methyl-*n*-butyl ketone, *n*-hexane)

SIGNS AND SYMPTOMS

- After acute exposure, symptoms of transient nausea, vomiting, and diarrhea, followed 5 to 10 days later by distal numbness and tingling, intense paresthesias, and burning pain, muscle tenderness, and weakness
- Neurologic signs include profound length-dependent sensory loss, weakness (sometimes progressing to quadriplegia with respiratory failure), areflexia, and dysautonomia. CNS signs include drowsiness, confusion, stupor, and coma. Signs reflect the magnitude of exposure and typically progress over several weeks after a single exposure.
- Additional signs include Mees lines (transverse bands in all nails) and pigmented dermatitis. Mees lines do not appear until about 1 month after acute ingestion, which limits their usefulness when the diagnosis is in question.

LABORATORY PROCEDURES

- Arsenic is readily absorbed and rapidly excreted in the urine (half-life in blood of about 60 hours). The amount of urinary excretion reflects the magnitude of exposure. A 24-hour collection is most reliable for establishing exposure. Abnormal excretion documents potential exposure, not intoxication. Transient increases are common after ingestion of some seafood items (the organic form of arsenic contained in seafood is not neurotoxic).
- Arsenic is rapidly cleared from the blood, so blood levels are helpful only when the blood is collected within several days of acute poisoning.
- Arsenic is bound to keratin, and remote exposures can be documented by the amount of arsenic present in hair or nails.
- CSF protein is elevated (150–300 mg/dL) early in the course of neuropathy.
- Other laboratory abnormalities reflect systemic involvement and include abnormal liver function studies, pancytopenia, and basophilic stippling of RBCs (a nonspecific but important indication of a toxic exposure).

IMAGING STUDIES

- There are no specific imaging abnormalities. Chest x-ray film may demonstrate cardiomegaly.

SPECIAL TESTS

- Nerve conduction studies (NCSs) at onset may suggest the presence of an acquired demyelinating neuropathy, with motor nerve evidence of abnormal temporal dispersion, partial conduction block, slowed conduction velocity, and prolonged distal latency. Sensory nerve responses may be of low amplitude or unobtainable.
- NCS and needle EMG findings progress to those of an axonal sensorimotor neuropathy, often with loss of distal responses and profuse fibrillation potentials.
- Sural nerve biopsy occasionally is required to exclude other considerations, such as vasculitis. Biopsy results in arsenic neuropathy are nonspecific and include a decreased number of myelinated fibers, with axons in varying stages of axonal degeneration.
- Toxicologic examination at autopsy (e.g., liver or kidney) can establish intoxication.

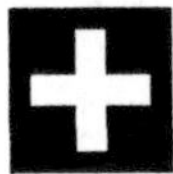

Management

GENERAL MEASURES

- Establish the diagnosis and remove the patient from exposure, although removal from exposure frequently is impossible because most cases involve single massive exposures.
- The treatment of acute arsenic poisoning is beyond the scope of this section but may include gastric lavage, hemodialysis, and chelation to increase arsenic excretion.
- Arsenic neurotoxicity progresses for weeks after a single toxic exposure. By the time neurologic signs develop, it is questionable whether chelation or related treatments, such as hemodialysis, influence the rate or extent of neurologic progression or recovery.

SURGICAL MEASURES

- Not applicable, other than sural nerve biopsy

SYMPTOMATIC TREATMENT

- Painful paresthesia may require symptomatic analgesic treatment.

ADJUNCTIVE TREATMENT

- Supportive care includes monitoring and management of respiratory function and prevention or treatment of infection, circulatory failure, and thromboembolism.
- Intubation is generally required when the forced vital capacity (FVC) approaches 15 mL/kg, but elective intubation should be considered when there is a rapid decline in FVC, independent of the absolute level.
- Autonomic dysfunction may require management of hypotension or cardiac dysrhythmia.
- Acute renal failure may require hemodialysis.
- Anecdotal reports suggest that therapeutic plasma exchange does not influence the course of neuropathy.

ADMISSION/DISCHARGE CRITERIA

- Admission criteria reflect the type and severity of the systemic involvement, as well as the magnitude and rate of progression of the neuropathy. All patients with progressive quadriparesis, respiratory decline, or evidence of dysautonomia require hospitalization and monitoring for progression.
- Discharge of patients with arsenical neuropathy is usually to a rehabilitation facility, depending on the magnitude of the residual impairment and deconditioning.

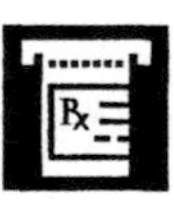

Medications

DRUG(S) OF CHOICE

- Despite a lack of evidence that chelation treatment influences the rate or extent of neurologic progression or recovery, standard treatment is chelation administration early in the course of the systemic intoxication.
- Chelation agents used for treatment of acute arsenic poisoning include DMPS (2,3-dimercapto-1-propanesulfonic acid), succimer (*meso* 2,3-dimercaptosuccinic acid, DMSA), and dimercaprol (British Anti-Lewisite, BAL). DMPS is preferred by some, but it is not widely available and is not FDA approved, which necessitates use of other agents in some cases. Succimer is the agent of choice for patients who can take PO medications. For those who cannot take PO succimer, BAL is recommended.

Contraindications

- Impaired renal or liver function, pregnancy, hypertension, prior hypersensitivity, or allergic reaction

Precautions

- The decision to proceed with chelation should be approached cautiously if treatment is being given only to treat the neurologic impairment (because of the lack of demonstrable efficacy).

ALTERNATIVE DRUGS

- Other chelating agents are available, but the relative advantages and risks are unspecified.

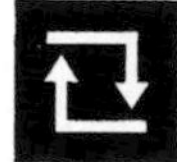

Follow-Up

PATIENT MONITORING

- Arsenic neuropathy may progress for many weeks after removal from exposure, so it is necessary to monitor patients for development of respiratory distress or dysautonomia until a plateau is reached or improvement is documented. Respiratory function should be monitored with interval measurement of FVC. Arterial blood gases are poor indicators of impending respiratory failure. Autonomic dysfunction requires monitoring of vital signs for hypotension or cardiac dysrhythmia. Systemic manifestations, such as renal failure or hepatic dysfunction, usually appear early in the course of intoxication, shortly after resolution of the acute gastrointestinal syndrome.

EXPECTED COURSE AND PROGNOSIS

- For patients who survive the acute systemic illness, including the complications of respiratory support, the prognosis for recovery is good. The systemic features of bone marrow suppression resolve rapidly, as do the chemical hepatitis and other non-neurologic features. The neuropathy becomes the most feared residual manifestation. The degree of axonal degeneration may be severe, and recovery typically is protracted. Patients who remain respirator dependent and nonambulatory for months require long-term rehabilitation. Neurologic improvement occurs over many years, but residual distal sensory and motor deficits, similar to those observed among patients with severe GBS or other forms of nonprogressive neuropathy, are common.

PATIENT EDUCATION

N/A

Miscellaneous

SYNONYMS

- Toxic neuropathy, arsenical polyneuropathy, neuropathy due to arsenic

ICD-9-CM: 357.7 Polyneuropathy, arsenical

SEE ALSO: N/A

REFERENCES

- Albers JW. Toxic neuropathies. In: Bleecker ML, ed. Continuum: lifelong learning in neurology. Baltimore: Lippincott Williams & Wilkins, 1999:27.
- Donofrio PD, Wilbourn AJ, Albers JW, et al. Acute arsenic intoxication presenting as Guillain-Barre-like syndrome. Muscle Nerve 1987;10:114.
- Mathieu D, Mathieu-Nolf M, Germain-Alonso M, et al. Massive arsenic poisoning—effect of hemodialysis and dimercaprol on arsenic kinetics. Intensive Care Med 1992;18:47.
- Rezuke WN, Anderson C, Pastuszak WT, et al. Arsenic intoxication presenting as a myelodysplastic syndrome: a case report. Am J Hematol 1991;36:291.
- Wax PM, Thornton CA. Recovery from severe arsenic-induced peripheral neuropathy with 2,3-dimercapto-1-propanesulphonic acid. J Toxicol Clin Toxicol 2000;38:777.
- Windebank AJ. Metal neuropathy. In: Dyck PJ, Thomas PK, Griffin JW, et al., eds. Peripheral neuropathy. Philadelphia: WB Saunders, 1993:1549.

Author(s): James W. Albers, MD, PhD; David H. Garabrant, MD, MPH

Attention Deficit Hyperactivity Disorder

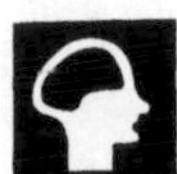

Basics

DESCRIPTION

- Attention deficit hyperactivity disorder (ADHD) is a common neurodevelopmental syndrome with symptom onset typically by age 7, most often between ages 3 and 5. It is primarily characterized by two symptoms: (i) inattention, and (ii) hyperactive and impulsive behaviors. The DSM-IV (1994) categorizes ADHD into three major subtypes: (i) predominantly inattentive type, (ii) predominantly hyperactive/impulsive type, and (iii) combined type.

EPIDEMIOLOGY

- Majority of studies report rates of 2%–5% within a school-aged population; therefore, 1–3 million children in the United States meet DSM-IV criteria for ADHD. ADHD occurs across cultures and genders. Boys seem to be affected at least three times more often than girls, and some statistics show the rates of boys to girls as high as 9:1. However, a recent epidemiologic study shows that girls are underdiagnosed and are diagnosed at a later age than boys. Differences in symptom expression may partially account for this. Boys tend to exhibit the more observable symptoms of hyperactivity and impulsivity, whereas girls tend to have the less obvious symptoms of inattention. About 60% of children will have residual symptoms into adulthood. In adulthood, the gender ratio of ADHD is 1:1.

ETIOLOGY

- Exact etiology of ADHD is not yet known, but recent research implicates both genetic and environmental factors. Growing evidence suggests that ADHD is genetically determined and primarily affects dopaminergic functions in the prefrontal cortex. Functional differences in the brains of ADHD patients are characterized by decreased prefrontal cortex dopaminergic activity and cerebral blood flow. Several twin studies demonstrate strong heritability. However, environmental contributions, such as premature birth, *in utero* exposure to substances, lead exposure, and psychosocial adversity, also are associated with ADHD symptoms in about 20%–30% of cases.

RISK FACTORS

- Family history of ADHD
- Significant environmental factors such as premature birth, *in utero* exposure to substances, lead exposure, and psychosocial adversity
- Traumatic brain injury
- Neurologic disorders such as Tourette's syndrome and seizure disorder

PREGNANCY

- Pregnant women who smoke, ingest alcohol or other illicit substances, or deliver prematurely are at higher risk for having a child with ADHD.

ASSOCIATED CONDITIONS

- Approximately 65% of children with ADHD will have a comorbid psychiatric condition. Most common are oppositional/defiant disorder (40%–50%; predominantly boys); anxiety and mood disorders (10%–35%; predominantly girls); learning disabilities (30%–40%), and conduct disorder (10%). Children with untreated ADHD are at high risk for developing significant comorbidities as they age. Children with seizure disorder (30%) and Tourette's syndrome (40%–70%) can have comorbid ADHD symptoms that warrant treatment.

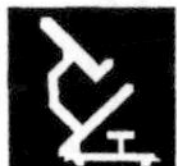

Diagnosis

DIFFERENTIAL DIAGNOSIS

- Because disruption of attention is a final common pathway affected by many psychiatric and neurologic disorders, the diagnosis of ADHD must be made in exclusion of other disorders that can account for the symptoms. Therefore, it is essential to rule out other psychiatric conditions, such as pervasive developmental disorders, obsessive-compulsive disorder, and other anxiety and mood disorders, especially bipolar disorder. Neurologic conditions, such as seizure disorder, head trauma, birth trauma, mental retardation, and Tourette's syndrome, must also be taken into consideration. The DSM-IV has very specific criteria for diagnosing ADHD, including symptom descriptions, time of symptom onset, symptom duration, and impairment criteria.

SIGNS AND SYMPTOMS

- The first signs of ADHD often are observed in a school setting, with teacher complaints initiating a referral. Children with ADHD can be excessively active, unable to sit still, disruptive to others, loud, inattentive, distractible, unable to focus on a task at hand, and impulsive. Due to these behaviors, academic performance often is below expected for their age and IQ. Peer and interpersonal interactions also are impaired. Depending upon the subtype and severity of ADHD in a particular child, a physician may not always be able to observe the symptoms in a brief office visit, and observational data from outside sources (e.g., teachers) are necessary for accurate diagnosis.

LABORATORY PROCEDURES

N/A

IMAGING STUDIES

- Imaging studies are not yet effective as diagnostic tools.

SPECIAL TESTS

- Observational data are obtained from teacher and parent rating scales of childhood behaviors. The most commonly used are the Conners' Parent (CPRS) and Teacher (CTRS) Rating Scales. These scales are easily completed and have excellent normative data based upon age and gender. Although these tests may be necessary to make the diagnosis of ADHD, they alone are not sufficient, nor are any other tests (cognitive, achievement, etc.) purported to "diagnose" ADHD.

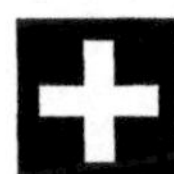

Management

GENERAL MEASURES

- Educational accommodations are almost always required in addition to medication management of symptoms. Psychoeducational evaluations and individual education programs should be pursued via the school system. Although behavioral therapy alone typically is not effective in fully controlling ADHD symptoms, behavioral treatments are a powerful adjunct to management with medication.

SURGICAL MEASURES

N/A

SYMPTOMATIC TREATMENT

- The most effective treatment of ADHD is multimodal and includes medication, academic accommodations, and behavioral interventions. The recent MTA (The Multimodal Treatment Study of Children with ADHD) demonstrated that when a multimodal approach to ADHD treatment was implemented, 68% of the subjects attained "normalized" behavior. Educational accommodations are necessary and implemented via the school system. For the vast majority of cases, drug "holidays" are neither necessary nor advisable.

ADJUNCTIVE TREATMENT

- Cognitive behavioral therapy, parent training, social skills groups, occupational and physical therapy, and academic interventions may be needed depending, upon the specifics of the case.

ADMISSION/DISCHARGE CRITERIA

- Admission for evaluation of ADHD is rarely needed, unless a comorbid neurologic or psychiatric condition requires inpatient evaluation.

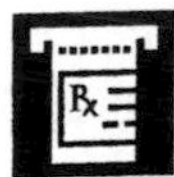

Medications

DRUG(S) OF CHOICE

- Stimulants are considered first-line therapy, with methylphenidate (MPH) therapies most commonly prescribed, followed by amphetamine-based therapies. Approximately 70% of children with ADHD will have a therapeutic response to stimulant treatment. Of the 30% who do not get a good response, switching to a different stimulant often will result in efficacy. Studies also demonstrate that, for the majority of ADHD patients, efficacy from stimulant therapy is not achieved until reaching a MPH dose of at least 15–20 mg/day.
- Long-acting methylphenidate products are now the treatment of choice and include Concerta (18–72 mg/day) and Metadate CD (20–60 mg/day). These medications are given once daily in the morning and last up to 9 hours (Metadate CD) to 12 hours (Concerta). The short-acting methylphenidate Ritalin (5–60 mg/day) is highly effective but wears off in 3–4 hours, necessitating multiple dosing and possibly causing rebound of symptoms during wear-off. A newer short-acting form of MPH, *d*-MPH, is now available under the name "Focalin". Focalin is MPH minus the *l*isomer and is purported to have fewer side effects than *d,l*-MPH. Ritalin SR was developed as a longer-acting form but has variable absorption and is not a preferred treatment. Ritalin LA, reportedly an improved version, will be available soon. Another form of MPH that will be available in the near future is the MethyPatch.
- Adderall (2.5–40 mg/day) and Adderall XR (10–40 mg/day), which are mixed-amphetamine salts compounds, are also commonly used long-acting stimulant therapies and last about 6 hours (Adderall) to 10 or more hours (Adderall XR). The side-effect profile for amphetamines, including Adderall, is higher than for MPH. Because of this, the amphetamine-based compounds Dexedrine and Dextrostat are currently used minimally.
- For children with comorbidities, combination pharmacotherapy often is necessary. Selective serotonin reuptake inhibitors, antidepressants, mood stabilizers, and α-adrenergic agonists are all commonly used in conjunction with stimulants to treat ADHD and associated comorbid conditions.

Contraindications

- Stimulants are contraindicated in children with a history of mania or bipolar disorder, psychosis and/or thought disorder, marked anxiety, high blood pressure, or glaucoma. Stimulants cannot be used in conjunction with monoamine oxidase inhibitors. Use with antiepileptic agents and anticoagulants must be closely monitored.
- Although MPH was once thought to be contraindicated in children with Tourette's syndrome and comorbid ADHD, a recent study demonstrated that this contraindication is not warranted.

Precautions

- The most common side effects of stimulants include loss of appetite, insomnia, headache, nausea, irritability, and depression. In general, stimulants are well tolerated, and side effects tend to be mild and wane over a few days after initiating treatment. Sleep disturbance and appetite loss should be carefully monitored and managed clinically if necessary (note: many children with ADHD have preexisting sleep disturbance unrelated to medication therapy). Little is known about the treatment response of preschoolers with ADHD. Long-term effects of stimulants are not well established. Abuse potential is limited with longer-acting agents.

ALTERNATIVE DRUGS

- α-Adrenergic agonists (clonidine, guanfacine) are second-line therapies that have a synergistic effect when used in conjunction with stimulants. Bupropion (Wellbutrin) has been touted as a treatment for ADHD, but data supporting its efficacy are limited. Imipramine and other tricyclics have been used in the past with modest efficacy, but use has been limited by concerns about cardiac toxicity and other side effects. Other alternative therapies are currently in development (e.g., atomoxetine).

Follow-Up

PATIENT MONITORING

- Patients should be monitored closely for side effects. The CTRS and CPRS can be used to monitor symptom response during treatment. Medication dosage can be titrated higher as long as the child is obtaining benefit without problematic side effects.

EXPECTED COURSE AND PROGNOSIS

- Highly variable, depending upon severity of comorbidities, environmental surroundings, and treatment compliance. For children with ADHD and minimal comorbidities, the prognosis with treatment is very good. For children with severe psychiatric or neurologic comorbidities, the prognosis is guarded. For children with ADHD who do not receive treatment, the prognosis is quite poor, and they are at risk for developing more severe psychiatric and behavior problems, becoming substance abusers, dropping out of school, being unemployed, and having unstable relationships.

PATIENT EDUCATION

- CHADD: National organization for children and adults with ADHD, providing educational materials, research updates, and national conferences. Website: *www.chadd.org*
- NIH/NIMH has a web page devoted to diagnosis and treatment of ADHD. Website: *www.nimh.nih.gov*

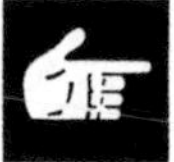

Miscellaneous

SYNONYMS

N/A

ICD-9-CM: 314.0 Attention deficit disorder; 314.00 ADD without hyperactivity; 314.01 ADD with hyperactivity

SEE ALSO: N/A

REFERENCES

- Greenhill LL. Diagnosing attention-deficit/hyperactivity disorder in children. J Clin Psychiatry 1998;59[Suppl 7]:31–41.
- Manuzza S, Gittelman Klein R, Bonagura N, et al. Hyperactive boys almost grown up. V. Replication of psychiatric status. Arch Gen Psychiatry 1991;48:77–83.
- Conners CK. Conners Rating Scales—Revised. Tonawanda, NY: Multi-Health Systems, 1997.
- The MTA Cooperative Group. A 14-month randomized clinical trial of treatment strategies for attention-deficit/hyperactivity disorder. Arch Gen Psychiatry 1999;56:1073–1086.
- The Tourette's Syndrome Study Group. Treatment of ADHD in children with tics: a randomized controlled trial. Neurology 2002;58:527–536.

Author(s): Donna Palumbo, PhD; Roger Kurlan, MD

Autism

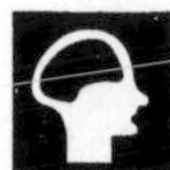

Basics

DESCRIPTION

- Autism is a condition characterized by delayed language, impaired social interaction, and stereotyped behavior with onset before age 3 years.

EPIDEMIOLOGY

- The incidence of autism is 2–5 cases per 10,000. There is no racial predilection known for autism, and the age of onset, by definition, is before age 3 years. There are 4–5 times as many males as females with autism.
- The incidence of autism is increased when a first-degree relative is affected. A small percentage has an inverted duplication on the proximal long arm of chromosome 15 (15q11-q13) that usually is maternally inherited.

RISK FACTORS

- Patients with fragile X syndrome or tuberous sclerosis have an increased incidence of autism. Otherwise, there is no confirmed risk factor for autism, although preliminary evidence suggests perinatal stressors may be a risk factor.

PREGNANCY

- There are no known issues specific to managing autism during pregnancy.

ASSOCIATED CONDITIONS

- There is a 75% incidence of mental retardation with autism. There is also an increased incidence of seizures in patients with autism. A variety of behavioral disturbances are also associated with autism. Although frank macrocephaly is uncommon, there is a tendency toward a larger head size in autism.

Diagnosis

DIFFERENTIAL DIAGNOSIS

- Asperger's syndrome resembles autism with relatively preserved language
- Pervasive developmental disorder—not otherwise specified (PDD-NOS) describes the condition where features of autism are present but the criteria for autism or Asperger syndrome are not met.
- Collectively, the related conditions of autism, Asperger's syndrome, and PDD-NOS are referred to by some specialists as "autism spectrum disorder."
- Rett's disorder consists of normal development for the first 5–48 months, followed by deceleration of head growth, stereotyped movements (typically midline hand movements), axial incoordination, loss of language skills, and retardation. Only females are affected.
- Fragile X syndrome is a genetic disorder that often can present with some autistic features.
- Landau-Kleffner syndrome consists of seizures originating in the language area, and occasionally this can resemble autism.
- Childhood-onset schizophrenia is characterized by early normal development followed by the development of schizophrenia, and can sometimes resemble autism.
- Mental retardation sometimes can be difficult to distinguish from autism with mental retardation when retardation is sufficiently severe.

SIGNS AND SYMPTOMS

- Signs and symptoms of autism develop by age 3 years, usually without a period of normal development previously (except in occasional patients in whom development is normal in the first 1–2 years), in three domains:
  - —*Impaired social interaction:* There is a lack of eye-to-eye gaze, blunted or abnormal facial expression, impaired use of social gesture, poor development of peer relationships (either lack of interest or lack of ability), lack of sharing enjoyment or interests with others, lack of social reciprocity, and inappropriate response to others' needs or distress.
  - —*Impaired communication:* There is a delay in verbal output, impaired ability to build a conversation, stereotypes or repetitive language, monotone or otherwise abnormal prosody to speech, idiosyncratic use of language, and inability to understand subtleties of language such as jokes and irony.
  - —*Restricted, repetitive, and stereotyped behavior:* There is preoccupation with strange interests, or interests held with an abnormal degree of intensity, inflexibility in rituals and routines, preoccupation with parts of objects, stereotyped motor behaviors, a restricted range of interests, and repetitive mimicry and a compulsion to line up objects or place them in a row.

LABORATORY PROCEDURES

- There are no specific laboratory procedures for the diagnosis of autism, except possibly testing to exclude fragile X syndrome. If pica is present, lead screening is indicated.

IMAGING STUDIES

- There are no imaging findings specific to autism, but some report cerebellar vermal hypoplasia.

SPECIAL TESTS

- Diagnosis is established by clinical evaluation by a child psychologist, child psychiatrist, pediatric neurologist, or behavioral neurologist. The Autism Diagnostic Interview-Revised and or the Autism Diagnostic Observation Schedule are considered the gold standard clinical evaluation tools.

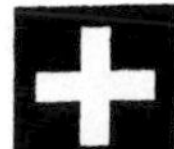

Management

GENERAL MEASURES

- Early and intensive behavioral intervention appears to be critical to optimizing development of functional ability in autism. This should be initiated as soon as possible after diagnosis and continued throughout schooling.
- Appropriate vocational rehabilitation services would be needed for those with sufficient cognitive ability to handle work.
- Medical treatment is directed at specific neuropsychiatric disturbances, such as obsessive-compulsive disorder, depression, agitation management, self-injurious behavior, anxiety, and sleep and eating disorders.
- No specific treatment for autism exists, but research on several agents is ongoing.

SURGICAL MEASURES

- There are no surgical measures specific to autism.

SYMPTOMATIC TREATMENT

- Behavioral therapy, sensory integration occupational therapy, auditory integration therapy, speech therapy, and cognitive therapy are options, as is vocational rehabilitation for older and higher functioning individuals.

ADJUNCTIVE TREATMENT

N/A

ADMISSION/DISCHARGE CRITERIA

- There are no admission/discharge criteria specific to autism, other than to ensure that the environment is safe and appropriate to the patient's level of functioning.

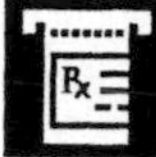

Medications

DRUG(S) OF CHOICE

- As of yet, there is no specific drug for autism (see Management-General Measures)

ALTERNATIVE DRUGS

N/A

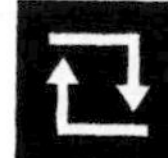

Follow-Up

PATIENT MONITORING

- Monitoring should include follow-up visits to monitor effects of drugs used to treat neuropsychiatric conditions associated with autism and to monitor for adequacy of behavioral intervention strategies.

EXPECTED COURSE AND PROGNOSIS

- Individuals with autism often slowly improve with regard to their impairments as they develop through school years and adolescence, but seldom improve to the point of independent functioning. Occasional patients will have a behavioral decline during adolescence, often associated with difficulty handling the increase in complexity of social interaction in adolescence. Improvement is greatest in individuals with better language skills and higher overall intelligence.

PATIENT EDUCATION

- Families should be informed of the importance of early intervention and should be given information on regional chapters of the Autism Society of America to help them locate other appropriate resources and support.
- Autism Society of America, 7910 Woodmont Avenue, Suite 300, Bethesda, MD 20814-3015. Phone: 1-800-3AUTISM, website: *www.autism-society.org*

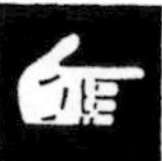

Miscellaneous

SYNONYMS

- Infantile autism
- Kanner's syndrome

ICD-9-CM: 299.00 Infantile autism current or active state

SEE ALSO: N/A

REFERENCES

- American Psychiatric Association. Diagnostic and Statistical Manual of Mental Disorders, 4th edition (DSM-IV). Washington, DC: American Psychiatric Association, 1995.
- Bauman ML, Kemper TL, eds. The neurobiology of autism. Baltimore, MD: The Johns Hopkins University Press, 1994:119–145.
- Filipek PA, Accardo PJ, Ashwal S, et al. Practice parameters: screening and diagnosis of autism. Report of the Quality Standards Subcommittee of the American Academy of Neurology and the Child Neurology Society. Neurology 2000;55:468–479.
- Naruse H, Ornitz EM, eds. Neurobiology of infantile autism. Amsterdam: Elsevier Science Publishers, 1992:43–57.
- Rapin I. Autism. N Engl J Med 1997;337: 97–104.

Author(s): David Q. Beversdorf, MD

Back Pain, Spondylosis, Lumbar Canal Stenosis

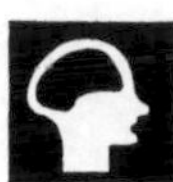

Basics

DESCRIPTION

- Lumbar spondylosis (LS) refers to degenerative changes including disc disease, osteophyte formation, facet joint disease, and ligamentous laxity, which can cause stenosis, segmental instability, and/or neurologic deficits. Lumbar canal stenosis (LCS) refers to a decrease in total area of spinal canal, lateral recess, or neural foramen. Other commonly used terms are spondylolisthesis (forward movement of one vertebral body in relation to the vertebral body below it) and spondylolysis (congenital or degenerative/posttraumatic absence of the pars interarticularis between the vertebral body and posterior bony spinal elements, frequently associated with spondylolisthesis).

EPIDEMIOLOGY

- About 80% of the adult population suffers from low back pain at some point during their lifetime. LS is one of the most frequent causes of low back and/or leg pain. The prevalence of LS by MRI studies ranges from 33% at age 20 to 95% in women >70. About 95% of males and 80% of females >65 show MRI evidence of LS. Plain radiographic evidence of LS is seen in about 80% of patients >65.
- Spondylosis is most frequent in the cervical and lumbar spine, the most mobile regions of the spinal column.
- LCS most commonly involves the L4-5 level, followed by L3-4, L2-3, L5-S1, and L1-2.

Age

- Both LS and LCS are seen with increasing frequency after the fifth decade of life.

Sex

- Males are affected more often than females.

ETIOLOGY

- LS results from a complex process of disc degeneration, bilateral facet joint arthropathy, and osteophyte formation. Facet joint cartilage destruction and capsular laxity lead to subluxation and segmental lumbar instability.
- LCS:
  —Congenital: idiopathic/achondroplastic
  —Acquired: degenerative stenosis
  -Iatrogenic: post lumbar fusion stenosis
  -Metabolic: Paget's disease, fluorosis
  -Posttraumatic
- Location of LCS: central canal/lateral recess/foraminal stenosis/far out foraminal stenosis (compression between L5 transverse process and sacral ala)
- Narrowing of spinal canal diameter in extension by hypertrophied facets, buckling of ligamentum flavum, and protruding intervertebral disc aggravates symptoms, which are relieved by flexion
- Etiology of neurogenic claudication: narrowed canal prevents vasodilation of blood vessels with activity, causing ischemic neuritis of the nerves

Genetics

N/A

RISK FACTORS

- Trauma

PREGNANCY

- Back pain is frequent during the third trimester of pregnancy (due to additional abdominal weight) and usually resolves postpartum.

ASSOCIATED CONDITIONS

- Cervical canal stenosis

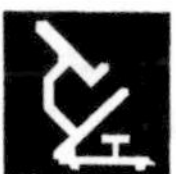

Diagnosis

DIFFERENTIAL DIAGNOSIS

- Vascular claudication
- Referred pain from leg, hip joint disease
- Lumbar disc disease
- Peripheral neuropathy (e.g., diabetes)
- Vertebral osteomyelitis
- Spinal tumors (bone tumors/metastasis)
- Myofascial syndromes

SIGNS AND SYMPTOMS

- Pain: midline low back pain (lumbar instability, paraspinal muscle spasm); radiculopathy (with lateral recess and foraminal stenosis); neurogenic claudication (pain; sensory and/or motor changes on standing and walking, relieved with rest and/or flexion)
- Absent or minimal neural signs. Neural deficits are reproducible with walking in LCS.
- Patients usually stoop forward to relieve symptoms (stoop sign) and may use a shopping cart to maintain flexion. Extension is limited and painful.
- Walking *down* stairs (i.e., extension) is more painful in LCS/neurogenic claudication; walking *up* stairs (i.e., flexion, exertion) is more painful in vascular claudication.
- Patients tend to walk with slight hip and knee flexion (simian stance).
- Straight-leg raising test usually is negative.
- Loss of lumbar lordosis is common.
- Examination of hip joints, abdomen, and peripheral vessels should be performed to rule out other etiologies or coexisting pathologies.

LABORATORY PROCEDURES

- CBC and differential; sedimentation rate; C-reactive protein to rule out infection or inflammatory process

IMAGING STUDIES

- Plain radiographs: Sagittal diameter of lumbar canal (normal 15–25 mm) is reduced below 12 mm in most patients with LCS. Lateral recess diameter (normal 3–5 mm) is reduced below 3 mm in patients with lateral recess stenosis. Foraminal height is reduced below 15 mm in patients with foraminal stenosis. Flexion-extension dynamic x-ray films may show subluxation of the involved spinal segments. Findings in LS include disc space narrowing, facet joint hypertrophy, LCS, foraminal stenosis, subluxation, and scoliosis.
- Myelography often reveals multiple areas of contrast compression (hourglass constriction). With lateral recess stenosis, myelography shows root sleeve cutoff. Complete block produces a characteristic paint brush appearance.
- CT with or without contrast provides details of the bony anatomy and may provide information necessary for complex cases. Patients with previous lumbar instrumentation may show less artifact on CT than MRI; those with implanted devices (e.g., cardiac pacemakers) may be limited to CT.
- MRI is the preferred imaging modality. It is noninvasive, highly sensitive, provides excellent soft-tissue resolution, and shows the extent of neural compression without risk of radiation. Asymptomatic degenerative changes may be seen in 60% of patients on MRI. Hypertrophied bone is low signal on T1 and T2 images, whereas hypertrophied ligamentum flavum is intermediate signal on T1 and T2 images.

SPECIAL TESTS

- Neurophysiologic studies (EMG and nerve conduction velocity [NCV]) can be very helpful in difficult cases of suspected peripheral neuropathy, nerve root compression, or paraspinous muscle syndromes. Somatosensory evoked potential recording also can be helpful, especially when performed before and after a walking stress test.

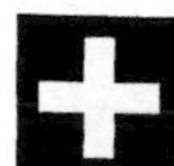

Management

GENERAL MEASURES

- Conservative measures are helpful in most patients with LS and about 50% of patients with LCS. Physical therapy (spinal exercises, traction, heat or cold pack application), weight reduction, or spinal epidural/foraminal injections can be tried in patients with LS or LCS. Flexion spinal exercises, which decrease lumbar lordosis, can be useful in patients with LCS. In LS patients with facet joint pain, facet joint injections are a useful option. A well-fitted lumbosacral corset can be helpful for low back pain secondary to instability.

SURGICAL MEASURES

- Indications for surgery include cauda equina syndrome, progressive neurologic deficits, and severe unrelenting pain. The onset of bowel or bladder dysfunction (incontinence or retention) is a surgical emergency, because permanent impairment in bowel or bladder function can quickly ensue. Surgery often is required in the presence of severe canal stenosis or segmental instability. Decompressive surgery (laminectomy, laminoforaminotomy, window laminotomy) of the stenotic segments by either open or endoscopic techniques is effective in most cases. Fusion should be considered for severe unrelenting back pain due to lumbar instability, or when stenosis requires complete excision of more than one facet joint at a particular level.

SYMPTOMATIC TREATMENT

- See General Measures

ADJUNCTIVE TREATMENT

- See General Measures and Surgical Measures

ADMISSION/DISCHARGE CRITERIA

- Emergent admission (and usually surgical treatment) is indicated for bowel or bladder dysfunction, sudden progressive neurologic deficits, or cauda equina syndrome.

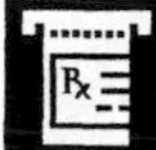

Medications

DRUG(S) OF CHOICE

- Nonsteroidal antiinflammatory drugs: ibuprofen, naproxen, celecoxib, rofecoxib

Contraindications

- Known history of gastrointestinal bleeding, hypersensitivity reaction to nonsteroidal antiinflammatory drugs, bronchial asthma

Precautions

- History of peptic ulcer, or renal, hepatic, or hematologic disease

ALTERNATIVE DRUGS

- Narcotic medications can be helpful for severe pain, and muscle relaxants for muscle spasms.

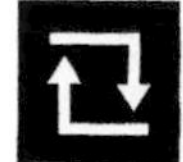

Follow-Up

PATIENT MONITORING

- Patients should be encouraged to keep a journal of activities performed and medication taken in order to have objective evidence of trends toward improvement or deterioration. Follow-up neurologic assessment should include, in addition to the standard motor and sensory examinations, the claudication distance in cases of LCS to assess progression of disease in functional terms. Serial EMG and/or NCV studies can be helpful to assess progression or improvement in selected cases.

EXPECTED COURSE AND PROGNOSIS

- About 50% of cases experience progressive worsening; 50% tend to be stationary or improve. About 80% of patients will have a satisfactory outcome after surgery; limited decompressive procedures (e.g., window laminotomy) have a quicker recovery time than more extensive decompressive surgery and/or fusion procedures. Operative morbidity ranges from 1%–2% up to 15%, depending upon the extensiveness of the procedure performed, initial versus reoperation, and the surgical risk status of the patient (e.g., age, medical conditions).

PATIENT EDUCATION

- Physical therapy can be very helpful in educating the patient about low back care, activities of daily living, risk avoidance, and use of walkers and other aids.

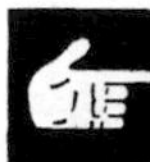

Miscellaneous

SYNONYMS

- Degenerative disc disease

ICD-9-CM: 724.02 Lumbar stenosis

SEE ALSO: N/A

REFERENCES

- An HS. Lumbar spinal stenosis. In: An HS, ed. Synopsis of spine surgery. Philadelphia: Lippincott Williams & Wilkins, 1998: 247–262.
- Beck CE, McCormack B, Weinstein PR. Surgical management of lumbar spinal stenosis. In: Schmidek HH, ed. Operative neurosurgical techniques, 4th ed. Philadelphia: WB Saunders, 2000:2207–2218.
- McColloch JA, Young PH. Microsurgery for lumbar spinal canal stenosis. In: McColloch JA, Young PH, eds. Essentials of spinal microsurgery. Philadelphia: Lippincott-Raven, 1998:453–486.
- Porter RW. Neurogenic claudication: its clinical presentations, differential diagnosis, pathology and management. In: Porter RW, ed. Management of back pain. New York: Churchill Livingstone, 1986: 110–121.
- Shields CB, Miller CA, Dunsker SB. Thoracic and lumbar spondylosis. In: Benzel E, ed. Spine surgery: techniques, complication avoidance and management. New York: Churchill Livingstone, 1999: 421–434.

Author(s): Raju S.V. Balabhadra, MD; Russell J. Andrews, MD

Bell's Palsy/Facial Palsy

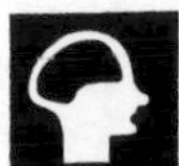

Basics

DESCRIPTION

- Facial palsy is a syndrome of weakness of the facial musculature that may be due to a number of causes. Bell's palsy was traditionally considered to be idiopathic.

EPIDEMIOLOGY

- Facial palsy is the most common of the cranial neuropathies. The majority of cases are Bell's palsy.

Incidence/Prevalence

- The incidence of Bell's palsy is estimated to be 23 per 100,000 annually. This disorder affects men and women equally. No differences in racial prevalence are known.

Etiology

- Significant evidence demonstrates that Bell's palsy is not idiopathic but rather due to infection with herpes simplex virus.

RISK FACTORS

- Diabetes mellitus

PREGNANCY

- Some studies show an increase in the incidence of Bell's palsy in the peripartum period.

ASSOCIATED CONDITIONS

- See Differential Diagnosis

Diagnosis

DIFFERENTIAL DIAGNOSIS

- The differential diagnosis of idiopathic facial palsy includes the numerous diseases that can injure the facial nerve by inflammation, infection, infiltration, compression, or trauma.
  —Neoplastic
    -Carcinomatous meningitis
    -Leukemic meningitis
    -Tumors (primary and metastatic) of the base of the skull
    -Parotid gland tumors
    -Cranial nerve VII (facial) neurinoma or cranial nerve VIII (acoustic) Schwannoma
  —Inflammatory or demyelinating
    -Sarcoidosis
    -Guillain-Barré syndrome
    -Multiple sclerosis
  —Infectious
    -HIV infection
    -Ramsey-Hunt syndrome (due to varicella-zoster infection)
    -Lyme disease
  —Idiopathic
    -Melkersson-Rosenthal syndrome (recurrent facial paralysis with facial edema, especially labial)
    -Idiopathic cranial polyneuropathy
    -Möbius syndrome
  —Trauma
    -Facial injuries
    -Basal skull fractures
    -Birth trauma
  —Metabolic
    -Diabetes mellitus
  —Pregnancy
  —Supranuclear facial palsy
    -Cerebrovascular accident
    -Pontine mass lesion

SIGNS AND SYMPTOMS

- Acute or subacute onset, often preceded by retroauricular pain and/or dysgeusia (impairment of taste)
- Half of patients reach maximal paralysis 48 hours after onset; the vast majority of cases by 5 days
- Followed by ipsilateral unilateral paralysis of facial muscles, partial or complete
- Subjective "numbness" or hypesthesia is present in branches of the trigeminal nerve on the same side
- Ipsilateral excess tearing or insufficient tearing
- Ipsilateral hyperacusis or distortion of sound indicating paralysis of the stapedius muscle (one third to one half)

LABORATORY PROCEDURES

- Complete blood count when infection is suspected
- Fasting blood glucose in the elderly population to screen for diabetes mellitus
- Lyme serology if history of tick bite, erythema migrans, or arthralgias

IMAGING STUDIES

- Routine imagine studies are not indicated for typical facial palsy with a normal otologic examination. CT and MRI of the temporal bone and posterior fossa should be considered in case of trauma, recurrent facial palsy, slowly progressive facial palsy, abnormal examination, or failure to show any improvement of paresis within 3 months.

SPECIAL TESTS

- Nerve conduction studies and EMG may help to distinguish a temporary conduction defect from denervation from axonal injury and may be useful in prognosis.

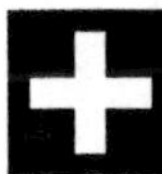

Management

GENERAL MEASURES

- General treatment includes treatment with a brief course of oral corticosteroids and oral acyclovir, reassurance regarding the generally favorable prognosis, and protection of the eye from drying and corneal exposure when eye closure is incomplete.

SURGICAL MEASURES

- Surgical decompression of the facial nerve is a standard approach to traumatic paralysis. Some recommend surgical exploration and decompression for idiopathic facial nerve palsy that does not improve after 3 months, but this is controversial and not well supported by evidence-based medicine.

SYMPTOMATIC TREATMENT

- Protection of the eye with lubricating agents and patching

ADJUNCTIVE TREATMENT

N/A

ADMISSION/DISCHARGE CRITERIA

N/A

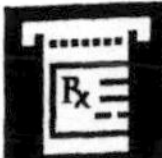

Medications

DRUG(S) OF CHOICE

- *Corticosteroids: prednisone.* Several different regimens proposed, all similar. May give 80 mg daily tapering in 20-mg increments over 10–12 days. Should be given in first 4 days but still is helpful after this time for relief of retroauricular pain.
- *Acyclovir* recommended at 400 mg five times per day for 10 days.

Contraindications

- Prednisone in known disseminated tuberculosis or fungal infections

Precautions

- Monitor blood glucose with prednisone use in diabetics; caution with acyclovir use in renal impairment or pregnancy.

ALTERNATIVE DRUGS

N/A

Follow-Up

PATIENT MONITORING

- Recheck after 1 month. Severe cases with poor eyelid closure should be seen monthly for 6–12 months to look for corneal abrasions.

EXPECTED COURSE AND PROGNOSIS

- High rate of spontaneous recovery (full, approximately 66%; moderate, 10%–12%; poor, 5%). Recovery typically begins in 3 weeks, may continue 6-9 months. Early recovery of some motor function within the first week is a very favorable prognostic sign.
- Better prognosis associated with incomplete paralysis, younger age group, nondiabetic
- Presence of pain has no prognostic value, but severe pain associated with Ramsay-Hunt syndrome
- Complications include facial weakness, aberrant regeneration with synkinesis, corneal abrasion, facial contractures, postparalytic hemifacial spasm (rare), tearing problems

PATIENT EDUCATION

- Eye protection
- Website: *www.ninds.nih.gor/patients/disorder/bells.htm*

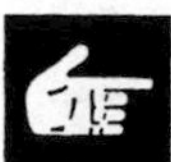

Miscellaneous

SYNONYMS

- Idiopathic facial palsy (questionable term now that there is significant evidence of viral causation)

ICD-9-CM: 351.0 Bell's palsy

SEE ALSO: N/A

REFERENCES

- Dyck PJ, Thomas PK, et al., eds. Peripheral neuropathy, 3rd ed. Philadelphia: WB Saunders, 1993.
- Jackson CG, von Doersten P. The facial nerve. Med Clin North Am 1999;83: 179–195.
- Roob G, Fazekas F, Hartung H. Peripheral facial palsy: etiology, diagnosis and treatment. Eur Neurol 1999;41:3–9.

Author(s): Ronnie Bergen, MD

Botulism

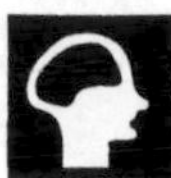

Basics

DESCRIPTION

- Botulism is an acute paralytic condition resulting from intoxication with a neuromuscular blocking agent that is produced by the anaerobic bacterium *Clostridium botulinum*. Currently, five clinical forms are recognized:
  - —Foodborne (adult)
  - —Infant
  - —Wound
  - —Hidden
  - —Inadvertent

EPIDEMIOLOGY

- Between 1973 and 1996, an annual median number of 24 cases of foodborne botulism, 3 cases of wound botulism, and 71 cases of infant botulism were reported to the CDC. Over the past decade, an increase in wound botulism has appeared among IV drug users. The numbers of cases of hidden and inadvertent botulism secondary to botulinum toxin injections remain very small.

ETIOLOGY

- Most potent toxin known
- Seven forms, A–G
- Neuromuscular blockade caused by irreversible binding of toxin to presynaptic terminal of acetylcholinergic neurons. This causes a decrease in number of acetylcholine quanta that are released.
- Number of quanta are insufficient for depolarization of adjacent nerve terminal and propagation of action potential.
- Most cases of foodborne caused by types A and B (E associated with seafood)
- Half of adult cases are caused by type A
- Infant botulism usually caused by types A and B
- Most cases of wound botulism caused by type A
- Botulinum toxin (BOTOX) for injection is purified type A

Genetics

N/A

RISK FACTORS

- Foodborne
  - —Ingestion of foods that contain preformed toxin
  - —Low-acid foods with anaerobic environment, e.g., poorly preserved meat, fish, potatoes, or vegetables
  - —Toxin is heat labile, but spores are heat resistant
- Wound
  - —Germination of spores and toxin formation in anaerobic wound environment
  - —Toxin may be absorbed through mucous membranes or inhalation
- Infant
  - —Immature infant GI tract can allow spores to germinate and produce toxin
  - —Honey often harbors *C. botulinum* spores
- Hidden botulism
  - —Occurs in adults with GI tract abnormality, e.g., achlorhydria or Crohn's disease
  - —Abnormal GI environment allows germination of spores and formation of toxin

PREGNANCY

- There is no evidence that maternal botulism can be transmitted to the fetus. The high molecular weight of botulinum molecule prevents it from diffusing across the placenta. The reported cases of maternal botulism did not indicate that the condition appeared in the fetus. Additionally, in reported cases of mothers who were given therapeutic injections of purified botulinum toxin there were no adverse effects on the fetus. It is not clear whether breast-feeding has a protective effect in cases of infant botulism.

ASSOCIATED CONDITIONS

N/A

Diagnosis

DIFFERENTIAL DIAGNOSIS

- Myasthenia gravis
- Landry-Guillain-Barré (LGB) syndrome
- Polio
- Tick bite paralysis
- Diphtheritic neuropathy
- Lambert-Eaton syndrome
- Hypokalemic periodic paralysis
- The clinical picture usually serves to differentiate among these disorders. Foodborne botulism is almost invariably preceded by prominent GI symptoms that are an important diagnostic clue. Botulism may be differentiated from LGB syndrome by the relative preservation of deep tendon reflexes and normal CSF in the former. Diphtheritic neuropathy occurs in the setting of a history of signs and symptoms of diphtheria, i.e., pharyngitis and tonsillar exudate. Both myasthenia and Lambert-Eaton syndrome are associated with autoimmune antibodies that can be assayed. Additionally, an edrophonium hydrochloride test in patients with botulism usually is negative. Poliomyelitis tends to present as an acute febrile syndrome with headache and meningismus.

SIGNS AND SYMPTOMS

- Incubation period several hours to 8 days
- Peak onset 18–36 hours after ingestion

GI Symptoms

- Nausea, vomiting
- Cramps, diarrhea
- Constipation is a later manifestation

Neurologic Symptoms

- Diplopia
- Ptosis
- Dysarthria
- Dysphagia
- Dysphonia
- Descending weakness
- Respiratory compromise
- Autonomic (xerostomia, pupillary dysfunction, postural hypotension, urinary retention)
- Neurologic presentation of wound botulism or hidden botulism is similar to that of foodborne botulism, except there is no prominent GI prodrome or history of ingestion of contaminated food. The incubation period for wound botulism is longer than that of foodborne intoxication, ranging from a few days to 2 weeks.

Infant Botulism

- Usually occurs in infants <6 months of age
- Early signs are constipation, weak cry, and poor sucking or feeding
- Progression to loss of head control, limb and bulbar weakness, respiratory distress
- Patients who develop inadvertent botulism from therapeutic injections of purified botulinum toxin can manifest generalized weakness and/or autonomic dysfunction similar to that seen in foodborne botulism.

LABORATORY PROCEDURES

- Clinical diagnosis is confirmed by the presence of botulinum toxin in the patient's blood, stool. or wound exudate. This is done via the mouse inoculation test, in which mice that received injections of samples of substances (e.g., foods, body fluids) thought to contain toxin are inoculated with type-specific botulinum antibodies. Clinical signs of botulism then develop in mice in which the toxin is not neutralized. Additionally, *C. botulinum* organisms may be isolated from the stool of about 60% of patients with botulism. In cases of foodborne botulism, toxin may be recovered from the contaminated food.

IMAGING STUDIES

- Neuroimaging studies in cases of botulism should be normal and help to differentiate from other causes of bulbar symptoms, such as brainstem stroke.

SPECIAL TESTS

- The most common EMG abnormality seen in muscles affected by botulism is a small muscle action potential in response to a single supramaximal nerve stimulus. The amplitude of the muscle action potential is reduced, but conduction velocities are normal. Some degree of posttetanic facilitation may be present, but not to the same degree as is seen in Lambert-Eaton syndrome. CSF analysis should be normal.

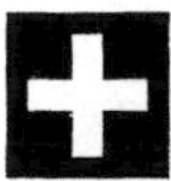

Management

GENERAL MEASURES

- Supportive treatment
- ICU monitoring until respiratory function is stable
- Assisted ventilation may be needed for several months, but usually only for a few weeks
- Gastric lavage may be useful if toxin ingestion was recent
- Pulmonary toilet
- Skin care
- Bowel and bladder protocol
- Report to state health agency and CDC (phone: 404-639-2206)

SURGICAL MEASURES

- Debride wound
- Antibiotics as needed

SYMPTOMATIC TREATMENT

- Dysphagia
  —Tube feedings
  —Swallowing therapy
  —Special diets
- Urinary retention and constipation
  —Intermittent straight catheterization
  —Stool softeners
  —Timed evacuation

ADJUNCTIVE TREATMENT

- May need to turn and position the patient frequently to prevent skin breakdown, and use decubitus-preventing mattresses or circulating fluid beds. Physical and occupational therapy should be instituted as early as possible to prevent contractures, promote mobility, and maximize function in activities of daily living.

ADMISSION/DISCHARGE CRITERIA

- All patients with suspected botulism should be admitted and monitored closely, particularly those with recent onset of symptoms. Patients may be discharged to home or a long-term care facility, depending upon degree of residual motor and/or respiratory deficit.

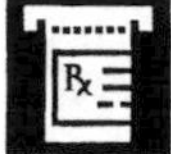

Medications

DRUG(S) OF CHOICE

- The only specific medications for treatment of botulism are antitoxins. Two botulinum antitoxins currently are available for treatment of adult botulism. The trivalent form has antibodies to toxin types A, B, and E; the bivalent only to types A and B. The antitoxin only neutralizes circulating toxin that has not yet bound to nerve terminals; thus, it is most effective when given as early as possible in the course of the illness. Current recommended dose is one vial of bivalent or trivalent antitoxin administered IV, with additional doses as needed. One vial also may be given intramuscularly to provide a reservoir of antitoxin. Antitoxin is distributed by the CDC through regional distribution stations. The bivalent and trivalent antitoxins are equine-derived products and are not recommended for treatment of infant botulism because of concerns with hypersensitivity reactions. A human-derived immune globulin is available from the California Department of Health Services (510-540-2646) for treatment of infant botulism.

Contraindications

- Antitoxin should not be administered to persons with known hypersensitivity to equine-derived products.

Precautions

- All patients should undergo skin or eye testing for hypersensitivity reactions prior to administration of antitoxin. Epinephrine solution should be available for immediate injection.

ALTERNATIVE DRUGS

N/A

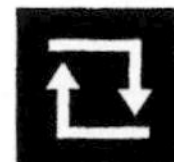

Follow-Up

PATIENT MONITORING

- Patients should be monitored in an ICU setting until respiratory function has stabilized. Respiratory care and rehabilitation in a long-term care facility may be required.

EXPECTED COURSE AND PROGNOSIS

- The majority of patients with botulism make a full functional recovery, but this may take several weeks to months, as recovery depends on the formation of new motor end plates at the neuromuscular junction. Current mortality rates are 5%–10%. Studies have reported shorter hospital stays and decreased mortality for patients who received botulinum antitoxin within the first 24 hours of symptom onset, compared to patients who received later administration or no antitoxin.

PATIENT EDUCATION

N/A

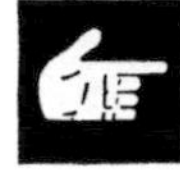

Miscellaneous

SYNONYMS

N/A

ICD-9-CM: 005.1 Botulism

SEE ALSO: N/A

REFERENCES

- Bakheit AMO, Ward CD, McLellan DL. Generalized botulism-like syndrome after intramuscular injections of botulinum type A: a report of two cases. J Neurol Neurosurg Psychiatry 1997;62:198.
- Boskamp JR, Kimura Y, Bomback FM. Breast feeding and infant botulism. J Pediatr 1982;102:1015.
- Cherington M. Clinical spectrum of botulism. Muscle Nerve 1998;21:701–710.
- Chia JK, Clark JB, Ryan CA, et al. Botulism in an adult associated with food borne intestinal infection with *Clostridium botulinum*. N Engl J Med 1986;315: 239–241.
- Robin L, Herman D, Redett R. Botulism in a pregnant woman. N Engl J Med 1996;335: 823–824.
- Shapiro R, Hatheway C, Swerdlow DL. Botulism in the US: a clinical and epidemiologic review. Ann Intern Med 1998;129:221–228.
- Tacket CO, Shandera WX, Mann JM, et al. Equine antitoxin use and other factors that predict outcome in type A foodborne botulism. Am J Med 1984;76:794–798.

Author(s): Barbara S. Giesser, MD

Brain Abscess

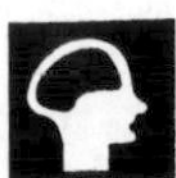

Basics

DESCRIPTION

- Brain abscesses begin as a localized area of cerebritis that develops into a focal parenchymal infection characterized by a capsularized collection of pus.

EPIDEMIOLOGY

- There are 1,500–2,500 cases diagnosed annually in the United States, with slight male predilection and median age of 30–40.

ETIOLOGY

- Brain abscesses arise by three main etiologies: local contiguous spread, hematogenous dissemination, and traumatic injury. The most common causes of brain abscesses are related to uncontrolled infections of the paranasal sinuses, middle ear, mastoid cells, and teeth. The cause is cryptogenic in 20%–30% of cases.
- For patients with a sinus source, aerobic and anaerobic streptococci, as well as *Haemophilus* sp, *Bacteroides* sp, and *Fusobacterium* sp, would be suspected. Prior otitis media or mastoiditis suggests *Bacteroides* sp, streptococci, Pseudomonaceae, or Enterobacteriaceae. Dental infections often predispose to brain abscesses with *Fusobacterium, Prevotella,* and *Bacteroides* spp and streptococci. Prior neurosurgery or penetrating head trauma would suggest Staphylococci, Enterobacteriaceae, *Clostridium* sp, or Pseudomonaceae.

Genetics

N/A

RISK FACTORS

- Risk factors include penetrating head trauma, neurosurgery, untreated bacterial otitis or sinusitis, dental infection, cyanotic congenital heart disease, and immunosuppression.

PREGNANCY

N/A

ASSOCIATED CONDITIONS

- Immunocompromised patients have a broadened differential diagnosis, including bacteria, fungi, protozoa, and helminths. Mucormycosis is classically seen in diabetics with acidemia who are severely systemically ill. *Nocardia* is associated with defects in cell-mediated immunity. Fungal infections are found more commonly in people who are immunosuppressed, taking corticosteroids, or have received broad-spectrum antibiotics. *Pseudallescheria boydii* or *Scedosporium apiospermum* often occurs after a near drowning. *Mycobacteria tuberculosis* brain abscesses occur in individuals with disseminated TB or those from endemic areas. *Aspergillus* brain abscesses may present as an acute cerebrovascular accident in an immunocompromised host. The most common cause of brain abscess in AIDS patients is toxoplasmosis.

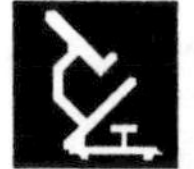

Diagnosis

DIFFERENTIAL DIAGNOSIS

- Conditions that mimic brain abscess include
  —Neoplasm
  —Cerebral hemorrhage
  —Acute cerebrovascular infarction

SIGNS AND SYMPTOMS

- The classic triad includes fever, headache, and focal neurologic deficit; however, it is present in <50% of patients. Presenting symptoms in order of decreasing frequency include
  —Headache
  —Mental status changes (disorientation, confusion, lethargy, neuropsychiatric complaints)
  —Focal neurologic deficits, depending upon the location of the abscess (motor, sensory or speech disorders, visual field defects, ataxia)
  —Fever
  —Seizures, focal and generalized
  —Nausea and vomiting
  —Nuchal rigidity
  —Papilledema
- Sudden worsening of a preexisting headache or new-onset meningismus may signal rupture of the abscess into the ventricles, an often fatal complication. Immunocompromised patients may have an occult presentation due to a decreased inflammatory response.

LABORATORY PROCEDURES

- Abscess aspirate should be sent for
  —Gram stain
  —Aerobic and anaerobic culture
  —Fungal stain and cultures
  —Acid-fast stain and culture
  —Modified acid-fast stain *(Nocardia)*
- Serum toxoplasmosis IgG titer should be obtained in immunocompromised patients. Routine blood cultures are infrequently positive but may be the only diagnostic data in patients requiring urgent antibiotics. Lumbar puncture is of low yield and risks brain herniation.

IMAGING STUDIES

- Imaging has improved the diagnosis of, and decreased the mortality from, brain abscesses. CT shows ring-enhancing lesion(s) with variable surrounding edema. Contrast-enhanced MRI is more sensitive and can differentiate abscess from early cerebritis. Radionuclide scans are sometimes of benefit when CT or MRI is inconclusive. PET scanning may be able to differentiate neoplasm from infection.

SPECIAL TESTS

- Sterotactic brain biopsy, aspiration, or excision may be necessary. The source of the brain abscess should be sought. Appropriate workup includes a thorough physical examination, with special attention to ears, mastoids, sinuses, and teeth. Consideration should be given to sinus imaging, chest x-ray film, dental x-ray film, or possibly echocardiography.

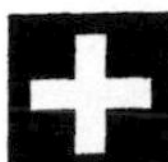

Management

GENERAL MEASURES

- Antimicrobial treatment is chosen to cover for predisposing conditions, presumed source, and gram stain. Therapy is then adjusted for culture data.

SURGICAL MEASURES

- Neurosurgical consultation should be obtained. Potential needs include radiographically guided aspiration, burr hole placement and aspiration, or craniotomy and excision (especially if the abscess is >2.5 cm).

SYMPTOMATIC TREATMENT

- Patients may require pain management and seizure precautions. Some experts recommend routine antiepileptic medications.

ADJUNCTIVE TREATMENT

- Steroids (e.g., dexamethasone 6–12 mg q6h) are indicated if the patient has significant edema or mass effect. Steroids may decrease response to antimicrobial treatment and should be tapered as soon as feasible. Elevated intracranial pressure may additionally require IV mannitol or induced hyperventilation.

ADMISSION/DISCHARGE CRITERIA

- The majority of patients with brain abscess will require inpatient admission for definitive diagnosis and initial treatment. Discharge is possible when the diagnosis is secure, the patient is stable or improving, and a plan for outpatient treatment has been finalized (i.e., IV or PO antimicrobials).

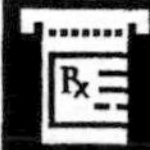

Medications

DRUG(S) OF CHOICE

- Treatment depends on the likely causative agent. In a bacterial abscess of unclear etiology, a third-generation cephalosporin (e.g., ceftriaxone 2 g IV q12h) and metronidazole (500 mg IV q6h) would be appropriate empiric therapy. Ceftazidime or cefepime would be used instead of ceftriaxone if *Pseudomonas aeruginosa* was suspected. Initial therapy in an immunocompromised patient should be chosen in consultation with an infectious disease specialist.
- Other predisposing conditions and suggested initial antibiotic regimens include
  - —Otitis media, mastoiditis, or sinusitis: metronidazole and a third-generation cephalosporin
  - —Dental source: penicillin (2–4 million units q4h) and metronidazole
  - —Penetrating trauma or neurosurgery: vancomycin (1 g q12h with dose adjustment to serum levels) and third-generation cephalosporin ± metronidazole

Contraindications

- Known hypersensitivity to a particular antibiotic
- Fluoroquinolones are not recommended due to a lack of data. Antimicrobials administered should penetrate the blood–brain barrier.

Precautions

- Use caution in choosing empiric therapy that may lower the seizure threshold (e.g., high-dose β-lactams).

ALTERNATIVE DRUGS

- Trimethoprim-sulfa 15 mg/kg divided tid would be added for a patient with concomitant lung pathology and suspected *Nocardia* sp infection.

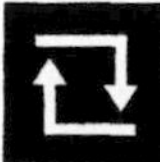

Follow-Up

PATIENT MONITORING

- Serial imaging is necessary to monitor for improvement or progression. Serial laboratory monitoring is determined by the specific toxicities of the antimicrobial agents chosen.

EXPECTED COURSE AND PROGNOSIS

- Prognosis depends on the rapidity of diagnosis and appropriate treatment, as well as the mental status of the patient upon presentation. If treatment is initiated while the patient is alert, expected mortality is 5%–10%. Mortality rises significantly to >50% if the patient is comatose when treatment is initiated. Approximately 30% of surviving patients have residual neurologic deficits such as focal epilepsy.

PATIENT EDUCATION

- Some experts recommend at least 3 months of antiepileptic therapy with a normal EEG prior to discontinuation. Driving may be affected.

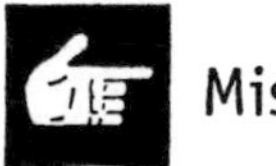

Miscellaneous

SYNONYMS

N/A

ICD-9-CM: 324.0 Brain abscess

SEE ALSO: N/A

REFERENCES

- Clafee DP, Wispelwey B. Brain abscess. Semin Neurol 2000;20:353–360.
- Mathisen GE, Johnson JP. Brain abscess. Clin Infect Dis 1997;25:763–781.
- Osenbach RK, Loftus CM. Diagnosis and management of brain abscess. Neurosurg Clin N Am 1992;3:403–420.
- Tunkel AR, Wispelwey B, Scheld WM. Brain abscess. In: Mandell GL, Bennett JE, Dolin R, eds. Mandell, Douglas and Bennett's principles and practice of infectious disease, 5th ed. Philadelphia: Churchill Livingstone, 2000:1016–1028.

Author(s): Ruth Mullowney-Agra, MD

Brain Death

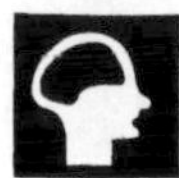

Basics

DESCRIPTION

- Brain death is defined as the irreversible loss of function of the entire brain, including the brainstem. Brain death was first proposed as a criterion of death in 1968 and was endorsed in 1981 by the President's Commission for the Study of Ethical Problems in Medicine and Biomedical and Behavioral Research. In the United States, properly documented brain death meets the legal standard for the declaration of death.

EPIDEMIOLOGY

Incidence/Prevalence

- Unknown

Race

- No ethnic predominance

Age

- May occur at any age. *Special criteria for determining brain death in children <5 years have been published.*

Sex

- No difference in males or females

ETIOLOGY

- Brain death resulting from a primary neurologic disease is most often caused by severe head trauma, hemorrhage, or ischemic strokes causing herniation. Infectious causes include severe cases of meningoencephalitis and abscesses resulting in herniation. The most common non-neurologic etiology is hypoxic-ischemic coma due to cardiorespiratory arrest, although other causes of severe encephalopathy, such as fulminant hepatic encephalopathy, also may cause brain death.

Genetics

N/A

RISK FACTORS

N/A

PREGNANCY

- Brain death occurring during pregnancy is a complex and controversial issue. There is a general consensus that attempts to maintain the brain-dead maternal body are appropriate if there is a reasonable possibility of delivering a healthy fetus. Who should make medical decisions is less clear: if the patient is married, the husband is generally considered the most appropriate surrogate decision maker; if unmarried, both the father of the fetus (if identified and involved) and the mother's immediate family should be included in the decision-making process. The basis for decision making also is controversial: many consider the interests of the fetus to be paramount, but others believe that the mother's interests are equally important.

ASSOCIATED CONDITIONS

N/A

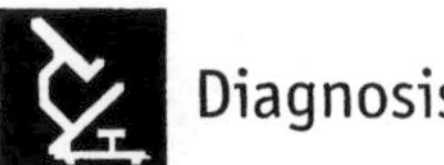

Diagnosis

DIFFERENTIAL DIAGNOSIS

- Conditions that resemble brain death
  - —Severe coma with minimal residual cortical or brainstem function
- Conditions that may interfere with diagnosing brain death
  - —Hypothermia (core temperature <32°C)
  - —Drug intoxication, poisoning, or severe metabolic derangements
- Conditions that interfere with the clinical diagnosis of brain death
  - —Severe facial trauma or preexisting pupillary abnormalities
  - —Sleep apnea or severe pulmonary disease; may preclude apnea testing

SIGNS AND SYMPTOMS

- Brain death is a clinical diagnosis. Confirmatory tests are optional unless the full clinical examination cannot be performed or provides ambiguous information, in which case the diagnosis will depend on appropriate confirmatory tests.
- Brain death is the absence of clinical brain function when the proximate cause is known and demonstrably irreversible. The diagnosis can be made only when the following are present:
  - —Clinical or neuroimaging evidence of an acute CNS catastrophe compatible with the diagnosis of brain death
  - —Exclusion of the following conditions
    - -Severe metabolic disturbances that may confound clinical assessment
    - -Drug intoxication or poisoning
    - -Hypothermia
- The three cardinal clinical findings in brain death are
  - —Unresponsiveness, including the absence of cerebral motor response to painful stimulation
  - —Absence of all brainstem reflexes, including pupillary response to bright light, oculocephalic and oculovestibular responses, corneal reflexes, jaw jerk, facial grimacing, gag reflex, and cough reflex to deep suctioning
  - —Apnea
    - -Apnea testing should be performed according to the AAN statement (Neurology 1995;45:1012–1014).
- The diagnosis of brain death requires two complete examinations consistent with brain death performed approximately 6 hours apart. The interval between examinations may be adjusted depending on the clinical situation.

LABORATORY PROCEDURES

- Blood and urine tests to exclude potentially reversible toxic/metabolic causes of severely diminished brain function
  - —Blood and urine toxicology screens
  - —Electrolytes, BUN, creatinine, glucose, liver function tests
  - —Additional laboratory tests may be appropriate when the etiology of coma is unclear after initial workup

IMAGING STUDIES

- Imaging studies to document the absence of intracerebral blood flow may be used to confirm the diagnosis of brain death.
  - —Cerebral radionuclide angiography demonstration of absence of intracerebral blood flow confirms the diagnosis. Conversely, the presence of intracerebral blood flow indicates that the individual is not brain dead. Minimal blood flow in a patient who meets clinical brain death criteria usually will disappear within 12–24 hours, so repeat testing may be appropriate.
  - —Conventional angiography: In brain death, intracerebral arterial blood flow will be absent, whereas external carotid circulation remains patent.

SPECIAL TESTS

- EEG documenting electrocerebral silence (ECS), i.e., a "flat EEG," for a minimum of 30 minutes utilizing appropriate recording technique as adopted by the American Electroencephalographic Society (AES) is consistent with the diagnosis of brain death. Because ECS may also be seen in patients with sedative overdose, hypothermia, or severe cerebral injury with residual brainstem function, the EEG must be interpreted in the context of the clinical evaluation.
- Transcranial Doppler ultrasonography may provide support for the diagnosis of brain death, but excellent technique and significant experience are required.
- Somatosensory evoked potentials (SSEPs) demonstrating bilateral absence of N20-P22 response with median nerve stimulation supports the diagnosis of brain death; however, the clinical value of SSEPs remains limited.

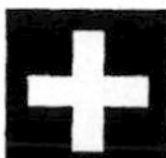

Management

GENERAL MEASURES

- Management must be separated into two phases: management of a patient who is being evaluated for possible brain death, but not yet declared brain dead; and management of a patient who has been declared brain dead. If the patient is a pregnant woman, this will influence the management of the patient.
- A pregnant woman who may be brain dead should be evaluated by an obstetrician to assess the gestational age, viability, and health of the fetus. Aggressive treatment should be continued while a decision is made as to how to manage the pregnancy. The involvement of a medical intensivist, an obstetrician, a neonatologist, and ethics consultant in the decision-making process is recommended.
- Nonpregnant patients being evaluated for possible brain death should be managed according to standard practice for their underlying neurologic or medical problems.
- Decisions about the aggressiveness of treatment, including establishing do-not-resuscitate (DNR) status, should made according to standard practice.
- The family should be informed when brain death evaluation is initiated. They should be advised of the severity of the neurologic injury, the possibility that the patient may be brain dead, and the fact that brain death is a legal definition of death throughout the United States.
  —In certain states (e.g., New York, New Jersey), if a family has a religious objection to using brain death criteria to determine death (e.g., some Orthodox Jews), the physician is legally obligated to respect this decision and use only the traditional cardiorespiratory criteria to determine death for such patients. In most states, although religious objections to brain death do not have legal support, sensitivity to these issues is important, and pastoral and ethics consultation should be obtained if the family indicates they have such an objection.
  —The possibility that a patient may qualify as an organ donor should not alter the medical care or decision-making process of the medical personnel.
  —Nevertheless, some families may strongly desire that their loved one, if brain dead, become an organ donor, and this may influence their decision-making process (e.g., continuing "futile" care to permit a nearly brain-dead patient to become brain dead).
  —Brain death determination itself should generally be performed by, or in consultation with, a physician experienced in the matter, usually a neurologist, neurosurgeon, or intensivist.
  —Pastoral care to provide support for the family often is helpful.
  —Ethics consultation may be beneficial if there are conflicts or disagreements between the family and the medical team.
  —Hospitals must contact their designated organ procurement organization (OPO) in a timely manner about individuals who die or whose death is imminent. It is optimal to contact the OPO when brain death evaluation is initiated or when the first examination is consistent with brain death.
- The time of death is the time of the second brain death evaluation.
  —The family should be immediately informed of the diagnosis.
- Hospitals must collaborate with the OPO to ensure that the family of every potential donor is informed of the option to donate organs or tissues.
  —If the family declines organ donation, all medical treatments should be discontinued and the patient should be extubated. It is not appropriate to ask the family's consent to discontinue treatment.
  —If the family consents to organ donation, medical treatment of the patient should continue according to the standard hospital protocol for an organ donor until the organs can be harvested.

SURGICAL MEASURES

N/A

SYMPTOMATIC TREATMENT

N/A

ADJUNCTIVE TREATMENTS

N/A

ADMISSION/DISCHARGE CRITERIA

- Brain death evaluation is generally performed in hospitalized patients.

Medications

DRUG(S) OF CHOICE

N/A

ALTERNATIVE DRUGS

N/A

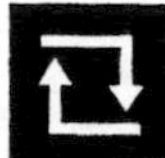

Follow-up

PATIENT MONITORING

N/A

EXPECTED COURSE AND PROGNOSIS

N/A

PATIENT EDUCATION

- Website: *www.organdonor.gov/*

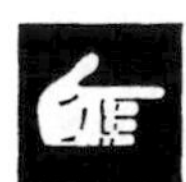

Miscellaneous

SYNONYMS

N/A

ICD-9-CM: N/A. The diagnosis should be coded according to the underlying process resulting in brain death.

SEE ALSO: N/A

REFERENCES

- Bernat JL, Culver CM, Gert B. On the definition and criterion of death. Ann Intern Med 1981;94:389–394.
- Field DR, Gates EA, Creasy RK, et al. Maternal brain death during pregnancy. JAMA 1988;260:816–822.
- Report of the Ad Hoc Committee of the Harvard Medical School to Examine the Definition of Brain Death. A definition of irreversible coma. JAMA 1968;205: 337–340.
- Report of the Medical Consultants on the Diagnosis of Brain Death to the President's Commission for the Study of Ethical Problems in Medicine and Biomedical and Behavioral Research. Guidelines for the Determination of Death. JAMA 1981; 246:2184–2186.
- Report of the Quality Standards Subcommittee of the American Academy of Neurology. Practice parameters for determining brain death in adults. Neurology 1995;45:1012–1014.
- Task Force for the Determination of Brain Death in Children. Guidelines for the determination of brain death in children. Neurology 1987;37:1077–1078.
- Wijdicks EFM. Determining brain death in adults. Neurology 1995;45:1003–1011.

Author(s): Robert M. Taylor, MD

Brain Tumor, Acoustic Schwannoma

Basics

DESCRIPTION

- Acoustic schwannomas are extraaxial benign neoplasms that arise from the vestibular branch of the eighth cranial nerve in the cerebellopontine angle (CPA) region, near the porus acusticus. They typically are slow growing, with a growth rate of 1–2 mm/year. In some cases, especially older patients, the tumor may remain dormant. There are three stages of growth: canalicular, cisternal, and brainstem compressive. In late stages of growth, the seventh cranial nerve becomes draped over the mass as it grows into the cistern toward the brainstem.

EPIDEMIOLOGY

Incidence/Prevalence

- Schwannomas account for 6%–8% of all primary brain tumors. The majority of schwannomas (85%–90%) are of the acoustic type and usually are unilateral (95%). The annual incidence is 1 per 100,000 persons. Bilateral tumors occur in patients with neurofibromatosis (NF) type II.

Race

- All races and ethnic groups equally affected.

Age

- Typical presentation is between 44 and 64 years.

Sex

- Females have a higher incidence than males (1.5:1).

ETIOLOGY

- The cells of origin of acoustic schwannomas are transformed Schwann cells from the eighth cranial nerve. In most cases, the initial genesis of transformation is unknown. The tumor appears as a discrete, rounded, encapsulated mass of a milky white color, arising from a nerve fascicle. Microscopically, schwannomas have biphasic architecture, with Antoni A and B regions. Antoni A is most common, with features of dense compact rows of elongated spindle-shaped cells; Antoni B regions demonstrate loosely organized areas of stellate cells, lipid, and microcystic change. Mitoses and nuclear pleomorphism may be seen. Abnormalities of chromosome 22 are common, including monosomy and alterations of the long arm (i.e., deletions, inversions, translocations).

Genetics

- The majority of acoustic schwannomas are sporadic and unilateral. Approximately 5% can develop in association with NF type I or II. In all NF-related tumors and between 65% and 70% of sporadic tumors, there are mutations of a tumor suppressor gene located at 22q12, the NF2 gene, which codes for a protein, schwannomin, which interacts with cytoskeletal proteins involved in regulation of cell adhesion and proliferation.

RISK FACTORS

- There are no known risk factors for acoustic schwannomas except for NF types I and II. Prior cranial radiation may be causally related in rare cases.

PREGNANCY

- Pregnancy has not been shown to affect the clinical course of acoustic schwannomas.

ASSOCIATED CONDITIONS

- NF type I, NF type II

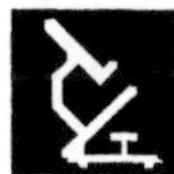

Diagnosis

DIFFERENTIAL DIAGNOSIS

- Acoustic schwannomas account for 80% of tumors in the CPA region. Differential diagnosis includes other masses or processes that can cause a progressive syndrome in the CPA: meningioma, epidermoid cyst, exophytic brainstem glioma, ependymoma, choroid plexus papilloma, schwannomas of other cranial nerves (V, VII, IX, X, XI), jugular foramen paraganglioma, metastatic tumor, vascular processes (aneurysm, arteriovenous malformation), and abscess.

SIGNS AND SYMPTOMS

- Common symptoms include unilateral sensory hearing loss (96%), unsteadiness (77%), tinnitus (71%), headache (29%), mastoid pain or otalgia (28%), facial numbness, diplopia, and vertigo. Mean time from onset of symptoms to diagnosis is 3.7 years. Loss of hearing and balance is slow and gradual in most cases. Tinnitus typically is unilateral, mild, and constant.
- Common neurologic signs include unilateral sensorineural hearing loss in 90%–95% of patients. Preserved hearing suggests the tumor will be <1.5 cm. In 50% of patients at presentation, hearing loss is the solitary neurologic sign. Gait is either normal or only mildly affected. Large tumors (>3 cm) can cause gait ataxia, dysmetria, nystagmus, facial hypesthesia, and papilledema.

LABORATORY PROCEDURES

- Screening tests that sometimes are used before MRI or CT in patients with hearing loss include pure tone audiometry, speech discrimination assessment, and auditory evoked brainstem responses (AEBR). In 60%–70% of patients, high-frequency loss is present on audiometry. Speech discrimination is abnormal in 45%–80% of cases. AEBR is the most sensitive nonimaging test and shows delayed latency or loss of wave V in approximately 95% of patients.

IMAGING STUDIES

- MRI, with and without gadolinium contrast, is the most critical diagnostic test; axial and coronal enhanced images should be obtained. MRI is more sensitive than CT for small intracanalicular tumors and vascular structures, although both modalities properly visualize large masses. The tumor usually is isointense to brain on T1 images but hyperintense on T2 images. Schwannomas enhance densely after administration of gadolinium. An MRI negative for an enhancing mass in the internal auditory canal rules out an acoustic schwannoma.

SPECIAL TESTS

- Intraoperative monitoring of cranial nerves V, VII, and XI during surgical resection is an excellent method for reducing morbidity of these nerves. Monitoring of cranial nerve VIII remains controversial; it may reduce morbidity during resection of tumors <2 cm.

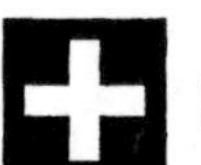

Management

GENERAL MEASURES

- In certain patient cohorts, tumors are followed conservatively after diagnosis, including patients in poor health, elderly patients with small lesions (<10 mm) or who are reluctant to proceed to surgery, and any patient with poor hearing in the contralateral ear. Tumors are likely to remain quiescent if they remain stable during the initial observation period (usually 6 months). Conservative approaches are unjustified in most young patients due to accelerated growth rates.

SURGICAL MEASURES

- Complete surgical resection is the treatment of choice in most patients. Tumors <1 cm in diameter are most likely to be completely resected while preserving cranial nerve function. Three surgical approaches are commonly used, the choice of technique depends on tumor size, depth of internal auditory canal penetration, hearing status, exposure of the facial nerve, and patient age.

The suboccipital or retrosigmoid approach allows for excellent exposure of the tumor and the CPA, and hearing may be preserved; this approach is excellent for large tumors. The translabyrinthine or anterosigmoid approach allows for good exposure of the internal auditory canal, CPA, and course of the facial nerve; although postoperative complications are reduced (especially facial nerve paralysis), hearing is abolished. The middle fossa or subtemporal approach does not give good exposure of the CPA, but it does allow for removal of intracanalicular or small cisternal tumors while sparing hearing and minimizing complications. Traction of the cerebellum during the suboccipital approach can cause dysmetria; traction of the temporal lobe during the middle fossa approach can cause epilepsy or dysphasia.

SYMPTOMATIC TREATMENT

- Evaluation for hearing aids in patients with residual hearing; physical therapy as needed (e.g., dysmetria, ataxia); facial nerve grafting and reconstruction can be of benefit in selected patients.

ADJUNCTIVE TREATMENTS

- Conventional external beam radiotherapy (RT) and stereotactic radiosurgery (linear accelerator, proton beam, gamma knife) can be adjunctive or alternative forms of treatment in selected patients. RT (30–50 Gy) should be considered in patients with large residual tumors after surgery, patients with large recurrent tumors, and patients with large tumors that are poor surgical candidates. RT can lengthen progression-free survival. Patients most appropriate for radiosurgery include those who are medically unstable, elderly (>65 years), contralaterally deaf, have failed previous surgery, or refuse surgical intervention; tumors <3 cm in diameter are most suitable. Dosing usually is between 16 and 18 Gy in a single fraction to the 50% isodense line; local control rates range from 90%–95%, with variable amounts of tumor shrinkage. Complications of radiosurgery include hearing loss, nausea and emesis, headaches, and delayed facial neuropathy.
- Currently, there is no role for chemotherapy in the treatment of acoustic schwannomas.

ADMISSION/DISCHARGE CRITERIA

- Admission is generally reserved for presurgical evaluation and surgical resection. Angiography may be included in the workup to assess regional vascular anatomy and rule out aneurysms and vascular malformations of the CPA. Patients with brainstem compression might benefit from admission for intravenous dexamethasone.

Medications

DRUG(S) OF CHOICE

- Dexamethasone 8–16 mg/day may be of benefit to reduce edema and swelling for patients in the brainstem compressive stage of growth. It also may improve transient symptoms of pressure and swelling after RT or radiosurgery.

Contraindications

N/A

Precautions

- All patients should be taking an H2-blocking drug while receiving chronic dexamethasone.

ALTERNATIVE DRUGS

N/A

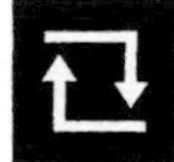

Follow-Up

PATIENT MONITORING

- Patients are followed with serial MRI scans and assessment of neurologic function every 6–12 months.

EXPECTED COURSE AND PROGNOSIS

- Overall prognosis for survival and neurologic function is good for sporadic tumors if diagnosed in the canalicular or cisternal phases. Recurrence rate after a gross total resection is 1%–2%. Surgical complications include mortality (0.5%–2%), hemorrhage, cerebellar injury, cranial nerve injury (V, VII, VIII, XI), headache, aseptic meningitis, and CSF leak. Incomplete resection will result in recurrent tumor within 7 years in 44% of patients. Almost two thirds of patients are able to return to work within 4 months after surgical resection.
- Complications of acoustic schwannomas and their treatment include partial or complete hearing loss, facial weakness, vertigo, and dysmetria. Less common sequelae include impairment of other cranial nerves, ataxia, and hydrocephalus.

PATIENT EDUCATION

- Acoustic Neuroma Association. Website: *www.anausa.org*
- National Institute of Health-Acoustic Neuroma. Website: *http://text.nml.nih.gov* (and search for "acoustic schwannoma")
- Braintumors.com. Website: *www.braintumors.com*
- Johns Hopkins Acoustic Neuroma Program-Textbook. Website: *www.med.jhu.edu/radiosurgery/braintumors/acoustic/textbook*

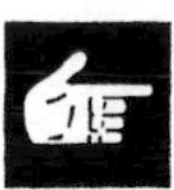

Miscellaneous

SYNONYMS

- Acoustic neuroma
- Vestibular neuroma or schwannoma
- Neurilemmoma
- Perineural fibroblastoma

ICD-9-CM: 225.1 Acoustic schwannoma

SEE ALSO: NEUROFIBROMATOSIS TYPES I AND II

REFERENCES

- Flickinger JC, Kondziolka D, Niranjan A, et al. Results of acoustic neuroma radiosurgery: an analysis of 5 years' experience using current methods. J Neurosurg 2001;94:1–6.
- Jackler RK, Pitts LH. Acoustic neuroma. Neurosurg Clin 1990;1:100–223.
- Jackler RK, Pitts LH. Selection of surgical approach to acoustic neuroma. Otolaryngol Clin North Am 1992;25:361–387.
- McKenzie JD. Magnetic resonance imaging of cerebellopontine angle masses. BNI Q 1994;10:9–18.
- Welling DB, Guida M, Goll F, et al. Mutational spectrum in the neurofibromatosis type 2 gene in sporadic and familial schwannomas. Hum Genet 1996; 98:189–193.

Author(s): Herbert B. Newton, MD

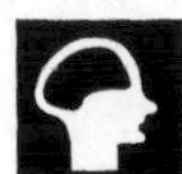

Basics

DESCRIPTION

- Ependymomas are gliomas that arise from cells forming the ependymal surfaces of the ventricles. As with other gliomas, the primary symptoms associated with ependymomas primarily reflect local compressive effects. By arising from the ependymal surface, frequently in the fourth ventricle, these tumors are more often associated with hydrocephalus and subarachnoid metastases than most gliomas, although less often than medulloblastoma/primitive neuroectodermal tumor (PNET). Childhood ependymomas usually are intracranial tumors; 60%–70% occur in the fourth ventricle. Most of these are histologically low grade, yet irrespective of grade there is a strong tendency for recurrence. Ependymomas in adults also are intracranial but occur with a higher frequency in the lateral ventricles.
- PNET with ependymal differentiation, ependymoblastoma, has biologic and clinical features that relate it to the medulloblastoma/PNET group of neoplasms. The prognosis and treatment are distinct from that of ependymomas.

EPIDEMIOLOGY

- Ependymomas represent 2%–8% of all neuroepithelial tumors but account for a higher percentage in children. They occur at all ages, with peaks in early childhood and again in young adult life. They represent 8.7% of gliomas in patients <19 years but only 1.3% in patients >65 years.

ETIOLOGY

- The etiology is uncertain, but an association with exposure to simian vacuolating virus no. 40 (SV40) through contaminated vaccines has been suggested. The SV40 large T antigen has been demonstrated in tumor samples from some patients, but some studies have failed to confirm this. Carcinogenic chemicals produce ependymomas and other gliomas in mice exposed *in utero*.

Genetics

- Ependymomas are observed with increased frequency in patients with neurofibromatosis (NF) type I and type II.

RISK FACTORS

- Family history of NF

PREGNANCY

- No specific relationship to pregnancy is known.

ASSOCIATED CONDITIONS

- Ependymomas are strongly associated with NF, especially type II, but they also can occur in NF type I.

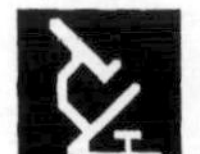

Diagnosis

DIFFERENTIAL DIAGNOSIS

- The differential diagnosis varies considerably based on site of the lesion and includes both neoplastic and progressive nonneoplastic disorders.
  —Astrocytoma
  —Medulloblastoma
  —Other mass lesions
  —Craniocervical junction anomalies and posterior fossa malformations

SIGNS AND SYMPTOMS

- Ataxia/dysequilibrium
- Headache
- Nausea and vomiting
- Rapidly increasing head circumference in children
- Diplopia, particularly related to cranial nerve (CN) VI palsies
- Cerebellopontine angle syndrome, including CN V, VII, and VIII
- Seizures
- Weakness

LABORATORY PROCEDURES

- CSF analysis for cytology is part of the extent of disease assessment in children. In adults this would be indicated only when clinical findings or neuroimaging studies suggested subarachnoid metastases.

IMAGING STUDIES

- MRI scanning usually demonstrates a well-demarcated, contrast-enhancing mass. Hydrocephalus is common with fourth ventricle ependymomas. In children, determining the extent of involvement by neoplasm (i.e., extent of disease or staging assessment) should include scanning the entire craniospinal axis to search for subarachnoid metastases. Rarely is this necessary for adults. If an ependymoma or other neoplasm with a propensity for subarachnoid dissemination (e.g., medulloblastoma/PNET) is suspected from the initial scans, it is preferable to perform the spine MRI studies prior to surgery because some postoperative artifacts may be difficult to distinguish from subarachnoid metastases. For patients who cannot undergo MRI scanning, myelography performed after surgery is used as an alternative for assessment of the spinal axis.
- CT scanning also is able to demonstrate intracranial ependymomas well, but MRI scanning tends to be more informative, particularly with regard to posterior fossa lesions and meningeal dissemination. Neither CT nor MRI scanning can distinguish ependymomas from other CNS neoplasms with sufficient certainty to be considered diagnostic.

SPECIAL TESTS

N/A

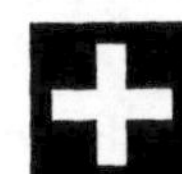

Management

GENERAL MEASURES

- Initial measures are aimed at controlling rapidly progressive neurologic symptoms and elevated intracranial pressure. Both cerebral edema and hydrocephalus may contribute to the increased pressure. Dexamethasone (Decadron) and occasionally osmotic diuretics such as mannitol are required for cerebral edema. Urgent surgical measures for tumor-related mass effect or hydrocephalus are sometimes needed.

SURGICAL MEASURES

- Emergency ventriculostomy may be needed for rapidly progressive hydrocephalus usually related to fourth ventricle neoplasms. Many patients will not require permanent shunting once the tumor is removed. If elevated intracranial pressure or hydrocephalus persists after tumor resection, a ventriculoperitoneal shunt may be needed.
- Tumor resection is the primary mode of antineoplastic therapy. Aggressive debulking is associated with improved long-term survival in children with ependymomas. Complete resection of histologically benign ependymomas in adults may result in long-term control without other therapy.

SYMPTOMATIC TREATMENT

- Corticosteroids are titrated to control symptoms arising from cerebral edema. Anticonvulsant therapy is used if seizures occur.

ADJUNCTIVE TREATMENT

- In very young children, multiagent chemotherapy is used and radiation is deferred to avoid the profound neurotoxicities associated with radiotherapy at this age. In older children, radiation therapy directed at the tumor bed is the main postoperative treatment. Craniospinal radiation is not advocated unless subarachnoid metastases are present. The addition of chemotherapy with radiation is not clearly beneficial but often is considered part of investigational protocols. In adults, radiation is used for incompletely resected ependymomas. Repeated resections and radiosurgery also are used for locally recurrent tumors. Chemotherapy is used as a second-line therapy for recurrence in adults.

ADMISSION/DISCHARGE CRITERIA

- Admit for signs of elevated intracranial pressure or rapidly progressive neurologic deficits.

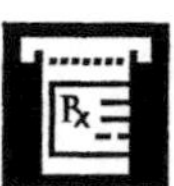

Medications

DRUG(S) OF CHOICE

- Corticosteroids, most often dexamethasone, are used to treat cerebral edema.
- A large number of chemotherapy agents have been tried, usually in multiagent combinations. Most of these are alkylating agents including the nitrosoureas (carmustine [BCNU], lomustine [CCNU]), platinum derivatives (cisplatin, carboplatin), and cyclophosphamide. Other agents including vincristine and etoposide are also commonly used.

Contraindications

- Chemotherapy is contraindicated in patients with persistent leukopenia (<2.0) or thrombocytopenia (<100,000).

Precautions

- Anticonvulsant therapy is indicated only when seizures have occurred. Perioperative prophylaxis is sometimes recommended, particularly if intracranial pressure is elevated. Anticonvulsants that are available in IV formulations are preferable, particularly in the perioperative period. Anticonvulsants with relatively common hematologic toxicities (carbamazepine, divalproex [Depakote]) should not be first-line choices for patients who will receive chemotherapy.
- Special care is required for sedation and pain control in patients suspected of having elevated intracranial pressure, especially if related to a posterior fossa mass where respiratory depression and loss of airway protection may rapidly develop.
- Severe encephalopathy and loss of brainstem reflexes may occur following resection of posterior fossa tumors in children. The exact cause is uncertain, but brainstem edema and ischemia due to vasospasm have been postulated. These symptoms may last for weeks or a few months, usually with slow improvement.

ALTERNATIVE DRUGS

N/A

Follow-Up

PATIENT MONITORING

- For children, MRI scans are obtained every 4 months during therapy and for the first year after, then every 6 months for 3–5 years. Less frequent scanning (every 6–12 months) is appropriate for histologically benign adult ependymomas.
- MRI scanning of the entire neuraxis may be required on a regular schedule for some patients. Clinical assessment must always include careful search for subarachnoid metastases, particularly spinal "drop metastases." CSF evaluation for cytology may be needed.

EXPECTED COURSE AND PROGNOSIS

- There is a high likelihood of recurrence in children. The site of recurrence is local in 90% of patients, although some patients will have concurrent subarachnoid metastases. Recurrence in the subarachnoid space without local recurrence is much less common. Metastasis outside of the neuraxis is rare. The 5-year survival rate is 50% in children. The median survival is considerably longer in adults than in children.

PATIENT EDUCATION

- American Brain Tumor Association, 2720 River Road Suite 146, Des Plaines, IL 60018. Phone: 708-827-9918, 800-886-2282, website: *www.abta.org*
- National Brain Tumor Foundation, 414 13th Street, Suite 700, Oakland, CA 94612. Phone: 510-839-9777, fax: 510-839-9779, website: *www.braintumor.org*

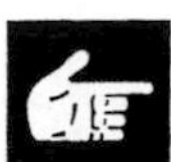

Miscellaneous

SYNONYMS

- Ependymoma
- Anaplastic ependymoma

ICD-9-CM: 191.9 Malignant neoplasm of the brain, unspecified; 237.5 Neoplasm of uncertain behavior of brain and spinal cord

SEE ALSO: N/A

REFERENCES

- Epstein FJ, Farmer J-P, Freed D. Adult intramedullary spinal cord ependymomas: the results of surgery in 38 patients. J Neurosurg 1993;79:204.
- Goldwein JW, Glauser TA, Packer RJ, et al. Recurrent intracranial ependymomas in children: survival, patterns of failure, and prognostic factors. Cancer 1990;66:557.
- Lyons MK, Kelly PJ. Posterior fossa ependymomas: report of 30 cases and review of the literature. Neurosurgery 1991;28:659.
- Pollack IF, Gerszten PC, Martinez AJ, et al. Intracranial ependymomas in childhood: long-term outcome and prognostic factors. Neurosurgery 1995; 37:655.
- Pollack IF. The role of surgery in pediatric gliomas. J Neurooncol 1999;42:271.
- Schild SE, Nisi K, Scheithauer BW, et al. The results of radiotherapy for ependymomas: the Mayo Clinic experience. Int J Radiat Oncol Biol Phys 1998;42: 953.
- Schwartz TH, Kim S, Glick RS, et al. Supratentorial ependymomas in adults. Neurosurgery 1999;44:721.
- Schweitzer JS, Batzdorf U. Ependymoma of the cauda equina region: diagnosis, treatment, and outcome in 15 patients. Neurosurgery 1992;30:202.
- Siffert J, Allen JC. Chemotherapy in recurrent ependymoma. Pediatr Neurosurg 1998;28:314.

Author(s): Paul L. Moots, MD

Brain Tumor, High-Grade Astrocytoma

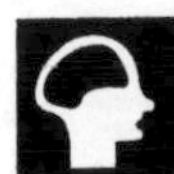

Basics

DESCRIPTION

- High-grade astrocytomas (HGAs) are a group of malignant neoplasms that typically occur in middle-aged and older adults. They have a high growth potential and are more infiltrative than low-grade gliomas. Survival is limited in most patients and ranges between 1 and 5 years.

EPIDEMIOLOGY

Incidence/Prevalence

- HGAs comprise approximately 33%–45% of primary brain tumors in adults, which corresponds to roughly 7,500 new cases of HGA each year in North America; 50%–80% of HGAs are glioblastoma multiforme (GBM); 20%–40% are anaplastic astrocytoma (AA). Gliosarcoma and mixed anaplastic oligoastrocytoma (AOA) occur less frequently.

Race

- All races and ethnic groups are affected. Caucasians are affected more commonly than blacks, Latinos, and Asians.

Age

- Typical presentation is between 50 and 65 years of age for GBM and gliosarcoma patients and between 30 and 50 years of age for AA and mixed AOA patients.

Sex

- Incidence is slightly higher in males than females (1.5:1).

ETIOLOGY

- The World Health Organization (WHO) classifies AA as grade III, GBM as grade IV, gliosarcoma as grade IV, and mixed AOA as grade III.
- HGAs are derived from transformed astrocytes. Pathologic evaluation of HGA reveals significant heterogeneity, with high cellularity, cellular and nuclear atypia, moderate-to-high mitotic rate, endothelial proliferation, and necrosis (GBM and gliosarcoma only). Gliosarcomas show regions of sarcomatous differentiation admixed with separate areas of neoplastic glial cells. Staining for glial fibrillary acidic protein is more variable in HGA and typically less than that of low-grade gliomas.
- Molecular genetic studies of HGA reveal frequent loss or mutation of the tumor suppressor gene p53, and amplification of MDM2 or CDK2. Deletion or mutation of the tumor suppressor genes p16 and retinoblastoma may be present. Primary GBMs have amplification of epidermal growth factor receptors and/or deletion of the primitive neuroectodermal tumor (PNET) tumor suppressor gene. Deletion of 1p and 19q may be noted in mixed AOA and is associated with improved survival.

Genetics

- HGAs usually are sporadic and do not have an underlying genetic predilection. Rarely, HGAs can manifest as part of a genetically mediated syndrome (i.e., neurofibromatosis [NF]).

RISK FACTORS

- The only known risk factors for HGA are prior cranial radiation exposure and genetic diseases with a predilection for astrocytomas, such as Turcot's syndrome, NF types I and II, and Li-Fraumeni syndrome. Rarely, HGA can be familial.

PREGNANCY

- Pregnancy does not affect the clinical course of HGA.

ASSOCIATED CONDITIONS

- NF type I, NF type II, Turcot's syndrome, Li-Fraumeni syndrome

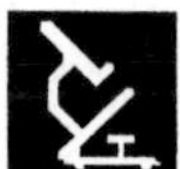

Diagnosis

DIFFERENTIAL DIAGNOSIS

- Other mass lesions that enhance should be considered, including mature abscess, subacute infarct, tumefactive regions of demyelination, and evolving hematoma.

SIGNS AND SYMPTOMS

- The median duration from onset of symptoms to diagnosis ranges from <6 months in GBM to 6–8 months for AA. The most common symptoms at presentation include headache (70%), seizure activity (54% overall; partial motor 23%; generalized tonic-clonic 20%; partial complex 9%), cognitive and personality changes (52%), focal weakness (43%), nausea and emesis (31%), speech disturbances (27%), and alterations of consciousness (25%).
- Common findings on neurologic examination include hemiparesis (57%), cranial nerve palsies (54%), papilledema (53%), cognitive deficits and confusion (45%), depressed sensorium (37%), hemianopsia (29%), and dysphasia (25%).

LABORATORY PROCEDURES

- Molecular analysis of chromosome 1p and/or 19q loss may be of prognostic significance for patients with mixed AOA.

IMAGING STUDIES

- MRI, with and without gadolinium contrast, is the most sensitive diagnostic test. MRI is more sensitive than CT for HGAs that are small or within the posterior fossa. On T1 images, the tumor usually is infiltrative and appears hypointense or isointense compared to brain; on T2 images, the mass is hyperintense. With gadolinium administration, most HGAs show either diffuse or ring-like enhancement. Peritumoral edema and mass effect usually are moderate to severe. Hemorrhage and regions consistent with necrosis may be noted. CT demonstrates an ill-defined region of hypodensity with moderate-to-severe enhancement, edema, and mass effect.

SPECIAL TESTS

- Fluorodeoxyglucose-positron emission tomography (FDG-PET) may be of benefit to assess the metabolism of HGA to differentiate from nonneoplastic lesions and to maximize targeting for biopsy. HGAs typically appear hypermetabolic on PET imaging. Magnetic resonance spectroscopy (MRS) also can be used for metabolic screening to differentiate HGA from other lesions. MRS of HGA often reveals an elevated choline peak, severely reduced *N*-acetylaspartate (NAA) peak, the presence of a lactate peak, and a reduced NAA/choline ratio.

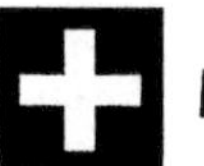

Management

GENERAL MEASURES

- The management of HGA requires a multimodality approach to cytoreduction that includes surgery, radiotherapy, and chemotherapy. Input from neurosurgeons, neuro-oncologists, and radiation oncologists is necessary for optimal treatment.

SURGICAL MEASURES

- Surgery should be considered in all patients to make a histologic diagnosis, reduce tumor bulk and intracranial pressure, and alleviate symptoms. Maximal surgical resection is the treatment of choice for accessible HGA, preferably by computer-assisted volumetric resection techniques (e.g., stealth apparatus). For patients with deep inaccessible lesions or tumors in eloquent cortex, stereotactic biopsy should be performed. Some studies suggest that overall and 1-year survival are improved with complete or subtotal resection versus biopsy.

SYMPTOMATIC TREATMENT

- Dexamethasone 4–16 mg/day IV may be of benefit to reduce peritumoral edema and swelling. In some patients, IV mannitol 12.5–25 g q3–6h may also be necessary to control severe edema, mass effect, and midline shift.

ADJUNCTIVE TREATMENT

- External beam radiation therapy (RT) should be considered for all HGAs after surgical resection. Phase III trials demonstrate that time to progression and overall survival are significantly improved with RT (overall survival 36 weeks with RT vs. 16 weeks with surgery alone). The recommended RT dose is 60 Gy over 6 weeks, in daily fractions of 180–200 cGy. Focal three-dimensional treatment planning and conformal techniques should be used whenever possible to minimize radiation exposure to normal brain, especially in younger patients. For elderly patients (>65 years) and those with poor Karnofsky performance status, a protracted course of RT may be appropriate: 30–40 Gy in 10 fractions over 3 weeks.
- Stereotactic radiosurgery (SRS) has been used for HGA, as a boost after initial RT and at recurrence, for tumors up to 4 cm in size; larger tumors will not benefit from SRS due to infiltration beyond the treatment field. Median doses range from 15–17 Gy in one fraction. SRS may improve survival in carefully selected patients with small HGA.
- Chemotherapy should be considered for all patients with HGA after RT and at recurrence. Clinical trials and meta-analyses suggest a modest survival benefit after RT (10%–15% extension in 1-year survival), especially in patients with AA and mixed AOA. For AA and GBM, the most active drugs and combinations include carmustine (BCNU), procarbazine, PCV (procarbazine, CCNU [lomustine], vincristine), cisplatin, carboplatin, temozolomide, and etoposide. Mixed AOA may respond well to chemotherapy with PCV or temozolomide if chromosome 1p and 19q deletions are noted. At recurrence, local chemotherapy with BCNU-impregnated wafers may add a modest survival benefit, as suggested by several phase III trials.

ADMISSION/DISCHARGE CRITERIA

- Patients with HGA often are admitted for seizure control or neurologic deterioration due to elevated intracranial pressure and tumor growth. Maximizing anticonvulsant doses, resolving metabolic disturbances, and reducing intracranial pressure are required before discharge.

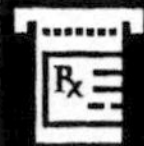

Medications

DRUG(S) OF CHOICE

- Seizures are a common problem in patients with HGA. Appropriate anticonvulsant choices (e.g., phenytoin, carbamazepine, levetiracetam) and management are critical. Dexamethasone is used at the lowest dose able to control symptoms related to intracranial pressure.

Contraindications

- Patients on chemotherapy must meet appropriate hematologic parameters before proceeding with the next cycle: WBC >2.0, hemoglobin >10.0, and platelets >100,000.

Precautions

- All patients should be taking H2-blocking drug while receiving chronic dexamethasone.

ALTERNATIVE DRUGS

N/A

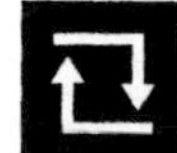

Follow-Up

PATIENT MONITORING

- Patients are followed with serial MRI scans and neurologic examinations every 4–8 weeks. Patients receiving chemotherapy may require more frequent follow-up. Anticonvulsant levels need to be monitored carefully.

EXPECTED COURSE AND PROGNOSIS

- Median survival after diagnosis of patients with HGA is 30–42 months for AA, 8–13 months for GBM and gliosarcoma, and 42–52 months for mixed AOA.
- Prognosis is improved with young age (<40 years), AOA or AA histology, and high Karnofsky performance status. Prognosis is worse with age >50 years, poor Karnofsky performance status, and GBM or gliosarcoma histology.

PATIENT EDUCATION

- Braintumors.com. Website: *www.braintumors.com*
- National Brain Tumor Foundation. Website: *www.braintumor.org*
- American Brain Tumor Association. Website: *www.abta.org*
- The Brain Tumor Society. Website: *www.tbts.org*
- Massachusetts General Hospital-Brain Tumor Center. Website: *brain.mgh.harvard.edu*
- Brain Tumor Treatment Options & Information. Website: *users.erols.com/colilla/index.htm*

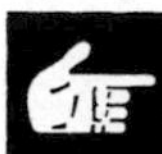

Miscellaneous

SYNONYMS

- High-grade astrocytoma
- Anaplastic astrocytoma
- Glioblastoma multiforme
- Gliosarcoma
- Mixed anaplastic oligoastrocytoma

ICD-9-CM: 191.8 Malignant astrocytoma of brain

SEE ALSO: BRAIN TUMOR, OLIGODENDROGLIOMA

REFERENCES

- Cokgor I, Friedman HS, Friedman AH. Chemotherapy for adults with malignant gliomas. Cancer Invest 1999;17:264–272.
- Maher EA, Furnari FB, Bachoo RM, et al. Malignant glioma: genetics and biology of a grave matter. Genes Dev 2001;15: 1311–1333.
- Newton HB. Primary brain tumors: review of etiology, diagnosis, and treatment. Am Fam Physician 1994;49:787–797.
- Salcman M. High-grade gliomas. In: Vecht CJ, ed. Handbook of clinical neurology, vol. 24 (68): neuro-oncology, part II. Amsterdam: Elsevier Science, 1997;4: 87–122.
- Shapiro WR, Shapiro JR. Biology and treatment of malignant glioma. Oncology (Huntingt) 1998;12:233–240.
- Wen PY, Fine HA, Black PM, et al. High-grade astrocytomas. Neurol Clin 1995;13:875–900.

Author(s): Herbert B. Newton, MD

Brain Tumor, Low-Grade Glioma

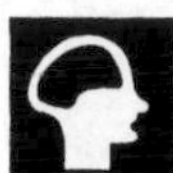

Basics

DESCRIPTION

- Low-grade gliomas (LGGs) are a diverse group of pathologically distinct neoplasms that usually occur in children and young adults. The most common LGGs are of astrocytic and oligodendroglial origin. These tumors have a reduced growth potential and often are less infiltrative compared to malignant gliomas. Survival typically is prolonged, >5 years in most patients.

EPIDEMIOLOGY

Incidence/Prevalence

- LGGs comprise approximately 10%–15% of primary brain tumors in adults, which corresponds to roughly 1,900 new cases of LGG each year in North America. The majority of LGGs consist of grade II astrocytomas, oligodendrogliomas, and mixed tumors.

Race

- All races and ethnic groups are equally affected.

Age

- Typical presentation is between 30 and 45 years (mean 37).

Sex

- Incidence is slightly higher in males than females.

ETIOLOGY

- LGGs are a heterogeneous group of neoplasms that include pilocytic astrocytoma (PCA; World Health Organization [WHO] grade I), diffuse astrocytoma (WHO grade II), WHO grade II oligodendroglioma, WHO grade II mixed oligoastrocytoma, subependymoma, subependymal giant cell astrocytoma, pleomorphic xanthoastrocytoma, ganglioglioma, central neurocytoma, and dysembryoblastic neuroepithelial tumors.
- Cells of LGG origin are variable, depending on tumor type. Pathologic evaluation of LGG reveals mild-to-moderate cellularity without anaplasia or severe nuclear atypia, minimal mitotic activity and endothelial proliferation, and no necrosis. Tumor cells often stain for glial fibrillary acidic protein. Diffuse astrocytomas can undergo anaplastic degeneration in up to 75% of cases.
- Molecular genetic studies of LGG reveal frequent allelic deletions of chromosome 17p, often with loss or mutation of the tumor suppressor gene p53. Presence of abnormal p53 protein in LGG is associated with shorter survival. Amplification of MDM2 or CDK2 and deletion of the tumor suppressors p16 and retinoblastoma (Rb) may be present in some tumors. Deletion of 1p and 19q may be noted in oligodendrogliomas and is associated with chemosensitivity and extended survival.

Genetics

- LGGs usually are sporadic and do not have an underlying genetic predilection. Rarely, LGGs can manifest as part of a genetically mediated syndrome (i.e., neurofibromatosis [NF]).

RISK FACTORS

- The only known risk factors for LGGs are prior cranial radiation exposure and genetic diseases with a predilection for gliomas, such as Turcot's syndrome, NF types I and II, Li-Fraumeni syndrome, basal cell nevus syndrome, and tuberous sclerosis. Rarely, LGGs can be familial.

PREGNANCY

- Pregnancy does not affect the clinical course of LGGs.

ASSOCIATED CONDITIONS

- NF type I, NF type II, Turcot's syndrome, Li-Fraumeni syndrome, basal cell nevus syndrome, tuberous sclerosis

Diagnosis

DIFFERENTIAL DIAGNOSIS

- Other mass lesions that may or may not enhance should be considered, including immature abscess, subacute infarct, tumefactive regions of demyelination, and evolving hematoma.

SIGNS AND SYMPTOMS

- The median duration from onset of symptoms to diagnosis ranges from 6–17 months. The most common symptom at presentation is seizure, which occurs in 60%–65% of patients. Focal seizures are more likely than generalized seizures. Headache and focal weakness each occurs in approximately one fourth of patients. Cognitive changes, speech deficits, and visual abnormalities are noted in $<15\%$ of patients.
- Neurologic examination is normal in about 50% of patients. Neurologic abnormalities may include focal motor deficits (45%), sensory alterations (40%), mental status alterations (25%), papilledema (20%), dysphasia (20%), and memory deficits (18%).

LABORATORY PROCEDURES

- Molecular analysis of chromosome 1p and/or 19q loss may be of prognostic significance in patients with oligodendroglioma. EEG should be considered in patients with atypical or unusual seizures.

IMAGING STUDIES

- MRI, with and without gadolinium contrast, is the most sensitive diagnostic test. MRI is more sensitive than CT for tumors that are small or within the posterior fossa. On T1 images, the tumor usually is somewhat circumscribed and appears hypointense or isointense compared to brain; on T2 images, the mass is hyperintense. Cystic regions are often present in PCA. With gadolinium administration, most LGGs show minimal or no enhancement. PCA can show variable enhancement, often within a cyst-associated mural nodule. Peritumoral edema and mass effect are usually mild to moderate. Calcification may be noted. CT demonstrates an ill-defined region of hypodensity with minimal enhancement. More than one third of tumors that appear to be LGGs by MRI/CT criteria are higher-grade tumors, usually anaplastic astrocytoma.

SPECIAL TESTS

- Fluorodeoxyglucose-positron emission tomography (FDG-PET) may be of benefit to assess the metabolism of the mass to differentiate it from nonneoplastic lesions. LGGs typically appear hypometabolic on PET imaging. Magnetic resonance spectroscopy (MRS) can also be used for metabolic screening to differentiate LGGs from other lesions. MRS of LGGs often reveals an elevated choline peak, reduced *N*-acetylaspartate (NAA) peak, the presence of a lactate peak, and a reduced NAA/choline ratio.

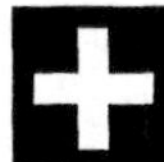

Management

GENERAL MEASURES

- The management of LGG remains controversial. Some authors recommend observation and serial MRI scans for proof of growth potential before initiation of treatment (i.e., surgery, irradiation); others suggest immediate tissue diagnosis with biopsy or resection, followed by irradiation or chemotherapy. Observation is most appropriate for small deep tumors that are asymptomatic except for seizure activity.

SURGICAL MEASURES

- Surgery should be considered in all patients to make a histologic diagnosis and alleviate symptoms. Maximal surgical resection is the treatment of choice for accessible LGGs, preferably by computer-assisted volumetric resection techniques (e.g., stealth apparatus). For patients with deep inaccessible lesions or tumors in eloquent cortex, stereotactic biopsy should be performed. Some studies suggest that overall and 5-year survival are improved with complete or subtotal resection versus biopsy.

SYMPTOMATIC TREATMENT

- Dexamethasone 4–16 mg/day may be of benefit to reduce peritumoral edema and swelling.

ADJUNCTIVE TREATMENT

- External beam radiation therapy (RT) should be considered for all nonpilocytic LGG after incomplete surgical resection. Postoperative RT can be postponed for patients with PCA until growth potential is demonstrated. Retrospective studies suggest that time to progression and overall survival are improved with RT (5-year survival 32% with RT vs. 10% with surgery alone). Timing of RT remains controversial; some authors advocate immediate postoperative treatment while others suggest waiting until the tumor progresses; however, the timing of RT does not appear to be critical, because overall survival is similar in the immediate and delayed treatment groups. RT for LGG is more beneficial for older patients (≥40 years). Conformal techniques should be used whenever possible to minimize radiation exposure to normal brain. Recommended RT doses are 50–55 Gy over 6 weeks. Irradiation should be delayed postoperatively in young children until proof of growth by MRI and/or neurologic examination.
- Stereotactic radiosurgery is a more recent RT option. Several studies have used doses of 15–50 Gy for LGGs up to 40 mm. Objective responses have been noted in >50% of patients, although follow-up has been brief.
- Chemotherapy does not have a clear role in most patients with LGG. Young children may respond to cisplatin-based regimens in order to delay the need for RT. A Southwest Oncology Group phase III trial of LGG in adults did not demonstrate a survival benefit for lomustine in combination with RT. Phase II studies suggest nitrosoureas (lomustine, carmustine), alone or in combination with platinum (cisplatin, carboplatin) drugs, may have benefit for patients with LGG. PCV (procarbazine, lomustine, vincristine) has demonstrated activity against LGG, especially oligodendrogliomas. Objective responses range from 30%–45% in some studies. Temozolomide has demonstrated activity similar to PCV against LGG in recent phase II studies. Progressive or recurrent PCA may respond to cisplatin-based multiagent chemotherapy regimens.

ADMISSION/DISCHARGE CRITERIA

- Patients with LGG are most often admitted for seizure control or to reduce elevated intracranial pressure. Maximizing anticonvulsant doses and resolving metabolic disturbances is required before discharge.

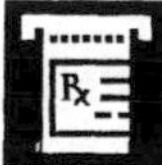

Medications

DRUG(S) OF CHOICE

- Seizures are a common problem in patients with LGG, so appropriate anticonvulsant choices and management are critical. Dexamethasone is used at the lowest dose able to control symptoms related to intracranial pressure.

Contraindications

- Patients on chemotherapy must meet appropriate hematologic parameters before proceeding with the next cycle. WBC should be >2.0, hemoglobin >10.0, and platelets >100,000.

Precautions

- All patients should be taking an H2-blocking drug while receiving chronic dexamethasone.

ALTERNATIVE DRUGS

N/A

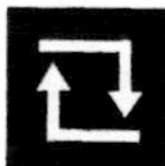

Follow-Up

PATIENT MONITORING

- Patients are followed with serial MRI scans and neurologic examinations every 4–6 months. Patients receiving chemotherapy will require more frequent follow-up; anticonvulsant levels will need to be monitored.

EXPECTED COURSE AND PROGNOSIS

- Median survival after diagnosis of patients with LGG is 4.7 years for diffuse astrocytomas, 7.1 years for mixed oligoastrocytomas, and 9.8 years for oligodendrogliomas. The 10-year survival in these cohorts is 17%, 33%, and 49%, respectively.
- Prognosis is improved with oligodendroglial or pilocytic histology, young age, and seizures at presentation. Prognosis is worse with age >40 years, poor performance status, and diffuse astrocytic histology.

PATIENT EDUCATION

- Braintumors.com. Website: *www.braintumors.com*
- National Brain Tumor Foundation. Website: *www.braintumor.org*
- American Brain Tumor Association. Website: *www.abta.org*
- The Brain Tumor Society. Website: *www.tbts.org*
- Massachusetts General Hospital-Brain Tumor Center. Website: *brain.mgh.harvard.edu*

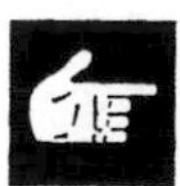

Miscellaneous

SYNONYMS

- Low-grade astrocytoma
- Low-grade oligodendroglioma
- Pilocytic astrocytoma
- Subependymoma
- subependymal giant-cell astrocytoma
- Low-grade mixed oligoastrocytoma
- Pleomorphic xanthoastrocytoma
- Ganglioglioma
- Central neurocytoma
- Dysembryoplastic neuroepithelial tumors

ICD-9-CM: 225.0 Benign neoplasm of brain

SEE ALSO: BRAIN TUMOR, OLIGODENDROGLIOMA

REFERENCES

- Brandes AA, Vastola F, Basso U. Controversies in the therapy of low-grade glioma: when and how to treat. Expert Rev Anticancer Ther 2002;2:529–536.
- Fuller CE, Perry A. Pathology of low- and intermediate-grade gliomas. Semin Radiat Oncol 2001;11:95–102.
- Henderson KH, Shaw EG. Randomized trials of radiation therapy in adult low-grade gliomas. Semin Radiat Oncol 2001;11:145–151.
- Lesser GJ. Chemotherapy of low-grade gliomas. Semin Radiat Oncol 2001;11: 138–144.
- Mason WP, MacDonald DR. Low-grade gliomas. In: Vecht CJ, eds. Handbook of clinical neurology, vol. 24 (68): neuro-oncology, part II. Amsterdam: Elsevier Science, 1997;2:33–62.
- Recht LD, Bernstein M. Low-grade gliomas. Neurol Clin 1995;13:847–859.
- Shaw EG, Scheithauer BW, O'Fallon JR. Management of supratentorial low-grade gliomas. Oncology (Huntingt) 1993;7: 97–107.

Author(s): Herbert B. Newton, MD

Brain Tumor, Medulloblastoma

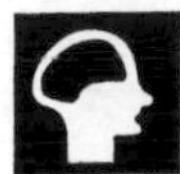

Basics

DESCRIPTION

- Medulloblastoma is the most common malignant primary brain tumor of childhood. It is an invasive embryonal neoplasm that arises in the midline cerebellum. Recent advances in multimodality treatment have led to significant improvements in local tumor control and survival.

EPIDEMIOLOGY

Incidence/Prevalence

- Medulloblastoma comprises approximately 20%–25% of all malignant primary brain tumors in children. The overall incidence in the United States is approximately 5 cases per million persons, which corresponds to roughly 350 new cases each year. Medulloblastoma is uncommon in adults, with an incidence of 1%. Adults account for 15%–20% of medulloblastoma cases.

Race

- All races and ethnic groups are affected. Caucasians are affected more commonly than blacks, Latinos, and Asians.

Age

- Typical presentation is between 7 and 9 years of age; 80% of patients present before age 20 years; a secondary peak occurs in adults between 26 and 30 years.

Sex

- Incidence in childhood is slightly higher in males than females (1.4–2.3:1). Males and females are equally affected in adulthood.

ETIOLOGY

- The World Health Organization classifies medulloblastoma as grade IV.
- The cell of origin of medulloblastoma remains controversial. The cells are derived from transformation of pluripotent cells that reside in either the external granular layer of the cerebellum or the subependymal matrix. In children they typically occur in the midline cerebellum, with variable extension into the brainstem; in adults, they are eccentrically located, with extension into one of the cerebellar hemispheres. Pathologic evaluation reveals a highly cellular tumor consisting of densely packed, small, poorly differentiated cells with hyperchromatic nuclei and scant cytoplasm, Homer-Wright rosettes, occasional ganglion cells, regions of necrosis, and frequent mitoses. Histologic variants include the desmoplastic, nodular, and large cell forms.
- Molecular genetic studies of medulloblastoma have noted frequent deletions of chromosomes 17p, 1q, and 10q. Three separate pathways have been implicated in the transformation process: amplification of the N- and C-myc genes, mutation of the PTCH gene, and dysfunction of the sonic hedgehog/PTCH signaling pathway, and dysregulation of the Wnt/APC/β-catenin signaling pathway. High expression of TrkC is associated with extended survival.

Genetics

- Medulloblastomas usually are sporadic. Medulloblastoma can arise as a manifestation of heritable disorders such as Turcot's syndrome, Li-Fraumeni syndrome, ataxia-telangiectasia, nevoid basal cell carcinoma syndrome, and Gorlin's syndrome. Rarely, medulloblastoma can be familial.

RISK FACTORS

- The only known risk factors for medulloblastoma are the above mentioned heritable syndromes and rare familial predilections.

PREGNANCY

- Pregnancy does not affect the clinical course of medulloblastoma.

ASSOCIATED CONDITIONS

N/A

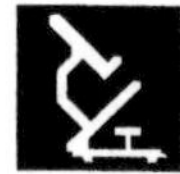

Diagnosis

DIFFERENTIAL DIAGNOSIS

- Other mass lesions of the cerebellum that may or may not enhance should be considered, including abscess, subacute infarct, tumefactive regions of demyelination, evolving hematoma, other primary brain tumors (e.g., astrocytoma), and metastasis.

SIGNS AND SYMPTOMS

- The median duration from onset of symptoms to diagnosis ranges from 3–6 months. Initial symptoms include irritability, loss of appetite, progressive headache, lethargy, and nausea and emesis (often in the morning). Later symptoms include double vision, truncal and/or limb ataxia, gait imbalance, neck stiffness, and dizziness.
- Common findings on neurologic examination include lethargy, papilledema, gait ataxia, nystagmus, and sixth nerve palsy. Less common findings include hemiparesis, internuclear ophthalmoplegia, dysphagia, and myelopathy.
- Unusual signs and symptoms, such as seizure activity, radicular pain, back pain, hemiparesis, internuclear ophthalmoplegia, dysphagia, and myelopathy, are suggestive of brainstem infiltration and/or leptomeningeal dissemination.
- Patients with persistent pain in the extremities or pelvis, or unexplained lymphadenopathy of the neck or axillae, should be suspected of having extraneural metastases.

LABORATORY PROCEDURES

- Evaluation of the CSF may be necessary in selected patients during the "extent of disease" workup (EODWU). CSF parameters should include cell count and differential, routine chemistries, lactate, β_2-microglobulin, and cytology.

IMAGING STUDIES

- MRI, with and without contrast, is the most sensitive diagnostic test. MRI is more sensitive than CT for tumors within the posterior fossa and has the advantage of midsagittal formatting. On T1 images, the tumor is mildly to moderately infiltrative and appears hypointense or isointense compared to brain; on T2 images, the mass is hyperintense. With gadolinium, medulloblastoma demonstrates patchy or dense enhancement (90%). Edema and mass effect are mild to moderate, with frequent compression of the fourth ventricle. Leptomeningeal metastases are noted in one third of patients. CT demonstrates an ill-defined region of hypodensity that has variable enhancement, mild edema, and mass effect. Hydrocephalus is common (75%–85%).

SPECIAL TESTS

- All patients require an EODWU to screen for leptomeningeal metastases and allow stratification into low-risk and high-risk groups. The EODWU involves a contrast-enhanced MRI scan of the spine. Patients with normal or equivocal MRI results require a lumbar puncture to evaluate CSF. Patients suspected of having extraneural metastases require a skeletal survey and nuclear medicine scan.

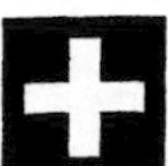

Management

GENERAL MEASURES

- Management of medulloblastoma involves a multimodality approach to cytoreduction that requires surgery, radiotherapy, and, in selected patients, chemotherapy.

SURGICAL MEASURES

- Surgery should be considered in all patients to make a histologic diagnosis, reduce tumor bulk and intracranial pressure, and alleviate symptoms. Maximal surgical resection is the treatment of choice for medulloblastoma, preferably by computer-assisted volumetric resection techniques. For patients with extensive infiltration of tumor into the brainstem or cerebellar hemispheres, an extensive subtotal resection should be performed. A ventriculoperitoneal shunt may be necessary if hydrocephalus persists after maximal tumor resection (35%–40%). Several studies suggest that overall and 5-year survival are improved with complete or subtotal resection versus biopsy. Postoperative CT or MRI should be performed within 24–72 hours to screen for residual tumor.

SYMPTOMATIC TREATMENT

- Dexamethasone 4–16 mg/day usually is necessary to reduce peritumoral edema, swelling, and mass effect.

ADJUNCTIVE TREATMENT

- External beam radiation therapy (RT) is recommended for all medulloblastoma patients. Standard RT involves treatment of the entire intracranial cavity and spine. RT to the posterior fossa consists of 50–55 Gy over 6–7 weeks in daily fractions of 180–200 cGy. RT to the brain and spinal neuraxis is administered concomitantly. Dosing for the brain ranges from 40–45 Gy; dosing for the spine ranges from 33–36 Gy. Patients receiving <30 Gy to the spine are at increased risk for early relapse and shorter survival time. RT is the sole initial treatment for low-risk patients. Recent attempts to reduce RT toxicity in pediatric patients have included using reduced doses in combination with multiagent chemotherapy. Focal RT may be necessary for patients with extraneural metastases (e.g., bone lesions). The role of radiosurgery remains unclear.
- Chemotherapy should not be used for low-risk medulloblastoma patients. Phase III trials have demonstrated a survival advantage for chemotherapy in the high-risk patient cohorts only when used during and after RT. Chemotherapy should be considered for all high-risk patients and for any patient with recurrent disease. The most active single agents include cisplatin, carboplatin, lomustine (CCNU), etoposide, and cyclophosphamide. The most active combination regimens include CCNU and vincristine, MOPP (mustard, vincristine, prednisone, procarbazine), cyclophosphamide and vincristine, and platinum-based regimens (e.g., cisplatin, CCNU, vincristine). Adult medulloblastoma patients have chemotherapy response profiles similar to those of pediatric patients.

ADMISSION/DISCHARGE CRITERIA

- Patients with medulloblastoma often are admitted for neurologic deterioration due to elevated intracranial pressure, tumor growth, seizures, leptomeningeal metastases, or infections. Maximizing anticonvulsant doses, reducing intracranial pressure, and treating infections are required before discharge. Some patients may require the initiation of new cytotoxic treatment (e.g., intrathecal chemotherapy).

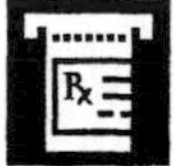

Medications

DRUG(S) OF CHOICE

- Seizures occasionally can be a problem. Appropriate anticonvulsant choices (e.g., phenytoin, carbamazepine, levetiracetam) and management are critical.

Contraindications

- Patients on chemotherapy must meet appropriate hematologic parameters before proceeding with the next cycle: WBC >2.0, hemoglobin >10.0, and platelets >100,000.

Precautions

- All patients should be taking an H2-blocking drug while receiving chronic dexamethasone.

ALTERNATIVE DRUGS

N/A

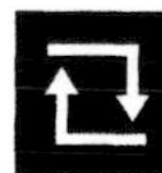

Follow-Up

PATIENT MONITORING

- Patients are followed with serial MRI scans and neurologic examinations every 4–8 weeks. Patients receiving chemotherapy may require more frequent follow-up.

EXPECTED COURSE AND PROGNOSIS

- Low-risk patients (complete resection, intact neurologic function, negative EODWU) have 5- and 10-year survival rates of 85% and 50%, respectively. High-risk patients (subtotal resection, brainstem infiltration, focal neurologic dysfunction, positive EODWU) have 5- and 10-year survival rates of 50% and 30%, respectively. Long-term survivors often develop impairment of memory and cognition.
- Prognosis is improved with adult onset, complete surgical resection, negative EODWU, intact neurologic function, and the presence of high TrkC expression. Prognosis is worse with young age, incomplete surgical resection, positive EODWU, and focal neurologic dysfunction.

PATIENT EDUCATION

- Braintumors.com. Website: *www.braintumors.com*
- National Brain Tumor Foundation. Website: *www.braintumor.org*
- American Brain Tumor Association. Website: *www.abta.org*
- The Brain Tumor Society. Website: *www.tbts.org*
- National Cancer Institute: Childhood Medulloblastoma. Website: *cancernet.nci.nih.gov/clinpdg/pif/Childhood_medulloblastoma_Patient.ht*

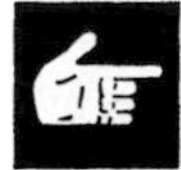

Miscellaneous

SYNONYMS

- Primitive neuroectodermal tumor (PNET) of the cerebellum

ICD-9-CM: 191.6 Malignant tumor of the cerebellum

SEE ALSO: N/A

REFERENCES

- Brandes AA, Palmisano V, Monfardini S. Medulloblastoma in adults: clinical characteristics and treatment. Cancer Treat Rev 1999;25:3–12.
- Newton HB. Review of the molecular genetics and chemotherapeutic treatment of adult and pediatric medulloblastoma. Expert Opin Invest Drugs 2001;10: 2089–2104.
- Paulino AC. Radiotherapeutic management of medulloblastoma. Oncology (Huntingt) 1997;11:813–823.
- Sutton LN, Phillips PC, Molloy PT. Surgical management of medulloblastoma. J Neurooncol 1996;29:9–21.
- Tomlinson FH, Scheithauer BW, Jenkins RB. Medulloblastoma: II. A pathobiologic overview. J Child Neurol 1992;7:240–252.
- Tomlinson FH, Scheithauer BW, Meyer FB, et al. Medulloblastoma: I. Clinical, diagnostic, and therapeutic overview. J Child Neurol 1992;7:142–155.
- Whelan HT, Krouwer HG, Schmidt MH, et al. Current therapy and new perspectives in the treatment of medulloblastoma. Pediatr Neurol 1998;18:103–115.

Author(s): Herbert B. Newton, MD

Brain Tumor, Meningioma

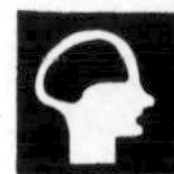

Basics

DESCRIPTION

- Meningiomas are extraaxial tumors that arise from the meninges of the intracranial dura mater. They can develop in any location that has continuity with the meninges. The most common locations are the parasagittal region (25%), cerebral convexities (20%), sphenoid wing (17%), posterior fossa (8.7%), olfactory groove (8%), and middle fossa (4%). Less common locations include the optic nerve or chiasmal region, cerebellopontine angle, and within the ventricles.

EPIDEMIOLOGY

Incidence/Prevalence

- Meningiomas comprise 18%–20% of all primary brain tumors in adults but only 2% in children. The incidence is 2–7 per 100,000 in women and 1–5 per 100,000 in men; this corresponds to approximately 3,500–4,500 newly diagnosed meningiomas in the United States each year.

Race

- All races and ethnic groups are equally affected.

Age

- Typical presentation is between 50 and 65 years of age.

Sex

- Females have a higher incidence than males (2:1).

ETIOLOGY

- The World Health Organization (WHO) grades typical low-grade meningiomas (e.g., meningothelial, fibrous, transitional, psammomatous, angiomatous) as WHO grade I; intermediate tumors (e.g., atypical, clear cell, chordoid) as WHO grade II; and malignant tumors (e.g., rhabdoid, papillary, anaplastic) as WHO grade III. The majority of meningiomas are WHO grade I; grade II and III tumors are uncommon.
- The cells of origin of meningiomas are transformed arachnoidal cap cells from the outer layer of the arachnoid membrane. Typical low-grade tumors demonstrate uniform sheets of spindle-shaped cells, minimal cellular and nuclear atypia, whirl formation, psammoma bodies, and no evidence for mitotic activity or brain infiltration. Higher-grade tumors have higher cellularity, more prominent nucleoli, high mitotic activity, necrosis, and brain invasion.
- Molecular genetic studies reveal frequent deletions of chromosomes 22q and 1p. The NF2 gene (located at 22q12.3) is mutated in up to 60% of meningiomas, with dysfunction of the merlin protein. The majority of meningiomas are positive for estrogen and progesterone receptors. Other receptors of importance include the epidermal growth factor (EGF) and platelet-derived growth factor (PDGF) receptors, both of which stimulate secretion of vascular endothelial growth factor. The ras signaling pathway is activated by stimulation by EGF and PDGF.

Genetics

- Meningiomas usually are sporadic tumors; less frequently, they can arise as part of a heritable syndrome such as neurofibromatosis (NF). In rare cases they can be familial.

RISK FACTORS

- Factors that increase the risk of meningioma include cranial radiation (≥10 Gy), focal head trauma (especially with dural penetration), breast cancer, heritable disorders (e.g., NF), and rare familial clusters.

PREGNANCY

- In some women, pregnancy can accelerate the growth and increase the clinical symptoms of meningiomas.

ASSOCIATED CONDITIONS

- NF type I, NF type II

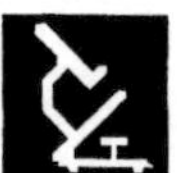

Diagnosis

DIFFERENTIAL DIAGNOSIS

- Includes other extraaxial enhancing masses, such as schwannoma, metastasis, choroid plexus papillomas, and abscess.

SIGNS AND SYMPTOMS

- Meningiomas are slow-growing tumors, with an insidious onset of symptoms. The time to diagnosis typically is prolonged (i.e., months to years). The presentation varies with tumor location, rate of growth, and amount of peritumoral edema. Common symptoms at presentation include headache, seizure activity (often focal), personality changes, speech abnormalities, cranial nerve dysfunction (e.g., double vision, facial numbness), visual field defects, and focal motor deficits. In some patients, meningiomas are asymptomatic at diagnosis.
- Common neurologic signs include monoparesis or hemiparesis, asymmetric reflexes, impairment of memory and cognition, visual loss (monocular or hemianopic), dysphasia, and cranial nerve palsies (i.e., V, VI, VII).

LABORATORY PROCEDURES

N/A

IMAGING STUDIES

- MRI, with and without gadolinium contrast, is the most critical diagnostic test; axial, coronal, and midsagittal enhanced images should be obtained. MRI is more sensitive than CT for small tumors and associated vascular structures, although both modalities properly visualize large masses. On T1 images, the tumor usually is isointense to brain; on T2 images, it is hyperintense. Meningiomas enhance densely after administration of gadolinium. On CT, meningiomas are isodense compared to brain and enhance densely with contrast. MRI and CT often demonstrate a site of dural attachment or a dural tail, as well as hyperostotic changes in nearby bone.

SPECIAL TESTS

- Angiography is performed in selected patients to assess vascular anatomy and collateral blood supply prior to surgery. It also may be useful as a prelude to presurgical embolization (to minimize intraoperative bleeding) or postoperative vascular reconstruction.

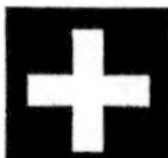

Management

GENERAL MEASURES

- In certain patient cohorts, meningiomas are followed conservatively after diagnosis, including patients with poor health, elderly patients with small lesions or who are reluctant to proceed to surgery, and patients with small tumors that do not correlate with symptoms. Observation should include an enhanced CT or MRI every 4–6 months to monitor for growth. Tumors may remain quiescent if they are stable during the initial observation period. Conservative approaches are unjustified in symptomatic patients and most young patients, especially if growth potential is demonstrated.

SURGICAL MEASURES

- Surgical resection is the treatment of choice for most symptomatic patients. The surgical approach will vary depending on the location of the tumor. Complete surgical extirpation is the goal whenever possible. Only subtotal removal is possible for tumors intimately associated with cranial nerves and/or vessels. After removal of the tumor, involved bone and dural attachments should also be resected, with a wide margin. Dural defects should be repaired with pericranium, temporalis fascia, or fascia lata grafts.

SYMPTOMATIC TREATMENT

- Consists of corticosteroids to control symptoms of intracranial pressure and anticonvulsants as required to control seizures.

ADJUNCTIVE TREATMENT

- Conventional external beam radiotherapy (RT) is of benefit for selected patients after subtotal removal, for recurrent or progressive tumors, and for all patients with malignant pathology (WHO grade III). Clinical trials demonstrate a survival advantage for patients given RT after subtotal removal versus surgery alone. Recommended RT doses for typical low-grade tumors are 50–55 Gy over 6 weeks, with 180–200 cGy fractions per day. More aggressive RT doses of 55–60 Gy may be appropriate for malignant meningiomas. Three-dimensional conformal treatment planning or intensity-modulated techniques should be used to minimize irradiation of normal brain. RT is not necessary for completely resected meningiomas with low-grade pathology.
- Stereotactic radiosurgery (linear accelerator, gamma knife) can be an adjunctive form of treatment in selected patients. Patients most appropriate for radiosurgery include those who are medically unstable, elderly (>65 years), have failed previous surgery, or refuse surgical intervention; tumors <3 cm in diameter are most suitable. Dosing is usually between 16 and 18 Gy in a single fraction to the 50% isodense line. Local control rates range from 90%–95%, with variable amounts of tumor shrinkage. Standard single-dose radiosurgery may be unsuitable for tumors in close proximity to the optic chiasm or brainstem. Fractionated radiosurgery (linear accelerator) may be a safer option for tumors near the optic apparatus or brainstem.
- Currently, chemotherapy has a limited role in the treatment of meningiomas. It should be considered for patients who cannot undergo surgical resection and for tumors that recur despite surgery and/or RT. Traditional cytotoxic chemotherapy has limited activity against meningiomas. Drugs with modest activity in phase II trials include mifepristone (RU-486; antagonist to progesterone receptors), hydroxyurea (induces apoptosis in meningioma cells), and interferon-α-2b. When active, chemotherapy usually induces tumor stabilization; shrinkage is uncommon.

ADMISSION/DISCHARGE CRITERIA

- Admission is generally reserved for presurgical evaluation and surgical resection. Angiography may be included in the workup to assess regional vascular anatomy. Patients with severe brain or brainstem compression might benefit from admission for IV dexamethasone.

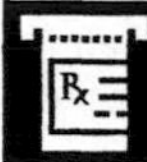

Medications

DRUG(S) OF CHOICE

- Dexamethasone 2–8 mg/day may be of benefit to reduce edema and swelling for patients with brain compression. It may improve transient symptoms of pressure and swelling after RT or radiosurgery.

Contraindications

N/A

Precautions

- All patients should be taking an H2-blocking drug while receiving chronic dexamethasone.

ALTERNATIVE DRUGS

N/A

Follow-Up

PATIENT MONITORING

- Patients are followed with serial MRI scans and assessment of neurologic function every 6–12 months.

EXPECTED COURSE AND PROGNOSIS

- The recurrence rate for completely resected tumors is 20% at 10 years. For incompletely resected tumors the rate is 55% at 10 years. For completely resected tumors the 5- and 10-year progression-free survival rates are 88% and 75%, respectively. For tumors that have undergone surgery plus RT, the 5- and 15-year progression-free survival rates are 95% and 86%, respectively. Survival is more limited for patients with malignant meningioma, with a 5-year survival rate of 63%.
- Factors that increase the probability for recurrence include incomplete removal of all dural attachments, invasion of bone, soft-tumor consistency, and malignant histology.

PATIENT EDUCATION

- Braintumors.com. Website: *www.braintumors.com*
- National Brain Tumor Foundation. Website: *www.braintumor.org*
- American Brain Tumor Association. Website: *www.abta.org*
- The Brain Tumor Society. Website: *www.tbts.org*
- MGH Neuro-Oncology–Meningiomas & Benign Brain Tumors. Website: *Neurosurgery.mgh.harvard.edu/BENIGNlk.htm#MGH*

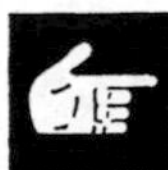

Miscellaneous

SYNONYMS

N/A

ICD-9-CM: 225.2 Benign neoplasm of cerebral meninges; 192.1 Malignant neoplasm of cerebral meninges

SEE ALSO: NEUROFIBROMATOSIS TYPES I AND II

REFERENCES

- Akeyson EW, McCutcheon IE. Management of benign and aggressive intracranial meningiomas. Oncology (Huntingt) 1996; 10:747–756.
- Black PM. Meningiomas. In: Vecht CJ, ed. Handbook of clinical neurology, 18:vol. 24 (68): neuro-oncology, part II. Amsterdam: Elsevier Science, 1997;401–420.
- De Monte F. Current management of meningiomas. Oncology (Huntingt) 1995;9:83–96.
- Newton HB, Slivka MA, Stevens C. Hydroxyurea chemotherapy for unresectable or residual meningioma. J Neurooncol 2000;49:165–170.
- Ojemannn R. Meningiomas. Neurosurg Clin N Am 1990;1:181–197.
- Stafford SL, Pollock BE, Foote RL, et al. Meningioma radiosurgery: tumor control, outcomes, and complications among 190 consecutive patients. Neurosurgery 2001;49:1029–1038.

Author(s): Herbert B. Newton, MD

Brain Tumor, Metastases

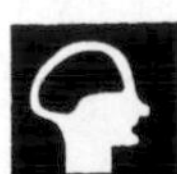

Basics

DESCRIPTION

- Metastatic brain tumors (MBTs) are the most common complication of systemic cancer. MBTs most often arise from tumors of the lung (50%–60%), breast (15%–20%), melanoma (5%–10%), and GI tract (4%–6%); however, they can develop from any systemic malignancy, including primary tumors of the prostate, ovary and female reproductive system, kidney, esophagus, soft-tissue sarcoma, bladder, and thyroid. In children and young adults, MBTs most often arise from sarcomas (e.g., osteogenic, Ewing's), germ cell tumors, and neuroblastoma. Postmortem studies suggest that melanoma, renal carcinoma, and testicular carcinoma have the greatest propensity for spread to the brain. In 65%–75% of patients, MBTs will present as multiple lesions. Multiple MBTs are most common with lung carcinoma and melanoma. Single MBTs are noted most often in patients with breast, colon, and renal cell carcinoma.

EPIDEMIOLOGY

Incidence/Prevalence

- Brain metastases develop in 20%–40% of adult and 6%–10% of children with systemic cancer. The annual incidence is 3.4–8.3 per 100,000 population. This corresponds to an estimated 125,000–170,000 new cases of MBT each year in the United States.

Race

- All races and ethnic groups are equally affected.

Age

- Typical presentation is 45–70 years in adults and 8–14 years in children; 40%–45% of MBTs present in patients $\geq$65 years.

Sex

- Males have a higher incidence than females (1.36:1).

ETIOLOGY

- Systemic tumor cells usually travel to the brain by hematogenous spread through the arterial circulation, most often originating from the lungs (primary or lung metastasis). The distribution of MBT follows the relative volume of blood flow to each area so that 80% of tumors arise in the cerebral hemispheres, 15% in the cerebellum, and 5% in the brainstem. Tumor cells typically lodge in small vessels at the gray-white junction and then spread into the brain parenchyma, where the cells proliferate and induce their own blood supply. MBTs are histologically similar to the primary tumor of origin.
- Neurologic function is disrupted by MBT through several mechanisms, including direct displacement of brain structures, perilesional edema, irritation of overlying gray matter, and compression of arterial and venous vasculature.
- Tumor cells more likely to metastasize to the brain have a more aggressive phenotype, with increased cell motility and angiogenic capacity. These changes are mediated by scatter factor, autocrine motility factor, activation of the ras signal transduction pathway, amplification of oncogenes, and loss or mutation of metastasis-suppressor genes (e.g., nm23, KiSS1).

Genetics

- Brain metastases are sporadic tumors without any specific genetic influence.

RISK FACTORS

- Risk factors that increase the probability of MBT include lung carcinoma and other primary malignancies with a predilection for the brain (i.e., melanoma, renal carcinoma, testicular carcinoma) and widespread aggressive disease, especially lung metastases.

PREGNANCY

- Pregnancy does not affect the clinical behavior of MBT.

ASSOCIATED CONDITIONS

- Include other common general and neurologic complications of cancer patients, such as infection and sepsis, metabolic encephalopathy, carcinomatous meningitis, and epidural spinal cord compression

Diagnosis

DIFFERENTIAL DIAGNOSIS

- Includes other enhancing solitary or multifocal masses, such as mature abscess or abscesses, primary brain tumor, acute infarct, and hemorrhage

SIGNS AND SYMPTOMS

- Symptoms caused by MBT usually are progressive over days to weeks. Any symptom can arise from MBT, depending on tumor location. The most frequent symptoms include headache (25%–40%), alterations of thinking and memory (20%–25%), focal weakness (20%–30%), and seizure activity (15%–20%). Less common symptoms consist of gait difficulty, visual loss, speech abnormalities, and sensory loss.
- Common neurologic signs include hemiparesis (55%–60%), impaired cognition (55%), papilledema (20%), dysphasia (15%–20%), gait disturbance (10%–20%), hemianopsia (5%), and hemisensory loss (5%).

LABORATORY PROCEDURES

N/A

IMAGING STUDIES

- MRI, with and without gadolinium contrast, is the most critical diagnostic test. Axial, coronal, and midsagittal enhanced images should be obtained. MBTs present as rounded, well-circumscribed, noninfiltrative masses surrounded by a large amount of edema. MRI is more sensitive than CT for small tumors and tumors in the posterior fossa and brainstem, although both modalities properly visualize large MBTs. On T1 images, the tumor usually is hypointense or isointense compared to brain; on T2 images, it is hyperintense. MBTs enhance densely after administration of gadolinium. On CT, MBTs are hypodense or isodense compared to brain and enhance densely with contrast.

SPECIAL TESTS

- Fluorodeoxyglucose-positron emission tomography (FDG-PET) may be of benefit to assess the metabolism of the suspected MBT to differentiate it from nonneoplastic lesions. MBT typically appear hypermetabolic on PET imaging. Magnetic resonance spectroscopy (MRS) also can be used for metabolic screening to differentiate MBTs from other lesions. MRS of MBT often reveals an elevated choline peak, reduced *N*-acetyl aspartate(NAA) peak, the presence of a lactate peak, and a reduced NAA/choline ratio.

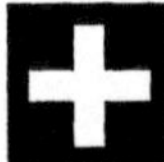

Management

GENERAL MEASURES

- Should include symptomatic treatment and consultation by radiation oncology, neurooncology, and neurosurgery for treatment evaluation

SURGICAL MEASURES

- Surgical resection is used for carefully selected patients with symptomatic accessible MBT and limited systemic disease. It is applied most frequently to patients with solitary MBT. Phase III trials have demonstrated a survival advantage for surgical resection plus irradiation versus irradiation alone (40 vs. 15 weeks) for patients with solitary lesions. Patients with multiple MBT can also be considered for resection if one or two accessible tumors are responsible for the majority of symptoms.

SYMPTOMATIC TREATMENT

- Consists of dexamethasone to control symptoms of intracranial pressure and anticonvulsants as required to control seizures. Anticonvulsants should not be used prophylactically; they should be implemented after documented seizure activity.

ADJUNCTIVE TREATMENT

- Conventional external beam radiotherapy (RT) to the whole brain is the most commonly used mode of treatment for patients with MBT. RT increases median survival to 12–24 weeks in most patients. RT is effective at palliation of neurologic symptoms (70%–80% rate of symptomatic improvement) and reduces the risk of death due to progression of MBT. Recommended RT doses are 30–45 Gy administered over 3–4 weeks, in fractions of 180–200 cGy. Addition of RT after surgical resection will prolong time to neurologic recurrence and reduce the risk of death from MBT.
- Stereotactic radiosurgery (linear accelerator, gamma knife) can be an adjunctive form of treatment in selected MBT patients. Although phase III trials have not been concluded, phase II data suggest that radiosurgery can extend survival and improve local tumor control. Appropriate patients have a good prognostic profile, including minimal neurologic dysfunction, three or fewer MBT that are <3 cm in size, stable systemic disease, and relatively young age. Recommended doses are 18–25 Gy in a single fraction.
- Chemotherapy has a limited role in the majority of patients with MBT. It is most beneficial for patients with stable systemic disease who have progressive MBT after RT or radiosurgery. Several approaches have been used (e.g., multiagent intravenous, intraarterial, oral) and demonstrated modest efficacy in phase II trials. The most active IV drugs are cisplatin, etoposide, and cyclophosphamide. Intraarterial carboplatin and oral temozolomide have been effective in some patients.

ADMISSION/DISCHARGE CRITERIA

- Admission usually is for exacerbation of cerebral edema and intracranial pressure or for excessive seizure activity. Maximizing anticonvulsant doses, resolving metabolic disturbances, and reducing intracranial pressure are required before discharge.

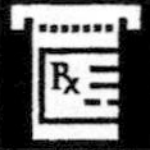

Medications

DRUG(S) OF CHOICE

- Dexamethasone 4–16 mg/day is of benefit to reduce edema and swelling and may improve transient symptoms of pressure and swelling after RT or radiosurgery. Seizures are a common problem in patients with MBT. Appropriate anticonvulsant choices (e.g., phenytoin, carbamazepine, levetiracetam) and management are critical.

Contraindications

- Patients on chemotherapy must meet appropriate hematologic parameters before proceeding with the next cycle: WBC >2.0, hemoglobin >10.0, and platelets >100,000.

Precautions

- All patients should be taking an H2-blocking drug while receiving chronic dexamethasone.

ALTERNATIVE DRUGS

N/A

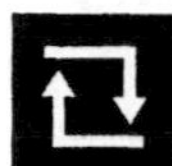

Follow-Up

PATIENT MONITORING

- Patients are followed with serial MRI scans and assessment of neurologic function every 2–4 months. Patients receiving chemotherapy may need more frequent monitoring of clinical and hematologic status. Anticonvulsant levels need to be monitored carefully.

EXPECTED COURSE AND PROGNOSIS

- Overall prognosis depends on the histologic tumor type, number and size of MBT, severity of neurologic dysfunction, and amount of systemic involvement. If left untreated, the expected survival of most patients with MBT is 4 weeks. Survival improves to 8 weeks with the addition of dexamethasone. Surgical resection and/or RT can extend survival another 8–20 weeks for most patients.
- The most important factors for extended survival are age <65 years, intact neurologic function, with a Karnofsky performance status >70, and well-controlled systemic disease. Patients with multiple MBTs have a reduced survival.

PATIENT EDUCATION

- Braintumors.com. Website: *www.braintumors.com*
- National Brain Tumor Foundation. Website: *www.braintumor.org*
- American Brain Tumor Association. Website: *www.abta.org*
- The Brain Tumor Society. Website: *www.tbts.org*
- Clinical Trials–Brain Metastases. Website: *www.bt-treatment.com/metstrials.htm*
- National Cancer Institute CancerNet. Website: *cancerweb.ncl.ac.uk/cancernet/103854.html*

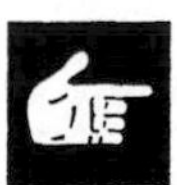

Miscellaneous

SYNONYMS

N/A

ICD-9-CM: 198.3 Secondary malignant neoplasm of brain and spinal cord

SEE ALSO: N/A

REFERENCES

- Berk L. An overview of radiotherapy trials for the treatment of brain metastases. Oncology (Huntingt) 1995;9:1205–1212.
- Boyd TS, Mehta MP. Stereotactic radiosurgery for brain metastases. Oncology (Huntingt) 1999;13:1397–1409.
- Lang FF, Sawaya R. Surgical management of cerebral metastases. Neurosurg Clin N Am 1996;7:459–484.
- Newton HB. Chemotherapy for the treatment of metastatic brain tumors. Expert Rev Anticancer Ther 2002;2: 495–506.
- Newton HB. Neurologic complications of systemic cancer. Am Fam Physician 1999; 59:878–886.
- Patchell RA. The treatment of brain metastases. Cancer Invest 1996;14: 169–177.
- Wen PY, Loeffler JS. Management of brain metastases. Oncology (Huntingt) 1999;13:941–961.

Author(s): Herbert B. Newton, MD

Brain Tumor, Oligodendroglioma

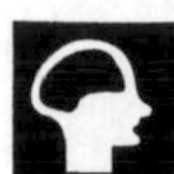

Basics

DESCRIPTION

- Oligodendrogliomas are an uncommon group of glial neoplasms that typically occur in young and middle-age adults. They have variable growth potential and can be quite infiltrative, depending on whether they are typical low-grade oligodendrogliomas (LGO) or the more aggressive anaplastic oligodendrogliomas (AO). Survival is prolonged in most patients and ranges between 4 and 10 years.

EPIDEMIOLOGY

Incidence/Prevalence

- Oligodendrogliomas comprise approximately 4%–5% of primary brain tumors in adults; this corresponds to roughly 700 new cases each year in North America. The incidences of LGO and AO are relatively equal, similar to the incidences of pure and mixed oligodendrogliomas.

Race

- All races and ethnic groups are affected. Caucasians are affected more commonly than blacks, Latinos, and Asians.

Age

- Typical presentation is between 40 and 50 years of age for all forms of oligodendrogliomas.

Sex

- Incidence is slightly higher in males than females (1.5:1).

ETIOLOGY

- The World Health Organization classifies LGO as grade II, AO as grade III, and mixed anaplastic oligoastrocytoma (AOA) as grade III.
- Oligodendrogliomas are most likely derived from transformed oligodendrocytes. They have a predilection for the subcortical white matter of the cerebral hemispheres. Pathologic evaluation of LGO reveals a moderately cellular tumor with rounded homogeneous cells that have a "fried-egg appearance" on paraffin sections. Other features include microcalcifications, dense branching capillaries, mild nuclear atypia, and low-level mitotic activity. AO will have similar features with the addition of higher cellular density, cellular and nuclear atypia, high mitotic rate, endothelial proliferation, and necrosis.
- Molecular genetic studies of oligodendrogliomas have noted that the two most common abnormalities are deletion of chromosomes 19q (50%–80%) and 1p (40%–65%). Loss of 1p and 19q are associated with chemosensitivity and prolonged survival of LGO and AO. Overexpression (without amplification) of epidermal growth factor receptors (EGFR) and platelet-derived growth factor receptors (PDGFR) is present in >50% of oligodendrogliomas. Other abnormalities include loss of chromosomal material on 9p and 10q, mutation or deletion of the tumor suppressor genes p53 and p16, and overexpression of vascular endothelial growth factor (VEGF).

Genetics

- Oligodendrogliomas usually are sporadic and do not have an underlying genetic predilection. Rarely, oligodendrogliomas can be familial.

RISK FACTORS

- The only known risk factors for oligodendrogliomas are prior cranial radiation exposure and those rare families in which oligodendrogliomas are genetically transmitted.

PREGNANCY

- Pregnancy does not affect the clinical course of oligodendrogliomas.

ASSOCIATED CONDITIONS

N/A

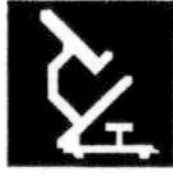

Diagnosis

DIFFERENTIAL DIAGNOSIS

- Other mass lesions that may or may not enhance should be considered, including abscess, subacute infarct, tumefactive regions of demyelination, and evolving hematoma.

SIGNS AND SYMPTOMS

- Median duration from onset of symptoms to diagnosis ranges from 6–12 months in AO and 18–30 months for LGO. The most common symptom at presentation is seizure activity (50%–70%). Seizures can be simple partial, complex partial, generalized tonic-clonic, or a combination. Other presenting symptoms include headache and other signs of increased intracranial pressure (e.g., nausea, emesis, diplopia), focal weakness, speech dysfunction, cognitive decline, and behavioral changes. Rarely, patients can have acute symptoms from intratumoral hemorrhage.
- Common findings on neurologic examination include hemiparesis, papilledema, dysphasia, impaired memory and cognition, hemianopsia, and sensory loss. Many patients with LGO have nonfocal neurologic examinations.

LABORATORY PROCEDURES

- Molecular analysis of chromosomes 1p and/or 19q loss is of prognostic significance in patients with AO and LGO.

IMAGING STUDIES

- MRI, with and without gadolinium contrast, is the most sensitive diagnostic test. MRI is more sensitive than CT for oligodendrogliomas that are small or within the posterior fossa. On T1 images, the tumor usually is infiltrative and appears hypointense or isointense compared to brain; on T2 images, the mass is hyperintense. Foci of hemorrhage or calcification may be noted. With gadolinium administration, most LGOs do not enhance, whereas AO/AOA show either patchy or ringlike enhancement. Peritumoral edema and mass effect usually are mild to moderate. CT demonstrates an ill-defined region of hypodensity with variable enhancement. Edema and mass effect are mild.

SPECIAL TESTS

- Fluorodeoxyglucose-positron emission tomography (FDG-PET) may be of benefit to assess the metabolism of oligodendrogliomas to differentiate from nonneoplastic lesions and to maximize targeting for biopsy. On PET imaging, LGOs appear hypometabolic and AOs appear hypermetabolic. Magnetic resonance spectroscopy (MRS) also can be used for metabolic screening to differentiate oligodendrogliomas from other lesions. MRS reveals an elevated choline peak, moderately reduced *N*-acetylaspartate (NAA) peak, the presence of a lactate peak, and a reduced NAA/choline ratio.

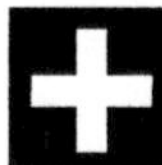

Management

GENERAL MEASURES

- The management of LGO and AO requires a multimodality approach to cytoreduction that may require surgery, radiotherapy, and chemotherapy. Treatment must be individualized. Input from neurosurgeons, neuro-oncologists, and radiation oncologists is necessary for optimal therapy. Patients with small indolent tumors (i.e., presentation with seizures, normal neurologic examination, no evidence on CT/MRI of increased intracranial pressure) may be followed without treatment for evidence of growth.

SURGICAL MEASURES

- Surgery should be considered in all patients to make a histologic diagnosis, reduce tumor bulk and intracranial pressure, and alleviate symptoms. Maximal surgical resection is the treatment of choice for accessible LGO and AO, preferably by computer-assisted volumetric resection techniques (e.g., stealth apparatus). For patients with deep inaccessible lesions or tumors in eloquent cortex, stereotactic biopsy should be performed. Several studies suggest that median and 5-year survival of LGO and AO are improved with complete or subtotal resection versus biopsy.

SYMPTOMATIC TREATMENT

- Dexamethasone 4–16 mg/day may be of benefit to reduce peritumoral edema and swelling.

ADJUNCTIVE TREATMENT

- External beam radiation therapy (RT) should be considered for carefully selected oligodendroglioma patients after subtotal resection or at progression. It is appropriate to consider delaying RT for patients with clean postoperative margins on follow-up MRI. Most patients with AO should be considered for RT after surgery, although it may be delayed until after chemotherapy in patients with deletion of 1p and 19q. The majority of phase II clinical trial data suggest an extension of median and 5-year survival by RT after subtotal resection and at recurrence. The recommended RT dose is 50–60 Gy over 6 weeks, in daily fractions of 180–200 cGy. Focal three-dimensional treatment planning and conformal techniques should be used whenever possible to minimize radiation exposure to normal brain.
- Stereotactic radiosurgery (SRS) has recently been used for recurrent oligodendrogliomas <4 cm. Larger tumors will not benefit from SRS due to infiltration beyond the treatment field. Median doses range from 15–17 Gy in one fraction. SRS may improve survival in carefully selected patients with small oligodendrogliomas.
- Oligodendrogliomas are the most chemosensitive type of primary brain tumor. Use of chemotherapy should be delayed until after complete surgical resection. Chemotherapy should be considered first-line treatment for subtotally resected LGO or AO with 1p/19q deletion status (100% response rate, survival >120 months) or 1p deletion/p53 mutation (100% response rate, survival >71 months). Patients with oligodendrogliomas that retain 1p and/or 19q may still respond to chemotherapy, but with lower response rates and shorter median survival. The most active regimens are PCV (procarbazine, CCNU [lomustine], vincristine), temozolomide, carmustine (BCNU), and melphalan.

ADMISSION/DISCHARGE CRITERIA

- Patients with LGO and AO often are admitted for seizure control or neurologic deterioration due to elevated intracranial pressure and tumor growth. Maximizing anticonvulsant doses, resolving metabolic disturbances, and reducing intracranial pressure are required before discharge.

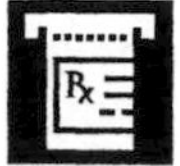

Medications

DRUG(S) OF CHOICE

- Seizures are a common problem for patients with LGO and AO. Appropriate anticonvulsant choices (e.g., phenytoin, carbamazepine, levetiracetam) and management are critical. Dexamethasone is used at the lowest dose able to control symptoms related to intracranial pressure.

Contraindications

- Patients on chemotherapy must meet appropriate hematologic parameters before proceeding with the next cycle: WBC >2.0, hemoglobin >10.0, and platelets >100,000.

Precautions

- All patients should be taking an H2-blocking drug while receiving chronic dexamethasone.

ALTERNATIVE DRUGS

N/A

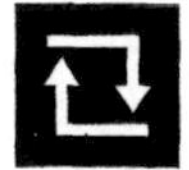

Follow-Up

PATIENT MONITORING

- Patients are followed with serial MRI scans and neurologic examinations every 4–6 months. Patients receiving chemotherapy may require more frequent follow-up. Anticonvulsant levels need to be monitored carefully.

EXPECTED COURSE AND PROGNOSIS

- Median survival of patients with LGO is 6–10 years, with a 5-year survival rate of 75%. Median survival of patients with AO is 3–4 years. Survival of AO patients is affected by 1p and 19q status. Tumors with deletion of both 1p and 19q are very chemosensitive, with patient survival of 8–10 years. Tumors that maintain both 1p and 19q are treatment resistant, with patient survival of 2–5 years.
- Prognosis is improved with young age (<40 years), LGO histology, high Karnofsky performance status, and deletion of 1p and/or 19q. Prognosis is worse with age >50 years, poor Karnofsky performance status, AO histology, and presence of 1p and 19q.

PATIENT EDUCATION

- Braintumors.com. Website: *www.braintumors.com*
- National Brain Tumor Foundation. Website: *www.braintumor.org*
- American Brain Tumor Association. Website: *www.abta.org*
- The Brain Tumor Society. Website: *www.tbts.org*
- Massachusetts General Hospital–Brain Tumor Center. Website: *brain.mgh.harvard.edu*
- Brain Tumor Treatment Options & Information. Website: *users.erols.com/colilla/index.htm*

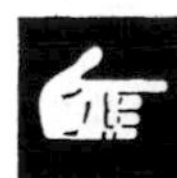

Miscellaneous

SYNONYMS

- Oligodendroglioma, anaplastic oligodendroglioma

ICD-9-CM: 191.8 Oligodendroglioma or anaplastic oligodendroglioma of brain

SEE ALSO: BRAIN TUMOR, HIGH-GRADE ASTROCYTOMA; BRAIN TUMOR, LOW-GRADE GLIOMA

REFERENCES

- Cairncross JG, Ueki K, Zlatescu MC, et al. Specific genetic predictors of chemotherapeutic response and survival in patients with anaplastic oligodendrogliomas. J Natl Cancer Inst 1998;90:1473–1479.
- Engelhard HH, Stelea A, Cochran EJ. Oligodendroglioma: pathology and molecular biology. Surg Neurol 2002;58: 111–00117.
- Hussein MR, Baidas S. Advances in diagnosis and management of oligodendroglioma. Expert Rev Anticancer Ther 2002;2:520–528.
- Perry JR, Cairncross JG. Oligodendrogliomas. In: Vecht CJ, ed. Handbook of clinical neurology, 5:vol. 24 (68): neuro-oncology, part II. Amsterdam: Elsevier Science, 1997;1223–1236.
- Perry JR, Louis DN, Cairncross JG. Current treatment of oligodendrogliomas. Arch Neurol 1999;56:434–436.
- Peterson K, Cairncross JG. Oligodendrogliomas. Cancer Invest 1996;14:243–251.

Author(s): Herbert B. Newton, MD

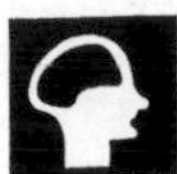

Basics

DESCRIPTION

- Pituitary tumors *(adenomas)* are benign monoclonal neoplasms that originate from the adenohypophysis (anterior pituitary gland). They can be classified as functional (secrete endocrinologically active hormones) or nonfunctional (nonsecretors). Based on their size, they can either be microadenomas (≤10 mm in greatest diameter) or macroadenomas (≥10 mm).

EPIDEMIOLOGY

Incidence

- Pituitary adenomas are among the most common adult intracranial neoplasms and account for 10%–15% of adult intracranial tumors. Microadenomas are far more common than macroadenomas and are detected in up to 27% of pituitaries in postmortem studies.

Age

- Pituitary tumors usually occur in adults (third to fifth decade of life), with only <10% diagnosed in children (comprising <2% of pediatric intracranial tumors).

Sex

- Prolactin-secreting and adrenocorticotropic hormone (ACTH)-secreting tumors are more common in females. Growth hormone-secreting and nonfunctioning adenomas predominate in males.

Race

- There is no evidence of racial predisposition.

ETIOLOGY

- One theory involves hormone regulatory dysfunction along the hypothalamic-pituitary axis, with regulatory peptides secreted by the hypothalamus leading to overstimulation and hyperplasia of the anterior lobe cells, followed by tumor proliferation. This implies that chronic pituitary hypertrophy or stimulation from a dysfunctional hypothalamus produces a distinctive population of mitogenic cells that has the potential to transform into a pituitary adenoma.

RISK FACTORS

- Multiple endocrine neoplasia (MEN) types I and II

PREGNANCY

- Pituitary adenomas can grow and become symptomatic during pregnancy. During pregnancy, the risk of symptomatic enlargement of a microadenoma is low (2%–4.5%) compared to the high risk (15%–25%) of symptomatic macroadenoma progression. For this reason, surgical debulking of pituitary macroadenomas is favored prior to conception, especially if they are nonfunctional.

ASSOCIATED CONDITIONS

- Cushing's syndrome
- Acromegaly

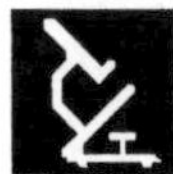

Diagnosis

DIFFERENTIAL DIAGNOSIS

- Pituitary hyperplasia
- Craniopharyngioma
- Empty sella syndrome
- Rathke cleft cyst
- Meningioma
- Germ cell tumors (germinoma)
- Chiasmatic/hypothalamic glioma
- Metastasis (lung, breast, prostate)
- Juxtasellar aneurysm
- Lymphocytic hypophysitis
- Hamartomas
- Chordomas
- Granulomas
- Langerhans' cell histiocytosis
- Sarcoidosis

SIGNS AND SYMPTOMS

- Microadenomas usually cause symptoms related to hormonal hypersecretion, but they also can be asymptomatic. Macroadenomas usually present with mass effect. The most common complaints are headache (vague, dull, and usually bifrontal and behind the eyes) and visual abnormalities (chiasmal compression with bitemporal field defect, blurred vision, decreased visual acuity).
- Approximately 75% of patients with functioning pituitary adenomas present with an endocrinopathy consistent with their underlying pathology. Prolactinomas present with amenorrhea and galactorrhea in women and impotence in men. A growth hormone-secreting adenoma presents with gigantism in children and acromegaly in adults. In addition to the acral changes, they have systemic hypertension and impaired glucose tolerance. ACTH-secreting pituitary tumors (Cushing's disease) typically present with Cushing's syndrome. Clinical signs and symptoms include central obesity with abdominal striae, buffalo hump, and moon facies, as well as menstrual irregularity, hirsutism, hypertension, and diabetes.
- Pituitary apoplexy is a syndrome that occurs as a result of hemorrhage and/or infarction within a pituitary adenoma and leads to acute and severe headache, nausea/vomiting, ocular paresis, meningeal signs, and altered sensorium. It can mimic an acute subarachnoid hemorrhage.

LABORATORY PROCEDURES

- Serum prolactin level, growth hormone level, insulin growth factor type I, serum TSH, T_4/T_3 levels, serum luteinizing hormone (LH), follicular stimulating hormone (FSH), estradiol and testosterone serum levels. Screen the pituitary adrenal axis with an AM cortisol and an ACTH level. Draw basic electrolyte panel if diabetes insipidus is suspected.
- When checking the prolactin serum levels, it should be noted that occasionally in giant invasive prolactinomas the laboratory should be instructed to dilute the samples before measuring them, otherwise a false low prolactin level may appear. This has the risk of denying the patient medical treatment with dopamine agonists and favoring a surgical approach when it is not indicated.

IMAGING STUDIES

- MRI is the radiologic study of choice. Pituitary microadenomas typically are hypointense to surrounding tissue on T1-weighted images, and isointense or hyperintense on T2-weighted images. These tumors typically enhance more slowly than normal pituitary tissue. Cavernous sinus invasion is suspected when the tumor encases the cavernous portion of the internal carotid artery. Pituitary macroadenomas enhance with gadolinium and may show heterogeneity due to necrosis, hemorrhage, or cyst formation. CT may be used for delineating the bony structures of skull base, especially when dealing with invasive adenomas.

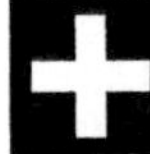

Management

GENERAL MEASURES

- The goals of treatment centers are
  - —Removing mass effect and associated neural compression
  - —Correcting any endocrinopathy
  - —Reestablishing normal hormonal functions in a preserved pituitary gland
- The decision of whether to proceed with a surgical or medical treatment depends on the hormonal evaluation. Prolactin-secreting pituitary adenomas are best treated with medical therapy using dopamine agonists.

- In some patients, however, a surgical approach with tumor debulking is indicated (e.g., for acute visual disturbances). Surgical intervention is also indicated in a small group of patients who do not respond to medical therapy or do not tolerate it. It is also offered to any female with a macroadenoma who may consider pregnancy in the future.
- Surgical therapy is the first-line treatment for ACTH-producing pituitary microadenomas, growth hormone-secreting tumors, and nonfunctional pituitary tumors. In case of failure to achieve cures or recurrence of these tumors, alternative treatment modalities are considered, such as pharmacotherapy and/or radiation therapy.

SURGICAL MEASURES

- Most pituitary adenomas can be approached via a transsphenoidal approach with low morbidity and mortality (complication rate 2%–4%). The sphenoid sinus is accessed via an endonasal or transnasal approach, followed by removal of the tumor from the sellar region. The most common surgical complications include transient CSF rhinorrhea, hypopituitarism, and diabetes insipidus. A cranial approach may be indicated for patients with tumor extension into the anterior and/or middle cranial fossa.

RADIATION THERAPY

- Radiation is effective in treating pituitary adenomas. Risks include damage to the optic nerve/chiasm, hypothalamus, and adjacent temporal lobe. Radiation therapy leads to permanent damage of the pituitary gland and hypopituitarism. Focused radiation therapy using radiosurgical techniques have the advantage of minimal exposure to radiation of the adjacent neural tissue and may be indicated in recurrent tumors that failed surgical resection.

SYMPTOMATIC TREATMENT

N/A

ADJUNCTIVE TREATMENT

N/A

ADMISSION/DISCHARGE CRITERIA

- Admission is warranted for surgical resection of adenomas.

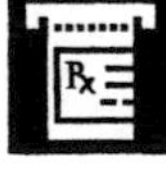

Medications

DRUG(S) OF CHOICE

- *Prolactinomas:* Bromocriptine is a dopamine agonist that suppresses prolactin secretion by binding the D2 receptors of the prolactin-producing cells in the anterior pituitary gland. Therapy is started 0.625–1.25 mg qhs and gradually increased up to 2.5 mg three times a day. This gradual increase avoids the possible side effects of headaches, nausea, and vomiting.
- *Growth hormone-secreting adenomas:* A somatostatin analog can be used as adjuvant therapy for patients with growth hormone-secreting pituitary adenomas. Octreotide has been given preoperatively to improve cardiovascular and endocrine function (100 μg SC tid).
- *ACTH-secreting adenomas:* Drugs that inhibit steroidogenesis, such as and ketoconazole and metyrapone, have been used in the perioperative period in Cushing's disease. These drugs are relevant before surgical intervention or in cases of recurrences that have been treated with radiation therapy.

Contraindications

- Bromocriptine should be discontinued if a female becomes pregnant.

Precautions

- Caution is indicated for use of octreotide in insulin-dependent diabetic patients because it can dramatically decrease the insulin requirement and cause hypoglycemia. Long-term use of octreotide carries the risk of cholesterol gallstones.

ALTERNATIVE DRUGS

- In case of intolerance to bromocriptine, cabergoline can be used.

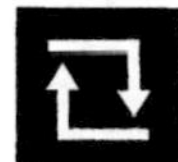

Follow-Up

PATIENT MONITORING

- A neuroendocrine nurse can contact these patients during the first 2 weeks regarding hormone replacement therapy. Desmopressin acetate (DDAVP) spray or tablets can be given to patients with a prolonged diabetes insipidus state.
- Patients are informed to call about any clear nasal drainage, fever, headaches, neck stiffness, or other signs of meningitis. Patients are then scheduled to come back to their first clinic visit in 4–6 weeks for follow-up MRI of the brain.

EXPECTED COURSE AND PROGNOSIS

- *Prolactinomas:* Surgical treatment of a prolactin-secreting microadenoma is very rewarding. Cure rates are estimated to be as high as 85%–90%. However, the medical treatment is as rewarding, and both options are excellent for patients with micro-adenomas. The cure rate is increased in patients with preoperative prolactin levels in the 200–300 range. The recurrence rate is as high as 10% over a 5- to 10-year period. Macroadenomas have lower cure rates with surgical treatment and respond optimally to medical therapy with dopamine agonists.
- *Growth hormone-secreting adenomas:* Up to 70% of patients with acromegaly are expected to achieve remission with surgical treatment (more common with microadenomas). The recurrence of these tumors is treated with either surgical exploration or medical therapy with octreotide. Radiation therapy also can be considered and is effective.
- *ACTH-secreting adenomas:* The ACTH-secreting adenomas are more likely to recur after remission is achieved by surgical removal. Approximately 70% of patients with a distinct microadenoma on MRI achieve remission. The recurrence rate of ACTH-producing adenomas is higher than the other secreting adenomas and occurs in up to 15%–20% of patients (40% following an initial resection).

PATIENT EDUCATION

- There are numerous support groups that provide assistance and information for patients and families with pituitary adenomas.
- Pituitary Tumor Network Association P.O. Box 1958 Thousand Oaks, CA 91358. Phone: (805) 499-9973. *www.pituitary.com*

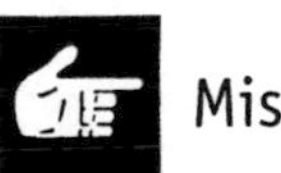

Miscellaneous

SYNONYMS

- Pituitary tumors

ICD-9-CM: 227.3 Benign neoplasm, pituitary

SEE ALSO: N/A

REFERENCES

- Izawa M, Hayashi M, Nakaya K, et al. Gamma knife radiosurgery for pituitary adenomas. J Neurosurg 2000;93[Suppl 3]: 19–22.
- Krisht A, Tindall GT. Pituitary disorders: comprehensive management. Baltimore, MD: Lippincott Williams & Wilkins, 1999:61–78,119–164,199–208,235–242, 349–360,407–415.
- Molitch ME. Pituitary diseases in pregnancy. Semin Pathol 1998;22:457–470.
- Osborn AG, Tong KA. Handbook of neuroradiology: brain and skull, 2nd ed. St. Louis: Mosby, 1996:280–284.
- Shimon I, Melmed S. Management of pituitary tumors. Ann Intern Med 1998;129:472–483.

Author(s): Said Elshihabi, MD; Ali F. Krisht, MD

Brain Tumor, Primary Central Nervous System Lymphoma

Basics

DESCRIPTION

- Primary CNS lymphoma (PCNSL) is a malignant non-Hodgkin's lymphoma limited to the cranial-spinal axis without systemic involvement. It originates in the brain and must be distinguished from metastatic systemic lymphoma. At the time of diagnosis, the leptomeninges (30%–35%) and eyes (25%) are frequently involved. PCNSL occurs most often in immunocompromised patients but also can arise in patients with intact immune function.

EPIDEMIOLOGY

Incidence/Prevalence

- The incidence of PCNSL is rising in immunocompetent patients and in those with HIV, with a 10-fold increase over the past 25 years. PCNSL now accounts for 2%–3% of all primary brain tumors in immunocompetent patients. For HIV patients, the lifetime incidence is in the range from 5%–10%. The annual incidence is currently 30 cases per 10 million persons.

Race

- All races and ethnic groups are affected. Caucasians are affected more commonly than blacks, Latinos, and Asians.

Age

- Typical presentation is between 50 and 55 years of age in immunocompetent patients and between 30 and 35 years in HIV patients.

Sex

- Incidence is slightly higher in males than females (3:2). HIV patients with PCNSL are predominantly male (7.3:1).

ETIOLOGY

- PCNSL is classified as a stage IE non-Hodgkin's lymphoma because the involvement is restricted to a single extranodal site—the brain. It is a clonal expansion of B cells in >97% of cases. T-cell PCNSL is uncommon (2%–3%). The World Health Organization does not have a specific classification scheme for PCNSL. Histologic subtyping of PCNSL suggests that diffuse large cell and diffuse large cell immunoblastic types are most common. However, subtyping has not been shown to have clinical relevance.
- It remains unclear how PCNSL arises in the brain, because the CNS is devoid of lymphoid tissue or lymphatics. Histologic evaluation reveals an angiocentric, diffusely infiltrative mass of neoplastic lymphoid cells, with extension into surrounding brain parenchyma. Isolated nodules of lymphoma cells can be observed at remote sites. Reactive astrocytosis and necrosis may be noted.
- Molecular genetic studies of PCNSL demonstrate clonal abnormalities of several chromosomes (1, 6, 7, 14) and translocations (e.g., 1;14, 6;14). Clonal rearrangements of the immunoglobulin and TcR genes are typically noted. The most common genetic alterations are mutations of the CDKN2A/p16 and CDKN2B/p15 tumor suppressor genes.

Genetics

- PCNSLs are sporadic and do not have an underlying genetic predilection, except for genetically mediated immunodeficiency states.

RISK FACTORS

- The most important risk factor for PCNSL is immunosuppression, usually in patients with HIV or after organ transplantation, less often in congenital immunodeficiency states such as ataxia-telangiectasia and Wiskott-Aldrich syndrome. Epstein-Barr virus (EBV) is involved in the pathogenesis of >95% of PCNSL from HIV patients. EBV is implicated in <5% of PCNSL from immunocompetent patients.

PREGNANCY

- Pregnancy does not affect the clinical course of PCNSL.

ASSOCIATED CONDITIONS

N/A

Diagnosis

DIFFERENTIAL DIAGNOSIS

- Other mass lesions that enhance should be considered, including other malignant brain tumors, mature abscess, subacute infarct, tumefactive regions of demyelination, and evolving hematoma.

SIGNS AND SYMPTOMS

- PCNSL is a highly aggressive tumor with a rapidly progressive course. Median time from onset of symptoms to diagnosis is only 4–12 weeks. The most common signs and symptoms at presentation include focal neurologic deficits (e.g., hemiparesis, dysphasia, cranial neuropathy; 50%–55%), mental status changes (e.g., reduced mentation, lethargy, confusion; 34%–50%), seizures (10%–25%), and evidence of increased intracranial pressure (e.g., headache, nausea, emesis, papilledema; 14%–30%). Patients with ocular involvement complain of blurred vision or floaters. Patients with spinal and/or leptomeningeal disease complain of neck or back pain, myelopathic weakness, and/or bowel and bladder dysfunction.

LABORATORY PROCEDURES

- Patients with suspected PCNSL require a lumbar puncture to assess CSF for cytology; HIV screening; CSF EBV DNA testing in AIDS patients, bone marrow evaluation for lymphomatous involvement

IMAGING STUDIES

- PCNSL usually presents in the periventricular region or among the deep nuclear structures. The tumor nodules are multifocal in 40% of cases (more so in HIV patients). MRI, with and without gadolinium contrast, is the most sensitive diagnostic test. On T1 images, the tumor usually is infiltrative and appears hypointense or isointense compared to brain. On T2 images, the mass is hyperintense. With gadolinium administration, most PCNSLs show either diffuse or ringlike enhancement. Peritumoral edema and mass effect are usually mild to moderate. Hemorrhage and regions consistent with necrosis are occasionally noted. CT demonstrates an ill-defined region of hypodensity with variable enhancement, and mild-to-moderate edema and mass effect. Spinal MRI is indicated in patients with spinal symptoms to screen for involvement of the spinal cord or leptomeninges.
- Chest x-ray film and CT of the abdomen and pelvis are necessary to screen for systemic lymphoma.

SPECIAL TESTS

- Fluorodeoxyglucose-positron emission tomography (FDG-PET) may be of benefit to assess the metabolism of PCNSL to differentiate it from nonneoplastic lesions. PCNSL typically appears hypermetabolic on PET imaging. PDG-PET is especially helpful in HIV patients to differentiate PCNSL from infection (i.e., toxoplasmosis). CSF evaluation reveals mild pleocytosis in 35%–60% of patients, with positive cytology in up to 30% of cases. Ophthalmologic evaluation (including slit-lamp testing) is necessary to screen for ocular lymphoma.

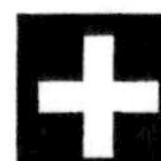

Management

GENERAL MEASURES

- Management of PCNSL requires a multimodality approach that involves input from neurosurgeons, neuro-oncologists, and radiation oncologists.

SURGICAL MEASURES

- Surgery should be considered in all patients to make a histologic diagnosis. Because extent of surgical resection has not been found to correlate with survival in PCNSL and most lesions are located deep in the brain, stereotactic biopsy is the recommended approach. Intraocular biopsy may be necessary to demonstrate lymphoma cells and justify ocular therapy. Ocular biopsy may be diagnostic of PCNSL in some patients.

SYMPTOMATIC TREATMENT

- Consists of reducing intracranial pressure, controlling seizures, and pain control. Corticosteroids should be used as sparingly as possible, because PCNSL may shrink transiently and make biopsy more difficult.

ADJUNCTIVE TREATMENT

- External beam radiation therapy (RT) should be considered, because PCNSL is radiosensitive in immunocompetent and HIV patients. Complete and partial responses can be noted; however, the responses are not durable, with relapse within 8–14 months. The recommended approach for immunocompetent patients is whole-brain RT, 45–50 Gy over 5 weeks in daily fractions of 180-cGy. HIV patients receive 40–45 Gy. Patients with ocular PCNSL may require RT to both orbits (40 Gy). Median survival with RT alone is 17 months in immunocompetent patients and 3 months in HIV patients. Lower-dose RT is sometimes combined with chemotherapy.
- Chemotherapy should be considered for all patients with PCNSL. The most active regimens use high-dose methotrexate (IV or intraarterial) in combination with other drugs (e.g., cyclophosphamide, etoposide, procarbazine, cytarabine). Intraarterial chemotherapy is combined with mannitol-induced blood-brain barrier disruption in some patients. Chemotherapy can be used alone (i.e., neoadjuvant) or in combination with RT. Younger patients with intact neurologic function and good performance status are the best candidates for neoadjuvant approaches. Median survival ranges from 40–45 months in patients treated with chemotherapy alone or in combination with RT. Intrathecal chemotherapy (methotrexate, cytarabine, cytarabine depofoam), preferably via an Ommaya reservoir, improves survival in PCNSL patients in combination with systemic chemotherapy. Intraocular chemotherapy (methotrexate) may be of benefit in selected patients with ocular PCNSL.

ADMISSION/DISCHARGE CRITERIA

- Patients with PCNSL often are admitted for seizure control, neurologic deterioration due to elevated intracranial pressure and tumor growth, or leptomeningeal metastases. Maximizing anticonvulsant doses, resolving metabolic disturbances, and reducing intracranial pressure are required before discharge. New therapeutic interventions may be necessary (e.g., intrathecal chemotherapy).

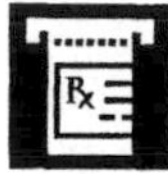

Medications

DRUG(S) OF CHOICE

- Seizures are a common problem in patients with PCNSL. Appropriate anticonvulsant choices (e.g., phenytoin, carbamazepine, levetiracetam) and management will be critical. Dexamethasone should be avoided, if possible, or used at the lowest dose able to control pressure-related symptoms.

Contraindications

- Patients on chemotherapy must meet appropriate hematologic parameters before proceeding with the next cycle: WBC >2.0, hemoglobin >10.0, and platelets $>100{,}000$.

Precautions

- All patients should be taking an H2-blocking drug while receiving chronic dexamethasone.

ALTERNATIVE DRUGS

N/A

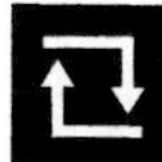

Follow-Up

PATIENT MONITORING

- Patients are followed with serial MRI scans and neurologic examinations every 4–8 weeks. Patients receiving chemotherapy may require more frequent follow-up. Anticonvulsant levels need to be monitored carefully.

EXPECTED COURSE AND PROGNOSIS

- The natural history of PCNSL is death within 8–14 weeks without treatment. With RT plus chemotherapy or chemotherapy alone, median survival ranges from 25–45 months in immunocompetent patients. For HIV patients, median survival is 6–18 months with treatment.
- Prognosis is improved with young age (<60 years), intact neurologic function, good performance status, and male sex. Prognosis is worse with age >60 years, poor neurologic function, female sex, and tumor involvement of the corpus callosum and/or brainstem.

PATIENT EDUCATION

- Braintumors.com. Website: *www.braintumors.com*
- National Brain Tumor Foundation. Website: *www.braintumor.org*
- American Brain Tumor Association. Website: *www.abta.org*
- The Brain Tumor Society. Website: *www.tbts.org*
- Update on Management of PCNSL. Website: *www.intouchlive.com/journals/oncology/o0002c.htm*

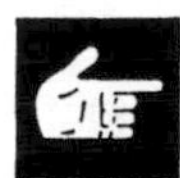

Miscellaneous

SYNONYMS

- Primary cerebral lymphoma
- Reticulum cell sarcoma
- Microglioma

ICD-9-CM: 191.8 Malignant neoplasm of brain

SEE ALSO: ACQUIRED IMMUNODEFICIENCY SYNDROME, FOCAL BRAIN LESIONS

REFERENCES

- Fine HA, Mayer RJ. Primary central nervous system lymphoma. Ann Intern Med 1993;119:1093–1104.
- Nasir S, DeAngelis LM. Update on the management of primary CNS lymphoma. Oncology (Huntingt) 2000;14:228–234.
- Nelson DF. Radiotherapy in the treatment of primary central nervous system lymphoma (PCNSL). J Neurooncol 1999;43:241–247.
- Newton HB, Fine HA. NCCN clinical practice guidelines for non-immunosuppressed primary CNS lymphoma. Oncology (Huntingt) 1999;13:153–160.
- Paulus W. Classification, pathogenesis and molecular pathology of primary CNS lymphoma. J Neurooncol 1999;43:203–208.
- Peterson K, DeAngelis LM. Primary cerebral lymphoma. In: Vecht CJ, ed. Handbook of clinical neurology, 11:vol. 24 (68): neuro-oncology, part II. Amsterdam: Elsevier Science, 1997;257–268.

Author(s): Herbert B. Newton, MD

Carcinomatous Meningitis

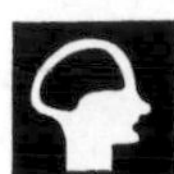

Basics

DESCRIPTION

- Carcinomatous meningitis (CAM) is a common neurologic complication of systemic cancer that is associated with severe mortality and morbidity. CAM is caused by the spread of cancer cells into the subarachnoid space and CSF, with subsequent access to the entire neuraxis. CAM has the capacity to affect every component of the CNS, including the brain, cranial nerves, spinal cord, spinal nerve roots, and cauda equina. It can develop in virtually any malignancy, but it is most common in leukemia, lymphoma, and solid tumors such as melanoma, breast carcinoma, and small cell lung carcinoma.

EPIDEMIOLOGY

Incidence/Prevalence

- The estimated incidence of CAM is 4%–15% of patients with solid tumors, 7%–15% of patients with lymphoma, 5%–15% of patients with leukemia, and 1%–2% of patients with primary brain tumors.

Race

- All races and ethnic groups are equally affected.

Age

- Typical presentation is between 45 and 60 years of age.

Sex

- Females have a higher incidence than males (1.6:1).

ETIOLOGY

- Systemic tumor cells gain access to the subarachnoid space and CSF through hematogenous spread to arachnoidal vessels, choroid plexus, or Batson's vertebral venous plexus; by direct extension from superficial regions of brain parenchyma, periventricular, or epidural metastases; and by perineural spread along spinal or cranial nerves. CAM is histologically similar to the primary neoplasm.
- Neurologic function is disrupted by CAM through several mechanisms, including elevation of intracranial pressure by the presence of diffuse tumor burden, direct invasion of neural tissues (brain, spinal cord, cranial and spinal nerves), ischemia due to obstruction of arterial blood flow, and regional metabolic alterations (e.g., lactic acidosis, low glucose concentration).
- Tumor cells most likely to metastasize to the CNS have a more aggressive and motile phenotype. These changes are mediated by scatter factor, autocrine motility factor, amplification of oncogenes, and mutation of metastasis-suppressor genes (e.g., nm23).

Genetics

- CAM is a sporadic process without any specific genetic influence.

RISK FACTORS

- Risk factors that increase the probability of CAM include tumor type (e.g., melanoma) and aggressive, widespread systemic disease.

PREGNANCY

- Pregnancy does not affect the clinical behavior of CAM.

ASSOCIATED CONDITIONS

- Include other common general and neurologic complications of cancer patients, such as infection and sepsis, metabolic encephalopathy, brain metastasis, and epidural spinal cord compression

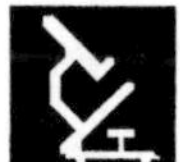

Diagnosis

DIFFERENTIAL DIAGNOSIS

- Includes other diseases that can involve the subarachnoid space, induce CSF inflammation, and cause enhancement of the leptomeninges on MRI, such as chronic bacterial or fungal meningitis, neurosarcoidosis, Guillain-Barré syndrome, and vasculitis

SIGNS AND SYMPTOMS

- Symptoms and signs of CAM can involve any region of the neuraxis, including the brain, cranial nerves, and spine. The symptoms usually are progressive over days to weeks. In 30%–40% of patients, more than one region of the neuraxis will be involved. Cerebral signs and symptoms include headache (60%), mental status changes (50%), gait alterations (25%), nausea and emesis (22%), seizures (11%), and hemiparesis (3%). Cranial nerve signs and symptoms include diplopia and ocular motor pareses of III, IV, and VI (30%), facial weakness (27%), impaired hearing (13%), facial numbness (8%), visual loss and optic neuropathy (8%), facial numbness (8%), and tongue weakness (8%). Spinal signs and symptoms include reflex asymmetry (85%), leg weakness (70%), paresthesias (40%), sensory loss (30%), back/neck pain (30%), radicular pain (26%), and bowel/bladder dysfunction (15%).

LABORATORY PROCEDURES

- The single most useful diagnostic test is examination of the CSF by lumbar puncture (LP). The CSF is always abnormal, even when the cytology is negative. In most patients, there is mild-to-moderate pleocytosis, elevated protein, reduced glucose level, and elevated lactate level. Tumor markers (e.g., β-glucuronidase, β_2-microglobulin, carcinoembryonic antigen) are adjunctive tests that can improve diagnostic accuracy if elevated; 50% of patients with CAM will have a positive cytology after one LP and 90% will be positive after the third LP. CSF cytology can remain negative in some patients.

IMAGING STUDIES

- MRI of the brain and/or spinal cord, with and without gadolinium contrast, is the most sensitive imaging test; axial, coronal, and midsagittal enhanced images should be obtained. Abnormal enhancement is noted in 70% of patients with CAM, along the surface of the brain, ventricular ependyma, cranial nerves, spinal cord, and cauda equina. Nodules of enhancement and hydrocephalus are noted in 38% and 7% of patients, respectively. CT reveals similar enhancement patterns, but in only 40% of patients with CAM. MRI or CT evidence of CAM can be diagnostic if CSF cytology is negative. However, a negative MRI or CT does not rule out CAM. Myelography, with or without CT followthrough, also can be diagnostic if MRI is unavailable.

SPECIAL TESTS

- Flow cytometry of the CSF may be diagnostic of CAM from leukemia and lymphoma if it is able to demonstrate a monoclonal population of cells. It also may demonstrate the presence of neoplastic aneuploid DNA populations. For CAM patients with diffuse bulky disease, a radionuclide CSF flow study may be necessary to demonstrate patency of the CSF pathways before intrathecal (IT) chemotherapy is administered through an Ommaya reservoir.

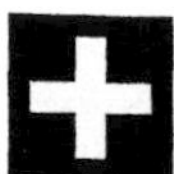

Management

GENERAL MEASURES

- Should include symptomatic treatment and consultation by radiation oncology, neuro-oncology, and neurosurgery for treatment evaluation.

SURGICAL MEASURES

- Surgical intervention is rarely necessary for treatment of CAM. Leptomeningeal biopsy may be of benefit in clinically suspicious patients with negative CSF and MRI testing. Ommaya reservoir placement should be considered for all patients receiving IT chemotherapy. Patients who develop hydrocephalus will require placement of a ventriculoperitoneal shunt. The shunt should contain an on/off valve to allow IT chemotherapy.

SYMPTOMATIC TREATMENT

- Consists of dexamethasone to control symptoms of intracranial pressure, anticonvulsants as required to control seizures, and pain control.

ADJUNCTIVE TREATMENT

- Conventional radiotherapy (RT) is of benefit to stabilize or palliate symptomatic regions of CAM. It is most often administered to the whole brain or to involved regions of the spinal axis with bulky disease. RT is more effective than IT chemotherapy for bulky disease, due to poor penetration of drug deeper than 2–3 mm. Pain-related symptoms often are improved with RT. Spinal neuraxis RT is generally avoided due to severe myelosuppression. The recommended dose to the brain or involved spine is 30 Gy in 10 fractions over 2 weeks. Patients with leukemic or lymphomatous CAM may improve neurologically after RT. Improvement is uncommon with CAM from solid tumors.
- Chemotherapy is the only therapeutic modality that can treat the whole neuraxis. It is best administered by the IT route, either by LP or Ommaya reservoir. Drug distribution is more even throughout the neuraxis when using the intraventricular route. Drugs that are approved for IT chemotherapy (usually once or twice weekly) include methotrexate, cytarabine, thiotepa, and depo-foam cytarabine. Systemic chemotherapy has not been as effective as IT, due to poor CSF penetration and low drug concentrations. High-dose intravenous methotrexate, cytarabine, and thiotepa have demonstrated modest efficacy in some patients.

ADMISSION/DISCHARGE CRITERIA

- Admission is usually for progression of neurologic dysfunction and/or seizure activity. Maximizing anticonvulsant doses and resolving metabolic disturbances are required before discharge. New modes of treatment may be required (e.g., RT, IT chemotherapy).

Medications

DRUG(S) OF CHOICE

- Dexamethasone 2–8 mg/day may be of benefit to reduce edema and swelling or to improve transient symptoms of pressure and swelling after RT. Seizures may be a problem in patients with CAM. Appropriate anticonvulsant choices (e.g., phenytoin, carbamazepine, levetiracetam) and management are critical. Narcotic analgesics may be necessary for adequate amelioration of pain.

Contraindications

- Patients on chemotherapy must meet appropriate hematologic parameters before proceeding with the next cycle: WBC >2.0, hemoglobin >10.0, and platelets >100,000.

Precautions

- All patients should be taking an H2-blocking drug while receiving chronic dexamethasone.

ALTERNATIVE DRUGS

N/A

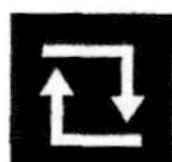

Follow-Up

PATIENT MONITORING

- Patients are followed with assessment of neurologic function and CSF evaluation every 4–8 weeks. MRI follow-up is required every 2–4 months. Patients receiving chemotherapy may need more frequent monitoring of clinical and hematologic status. Anticonvulsant levels need to be monitored carefully.

EXPECTED COURSE AND PROGNOSIS

- CAM is a virulent complication of cancer with a natural history of death in 4–8 weeks without treatment. Median overall survival is poor and ranges from 4–6 months with treatment. Survival is most limited for patients with solid tumors, except for those with breast cancer, who may survive 6–12 months. Patients with leukemia and lymphoma may respond well to therapy.
- The most important factors for extended survival are early diagnosis with low subarachnoid tumor burden, good performance status, mild neurologic dysfunction, female sex, longer duration of symptoms, and treatment with IT chemotherapy. Factors contributing to brief survival include high CSF protein levels, severe neurologic dysfunction, male sex, poor performance status, and clinical involvement of the supratentorial leptomeninges.

PATIENT EDUCATION

- Carcinomatous/neoplastic meningitis: *www.neuro-oncology.org/neomen1.htm; www.bt-treatment.com/neomen1.htm; www.uscneurosurgery.com/glossary/c/carcinomatous%20meningitis.htm*
- Carcinomatous meningitis clinical resources. Website: *www.slis.ua.edu/dis/cchs/main/clinical/oncology/neurological/cns/spine*

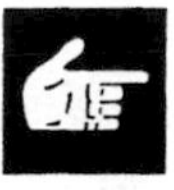

Miscellaneous

SYNONYMS

- Leptomeningeal metastases
- Neoplastic meningitis
- Leptomeningeal carcinomatosis

ICD-9-CM: 198.3 Secondary malignant neoplasm of brain and spinal cord; 198.4 Secondary malignant neoplasm of other parts of CNS

SEE ALSO: N/A

REFERENCES

- Balm M, Hammack J. Leptomeningeal carcinomatosis: presenting features and prognostic factors. Arch Neurol 1996; 53:626–632.
- Chamberlain MC. Leptomeningeal metastases. In: Vecht CJ, eds. Handbook of clinical neurology, 10:vol. 25 (69): neuro-oncology, part III. Amsterdam: Elsevier Science, 1997;151–165.
- Cokgor I, Friedman AH, Friedman HS. Current options for the treatment of neoplastic meningitis. J Neurooncol 2002;60:79–88.
- DeAngelis LM. Current diagnosis and treatment of leptomeningeal metastasis. J Neurooncol 1998;38:245–252.
- Gomori JM, Heching N, Siegal T. Leptomeningeal metastases: evaluation by gadolinium enhanced spinal magnetic resonance imaging. J Neurooncol 1998;36:55–60.
- Newton HB. Neurologic complications of systemic cancer. Am Fam Physician 1999;59:878–886.

Author(s): Herbert B. Newton, MD

Cardioembolic Stroke

Basics

DESCRIPTION

- Cardioembolic infarction is defined as rapidly developing clinical signs of focal or sometimes global disturbance of cerebral function lasting >24 hours caused by embolism originating from a cardiac source of thrombus.

EPIDEMIOLOGY

Incidence

- Frequency of cardiac embolism ranges from 15%–30% of all cases of stroke.

Age

- Affects all ages

Sex

- Males and females equally affected

Race

- No difference

ETIOLOGY

- Cardiac disorders that lead to the formation of a thrombus with subsequent brain embolism can be divided into six groups:
  - —*Arrhythmias:* Atrial fibrillation is one of the most common cardiac disorders. It is more common as patients age. It accounts for approximately 70% of emboli of cardiac origin. Sick sinus syndrome is another condition that is associated with brain embolism.
  - —*Valvular heart diseases:* This group especially includes mitral stenosis, prosthetic heart valves, infective endocarditis, and marantic endocarditis. Other valvular diseases shown to be associated with cardiac embolism include mitral valve prolapse, aortic valve disease, and mitral annulus calcification.
  - —*Ventricular myocardial abnormalities* related to coronary artery disease, myocarditis, or other dilated cardiomyopathy.
  - —*Lesions within the cavity of the ventricles* such as tumors (myxomas) or thrombi
  - —*Shunts:* Intraatrial septal defects and patent foramen ovale (PFO) allow emboli formed in the peripheral veins to enter the systemic circulation causing paradoxical embolism.
  - —*Atrial lesions* such as dilated atria, atrial infarcts and thrombi, and atrial septal aneurysms.
- Many times the development of thrombi within the heart is triggered by a superimposed hypercoagulable state.

Genetics

- Some hypercoagulable states are inherited.

PREGNANCY

- Cardioembolic stroke is relatively common in pregnancy. Atrial septal defects or PFO in association with pelvic or leg vein thrombosis, which is more frequent in pregnancy, may cause stroke during delivery. This is due to the transient rise in right atrial pressure above left atrial pressure during the Valsalva maneuver, causing right to-left shunting of embolic material.
- Postpartum cardiomyopathy is a less common cause of cardioembolic stroke in pregnancy and occurs typically in older African-American women.

ASSOCIATED CONDITIONS

- See Etiology

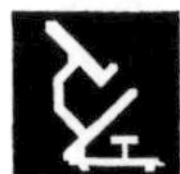

Diagnosis

DIFFERENTIAL DIAGNOSIS

- Large artery atherosclerosis with *in situ* thrombosis and occlusion or artery-to-artery emboli
- Arterial dissection with occlusion or artery-to-artery emboli
- Vasculitis
- Fat, air, tumor, or foreign body embolism

SIGNS AND SYMPTOMS

- The neurologic picture depends on the area infarcted. The most common and most characteristic time course in patients with cardiac embolism to the brain is the sudden onset of neurologic signs that are maximal at onset without warning episodes.
- Another pattern quite characteristic of brain embolism has been called the *spectacular shrinking deficit,* which is described as sudden, complete or nearly complete clearing of the neurologic deficit.
- Transient ischemic attacks do occur in some patients with brain embolism. Headache is common. Seizures are uncommon; however, they are more frequent in cardiac origin embolism compared to nonembolic causes of ischemic stroke.
- Cardiac origin embolism should be suspected in young patients in whom atherosclerosis is unlikely.

LABORATORY PROCEDURES

- Blood test should include lipid profile, RPR, BUN, creatinine, CBC and platelet, PT, PTT, and INR.
- Hypercoagulability can contribute to cardioembolic strokes, so a hypercoagulable profile should be requested in young patients.
- Serial blood cultures should be obtained when infective endocarditis is suspected.

IMAGING STUDIES

- *Chest x-ray film* should be obtained to look for cardiomegaly.
- *CT scan* must be performed in all patients presenting with suspected stroke because it is very sensitive in detecting intracranial hemorrhage. It is also inexpensive, quick, and readily available. When CT shows strokes in multiple vascular distribution, then cardiac source of emboli must be suspected.
- *MRI:* MRI of the brain (especially diffusion water imaging and FLAIR) is more sensitive in detecting early infarction, and infarcts in the cerebellum, brainstem, and inferior temporal lobes.
- *MR angiography* is a noninvasive test and is accurate for assessing the major extracerebral and intracerebral arteries, but it may overestimate the severity of the stenosis.
- *Transthoracic echocardiography (TTE)* is indicated in all patients suspected of having a potential cardiac source of ischemic stroke. If the TTE is negative and a cardiac source is still suspected, then transesophageal echocardiography (TEE) must be performed. TEE is more accurate than TTE in showing atrial and ventricular thrombi, vegetations, and left atrial enlargement; detecting shunts; and evaluating the proximal aorta.
- *Angiography* is the gold standard for an accurate assessment of both the extracranial and intracranial vasculature. However, it is an invasive procedure and should be reserved for use in patients in whom noninvasive testing has not shown a source of embolism and an arterial source is suspected.
- *Ultrasound* is safe, portable, and less expensive. It includes transcranial Doppler to look for intracranial disease and carotid duplex to assess for extracranial carotid and vertebral artery disease.
- *ECG* and *cardiac monitoring* should be performed to evaluate for arrhythmias.

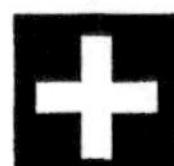

Management

GENERAL MEASURES

- General treatment of stroke includes acute supportive care, management of contributory cardiac lesions, and secondary stroke prevention.

SURGICAL MEASURES

- Some cardiac lesions require surgical or radiologic interventions, such as valve replacement for infected prosthetic valve, resection of cardiac tumors (myxoma), occasionally closure of PFO or atrial septal defect, removal of mobile protruding aortic arch atheroma, and pacemaker placement for sick sinus syndrome.

SYMPTOMATIC TREATMENT

- Includes treatment of hyperglycemia, fever, and infection; deep vein thrombosis prophylaxis; aspiration precaution; adequate hydration and nutrition; judicious control of blood pressure with avoidance of excessive reduction in the acute setting and adequate control in the long run; avoidance of prolonged use of indwelling catheter to prevent urinary tract infection
- Amitriptyline or gabapentin for pain related to thalamic strokes; antidepressants for the cortical strokes with resultant depression; muscle relaxant with baclofen for residual spasticity; stool softener for constipation

ADJUNCTIVE TREATMENT

- Physical, occupational, speech, and cognitive therapy may be needed.

ADMISSION/DISCHARGE CRITERIA

- In general, any patient presenting with acute ischemic stroke should be admitted to the hospital for evaluation of etiology and appropriate prevention measures; prevention and management of stroke complications; early initiation of physical, occupational, and speech therapy; evaluation for eligibility for inpatient rehabilitation; assistance with appropriate placement; and patient and caretaker education.

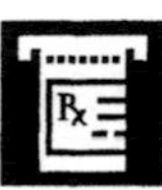

Medications

DRUG(S) OF CHOICE

- *Recombinant tissue plasminogen activator (r-tPA)* is indicated for acute ischemic strokes, including those with cardiac source, and must be given within 3 hours of the onset of symptoms. The dose is 0.9 mg/kg up to a maximum of 90 mg; 10% of the dose is given as an IV bolus over 1 minute and the rest as IV drip over 1 hour.
- *Antiplatelet agents* are indicated for stroke prevention in irregular nonstenotic valve surfaces and in patients who are not warfarin (Coumadin) candidates. *Aspirin: clopidogrel (Plavix)* (75 mg qd) or *Aggrenox* (combination aspirin 25 mg/extended release dipyridamole 200 mg one tablet bid)
- *Anticoagulants (warfarin)* are indicated for atrial fibrillation, especially when associated with other cardiac lesions or other stroke risk factors; intracardiac thrombi; myocardial aneurysm; prosthetic valves; noninfective endocarditis; and sometimes PFO.

Contraindications

- *r-tPA:* suspicion of subarachnoid hemorrhage; recent (within 3 months) intracerebral or intraspinal surgery; recent head trauma; recent previous stroke; history of intracerebral hemorrhage; uncontrolled hypertension at time of treatment (SBP >185 mm Hg or DBP >110 mm Hg); seizure at the onset of stroke; active internal bleeding; intracranial neoplasm, arteriovenous malformation, or aneurysm; known bleeding diathesis, including but not limited to current use of oral anticoagulants (e.g., warfarin sodium) or INR >1.7 or PT >15 seconds; administration of heparin within 48 hours preceding the onset of stroke and elevated aPTT at presentation; platelet count <100,000/mm^3
- *Aspirin/Aggrenox:* mainly known allergic reaction to salicylic acid, active systemic bleeding, or active gastric ulcer
- *Clopidogrel:* mainly active systemic bleeding
- *Warfarin:* mainly active bleeding, bleeding tendency, noncompliance, and gait difficulty with increased falling risk

Precautions

- *r-tPA:* Noncompressible arterial or venous punctures must be avoided. Blood pressure must be monitored closely during administration of the medicine and treated if elevated. If serious bleeding is suspected, it must be stopped immediately. Watch for allergic reaction.
- *Clopidogrel:* Monitor for any TTP symptoms at the beginning of treatment.
- *Warfarin:* Watch for compliance, bleeding events, and falling events.

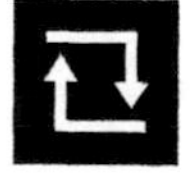

Follow-Up

PATIENT MONITORING

- Close monitoring of INR is important for treatment with warfarin. Therapeutic range is usually 2–3. Mechanical prosthetic valves require a higher INR. If follow-up shows noncompliance with the medication, bleeding events, or falling episodes, discontinuation of warfarin must be considered.

EXPECTED COURSE AND PROGNOSIS

- Most important predictor of recovery from brain embolism is whether or not ischemic brain is reperfused and how quickly. Most patients survive the initial insult. In 80% of cases, the first episode will be followed by another event, frequently with more severe damage. Appropriate prophylactic treatment significantly decreases the recurrence rate. However, patients will still be at increased risk for recurrent events despite appropriate measures. If recurrent events occur, the combination of platelet antiaggregants and warfarin is a reasonable alternative to either agent alone.

PATIENT EDUCATION

- American Stroke Association, National Center 7272 Greenville Avenue, Dallas TX, 75231. Phone: 1-888-478-7653, website: *www.strokeassociation.org*

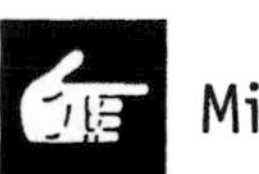

Miscellaneous

SYNONYMS

N/A

ICD-9-CM: 436 Cerebrovascular accident

REFERENCES

- Bogousslavsky J, Cachin C, Regli F, et al. Cardiac sources of embolism and cerebral infarction. Clinical consequences and vascular concomitants. Neurology 1991; 41:855–859.
- Mohr JP, Caplan LR, Melski JW, et al. The Harvard Cooperative Stroke Registry: a prospective registry. Neurology 1978; 28:754–762.
- Caplan LR Brain embolism. In: Caplan LR, Hurst JW, Chimowitz MI, eds. Clinical neurocardiology. New York: Marcel Dekker, 1999:35–157.
- Minematsu K, Yamaguchi T, Omae T. Spectacular shrinking deficit : rapid recovery from a major hemispheric syndrome by migration of an embolus. Neurology 1992;42:157–162.
- Stroke Prevention in Atrial Fibrillation Investigators. Warfarin versus aspirin for prevention of thromboembolism in atrial fibrillation: Stroke Prevention in Atrial Fibrillation II Study. Lancet 1994;343: 687–691.

Author(s): Roula al-Dahhak, MD; Yousef Mohammad, MD, MSc

Carpal Tunnel Syndrome

Basics

DESCRIPTION

- Carpal tunnel syndrome is a compression injury of the median nerve as it traverses the carpal tunnel in the wrist, with resultant pain, numbness, and/or weakness in a median nerve distribution.

EPIDEMIOLOGY

- Most common nerve entrapment syndrome
- Lifetime individual risk of 10%
- Incidence of 200–500 per 100,000 individuals over a 1-year period
- As many as 50% may have an occupational etiology
- May be bilateral in >50% of patients

Race

- No ethnic predominance

Age

- Frequency increases with advancing age

Sex

- Pregnancy and perimenopausal state may predispose

ETIOLOGY

- The etiology of carpal tunnel syndrome is multifactorial. As the median nerve enters the wrist, it traverses the carpal tunnel, a narrow anatomic pathway bounded by carpal bones on its floor and sides and the transverse carpal ligament as its roof. The nerve is accompanied by nine flexor tendons in this space; any activity or metabolic derangement that causes edema may increase pressure on the nerve or compress it.

Genetics

- Patients with hereditary neuropathy with predisposition to pressure palsies (HNPP) are more susceptible to carpal tunnel.
- HNPP is due to a deletion on chromosome 17 in the region that codes for the PMP22 gene (a component of peripheral nerve myelin).

RISK FACTORS

- Metabolic disorders
  - —Diabetes
  - —Renal disease
  - —Thyroid dysfunction
  - —Amyloidosis
  - —Monoclonal gammopathy
- Underlying peripheral neuropathy
- Occupational
  - —Individuals with repetitive manual tasks, such as keyboarding, carpentry, knitting, or food handling
- Perimenopausal state
- Pregnancy
- Connective tissue disorders, e.g., rheumatoid arthritis
- Acromegaly
- Osteoarthritis
- Trauma

PREGNANCY

- Carpal tunnel syndrome may present during pregnancy, especially in the last trimester when peripheral edema may develop.

ASSOCIATED CONDITIONS

- Peripheral neuropathy
- Other entrapment syndromes

Diagnosis

DIFFERENTIAL DIAGNOSIS

- Cervical radiculopathy
- Brachial plexopathy
- Proximal median nerve injury
- Motor neuron disease
- Arthritis
- Tendonitis
- Peripheral neuropathy

SIGNS AND SYMPTOMS

- Paresthesias of the hand and fingers; patient may not be able to localize to the median nerve distribution (first three digits and the lateral aspect of the fourth digit)
- Pain in the wrist, sometimes radiating to the shoulder and even the scapula
- Weakness is a late presentation; may involve thumb abduction and opposition
- *Tinel's sign* is elicited by gently tapping over the median nerve at the wrist. A positive finding includes reproduction of paresthesias in the fingertips or traveling through the hand. It should be noted that this is not diagnostic for carpal tunnel entrapment, as there is a high false-positive rate.
- *Phalen's sign* is elicited by placing the wrists in flexion for 30–60 seconds. A positive finding is the reproduction or exacerbation of symptoms. Again the false-positive rate is high.

LABORATORY PROCEDURES

- Nerve conduction studies
  - —Sensory nerve testing is the most sensitive
  - —Demonstration of slowing across the carpal tunnel
  - —May be accompanied by loss of amplitude or response
- Motor conductions are also useful
  - —Prolonged distal latency
- Electromyography
  - —Usually normal in mild cases
  - —Useful to determine extent of injury
  - —Important to differentiate carpal tunnel from other entities such as cervical radiculopathy, peripheral neuropathy, and brachial plexopathy
- Blood work
  - —Screening for predisposing conditions should be based on degree of clinical suspicion

IMAGING STUDIES

- A history of trauma (especially a Colles fracture) or fullness in the wrist or palm (ganglion, lipoma, schwannoma) is an indication for CT or MRI.

SPECIAL TESTS

N/A

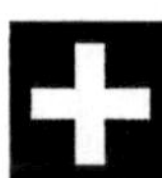

Management

GENERAL MEASURES

- Conservative therapy is successful for patients with mild-to-moderate symptoms and findings on clinical examination.
  - —Immobilization ideally done with a *custom-made, neutral position, rigid splint* worn primarily at night or after activities that precipitate symptoms
  - —Nonsteroidal antiinflammatory agents
  - —If possible, avoidance of predisposing activities is beneficial
  - —Consider ergonomic redesign of the workplace to avoid repetition injury (although data supporting this approach are not available)
  - —90% of mild-to-moderate cases should improve in 4–6 weeks
  - —Therapy should continue for at least 2 months
  - —If no response to above measures, consider steroid injections, particularly if pain is a significant feature
  - —Training in steroid injections is essential, as complications can include infection, tendon rupture, and scarring of the nerve

SURGICAL MEASURES

- Surgery is considered if
  - —There is no response to conservative measures
  - —Symptoms significantly limit the patient's activity
  - —Findings on examination demonstrate significant axon loss (atrophy or denervation by EMG)
- Traditionally, surgery for carpal tunnel syndrome was performed through an open release technique (palmar incision).
- More recently, endoscopic techniques have been developed.
- There is no significant difference in the outcomes of the two types of surgeries; however, the endoscopic approach requires significant surgical experience to avoid possible complications.

SYMPTOMATIC TREATMENT

- Nonsteroidal antiinflammatory agents may provide symptomatic relief of pain and swelling.
- Occasionally, diuretics are useful to decrease edema around the carpal tunnel.

ADJUNCTIVE TREATMENT

N/A

ADMISSIONS/DISCHARGE CRITERIA

N/A

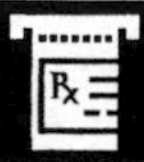

Medications

DRUG(S) OF CHOICE

- Symptoms may respond to nonsteroidal antiinflammatory medications.

ALTERNATIVE DRUGS

N/A

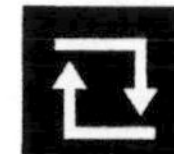

Follow-Up

PATIENT MONITORING

- For those patients treated conservatively, follow-up should be performed within 2 months. If symptoms persist or if there is evidence of disease progression, consider surgical treatment.

EXPECTED COURSE AND PROGNOSIS

- Most patients will do well with conservative therapy and avoidance of exacerbating activities.
- For patients with mild-to-moderate signs and symptoms, neurologic function should return to near normal after surgery.
- Patients with moderate-to-severe neurologic dysfunction can avoid progression of nerve injury with surgery and, at best, may demonstrate minimal improvement in nerve function.

PATIENT EDUCATION

- Involves avoidance of activities, behaviors, or postures that might exacerbate symptoms

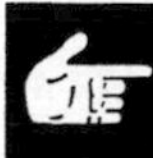

Miscellaneous

SYNONYMS

N/A

ICD-9-CM: 354.0 Carpal tunnel syndrome

SEE ALSO: N/A

REFERENCES

- Dawson DM. Entrapment neuropathies of the upper extremities. N Engl J Med 1993;329:2013–2018.
- Dawson DM, Hallet M, Wilbourn AJ, eds. Entrapment neuropathies, 3rd ed. Philadelphia: Lippincott-Raven, 1999.
- The Quality Standards Subcommittee for the American Academy of Neurology. Practice parameters for carpal tunnel syndrome: summary statement. Neurology 1993;43:2406–2409.
- Stevens JC. AAEM minimonograph #26: the electrodiagnosis of carpal tunnel syndrome. Muscle Nerve 1997;20: 1477–1486.

Author(s): Miriam L. Freimer, MD

Cauda Equina Syndrome

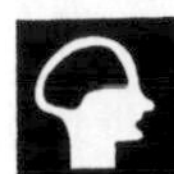

Basics

DESCRIPTION

Cauda equina syndrome occurs with lesions of the "tail" of the spinal cord. Secondary to the foreshortening of the spinal cord, which ends in the conus medullaris at approximately the L2 vertebral level, the nerve roots from the lumbar and sacral spinal cord must travel for a variable length within the spinal canal before they exit through their respective neural foramina. This produces a bundle of nerve roots descending within the spinal canal, resembling a horse's tail (cauda equina).

Compression of the lower spinal canal may variably injure these nerve roots while they remain in the canal. Lesions of the lower nerve roots produce sensory and motor dysfunction of the lower extremities, as well as sacral dysfunction. Asymmetric pain, asymmetric sensory loss or hyperesthesia, and asymmetric motor weakness will develop. The asymmetry results because the lesion rarely compresses nerve roots equally; that is, some nerve roots are involved more than others and one side may be more affected than the opposite. Patients may have bowel and bladder dysfunction as well as numbness and paresthesias of the sacral area. If the conus medullaris is involved, or any more proximal part of the spinal cord, signs and symptoms of myelopathy, or upper motor neuron dysfunction, may additionally be seen. Thus, cauda equina primarily produces a lower extremity and sacral lower motor neuron dysfunction; but upper motor neuron signs and symptoms, such as hyperreflexia and spasticity are sometimes seen.

EPIDEMIOLOGY

Cauda equina syndrome is uncommon, being rarer than other lumbar spine compressive syndromes.

The distribution is unaffected by race, sex, and age.

ETIOLOGY

Causes of cauda equina syndrome are any compressive lesion within the spinal canal, not just a single spinal neural foramina. Thus, a central disc herniation may cause cauda equina syndrome, but not a paracentral disc herniation, which compresses a neural foramina, resulting in a radiculopathy. Infectious processes that produce a mass effect, either through inflammation (bacterial, CMV) or granuloma (TB, sarcoid) may result in a cauda equina presentation. Any structural abnormality (disc, abscess, hematoma, metastasis) in the lower spinal canal will compress multiple nerve roots. Other, less easily identifiable causes, include carcinomatous meningitis, in which cancerous cells coat the nerve roots, may also cause a cauda equina syndrome.

Tethered cord syndrome may present as a cauda equina syndrome, by presenting subacutely in an adult rather than an infant or child.

PREGNANCY

Little is known regarding the relationship of cauda equina and pregnancy.

ASSOCIATED CONDITIONS

- Conus medullaris syndrome
- Tumors of the base of the spinal cord
- Multiple lumbosacral radiculopathies
- Tethered cord syndrome

Diagnosis

DIFFERENTIAL DIAGNOSIS

- Spinal cord compression
  - —Tumors of the lower spinal cord, especially ependymoma
  - —Epidural abscess or hematoma
  - —Central disc herniation
  - —Metastasis
  - —Spinal stenosis
- Infections of the CNS
  - —Syphilis
  - —Tuberculosis
  - —Cryptococcus
  - —Bacterial abscess
  - —Cytomegalovirus (CMV) infection
  - —HIV (with or without CMV)
- Sarcoidosis
- Carcinomatous meningitis
- Radiculopathies
- Acute inflammatory demyelinating polyradiculopathy (AIDP)

SIGNS AND SYMPTOMS

The symptoms of cauda equina syndrome may develop acutely, subacutely, or chronically, depending on the underlying etiology. Typically, there is a patchy disturbance, as various nerve roots within the spinal canal are involved.

In addition, there may be significant asymmetry between the right and left extremities. Most of the symptoms are lower motor neuron signs, such as weakness and sensory loss. Some upper motor neuron signs may rarely be seen, if the conus medullaris is involved. Bowel incontinence and bladder retention indicate sacral nerve root involvement. Radicular pain may occur in the territory of affected nerve roots.

LABORATORY PROCEDURES

Blood work should be checked with a view to diagnosing the underlying abnormality. HIV, RPR, ACE level may all be warranted. PT/PTT and CBC with platelets should be performed if a lumbar puncture is under consideration.

IMAGING STUDIES

MRI of the lumbosacral spine, with gadolinium, should be performed immediately to evaluate for a compressive lesion that requires emergent surgery. Inflammation and infiltration of the cauda equina may be seen as high signal and thickening of the nerve roots.

SPECIAL TESTS

If there is no contraindication, a lumbar puncture should be performed, checking glucose, protein, all cultures, including fungal, and cytology, if cancer is suspected. CXR should be checked if sarcoid or TB is suspected. An EMG/NCS may be useful to distinguish this lesion from a more peripheral nerve root lesion, such as radiculopathies or AIDP (Guillain-Barré syndrome).

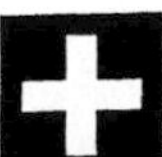

Management

GENERAL MEASURES

Treatment is aimed at the underlying cause. If the lesion is mechanical, then urgent surgery is required. If the lesion is infectious, then the appropriate antimicrobial therapy should be initiated. Sarcoid requires immunosuppression, usually initially with steroids. Fungal and tuberculous CNS infections may also require steroids in addition to antimicrobial therapy. If cancer is the etiology, then radiation therapy provides the quickest, but not necessarily permanent, relief. Consultation with an oncologist should be undertaken.

SURGICAL MEASURES

If a compressive lesion is seen on MRI, neurosurgical consultation should be obtained immediately. This is imperative for epidural abscesses and hematomas. Disc disease and intrinsic cord tumors are urgent but do not require immediate intervention. Some compressive lesions may be better served by an initial course of steroids before surgery.

SYMPTOMATIC TREATMENT

Supportive care should include bowel and bladder management, if they are involved. Straight catheterization is performed every 4 to 6 hours as needed, if the bladder has greater than 200 cc postvoid residuals. Stool softeners and other bowel management (such as digital rectal stimulation, qd) are indicated to prevent significant constipation. Physical therapy should be initiated early to avoid sequelae from prolonged bed rest. If the patient is profoundly weak, then an egg-crate mattress and appropriate turning of the patient may prevent decubitus ulcers. The patient should be out of the bed at least two times per day to prevent atelectasis of the lungs. DVT prophylaxis should be composed of either 5,000 units of heparin SC, or SCD compression hose, worn at all times.

ADJUNCTIVE TREATMENT

Radiation therapy: if a metastatic lesion is found to be the underlying etiology on MRI, then an urgent radiation therapy consult is required. Return of function is best seen if radiation begins immediately.

ADMISSION/DISCHARGE CRITERIA

Patients are generally admitted for acute evaluation and treatment. If significant symptoms persist after initial therapy, consider inpatient rehabilitation. Discharge depends on the stability of the patient's clinical exam, adequacy of treatment, and stabilization of the underlying cause.

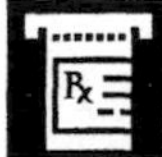

Medications

DRUG(S) OF CHOICE

Steroids are often used to reduce initial inflammation. If the cauda equina syndrome has developed chronically and is due to a slowly compressive lesion, such as spinal stenosis, then steroids are of little benefit. Steroids, such as methylprednisolone 1 g/d for 5 days (or dexamethasone 4 mg q6h for 4–5 days), provide the most benefit for acute, rapidly progressive lesions, most often due to infectious or carcinomatous causes.

Contraindications

Hypersensitivity to specific corticosteroid—use alternative medication.

Precautions

Assess patient for peptic ulcers, hyperglycemia, steroid-induced behavioral changes, and hypokalemia during steroid therapy.

ALTERNATIVE DRUGS

N/A

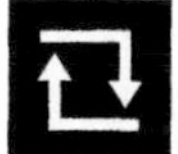

Follow-Up

PATIENT MONITORING

Monitoring over the long-term depends entirely on the underlying cause. In patients with a compressive lesion from a disc, or tethered cord syndrome, no follow-up may be necessary. In people with an underlying neoplasm, appropriate tumor management is indicated. In patients with a chronic infection, occasional reevaluations are necessary to ensure that no relapses occur.

EXPECTED COURSE AND PROGNOSIS

Recovery depends entirely on the underlying etiology and length of symptoms. Acute-onset lesions recover better than do chronic ones. Lesions due to a structural defect, such as a herniated disc, do better than a diffuse, systemic process, such as cancer. Patients with subtle or partial deficits recover more function than patients with complete paralysis and neurogenic bladder.

PATIENT EDUCATION

N/A

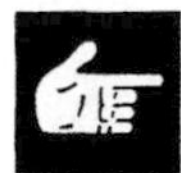

Miscellaneous

SYNONYMS

None

ICD-9-CM: 344.6 Cauda equina syndrome; 344.60 Without mention of neurogenic bladder; 344.61 With neurogenic bladder; 336.3 Myelopathy in other diseases classified elsewhere; 13.4 Tuberculoma of spinal cord; 115.9 Histoplasmosis, other; 135 Sarcoidosis; 192.2 Malignant neoplasm of other and unspecified parts of the nervous system, spinal cord

SEE ALSO: SPINAL CORD TUMOR; RADICULOPATHY, LUMBOSACRAL

REFERENCES

- A 67-year-old woman with the cauda equina syndrome. N Engl J Med 1997; 337:1829–1837.
- Brazis P, Masdeu J, Biller J. Localization in Clinical Neurology, 3rd ed. Boston: Little, Brown, 1996.
- Haerer A. DeJong's the neurologic examination, 5th ed. Philadelphia: Lippincott, 1992.
- Jaradeh S. Cauda equina syndrome: a neurologist's perspective. Reg Anaesth 1993;18:473–480.
- Rydevik B. Neurophysiology of cauda equina compression. Acta Orthop Scand 1993;suppl 251:52–55.
- Shapiro S. Cauda equina syndrome secondary to lumbar disc herniation. Neurosurgery 1993;32:743–747.

Author(s): Holli Horak, MD

Cavernous Sinus Thrombosis

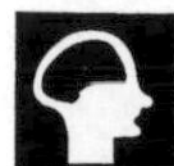

Basics

DESCRIPTION

- Cavernous sinus thrombosis (CST) is a rare disorder characterized by clot formation in the cavernous sinuses. Although typically due to hematogenous spread of infection, aseptic and chronic forms also exist.

EPIDEMIOLOGY

Incidence/Prevalence

- Only a few hundred cases have been reported in the literature. The incidence has declined dramatically since the advent of antibiotics.

Race

- No known difference

Age

- This disorder typically affects young adults.

Sex

- No known difference

ETIOLOGY

- The cavernous sinuses are paired, interconnected, venous structures located on either side of the sella turcica, superior to the sphenoid sinus and posterior to the optic chiasm. They drain veins of the face, orbits, sinuses, and brain via the superior ophthalmic, inferior ophthalmic, central retinal, superficial middle cerebral, and inferior cerebral veins, as well as the sphenoparietal sinus. The carotid artery and abducens nerve lie medially within the sinuses, whereas the oculomotor nerve, trochlear nerve, and ophthalmic and maxillary branches of the trigeminal nerve lie within the lateral wall of the sinuses.
- In the septic form of CST, infection in structures with venous drainage to the cavernous sinuses propagates through valveless veins over 5–10 days. Once the organisms are caught in the trabeculations of the sinuses, inflammation and secretion of coagulase may lead to clot formation and thrombosis.
- In the aseptic form, surgical or blunt trauma or hypercoagulable state leads to thrombosis of the cavernous sinus and often to bacterial superinfection.
- In the rare chronic form, slow thrombosis of the sinuses allows time for formation of venous collaterals.
- Coagulase-positive *Staphylococcus aureus* is the most common organism isolated. Other commonly encountered organisms include streptococcal species, pneumococcal species, Gram-negative bacilli, *Rhizopus, Aspergillus,* and *Mucor.*

Genetics

N/A

RISK FACTORS

- Septic form: infection of the middle third of the face, paranasal sinuses, pharynx, maxilla, middle ear, or mastoid process
- Aseptic form: otolaryngologic surgery, trauma, subarachnoid hemorrhage, malignancy, pregnancy, oral contraceptive use, and other hypercoagulable states
- Chronic form: diabetes mellitus, chronic sinusitis

PREGNANCY

- Pregnancy is a risk factor for the aseptic form of CST.

ASSOCIATED CONDITIONS

N/A

Diagnosis

DIFFERENTIAL DIAGNOSIS

- Contralateral spread of signs and symptoms within 48 hours is virtually pathognomonic for CST. In contrast to the most significant disorder in the differential diagnosis, postseptal orbital cellulitis, in CST there is a source of sepsis remote from the eye, systemic illness out of proportion to local signs, positive blood cultures, meningismus, ophthalmoplegia, visual impairment, papillary defect, funduscopic abnormality, and inflammatory CSF. Other disorders in the differential diagnosis include postseptal orbital cellulitis, periorbital cellulitis, sinusitis, orbital apex syndrome, superior orbital fissure syndrome, intraorbital abscess, orbit or optic nerve tumor, rhinocerebral mucormycosis, intracavernous carotid artery aneurysm, carotid-cavernous fistula, intraorbital pseudotumor, Tolosa-Hunt syndrome, and exophthalmic goiter.

SIGNS AND SYMPTOMS

- *Categories:* signs and symptoms of the primary infection, venous congestion, sepsis, retro-orbital inflammation, and cranial nerve irritation
  —Fever
  —Ptosis
  —Chemosis of bulbar conjunctiva
  —External ophthalmoplegia
  —Proptosis and periorbital edema
  —Headache
  —Internal ophthalmoplegia
  —Meningismus
  —Decreased visual acuity
  —Altered mental status
  —Retinal edema and retinal vein dilation

LABORATORY PROCEDURES

- CST is primarily a clinical diagnosis. The presence of peripheral leukocytosis on CBC confirms an infectious etiology. Identification of the infectious agent with blood cultures is necessary as CSF Gram stain rarely demonstrates organisms.

IMAGING STUDIES

- MRI and contrast-enhanced CT of the head are the most sensitive and specific imaging studies. In addition to aiding in diagnosis, they evaluate for contraindications to anticoagulation. Angiography and venography are only indicated for suspected carotid-cavernous fistula or intracavernous aneurysm.

SPECIAL TESTS

- Lumbar puncture: CSF is typically inflammatory but aseptic.
- Funduscopic examination

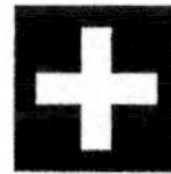

Management

GENERAL MEASURES

- Treatment of CST involves eradicating the infection, halting progression of thrombosis, and reducing inflammation. Rapid diagnosis and instigation of treatment are essential.

SURGICAL MEASURES

- Surgical interventions are limited to drainage of refractory infections in the paranasal sinuses.

SYMPTOMATIC TREATMENT

- Routine pain control

ADJUNCTIVE TREATMENT

N/A

ADMISSION/DISCHARGE CRITERIA

- Patients with diagnosed or suspected CST are admitted to an intensive care unit.

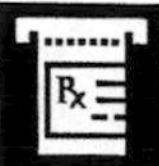

Medications

DRUG(S) OF CHOICE

- Antibiotics
  - —High-dose, broad-spectrum antibiotic coverage begun within 7 days of hospitalization improves outcome. Antibiotic spectrum should cover Gram-positive, Gram-negative, and anaerobic organisms. Antifungals should be added if the patient is in diabetic ketoacidosis, is neutropenic, or is otherwise immunosuppressed.
  - —A regimen including intravenous oxacillin or nafcillin at a dose of 2 g every 4 hours plus a third-generation antipseudomonal cephalosporin such as intravenous ceftazidime 2 g every 8 hours or IV imipenem 2 g every 6 hours should cover relevant Gram-positive and Gram-negative organism. IV metronidazole at 500 mg every 6 hours should be added for anaerobic coverage. Treatment should continue at least 2 weeks beyond clinical resolution as the infection may be sequestered within the thrombus.
- Anticoagulation
  - —Although there are no prospective studies, the current literature demonstrates a reduction in morbidity and mortality from early anticoagulation. Anticoagulation prevents propagation and septic embolization, and enhances recanalization.
  - —Dose heparin at 80 units/kg IV bolus then 18 units/kg/hour, following aPTT ratio with a goal between 1.5 and 2.5 times normal. Whereas low-molecular-weight heparin is not recommended in the acute stage, either coumadin (goal INR 2-3) or low-molecular-weight heparin may be used for anticoagulation after the patient is stabilized. The duration of anticoagulation is controversial, but the general consensus is between 3 and 9 months depending on the severity of symptoms and the clinical course.

Contraindications

- Antibiotics: known sensitivity to the agent
- Anticoagulation: intracerebral hemorrhage, subarachnoid hemorrhage, bleeding diathesis

Precautions

- Anticoagulation: cortical venous infarction, intracavernous carotid artery necrosis, intraorbital hemorrhages, epistaxis

ALTERNATIVE DRUGS

- Vancomycin 1 g IV q12 plus meropenem 1 g IV q8
- Corticosteroids: anecdotal benefit only in the absence of pituitary dysfunction. A recent study demonstrates benefit in meningitis. Indicated for addisonian crisis.

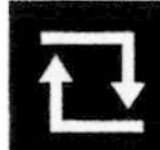

Follow-Up

PATIENT MONITORING

- Follow clinical course rather than normalization of imaging studies. Late sequelae include meningitis, encephalitis, brain abscess, pituitary infection, subdural empyema, epidural abscess (consider if not responding to therapy), dural sinus thrombosis, cortical vein thrombosis and hemorrhagic infarction, hydrocephalus, and carotid stenosis or occlusion (leading to dysphasia or hemiparesis).

EXPECTED COURSE AND PROGNOSIS

- Signs typically develop unilaterally 5-10 days after instigating infection elsewhere in the head. Bilateral spread occurs within 48 hours in most cases. In the absence of treatment, meningitis, intracranial spread, and death follow universally. With treatment, modern mortality is 30%. Greater than 50% have morbidity including blindness, visual impairment, diplopia, pituitary insufficiency, hemiparesis, seizure disorder, or vascular steal syndrome. Due to sequestration of bacteria within thrombus, relapses have been reported within 6 weeks and intracranial abscesses up to 8 months. Thus, patients should be followed for several months after antibiotics are stopped.

PATIENT EDUCATION

N/A

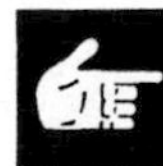

Miscellaneous

SYNONYMS

- Cavernous sinus phlebitis
- Cavernous sinus thrombophlebitis
- Cavernous sinus phlebothrombosis
- Septic cavernous sinus thrombosis
- Aseptic thrombosis of the cavernous sinuses

ICD-9-CM: 325.0 Phlebitis and thrombophlebitis of intracranial venous sinuses

SEE ALSO: N/A

REFERENCES

- Bhatia K, Jones N. Septic cavernous sinus thrombosis secondary to sinusitis: are anticoagulants indicated? A review of the literature. J Laryngol Otol 2002;116: 667–676.
- DiNubile M. Septic thrombosis of the cavernous sinuses. Arch Neurol 1988; 45:567–572.
- Ebright J, Pace M, Niazi A. Septic thrombosis of the cavernous sinuses. Arch Intern Med 2001;161:2671–2676.
- Karlin R, Robinson W. Septic cavernous sinus thrombosis. Ann Emerg Med 1984; 13:449–455.
- Levine S, Twyman R, Gilman S. The role of anticoagulation in cavernous sinus thrombosis. Neurology 1988;38:517–522.
- Migirov L, Eyal A, Kronenberg J. Treatment of cavernous sinus thrombosis. Isr Med Assoc J 2002;4:468–469.
- Southwick F, Richardson E, Swartz M. Septic thrombosis of the dural venous sinuses. Medicine 1986;65:82–106.
- Zahller M, Spector R, Skoglund R, et al. Cavernous sinus thrombosis. West J Med 1980;133:44–48.

Author(s): Richard E. Burgess, MD, PhD

Central Pontine Myelinolysis

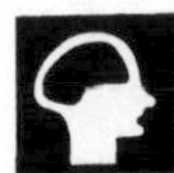

Basics

DESCRIPTION

Central pontine myelinolysis (CPM) is an acute demyelination of the central basis pontis. The characteristic presentation includes spastic tetraparesis, pseudobulbar paralysis, and decreased level of consciousness.

EPIDEMIOLOGY

The precise incidence is unknown. Autopsy data suggest a prevalence of approximately 0.25%. The peak incidence occurs between the ages of 30 and 50 years, although pediatric cases have been reported. A slight male predominance has been noted.

ETIOLOGY

- The pathogenesis underlying CPM remains unknown. CPM is most often associated with rapid correction of hyponatremia. One hypothesis suggests that the increase in sodium leads to endothelial injury and osmotic disruption of the blood–brain barrier, which cause edema and leakage of myelinotoxic factors. Mechanisms of controlling osmotic balance may not respond quickly enough, leading to cerebral edema that destroys the neighboring myelin sheaths and blood vessels. Others propose that osmotic imbalance may dehydrate the brain such that the myelin sheaths are stripped away from the axons, and oligodendrocytes are injured. Others have argued for an autoimmune etiology.
- Those with underlying medical illness may be more susceptible to CPM, because of decreased ability to generate the necessary osmoles to protect against the above processes. Alternatively, it may be that those with other medical conditions are more likely to be hospitalized, where iatrogenic fluctuations in osmolality can occur.
- The pons is particularly affected by demyelination. This selective vulnerability may be due to the proximity of oligodendrocytes to vascular gray matter, where they are susceptible to injury from edema and myelinotoxic substances. Another hypothesis proposes that the close apposition of gray to white matter allows gray matter to "steal" nutrients from oligodendrocytes, resulting in demyelination.

Genetics

N/A

RISK FACTORS

- CPM is commonly associated with rapid correction of hyponatremia. Varying susceptibility to myelinolysis makes establishment of protective guidelines difficult. The general recommendation is that sodium correction rates should not exceed 12 mEq/L within the first 24 hours or 20 mEq/L within the first 48 hours. Others advocate more rapid rates of sodium delivery. CPM, however, can occur with modest levels of hyponatremia and rates of correction, indicating that more conservative guidelines may be needed. Some argue that a greater risk of CPM occurs with chronic hyponatremia and that rates of sodium replacement should depend on the chronicity of the deficit. They recommend a minimum rate of correction of 1 mm/L/h for acute hyponatremia and a maximum rate of correction of 0.5 mmol/L/h for chronic hyponatremia.
- Hypokalemia is an additional risk factor for CPM, and should be addressed prior to treatment of hyponatremia.

PREGNANCY

CPM is associated with hyperemesis gravidarum and pregnancy.

ASSOCIATED CONDITIONS

- Almost all cases of CPM occur with severe comorbid medical conditions.
  - —Alcoholism (39.4–78%). Alcohol blocks antidiuretic hormone (ADH). During alcohol withdrawal, ADH function may be overactive, resulting in hyponatremia.
  - —Rapid correction of hyponatremia (21.5–61%).
  - —Liver transplants (17.4%). Incidence of CPM among liver transplant patients is 0.29%. Onset is usually within the first 30 days after transplant. Liver transplant-associated CPM occurs more commonly in children and those with sepsis, metabolic disorders, hepatic encephalopathy, and hypoxia, and cyclosporine use.
  - —Other liver disease, including cirrhosis (4.8%) and Wilson's disease
  - —Burns (2.5%). CPM occurs in 7% of burn patients.
  - —Diabetes (2%)
  - —AIDS (1.4%)
  - —Pregnancy (0.5%) and hyperemesis gravidarum (1.4%)
  - —Other electrolyte disturbances and abnormalities in osmolality (0.7%), including hypernatremia, hypokalemia, lithium toxicity, and correction of hypoglycemia
  - —Neoplasms (0.5%), particularly of lung or GI tract; Hodgkin's disease
  - —Cerebral infarct (0.5%) and other CNS diseases
  - —Schizophrenia (0.5%)
  - —Acute porphyria (0.5%)
- Pulmonary infections
- Eating disorders, malnutrition, folate deficiency
- Hypoxia
- Sepsis
- ADH deficiency, adrenal insufficiency, pituitary surgery
- Heat stroke
- Hemorrhagic pancreatitis
- Trauma
- Isaacs' syndrome
- Ornithine-carbamoyl-transferase deficiency
- Arginine hydrochloride deficiency
- Sjögren's syndrome
- Extrapontine myelinolysis (EPM) occurs in 10% to 15% of patients with CPM. The demyelinating lesions are typically located in the cerebellum, lateral geniculate body/thalamus, putamen, cerebral cortex, and subcortical white matter.

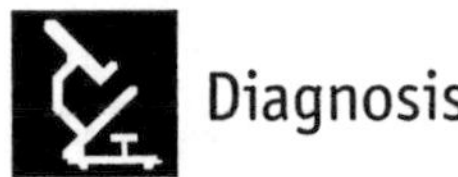

Diagnosis

DIFFERENTIAL DIAGNOSIS

The differential diagnosis includes any acute neurologic process that localizes to the pons. Other demyelinating diseases, such as multiple sclerosis and acute disseminated encephalomyelitis, should be considered. Comorbid conditions such as Wernicke's encephalopathy and hepatic encephalopathy may have symptoms that overlap with CPM.

SIGNS AND SYMPTOMS

Symptoms of CPM vary widely and may reflect damage to the pons and ascending and descending tracts of the brainstem. Presentation can range from no deficit to devastating neurologic injury. Pseudobulbar paralysis, spastic tetraparesis, and coma are characteristic of CPM. Pseudobulbar paralysis includes dysphagia, dysarthria, tongue weakness, and emotional lability, and occurs in approximately 40% of cases. Tetraparesis, paraparesis, or the locked-in syndrome occurs in 33% of patients. Alternative presentations include hemiparesis or weakness more pronounced in the upper extremities. Alterations in consciousness occur in 70% of cases, and can range from lethargy to coma. Ocular findings may include miosis or sixth nerve palsies. Patients may also present with seizures (25% of cases), hyporeflexia, hypotension, respiratory depression, and bowel or bladder dysfunction. In 25% of cases, the only manifestations of CPM are psychiatric such as pseudobulbar laughing and crying, agitated delirium, akinetic mutism, or catatonia. Patients can also have cognitive deficits affecting speech, judgment, insight, attention, and memory. Ataxia and other cerebellar signs rarely occur in isolation and may be masked by weakness.

LABORATORY PROCEDURES

Electrolytes.

IMAGING STUDIES

- MRI is the study of choice. Characteristic images show a symmetric, non-space-occupying lesion located in the central pons. The lesion is hypointense on T1 and hyperintense on T2 images. The demyelinated area is more visible on T2 sequences. The shape of the affected area typically looks like a "bat's wing" on coronal views, appears triangular on axial views, and has an oval shape on sagittal views.
- The CT finding in CPM is usually a symmetric central pontine hypodense lesion, similar to that demonstrated on MRI. CT is not as sensitive as MRI.
- Findings on neuroimaging lag behind clinical symptoms. Hence, it is recommended to repeat imaging in suspicious cases in 10 to 14 days if early scans are unrevealing. A time lag also exists, however, between clinical improvement and the resolution of MRI changes, in that radiologic findings may persist for months or longer after neurologic recovery. Some propose that early CT and MRI changes are secondary to edema and will often resolve, while later changes are secondary to demyelination itself and are more likely to be permanent. The severity of clinical manifestations does not necessarily correlate with the radiographic evidence of disease.

SPECIAL TESTS

- Positron emission tomography (PET) studies have shown the demyelinated patches to have increased metabolic activity early and decreased metabolic activity as CPM progresses. PET, however, is not routinely used in the evaluation of CPM.
- Auditory evoked potentials may be abnormal, with prolongation of the latency period between waves I and V, secondary to demyelination of auditory pathways in the pons. This finding, however, is nonspecific and inconstant.

Pathology

- Autopsy studies demonstrate a single, symmetric region of demyelination in the central basis pontis, grossly seen as a triangular region of soft, discolored tissue.
- Microscopic examination reveals demyelination with loss of oligodendrocytes, myelin-filled phagocytes, astrocytic gliosis, and fat decomposition. Evidence of inflammation is notably absent. Axons, nuclei, and blood vessels are relatively spared.

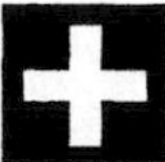

Management

GENERAL MEASURES

No consensus guidelines have been established for the treatment of CPM. It remains unclear whether early initiation of treatment improves prognosis.

SURGICAL MEASURES

N/A

SYMPTOMATIC TREATMENT

Rehabilitation programs including cognitive, speech, occupational, and physical therapy may be helpful.

ADJUNCTIVE TREATMENT

N/A

ADMISSION/DISCHARGE CRITERIA

Initial treatment should take place in an ICU setting.

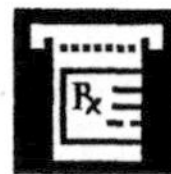

Medications

DRUG(S) OF CHOICE

There is no accepted treatment for CPM. Case reports of anecdotal successful treatment regimens have included:

- Varying regimens of corticosteroids, plasma exchange, and IVIG
- Thyrotropin-releasing hormone (TRH) (0.6 mg IV daily for 6 weeks)
- Methylphenidate, titrated to a final dose of 10 mg bid, for treatment of neuropsychiatric symptoms

Contraindications

N/A

Precautions

N/A

ALTERNATIVE DRUGS

N/A

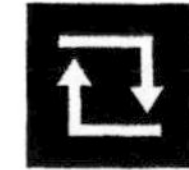

Follow-Up

PATIENT MONITORING

After stabilization of electrolyte abnormalities, patients should be monitored for swallowing dysfunction and progress in PT, OT, and speech therapy.

EXPECTED COURSE AND PROGNOSIS

- In cases of hyponatremia, symptoms of CPM typically manifest 2 to 6 days after correction of sodium levels. The course may range from death to nearly complete recovery. Symptoms typically worsen over the first week, then stabilize or improve. Improvement may be seen over the span of weeks to months, and even those with severe symptoms may survive. Recurrence is possible.
- Electrophysiologic studies, MRI, and CT are not particularly useful for establishing prognosis. Nor does the associated disease process, e.g., alcoholism or hyponatremia, help to predict outcome. Mortality depends in large part on effective prevention and treatment of complications such as pulmonary emboli and pneumonia. The majority of those who survive CPM have remaining neurologic deficits, such as ataxia and dysarthria. The cognitive effects of CPM may be most persistent.

PATIENT EDUCATION

N/A

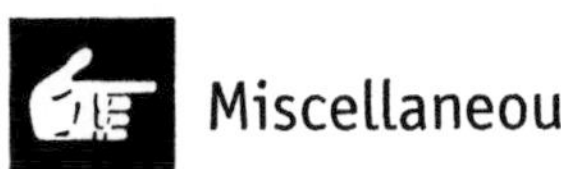

Miscellaneous

SYNONYMS

Osmotic demyelinization syndrome refers to pontine and extrapontine myelinolysis.

ICD-9-CM: 341.8 CNS demyelination NEC

SEE ALSO: N/A

REFERENCES

- Bridgeford D, Arciniegas DB, Batkis M, et al. Methylphenidate treatment of neuropsychiatric symptoms of central and extrapontine myelinolysis. J Stud Alcohol 2000;61:657–660.
- Lampl C, Yazdi K. Central pontine myelinolysis. Eur Neurol 2002;47(1):3–10.
- Laubenberger J, Schneider B, Ansorge O, et al. Central pontine myelinolysis: clinical presentation and radiologic findings. Eur Radiol 1996;6(2):177–183.
- Norenberg MD. A hypothesis of osmotic endothelial injury: a pathogenetic mechanism in central pontine myelinolysis. Arch Neurol 1983;40:66–69.
- Pirzada NA, Ali II. Central pontine myelinolysis. Mayo Clin Proc 2001;76: 559–562.

Author(s): Beth A. Leeman, MD

Cerebral Palsy

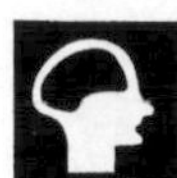

Basics

DESCRIPTION

Cerebral palsy is the term used to describe the neurologic disorder of motor dysfunction that occurs as a direct result of injury to the developing brain. The insult is nonprogressive and occurs before the age of 3 to 5 years and manifests as abnormalities of tone, posture, or motion. Although the insult is nonprogressive, the manifestations of motor dysfunction may subtly change with time, as the injured brain matures. However, by definition this condition does not involve true neurologic regression.

EPIDEMIOLOGY

Prevalence

The prevalence of cerebral palsy among children at school entry is about 2 per 1,000 live births.

ETIOLOGY

It is known that many conditions can injure the developing brain and lead to cerebral palsy. Yet, approximately one quarter of all cases have no definable cause.

Causes of Cerebral Palsy

- Prenatal
  - —First trimester (44%): teratogens, genetic syndromes, brain malformations, chromosomal abnormalities
  - —Second and third trimesters: intrauterine infections, fetal/placental dysfunction
- Labor and delivery (19%): Preeclampsia/eclampsia, complications of labor and delivery
- Perinatal (8%): Sepsis/CNS infections, asphyxia, prematurity
- Childhood (5%): Meningitis/encephalitis, traumatic brain injury, toxins
- No obvious cause (24%)

Note: Cerebral palsy occurring repeatedly in a family that is not due to a definable genetic syndrome or chromosomal abnormality should raise the concern that the diagnosis of cerebral palsy is inaccurate. In these cases, an underlying neurometabolic or neurodegenerative disorder should be sought.

RISK FACTORS

Prematurity is a risk factor for cerebral palsy. The risk of cerebral palsy rises steadily as birth weight declines. The risk is approximately 3.4 per 1,000 in infants 2,500 g and over, 13.9 per 1,000 in infants 1,501 to 2,500 g, and 90.4 per 1,000 in infants less than or equal to 1,500 grams. Infants of normal birth weight with a 5-minute Apgar score of 3 or less had a 5% probability of developing cerebral palsy. Similar scores at 10 minutes increased the risk to 17%, and scores of 3 or less at 20 minutes were associated with a 57% risk of cerebral palsy.

PREGNANCY

See above.

ASSOCIATED CONDITIONS

Many children with cerebral palsy have at least one additional disability associated with damage to the CNS. The most common associated deficits are:

- Cognitive impairment
- Sensory deficits
- Communication disorders
- Seizures
- Feeding problems
- Behavioral and emotional problems

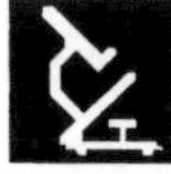

Diagnosis

Cerebral palsy is a clinical diagnosis. To make the diagnosis there has to be motor dysfunction that localizes to the brain as opposed to the peripheral nervous system. Motor dysfunction can manifest as failure to attain motor milestones at the appropriate age, or abnormalities in tone. Clinical examination should localize the lesion to the brain. Clues on physical examination that raise the suspicion of peripheral nervous system dysfunction include difficult-to-elicit or absent reflexes. Neurologic regression or loss of neurologic skills either in the area of motor dysfunction or in other areas of development makes the diagnosis of cerebral palsy suspect.

CLASSIFICATION OF CEREBRAL PALSY

Multiple classifications have been proposed for cerebral palsy.

Swedish Classification of Cerebral Palsy

Spastic: Quadriparesis, hemiparesis, diparesis
Dyskinetic: choreoathetosis, dystonia
Ataxic
Mixed type
Spastic cerebral palsy: abnormalities of the pyramidal tract, increased tendon reflexes, increased muscle tone.
Dyskinetic: choreoathetosis or dystonia with variable tone and rigidity.
Ataxic cerebral palsy: truncal ataxia, limb dysmetria and tremor.

DIFFERENTIAL DIAGNOSIS

Differential diagnosis includes progressive brain diseases that initially manifest as delayed motor milestones. Aspects of the history and physical examination in a child with motor dysfunction that would steer the clinician away from the diagnosis of cerebral palsy toward a diagnosis of a progressive neurometabolic or neurodegenerative disorder would include:

- Regression of previously acquired skills
- Strong family history of similar conditions
- Family history of sudden infant death
- Repetitive episodes of unexplained vomiting, shock, or metabolic acidosis
- Unusual body odors
- Hypotonia with absent or diminished reflexes
- Abnormal movements
- Ataxia
- Pigmentary retinopathy

Some of the mimickers of the various types of cerebral palsy are listed below.

- Spastic quadriparesis
  - —Leukodystrophies occurring in infancy such as Krabbe's disease, congenital adrenoleukodystrophy, and Pelizaeus-Merzbacher disease
  - —Other hereditary metabolic diseases
- Spastic diparesis
  - —Arginase deficiency
  - —Familial spastic paraparesis
  - —Tethered cord syndrome
- Ataxic cerebral palsy
  - —Vitamin E deficiency
  - —Ataxia telangiectasia
  - —Late infantile sphingolipidoses
  - —Late infantile ceroid lipofuscinoses
  - —Abetalipoproteinemia
  - —Hypobetalipoproteinemia
  - —Spinocerebellar ataxias (SCAs)
- Dyskinetic cerebral palsy
  - —Mitochondrial disorder
  - —Fahr syndrome
  - —Hallervorden-Spatz disease
  - —Lesch-Nyhan disease
  - —Segawa syndrome or dopa-responsive dystonia
  - —Dystonia musculorum deformans
  - —Glutaric aciduria
  - —Rett syndrome

LABORATORY PROCEDURES

Laboratory testing in patients suspected of having cerebral palsy is undertaken to delineate extent of neurologic impairment and the presence of other associated deficits, as well as in selected cases a thorough evaluation for progressive disorders mimicking cerebral palsy. Testing that may be helpful includes:

- Hearing evaluation
- Eye examination including dilated eye examination
- Swallowing evaluation
- X-rays when scoliosis or dislocation of hips are suspected
- Serial developmental assessments
- EEG when spells suspicious of seizures are present

IMAGING STUDIES

Imaging studies are helpful with regard to pattern recognition. Certain patterns are recognized as occurring in static disorders:

- Developmental abnormalities such as migrational disorders
- Patterns of previous insult such as periventricular leukomalacia, multicystic encephalomalacia, and porencephalic cysts.

Certain imaging abnormalities are specific in pointing away from cerebral palsy to a neurodegenerative disorder such as white matter changes indicative of leukodystrophy. In a portion of children with cerebral palsy, the MRI of the brain reveals no radiographic abnormality.

In general the MRI is a better tool for assessing brain parenchyma, whereas the CT is a better test for evaluation of the size of the ventricles.

SPECIAL TESTS

Evaluation for a neurometabolic or neurodegenerative disease should be undertaken in any child with motor dysfunction with neurologic regression.

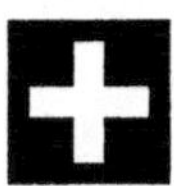

Management

GENERAL MEASURES

Once the clinical diagnosis has been made, a comprehensive evaluation should be undertaken to define the extent of motor disability, and to determine the presence of associated conditions. Early and aggressive physical and occupational therapy is recommended, with enrollment in an early intervention program. Speech therapy should be instituted if speech is delayed as well. Treatment, by medications and surgical measures, is aimed at maximizing motor function, treatment of associated conditions, and monitoring and treatment of complications.

SURGICAL MEASURES

- Dorsal rhizotomy to decrease spasticity
- Tendon lengthening and transplant measures to decrease impact of contractures

SYMPTOMATIC TREATMENT

See Medications, below.

ADJUNCTIVE TREATMENT

N/A

ADMISSION AND DISCHARGE CRITERIA

N/A

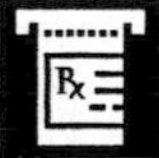

Medications

DRUG(S) OF CHOICE

There are no specific medications for cerebral palsy. Medications used for spasticity include baclofen (Lioresal), diazepam (Valium), or tizanidine (Zanaflex). Dosages depend on age and body weight.

Contraindications

Baclofen, diazepam, or tizanidine is contraindicated if there is a history of prior hypersensitivity to these or similar agents.

Precautions

Baclofen may in higher doses cause reversible muscular weakness or sedation. Diazepam may be habit forming, and cause sedation and respiratory compromise in higher doses. Tizanidine may cause fatigue or hypotension.

ALTERNATIVE DRUGS

Danazol is occasionally used for syndromes of muscular spasticity.

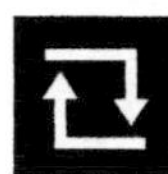

Follow-Up

PATIENT MONITORING

Patient monitoring should target the following:

- Efficacy and adequacy of therapies, e.g., physical therapy
- Monitoring of musculoskeletal system, e.g., bones/joints
- Adequacy of nutrition and growth
- Treatment of associated conditions such as seizures
- Adequacy of daily programs in the school or preschool systems
- Serial monitoring to determine that there is no true regression

EXPECTED COURSE AND PROGNOSIS

Although cerebral palsy is a static condition, the clinical symptoms can subtly change with time. Usually infants who are hypotonic with increased reflexes eventually become hypertonic within a few years. Athetosis or chorea in dyskinetic cerebral palsy may gradually appear toward the end of the first year of life. Ataxia may be noted only when the child begins to sit or reach for objects. Contractures tend to develop over time in patients with spasticity. In general, a number of factors affect prognosis: the type of cerebral palsy, the degree of delay in motor milestones, and the degree of associated deficits in intelligence, sensation, and emotional adjustment. The following are general guidelines:

- Children with hemiplegia and no other problems have a good chance of walking at about the age of 2 years.
- More than 50% of children with spastic diplegia learn to walk by about the age of 3 years.
- Of children with quadriplegia, 25% require total care, approximately 33% walk—usually after age 3 years.
- Few children who do not sit by age 4 years will learn to walk.

PATIENT EDUCATION

Educating parents of children with cerebral palsy, demonstrating how positioning can be an effective way of helping the child with mobility, encouraging the parent-child interaction, and muscle stretching should be part of the teaching given to parents. Counseling on the need to monitor for associated conditions and complications is also an important aspect of treatment.

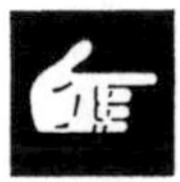

Miscellaneous

SYNONYMS

Static encephalopathy manifested by motor dysfunction.

ICD-9-CM: 343.9 Cerebral palsy NOS

SEE ALSO: N/A

REFERENCES

- Dormans JP, Orthopedic management of children with cerebral palsy. Pediatr Clin North Am 1993;40(3):645–656.
- Kuban KCK, Leviton A. Cerebral palsy. N Engl J Med 1994;330(3)188–195.
- Mutch L, Alberman E, Hagberg B, et al. Cerebral palsy epidemiology: where are we now and where are we going? Dev Med Child Neurol 1992;34:547–555.
- Peacock WJ, Staudt LA. Selective posterior rhizotomy: evolution of theory and practice. Pediatr Neurosurg 1991; 92(17):128–134.
- Swaiman KF, Russman BS. Cerebral palsy. In: Swaiman KF, Ashwal S, eds. Pediatric neurology principles and practice, vol 1. St. Louis: Mosby, 1999.
- Volpe J. Value of MR in definition of the neuropathology of cerebral palsy in vivo. AJNR 1992;13:79–83.
- Wossum DJ. Neuropsychologic issues in children with disabilities. Compr Ther 1994;20(2):79–83.

Author(s): S. Anne Joseph, MD

Cerebrovascular Disease, Arteriovenous Malformation

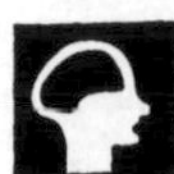

Basics

DESCRIPTION

Arteriovenous malformations (AVMs) are congenital masses of arteries and veins with no intermediate capillaries. They appear as well-circumscribed tangles of vessels fed directly by arteries. AVMs exert pressure on draining veins and prevent adequate extraction of nutrients and oxygen by adjacent tissues. Most are asymptomatic; but left untreated, AVMs can cause hemorrhage, hypoperfusion, and/or mass effect, resulting in minimal symptoms, focal deficits, or catastrophic neurologic injury. AVMs can cause seizures by directly irritating surrounding brain.

EPIDEMIOLOGY

- Several autopsy studies reflect a 0.01% to 0.50% prevalence of sporadic AVMs. About 300,000 Americans are believed to have intracranial or intraspinal AVMs; 85% are supratentorial, and 15% are infratentorial.
- The natural history is not well known as most symptomatic lesions are treated and most asymptomatic lesions are undetected; however, it is estimated that 12% of patients harboring AVMs are symptomatic. Most patients present with hemorrhage.
- Best evidence suggests a 1.3% to 4%/year cumulative hemorrhage risk with 10% to 17.6% mortality and 53% to 81% significant neurological morbidity per hemorrhage. The risk of rehemorrhage in the first year after a hemorrhage increases to 6% to 6.9%. There is a 22% risk of hemorrhage-induced epilepsy. About 2% of hemorrhagic strokes in adults and up to 40% in children are attributed to AVMs. Very rare spontaneous obliteration has been reported.

Age

Patients are generally 20 to 40 years of age; most are diagnosed before 30.

Race/Sex

Males and females of all races and ethnic groups are equally affected.

ETIOLOGY

Current evidence suggests that AVMs result from dysregulated angiogenesis producing persistent primitive arteriovenous connections or redevelopment of such connections after initial closure. Trauma to developing vessels may also contribute. The lack of normal capillaries results in a high-flow, high-pressure arteriovenous shunt. High flow produces vascular steal, and high pressure promotes growth of the AVM, formation of aneurysms, and rupture. Persistent high pressure also causes feeding arteries to swell and distort and draining veins to stenose. Vessels become progressively thinner and weaker. Multiple AVMs are very rare.

Genetics

Sporadic AVMs have no known genetic susceptibility. AVMs have been associated with hereditary hemorrhagic telangiectasia (Osler-Weber-Rendu disease) and other rare neurologic syndromes (Wyburn-Mason syndrome, Sturge-Weber syndrome, von Hippel-Lindau disease).

RISK FACTORS

The risk of hemorrhage cannot be accurately predicted. Irregular growth of AVMs complicates this further. Several factors may increase the risk of hemorrhage: deep venous drainage, high feeding artery pressure, hypertension, prior hemorrhage, related aneurysms, smaller size, and venous stasis.

PREGNANCY

Current evidence indicates that pregnancy and method of delivery do not increase the risk of hemorrhage. Pregnancy-related hemodynamic changes have been postulated potentially to increase hemorrhage risk or to exacerbate symptoms. Treatment should be considered before pregnancy. During pregnancy, the risk of treatment should be carefully considered against the risk of hemorrhage.

ASSOCIATED CONDITIONS

Aneurysms may be present within, near, or far from the AVM (17–48%). These aneurysms behave like non-AVM-related aneurysms. As aneurysms are much more likely to hemorrhage, they should be sought in any patient with an AVM-related hemorrhage and may need to be treated before or at the same time as the AVM.

Diagnosis

DIFFERENTIAL DIAGNOSIS

- Non-AVM-related intraparenchymal hemorrhage (IPH)
- Cavernous malformation—an abnormal collection of low-flow blood-filled channels with no intervening neural tissue. These can hemorrhage and are more likely to be multiple.
- Cerebral aneurysm
- Venous angioma (developmental venous anomaly, DVA), the most common vascular malformation of the brain—multiple abnormally enlarged veins near a ventricular surface confluence into a larger vein toward the cortex forming a "caput medusa" appearance on angiography. These generally do not impair neural function, and rarely, if ever, hemorrhage.
- Arteriovenous fistula (AVF)—an abnormal acquired arteriovenous shunt sometimes resulting from trauma involving the external and internal cranial vasculature.
- Tumor—rarely, an AVM may resemble a tumor by its mass effect and edema.

SIGNS AND SYMPTOMS

Most AVMs are asymptomatic. The most common symptom is hemorrhage (50%) with varying neurologic deficits related to the location and extent of hemorrhage. Other common symptoms are seizures (25%) and headache (15%) of no characteristic pattern. Focal neurologic deficits can also occur (5%), including aphasia, apraxia, ataxia, cognitive dysfunction, memory difficulties, papilledema, paresthesias, vertigo, visual disturbances, and weakness. Asymptomatic adult patients have a higher incidence of learning disabilities. A rare sign may be a cranial bruit.

LABORATORY PROCEDURES

N/A

IMAGING STUDIES

- CT has low sensitivity but may demonstrate calcifications (25–30%).
- MRI is very sensitive and demonstrates a characteristic honeycomb tangle of flow voids. Large arteries, arterialized veins, and the relation of the AVM to intracranial structures can often be seen. Areas of hemorrhage, blood products of various ages, and local edema may be present.
- MRI and MRA can noninvasively create 3D representations of the AVM.
- Cerebral angiogram best demonstrates blood vessel architecture. Superselective angiogram is recommended to delineate the internal architecture of an AVM. Associated aneurysms should also be identified.
- MRI and cerebral angiography are recommended prior to surgery.

SPECIAL TESTS

The Wada test and functional imaging techniques can be useful in localizing eloquent areas prior to treatment.

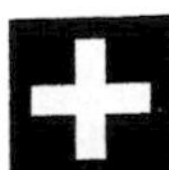

Management

GENERAL MEASURES

Indications for treatment include prevention of hemorrhage, treatment of seizures, enhancement of local perfusion, and treatment of hemorrhage. Hemorrhage risk is unchanged as long as an AVM is present; early treatment to achieve angiographic obliteration while mitigating neurologic risk is usually recommended. Incomplete treatment is generally not recommended.

There are four treatment options: observation, surgery, radiosurgery, and endovascular therapy. Treatment planning considers the lowest risk of injury with the highest chance of lesion obliteration. Many centers treat AVMs with a combination of interventions.

SURGICAL MEASURES

- Surgery: surgical removal of the entire AVM while limiting brain injury is the treatment of choice. Spetzler and Martin devised a grading system of AVMs, based on size, location, and venous drainage, to estimate the risk of surgical intervention (grades 1 to 5). Low surgical risk lesions (grades 1 to 3) are treated with 94% to 100% efficacy and negligible morbidity. High surgical risk lesions (grades 4 to 5) can be treated but with 17% to 22% morbidity.
- Radiosurgery: conventional radiotherapy is not considered effective, but stereotactic radiosurgery can treat high surgical risk lesions. Radiosurgical treatment through vessel wall injury takes years, during which the risk of hemorrhage remains unchanged. Angiographic cure occurs in 65% to 85% of lesions <3 cm in size at 3 years, but is significantly less for larger lesions. There is radiation exposure and a small risk of recurrence. Still, treatment-related risks are low, and outpatient treatment is employed.

ADJUNCTIVE TREATMENT

Embolization: current techniques of plugging vessels intravascularly are generally inadequate as sole therapy (<10%), but embolization can reduce the flow or size of a lesion to facilitate surgery or radiosurgery. Functional tests can also be performed by injecting barbiturates through the AVM. This technique is invasive but less so than surgery and carries modest treatment-related risks. Multiple procedures may be required.

SYMPTOMATIC TREATMENT

No medical management can completely mitigate AVM hemorrhage risk. Acute hemorrhage should be treated like any intracranial hemorrhage. Seizures can be treated with surgery. Focal neurologic deficits may or may not improve with treatment. Surgery should be strongly considered for low surgical risk lesions that are easily accessible. Small lesions that cannot be easily accessed may be treated with radiosurgery. A combined embolization and surgery approach may be suggested for moderate surgical risk lesions. High surgical risk and unresectable lesions may be treated by radiosurgery with or without embolization. Some centers may attempt palliative partial embolization of very high risk lesions, but long-term results are poor.

ADMISSION/DISCHARGE CRITERIA

The decision to treat an AVM is based on age, neurologic status, hemorrhage risk factors, medical condition, and the architecture of the lesion. Carefully planned treatment with multiple preoperative visits for testing and counseling affords the best possible outcome. Due to the lifetime risk of hemorrhage, more aggressive treatment is warranted in younger patients.

Medications

DRUG(S) OF CHOICE

Medications treat symptoms (e.g., headaches, seizures) and the side effects of treatment (e.g., antihypertensives, antiemetics, steroids).

Contraindications

N/A

Precautions

Monitor blood glucose with steroids.

ALTERNATIVE DRUGS

N/A

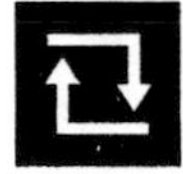

Follow-Up

PATIENT MONITORING

After surgery, standard postcraniotomy care, including control of intracranial pressure and blood pressure, is warranted. Rapid neurologic decline after AVM resection due to the increased perfusion to previously hypoperfused tissue (normal perfusion pressure breakthrough) may occur. Angiography should be performed after surgery to confirm AVM obliteration. Serial angiography should be performed in patients electing observation or radiosurgery. Some centers may employ MRA and CTA in serial follow-up of treated and untreated lesions.

EXPECTED COURSE AND PROGNOSIS

A surgically excised AVM can be considered cured with no further risk of hemorrhage and recurrence. Rarely, recurrence has been described in radiosurgically obliterated AVMs. Incompletely treated lesions do not reduce the risk of hemorrhage.

PATIENT EDUCATION

- No restrictions on activity or diet are recommended to prevent hemorrhage. Aspirin and other nonsteroidal antiinflammatory drugs (NSAIDs) may promote a more serious hemorrhage.
- Web site: National Institute of Neurological Disorders and Stroke, *ww.ninds.nih.gov/health_and_medical/disorders/avms_html.htm.*
- Organization: The AVM Support Group Toronto Hospital, Western Division 399 Bathurst St. Toronto, Ontario, MST 258. Phone: (416) 603-2197. *www.radsci.ucla.edu:8000/avm/index.html*

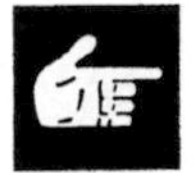

Miscellaneous

SYNONYMS

Vascular malformation

ICD-9-CM: 747.81 AVM, brain

SEE ALSO: CEREBROVASCULAR DISEASE, INTRACEREBRAL HEMORRHAGE; CEREBROVASCULAR DISEASE, INTRACRANIAL ANEURYSMS AND SUBARACHNOID HEMORRHAGE

REFERENCES

- The Arteriovenous Malformation Study Group. Arteriovenous malformations of the brain in adults. N Engl J Med 1999;340: 1812–1818.
- Fleetwood IG, Steinberg GK. Arteriovenous malformations. Lancet 2002;359:863–873.
- Hofmeister C, Stapf C, Hartmann A. Demographic, morphological, and clinical characteristics of 1289 patients with brain arteriovenous malformation. Stroke 2000; 31:1307–1310.
- Mast H, Young WL, Koennecke HC. Risk of spontaneous haemorrhage after diagnosis of cerebral arteriovenous malformation. Lancet 1997;350:1065–2068.
- Ogilvy CS, Stieg PE, Awad I, et al. Recommendations for the management of intracranial arteriovenous malformations: a statement for healthcare professionals from a special writing group of the Stroke Council, American Stroke Association. Circulation 2001;103:2644–2657.

Author(s): Stephen I. Ryu, MD; Robert L. Dodd, MD, PhD; Gary K. Steinberg, MD, PhD

Cerebrovascular Disease, Intracerebral Hemorrhage

Basics

DESCRIPTION

Intracerebral hemorrhage (ICH) results from bleeding directly into the brain substance.

EPIDEMIOLOGY

Approximately 10% of all strokes in North America.

Incidence/Prevalence

Incidence in the general population is 12–29/100,000.

Race

African Americans have an approximate twofold increase in the risk for ICH with incidence rates up to 50/100,000. Asian populations also have higher rates of ICH.

Age

Incidence rates increase with age.

Sex

Males and females affected equally.

ETIOLOGY

Frequently associated with location of hemorrhage and patient age.

- Hypertension: implicated in over 50% of ICH. Most commonly located in the basal ganglia, thalamus, deep subcortical white matter, pons, or cerebellum. Lobar hypertensive ICH occurs much less frequently.
- Vascular malformations: account for 4% to 8% of ICH and include arteriovenous malformations, cavernous malformations, and venous angiomas. Frequently located at the cerebral convexity or in the subcortical white matter. More common in younger patients.
- Aneurysm: accounts for 3% to 4% of ICH. Usually associated with subarachnoid hemorrhage (SAH), but rupture into the parenchyma may occur when located in the intrahemispheric or sylvian fissures.
- Cerebral amyloid angiopathy: results from deposition of amyloid protein in leptomeningeal and cortical arterioles. Common cause of lobar ICH in the elderly (>50% in patients over 75 years old).
- Bleeding diathesis: anticoagulant therapy implicated in 5% to 20% of all ICH, especially in patients treated with warfarin with the international normalized ratio (INR) >4.0. Symptomatic ICH rates with thrombolytic therapy are 1% with treatment for acute myocardial infarction and 6.4% for acute ischemic stroke (AIS). Also occurs in disseminated intravascular coagulopathy, thrombocytopenia, specific clotting factor deficiencies, polycythemia/hyperviscosity syndromes, leukemias (especially promyelocytic), von Willebrand disease, and sickle cell anemia.
- Neoplasms: bleeding into brain tumors accounts for 2% to 7% of ICH. Occurs with primary brain tumors or metastatic tumors, especially melanoma, renal cell, breast or lung cancers.
- Drug-related: use of cocaine, amphetamines, and over-the-counter sympathomimetic agents found in cold remedies and diet pills, and heavy alcohol use.
- Cerebral venous occlusive disease (CVOD): venous infarction resulting from venous occlusive disease may undergo hemorrhagic transformation. Associated with pregnancy and the postpartum period, contiguous air space infections, hypercoaguable disorders, and dehydration.
- Hemorrhagic transformation of ischemic arterial infarct: up to 50% of ischemic infarctions undergo some amount of hemorrhagic transformation within 1 to 3 weeks of the original event. Symptomatic transformation is much less frequent.
- Arteritis/arteriopathies: infectious vasculitis, multisystem vasculitis, isolated CNS angiitis, or moyamoya disease.
- Other: trauma, after carotid endarterectomy or other neurosurgical procedures, postmyelography.

RISK FACTORS

As above.

PREGNANCY

Increased risk of vascular malformation hemorrhage or aneurysmal rupture during pregnancy and labor. CVOD more frequent during pregnancy and the puerperium.

ASSOCIATED CONDITIONS

N/A

Diagnosis

DIFFERENTIAL DIAGNOSIS

Acute ischemic stroke, SAH, epidural hematoma, seizure, migraine.

SIGNS AND SYMPTOMS

Abrupt onset and rapid evolution of signs and symptoms over minutes. Over half of patients complain of headache, and almost half have nausea and vomiting. Focal neurologic symptoms reflect location of ICH. Decreased level of consciousness (LOC) found with large or rapidly expanding ICH and when structures regulating consciousness are involved (e.g., brainstem). Seizures occur in 10% to 15% of cases, especially in lobar ICH.

LABORATORY PROCEDURES

No specific blood work to diagnose ICH. The following studies should be obtained to help establish etiology or in preparation for further diagnostic testing:

- CBC and platelet count
- Coagulation studies (prothrombin time/INR, activated partial thromboplastin time)
- Electrolyte panel, including renal function studies
- Urine drug screen
- Blood typing/cross-matching, if delivery of blood products or surgical intervention is planned
- Other testing may include liver function tests, sedimentation rate, antinuclear antibodies, blood cultures, fibrinogen, fibrin split products, bleeding time, hemoglobin electrophoresis.

IMAGING STUDIES

- CT: Noncontrasted CT should be performed immediately to provide rapid information about hemorrhage location and size, presence of mass effect, and intraventricular extension. No further imaging study required if ICH is found in a location typical for hypertensive hemorrhage in a patient with known hypertension.
- MRI: Generally not useful in acute imaging of ICH, but should be used acutely in suspected cases of CVOD. Useful in diagnostic workup of ICH to search for underlying neoplasm or vascular malformation. Timing of MRI controversial; acute hematoma can obscure underlying lesions. Typically delayed for 4 to 6 weeks but can be used sooner to identify other previous hemorrhagic lesions, as seen with amyloid angiopathy or multiple cavernous malformations.

SPECIAL TESTS

- Cerebral angiography: indicated when a primary vascular abnormality such as aneurysm, vascular malformation, or vasculitis is suspected, based on hemorrhage location or patient characteristics. Should be performed in young, nonhypertensive patients and in those with atypical location for hypertensive hemorrhage. If angiography negative in young patient with lobar hemorrhage, should be repeated in 1 to 2 months, as large hematomas may compress underlying vascular malformations in the acute phase.

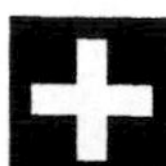

Management

GENERAL MEASURES

- Rapid assessment of LOC, airway, and adequacy of ventilation. Patients with inability to protect the airway or with respiratory depression should be intubated immediately and mechanically ventilated.
- Increased intracranial pressure (ICP) may be treated with hyperventilation to a $Paco_2$ of about 30 mm Hg. Medical and surgical management of increased ICP discussed below.
- Correction of any underlying coagulopathy.
- Seizures generally occur within 72 hours of the ictus. Prophylactic use of anticonvulsant agents reserved for patients with cortical involvement.
- Prophylaxis for deep venous thrombosis with pneumatic sequential compression devices.

SURGICAL MEASURES

- Supratentorial ICH: comatose patients with massive ICH and neurologically stable patients with small hemorrhages are not considered surgical candidates. For other cases, surgical evacuation remains controversial. Older randomized trials of surgery found no benefit for surgery, but the largest were performed in the pre-CT era and before development of modern neurosurgical techniques. Endoscopic evacuation, as compared to open craniotomy, is currently being explored. Cortical ICH is more often evacuated than are deeper, ganglionic hemorrhages. Timing of surgery is also controversial, with some authors arguing for early evacuation to prevent primary hematoma expansion and neurologic decompensation and also to prevent secondary brain injury from toxic blood products.
- Cerebellar ICH: surgical evacuation indicated for cerebellar hemispheric ICH >3 cm in diameter or for decreased LOC.
- Ventricular drainage: associated intraventricular hemorrhage may result in communicating or noncommunicating hydrocephalus. Ventriculostomy performed to drain CSF and also to monitor ICP. Intraventricular instillation of thrombolytic agents to aid in dissolution of clot remains investigational.
- ICP monitoring: not proven to improve survival or outcome, but may be used to help direct therapy.

SYMPTOMATIC TREATMENT

Physical therapy, occupational therapy, and speech therapy are often helpful once the patient is stable.

ADJUNCTIVE TREATMENT

N/A

ADMISSION/DISCHARGE CRITERIA

All patients admitted for acute evaluation and management. ICU admission often required. Depending on residual symptoms, patients may need inpatient rehabilitation.

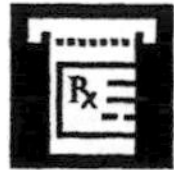

Medications

DRUG(S) OF CHOICE

No medical therapies have been shown to decrease mortality or improve recovery. Randomized studies of dexamethasone and glycerol for ICH were negative. Medical intervention is currently directed at conditions that result from ICH.

- Increased ICP
  - —Mannitol 20% solution
    - -Initial IV bolus 1 g/kg over 30 minutes and maintenance dose of 0.25–0.5 g/kg every 4 to 6 hours. Dosing adjusted to clinical status, ICP values, and serum osmolarity (300–310 mOsm/L).
  - —Intravenous barbiturate use limited by hypotension and not shown to improve outcome.
- Acute hypertension
  - —Control of acute hypertension has never been proven to prevent recurrent bleeding or improve outcome, but recommendations to keep mean arterial pressure <130 mm Hg are reasonable. Short-acting, easily titratable agents are preferred. Precipitous lowering of blood pressure should be avoided.
    - -Labetalol: 10–20 mg IV bolus, then 20 mg IV boluses every 10 to 15 minutes or IV infusion 0.5–1.0 mg/min (maximum 300 mg/day).
    - -Enalaprilat: 1.25 mg IV bolus over 5 minutes every 6 hours. For elderly or hypotensive patients, a starting dose of 0.625 mg is recommended.
    - -Nitroprusside: 0.2–0.5 μg/kg/min IV, titrated to desired blood pressure.

Contraindications

- Sublingual nifedipine contraindicated in all stroke syndromes.
- Labetalol not recommended for patients with asthma, chronic obstructive pulmonary disease, congestive heart failure, heart block, hypotension, or severe bradycardia (due to beta-blockade properties).
- Nitroprusside not recommended in pregnancy.

Precautions

- Nitroprusside and other vasodilators should be used with care as they may increase ICP.

ALTERNATIVE DRUGS

N/A

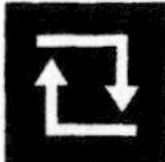

Follow-Up

PATIENT MONITORING

Monitor vital signs and neurologic status closely. Worsened neurologic status may arise from increased intracranial pressure, hydrocephalus, or rebleeding.

EXPECTED COURSE AND PROGNOSIS

Outcome is poor with 6-month mortality rate of 43%. Only 12% of patients are left with minor or no disability. Predictors of poor outcome include hemorrhage volume >60 cc, Glasgow Coma Scale score less than 9 at presentation, brainstem ICH, and intraventricular extension.

PATIENT EDUCATION

Given poor outcome once ICH occurs, educational efforts should be directed at prevention through risk factor modification. Further information may be obtained by contacting the American Stroke Association at 1-888-4STROKE or visiting *www.strokeassociation.org*.

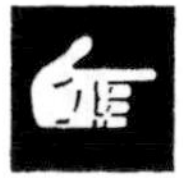

Miscellaneous

SYNONYMS

Intraparenchymal hemorrhage (IPH)
Parenchymatous hemorrhage (PH)

ICD-9-CM: 431 Intracerebral hemorrhage; Code for etiology (e.g., 437.6 Nonpyogenic thrombosis of intracranial venous sinus, 747.81 Anomalies of cerebrovascular system including arteriovenous malformation of brain); 674.0 Intracerebral hemorrhage occurring during pregnancy, childbirth, or the puerperium; 671.5 Cerebral venous thrombosis as a complication in pregnancy and the puerperium

SEE ALSO: N/A

REFERENCES

- Broderick JP, Brott T, Zuccarello M. Management of intracerebral hemorrhage. In: Batjer HH, Caplan LR, Freiberg L, et al., eds. Cerebrovascular disease. Philadelphia: Lippincott-Raven Publishers, 1996: 611–628.
- Qureshi AI, Giles WH, Croft JB. Racial differences in the incidence of intracerebral hemorrhage. Effects of blood pressure and education. Neurology 1999;52:1617–1621.
- Seestedt RC, Frankel MR. Intracerebral hemorrhage. Curr Treat Options Neurol 1999;1:127–137.
- Shah MV, Biller J. Medical and surgical management of intracerebral hemorrhage. Semin Neurol 1998;18:513–519.

Author(s): Susan L. Hickenbottom, MD

Cerebrovascular Disease, Intracranial Aneurysms, and Subarachnoid Hemorrhage

Basics

DESCRIPTION

Saccular aneurysms, the most common type of intracranial aneurysms, are focal protrusions arising from vessel wall weaknesses at major arterial bifurcations along the base of the brain. Their rupture results in hemorrhage into the subarachnoid spaces in which they reside, and is the second most common cause of hemorrhagic stroke.

EPIDEMIOLOGY

Incidence/Prevalence

The prevalence of unruptured aneurysms is controversial; however, most reports estimate their occurrence to be 1% to 6% in the general population. Incidence of aneurysmal subarachnoid hemorrhage (SAH) is approximately 10 to 15 per 100,000 people per year of which 80% to 90% are from ruptured saccular aneurysms.

Race

No known racial predisposition.

Age

The age distribution of patients with ruptured aneurysms is bell-shaped, occurring most frequently between the ages of 35 and 65, with the highest incidence between 55 and 60 years of age.

Sex

Approximately 60% of ruptured aneurysms occur in women.

ETIOLOGY

Almost all intracranial aneurysms are acquired, and while some occur after trauma and infection, most arise spontaneously. Saccular aneurysms are believed to result from prolonged hemodynamic stress and resultant local arterial degeneration at branch points and bifurcations of major cerebral arteries.

Genetics

Familial occurrence of intracranial aneurysms is uncommon; however, a small percentage of patients have a striking family history of inherited factors. Furthermore, the incidence of aneurysms is increased in patients with aortic coarctation and polycystic kidney disease, indicating a genetic predisposition in some patients.

RISK FACTORS

Hypertension, cigarette smoking, oral contraceptives, alcohol consumption, pregnancy, and cocaine use are all known risk factors for SAH and probably increase the risk of aneurysmal rupture. Other risk factors include trauma, atherosclerosis, and infection (bacterial endocarditis).

PREGNANCY

Intracranial hemorrhage during pregnancy is rare (incidence: 0.01–0.05% of all pregnancies). However, over half are SAH and most of these are aneurysmal, representing an increased incidence of aneurysmal SAH in pregnant women relative to the general female population. While the increased blood volume and pressure during pregnancy and late gestation are believed to contribute, the exact pathophysiologic and hormonal factors associated with the increased risk remain unknown. Mortality and morbidity of aneurysmal SAH during pregnancy is high, with a maternal mortality rate of 13% to 35% (accounting for about 1 in 25 maternal deaths during pregnancy) and a fetal mortality rate of 7% to 25%.

ASSOCIATED CONDITIONS

Aneurysms have been associated with a number of conditions including polycystic kidney disease (PKD), arteriovenous malformations (AVMs), moyamoya disease, fibromuscular dysplasia (FMD), and other hereditary connective tissue disorders.

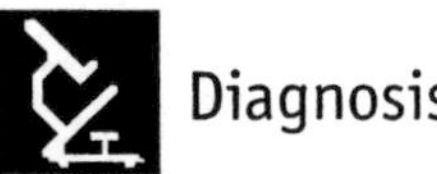

Diagnosis

DIFFERENTIAL DIAGNOSIS

The differential diagnosis of aneurysmal SAH narrows considerably following the confirmation of blood in the subarachnoid spaces:

- Arteriovenous malformations
- Dural arteriovenous fistula
- Vasculopathy (amyloid angiopathy, systemic lupus erythematosus, polyarteritis nodosa)
- Carotid dissection
- Pituitary apoplexy
- Hemorrhage from a tumor
- Benign perimesencephalic hemorrhage

SIGNS AND SYMPTOMS

The clinical presentation of aneurysmal SAH is usually characterized by the acute onset of severe headache that may initially be localized, but often generalizes quickly. Headache is the most common symptom in over 90% of cases and is classically described as "the worst headache of my life." Nausea and vomiting are frequent, and loss of consciousness may occur. Signs of meningeal irritation, including nuchal rigidity (especially to flexion) and photophobia, are often present within 4 to 8 hours after the onset of SAH. Focal neurologic signs and symptoms may also be present, depending on the size and location of the aneurysm, and the severity and location of the hemorrhage. Ocular hemorrhages may cause blurred vision and are frequently found on funduscopic examination, the most common of which are subhyaloid (preretinal) hemorrhages, seen in approximately 25% of patients.

LABORATORY PROCEDURES

- Lumbar puncture (LP) is the most sensitive test for SAH, and should be performed in cases where the head CT is negative but there remains a high clinical suspicion. Typical CSF findings in SAH are an elevated opening pressure, nonclotting bloody fluid that fails to clear with sequential tubes, xanthrochromia of the supernatant, a RBC count of usually $>$100,000 cells/mL, elevated protein, and normal glucose.
- Serum electrolyte abnormalities are frequent, with hyponatremia found in about one third of patients.

IMAGING STUDIES

The sequence of evaluation for suspected aneurysmal SAH begins with a high-resolution noncontrast CT scan. A good-quality head CT will detect SAH in over 95% of patients who undergo the study within 24 hours of the hemorrhage. The scan will also demonstrate the extent and location of the hemorrhage, as well as the presence of hydrocephalus. MRI provides a noninvasive method of evaluating patients who present several weeks after acute symptoms, since subacute or remote hemorrhages can be differentiated by their signal characteristics long after CT findings have normalized. Cerebral digital subtraction angiography (DSA) is the "gold standard" for diagnostic evaluation of aneurysms, and should be performed in CT- or LP-confirmed nontraumatic SAH and in patients in whom the clinical suspicion remains high despite negative CT scan and/or inconclusive LP. Magnetic resonance angiography (MRA) and rapid spiral CT angiography (CTA) are both noninvasive methods to evaluate the cerebral circulation that are increasingly being used for both screening and diagnosis.

SPECIAL TESTS

Transcranial Doppler ultrasonography (TCD) can be used to evaluate for the development of cerebral vasospasm, which is the leading cause of death and morbidity following successful treatment of the ruptured aneurysm.

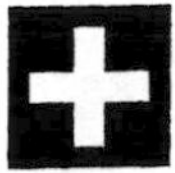

Management

GENERAL MEASURES

Early diagnosis and treatment is imperative for the best possible outcome. Treatment of intracranial aneurysms centers on efforts to exclude the aneurysm from the intracranial circulation while maintaining patency of the normal vasculature, restoring and maintaining normal cerebral blood flow.

SURGICAL MEASURES

- *Microsurgery clip ligation:* Most cerebral aneurysms are now treated with clip ligation, where a craniotomy is performed and a clip is placed, occluding the aneurysmal neck. Following adequate placement, long-term data suggest that this treatment is curative.
- *Endovascular coil embolization:* Intraarterial microcatheters can be used to place detachable, thrombogenic platinum coils (GDC coils) into saccular aneurysms, promoting their exclusion from the normal vasculature and reducing the risk of hemorrhage. Recent data suggest this treatment is safe and effective in preventing short-term rebleeding for some aneurysms, but long-term recanalization rates and efficacy are not yet known.

SYMPTOMATIC TREATMENT

The natural history of aneurysmal SAH carries an extremely high risk of death and/or disability, and medical management alone does little to change this outcome.

ADJUNCTIVE TREATMENT

Following elimination of the aneurysm via surgery, the remainder of therapeutic intervention focuses on preventing cerebral vasospasm and treating associated hydrocephalus. Treatment of vasospasm consists of the combination of calcium channel blockers, hypervolemic-hypertensive therapy, and endovascular angioplasty. Treatment of hydrocephalus includes either temporary CSF drainage or placement of a permanent ventriculoperitoneal (VP) shunt.

ADMISSION/DISCHARGE CRITERIA

All patients suspected of harboring a ruptured cerebral aneurysm should be admitted and urgently evaluated by a neurosurgeon.

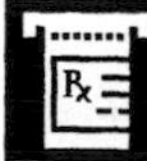

Medications

DRUG(S) OF CHOICE

- Antihypertensive medications, to control blood pressure.
- Nimodipine, a calcium channel antagonist used to treat vasospasm, has been demonstrated in prospective, randomized, placebo-controlled clinical trials to improve the outcome after aneurysmal SAH, and should be routinely administered during the first 21 days following SAH.
- Anticonvulsant medications should be administered if seizures occur.
- Analgesics to treat headaches.

Contraindications

Known hypersensitivity to particular medication.

Precautions

None

ALTERNATIVE DRUGS

None

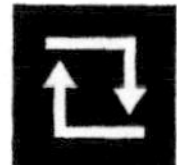

Follow-Up

PATIENT MONITORING

Survival from and successful treatment of a ruptured aneurysm does not provide cure of the disease. Patients who have had a previous SAH from an aneurysm are at increased risk for the development of new aneurysms. For this population, there is a 2% annual rate of new aneurysm development and the incidence of aneurysmal rupture is five times higher than the general aneurysmal population. Therefore, periodic follow-up with imaging is recommended not only for the treated lesion, but also to evaluate development of new ones.

EXPECTED COURSE AND PROGNOSIS

Despite advances in recognition, diagnosis, and treatment, the natural history of ruptured saccular aneurysms remains poor, with approximately one third of patients left dead or severely disabled by the initial hemorrhage. Another third of those who reach treatment die or are severely disabled because of rehemorrhage or cerebral vasospasm, leaving only one in three patients as functional survivors following aneurysmal SAH. Furthermore, some reports suggest that as many as 66% of the functional survivors never return to the same quality of life before the SAH because of mild cognitive or other neurologic deficits.

PATIENT EDUCATION

American Association of Neurological Surgery (AANS)/Congress of Neurological Surgery(CNS) Web site: *NEUROSURGERY//ON-CALL: www.neurosurgery.org/health/patient/detail.asp?DisorderID = 34, www.neurosurgery.org/health/patient/detail.asp?DisorderID = 87*

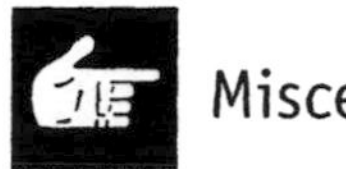

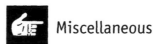

Miscellaneous

SYNONYMS

None

ICD-9-CM: 430.0 Aneurysm, ruptured

SEE ALSO: N/A

REFERENCES

- Dodd RL, Steinberg GK. Intracranial aneurysms. In: Aminoff MJ, Daroff RB, eds. Encyclopedia of neurological sciences. St. Louis: Academic Press, Elsevier, 2003.
- Hop JW, Rinkel GJ, Algra A, et al. Case-fatality rates and functional outcome after subarachnoid hemorrhage: a systematic review. Stroke 1997;28(3): 660–664.
- Molyneux A, Kerr R, Stratton I, et al. International Subarachnoid Aneurysm Trial (ISAT) of neurosurgical clipping versus endovascular coiling in 2143 patients with ruptured intracranial aneurysms: a randomized trial. Lancet 2002;360(9342): 1267–1274.
- Nishioka H, Torner JC, Graf CJ, et al. Cooperative study of intracranial aneurysms and subarachnoid hemorrhage: a long-term prognostic study. II. Ruptured intracranial aneurysms managed conservatively. Arch Neurol 1984;41(11):1142–1146.
- Stoodley MA, Macdonald RL, Weir B. Pregnancy and intracranial aneurysms. In: LeRoux PD, Winn HR, eds. Neurosurgery clinics of North America. 9(3):Philadelphia: WB Saunders, 1998;549–556.
- Teunissen LL, Rinkel GJ, Algra A, et al. Risk factors for subarachnoid hemorrhage: a systematic review. Stroke 1996;27: 544–549.
- Unruptured intracranial aneurysms—risk of rupture and risks of surgical intervention. International Study of Unruptured Intracranial Aneurysms Investigators. N Engl J Med 1998;339:1725–1733.

Author(s): Robert L. Dodd, MD, PhD; Stephen I. Ryu, MD; Gary K. Steinberg, MD, PhD

Cerebrovascular Disease, Ischemic Infarcts

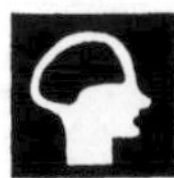

Basics

DESCRIPTION

Ischemic stroke is defined as an irreversible focal, and sometimes multifocal, brain damage caused by blood disruption to the affected area.

EPIDEMIOLOGY

Incidence/Prevalence

There are approximately 700,000 new strokes every year; 80% of these are ischemic in nature.

Age

It is more common in the elderly, though a significant portion occurs in individuals over 40 years of age.

Sex

It is more common in males.

Race

It is more common in African Americans and Hispanics.

ETIOLOGY

- Hypercoagulable state: includes deficiencies of protein C, S, or antithrombin III, factor V mutation, factor II mutation; antiphospholipid antibody syndrome; sickle cell anemia; mucin-secreting carcinomas.
- Cardiac emboli: conditions that predispose to the formation of cardiac emboli include atrial fibrillation, mitral valve stenosis, sick sinus syndrome, prosthetic heart valve, infective endocarditis, marantic endocarditis, congestive heart failure, dilated cardiomyopathy, myxomas, intraatrial septal defect, patent foramen ovale, dilated atria, and atrial septal aneurysm.
- Large artery disease: the extracranial carotid, intracranial carotid, extracranial vertebral, intracranial vertebral, middle cerebral, basilar, anterior cerebral, and posterior cerebral are all large arteries. Disease in these vessels can lead to ischemic stroke. The most common is atherosclerosis. Other diseases include dissection, vasculitis, moyamoya, and fibromuscular dysplasia.
- Small vessel disease: the most common cause of small vessel disease is hypertension. Other etiologies include diabetes, vasculitis, and rare genetic conditions like mitochondrial encephalopathy, lactic acidosis, and stroke-like episodes (MELAS) and cerebral autosomal-dominant arteriopathy with subcortical infarcts and leukoencephalopathy (CADASIL). The stroke caused by small vessel disease is small and frequently called a lacunar stroke.

Genetics

MELAS and CADASIL are rare genetic conditions that lead to ischemic stroke.

PREGNANCY

Pregnancy increases the risk of ischemic stroke. Conditions peculiar to pregnancy that lead to stroke include paradoxical emboli from the legs or pelvic veins, cardiomyopathy of pregnancy, cervical arterial dissection during labor and delivery, hypercoagulable state, amniotic fluid embolism, and vasoconstrictive medications like ergotamines.

ASSOCIATED CONDITIONS

Coronary artery disease and peripheral artery diseases.

Diagnosis

DIFFERENTIAL DIAGNOSIS

- Intracerebral hemorrhage
- Multiple sclerosis
- Migraine aura
- Seizures (Todd's paralysis)
- Intracranial structural lesions
- Intracranial infections
- Metabolic disorders
- Somatization disorders
- Labyrinthine disorders

SIGNS AND SYMPTOMS

Stroke symptoms are usually sudden and abrupt. The clinical features depend on the brain area infarcted. Common symptoms include:

- Hemiparesis
- Hemisensory loss
- Visual field defects
- Ataxia and incoordination
- Aphasia
- Dysarthria
- Dysphagia
- Diplopia
- Vertigo

LABORATORY PROCEDURES

- All patients with ischemic stroke should have blood for fasting lipid profile, RPR, BUN, creatinine, CBC and platelets, PT, PTT, and INR.
- Hypercoagulable profile, including protein C, protein S, antithrombin III, factor V, factor II, lupus anticoagulant, antiphospholipid antibodies, and homocysteine should be requested in young patients.
- Serial blood cultures should be sent when infective endocarditis is suspected.

IMAGING STUDIES

- Chest x-ray to evaluate for cardiomegaly.
- CT scan must be performed in all patients presenting with suspected stroke because it is very sensitive in detecting intracranial hemorrhage, which can easily mimic ischemia. It is also cheap, quick, and readily available.
- MRI of the brain (especially diffusion weighted imaging and FLAIR) is more sensitive than CT scan in detecting early infarction, and infarcts in the cerebellum, brainstem, and inferior temporal lobes.
- MR Angiography is a noninvasive test, and is accurate for assessing the major extracerebral and intracerebral arteries, though it may overestimate the severity of the stenosis.
- Transthoracic echocardiogram (TTE) is indicated in most patients with ischemic stroke. If the TTE is negative and a cardiac source is still suspected, then transesophageal echocardiogram (TEE) must be performed. TEE is also indicated in all young patients. TEE is more accurate than TTE in showing atrial and ventricular thrombi, vegetations, and left atrial enlargement, detecting shunts, and evaluating the proximal aorta.
- Angiography: the gold standard for an accurate assessment of both the extra- and intracranial vasculature. However, it is an invasive procedure and should be reserved for patients in whom noninvasive testing has not definitely shown the source of stroke, and to assess accurately the degree of stenosis.
- Ultrasound is safe, portable, and less expensive. It includes transcranial Doppler to look for intracranial disease and carotid duplex to assess for extracranial carotid and vertebral artery disease.

SPECIAL TESTS

ECG and cardiac monitoring to evaluate for arrhythmias.

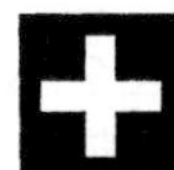

Management

GENERAL MEASURES

General treatment of stroke includes acute supportive care, management of coexisting medical illnesses and secondary stroke prevention.

SURGICAL MEASURES

- Carotid endarterectomy (CEA) is indicated for significant (>50%) symptomatic carotid artery stenosis. For those patients who are considered high risk for surgery, carotid angioplasty with stent placement is performed in a few medical centers. Intracranial large artery (basilar, vertebral, middle cerebral, and internal carotid) angioplasty with or without stent placement is occasionally performed in a few academic centers for those patients who fail maximal medical therapy.
- Intraarterial thrombolysis for acute ischemic stroke, only within 6 hours from the onset of symptoms, is being provided in few experienced centers.

- Some cardiac lesions require surgical or radiologic interventions.

SYMPTOMATIC TREATMENT

- Includes treatment of hyperglycemia, fever, and infection; deep vein thrombosis prophylaxis; aspiration precaution; adequate hydration and nutrition; judicious control of blood pressure with avoidance of excessive reduction in the acute setting and adequate control in the long run, and avoidance of prolonged use of indwelling catheter to prevent urinary tract infection.
- Amitriptyline or gabapentin for pain related to thalamic strokes; antidepressants for the depression that may accompany some cortical strokes; muscle relaxants such as baclofen for residual spasticity; and stool softeners for constipation.

ADJUNCTIVE TREATMENT

Physical, occupational, speech, and cognitive therapy may be needed.

ADMISSION/DISCHARGE CRITERIA

In general any patient presenting with acute ischemic stroke should be admitted to the hospital for the evaluation of etiology and appropriate prevention measures; prevention and management of stroke complications; early initiation of physical, occupational, and speech therapy; evaluation for eligibility for inpatient rehabilitation; assistance with appropriate placement; and patient and caregiver education.

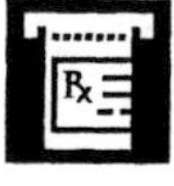

Medications

DRUG(S) OF CHOICE

- Recombinant tissue plasminogen activator (rt-PA) is the only FDA-approved medication for acute ischemic stroke and must be given within 3 hours from the onset of symptoms. The dose is 0.9 mg/kg up to a maximum of 90 mg; 10% of the dose is given as an IV bolus over 1 minute and the rest as an IV drip over 1 hour.
- Antiplatelet agents: indicated for stroke prevention in small vessel disease, intracranial large artery disease, mild (<50%) extracranial carotid artery disease, extracranial vertebral artery disease, aortic arch disease without mobile plaque, irregular nonstenotic valve surfaces, and in patients who are not Coumadin candidates.
  - —Aspirin: 50–325 mg qd
  - —Plavix: 75 mg qd
  - —Aggrenox (combination aspirin 25 mg/extended release dipyridamole 200 mg one tablet bid)
- Anticoagulants
  - —Warfarin (Coumadin): indicated in hypercoagulable states; cardiac sources like atrial fibrillation, intracardiac thrombi, etc.; and intracranial large artery stenosis.

Contraindications

- rtPA: suspicion of subarachnoid hemorrhage; recent (within 3 months) intracerebral or intraspinal surgery; recent head trauma; recent previous stroke; history of intracerebral hemorrhage; uncontrolled hypertension at time of treatment (SBP >185 mm Hg or DBP >110 mm Hg); seizure at the onset of stroke; active internal bleeding; intracranial neoplasm, arteriovenous malformation, or aneurysm; known bleeding diathesis including but not limited to current use of oral anticoagulants (e.g., warfarin sodium), or an international normalized ratio (INR) >1.7, or a prothrombin time (PT) >15 seconds; administration of heparin in the preceding 48 hours and an elevated activated partial thromboplastin time (aPTT) at presentation; platelet count <100,000/mm^3.
- Aspirin/Aggrenox: mainly known allergic reaction to salicylic acid, active systemic bleeding, or active gastric ulcer.
- Clopidogrel: mainly active systemic bleeding.
- Warfarin: mainly active bleeding, bleeding tendency, noncompliance, and gait difficulty with increased falling risk.

Precautions

- rtPA: Noncompressible arterial or venous punctures must be avoided. Blood pressure must be monitored closely during administration of the medicine and treated if elevated. If serious bleeding is suspected, then it must be stopped immediately. Watch for allergic reaction.
- Clopidogrel: monitor for any TTP symptoms at the beginning of treatment.
- Warfarin: watch for compliance, bleeding events, and falling events.

ALTERNATIVE DRUGS

N/A

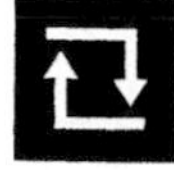

Follow-Up

PATIENT MONITORING

- Frequent follow-up visits are important to assess patients for recurrent events, compliance with treatment and recommendations, and adverse reactions from the treatment medications.
- Close monitoring of INR is crucial for treatment with Coumadin.

EXPECTED COURSE AND PROGNOSIS

Appropriate preventive secondary measures significantly decrease the risk of recurrent stroke. However, despite these measures patients continue to be at increased risk. If recurrent events occur, reevaluation for the etiology and modification of the management is important.

PATIENT EDUCATION/ORGANIZATIONS

American Stroke Association, National Center, 7272 Greenville Avenue, Dallas TX, 75231, 1-888-478-7653, *www.strokeassociation.org.*

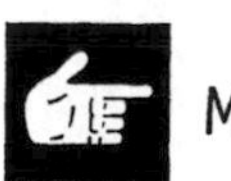

Miscellaneous

SYNONYMS

N/A

ICD-9-CM: 436 CVA

SEE ALSO: CEREBROVASCULAR DISEASE, TRANSIENT ISCHEMIC ATTACK; CARDIOEMBOLIC STROKE

REFERENCES

- Albers GW, Easton JD, Sacco RL, et al. Antithrombotic and thrombolytic therapy for ischemic stroke. Chest 1998;114 (suppl 5):683S–698S.
- Antiplatelet Trialists' Collaboration. Collaborative overview of randomized trials of antiplatelet therapy-I: prevention of death, myocardial infarction, and stroke by prolonged antiplatelet therapy in various categories in patients. BMJ 1994;308: 81–106.
- Barnett HJ, Taylor DW, Eliasziw M, et al. , for the North American Symptomatic Carotid Endarterectomy Trial Collaborators. Benefit of carotid endarterectomy in patients with symptomatic moderate or severe stenosis. N Engl J Med 1998;339: 1415–1425.
- Mohr JP, Caplan LR, Melski JW, et al. The Harvard Cooperative Stroke Registry: a prospective registry. Neurology 1978;28: 754–762.
- National Institute of Neurological Disorders and Stroke rt-PA Stroke Study Group. Tissue plasminogen activator for acute ischemic stroke. N Engl J Med 1995; 333:1581–1587.

Author(s): Yousef Mohammad, MD, MSc

Cerebrovascular Disease, Transient Ischemic Attack

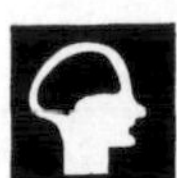

Basics

DESCRIPTION

Transient ischemic attack (TIA) is defined as a transient focal, and sometimes multifocal, brain ischemia from disrupted blood supply that completely resolves within 24 hours.

EPIDEMIOLOGY

Incidence/Prevalence

The annual incidence of TIA in the United States is estimated to vary from 1 in 200,000 to 1 in 500,000. However, the accurate incidence is probably much higher because many of these attacks are not reported by the patients.

Age

It is more common in the elderly, as is stroke.

Sex

It is more common in males, as is stroke.

Race

It is probably more common in African Americans and Hispanics, given the increased incidence of stroke in these populations.

ETIOLOGY

It is the same as ischemic stroke. This includes the following:

- Hypercoagulable state: deficiencies in protein C, S, or antithrombin III, factor V mutation, factor II mutation, antiphospholipid antibody syndrome, sickle cell anemia, mucin-secreting carcinomas.
- Cardiac emboli: conditions that predispose to the formation of cardiac emboli include atrial fibrillation, mitral valve stenosis, sick sinus syndrome, prosthetic heart valve, infective endocarditis, marantic endocarditis, congestive heart failure, dilated cardiomyopathy, myxomas, intraatrial septal defect, patent foramen ovale, and dilated atria.
- Large artery disease: the extracranial internal carotid, intracranial internal carotid, extracranial vertebral, intracranial vertebral, middle cerebral basilar, anterior cerebral, and posterior cerebral are all large arteries in the cerebrovascular circulation. Disease in these vessels can lead to TIA. The most common is atherosclerosis. Other diseases include dissection, vasculitis, moyamoya, and fibromuscular dysplasia.
- Small vessel disease: an uncommon cause of TIA.

Genetics

Mitochondrial encephalopathy, lactic acidosis, and stroke-like episodes (MELAS), cerebral autosomal-dominant arteriopathy with subcortical infarcts and leukoencephalopathy (CADASIL), factor II, and factor V mutations are all genetic conditions that can present with TIA.

RISK FACTORS

Risk factors include hypertension, diabetes mellitus, hyperlipidemia, tobacco, sedentary life, obesity, family history of stroke, and history of coronary or peripheral vascular disease.

PREGNANCY

It is likely that there is an increased incidence of TIA in pregnancy, as there is an increased incidence of ischemic stroke in pregnancy.

ASSOCIATED CONDITIONS

Ischemic stroke, coronary artery disease, and peripheral artery disease.

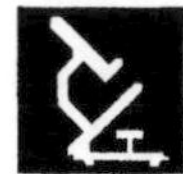

Diagnosis

DIFFERENTIAL DIAGNOSIS

- Ischemic stroke
- Migraine aura
- Multiple sclerosis
- Seizures (Todd's paralysis)
- Labyrinthine disorders
- Syncope
- Metabolic disorders
- Intracerebral hemorrhage
- Subdural hematoma
- Somatization disorders

SIGNS AND SYMPTOMS

By definition a TIA must resolve within 24 hours; otherwise it is considered a stroke. However, it usually resolves within 1 hour. As in ischemic stroke, the symptoms are typically sudden and abrupt. The clinical features depend on the brain area affected. Common symptoms include:

- Hemiparesis
- Hemisensory loss
- Visual field defects
- Ataxia and incoordination
- Aphasia
- Dysarthria
- Dysphagia
- Diplopia
- Vertigo

LABORATORY PROCEDURES

- All patients with TIA should have blood drawn for fasting lipid profile, RPR, BUN, creatinine, CBC and platelets, PT, PTT, and INR.
- Hypercoagulable profile, including protein C, protein S, antithrombin III, factor V mutation, factor II mutation, lupus anticoagulant, antiphospholipid antibodies, and homocysteine should be requested in young patients.
- Serial blood cultures should be done when infective endocarditis is suspected.

IMAGING STUDIES

- Chest x-ray to evaluate for cardiomegaly.
- CT scan must be performed in all patients with suspected TIA because it is very sensitive in detecting intracerebral hemorrhage or subdural hematoma, which can mimic TIA. Also, it can be performed quickly and is cheap and readily available.
- MRI of brain is more sensitive than CT scan in detecting small or early infarction. The infarction is sometimes shown despite the resolution of the symptoms within 24 hours, a fact that urged the stroke community to work on redefining TIA, which is currently in process.
- MR angiography is a noninvasive test, and is accurate for assessing the major extracranial and intracranial arteries, though it may overestimate the degree of stenosis.
- Transthoracic echocardiogram (TTE) is indicated in most patients with TIA. If the TTE is negative and a cardiac source is still suspected, the transesophageal echocardiogram (TEE) must be performed. TEE is also indicated in almost all young patients.
- TEE is more accurate than TTE in showing atrial and ventricular thrombi, vegetations, and left atrial enlargement, detecting shunts, and evaluating the proximal aorta.
- Angiography is the gold standard for an accurate assessment of both the extra- and intracranial vasculature. However, it is an invasive procedure and should be reserved for patients in whom noninvasive testing has not definitely shown the source of TIA, and to assess precisely the degree of stenosis.
- Ultrasound is a safe, portable, and less expensive. It includes transcranial Doppler to look for intracranial disease and carotid duplex to assess for extracranial carotid disease.

SPECIAL TESTS

ECG and cardiac monitoring to evaluate for arrhythmias.

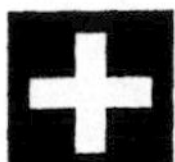

Management

GENERAL MEASURES

Management of coexisting medical illnesses and secondary stroke prevention.

SURGICAL MEASURES

- Carotid endarterectomy (CEA) is indicated for significant (>50%) symptomatic carotid artery stenosis. For those patients who are considered high risk for surgery, carotid angioplasty with stent placement is performed in a few medical centers. Intracranial large artery (basilar, vertebral, middle cerebral, and internal carotid) angioplasty with or without stent placement is occasionally performed in a few academic centers for those patients who fail maximal medical therapy.
- Some cardiac lesions require surgical or radiologic interventions.

SYMPTOMATIC TREATMENT

This includes prophylaxis for deep vein thrombosis and judicious control of blood pressure with avoidance of excessive reduction in the acute setting and adequate control in the long run.

ADJUNCTIVE TREATMENT

None needed since symptoms resolve completely within 24 hours.

ADMISSION/DISCHARGE CRITERIA

In general any patient presenting with TIA, within 1 week from the onset of symptoms should be admitted to the hospital for the evaluation of etiology and appropriate stroke prevention measures.

Medications

DRUG(S) OF CHOICE

- Antiplatelet agents: indicated for stroke prevention in small vessel disease, intracranial large artery disease, mild (<50%) extracranial carotid artery disease, extracranial vertebral artery disease, aortic arch disease without mobile plaque, irregular nonstenotic valve surfaces, and in patients who are not coumadin candidates.
  —Aspirin: 50–325 mg qd
  —Plavix: 75 mg qd
  —Aggrenox: combination aspirin 25 mg/ extended release dipyridamole 200 mg one tablet bid
- Anticoagulants
  —Warfarin (Coumadin): indicated in hypercoagulable states, cardiac sources like atrial fibrillation, intracardiac thrombi, and intracranial large artery stenosis.

Contraindications

- Aspirin/Aggrenox: mainly known allergic reaction to salicylic acid, active systemic bleeding, or active gastric ulcer.
- Clopidogrel: mainly active systemic bleeding.
- Warfarin: mainly active bleeding, bleeding tendency, noncompliance, and gait difficulty with increased falling risk.

Precautions

- Clopidogrel: monitor for any TTP symptoms at the beginning of treatment.
- Warfarin: watch for compliance, bleeding events, and falling events.

ALTERNATIVE DRUGS

None

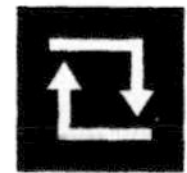

Follow-Up

PATIENT MONITORING

- Frequent follow-up visits are important to assess patients for recurrent ischemic events, compliance with treatment and recommendations, and adverse reactions from the treatment medications.
- Close monitoring of INR is crucial for the patients maintained on coumadin.

EXPECTED COURSE AND PROGNOSIS

- TIA is a precursor for a stroke or vascular death. The risk of stroke or death in untreated patients, after a TIA, is about 10% a year. The risk of stroke is highest within the first few weeks and month after the TIA.
- Appropriate secondary preventive measures significantly decrease the risk of stroke.

PATIENT EDUCATION

American Stroke Association, National Center, 7272 Greenville Avenue, Dallas TX, 75231, 1-888-478-7653, *www.strokeassociation.org.*

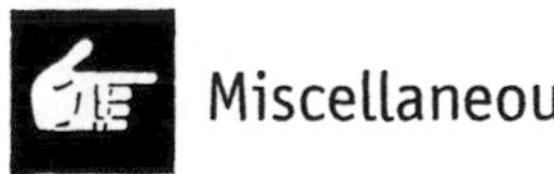

SYNONYMS

None

ICD-9-CM: 435.9 Transcerebral ischemia NOS

SEE ALSO: CEREBROVASCULAR DISEASE, ISCHEMIC INFARCT

REFERENCES

- Adams HP, Kassell NF, Mazuz H. The patient with transient ischemic attacks—is this the time for a new therapeutic approach? Stroke 1984;15:371–375.
- Bernstein RA, Alberts MJ. Transient ischemic attack—proposed new definition. N Engl J Med 2003;348(16):1607–1609.
- Johnston SC. Transient ischemic attack. N Engl J Med 2002;347(21):1687–1692.
- Rothwell PM. Incidence, risk factors and prognosis of stroke and TIA: the need for high quality, large scale epidemiological studies and meta-analysis. Cerebrovascular Dis 2003;16(suppl 3):2–10.
- Toole JF, Yuson CP, Janeway R, et al. Transient ischemic attacks: a prospective study of 225 patients. Neurology 1978; 28:746–753.
- Werdelin L, Juhler M. The course of transient ischemic attacks. Neurology 1988;38:677–680.

Author(s): Yousef Mohammad, MD, MSc; Umesh Sharma, MD

Cerebrovascular Disease, Venous Thrombosis

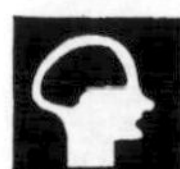

Basics

DESCRIPTION

Thrombosis of the cerebral veins and sinuses is an uncommon but important cause of stroke whose diagnosis is often missed or delayed.

EPIDEMIOLOGY

Incidence/Prevalence

Unknown in the general population. The incidence in the peripartum period in India is 4.5 cases per 1,000 obstetric admissions compared to less than 1 in 3,000 in Western countries.

Age

Can occur in any age group.

Sex

It is more common in females.

ETIOLOGY

- Infections of the head and neck
- Pregnancy and puerperium
- Severe dehydration
- Hypercoagulable state
- Disseminated intravascular coagulation
- Sickle cell disease
- Polycythemia rubra vera
- Paroxysmal nocturnal hemoglobinuria
- Oral contraceptive pills
- L-asparaginase
- Nephrotic syndrome
- Liver disease
- Head trauma
- Intracranial operations
- Systemic lupus erythematosus
- Behçet's disease
- Sarcoidosis
- Wegner's granulomatosis
- Cancer
- Idiopathic

PREGNANCY

Pregnancy and the peripartum period are times of significantly higher risk for the development of cerebral venous thrombosis (CVT). Almost 50% of adult cases occur in this group.

ASSOCIATED CONDITIONS

Venous thrombosis of the pelvic and lower extremities veins.

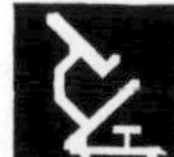

Diagnosis

DIFFERENTIAL DIAGNOSIS

Pseudotumor cerebri
Arterial stroke
Hemorrhagic stroke
Migraine
Preeclampsia
Eclampsia
Encephalitis
Meningitis

SIGNS AND SYMPTOMS

CVT is associated with a wide range of signs and symptoms, depending on the specific cerebral venous structures involved. Common symptoms include:

- Headache
- Nausea
- Vomiting
- Focal neurologic deficit (weakness, sensory loss, visual changes, and aphasia)
- Focal or generalized seizures
- Altered conscious level
- Coma
- Papilledema
- Chemosis*
- Proptosis*
- Painful ophthalmoplegia*

LABORATORY PROCEDURES

All patients should have blood tests for CBC and platelet count, PT, PTT, and INR, renal and liver panels, hypercoagulable profile (including protein C, protein S, antithrombin III, factor V Leiden mutation, factor II, lupus anticoagulant, antiphospholipid antibodies and homocysteine), sedimentation rate, rheumatoid factor, and antinuclear antibodies.
Blood cultures if infection is suspected.

IMAGING STUDIES

- CT scan of the brain might show hemorrhagic or ischemic changes. In some of the patients, contrast study demonstrates the empty delta sign, which is consistent with sagittal sinus thrombosis.
- MR imaging and MR venogram (MRV) help to define the anatomy of the cerebral venous system and have a better sensitivity to detect CVT.
- Conventional cerebral angiography is the gold standard to fully evaluate the venous anatomy and the clot burden.

SPECIAL TESTS

Lumbar puncture should be performed if meningitis is a consideration but should be deferred if the patient has mass effect on brain CT or MRI.
EEG should be obtained in patients with recurrent seizures or in coma.

*Seen in cavernous sinus thrombosis.

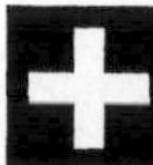

Management

GENERAL MEASURES

General measures include acute supportive care and management of coexisting illnesses and underlying cause if established.

SURGICAL MEASURES

N/A

SYMPTOMATIC TREATMENT

Includes aggressive treatment of seizures and metabolic derangements, adequate hydration and nutrition, aspiration precautions, DVT prophylaxis, elevation of the head of the bed by 15 to 30 degrees; other measures to reduce intracranial pressure as dictated by the clinical situation. Use of antibiotics if infection is suspected. Discontinuation of oral contraceptive pills.

ADJUNCTIVE TREATMENT

Physical, occupational, speech, and cognitive therapy may be needed. Prenatal or postpartum care when appropriate for women who present with this condition.

ADMISSION/DISCHARGE CRITERIA

Any patient who presents with CVT should be admitted for treatment, evaluation, and management of the cause; early initiation of physical, occupational, and speech therapy; evaluation of eligibility for inpatient rehabilitation; assistance with appropriate placement; and patient and caregiver education.

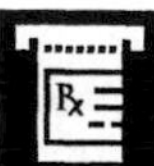

Medications

DRUG(S) OF CHOICE

- Anticoagulants: though there was a history of controversy regarding its role, there is a strong evidence that anticoagulation can prevent further thrombus formation and larger venous infarction. Most authors recommend its use in the absence of radiologic evidence of significant hemorrhage. It should be used with extreme caution in patients with evidence of intracerebral hemorrhage because of the risk of further intracerebral bleeding. After the use of heparin in the acute stage, oral anticoagulation with Coumadin is used for 3 to 6 months.
  Patients with an underlying hypercoagulable state might require prolonged period of coumadin intake.
- Thrombolytics: Limited data available. Local infusion of thrombolytics into the dural sinus thrombosis is reported to be effective and safe in small series. This should be reserved for rapidly declining patients despite anticoagulation.

Contraindications

Anticoagulants: significant intracerebral hemorrhage or significant active systemic bleeding.

Precautions

Warfarin: watch for compliance, bleeding events, and falling events.

ALTERNATIVE DRUGS

N/A

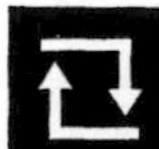

Follow-Up

PATIENT MONITORING

Frequent follow-up visits are important to assess patients for recurrence, control of the underlying etiology, compliance with treatment and recommendations, and adverse reactions from the medications.
Close monitoring of the INR is crucial for the patients who are maintained on warfarin.

EXPECTED COURSE AND PROGNOSIS

Mortality from CVT is estimated to be 6% to 30%. Poor outcome is expected in patients with involvement of the deep cerebral veins, coma, large intracerebral hemorrhage, and if sepsis is the underlying cause.

PATIENT EDUCATION

American Stroke Association, National Center, 7272 Greenville Avenue, Dallas TX, 75231, 1-888-478-7653, *www.strokeassociation.org.*

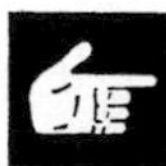

Miscellaneous

SYNONYMS

Venous thrombosis of the brain
Cerebral vein thrombosis

ICD-9-CM: 453.9 Venous thrombosis NOS

SEE ALSO: N/A

REFERENCES

- Ameri A, Bousser M-G. Cerebral venous thrombosis. Neurol Clin 1992;10:87–111.
- Benamer HT, Bone I. Cerebral venous thrombosis; anticoagulants or thrombolytic therapy? J Neurol Neurosurg Psychiatry 2000;69:427–430.
- Bousser M-G. Cerebral venous thrombosis: diagnosis and management. J Neurol 2000;247:252–258.
- Bousser MG. Cerebral venous thrombosis: nothing, heparin or local thrombolysis? Stroke 1999;30:481–483.
- Cantu C, Barinagarrementeria F. Cerebral venous thrombosis associated with pregnancy and puerperium. Stroke 1993;24:1880–1884.
- De Braijn SF. et al. CVST study group. Randomized placebo controlled trial of anticoagulant treatment with low molecular weight heparin for cerebral sinus thrombosis. Stroke 1999;30:484–488.
- Einhaupl K, Villringer A, Meister W, et al. Heparin treatment in sinus venous thrombosis. Lancet 1991;338:597–600.
- Lewis MB. Cerebral venous thrombosis: nothing, heparin or local thrombolysis? Stroke 1999;30:1729.

Author(s): Yousef Mohammad, MD, MSc; Bakri Elsheikh, MBBS, MRCP (UK)

Cerebrovascular Disease, Young Patient Evaluation for Ischemic Stroke

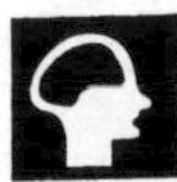

Basics

DESCRIPTION

The evaluation of suspected cerebrovascular disease in the young patient should be undertaken in patients between the ages of 15 and 44 who present with the clinical presentation of ischemic stroke. While this age range is somewhat arbitrary, the consideration of ischemic stroke in the young patient suggests a specific diagnostic strategy, which includes the evaluation of those causes of stroke seen in the older population as well as additional etiologies found in young persons.

EPIDEMIOLOGY

Incidence/Prevalence

The incidence is 3 to 9 per 100,000 in the 15- to 44-year-old age group.

Race

Higher incidence of up to 20 per 100,000 has been reported in the African-American population.

Sex

Overall, males and females are affected equally; however, females have a higher incidence during the childbearing years. The relative risk for ischemic stroke is 0.7 during pregnancy and increases to 9.7 for the postpartum period.

ETIOLOGY

While some causes of ischemic stroke in the young are similar to causes of stroke in the elderly, the list of potential etiologies is longer and more consideration needs to be given to unusual causes of stroke. The specific etiology of stroke in the young remains unclear (cryptogenic) in up to 40% of patients even after extensive evaluation.

- Large artery atherosclerosis
  - —Accelerated atherosclerosis may be associated with hyperlipidemia, elevated serum lipoprotein (a), or homocysteine levels
- Nonatherosclerotic large artery disease
  - —Arterial dissection
  - —Fibromuscular dysplasia
  - —Angiitis associated with underlying immune disease: polyarteritis nodosa, Wegener's granulomatosis, systemic lupus erythematosus, giant cell arteritis, Takayasu's disease, or primary angiitis of the central nervous system
  - —Moyamoya disease
  - —Other infectious/immune vasculopathies: bacterial meningitis, syphilis, herpes zoster, fungal, tuberculosis, cysticercosis, sarcoid
- Small vessel atherosclerosis
- Cardioembolism
  - —Bacterial endocarditis
  - —Atrial fibrillation
  - —Intracardiac shunt (patent foramen ovale) with associated deep venous thrombosis
  - —Left atrial thrombus or spontaneous echo contrast, intraatrial septal aneurysm
  - —Acute myocardial infarction
  - —Prosthetic valve
  - —Mitral stenosis
- Hypercoaguable states
  - —Antiphospholipid antibody syndrome
  - —Sickle cell disease
  - —Thrombotic thrombocytopenic purpura
  - —Disseminated intravascular coagulation
  - —Polycythemia vera, essential thrombocytosis, and other hyperviscosity syndromes
  - —Protein C deficiency, protein S deficiency, antithrombin III deficiency
  - —Factor V mutation resulting in resistance to activated protein C
  - —Prothrombin 20210 G→A mutation
  - —Dysfibrinogenemia and disorders of fibrinolysis
- Other causes
  - —Systemic infection/inflammation: cytomegalovirus, chlamydia, herpes simplex virus
  - -Substance abuse: cocaine, amphetamines
  - —Migraine headache
  - —Pregnancy- and puerperium-related causes
  - —Oral contraception

Genetics

Multiple genetic factors increase the risk of ischemic stroke, including those associated with hyperlipidemia, early-onset diabetes, and severe hypertension. Several hereditary disorders are specifically related to stroke in the young: sickle cell disease; neurofibromatosis (moyamoya-like syndrome); cerebral autosomal-dominant arteriopathy with subcortical infarcts and leukoencephalopathy (CADASIL); mitochondrial encephalopathy, lactic acidosis and stroke-like episodes (MELAS); epidermal nevus syndrome; Sneddon's syndrome.

RISK FACTORS

- Atherosclerotic: family history of early cerebrovascular or cardiovascular disease, cigarette smoking, hypertension, hyperlipidemia, diabetes mellitus, elevated serum homocysteine levels, radiation therapy to neck
- Dissection: trauma, chiropractic manipulation
- Cardiogenic: intravenous drug use, valve replacement
- Hematologic: inherited or acquired hypercoaguable state, deep venous thrombosis, pregnancy

PREGNANCY

Pregnancy and the puerperium are associated with increased risk of stroke and suggest a specific differential diagnosis, depending on the time of presentation.

- Third trimester: cardiogenic embolus, venous infarction secondary to cerebral venous occlusive disease (CVOD), eclampsia
- Labor/delivery: amniotic, air or fat embolus.
- Postpartum: same as labor/delivery, also cardiogenic embolus, CVOD, postpartum eclampsia, trophoblastic disease, or arterial occlusions.

ASSOCIATED CONDITIONS

As above.

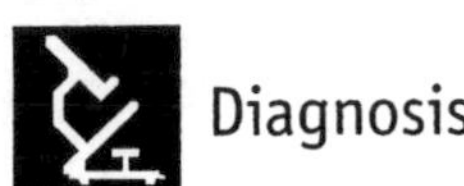

Diagnosis

DIFFERENTIAL DIAGNOSIS

As with ischemic stroke in the general population, may include intracerebral hemorrhage, subarachnoid hemorrhage, generalized/focal seizure with Todd's phenomenon, complicated migraine, conversion disorder.

SIGNS AND SYMPTOMS

Identical in clinical presentation to ischemic stroke in the general population, with focal neurologic signs and symptoms relating to the affected anatomy.

LABORATORY PROCEDURES

- Initial blood work: CBC with platelets, chemistry profile, sedimentation rate, fasting glucose, prothrombin time, partial thromboplastin time, lipid profile, fluorescent treponemal antibody, anticardiolipin antibodies, toxicology screen, pregnancy screen, serum homocysteine, and lipoprotein (a) levels. If infection is suspected, blood cultures and CSF analysis are warranted. African-American patients should have hemoglobin electrophoresis.
- Additional blood work: if etiology is elusive, evaluation should be expanded to include antithrombin III, protein C antigen and activity, protein S antigen and activity, D-dimer, fibrin split products, fibrinogen, other antiphospholipid antibodies, factor V Leiden mutation, prothrombin 20210 G→A mutation, Russell viper venom time, and HIV screen.

IMAGING STUDIES

- Brain imaging: noncontrasted CT is performed initially to rule out an acute hemorrhage. Otherwise, MRI with diffusion-weighted imaging is preferable.
- Vascular imaging: initial investigation should include noninvasive imaging with carotid and/or transcranial Doppler ultrasound. Magnetic resonance angiography can also be used. If the clinical suspicion of intracranial disease is high, or initial evaluation is inconclusive, cerebral angiography is warranted. Magnetic resonance venography should be used when CVOD is suspected.

SPECIAL TESTS

- Electrocardiogram
- Transesophageal echocardiogram (TEE) if infection is suspected or routine evaluation does not provide an etiology. Transesophageal with bubble contrast rather than transthoracic echocardiogram is preferred to increase the sensitivity and specificity for detecting an atrial septal defect, septal aneurysm, vegetation, or left atrial "smoke."

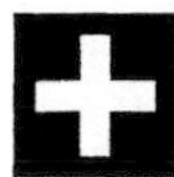

Management

GENERAL MEASURES

General management is identical to that of the general ischemic stroke patient.

SURGICAL MEASURES

Identical to those for the general ischemic stroke patient, e.g., carotid endarterectomy when appropriate.

SYMPTOMATIC TREATMENT

- Speech therapy
- Physical therapy

ADJUNCTIVE TREATMENT

N/A

ADMISSION/DISCHARGE CRITERIA

Patients should be admitted for evaluation and treatment using the same criteria for the general ischemic stroke patient.

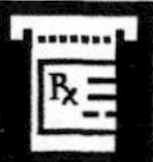

Medications

DRUG(S) OF CHOICE

Overall, medications and indications/ contraindications for the young stroke patient are identical to those used for the general stroke patient. However, many of the conditions associated with stroke in the young patient are reported to be more effectively treated with long-term anticoagulation with warfarin. These conditions include arterial dissection, hereditary and acquired hypercoaguable disorders, patent foramen ovale, and other atrial abnormalities discovered on TEE. Levels of evidence and resulting recommendations for anticoagulation for these conditions varies according to the condition.

ALTERNATIVE DRUGS

N/A

Follow-Up

PATIENT MONITORING

Acute ischemic stroke patients require frequent monitoring of vital signs and neurologic status and may require admission to an intensive care setting.

EXPECTED COURSE AND PROGNOSIS

Course and prognosis, including recurrence rates, vary widely depending on the underlying etiology of the stroke.

PATIENT EDUCATION

The importance of aggressive management of the modifiable stroke risk factors should be stressed, as well as the need for medical compliance. Patients and their families should begin the self-education process by contacting the American Stroke Association at 1-888-4STROKE or visiting *www.strokeassociation.org.*

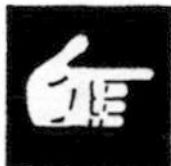

Miscellaneous

SYNONYMS

Stroke in the young
Young stroke

ICD-9-CM: 433.0 Occlusion and stenosis of precerebral arteries (with or without cerebral infarction); 434.0 Occlusion of cerebral arteries (with or without cerebral infarction); 435.0 Transient cerebral ischemia; 436.0–437.9 Other and ill-defined cerebrovascular disease; 674.0 Cerebrovascular disorders occurring during pregnancy, childbirth, or the puerperium; 671.5 Cerebral venous thrombosis as a complication in pregnancy and the puerperium

SEE ALSO: THE OTHER CEREBROVASCULAR DISEASE TOPICS

REFERENCES

- Bogousslavsky J, Pierre P. Ischemic stroke in patients under age 45. Neurol Clin 1992;10:113–124.
- Calabrese LH, Furlan AJ, Gragg LA, et al. Primary angiitis of the central nervous system: Diagnostic criteria and clinical approach. Cleve Clin J Med 1992;59: 293–306.
- Chimowitz MI. Ischemic stroke in the young. In: Welch KMA, Caplan LR, Reis DJ, et al., eds. Primer on cerebrovascular diseases. San Diego: Academic Press, 1997:330–332.
- DeGraba TJ, Penix L. Genetics of ischemic stroke. Curr Opin Neurol 1995;8:24–29.
- Kittner SJ, Stern BJ, Wozniak M, et al. Cerebral infarction in young adults: the Baltimore-Washington Cooperative Young Stroke Study. Neurology 1998;50:890–894.
- Qureshi AI, Safdar K, Patel M, et al. Stroke in young black patients. Risk factors, subtypes, and prognosis. Stroke 1995;26:1985–1988.
- Williams LS, Garg BP, Cohen M, et al. Subtypes of ischemic stroke in children and young adults. Neurology 1997;49:1541–1545.

Author(s): Susan L. Hickenbottom, MD; Jeffrey S. Kutcher, MD

Cervical Stenosis/Spondylosis/Spondylotic Myelopathy

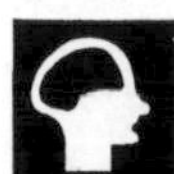

Basics

DESCRIPTION

Cervical spondylosis refers to intervertebral disc degeneration, disc space narrowing, and spur formation associated with age-related changes of the cervical spine. Cervical stenosis is the narrowing of the cervical spinal canal. Cervical spondylotic myelopathy (CSM) refers to the clinical presentation resulting from the degenerative processes leading to neural canal compromise and subsequent myelopathy. CSM is the most common cause of spinal cord dysfunction in adults over the age of 55.

EPIDEMIOLOGY

Incidence/Prevalence

Degenerative changes of cervical spine have been observed in up to 95% of asymptomatic individuals over 65 years old. Up to 20% of individuals with evidence of spondylosis are thought to progress to myelopathy.

Race

There is no known racial or ethnic predilection.

Age

The disease process is associated with natural aging, and individuals over 65 years old have a much higher rate of spondylosis, and therefore a higher rate of CSM.

Sex

Males are more commonly affected. Some Scandinavian studies estimate that males may be affected twice as often as females. Most investigators believe there is at least a 1.5:1 male to female ratio.

ETIOLOGY

The pathophysiologic hallmark is cord dysfunction brought on by a combination of mechanical compression and degenerative instability. With aging, the intervertebral disc degenerates and collapses, leading to spur formation. This process tends to begin at C5-6 and C6-7. There is a relative decrease in spinal motion at these levels with a concomitant increase in spinal motion at C3-4 and C4-5. At these higher levels, the resultant degeneration and motion leads to instability with antero- or retrolisthesis (subluxation of vertebral bodies out of the normal cervical alignment). Therefore, at C5-6 and C6-7 the cord tends to be compressed from spur formation, and at C3-4 and C4-5 from listhesis. Anterior cord compression from degenerated discs and spurs is often accompanied by posterior compromise from ligamentum flavum hypertrophy. In addition to the static compressive forces, the cord is subject to further injury from repetitive dynamic injury during normal neck movements. These static and dynamic compressive forces on the cord lead to spinal cord injury and the clinical myelopathic syndrome.

Genetics

The disease is sporadic with no known genetic factors involved.

RISK FACTORS

Male sex, older age (>55), repetitive neck trauma, congenitally narrow cervical canal (less than 12-mm diameter).

PREGNANCY

There is no additional risk with pregnancy.

Diagnosis

DIFFERENTIAL DIAGNOSIS

Alternative diagnoses should be considered in patients without risk factors (young, female, no history or cervical stenosis) or if there is findings on the exam that are inconsistent with CSM (e.g., cranial nerve palsy). However, many of the following present with similar clinical findings:

- Tumor
- Amyotrophic lateral sclerosis
- Syringomyelia
- Multiple sclerosis
- Transverse myelitis
- Herniated disc
- Ossified posterior longitudinal ligament
- Spinal arteriovenous malformation
- Subacute combined degeneration
- Neurosyphilis
- Rheumatoid arthritis with subluxation

SIGNS AND SYMPTOMS

- Initial symptoms may be subtle. Loss of hand dexterity, painless weakness of the upper extremities, and ambulatory difficulty may be present. There is often a history of progressive difficulty with the hands. Pain may or may not be a significant complaint. If pain is present, it is usually neck pain with or without some radicular component down the arm. Loss of fine motor control in the hands, such as difficulty with writing, buttoning, or painting, is a usual complaint. Walking difficulty is usually present but may initially be subtle.
- The exam usually shows bilateral (or initially unilateral) weakness of the hands and arms with varying degrees of lower extremity weakness. Long tract signs resembling an anterior cord syndrome may be present. Initially the strength may not be affected, but spastic quadriparesis is seen as patients experience clinical progression. Disturbances of bowel and bladder are rarely caused by CSM, although these symptoms are common in the elderly. Hyperreflexia in all four extremities and pathologic reflexes such as bilateral Hoffmann's, clonus, and even Babinski's may be present.
- Paresthesias in the fingertips signaling posterior column dysfunction are less common than anterior cord signs. Rarely patients may present with Brown-Séquard syndrome with the development of a crossed motor and sensory deficits presumably arising from unilateral cord compression. Some patients also complain of Lhermitte's phenomenon with electric shocks going down the spine or into the arms. This may be most apparent in certain neck positions, especially extension, which decreases the width of the spinal canal.
- Of the five clinical syndromes characterized by Crandall (1966), the most common are brachialgia cord syndrome (upper extremity radiculopathy from nerve root compression combined with myelopathy) and motor system syndrome (corticospinal tract compromise by anterior compressive pathology producing spastic quadriparesis with minimal sensory complaints).

LABORATORY PROCEDURES

No specific laboratory tests have been identified.

IMAGING STUDIES

MRI is the most useful diagnostic tool in evaluating cord compression, canal diameter, and most of the other causes of myelopathy. Plain x-ray films may demonstrate disc degeneration, loss of vertebral height, subluxation, and loss of lordotic curvature. CT with myelography is recommended in cases where MRI is contraindicated or unavailable.

SPECIAL TESTS

Electrophysiologic studies may be useful in confirming dysfunction at the root or cord level. A majority of patients with CSM have abnormal findings on EMG and nerve conduction velocity (NCV) testing. These studies also offer a useful method to follow the progression of CSM in the absence of obvious changes on MRI or the neurologic examination.

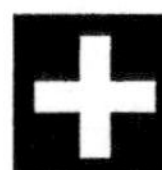

Management

GENERAL MEASURES

- Immobilization with a rigid neck brace: there is no well-recognized nonsurgical therapy for CSM other than this.
- Cervical traction under the supervision of a physician and physical therapist for severe pain (radiculopathy). This may have associated risks in patients with narrow cervical canal, and should be used with caution in patients with myelopathy.
- Ultrasound with electronic stimulation for severe neck/shoulder pain.

- Discriminate use of antiinflammatory medication and analgesics.
- Avoidance of excessive neck motion and trauma

SURGICAL MEASURES

- Because patients with CSM may deteriorate, surgery to alleviate the compression and instability has been the primary treatment of this condition. Laminectomy alone has been used extensively and is excellent at spinal cord decompression, but it does not address the dynamic forces in CSM. Its use is limited to lordotic spines, and there is associated risk of postoperative instability and late deterioration.
- Anterior discectomies and corpectomies combined with fusion and fixation can be performed on kyphotic spines and address the compressive and dynamic forces leading to CSM. However, they can be associated with high morbidity and complications, especially when deployed over a long segment (three or more vertebral levels). Laminoplasty had been performed in different fashions to decompress the cord and minimize postoperative instability. Recent studies of laminectomy with fusion appear to have promising results and low morbidity in straight or lordotic cervical spines. A lordotic spine can be treated with a decompressive laminectomy alone in a patient with advanced age (>75 years).

SYMPTOMATIC TREATMENT

Refer to general measures.

ADJUNCTIVE TREATMENT

Body mechanics emphasizing optimal posture (easier with rigid collar) with avoidance of neck twisting and excessive flexion and extension are recommended. Rest, isometric exercise, and application of ice or heat for symptomatic relief can be prescribed.

ADMISSION/DISCHARGE CRITERIA

Patients with new neurologic deficit, progressive myelopathy, new gait or bowel/ bladder disturbance, or uncontrollable pain should be admitted for serial evaluations. Significant neck trauma in a patient with known CSM also warrants an evaluation.

Medications

DRUG(S) OF CHOICE

- NSAIDs: must be used with caution in patients over 65 years of age and in patients with history of gastrointestinal problems or renal insufficiency.
- Oral steroids: very short course (a few days) only, and must consider the additional risk imposed by steroid use in patients with diabetes mellitus, immunocompromised patients, or those with history of infection. This seems to be effective only in the treatment of radiculopathic pain. Steroids may exacerbate NSAIDs' gastrointestinal side effects and should not be routinely used in conjunction with other antiinflammatory medications.
- Muscle relaxants: no benefit seen for use longer than 3 weeks.

ALTERNATIVE DRUGS

N/A

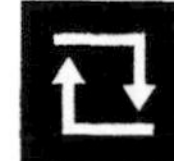

Follow-Up

PATIENT MONITORING

- Frequent evaluation of patients with overt myelopathy is recommended due to probability of deterioration. All patients should undergo complete radiologic evaluation. In the most severe cases, MRI will reveal evidence of cord injury. After serial examinations depicting a stable neurologic status, the frequency of clinical monitoring may be gradually decreased. All patients with CSM should undergo a neurosurgical evaluation for consideration of surgical intervention.
- Patients who opt for nonsurgical therapy should be followed by periodic MRIs to evaluate the extent of spinal cord deformation and spinal alignment. Patients with clear CSM who do not undergo surgery should wear a cervical collar at all times to minimize further injury associated with normal motion.

EXPECTED COURSE AND PROGNOSIS

The natural history of CSM is difficult to elucidate, because early investigations combined patients with cervical stenosis, cervical spondylosis, and CSM. Up to 75% of patients with myelopathy show episodic deterioration; 20% are thought to show steady deterioration. Spontaneous, rapid progression is seen in only 5% of patients. Useful indicators of poor prognosis are duration of symptoms, severity of myelopathy, presence of high-intensity cord lesion on MRI, and multilevel compression. These patients should be strongly considered for surgery.

PATIENT EDUCATION

The Congress of Neurological Surgeons has ample educational material on this subject on the Web at Neurosurgery-On-Call (*www.neurosurgery.org*). The Cervical Spine Research Society provides useful educational material as well as in depth research on the pathophysiology and management of CSM (*www.csrs.org*).

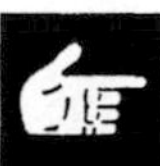

Miscellaneous

SYNONYMS

Refer to basic descriptions.

ICD-9-CM: Stenosis: 724.00 Spinal—unspecified region; 723.0 Cervical. Disc: 722.71 Cervical—with myelopathy; 722.70 Displacement—with myelopathy (unspecified site); 722.0 Cervical—without myelopathy

SEE ALSO: N/A

REFERENCES

- Benner BG. Etiology, pathogenesis, and natural history of discogenic neck pain, radiculopathy, and myelopathy. In: Clark CR, ed. The cervical spine, The Cervical Spine Research Society Editorial Committee, 3rd ed. Philadelphia: Lippincott-Raven, 1998:735–740.
- Bernhardt M, Hynes RA, Blume HW, et al. Current concepts review, cervical spondylotic myelopathy, J Bone Joint Surg 1993;75A(1):119–128.
- Brouer RS, et al. Cervical disc disease. In: Herkowitz H, et al., eds. Rothman-Simeone: The spine, 4th ed, vol. 1. Philadelphia: WB Saunders, 1999:455–496.
- Crandall PH, Batzdorf U. Cervical spondylotic myelopathy. J Neurosurg 1966;25:57–66.
- Fessler RG, Steck JC, Giovanni MA. Anterior cervical corpectomy for cervical spondylotic myelopathy. Neurosurgery 1998;43(2):257–267.
- Kohno K, Kumon Y, Oka Y, et al. Evaluation of prognostic factors following expansive laminoplasty for cervical spinal stenotic myelopathy. Surg Neurol 1997;48:237–245.
- Kumar VGR, Rea GL, Mervis LJ, et al. Cervical spondylotic myelopathy: functional and radiographic long-term outcome after laminectomy and posterior fusion. Neurosurgery 1999;44(4):771–778.
- Sachs B. Differential diagnosis of neck pain, arm pain, and myelopathy. In: Clark CR, ed. The cervical spine, The Cervical Spine Research Society Editorial Committee, 3rd ed. Philadelphia: Lippincott-Raven, 1998:741–753.
- Sidhu KS, Herkowitz H, et al. Surgical management of cervical disc disease. In: Herkowitz H, et al., eds. Rothman-Simeone: The spine, 4th ed, vol 1. Philadelphia: WB Saunders, 1999:497–564.

Author(s): Amir Vokshoor, MD; Gary L. Rea, MD, PhD

Cervical Trauma

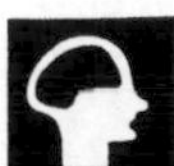

Basics

DESCRIPTION

Cervical trauma constitutes the broad spectrum of soft tissue, bony, and spinal cord injury (SCI) involving the cervical spine. Cervical trauma includes:

- Musculotendinous injuries: strain/sprain
- Bony injuries: flexion/extension/vertical compression/distractive flexion/distractive extension/lateral flexion injuries
- Spinal cord injury without radiologic abnormality (SCIWORA)
- Transient cervical cord injury—central cord syndrome

EPIDEMIOLOGY

Incidence/Prevalence

Incidence of SCI is 10,000 cases per year in the United States. Cervical spine injuries constitute 50% of all SCI, i.e., the incidence of cervical SCI is 5,000 cases per year. Midcervical spine—levels C4 to C6—are the most commonly involved levels.

Age

Young adults (less than age 40) are most commonly affected.

Sex

Males (80%) are more commonly affected than females.

ETIOLOGY

- Motor vehicular injuries are the most common cause.
- Sports injuries, e.g., horseback riding, gymnastics, diving injuries
- Falls
- Penetrating spinal injuries—missile (gunshot) or nonmissile (stabbing) injuries constitute 12% of all traumatic SCIs.
- Industrial and domestic injuries

Genetics

See Risk Factors.

RISK FACTORS

Patients with osteoporosis or ankylosing spondylitis are at high risk of spinal fractures even with minor trauma. Patients with preexisting spinal stenosis (congenital or acquired) are at increased risk of neurologic deficits with minor trauma. Children younger than 10 years of age are at risk of SCIWORA, although recent use of high-field MRI has shown soft tissue injury in many cases previously thought to be SCIWORA.

PREGNANCY

N/A

ASSOCIATED CONDITIONS

Cervical canal stenosis.

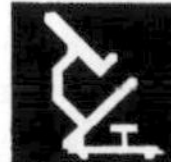

Diagnosis

DIFFERENTIAL DIAGNOSIS

- Polytrauma with head injuries.
- Missed lesions are common: (a) intoxicated or comatose patients; (b) multilevel noncontiguous spinal injuries; (c) upper cervical injuries (e.g., odontoid fractures) where neurologic deficits are frequently absent.

SIGNS AND SYMPTOMS

- Pain: neck pain, radicular arm pain, occipital headache
- Neurologic deficits due to SCI, which can be complete or incomplete
- Complete injury: no motor or sensory function below the level of injury
- Incomplete injury: partial preservation of motor or sensory function below the level of injury. It may present as:
  —Central cord syndrome: upper extremity more than lower extremity weakness, with sacral sparing
  —Anterior cord syndrome: motor paralysis, hypesthesia, loss of pain and temperature, preservation of posterior columns (position, proprioception, and vibration)
  —Brown-Séquard syndrome: ipsilateral loss of motor function and posterior column sensation, contralateral loss of pain and temperature sensation
  —Mixed syndromes: combination of the above syndromes
- Spinal shock may be seen immediately after injury. Total loss of neurologic function (sensory, motor, reflexes) plus hypotension without tachycardia.
- Persisting hypotension and bradycardia after cervical SCI indicate a poor prognosis.
- High cervical spine injuries (at or above C4) often present with respiratory insufficiency due to phrenic nerve involvement.
- Neurologic status is often assessed by Frankel grading or the American Spinal Injury Association (ASIA) scale.
- Frankel grading:
  —Type A—no motor or sensory function below the injury level
  —Type B—sensory preservation without motor function
  —Type C—motor function useless
  —Type D—motor function useful
  —Type E—normal motor and sensory function
- ASIA scale:
  —Total motor score (normal = 100). Strength is graded from 0 to 5 in (a) five upper extremity muscles groups (elbow flexors and extensors, wrist extensors, finger flexors of middle phalanx, finger abductors of the little finger), and (b) five lower extremity muscle groups (hip flexors, knee extensors, ankle dorsiflexors and plantar flexors, long toe extensors) bilaterally.
  —Total sensory score (normal = 224). Sensation (pain + light touch) is graded from 0 to 2 (0 = absent, 1 = impaired, 2 = normal) by testing 28 dermatomes (C2 to S5) bilaterally.
  —The ASIA score more accurately predicts neurologic recovery than Frankel grading.
- Ascending neurologic deficits can occur a few days after injury, likely due to vascular compromise.
- Autonomic dysreflexia may result in headache, sweating, nasal congestion, etc.

LABORATORY PROCEDURES

N/A

IMAGING STUDIES

- Plain radiographs may show an increase in prevertebral soft tissue (normal soft tissue less than 5 mm at C2 to C4, and up to 15 mm at C4 to C7). Dynamic radiographs (flexion and extension) can identify instability due to ligamentous injuries. Open-mouth view and swimmer's views are important to evaluate odontoid fractures and the cervicothoracic junction, respectively.
- CT often detects fractures not evident on plain radiographs or MRI. It can delineate the fracture geometry and the extent of spinal canal encroachment. CT with coronal and sagittal reconstructions is recommended to rule out cervical spine injuries in all unconscious trauma patients. It is useful in the evaluation of penetrating spinal injuries due to gunshot wounds (the metallic bullet fragments prevent evaluation by MRI).
- MRI is the imaging modality of choice for direct SCI and cord compression. It can detect soft tissue and ligamentous injuries as well as traumatic disc lesions. Because it can differentiate cord edema from cord contusion, it can provide prognostic information. Dynamic MRI may demonstrate instability due to ligamentous injuries (e.g., atlantoaxial dislocations).

SPECIAL TESTS

Neurophysiological studies—somatosensory evoked potential recording (SSEP)—can be of prognostic value after SCI.

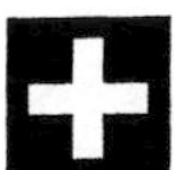

Management

GENERAL MEASURES

As in all trauma cases, assessment of patient's airway, breathing, and circulation are the initial priority. All comatose and polytrauma patients should be considered to have a cervical spine injury until ruled out by radiologic evaluation, and kept in cervical immobilization (back board, hard cervical collar). In-line emergency intubation or tracheostomy should be performed if the patient presents with respiratory distress. Cervical SCI is often complicated by hypotension and bradycardia due to sympathetic insufficiency. Maintenance of normal to high-normal blood pressure is essential to avoid worsening of SCI. Soft tissue injuries can be managed with rest, cervical collar, physical therapy, analgesics, and muscle relaxants.

SURGICAL MEASURES

Surgery is clearly indicated in the presence of spinal cord compression, spinal instability, neurologic deficits (especially incomplete SCI), and certain cases of penetrating SCI. The goals of surgery include (a) correction of deformity and restoration of normal spinal alignment, (b) decompression of spinal cord and nerve roots, and (c) rigid internal fixation for early mobilization and rehabilitation with minimal orthotic supports. Though the timing of surgery is controversial, early surgery may afford greater neurologic recovery. Halo fixation may be an alternative to surgical stabilization, especially in upper cervical spine injuries and high-risk surgical patients, or as an adjunct to surgery where the strength of the internal stabilization is questionable in the early healing period.

SYMPTOMATIC TREATMENT

Pain control by nonsteroidal antiinflammatory drugs, narcotics, and/or muscle relaxants is often required.

ADJUNCTIVE TREATMENT

Cervical traction may reduce dislocations, restore normal alignment, and stabilize the spine. In the presence of respiratory insufficiency, ventilatory support by endotracheal intubation or tracheostomy is mandatory. Patients with permanent respiratory insufficiency can be treated by phrenic nerve pacemaker implantation or domiciliary mechanical ventilatory support. Patients with SCI benefit from comprehensive multidisciplinary rehabilitation. This is best achieved in a SCI unit. Patients with SCI require appropriate bladder, bowel, and skin care. Psychological counseling and support are essential to make necessary mental adjustments to the residual disability.

ADMISSION/DISCHARGE CRITERIA

Admission should be considered in all patients with severe neck pain, neurodeficits, and severe trauma with suspected spinal instability. It is imperative to rule out unequivocally any cervical spine injury before discharge.

Medications

DRUG(S) OF CHOICE

Methylprednisolone has been shown to be of some benefit in improving neurologic outcome when given within 8 hours after SCI. It is given as an intravenous bolus of 30 mg/kg followed by 5.4 mg/kg/h for 23 hours when begun within 3 hours (or for 48 hours when begun 3 to 8 hours) after SCI.

Contraindications

Known history of gastrointestinal bleeding.

Precautions

History of peptic ulcer/immunosuppression.

ALTERNATIVE DRUGS

There is evidence suggesting that antioxidants (e.g., tirilazad mesylate, G_{M1} ganglioside) may be of some benefit in improving neurologic outcome after SCI in human studies.

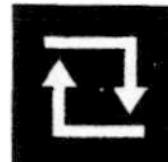

Follow-Up

PATIENT MONITORING

Follow-up neurologic assessment with the ASIA scale provides objective evidence of neurologic improvement. Radiologic assessment is required for evaluation of fusion progression and to rule out delayed spinal deformity, instability, or a posttraumatic syrinx. Delayed neurologic deterioration should prompt an MRI of the cervical spine to rule out a posttraumatic syrinx—a treatable cause of delayed neurologic deterioration (e.g., by syringosubarachnoid or syringoperitoneal shunting).

EXPECTED COURSE AND PROGNOSIS

Neck pain usually resolves, or decreases significantly, in the initial weeks to months postinjury. Patients with complete SCI usually remain complete except for one or two cervical root level recovery. Incomplete cord injuries (especially Brown-Séquard or central cord syndromes) may show significant recovery, especially with surgical decompression of the cord. Patients with penetrating wounds usually experience limited recovery, unless the spinal canal has not been violated (e.g., ricochet gunshot injury).

PATIENT EDUCATION

Patients with SCI and their families require education and psychological support to facilitate rehabilitation and for reintegration into the social environment.

- National Spinal Cord Injury Association
  8701 Georgin Avenue-Suite 500
  Silver Spring, MD 20910
  1-800-962-9629
  www.spinalcord.org
- Paralyzed Veterans of America
  801 18th Street NW
  Washington, DC 20006
  1-800-424-8200
  www.pva.org

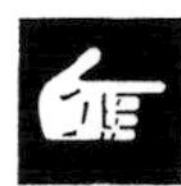

Miscellaneous

SYNONYMS

Cervical spine injuries
Cervical spinal cord injuries

ICD-9-CM: 805.00 Cervical fracture; 847.0 Cervical strain

SEE ALSO: N/A

REFERENCES

- An HS. Cervical spine injuries. In: An HS, ed. Synopsis of spine surgery, 1st ed. Philadelphia: Williams & Wilkins, 1998: 263–282.
- D'Alise MD, Benzel E, Hart BL, et al. Evaluation of the cervical spine after trauma. In: Benzel E, ed. Spine surgery: techniques, complication avoidance and management, 1st ed. New York: Churchill Livingstone, 1999:815–824.
- Rosner MJ, Halliday AL, Ball PA. Medical management of the patient with spinal cord injury. In: Benzel E, ed. Spine surgery: techniques, complication avoidance and management, 1st ed. New York: Churchill Livingstone, 1999:1303–1321.
- Takhtani D, Melhem ER. MR Imaging in cervical spine trauma. Clin Sports Med 2002;21:49–75.

Author(s): Raju S. V. Balabhadra, MD; Russell J. Andrews, MD

Chiari Malformation

Basics

DESCRIPTION

Chiari malformations consist of four congenital hindbrain malformations, probably mechanistically unrelated to each other. These malformations can involve only the mesenchymal elements of the posterior fossa (bone, dura, muscle, and skin) or include the cerebellum and brainstem. Patients with Chiari malformation can exhibit symptoms of headache, fatigue, cerebellar or brainstem dysfunction, and sometimes hydrocephalus and syringomyelia depending on the type. The vast majority of Chiari malformations are types I or II, and only a small subset of cases represent the other Chiari types.

- Chiari type I: abnormal development of the posterior fossa resulting in ectopic descent of the cerebellar tonsils and medial inferior cerebellar lobes into the upper cervical spinal canal. The basis for diagnosis is dependent on evaluation of the posterior fossa and identification of the foramen magnum. Chiari I malformations are the cause of approximately 70% of adult syringomyelia.
- Chiari type II: an anomaly of the hindbrain, possibly a failure of pontine flexure during embryogenesis, resulting in elongation of the fourth ventricle. Type II has type I features, along with displacement of the inferior vermis, and caudal displacement of the pons and medulla. These patients also have an elongated fourth ventricle and often an associated lumbar meningomyelocele.
- Chiari type III: the suggested mechanism for type III is defective closure of the roof plate resulting in displacement of the entire cerebellum and medulla into an infratentorial meningoencephalocele. This is usually incompatible with life.
- Chiari type IV: complete cerebellar hypoplasia is referred as type IV Chiari, also known as Dandy-Walker malformation. This type consists of a cystic expansion of the fourth ventricle in the posterior fossa, due to a developmental failure of the 4th ventricle roof.

EPIDEMIOLOGY

- Chiari I: average age at presentation is 41 years, with a slight female predilection.
- Chiari II: most common serious malformation of the posterior fossa, with a frequency of approximately 1 case per 1,000 population in the United States.
- Chiari III and IV: very rare

ETIOLOGY

Chiari malformations are congenital anomalies of the hindbrain and associated tissues.

RISK FACTORS

Myelomeningocele has been associated with folic acid deficiency during early pregnancy. Chiari type II is commonly associated with myelomeningocele.

PREGNANCY

Patients with headache associated with Chiari malformations may experience more headache during the active stage of labor. Otherwise, there are no major issues related to pregnancy and Chiari malformations.

ASSOCIATED CONDITIONS

- Chiari type I is associated with syringomyelia.
- Chiari type II is associated with myelomeningocele.
- Chiari type IV is associated with hydrocephalus.

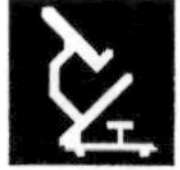

Diagnosis

DIFFERENTIAL DIAGNOSIS

A variety of chronic conditions affecting the cerebellum, brainstem, and foramen magnum region may mimic the findings of Chiari malformations. Cerebellar degenerations or mass lesions may cause slowly progressive ataxia with gait disorder. Brainstem gliomas and other brainstem tumors may present with nystagmus, vertigo, ataxia, and headache. Mass lesions at the foramen magnum may cause downbeat nystagmus with four-limb weakness, spasticity, and headache.

SIGNS AND SYMPTOMS

- Chiari type I: the most common initial presenting symptoms are headaches, gradual dysphagia, cervical pain, vertigo, weakness, paresthesias and ataxia. Symptoms of Chiari type I are divided into early and late symptoms. Early symptoms consist of headache, fatigue, vertigo, intermittent nausea, dysphagia, and tinnitus. Headache may occur with exercise or coughing. Late symptoms are generally associated with syringomyelia, and consist of a dissociated sensory examination with a cape-like distribution of hypesthesia over the shoulders and upper back. In addition, patients can become myelopathic, with prominent upper extremity dysfunction. Signs may include ataxia, spastic quadriparesis, syringomyelic signs, and downbeating nystagmus. Lower cranial nerve palsies are often seen (absent gag, tongue wasting, etc.).
- Chiari type II: patients are usually diagnosed in early childhood along with the diagnosis of myelomeningocele. Symptoms of Chiari type II can be mild or severe, and can include head lag, apnea, respiratory distress, stridor, and dysphagia. Patients may develop progressive hydrocephalus.
- Chiari type III: these malformations are usually incompatible with life.
- Chiari type IV: patients with Dandy-Walker syndrome can present with headaches and symptoms of raised intracranial pressure due to hydrocephalus.

Chiari type I patients present in late childhood to early adulthood and commonly have multiple and variable clinical manifestations. This often results in delay or incorrect diagnosis until imaging is obtained. The systems involved include, but are not limited to, the lower brainstem, lower cranial nerves, and the otologic, cerebellar, sensory, and motor systems.

Chiari type II patients present as neonates and infants. When symptomatic, these patients most often have an associated myelomeningocele and exhibit signs of neurogenic dysphagia, stridor, apneic spells and opisthotonia.

Chiari III patients present as neonates on the basis of their meningomyelocele.

Chiari IV patients often present with symptoms of hydrocephalus. Most patients with this type of Chiari malformation have normal development and normal intelligence.

LABORATORY PROCEDURES

No specific laboratory studies are helpful in the diagnosis and treatment of the Chiari malformations.

IMAGING STUDIES

- Chiari type I: MRI is used to diagnose Chiari type I. The hallmark imaging finding is pointed cerebellar tonsils that lie greater than 5 mm below the foramen magnum.
- Chiari type II: MRI is the imaging study of choice and will show displacement of the inferior vermis, and caudal displacement of the pons and medulla causing descent of the cerebellar tonsils below the foramen magnum. These patients also have an elongated fourth ventricle and may have other abnormalities of the hindbrain and brainstem including beaked tectum, absence of the septum pellucidum, poorly myelinated cerebellar folia, hydrocephalus, heterotopias, hypoplasia of falx, microgyria, and degeneration of lower cranial nerve nuclei.
- Chiari III: MRI imaging shows a high cervical or occipitocervical meningomyelocele with cerebellar herniation.
- Chiari IV: MRI imaging classically shows hypoplasia or absence of the cerebellar vermis, extension of the fourth ventricle into the posterior fossa, and cerebellar hypoplasia.

SPECIAL TESTS

N/A

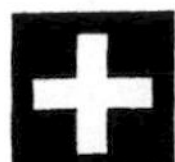

Management

GENERAL MEASURES
N/A

SURGICAL MEASURES
Surgery is the only treatment for symptomatic Chiari type I malformations. Surgical therapy is usually reserved for progressive and debilitating symptoms. The surgery involves a craniectomy to remove the suboccipital bone and foramen magnum along with an upper cervical laminectomy of C1, C2, and sometimes C3. The decompression is further augmented by a duraplasty, which is patched using a dural substitute. If there is an associated syrinx, serial MRIs are used to assess the progression of syringomyelia. In most cases, an adequate posterior fossa decompression will halt the progression of syringomyelia. If the syrinx persists and becomes more symptomatic, a syringo-subarachnoid shunt may be placed.

For Chiari type II, correction of associated malformations is performed first, with the closure of a myelomeningocele and ventriculoperitoneal shunting if hydrocephalus is present. Surgical therapy for type II Chiari malformations is reserved for patients with critical warning signs of neurogenic dysphagia, stridor, and apnea. The operative results for posterior fossa decompression in type II Chiari malformation are poor, partly due to inherent uncorrectable brainstem and cerebellar abnormalities.

Chiari IV patients who develop hydrocephalus must be treated with conventional ventricular shunting procedures. Often, there is little communication of the lateral ventricular system with the Dandy Walker cyst. In these patients, it may be necessary to place a shunt to decompress the posterior fossa cyst as well.

SYMPTOMATIC TREATMENT
Headache may be treated in a similar fashion to migraine. Beta-blockers, tricyclic anti-depressants, or nonsteroidals may be useful in therapy for headache related to Chiari I malformations.

ADJUNCTIVE TREATMENT
N/A

ADMISSION/DISCHARGE CRITERIA
Patients usually require admission for surgery, often on the day of surgery. Discharge depends on postoperative status and course in hospital.

Medications

DRUG(S) OF CHOICE
N/A

ALTERNATIVE DRUGS
N/A

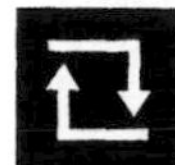

Follow-Up

PATIENT MONITORING
Patients with Chiari type I and associated syringomyelia must be monitored on a yearly basis for progression of the syrinx. For Chiari type II patients, close follow-up by a pediatric neurologist is critical in identifying progressive symptoms and the need for operative or reoperative therapy.

EXPECTED COURSE AND PROGNOSIS
Surgical management may stabilize progressive symptoms of Chiari I malformation, and improve headache symptoms. Patients may continue to have neurologic symptoms of gait disorders and dysphagia depending on the extent of prior injury.

PATIENT EDUCATION
Patients should be made aware of the congenital nature of these abnormalities, the usual symptoms, the potential for progression, and the options for treatment. They should inform their doctor about any progression of symptoms.

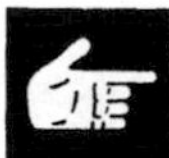

Miscellaneous

SYNONYMS
Arnold-Chiari malformation

ICD-9-CM: 348.4 Chiari type 1; 741.0 Chiari type 2; 742.0 Chiari type 3; 742.2 Chiari type 4

SEE ALSO: SYRINGOMYELIA

REFERENCES

- Bejjani GK, Cockerham KP. Adult Chiari malformation. Contemp Neurosurg 2001;23(26):1–8.
- De Reuck J, Thienpont L. Fetal Chiari's type III malformation. Childs Brain 1976;2:85–91.
- Elster AD, Chen MY. Chiari I malformations: clinical and radiologic reappraisal. Radiology 1992;183:347–353.
- Gilbert JN, Jones KL, Rorke LB, et al. Central nervous system anomalies associated with myelomeningocele, hydrocephalus and the Arnold-Chiari malformation: reappraisal of theories regarding the pathogenesis of posterior neural tube closure defects. Neurosurgery 1986;18:559–564.
- Golden JA, Bonnemann CG. Developmental structural disorders. In: Goetz CG, ed. Textbook of neurology, 1st ed. Philadelphia: WB Saunders, 1999:510–538.
- Haslam RHA. Congenital anomalies of the central nervous system. In: Behrman RE, ed. Nelson textbook of pediatrics, 16th ed. Philadelphia: WB Saunders, 2000:1803–1813.
- Osenbach RK, Menezes AH. Diagnosis and management of the Dandy-Walker malformation: 30 years of experience. Pediatr Neurosurg 1992;18:179–189.
- Paul KS, Lye RH, Strang FA, et al. Arnold-Chiari malformation: review of 71 cases. J Neurosurg 1983;58:183–187.

Author(s): P. Mark Li, MD

Chorea

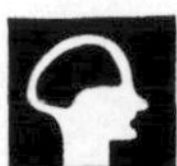

Basics

DESCRIPTION

Chorea is a hyperkinetic movement disturbance typically characterized by rapid, non-stereotyped, semipurposeful movements that flow from one body part to another. Clinical manifestations exist along a wide spectrum.

EPIDEMIOLOGY

Incidence/Prevalence

Incidence and prevalence is variable, depending on etiology.

ETIOLOGY

- The etiologies of chorea number well over 100.
- A classification of potential etiologies of chorea:
  - —As a distinct neurologic entity, e.g., benign hereditary chorea, senile chorea
  - —As a feature of an inherited neurologic disease, e.g., Huntington's disease (HD)
  - —As a sign/symptom of underlying neurologic disease, systemic disease, or insult to the nervous system
  - —See Associated Conditions, below, for further description of these etiologies.

RISK FACTORS

- Family history of chorea, progressive neurologic condition, or other movement disorder.
- Some medications or drug use; see Associated Conditions, below.

PREGNANCY

Chorea can occur during pregnancy, i.e., chorea gravidarum (CG), and typically resolves following delivery. However, the occurrence of CG may be the initial manifestation of systemic lupus erythematosus, HD, and the antiphospholipid antibody syndrome.

ASSOCIATED CONDITIONS

Distinct Neurologic Entities

- Benign hereditary chorea: characterized by the onset of chorea in childhood, which is nonprogressive through adult life, with no impairment of cognition; demonstrates autosomal-dominant inheritance. HD should be excluded if any suspicion exists.
- Senile chorea: chorea appearing in late life without dementia, psychiatric disturbance, or a family history of chorea and no other identifiable cause. HD should be excluded if any suspicion exists.

Inherited Neurologic Disorders

- Autosomal dominant
  - —HD: a neurodegenerative disease characterized by onset of chorea in mid-adulthood, followed by dementia and psychiatric disturbances. The genetic basis is an expansion of unstable stretch of CAG trinucleotide repeats in the Huntington gene on chromosome 4p. See chapter on Huntington's Disease.
  - —Dentatorubropallidoluysian atrophy (DRPLA): a rare neurodegenerative disease most prevalent in Japan. Like HD, it is also a trinucleotide repeat disorder; an expansion of unstable CAG trinucleotide repeats occurs in the "atrophin" gene on chromosome 12p to give rise to a variable phenotype that has been categorized into three types: (a) an ataxo-choreoathetoid type, (b) a pseudo-Huntington type, and (c) a myoclonic-epileptic type.
- Autosomal recessive
  - —Wilson's disease (WD): the underlying defect is impaired biliary excretion of copper due to a defect in the WD gene, *Wc1*, on chromosome 13q, which encodes for a copper transporting adenosine triphosphatase (ATPase). The resulting copper toxicity results in the deposition of copper initially in the liver and then the CNS. Neurologic manifestations are varied, often resulting in a movement disorder. Tremor is the most common, though chorea, dystonia, tics, myoclonus, parkinsonism, and ataxia are not infrequent.
- Neurologic syndromes associated with acanthocytes: there are three such syndromes, the latter of which is X-linked recessive
  - —Bassen-Kornzweig syndrome: Abetalipoproteinemia, very low cholesterol (<1.5 mmol/L) and triglycerides (<0.1 mmol/L). Clinically, these patients present with a progressive spinocerebellar syndrome, pigmentary retinopathy, and areflexia. Involuntary movements are typically not part of the clinical picture, although severe position sense loss can result in pseudoathetosis. There is absent apolipoprotein B with resultant fat malabsorption, including the fat-soluble vitamins; it is the absence of vitamin E that is responsible for the clinical features and are reversible with vitamin E supplementation.
  - —Chorea-acanthocytosis: normal lipoprotein study in association with acanthocytosis. Clinical features consist of chorea, orofacial dyskinesias with tongue and lip biting, motor tics, peripheral neuropathy, amyotrophy, and vocalizations.
  - —McLeod phenotype: normal lipoproteins and acanthocytosis with weak expression of the Kell system blood group antigens. X-linked recessive condition, occurring only in males. Features consistently noted include elevated creatine kinase, a slowly progressive myopathy, and evidence of cardiomyopathy. However, there are reports of male patients developing a clinical picture of chorea-acanthocytosis but were found to have the McLeod phenotype.

Other Causes of Chorea

- Medications:
  - —Dopamine receptor blockers—antipsychotics, antiemetics
  - —Levodopa
  - —Anticonvulsants—phenytoin, valproic acid
  - —Stimulants—amphetamines, theophylline, cocaine
  - —Lithium
  - —Oral contraceptives
- Metabolic disturbances
  - —Abnormalities in glucose, sodium, calcium, or magnesium
- Hematologic disturbances
  - —Polycythemia vera
- Structural lesions
  - —Vascular—infarction, hemorrhage, subdural hematoma
  - —Neoplastic—primary or metastatic lesions
  - —Congenital—cerebral palsy
- Endocrine disturbances
  - —Hyperthyroidism
  - —Hypoparathyroidism
  - —Hyperparathyroidism
- Immunologic conditions
  - —Systemic lupus erythematosus (SLE)
  - —Sydenham's chorea
  - —Antiphospholipid antibody syndrome (APAS)
  - —Multiple sclerosis
- In infants and children:
  - —Kernicterus
  - —Lesch-Nyhan syndrome
  - —Post-pump chorea following cardiac bypass surgery for congenital heart disease

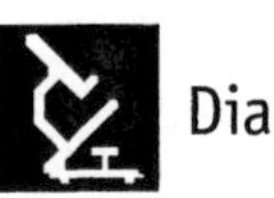

Diagnosis

DIFFERENTIAL DIAGNOSIS

Other Hyperkinetic Movement Disorders

- Tics—rapid, nonrhythmic movements or sounds that are suppressible for a short time
- Myoclonus—random, irregular movements caused by rapid muscle contractions
- Dystonia—characterized by sustained muscle contractions, resulting in twisting, repetitive, and patterned movements, or abnormal postures
- Tremor—regular, rhythmic movement

- Apseudochoreoathetosis—due to proprioceptive sensory loss
- Paroxysmal kinesigenic choreoathetosis

SIGNS AND SYMPTOMS

The clinical manifestations of chorea exist along a wide spectrum. In its mildest expression, the patient may simply appear to be fidgety or restless; in its most extreme fashion, chorea can exist as large amplitude flinging movements of the proximal extremities, i.e., ballistic movements. Chorea may be present with other neurologic findings, in particular athetosis, which can be thought of as a slow form of chorea and consists of slow writhing movements. Dystonia may occur also.

LABORATORY PROCEDURES

- Serum and urine for drug/medication screen
- Serum glucose, sodium, calcium, phosphate, magnesium
- CBC and smear for acanthocytes
- Lipid profile (including lipoproteins)
- Endocrine studies: thyroid function studies; PTH level
- For suspected WD: serum total and free copper; ceruloplasmin level; 24-hour urine collection for copper
- For suspected SLE: ANA, anti-double-stranded DNA antibodies, anti-Smith antibodies
- For suspected rheumatic chorea: antistreptolysin O titer, ESR, nose/throat culture, ECG, or echocardiogram
- For suspected APAS: VDRL (false positive); platelet count (thrombocytopenia); aPTT (prolonged by at least 5 seconds and that does not correct with 1:1 dilution of the patient's plasma with normal or control plasma); lupus anticoagulant; and anticardiolipin antibody

IMAGING STUDIES

Brain MRI: caudate atrophy in HD; focal structural lesions; multiple sclerosis

SPECIAL TESTS

- Genetic testing for suspected HD and DRPLA; both are CAG repeat expansion disorders
- Slit-lamp examination for Kayser-Fleischer rings
- CSF exam and evoked potentials for suspected multiple sclerosis

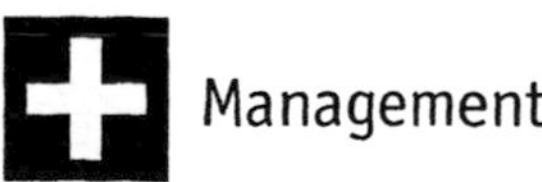

Management

GENERAL MEASURES

Management of the patient with chorea is dependent on the etiology. In all patients, any underlying treatable or reversible condition should be ruled out, e.g., metabolic or endocrine disturbance, adverse effect of medications, structural lesion, stroke, multiple sclerosis. If female, the possibility of pregnancy should be investigated. Wilson's disease should be ruled out in every child, adolescent, or young adult presenting with chorea or other movement disorder for which no cause can be found. Immunologic etiologies should be identified and treated as indicated.

SURGICAL MEASURES

N/A

SYMPTOMATIC TREATMENT

N/A

ADJUNCTIVE TREATMENT

N/A

ADMISSION/DISCHARGE CRITERIA

N/A

Medications

DRUG(S) OF CHOICE

Dopamine-Receptor Antagonists—Antipsychotic Medications

- Mechanism: the high-potency antipsychotic medications have strong affinity for blockade of the D2 dopamine receptor; these include haloperidol, fluphenazine, perphenazine, trifluoperazine, and pimozide.
- Dose: initially with a small nightly dose (0.5–2 mg); titrate as needed for symptom control.
- Adverse effects: extrapyramidal side effects—acute dystonic reaction, neuroleptic malignant syndrome, parkinsonism, tardive dyskinesia, akathisia.
- Precautions: an ECG should be obtained prior to the use of pimozide; pimozide slows cardiac conduction and can result in arrhythmias (heart block, torsades de pointes ventricular tachycardia).

ALTERNATIVE DRUGS

Tetrabenazine

Tetrabenazine is not approved by the FDA; available only as an investigational drug in the U.S.

- Mechanism: reversible depletion of presynaptic monoamines and postsynaptic dopamine receptor antagonist.
- Dose: 12.5–200 mg/d
- Only rarely associated with acute dystonic reaction; tardive dyskinesia has not been seen.

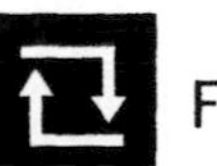

Follow-Up

PATIENT MONITORING

N/A

EXPECTED COURSE AND PROGNOSIS

- Dependent on etiology:
  - —BHC and senile chorea—benign course, life span is not threatened
  - —Inherited neurologic disorders—typically a more malignant disease course with shortened life span
  - —Chorea secondary to medications may be transient or persistent
  - —Chorea can recur in Sydenham's chorea, SLE, and APAS

PATIENT EDUCATION

www.wemove.org: a comprehensive resource for movement disorder information.

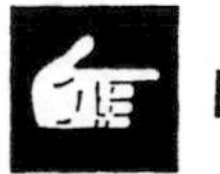

Miscellaneous

SYNONYMS

Huntington's chorea/Huntington's disease
Sydenham's chorea/rheumatic chorea/St. Vitus' dance

ICD-9-CM: 333.5 Chorea/choreoathetosis; 392.9 Sydenham's chorea; 333.4 Huntington's disease/hereditary/chronic

SEE ALSO: HUNTINGTON'S DISEASE, WILSON'S DISEASE, SYSTEMIC LUPUS ERYTHEMATOSUS, SYDENHAM CHOREA, ANTIPHOSPHOLIPID ANTIBODY SYNDROME

REFERENCES

- Bruyn GW, Padberg G. Chorea and systemic lupus erythematosus. Eur Neurol 1984;23:278–290.
- Levine SR, Welch KMA. The spectrum of neurologic disease associated with antiphospholipid antibodies. Arch Neurol 1987;44:876–883.
- Nausieda PA, Grossman BJ, Koller WC, et al. Sydenham chorea: an update. Neurology 1980;30:331–334.
- Padberg G, Bruyn GW. Chorea: differential diagnosis. In: Vinken PR, Bruyn GW, Klawans HL, eds. Handbook of clinical neurology, vol 49. Amsterdam: Elsevier, 1986:549–564.
- Walshe JM, Yealland M. Wilson's disease: the problem of delayed diagnosis. J Neurol Neurosurg Psychiatry 1992;55:692–696.

Author(s): Paul G. Wasielewski, MD

Chronic Inflammatory Demyelinating Polyneuropathy

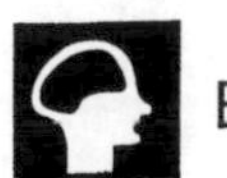

Basics

DESCRIPTION

Chronic inflammatory demyelinating polyneuropathy (CIDP) is an acquired disorder of the peripheral nervous system with a chronic, subacute, or relapsing course.

EPIDEMIOLOGY

Incidence/Prevalence

CIDP has a prevalence of 1–2 per 100,000.

Age

Maximum occurrence is in 70- to 79-year-olds. The mean age of onset of 48. CIDP may occur in children.

Sex

The male/female ratio is 1.3:1.

ETIOLOGY

CIDP is an autoimmune demyelinating low-grade inflammatory polyneuropathy, but its triggers are unknown. Unlike its acute cousin, Guillain-Barré syndrome (GBS; acute inflammatory demyelinating polyneuropathy), it generally does not follow a flu-like illness or vaccination. While the primary pathologic change in CIDP is that of segmental and paranodal demyelination, loss of axons may also occur. Repeated bouts of demyelination and remyelination may lead to the formation of concentric whorls of Schwann cells and fibroblasts surrounding fibers, resulting in structures known as "onion bulbs." CIDP patients may have autoantibodies to protein zero (P0), a peripheral myelin protein.

RISK FACTORS

None known.

PREGNANCY

CIDP may have onset or worsen during pregnancy or postpartum.

ASSOCIATED CONDITIONS

CIDP has been associated with benign monoclonal gammopathy. Monoclonal immunoglobulin M (IgM) κ subtype, associated with an autoantibody directed to myelin-associated glycoprotein (anti-MAG), has more prominent distal motor nerve fiber demyelination (very prolonged distal motor latencies on nerve conduction studies), and inappropriate separation and widening of the spaces between myelin spaces (widened myelin lamellae) with abnormal deposition of the monoclonal protein in these widened spaces. There are sporadic reports of CIDP-like polyneuropathies associated with malignancy with and without gammopathy. Overall, uncommon associations with CIDP are Charcot-Marie-Tooth disease, lymphoma, melanoma, carcinoma, diabetes mellitus, collagen vascular disease, thyrotoxicosis, chronic hepatitis, inflammatory bowel disease, HIV infection, hepatic transplantation, glomerulonephritis, alopecia universalis, and the medication procainamide.

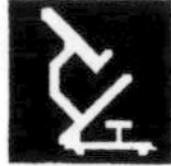

Diagnosis

DIFFERENTIAL DIAGNOSIS

In examining patients with prominent upper limb weakness, the clinician should consider motor neuron disease, multifocal motor neuropathy, hand wasting from a high cervical myelopathy, cervical radiculopathy, paraneoplastic motor and sensory polyneuropathy, plexopathy from infiltrative tumor or radiation, and others. Some polyneuropathies that do not fulfill CIDP criteria may be milder versions of CIDP, while others are axonal polyneuropathies with superimposed demyelinating change. In diabetes, for example, there may be segmental demyelination especially at sites of entrapment, but sensory loss is more prominent than the motor weakness of CIDP. Hereditary neuropathy with sensitivity to pressure palsy (HNPP) is an autosomal-dominant inherited deletion of the peripheral nerve myelin protein gene. HNPP is a generalized polyneuropathy with focal demyelination at sites of entrapment and it may sometimes resemble CIDP in patients without a family history. CIDP progresses to peak disability by at least 8 weeks compared to 4 weeks in GBS.

SIGNS AND SYMPTOMS

CIDP presents with motor weakness and incoordination especially of the hands, impaired walking, and foot drop. There may be muscle cramps and fasciculations. Sensory symptoms may include loss of sensation (numbness), paresthesias (tingling, prickling, "pins and needles," "asleep" sensations), and sometimes pain. Tremor may be prominent during recovery from an exacerbation. Cranial nerves, respiration, and autonomic function are usually not involved. In long-standing untreated CIDP there may be intrinsic hand or foot wasting, but usually there is an absence of wasting in the setting of prominent weakness. Weakness is usually symmetrical and may be proximal and distal, and especially involves intrinsic hand muscles, and foot and toe dorsiflexors. Some patients may be quadriparetic. Deep tendon reflexes are frequently absent or reduced. Sensory loss may be minimal or there may be stocking and glove distribution loss to pinprick, thermal appreciation, light touch, vibration perception, and joint position sense. In many patients, however, the sensory loss to light touch, vibration, and position is more prominent, reflecting the greater involvement of large myelinated sensory fibers. Additional features are gait ataxia and rombergism or a flopping gait reflecting bilateral foot drop. The peripheral nerves are sometimes palpably enlarged, reflecting nerve hypertrophy from repeated cycles of demyelination with remyelination.

LABORATORY PROCEDURES

On nerve conduction studies features of demyelination include prolonged distal latencies, motor and sensory conduction velocity slowing, temporal dispersion of compound muscle action potentials (CMAPs), and conduction block in motor nerve territories. Sensory nerve action potentials are reduced or absent. Needle EMG of weak muscles may identify abnormal recruitment of motor unit potentials, but infrequent fibrillations. Some patients with CIDP have axonal damage with reduced distal CMAP amplitudes and fibrillations.

CSF protein is usually elevated without pleocytosis. If present, pleocytosis may suggest associated HIV infection. Serum protein electrophoresis, immunoelectrophoresis, and immunofixation may identify a monoclonal spike. Patients with IgMκ monoclonal gammopathy may have elevated anti-MAG antibodies. Nerve biopsy is not routinely required to make the diagnosis. IgA deficiency, associated with anaphylaxis after IVIG, should be excluded. Inquiring about a history of TB or a TB skin test is important if prednisone is to be offered (see below).

IMAGING STUDIES

Nerve root hypertrophy and enhancement may occur on spinal MRI studies. Rarely, brain MRI has identified concurrent CNS demyelination.

SPECIAL TESTS

Sural nerve or deep and superficial peroneal nerve biopsies are reserved for "atypical" instances of CIDP, for example patients who do not fulfill its strict electrodiagnostic criteria or have normal CSF protein. Biopsies may identify myelinated fiber loss, axonal degeneration, regenerative clusters, segmental and paranodal demyelination, remyelination, and sometimes infiltrates of inflammatory cells. It is important that nerves are harvested, processed, and interpreted by specialized laboratories with expertise in peripheral nerve pathology.

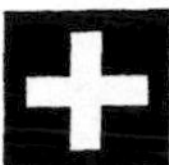

Management

GENERAL MEASURES

Patients with CIDP may be unable to work, may need the input of an occupational therapist to help prevent falls at their homes and to provide other types of assistance with activities of daily living.

SYMPTOMATIC TREATMENT

Pain may be treated with simple analgesics; more severe pain may be treated with tricyclic antidepressants and anticonvulsants such as gabapentin, carbamazepine, or phenytoin. Patients with foot drop should be prescribed a custom-fitted ankle-foot orthosis.

ADMISSION/DISCHARGE CRITERIA

Quadriparetic and rapidly deteriorating patients can require hospitalization for investigation and therapy. Most management, however, is carried out in an outpatient setting.

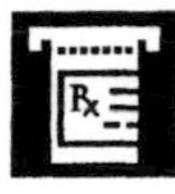

Medications

DRUG(S) OF CHOICE

Level 1 evidence supports the use of high-dose chronic prednisone in CIDP starting at 80 mg daily or 120 mg alternating with 7.5 mg. High doses are required for the first 1 to 3 months followed by very slow tapering, depending on the clinical response. Patients should receive osteoporosis prophylaxis (e.g., etidronate and calcium). Complications can include hypertension, diabetes, susceptibility to infection, peptic ulceration, weight gain, edema, osteoporosis, and hip necrosis. All are relative contraindications/precautions.
Intravenous gamma globulin may be used in lieu of or together with prednisone. The dose is 0.4 g/kg/d for 5 days monthly, although higher doses over fewer numbers of days or more frequent treatment courses can be given in stable patients. This is expensive therapy. Anaphylaxis is a contraindication. Headaches, chills, and nausea are benign side effects, though aseptic meningitis, hyperviscosity, susceptibility to thrombosis, and transmission of viral infections have been reported rarely. Patients may require ongoing treatments over years.
Plasma exchange is of benefit in CIDP but less commonly used now because of the difficulties obtaining venous access and less common availability of appropriate facilities.

Contraindications

See above.

Precautions

See above.

ALTERNATIVE DRUGS

Azathioprine, with careful monthly monitoring of blood counts and hepatic function, is equally effective compared to prednisone and may be used in some patients with steroid side effects or inadequate response to the above therapies.

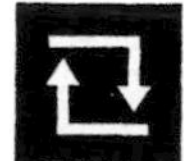

Follow-Up

PATIENT MONITORING

Patients require follow-up by primary care physicians to monitor steroid or azathioprine side effects and by their neurologist to monitor the need for and dose of therapy. Periodic electrophysiologic monitoring may add to the precision of clinical monitoring.

EXPECTED COURSE AND PROGNOSIS

Patients may experience long-term remissions after a prolonged course of prednisone, or may require ongoing IVIG to maintain their functional status. There may be relatively rapid downhill relapses in CIDP that require urgent therapy.

PATIENT EDUCATION

Excellent educational and support services are offered through the Peripheral Nerve Association patient group: *www.neuropathy.org*.

Miscellaneous

SYNONYMS

Chronic relapsing polyneuropathy
Chronic inflammatory radiculoplexus neuropathy
Chronic inflammatory demyelinating radiculoneuropathy
Chronic Guillain-Barré syndrome (this term is discouraged)

ICD-9-CM: 357.8 Inflammatory and toxic neuropathy—other

SEE ALSO

N/A

REFERENCES

- Ad Hoc Subcommittee of the American Academy of Neurology AIDS Taskforce. Research criteria for diagnosis of chronic inflammatory demyelinating polyneuropathy (CIDP). Neurology 1991;41:617–618.
- De Silva RN, Willison HJ, Doyle D, et al. Nerve root hypertrophy in chronic inflammatory demyelinating polyneuropathy. Muscle Nerve 1994;17(2):168–170.
- Dyck PJ, Lais AC, Ohta M, et al. Chronic inflammatory polyradiculoneuropathy. Mayo Clin Proc 1975;50:621–637.
- Dyck PJ, O'Brien PC, Oviatt KF, et al. Prednisone improves chronic inflammatory demyelinating polyradiculoneuropathy more than no treatment. Ann Neurol 1982;11:136–141.
- Dyck PJ, O'Brien P, Swanson C, et al. Combined azathioprine and prednisone in chronic inflammatory demyelinating polyneuropathy. Neurology 1985;35: 1173–1176.
- Hahn AF, Bolton CF, Zochodne DW, et al. Intravenous immunoglobulin treatment in chronic inflammatory demyelinating polyneuropathy. A double-blind, placebo-controlled, cross-over study. Brain 1996;119:1067–1077.
- Kaku DA, England JD, Sumner AJ. Distal accentuation of conduction slowing in polyneuropathy associated with antibodies to myelin-associated glycoprotein and sulphated glucuronyl paragloboside. Brain 1994;117:941–947.
- McCombe PA, McManis PG, Frith JA, et al. Chronic inflammatory demyelinating polyradiculoneuropathy associated with pregnancy. Ann Neurol 1987;21:102–104.
- McLeod JG, Pollard JD, Macaskill P, et al. Prevalence of chronic inflammatory demyelinating polyneuropathy in New South Wales, Australia. Ann Neurol 1999;46:910–913.
- Yan WX, Archelos JJ, Hartung HP, et al. P0 protein is a target antigen in chronic inflammatory demyelinating polyradiculoneuropathy. Ann Neurol 2001;50:286–292.

Author(s): Douglas W. Zochodne, MD

Conversion Disorder

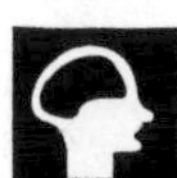

Basics

DESCRIPTION

Conversion disorder is a somatoform disorder defined as a condition characterized by symptoms or deficits affecting voluntary motor or sensory function in which there is a loss or alteration in physical functioning. These symptoms are suggestive of a physical disorder but are in fact the expression of an underlying psychological conflict. By definition, the symptoms are *not* voluntarily produced.

EPIDEMIOLOGY

Incidence/Prevalence

- The incidence of conversion symptoms varies widely depending on the population being studied; it is common on a general medical service where prevalence is estimated at 20% to 25%. It is estimated that conversion symptoms account for 5% to 14% of all psychiatric consultations for hospitalized medical or surgical patients.
- Conversion symptoms are more common in rural areas, and lower socioeconomic groups (less psychologically sophisticated populations). These symptoms are also more common in military personnel exposed to combat situations.

Sex

Conversion symptoms are more frequently diagnosed in women, although some authorities suggest that the disorder is probably gender-equal.

Age

Conversion symptoms may present at any age, although onset is rare before age 5 or after age 35. Typically conversion symptoms are first seen in adolescence or early adulthood.

ETIOLOGY

Conversion symptoms are caused by the conversion of psychological stress or conflict into somatic symptoms. There is still disagreement about whether the conversion phenomenon reflects primarily:

- An intrapsychic conflict. The patient may experience conflict over an unconscious, unacceptable, sexual, aggressive, or dependency wish. The somatic symptom maintains the unacceptable wish out of awareness and often resolves the conflict by "punishing or not rewarding" the wish (primary gain).
- An interpersonal communication motivated by obtaining gratification from the environment. In this model, patients who have great dependency needs use their conversion symptoms to obtain attention and to influence their environment (secondary gain). The patient's disability and "helplessness" can become powerful tools in controlling friends, family, or physicians.
- Recently some studies have indicated that there may be cerebral dysfunction in patients with conversion disorder. According to this hypothesis, conversion may reflect certain neurophysiologic vulnerabilities in these patients.

Genetics

No information is available.

PREGNANCY

No association described.

ASSOCIATED CONDITIONS

- Conversion is probably multidetermined and represents a common pathway for a variety of etiologic factors. High rates of concomitant psychopathology have been found in patients with conversion symptoms. Depression and antisocial personality disorder are the most commonly reported. Patients with dissociative disorders have relatively high rates of conversion symptoms. Hysterical personality features are found in less than half of patients with conversion symptoms.
- A number of studies have found that patients with conversion symptoms also have high rates of medical and neurologic illness. Physical trauma, temporal lobe abnormalities, and multiple sclerosis may predispose to the development of conversion symptoms. Long-term follow-up studies up to 10 years past diagnosis of conversion disorder found a 25% to 62% incidence of false positives. It is extremely important to keep an open mind regarding the possibility of an organic etiology when making a diagnosis of conversion disorder and to seek appropriate consultations in order to rule out an organic etiology.

Diagnosis

DIFFERENTIAL DIAGNOSIS

The list of differential diagnoses may cover a good portion of a neurologic textbook. Diagnoses that may be more problematic to exclude are:

- Multiple sclerosis
- Myasthenia gravis
- Periodic paralysis
- Polymyositis
- Guillain-Barré syndrome
- Transient ischemic attack
- Stroke
- Mercury toxicity

The DSM-IV diagnostic criteria for conversion disorder are:

1. One or more symptoms or deficits affecting voluntary motor or sensory function that suggest a neurologic or other general medical condition.
2. Psychological factors are judged to be associated with the symptom or deficit because the initiation or exacerbation of the symptom or deficit is preceded by conflicts or other stressors.
3. The symptom or deficit is not intentionally produced or feigned (as in factitious disorder or malingering).
4. The symptom or deficit cannot, after appropriate investigation, be fully explained by a general medical condition, or by the direct effects of a substance, or as a culturally sanctioned behavior or experience.
5. The symptom or deficit causes clinically significant distress or impairment in social, occupational, or other important areas of functioning or warrants medical evaluation.
6. The symptom or deficit is not limited to pain or sexual dysfunction, does not occur exclusively during the course of somatization disorder, and is not better accounted for by another mental disorder.

The diagnosis of a conversion symptom can be made only when the symptom in question cannot be adequately explained on the basis of a medical condition. What complicates the diagnosis is the fact that conversion symptoms and physical illness frequently coexist. The history is most helpful in diagnosing conversion reactions. It should include information about the patient's family, work, other possible stressors, as well as the possibility of secondary gain.

SIGNS AND SYMPTOMS

- Weakness, paralysis, sensory disturbances, pseudoseizures, blindness, deafness, and aphonia are the most frequent complaints.
- Patients often show a puzzling lack of concern about their deficits. This characteristic lack of concern has been termed "la belle indifference." Neurologic abnormalities usually lack an anatomic distribution on physical exam.

LABORATORY PROCEDURES

Laboratory testing should be considered to rule out an organic etiology. There are no specific tests to diagnose or rule out conversion disorder. Laboratory studies that are inconsistent with the presenting symptom(s) may help with diagnosis of conversion disorder.

IMAGING STUDIES

A CT scan or MRI of the head or spinal cord should be considered to rule out a lesion in these areas.

SPECIAL TESTS

No psychological test can provide a definitive diagnosis of conversion disorder. An EEG or prolonged EEG monitoring may be helpful in differentiating a true seizure disorder from pseudoseizures. Evoked potentials should be considered in the case of conversion blindness. A spinal tap to rule out an infection or a neurologic illness should be considered when appropriate.

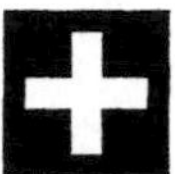

Management

GENERAL MEASURES

- Many conversion symptoms are fleeting and half to almost all symptoms remit by the time of hospital discharge. Prompt resolution is important since a number of studies have shown that there is a direct relationship between duration of conversion symptoms and chronic disability.
- In acute cases the initial aim is to remove the symptom. Direct confrontation of the patient regarding the psychological nature of the symptom is not recommended. A simple approach of reassurance, relaxation, and suggestion is indicated. Patients are reassured that their symptoms will disappear and are encouraged to discuss any stressful events or feelings that most likely have been on their mind. No relationship to the conversion symptoms should be suggested.
- Most patients respond to a course of brief supportive psychotherapy. The focus is on developing a solid working alliance in an environment of mutual trust, respect, and acceptance. The aim of this treatment is to help patients explore various areas of conflict or stress and to help them develop better coping mechanisms. The focus generally shifts from the conversion symptoms to the psychological makeup of the individual. Behavioral therapy, focusing on the development of adaptive behaviors at the expense of maladaptive conversion reactions, is also helpful.

Hypnosis

Hypnotherapy has been found beneficial, especially in patients with acute symptoms. While patients are under hypnosis, it is suggested to them that their symptoms will gradually improve posthypnotically. Patients are also encouraged to discuss areas of conflict or stress.

SURGICAL MEASURES

N/A

SYMPTOMATIC TREATMENT

N/A

ADJUNCTIVE TREATMENT

N/A

ADMISSION/DISCHARGE CRITERIA

Admission should be considered to rule out any serious medical condition and when the severity of the conversion disorder prevents patients from caring for themselves.

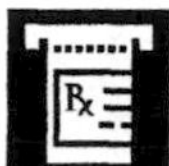

Medications

DRUG(S) OF CHOICE

- Medication has not been found to be effective for conversion disorder with the exception of narcoanalysis in acute cases. In narcoanalysis, the patient is given amobarbital IV to the point of drowsiness. The patient, who is in a relaxed state, is encouraged to discuss recent stresses or conflicts.
- Amobarbital IV is given at a rate no faster than 50 mg/min. Infusion is continued until drowsiness, slurring of speech, or sustained lateral nystagmus occur. It is very uncommon to need to use 500 mg or more of Amytal.

Contraindications

- Any condition in which pharmacologic respiratory depression would be likely to cause respiratory failure.
- A history of porphyria.

Precautions

Narcoanalysis must be administered with close monitoring for respiratory depression.

ALTERNATIVE DRUGS

None

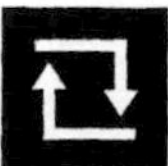

Follow-Up

PATIENT MONITORING

Following discharge, patients should be referred to a psychiatrist for individual treatment (brief psychotherapy or hypnotherapy).

EXPECTED COURSE AND PROGNOSIS

- Good prognostic indicators include:
  - —Acute symptoms (less than 30 days)
  - —Fewer symptoms
  - —Absence of psychiatric comorbid conditions
  - —An identifiable stressor
  - —Good premorbid health
  - —Good intelligence
- Chronic conversion symptoms (over 1 year) have a much poorer prognosis and may require long-term psychotherapy.
- Even though individual conversion symptoms are generally self-limited and remit quickly, a study found that symptoms relapse within 1 year in 20% to 25% of patients.
- Aphonia, blindness, and paralysis are associated with a better prognosis than pseudoseizures and conversion tremor.

PATIENT EDUCATION

Patients should be educated about the possibility of recurrent symptoms under stress.

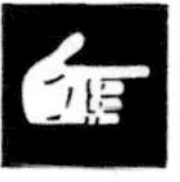

Miscellaneous

SYNONYMS

Conversion hysteria

ICD-9-CM: 300.11 Conversion disorder

SEE ALSO: N/A

REFERENCES

- Folks DG, Ford CV, Regan WM. Conversion symptoms in a general hospital. Psychosomatics 1984;25(4):285–295.
- Ford CV. The somatoform disorders. In: Michels R, ed. Psychiatry, vol 2(1). Philadelphia: JB Lippincott, 1990:3–11.
- Martin RL, Yutzy SH. Somatoform disorder. In: Tasman A, ed. Psychiatry, vol 2. Philadelphia: WB Saunders, 1997: 1135–1140.
- Putnam FW. Conversion symptoms in movement disorders. In: Joseph AB, Young RR, eds. Neurology and neuropsychiatry, 2nd ed. Malden, MA: Blackwell Science, 1998:397–403.
- Viederman M. Somatoform and factitious disorders. In: Michels R, ed. Psychiatry, vol 1.Philadelphia: JB Lippincott, 1990: 1–20.

Author(s): Radu V. Saveanu, MD

Creutzfeldt-Jakob Disease

Basics

DESCRIPTION

The triad of rapidly progressive dementia, myoclonus, and a characteristic EEG define classical Creutzfeldt-Jakob disease (CJD). It occurs in sporadic and familial/community clusters. CJD is the most common of the prion diseases, or transmissible spongiform encephalopathies (TSEs). The histologic hallmarks in the brain are neuronal loss (by apoptosis), gliosis, and vacuolization of gray matter (microscopic spongiform change) without significant inflammation.

EPIDEMIOLOGY

Incidence

About 1 per million per year.

Age

Peak incidence in sixth decade. Rare in children.

Sex

No sex preference.

Special Populations

Butchers and farmers have been reported to have an increased incidence. Variant CJD (vCJD) is a special cross-species transmitted form of CJD associated with the epidemic of bovine spongiform encephalopathy (BSE), largely confined to Great Britain. Clusters of cases are usually associated with the inherited form.

ETIOLOGY

- Sporadic: caused by a change in structure or conformation in the protease resistant protein (PrP-C going to PrP-SC), creating a preference for PRP-SC to form an amyloid (beta pleated sheet) protein. This protein is then deposited in the CNS, and is the presumed toxic agent. In sporadic CJD, the event that triggers the first PRP-C molecules to change structure is unknown, but it is then apparently autocatalytic. Alternatively, there may be a primary somatic cell mutation leading to a PrP with increased predilection to form PrP-SC. PrP is a membrane-bound glycoprotein whose exact function is unknown. About 85% of cases are sporadic.
- Inherited: several mutations in PrP cause it to be more amyloidogenic. The disease is usually inherited as an autosomal-dominant disease with incomplete penetrance. The gene is located on the short arm of chromosome 20. Specific mutations may be associated with specific clinical symptoms or variants, but these findings are not absolute. About 10% of cases are inherited.
- Transmitted: disease can be induced by introducing PrP-SC directly to the bloodstream (thus transmissible) or CSF. This forms the basis for the general term *transmissible spongiform encephalopathy* (TSE). The incubation time for this process to become clinically evident in humans is usually several years. Less than 5% of cases are documented as transmitted.

RISK FACTORS

Consuming tissue known to be contaminated with an agent of an animal TSE is a risk. This is the presumed cause of BSE. The TSE Kuru was shown to be associated with ritual cannibalism. Iatrogenic disease from cornea or dura mater transplant, invasive EEG leads, contaminated neurosurgical equipment, and through giving contaminated growth hormone extracts are known risks.
Receiving a blood transfusion from a patient with CJD is a theoretical risk, which has led to changes in blood collection and distribution policies.

PREGNANCY

No known risk.

ASSOCIATED CONDITIONS

- Variants
  - —Heidenhain—cortical blindness, occipital lobe involvement
  - —Brownell-Oppenheimer—cerebellar predominant
  - —Stern-Garcia—basal ganglia and thalamus predominant
  - —Panencephalitic—white matter involvement; more common in Japan
- Gerstmann-Strausler syndrome (GSS) is a variant of inherited CJD with prominent cerebellar signs. Pathologic changes predominate in the cerebellum.
- Familial fatal insomnia (FFI) is an inherited form of CJD in which insomnia, autonomic, and behavioral abnormalities predominate. Pathologic changes are most prominent in the thalamus and basal ganglia.
- Variant CJD (vCJD) is a rare form of the disease, seen predominantly in young adults in Great Britain, associated with the BSE epidemic in that country.
- Kuru is the form of the disease associated with ritual cannibalism in New Guinea. Cerebellar signs predominate. Amyloid plaques in the cerebellum ("Kuru plaques") are characteristic.

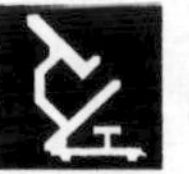

Diagnosis

DIFFERENTIAL DIAGNOSIS

Several weeks or months into the disease, the rapid progression of the dementia and appearance of myoclonus make the diagnosis certain.
Early CJD may resemble any adult dementing illness—degenerative, infectious, metabolic, or reversible in etiology. Most can be ruled out by appropriate laboratory and radiologic testing.

- Alzheimer disease
- Parkinson disease
- Amyotrophic lateral sclerosis
- Frontotemporal dementia
- Vascular dementia
- CNS vasculitis
- AIDS dementia
- Progressive multifocal leukoencephalopathy
- Progressive supranuclear palsy
- Tertiary syphilis
- Subacute sclerosing panencephalitis
- Infectious encephalitis
- Toxic encephalopathy—bismuth, bromides, lithium
- Adult-onset leukodystrophies
- Brain tumor, particularly frontal or diffuse

SIGNS AND SYMPTOMS

- Early
  - —Asthenia, insomnia, mild anorexia, fatigue
  - —Rapidly progressive dementia
  - —Cerebellar signs—ataxia, incoordination
  - —Extrapyramidal signs—rigidity, choreoathetoid movements
  - —Behavioral problems
  - —Myoclonus, with startle and persisting during sleep
  - —Visual difficulties—blurring or decreased acuity
- Late
  - —Akinetic mutism
- Occasional signs
  - —Fasciculations, muscle atrophy, focal cortical signs

LABORATORY PROCEDURES

No standard laboratory test assists in the diagnosis, although the lack of abnormalities may help to rule out other conditions.
CSF analysis of the 14-3-3 protein and neuron-specific enolase are gaining popularity, and elevated levels correlate with disease, although the tests may be positive in other degenerative brain disorders.
The diagnostic surgical biopsy is still the gold standard, but small biopsies away from areas of clinical involvement may yield equivocal or negative results.
Autopsy confirmation may be necessary, or requested by the family.

IMAGING STUDIES

- Nonspecific cerebral atrophy may be seen on CT late in the disease.
- MRI may show high signal intensities in the basal ganglia or other gray matter in T2-weighted images.
- SPECT scan shows an irregular decrease in metabolic activity predominantly in gray matter.

SPECIAL TESTS

EEG will show characteristic periodic high-voltage sharply contoured discharges, particularly as the disease progresses. It may be normal early in the disease.

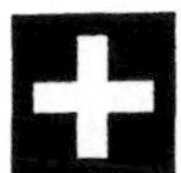

Management

GENERAL MEASURES

- Support, particularly of family.
- Counsel family on noninfectious nature of disease.
- Hospice care

SURGICAL MEASURES

Diagnostic biopsy is reserved for unusual cases, or where antemortem confirmation is required.

SYMPTOMATIC TREATMENT

See medications, below.

ADJUNCTIVE TREATMENT

None

ADMISSION/DISCHARGE CRITERIA

Rarely a cause for admission to hospital, except for complicating comorbidities. Consider hospice admission later in disease when patient cannot be cared for at home.

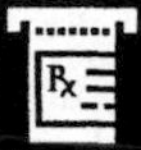

Medications

DRUG(S) OF CHOICE

There is no known treatment to reverse the disease in humans. Phenothiazine derivatives, quinacrine, and chlorpromazine have been shown to inhibit the production of prion proteins in cell culture; they are unproven to date in humans. Clinical trials are in process.

ALTERNATIVE DRUGS

Myoclonus may be treated with clonazepam (0.5–1 mg tid) if necessary. Consider antidepressant therapy or antianxiety therapy as needed.

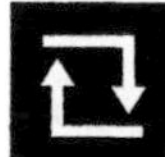

Follow-Up

PATIENT MONITORING

Prior to definitive diagnosis, careful workup to exclude all treatable causes of disease is necessary.

EXPECTED COURSE AND PROGNOSIS

The median survival is 4 to 8 months, with almost all patients dead within 2 years.

PATIENT EDUCATION

The primary education is for the family, preparing them for the devastating course of the disease. Careful counseling on the nature of transmissible as opposed to infectious disease is necessary, to allow proper home or hospice care. Health care workers performing EEGs or invasive testing should be informed of the diagnosis. Funeral directors should be notified of the diagnosis. Autopsy should be requested to confirm the diagnosis in all cases.

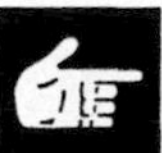

Miscellaneous

SYNONYMS

Jakob-Creutzfeldt disease

ICD-9-CM: 046.1 Creutzfeldt-Jakob disease; 294.10 CJD with dementia; 294.11 CJD with behavioral disturbance

SEE ALSO: N/A

REFERENCES

- Brown P, Preece M, Brandel JP, et al. Iatrogenic Creutzfeldt-Jakob disease at the millennium. Neurology 2000;55: 1075–1081.
- Burkhard PR, Sanchez JC, Landis T, et al. CSF detection of the 14-3-3 protein in unselected patients with dementia. Neurology 2001;56:1528–1533.
- Collinge J. Variant Creutzfeldt Jakob disease. Lancet 1999;354:217–323.
- Korth C, May BCH, Cohenm FE, et al. Acridine and phenothiazine derivatives as pharmacotherapeutics for prion diseases. Proc Natl Acad Sci USA 2001;98: 9836–9841.
- Pruisner SB. Shattuck Lecture–neurodegenerative disorders and prions. N Engl J Med 2001;344:1516–1526.
- Schroter A, Serr I, Henkel K, et al. Magnetic resonance imaging in the clinical diagnosis of Creutzfeldt-Jakob disease. Arch Neurol 2000;57:1751–1757.

Author(s): Brian W. Little, MD, PhD

Decompression Sickness

Basics

DESCRIPTION

Decompression sickness (DCS) develops when nitrogen gas, in solution at an elevated concentration within the bloodstream and tissues at depth, forms bubbles after rapid lowering of ambient pressure, with subsequent ischemia, inflammation, and mechanical disruption of the nervous system.

EPIDEMIOLOGY

Incidence/Prevalence

Estimated incidence of DCS is 1 case per 5,000 to 10,000 dives for recreational scuba divers; 1 case per 500 to 1,000 dives for commercial divers.

Race

No studies have demonstrated any ethnic predominance.

Age

Adults of all ages are at risk for DCS; risk is increased in older patients. The peak incidence of DCS is in the fourth and fifth decades.

Sex

Reported more often in men than women (due to the substantially lower number of women engaged in diving). Women may be at increased risk for DCS.

ETIOLOGY

Exposure to elevated ambient pressure causes partial pressures of the gases in the breathing mixture to increase proportionately and reach a new equilibrium within the tissues. Although oxygen is actively metabolized within tissues, nitrogen is an inert gas that will become dissolved in tissues and body fluids until saturation, proportional to the ambient pressure. The diver will be at risk for DCS only if there is a sudden reduction of the ambient pressure. If the ambient pressure is decreased slowly (i.e., careful, slow ascent to the surface), the nitrogen can be passively transferred down concentration gradients from tissues into the bloodstream and then to the lungs, where off-gassing can occur. In cases where ambient pressure is reduced rapidly, the potential for bubble formation will depend on the depth of the dive, length of time at depth, and the rate of ascent. If the ambient pressure is released too quickly, nitrogen dissolved in tissues will need to reach a new equilibrium, such that excess gas that cannot remain in solution will form bubbles. In type II neurologic DCS, the brain, spinal cord, cranial and peripheral nerves, and/or neural vasculature are affected by bubble formation. If the concentration of bubbles reaches a certain threshold, nervous system structures may be damaged by mechanical disruption, tissue compression, vascular stenosis or obstruction, and activation of inflammatory pathways (e.g., leukocyte cytokines, complement). Cerebral DCS (30–40% of cases) most often involves the arterial circulation, while spinal cord DCS (50–60% of cases) more typically involves obstruction of venous drainage from the cord.

Genetics

Genetic factors have not been identified.

PREGNANCY

Pregnancy may increase the risk for developing DCS. If DCS were to occur in a pregnant diver, the fetus would be at risk for significant damage from bubble formation. In general, it is recommended that pregnant women refrain from diving.

ASSOCIATED CONDITIONS

Air gas embolism (AGE): DCS and AGE can occur together and the combined syndrome is referred to as decompression illness.

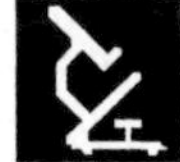

Diagnosis

DIFFERENTIAL DIAGNOSIS

An alternative diagnosis to DCS should be considered if severe symptoms begin more than 6 hours after return to atmospheric pressure without altitude exposure, if any symptom develops more than 24 hours after surfacing, or if a diver fails to improve despite prompt recompression treatment.

- Contaminated breathing gas (carbon monoxide)
- Near drowning and hypoxic brain injury
- Ingestion of toxic seafood—ciguatera, puffer fish, paralytic shellfish
- Envenomation—sea snake, cone shell
- Migraine
- Guillain-Barré syndrome
- Porphyria
- Multiple sclerosis
- Transverse myelitis
- Spinal cord compression
- Middle ear or sinus barotrauma with cranial nerve compression
- Inner ear barotrauma
- Oxygen toxicity with seizure
- Unrelated seizure
- Ischemic or hemorrhagic stroke
- Subarachnoid hemorrhage

SIGNS AND SYMPTOMS

Greater than 50% of patients with neurologic DCS have onset of symptoms within 1 hour of returning to atmospheric pressure. Within 6 hours, more than 90% of patients will have become symptomatic. The thoracic spinal cord is the most commonly affected region of the nervous system. The most frequent symptoms are numbness and paresthesias of the trunk that often begin in a band-like pattern and then progressively worsen, ascending weakness of the lower extremities that may progress to paralysis, and bowel and bladder dysfunction. Less often, patients develop cervical cord involvement with quadriparesis or quadriplegia. General cerebral symptoms can manifest as headache, confusion, fatigue, lethargy, change in personality, or poor concentration. Focal symptoms and signs are numerous and may include hemiparesis, hemisensory loss, ataxia, loss of vision or hemianopsia, dysphasia, and gait disturbance. When DCS involves the inner ear, patients usually complain of vertigo, sensorineural hearing loss, nausea, emesis, and tinnitus. On neurologic examination, the most common findings are weakness (legs more often than arms), sensory deficits, gait disturbance, ataxia, visual dysfunction, and alterations of consciousness.

LABORATORY PROCEDURES

N/A

IMAGING STUDIES

CT scans are relatively insensitive to the structural changes induced by DCS. MRI T2-weighted images may show high-signal abnormalities within the brain or spinal cord. Regions of injury are often swollen and edematous, but usually do not enhance with administration of contrast. MRI of the brain correlates with the clinical symptoms in approximately 55% of neurologic DCS patients, while imaging of the spinal cord correlates in one third of patients.

SPECIAL TESTS

- EEG and evoked potentials may be helpful to determine the extent of injury and follow recovery from neurologic DCS. However, these tests are not sensitive enough to recommend routine use, especially in the acute setting. Neuropsychological testing may be helpful to screen for subtle cognitive and motor deficits that may not be detectable on the bedside neurologic examination.
- Audiography and electronystagmography are sensitive tests that may be helpful in cases of vestibular DCS.

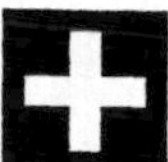

Management

GENERAL MEASURES

- Initial management of DCS occurs in the field, most often at some form of dive site (e.g., lake, dive boat, ocean beach). The patient should be assessed for adequacy of the airway, ventilation, pulse, and blood pressure. Cardiopulmonary resuscitation should be initiated in appropriate patients. In all cases, 100% oxygen should be started immediately. The patient should be placed in the supine position and prepared for transport to a medical facility with a recompression chamber.
- During transport the patient should be monitored carefully for further deterioration (e.g., shock). If the patient is unconscious or apneic, intubation and mechanical ventilation should be initiated. Proper ventilation with 100% oxygen should continue. Intravenous fluids should be started, since dehydration is common in DCS. In patients suspected of spinal cord DCS, the bladder should be catheterized and the urine output monitored.

SURGICAL MEASURES

There are no beneficial surgical procedures for DCS.

SYMPTOMATIC TREATMENT

- The definitive treatment for DCS is recompression therapy, using algorithms established by the United States Navy (USN). The treatment algorithm used most often for patients with neurologic DCS is USN Table 6. The patient is recompressed to 60 FsW, breathing 100% oxygen, for a total of 60 minutes. Three brief periods of air breathing (5 minutes each) are interposed during this initial recompression to reduce the risk of oxygen toxicity. The patient is then decompressed to 30 FsW for two additional periods each of breathing pure oxygen (60 minute sessions) and air (15 minute sessions). The total treatment takes 4 ¾ hours. For patients with incomplete resolution of symptoms and signs, the treatment may be extended to as long as 12 hours. More complex treatment algorithms can be used for severely ill patients.
- Recompression therapy reduces the bubble volume in tissues and body fluids by allowing easier reabsorption and dissipation of the bubbles.

ADJUNCTIVE TREATMENT

- Aggressive hydration with isotonic fluids may accelerate off-gassing of nitrogen and is recommended for all patients. Because neurologic injury can be exacerbated by hyperglycemia, intravenous solutions should not contain glucose. Blood glucose levels should be monitored and kept at or below 200 mg/dL. Some form of prophylaxis against deep vein thrombosis is recommended for patients with spinal or severe cerebral DCS, in which there may be a risk for venous thrombosis and pulmonary embolism. Fevers should be treated aggressively, since hyperthermia may aggravate neurologic injury.
- Rehabilitation and physical therapy are helpful in DCS patients with residual neurologic deficits. Function may slowly improve for several months to years after the effects of recompression therapy have plateaued.

ADMISSION/DISCHARGE CRITERIA

Patients are generally admitted for acute evaluation and recompression therapy as outlined above. Patients with significant residual neurologic deficits following treatment should be considered for inpatient or aggressive outpatient rehabilitation.

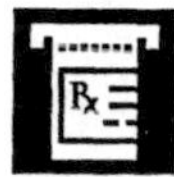

Medications

DRUG(S) OF CHOICE

There are no medications specific for DCS. Other than recompression therapy, oxygen is the only specific therapeutic intervention that expedites and enhances recovery. Aspirin and corticosteroids are often used; however, there is no conclusive evidence for benefit.

ALTERNATIVE DRUGS

N/A

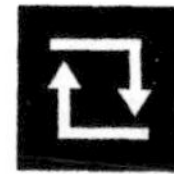

Follow-Up

PATIENT MONITORING

Follow-up of neurologic status is required.

EXPECTED COURSE AND PROGNOSIS

Prognosis for complete recovery following neurologic DCS is good for military and commercial divers, with relief of all symptoms reported in 95% and 70% of patients, respectively, after prompt recompression therapy. For recreational divers, the prognosis is more guarded. Recent data indicate that residual symptoms exist after treatment in 75% of recreational divers with severe DCS and 46% of those with mild to moderate cases of DCS. The poorer outcomes in recreational divers are likely related to delays in the initiation of recompression therapy and less frequent utilization of surface oxygen at the dive site.

PATIENT EDUCATION/ORGANIZATIONS

The Divers Alert Network (DAN), at Duke University Medical Center in Durham, North Carolina, maintains a database of information related to diving injuries, including the location of recompression facilities around the world. They are able to provide instant referral for potentially injured divers to the nearest facility that can properly manage DCS. DAN also has a 24-hour hotline for consultation on suspected dive injuries: 919-684-8111.

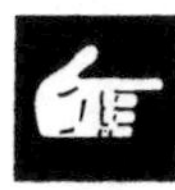

Miscellaneous

SYNONYMS

N/A

ICD-9-CM: 434.1 Embolism to brain, unspecified; 336.1 Embolism to spinal cord, unspecified; 386.9 Unspecified vertiginous syndromes and labyrinthine disorders.

SEE ALSO: N/A

REFERENCES

- Aharon-Peretz J, Adir Y, Gordon CR, et al. Spinal cord decompression sickness in sport diving. Arch Neurol 1993;50:753–756.
- Dutka AJ, Francis TJ. Pathophysiology of decompression sickness. In: Bove AA, ed. Bove and Davis' diving medicine, 3rd ed. Philadelphia: WB Saunders, 1997:159–175.
- Greer HD, Massey EW. Neurologic injury from undersea diving. Neurol Clin 1992;10:1031–1045.
- Moon RE. Treatment of decompression sickness and arterial gas embolism. In: Bove AA, ed. Bove and Davis' diving medicine, 3rd ed. Philadelphia: WB Saunders, 1997:184–204.
- Warren LP, Djang WT, Moon RE, et al. Neuroimaging of scuba diving injuries to the CNS. Am J Radiol 1988;151:1003–1008.

Author(s): Herbert B. Newton, MD

Dementia, General

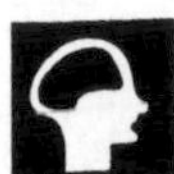

Basics

DESCRIPTION

Dementia is progressive impairment of memory and cognition that interferes with a patient's work and social relationships. Level of consciousness and attention are preserved in dementia. It is important to recognize that although Alzheimer's disease is the most common form of dementia, there are many other types that can be diagnosed premorbidly by careful clinical evaluation. Frequently, prominent presenting symptoms such as personality changes, or associated neurologic complaints such as gait change, or clinical course such as rate of progression can direct the differential diagnosis.

EPIDEMIOLOGY

Incidence/Prevalence

Alzheimer's disease affects 5% to 10% of elderly Caucasian Americans. Similar prevalence in blacks, Hispanics, and Americans of Japanese descent when corrected for age and level of education. Prevalence increases exponentially with age. Prevalence doubles with every 5-year increase in age. It is estimated in people age 90 to 95 years old, the prevalence is possibly as high as 30% to 40%. It is unknown if the prevalence continues to increase after age 95. Incidence is estimated at 0.6% in patients 65 years old and older per year in one study where mild to severely demented cases were included.

Age

Alzheimer's disease increases with age; see above.

Sex

Females are affected more than males, even when corrected for life span.

ETIOLOGY

The following is a list of causes of dementia by disease category.

- Trauma: dementia pugilista; diffuse axonal injury, hemorrhage; chronic subdural hematoma; postconcussion syndrome
- Inflammation/infection: chronic meningitis (tuberculosis, cryptococcus)
- Syphilis
- Post-herpes simplex encephalitis
- Focal cerebritis/abscess
- HIV dementia and opportunistic infections
- Progressive multifocal leukoencephalopathy
- Creutzfeldt-Jakob disease
- Lyme encephalopathy
- Sarcoidosis
- Subacute sclerosing panencephalitis
- Whipple's disease of the brain
- Neoplastic: tumor—benign; tumor—malignant, primary or metastatic; paraneoplastic limbic encephalitis
- Metabolic: hypothyroidism; vitamin B_{12} deficiency; vitamin B_1 deficiency; vitamin E deficiency; nicotinic acid deficiency; uremia/dialysis dementia; chronic hepatic encephalopathy; chronic hypoglycemia encephalopathy
- Chronic hypercapnia/hyperviscosity/hypoxemia
- Addison's/Cushing's diseases
- Hartnup disease
- Vascular: multiinfarct dementia; Binswanger's encephalopathy; amyloid dementia; strokes in particular brain locations (thalamic, bifrontal, infratemporal); diffuse hypoxic/ischemic injury; mitochondrial encephalopathy, lactic acidosis, and stroke-like episodes (MELAS); and cerebral autosomal-dominant arteriopathy with subcortical infarcts and leukoencephalopathy (CADASIL)
- Autoimmune: systemic lupus erythematosus; isolated angiitis of the CNS
- Drugs/toxins: medications (beta blockers, neuroleptics, antidepressants, anticonvulsants); substance abuse (alcohol, marijuana, PCP); toxins (lead, mercury, arsenic)
- Demyelinating
- Multiple sclerosis, Schilder's, Balo's sclerosis
- Decompression sickness with demyelination
- Adrenoleukodystrophy
- Metachromatic leukodystrophy
- Obstructive: normal pressure hydrocephalus; obstructive hydrocephalus
- Degenerative—adult: Alzheimer's disease; Pick's disease; Parkinson's disease; Huntington's disease; frontotemporal dementia; progressive supranuclear palsy; diffuse cortical Lewy body disease; multisystem atrophy/spinocerebellar ataxias; primary progressive aphasia; corticobasal degeneration; Wilson's disease; Hallervorden-Spatz disease

Genetics

Genetics are applicable in some forms of Alzheimer's disease.

RISK FACTORS

These vary depending on the cause of dementia, for example:

- Vascular dementia: hypertension, diabetes, hypercholesterolemia
- Alzheimer's disease: age, sex, Apo-E genotype, prior history of head trauma, family history

PREGNANCY

N/A

ASSOCIATED CONDITIONS

Some dementias have associated neurologic symptoms (e.g., parkinsonian symptoms, cerebellar degeneration, motor neuron disease, etc.), or medical conditions. These depend on the specific diagnosis.

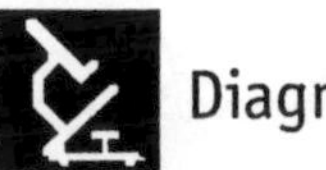

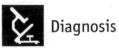

Diagnosis

DIFFERENTIAL DIAGNOSIS

- Normal aging
- Mild cognitive impairment (excessive, predominant memory loss with preservation of daily function)
- Psychiatric disorders (mood is affected predominantly)
- Toxic/confusional states or encephalopathy (level of attention and/or impaired consciousness present)

SIGNS AND SYMPTOMS

Once it has been established that the patient meets the criterion for dementia, the history of present illness should be directed toward soliciting presenting symptoms and associated medical conditions that suggest a specific diagnosis. These include the symptoms noted below, as well as speed of progression, mode of onset, associated focal neurologic deficits, presence or absence of headache, and incontinence. A thorough review of the patient's medications, assessment of patients vascular and HIV risk factors, alcohol use, and family history of dementia should be obtained. A review of systems that includes complaints that suggest associated medical illnesses is useful. Symptoms vary depending on the cause of dementia. They can include but are not limited to the following:

- Memory loss
- Personality changes
- Incontinence
- Language and naming difficulties
- Difficulty using everyday objects
- Disorientation
- Poor judgment
- Poor logic
- Hallucinations or delusions
- Wandering
- Abnormalities on a detailed neurologic exam can suggest a specific cause, such as asymmetric reflexes in vascular dementia or extraocular movement abnormalities in progressive supranuclear palsy.

LABORATORY PROCEDURES

- Initial evaluation should include CBC, liver function tests, sodium, calcium, thyroid stimulating hormone, RPR, vitamin B_{12} level.
- In appropriate circumstances, consider HIV testing or Lyme serology.
- Atypical presentations of dementia may require one of the following: ceruloplasmin and copper levels (Wilson's disease), plasma levels of very long chain fatty acids (adrenoleukodystrophy), WBC arylsulfatase A (metachromatic leukodystrophy), vitamin E and B_1 levels, porphyrins, blood gas, hemoglobin A_{1C}, tumor markers (anti-Hu/Yo/Ri), ANA/vasculitis workup, urinary heavy metals, thyroid antibodies, toxicology screen.

IMAGING STUDIES

- CAT scan of head without contrast; consider brain MRI especially in dementias not typical of Alzheimer's disease or suspected vascular dementia.
- PET/SPECT can be useful in diagnosing Alzheimer's disease.
- Tumor screen if limbic encephalitis is considered.

SPECIAL TESTS

- EEG and cerebral arteriography are appropriate in certain circumstances. Examples include Creutzfeldt-Jakob disease and CNS vasculitis, respectively.
- Bedside neuropsychologic testing
  - —Standardized testing including the Mini-Mental Status Exam and the Clinical Dementia Rating Scale. These provide objective, reproducible scores for future comparison.
  - —Tests of memory, orientation, attention, calculation, reading, writing, naming, drawing, abstraction, praxis
  - —Observation of comportment, judgment, and insight
- Formal neuropsychological testing: can be used to aid in diagnosis, assess severity, dissect out superimposed depression, and provide formal documentation of impairment for disability applications and legal purposes.
- The following biomarkers are available but not yet generally accepted for clinical diagnosis:
  - —Genetic tests such as serum apoE-4, and tests for the presenilin gene
  - —CSF analysis for the A beta form of the amyloid precursor protein and tau

Diagnostic Procedures

- Lumbar puncture should be considered in the following circumstances:
  - —Age <60
  - —Rapid progression
  - —Immunocompromised patient
  - —Cancer
  - —Reactive syphilis or Lyme serology
  - —Unusual clinical presentation
  - —CNS infection
  - —Systemic infection
  - —Connective tissue diseases
  - —CNS vasculitis
  - —For 14-3-3 (Creutzfeldt-Jakob protein) testing
- Brain biopsy should be considered in unusual cases as follows:
  - —Focal, relevant lesions of undetermined cause, after extensive evaluation
  - —CNS vasculitis
  - —Subacute sclerosing panencephalitis
  - —Progressive multifocal leukoencephalopathy where lymphoma cannot be conclusively ruled out by neuroimaging or spinal fluid analysis
  - —Degenerative neurologic illnesses such as Kufs' disease, Alexander's disease.
- Muscle biopsy in suspected mitochondrial disorders

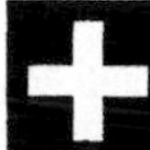

Management

GENERAL MEASURES

- Treat any reversible causes of dementia.
- Evaluate for superimposed illnesses or depression and treat them.
- Establish an etiologic diagnosis and institute therapy for specific cause.
- Determine if specific pharmacologic intervention is appropriate, such as centrally acting acetylcholinesterase inhibitors in Alzheimer's disease.
- Identify and address symptoms that brought the patient to medical attention, e.g., patient's and/or caregivers' primary concerns.
- Suggest to patients that they may want to consider designating a family member who will help with future legal and financial decisions.
- Assess patients' personal security (for instance, in regard to wandering, judgment, and monitoring their own medications) as well as possible threats to public safety (driving).

SURGICAL MEASURES

N/A

SYMPTOMATIC TREATMENT

Depends on the specific diagnosis. Risperidone has been shown to reduce psychotic symptoms and aggression in demented patients. Selective serotonin reuptake inhibitors (SSRIs) may be useful in depressed patients with dementia.

ADJUNCTIVE TREATMENT

- Activity: low levels of exercise may aid in behavioral management in agitated, demented patients.
- Diet: anorexia may complicate dementia or be a side effect of its treatment, so weight should be monitored and it may be appropriate to eliminate dietary restrictions.

ADMISSION/DISCHARGE CRITERIA

Usually managed as an outpatient, may require admission for evaluation of rapid decline, advanced workup (biopsy), or caregiver's inability to care for the patient at home.

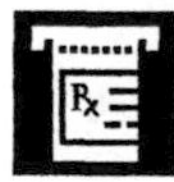

Medications

DRUG(S) OF CHOICE

Depends on the specific cause of dementia. Refer to the chapters on specific causes of dementia for information on their treatment. Gingko biloba has been found to improve cognition and is well tolerated in studies where multiple causes of dementia were included; the largest effect is seen in Alzheimer's patients.

ALTERNATIVE DRUGS

N/A

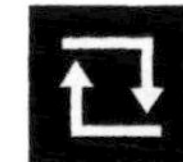

Follow-Up

PATIENT MONITORING

Depends on the specific cause of dementia.

EXPECTED COURSE AND PROGNOSIS

Generally, relentless decline, although with periods of stability; fluctuations in severity and speed of progression vary depending on type.

PATIENT EDUCATION

- Discussion of patient's diagnosis and prognosis.
- Explain necessity of changing routines and expectations in response to the disease.
- Educate family about stages of disease and changes in patient's daily function.
- Educate about risk of stress, enlisting the help of friends and family and need for occasional respite. The NIH's Web site has information on experimental research trials in various aspects and causes of dementia: *www.ninds.nih.gov//nindsnotes2000.htm#ad.*

Miscellaneous

SYNONYMS

None. Consider specific diagnosis.

ICD-9-CM: 294.8 Dementia; 294.1 Dementia in conditions classified elsewhere; 331.0 Alzheimer's disease; 046.1 Jakob-Creutzfeldt disease; 290.4 Dementia—arteriosclerotic (simple type) (uncomplicated); 331.3 Communicating hydrocephalus; 331.1 Pick's disease

SEE ALSO: ALZHEIMER'S DISEASE

REFERENCES

- Kukull WA, Ganguli M. Epidemiology of dementia: concepts and overview. Neurol Clin 2000;18(4):923.
- Morris JC. The nosology of dementia. Neurol Clin 2000;18(4):773.
- Peterson RC. Aging, mild cognitive impairment, and Alzheimer's disease. Neurol Clin 2000;18(4):789.
- Schmahmann J. Clinical profiles and differential diagnosis of dementia. Presented at May 2001 Comprehensive Update on Dementia, Harvard Medical School, Department of Continuing Medical Education.
- Warner J, Butler R. Alzheimer's disease. Clin Evidence 2001;5:630–641.

Author(s): Lorraine Spikol, MD

Dementia, Alzheimer's Disease

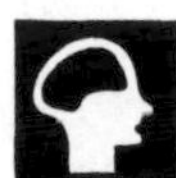

Basics

DESCRIPTION

Alzheimer's disease (AD) is the most common form of degenerative dementia. It is characterized pathologically by neurofibrillary tangles, neuritic plaques, and neuronal loss starting first in the entorhinal cortex, hippocampus, and the temporal and parietal association cortex before affecting frontal association cortex.

EPIDEMIOLOGY

Incidence/Prevalence

Age-specific incidence of 0.5%, 2%, and 5% at age 70, 80, and 90, respectively. Age-specific prevalence of 3% at ages 65 to 74, 18% at ages 75 to 84, and 30% to 47% at ages 85 and over.

Age

Typically >60 but some genetic cases as young as the late thirties.

Sex

Female/male ratio of 2:1.

Race

Higher rates reported in African Americans and Hispanics, but effect wanes when controlling for education level. Rural Chinese and Nigerians have lower prevalence rates.

ETIOLOGY

- Genetic and sporadic forms
- Amyloid hypothesis: either overproduction or decreased metabolism of amyloid beta peptide lead to a toxic state causing degeneration of neuronal processes, neuritic plaque formation, and eventually neuronal loss and clinical dementia.
- Tau hypothesis: abnormally phosphorylated tau proteins (tauopathy) accumulate in neurons as neurofibrillary tangles and ultimately cause neuronal death.
- Other suggested etiologies: disorder of immune function, oxidative stress, excitatory amino acid toxicity, and primary mitochondrial abnormality.
- There is little evidence for aluminum intoxication, viral infections, or prion diseases as causes of AD.

Genetics

- Autosomal dominant with age-dependent penetrance: 40% to 50%.
- 2% have known mutations on chromosomes 21, 14, or 1 with onset late 30s to early 50s.
- Trisomy 21 (Down syndrome) individuals develop AD pathology after age 35 and clinical AD symptoms by age 50.
- Chromosome 19 carries the apolipoprotein E gene, a cholesterol transport and AD susceptibility gene. The $\epsilon 4$ allele is a risk factor for AD, while the $\epsilon 2$ allele appears to be protective.

RISK FACTORS

- Definite risk factors: increasing age, being female, increased apolipoprotein E $\epsilon 4$ allele load, and family history of AD, dementia, or Down syndrome.
- Possible risk factors: history of significant head trauma with loss of consciousness, myocardial infarction, coronary artery disease, and cerebral white matter disease.
- Protective factors: higher educational achievement, increased apolipoprotein E $\epsilon 2$ allele load, use of estrogens in postmenopausal women, use of cholesterol-lowering statin medications, rheumatoid arthritis, and taking nonsteroidal antiinflammatory drugs for longer than 2 years.

PREGNANCY

No relationship known.

ASSOCIATED CONDITIONS

N/A

Diagnosis

DIFFERENTIAL DIAGNOSIS

- Acute confusional states and delirium
- Vascular dementia
- Frontotemporal degenerations (i.e., Pick's disease)
- Dementia with Lewy bodies
- Parkinson plus syndromes
- Huntington's disease
- Traumatic dementias
- Neoplastic and paraneoplastic dementias
- Hydrocephalic dementias
- CNS vasculitis
- Toxic dementias
- Uremia
- Hepatic encephalopathy
- B_{12}, folate, or niacin deficiencies
- Thyroid, parathyroid, or adrenal conditions
- Hypoxic encephalopathy
- Infectious dementias
- Multiple sclerosis
- Depression

SIGNS AND SYMPTOMS

- Course: insidious onset, gradually progressive over years.
- Elemental neurologic examination: normal until very late.
- Mild-stage AD: disorientation to date, mild anomia, low verbal fluency, impaired delayed recall, difficulties copying 3-D figures (cube), trouble with bill paying and complicated financial transactions, diminished insight, irritability, and apathy.
- Moderate-stage AD: disorientation (time and place), fluent aphasia, difficulties with comprehension, impaired delayed recall, impaired recognition memory, getting lost in familiar areas, difficulties in copying 2-D figures, impaired calculations, concrete abstractions, poor judgment, trouble with instrumental activities of daily living (cooking, shopping, and handiwork), and increased behavioral symptoms (aggression, restlessness, psychosis, sleep disturbance, and dysphoria).
- Severe-stage AD: unable to use language effectively, may become mute, memory only for the moment, unable to find one's way around one's home, need assistance with basic ADLs (bathing, dressing, and toileting) due to increasing apraxia, urinary and fecal incontinence, and often troublesome behavioral symptoms.

LABORATORY PROCEDURES

- Lab tests are used to rule out other dementias.
- Apolipoprotein E genotyping is seldom useful.
- Genetic markers for known chromosome mutations are only useful to consider in patients in their early 50s or younger with a significant family history of dementia.
- Biomarkers for AD including reduced beta amyloid peptide and elevated tau protein in CSF, and increased neural thread proteins in urine and CSF need to be more sensitive before they are recommended for routine use.

IMAGING STUDIES

- CT or MRI scans show atrophy in AD and can rule out other conditions.
- MRI volumetric measurement of hippocampus and entorhinal cortex atrophy is 95% sensitive but only 40% specific for AD.
- Functional imaging using single photon emission computed tomography (SPECT) and positron emission tomography (PET) may be helpful for early diagnosis and typically shows bilateral temporal and parietal hypoperfusion and hypometabolism respectively. These patterns on SPECT and PET predict the risk of progression to AD in mild cognitive impairment (MCI) subjects in 83% and 94%, respectively.
- Functional MRI (fMRI) shows increased activation during memory tasks in individuals at high risk for AD.
- Functional imaging techniques are not routinely recommended at this time.

SPECIAL TESTS

- Mental status examination or neuropsychological testing profiles a patient's cognitive functioning and should be done in every suspected AD case. It is the most sensitive tool we have for early diagnosis.
- The earliest changes on mental status examination include difficulties with memory, language, visuospatial skills, orientation, and problem-solving abilities.

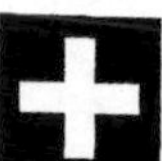

Management

GENERAL MEASURES

- AD patients underreport symptoms of coincidental illness, infection, dehydration, and pain that cause increased disability if not discovered and treated.
- Minimize adverse drug effects and drug interactions. Avoid anticholinergic and benzodiazepine medications.
- Provide adequate supervision for medication compliance, proper nutritional intake, and accident prevention.
- Minimize sensory deprivation by social stimulation, vision and hearing care.
- Watch for overstimulation that may cause agitation.
- In early stages, limit driving to local areas during daytime and good weather. Caregivers should ride with patients monthly to ensure they are driving safely with good judgment.

SURGICAL MEASURES

None available.

SYMPTOMATIC TREATMENT

- Cholinesterase inhibitors are the only approved drugs for AD treatment in the U.S., providing, in mild to moderate disease, efficacy for cognitive and functional impairments compared to placebo. Most also show behavioral symptom improvement. Typically, these medications stabilize symptoms for 1 year but continue to offer advantages over no treatment for another 5 years.
- Vitamin E and selegiline showed disease-modifying benefits in one study.

ADJUNCTIVE TREATMENT

- The behavioral abnormalities seen with AD are treated with symptom-specific agents including antidepressants, antipsychotics, and mood stabilizers.
- Antiinflammatory drugs, estrogen in women, and statin (lipid-lowering) medications may reduce the risk or delay the onset of AD.

ADMISSION/DISCHARGE CRITERIA

- Patients are occasionally admitted for wandering or aggressive behaviors.
- Provide a sitter to ensure patient safety when delirium or acute confusional states occur.
- Low-dose antipsychotics are the most effective and tolerated agents for acute agitation.

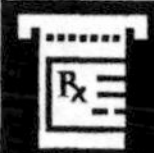

Medications

DRUG(S) OF CHOICE

Cognitive Therapy

- Cholinesterase inhibitors (strive for highest recommended dose): donepezil 5 mg/d for 6 weeks then 10 mg/d; or galanthamine 4 mg bid for 4 weeks then 8 mg bid for 4 weeks then 12 mg bid; or rivastigmine 1.5 mg bid for 4 weeks then 3 mg bid for 4 weeks then 4.5 mg bid for 4 weeks then 6 mg bid
- Antioxidants: Vitamin E 1000 IU bid

Behavioral Therapy

- Depression or anxiety: selective serotonin reuptake inhibitors (SSRIs)
- Psychosis: quetiapine 25 mg qhs to 75 mg bid or risperidone 0.25 mg qd to 1.0 mg bid or olanzapine 2.5 to 10 mg qd
- Sleep disturbance: trazodone 50 to 150 mg qhs
- Restless behaviors: citalopram 20 to 40 mg qd or divalproex sodium 125 to 500 mg bid
- Aggression: SSRIs or antipsychotics or mood stabilizers (divalproex sodium, carbamazepine)

Contraindications

- SSRIs: avoid monoamine oxidase inhibitors.
- Divalproex sodium: avoid in patients with hepatic dysfunction.
- Carbamazepine: avoid monoamine oxidase inhibitors and in patients with previous bone marrow depression.

Precautions

- Cholinesterase inhibitors: avoid medications with anticholinergic effects including: antihistamines, certain psychotropics.
- SSRIs: may cause hyponatremia and SIADH.
- Atypical antipsychotics: may lower seizure threshold; watch for orthostatic hypotension.
- Divalproex sodium: may cause hepatotoxicity, thrombocytopenia, teratogenicity, pancreatitis, and hyperammonemia; liver tests and platelet counts should be monitored.
- Carbamazepine: may cause aplastic anemia, hepatotoxicity; CBC and liver tests should be monitored.

ALTERNATIVE DRUGS

Cognitive Therapy

- Antioxidants: selegiline 10 mg qd

Behavioral Therapy

- Depression: venlafaxine, bupropion, nefazodone, nortriptyline, or mirtazapine
- Anxiety: buspirone, propranolol, or lorazepam
- Psychosis: haloperidol or clozapine
- Sleep disturbances: zolpidem
- Restless behaviors: other SSRIs
- Aggression: propranolol or buspirone

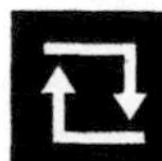

Follow-Up

PATIENT MONITORING

- Every 6 months measure cognitive status and ask about behavioral and functional abilities.
- Mini-Mental Status Examination (MMSE), the most commonly used evaluation tool, will decline 3 points per year on the average in untreated mild to moderate patients.

EXPECTED COURSE AND PROGNOSIS

Gradually progressive cognitive and functional declines leading to death.

PATIENT EDUCATION

Provide information about the disease, local Alzheimer's Association (*www.alz.org*), support groups, family counseling, social services, day-care services, in-home health care assistance, assisted living, long-term-care facilities, legal services, advanced directives, and financial planning.

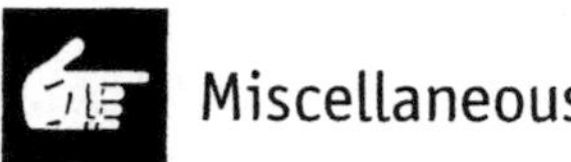

Miscellaneous

SYNONYMS

Senile or presenile dementia
Dementia of the Alzheimer's type

ICD-9-CM: 331.0 Alzheimer's disease; 290.0 Senile dementia; 290.1 Presenile dementia

SEE ALSO: DEMENTIA, GENERAL

REFERENCES

- Knopman DS, DeKosky ST, Cummings JL, et al. Practice parameter: diagnosis of dementia (an evidence-based review). Report of the Quality Standards Subcommittee of the American Academy of Neurology. Neurology 2001;56:1143–1153.
- Lautenschlager NT, Cupples LA, Rao VS, et al. Risk of dementia among relatives of Alzheimer's disease patients in the MIRAGE study. Neurology 1996;46:641–650.
- McKhann G, Drachman D, Folstein M, et al. Clinical diagnosis of Alzheimer's disease: report of the NINCDS-ADRDA work group under the auspices of the Department of Health and Human Services Task Force on Alzheimer's disease. Neurology 1984;34:939–944.
- Parks RW, Zec RF, Wilson RS, eds. Neuropsychology of Alzheimer's disease and other dementias. New York: Oxford University Press, 1993.
- Schneider LS. Treatment of Alzheimer's disease with cholinesterase inhibitors. Clin Geriatr Med 2001;17:337–358.

Author(s): Douglas W. Scharre, MD

Dermatomyositis

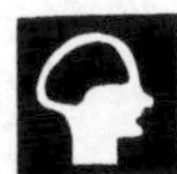

Basics

DESCRIPTION

An idiopathic inflammatory myopathy characterized by proximal muscle weakness and a characteristic rash. Dermatomyositis (DM) is epidemiologically, histologically, and immunologically distinct from the other idiopathic inflammatory myopathies, polymyositis (PM), and inclusion body myositis.

EPIDEMIOLOGY

Incidence/Prevalence

Uncommon, with an annual incidence of less than 1:100,000.

Age

Unique in that it can present at any age from infancy to adult. Juvenile form presents most commonly at ages 5 to 15.

Sex

Affects both males and females, with female preponderance.

Race

No known racial predominance.

ETIOLOGY

Based on histologic and immunologic studies of muscle biopsy, DM appears to result from a humorally mediated microangiopathy. The inciting event for this autoimmune phenomenon is not known. Deposits of IgM, IgG (less common), C3, C9, and the C5b-9 membrane attack complex (MAC) have been demonstrated in the perifascicular microvasculature and at the dermal–epidermal junction. The immunologic destruction of the microvasculature causes ischemic damage to perifascicular muscle fibers and recruitment of $CD4^+$ T cells, B cells, and macrophages. This secondary perimysial and perivascular infiltration by inflammatory cells then leads to further muscle damage.

Genetics

At this time, no genetic predisposition has been conclusively determined, although some investigators have proposed an association with certain human leukocyte antigen (HLA) haplotypes.

RISK FACTORS

None are known for idiopathic DM. Secondary DM is associated with the several overlap connective tissue diseases (see Associated Conditions, below).

PREGNANCY

There is no known relationship to pregnancy.

ASSOCIATED CONDITIONS

Autoimmune Diseases

Systemic lupus erythematosus, rheumatoid arthritis, scleroderma, mixed connective tissue disease, Sjögren's syndrome.

Neoplasia

Ovarian, lung, pancreatic, and colorectal (seen particularly in adults over 40 and peak incidence within 5 years of DM diagnosis).

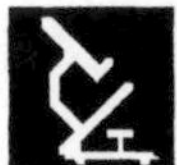

Diagnosis

DIFFERENTIAL DIAGNOSIS

Polymyositis
Inclusion body myositis
Connective tissue disease (sarcoidosis, SLE, mixed connective tissue disease)
Infectious myositis (viral, bacterial, helminthic, protozoan, fungal)
Toxic myopathy (illicit drugs and medications)
Eosinophilic myopathies
Endocrinopathies (hypothyroidism, hypercalcemia)

SIGNS AND SYMPTOMS

Classic DM presents with subacute (over weeks) proximal weakness and characteristic heliotrope (purple) rash over the eyes. Weakness predominantly involves the neck flexors, hip flexors/extensors, and shoulder girdle. Dysphagia is reported in up to one third of patients, but respiratory muscle involvement is rare. Sensation is unaltered and muscle stretch reflexes are maintained until severe involvement occurs. In addition to the heliotrope rash, sun-sensitive erythema, scaling, and telangiectasias may be found over the malar region and over the chest (V-sign), shoulders (shawl sign), knees, and elbows. Gottron's papules (red, scaly lesions) may be found over the joints of the dorsal hand; dilated capillaries may be seen in the nailfold bed. Cutaneous calcifications can be found over pressure points, especially in children with severe, long-standing disease.

Less common manifestations include:

- Arthropathy: joint contractures, arthralgias
- Cardiac involvement with cardiomegaly, dyspnea, arrhythmias
- Pulmonary: aspiration pneumonia in patients with significant pharyngeal and upper esophageal weakness, interstitial lung disease (5–10%)
- Necrotizing vasculitis: skin, muscle, gastrointestinal tract, retina, and kidney especially in childhood DM

LABORATORY PROCEDURES

Serum creatine kinase (CK) is the most sensitive and specific marker for muscle destruction and necrosis. CK is elevated in nearly 90% of patients at some point in disease progression and may be as high as 50 times normal; however, a random CK may be normal in approximately 30% of DM and persistently normal in 10%. Antinuclear antibodies (ANAs) may be found in 24% to 60% of DM but are more common when DM is associated with the overlap connective tissue diseases. The same is true for the ESR, which is usually normal or only mildly elevated in idiopathic DM. Certain myositis-specific antibodies may be found, including anti-Jo-1 and anti-Mi-2. Anti-Jo-1 is found in approximately 20% of the cases of PM and DM, and may predict a subset of patients destined to have interstitial lung disease and/or arthritic complications. CBC, chemistry panel, PSA, urinalysis, and stool for occult blood may also be checked for underlying malignancy. Referral for breast and pelvic examination for women and testicular and prostate for men may also be needed in malignancy workup.

IMAGING STUDIES

MR of affected muscles may show edema and inflammation, although this is not used routinely in evaluation. Chest radiography and mammography are useful in malignancy workup.

SPECIAL TESTS

- EMG is a good screening test for inflammatory myopathy and reveals increased insertional activity with polyphasic, short duration, and low-amplitude motor unit potentials and complex repetitive discharges. Also, positive sharp waves, fibrillations, and early recruitment are found.
- Muscle biopsy is the best test for pathologic confirmation of the disease and should be performed in the vast majority of cases. The typical pathology is that of perifascicular muscle fiber atrophy and decreased capillary density. Perimysial and perivascular inflammation with B cells and T-helper cells is present. Microvascular deposits of immunoglobulin and MAC, relatively specific to DM, are also found.

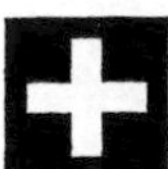

Management

GENERAL MEASURES

Medical therapy is primarily immunomodulation with corticosteroids or IVIG. High-dose oral prednisone (1.5 to 2 mg/kg/d) or IV methylprednisolone (1 g/d) is the initial treatment. In severe cases, however, some centers also consider IVIG for young patients to spare the steroid side effects. Steroids are slowly transitioned to alternate-day dosing over 2 to 4 weeks and maintained until strength returns to normal, plateaus, or shows no response after 3 to 6 months. Adjuvant medications are considered if there is little or no response to steroids, disease relapse upon tapering, or if side effects are intolerable.

SURGICAL MEASURES

Biopsy may be required for diagnosis. Surgical excision may be necessary for cutaneous calcinosis.

SYMPTOMATIC TREATMENT

Cardiac disease and hypertension secondary to steroid therapy require treatment. Arthritis can be managed with NSAIDs. An exacerbation of weakness during steroid taper requires immediate increased to double current dose (max 100 mg) daily for 2 to 3 weeks, followed by another taper.

ADJUNCTIVE TREATMENT

Physical, occupational, and speech therapy may be needed, depending on the affected muscle groups. Referral to dermatology for the rash and to ophthalmology may be necessary.

ADMISSION/DISCHARGE CRITERIA

Patients are admitted for severe weakness and/or respiratory compromise. Certain institutions may require admission for IV methylprednisolone or IVIG.

Medications

DRUG(S) OF CHOICE

- Prednisone: 1.5–2.0 mg/kg/d (maximum dose 100 mg) PO qAM for 2 to 4 weeks then switched over 2 to 4 weeks to qod regimen. Treat until maximum response or for 3 to 6 months and then slowly taper.
- A pulse of high-dose intravenous corticosteroids may be needed for severe presentations or exacerbations.
- Methylprednisolone (fulminant disease): 1 g IV qd × 3 to 6 doses followed by 1.5 mg/kg/d PO for 3 to 4 weeks
- IVIG: 2.0 g/kg over 2 days per month for 3 months. May need periodic booster infusions.

Contraindications

Immunosuppression should be avoided or minimized if an infection is identified. Prior history of hypersensitivity or allergic reaction to any of the above drugs may preclude their use.

Precautions

Corticosteroid therapy is associated with hypertension, gastric ulcers, hyperglycemia, cataracts, glaucoma, sodium retention, hypokalemia, osteopenia, and aseptic necrosis. Prophylaxis with H2 antagonists, calcium carbonate 1,200 to 1,500 mg qd, calcitriol 0.25 μg qd, bisphosphonate, and hormone replacement in postmenopausal women is recommended. A tuberculin skin test should be performed to screen for tuberculosis exposure before starting chronic corticosteroid treatment. Isoniazid may be necessary for those with positive PPD or history of tuberculosis. Bactrim should be given tiw for those on chronic oral prednisone (over 2 to 3 months). For IVIG, blood pressure, heart rate, and BUN/Cr should be monitored during and after infusion. Azathioprine and methotrexate require monthly liver enzyme and CBC, as leukopenia, anemia, and hepatotoxicity are dangerous side effects. All of these drugs should be prescribed only by individuals experienced with their potential toxicity.

ALTERNATIVE DRUGS

- The next best drugs:
  - —Azathioprine—1.5–2.0 mg/kg/d PO, or
  - —Methotrexate—7.5–15.0 mg PO once a week
- Other immunosuppressive drugs may be useful in steroid failures: cyclosporine, mycophenolate mofetil, tacrolimus, cyclophosphamide, and chlorambucil.

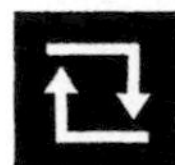

Follow-Up

PATIENT MONITORING

Patients are followed to monitor progression of symptoms, efficacy of therapy, and drug side effects.

EXPECTED COURSE AND PROGNOSIS

Partial response (improved strength) to corticosteroids is reported to be 58% to 100% and complete response of 30% to 66% within 6 months. Poor prognostic features include coexisting malignancy, cardiac involvement, lung involvement, and older age. Some patients may require 10 to 30 mg of prednisone qod for 2 or more years to achieve remission.

PATIENT EDUCATION

Myositis Association of America, 755 Cantrell Avenue, Suite C, Harrisonburg, VA 22801, *www.myositis.org.*
Muscular Dystrophy Association, 3300 E Sunrise Dr, Tucson, AZ 85718-3208, Phone 1-800-572-1717, *www.mdausa.org.*
NINDS Dermatomyositis Information Page Fact Sheet: *www.ninds.nih.gov/health_and_medical/disorders/dermato_doc.htm.*

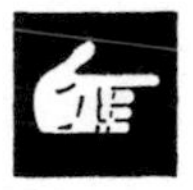

Miscellaneous

SYNONYMS

Idiopathic inflammatory myopathy

ICD-9-CM: 729.1 Myositis

SEE ALSO: POLYMYOSITIS, INCLUSION BODY MYOSITIS

REFERENCES

- Amato AA, Barohn RJ. Idiopathic inflammatory myopathies. Neurol Clin 1997;15:615–648.
- Choy EH, Isenberg DA. Treatment of dermatomyositis and polymyositis. Rheumatology 2002;41:7–13.
- Griggs RC, Mendell JR, Miller RG. Evaluation and treatment of myopathies. Philadelphia: F. A. Davis, 1995:154–167.
- Kissel JT. Misunderstandings, misinterpretations, and mistakes in the management of the inflammatory myopathies. Semin Neurol 2002;22:41–51.

Author(s): Ted Woodruff, MD

Developmental Delay

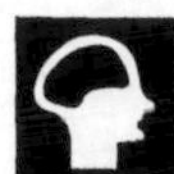

Basics

DESCRIPTION

Developmental delay is a common problem presenting to pediatricians and family physicians. Children with delayed development are usually identified in the preschool years. This review focuses on conditions that have symptoms affecting cognition or language development. Motor delays may be found as part of a global developmental dysfunction or be recognized as a form of cerebral palsy. Although the term *mental retardation* is little used by the lay public and educators, it is currently synonymous with *global developmental delay* in the medical literature.
Developmental delay is nonspecific, seldom provides an accurate diagnostic description of a child's disability, and should have restricted formal use as a presenting symptom or in situations where assessment and investigations have failed to yield a definitive diagnosis.

EPIDEMIOLOGY

Incidence/Prevalence

Mental retardation has an incidence of 2% to 3%, with the prevalence of mild retardation being inversely related to family socioeconomic status. Mild retardation affects 85% to 89%. An organic cause can be found in 55% to 75% of children with severe retardation who represent the smaller remaining proportion.

Sex

Twice as many males as females are affected.

ETIOLOGY

It is recognized that some children have delayed milestones or exhibit variations from normal. The norms and standard deviations from normal are well documented but, particularly in language development, are variable and broad (for example, lack of speech development in the hearing child may be acceptable to 2 to 3 years of age depending on a variety of factors if receptive language is age appropriate).
Disorders of cognition, language, and social development may have many different causes, the common factor being nonprogressive pathology affecting the CNS, including fetal environmental syndromes (*in utero* infection or toxic exposure), disorders of chromosomal or molecular genetics (Down syndrome and fragile X syndrome), and major brain dysgenesis or malformation. More severely affected children are usually identified in the first year of life.
Prenatal factors (including genetic conditions, neurometabolic disorders, neurocutaneous syndromes, and nonchromosomal dysmorphic syndromes) account for 60% to 70% of cases. Perinatal problems (prematurity, birth asphyxia, or injury) cause 10%, with postnatal brain injury (meningitis/encephalitis or trauma) being somewhat less than 10%.

RISK FACTORS

N/A

PREGNANCY

As a significant percentage of conditions with delayed development are prenatal in origin, the pregnancy history is critical to obtain information related to toxin exposures (fetal alcohol syndrome), teratogens (anticonvulsant and other medical treatment), infections (cytomegalovirus), and maternal trauma.

ASSOCIATED CONDITIONS

- Children with developmental delay may present with other disorders affecting brain growth and development. Motor delays may represent the initial symptoms of cerebral palsy (a nonprogressive disorder of movement and posture).
- Language disorders indicate that communication skills are significantly behind cognitive development; subtypes are mixed receptive and expressive disorders, expressive disorders, and conditions in which higher order language processing is affected.
- Autistic spectrum disorders including "classical" autism, pervasive developmental disorders, and Asperger syndrome are characterized by impaired social interactions and communication.
- Other common associated conditions are vision and hearing problems as well as attention deficit and hyperactivity disorders.

Diagnosis

DIFFERENTIAL DIAGNOSIS

- Developmental delay/mental retardation must be distinguished from primary speech and language disorders and autistic spectrum conditions. Children with isolated motor delays require evaluation for neuromuscular disorders (muscular dystrophy, congenital myopathies).
- Broad categories of etiologic diagnosis include malformations of brain development, prenatal infections, or exposure and neurogenetic disorders.
- A careful history is necessary to distinguish delayed development from disorders in which there is a loss of acquired skills and developmental regression (the neurodegenerative disorders of childhood).

SIGNS AND SYMPTOMS

- Development may be globally delayed with involvement of gross and fine motor skills, speech and language acquisition, social or daily adaptive skills. Motor delay is usually noted early in the first year or two of life as a child fails to meet sitting and walking milestones; early identification of delay generally implies a more severe disorder of brain development.
- As the etiology of developmental delay/mental retardation is related to various environmental and genetic processes, the clinical and laboratory investigations must be based on a careful history, and neurologic and developmental examination of the child.
- The pregnancy history may reveal risk factors for poor fetal growth and development. The prenatal, labor, and delivery records should be obtained whenever possible. The results of fetal ultrasound and newborn growth measurements, particularly head circumference, are invaluable in assessing a child who has failed to thrive or has micro- or macrocephaly.
- The comprehensive evaluation of the child's current level of functioning should include physical motor, cognitive, communication (speech and language), and social and play development. It is useful to ask parents to bring photographs or videotapes that will demonstrate previous developmental skills.
- Family history must be reviewed in detail; it is essential to complete a three-generation pedigree.
- Physical examination is focused on detection of dysmorphic features, major and minor anomalies and organomegaly. Findings on neuromotor examination should clearly localize to the CNS, and rule out myopathic or dystrophic disorders.

LABORATORY PROCEDURES

There is no consensus on the choice of laboratory investigations for developmental delay. The decision to perform diagnostic imaging and laboratory procedures is based on the comprehensive historical and physical examination described above (and should include ophthalmology and audiology assessments).
A stepwise approach to minimize unnecessary investigations, should begin with a clinical and neuroimaging workup followed by thoughtful and careful choice of metabolic and cytogenetic/molecular genetic studies.
The following are considered screening investigations:
- Cytogenic/molecular genetic
  - —Karyotype (standard)
  - —Fragile X
- Metabolic screening
  - —Serum amino acids, lactate, ammonia, and very-long-chain fatty acids
  - —Urine amino acids, organic acids, oligosaccharides, and mucopolysaccharides

- Neurophysiology
  —Electroencephalogram
  —Evoked potentials

The causal yield is low, about 40%, if there is a necessity for general screening. The most cost-effective studies yielding diagnosis are MRI scanning and fragile X studies.

IMAGING STUDIES

Screening imaging evaluation includes:

- MRI
- CT
- Skeletal survey

SPECIAL TESTS

Children with developmental delay also need neuropsychological evaluation. Program recommendations and current level functioning are provided by educational, speech, physical, and occupational therapy assessment.

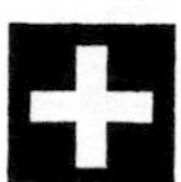

Management

GENERAL MEASURES

As there are many diverse origins for developmental disorders, management is based on thorough assessment and program planning; for example, the child with an isolated speech delay requires audiology evaluation, communication testing, and focused speech and language treatment programming.

SYMPTOMATIC TREATMENT

- General treatment and rehabilitation measures are necessary following assessment recommendations, with educational programming provided in structured classroom environment for the older child.
- The multidisciplinary team approach is considered the most comprehensive assessment and treatment model. Management is usually best arranged and supervised at a special children's treatment center.

SURGICAL MEASURES

N/A

ADJUNCTIVE TREATMENTS

Parents who have children with developmental disorders may be assisted in caring for their child through the provision of a variety of nonmedical services, for example, behavioral counseling and respite care.

ADMISSION/DISCHARGE CRITERIA

N/A

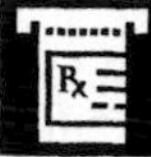

Medications

DRUG(S) OF CHOICE

There are no specific pharmacologic treatments for children with developmental delay, although if situations arise when behavioral management methods fail, then psychotropic medication options can be cautiously considered.

ALTERNATIVE DRUGS

Many alternative treatments for developmental disorders are available: multivitamins, craniosacral therapy, and pattering treatment. There are no evidence-based studies to support the use of alternative treatment methods.

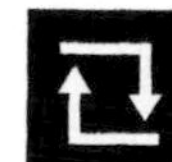

Follow-Up

PATIENT MONITORING

- After a comprehensive diagnostic evaluation and arrangements made for developmental and rehabilitation treatment carried out by a appropriate members of the multidisciplinary team, medical follow-up can focus on general monitoring of expected progress in providing anticipatory counseling. Such issues as the need for formal genetic counseling (in defined disorders) and assessment for requirement for medication intervention with behavioral problems may need to be addressed.
- In cases in which no specific diagnosis is made, a thoughtful tailored reinvestigation should be conducted every 2 to 3 years.

EXPECTED COURSE AND PROGNOSIS

N/A

PATIENT EDUCATION

Parents of children who have a defined developmental diagnosis should be referred to the appropriate family association and provided with a list of Internet resources.

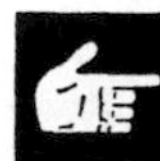

Miscellaneous

SYNONYMS

Developmental delay
Mental retardation
Developmental disability

ICD-9-CM: 319 Unspecified mental retardation; 315 Specific delays in development; 343 Cerebral palsy

SEE ALSO: N/A

REFERENCES

- Battaglia A, Bianchini E, Carey JC. Diagnostic yield of the comprehensive assessment of developmental delay/mental retardation in an institute of child neuropsychiatry. Am J Med Genet 1999;82:60–66.
- Bosch JJ. Use of directed history and behavioral indicators in the assessment of the child with a developmental disability. J Pediatr Health Care 2002;16:170–179.
- Dorling J, Salt A. Evidence based case report: assessing developmental delay. BMJ 2001;323:148–149.
- Hartley L, Salt A, Dorling J, et al. Investigation of children with "developmental delay." West J Med 2002;176(1):29–33.
- Papavasiliou AS, Bazigou H, Paraskevoulakos E, et al. Neurometabolic testing in developmental delay. J Child Neurol 2000;15(9):620–622.
- Shevell MI, Majnemer A, Rosenbaum P, et al. Etiologic determination of childhood developmental delay. Brain Dev 2001;23(4):228–235.
- Simms MD, Schum RL. Preschool children who have atypical patterns of development. Pediatr Rev 2000;21(5):147–158.
- Young PT, Barnes PD. Imaging of the developmentally delayed child. Magn Reson Imaging Clin North Am 2001;9(1):99–119.

Author(s): Daune L. MacGregor, MD

Diffuse Lewy Body Disease

Basics

DESCRIPTION

Diffuse Lewy Body Disease (DLBD) shares a classic pathological feature with idiopathic Parkinson's disease (IPD), the eosinophilic, cytoplasmic intraneuronal inclusion bodies (precipitates) known as Lewy bodies, but with additional brain regions affected. These two diseases may be difficult to differentiate in the early stages of disease. Neurodegeneration and Lewy body formation are seen in the substantia nigra, locus ceruleus, the nucleus basalis of Meynert, dorsal motor nucleus of the vagus, and cortical regions, including limbic, neocortex, hippocampus and amygdala. There may be coexistent senile plaques.

EPIDEMIOLOGY

The incidence, prevalence and other population features (Age, Race) of DLBD are unknown. It has been suggested that this disease is the most common form of dementia with extrapyramidal features and represents the second most common form of dementia after Alzheimer's disease.

ETIOLOGY

DLBD is thought to be a disorder on a continuum between PD and Alzheimer's disease.

RISK FACTORS

None known

PREGNANCY

N/A

ASSOCIATED CONDITIONS

N/A

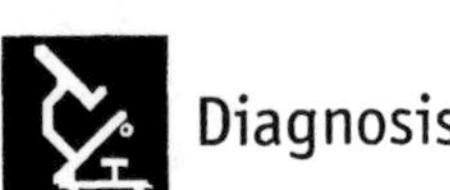

Diagnosis

DIFFERENTIAL DIAGNOSIS

Includes both disorders of extrapyramidal type and dementing illnesses.

- Essential or Familial tremor
- Parkinson's disease (IPD)
- Drug-induced parkinsonism (e.g. anti-psychotics, anti-emetics, and other dopamine blocking agents)
- Multiple System Atrophy (MSA)
- Progressive Supranuclear Palsy (PSP)
- Vascular parkinsonism
- Post-traumatic parkinsonism
- Wilson's disease
- Frontotemporal dementia with parkinsonism
- Alzheimer's with extrapyramidal features (probably a DLBD variant)
- Creutzfeldt-Jakob disease

SIGNS AND SYMPTOMS

The clinical symptoms of diffuse Lewy body disease have not been fully characterized. There is extensive clinical overlap with primary dementing disorders and IPD, as well as with other parkinsonian disorders. A combination of parkinsonian manifestations (bradykinesia, tremor, mask facies, gait disorder, rigidity) and early dementia suggest the possible diagnosis of DLBD. Symptoms more characteristic of DLBD include dramatic fluctuations in motor function and mentation that do not coincide with their medication dosing schedule. Patients may have syncope-like spells. Visual hallucinations (sometimes prior to the administration of dopaminergic medication) are common in DLBD. A characteristic sleep disturbance, REM sleep behavior disorder, is very common in DLBD patients and may precede cognitive and motor changes by years. Patients may demonstrate exquisite sensitivity (unresponsiveness, severe rigidity) to conventional neuroleptics, prohibiting their use. Patients with DLBD may also develop myoclonus.

LABORATORY PROCEDURES

There are no specific blood tests to diagnose DLBD, but the following tests should be considered to identify potential underlying secondary causes of parkinsonism: serum vitamin B12 level, thyroid function tests, serum ceruloplasmin, 24 hour urine copper excretion.

IMAGING STUDIES

There is no evidence to suggest that structural imaging studies (CT, MRI) can assist in the diagnosis of DLBD. PET or SPECT scanning are not specific for DLBD, although some studies have suggested hypometabolism in parietal and occipital regions of DLBD patients in contrast to parietal and temporal hypometabolism in Alzheimer's patients. MRI imaging may reveal evidence of other causes of parkinsonism and/or dementia such as vascular insults, mass lesions, communicating hydrocephalus, calcium or iron deposition in the striatum, atrophy in the posterior fossa suggestive of multiple system atrophies, and cortical atrophy patterns suggestive of other dementing illnesses.

SPECIAL TESTS

A therapeutic trial of Sinemet, a combination of carbidopa and levodopa, at doses of up to 600–800 mg of levodopa equivalents in 24 hours, is sometimes considered diagnostic of true idiopathic PD when the patient responds with dramatic symptomatic improvement. Patients with DLBD usually have only partial results with anti-parkinsonian agents.

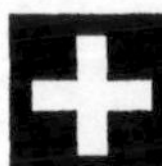

Management

GENERAL MEASURES

The management of DLBD is complicated by cognitive decline, behavioral changes, and frequent delusions and hallucinations. Management of the parkinsonian symptoms in DLBD is best managed by single agent therapy using carbidopa/levodopa formulations. Cholinesterase inhibitors for the cognitive decline and atypical anti-psychotics for the symptoms of psychosis are useful tools for the management of these difficult cases.

SURGICAL MEASURES

Not presently an option for DLBD.

SYMPTOMATIC TREATMENT

See section below under Medications for a complete discussion of pharmacological therapy of DLBD.

ADJUNCTIVE TREATMENT

See section below under Medications for a complete discussion of pharmacological therapy of DLBD.

ADMISSION/DISCHARGE CRITERIA

DLBD is usually managed in an outpatient setting. Rarely, concomitant illnesses (e.g., pneumonia, UTI) can lead to an acute exacerbation of parkinsonian or cognitive symptoms, requiring hospitalization for dysphagia, airway management, confusion and issues of decreased mobility. Psychosis frequently precipitates hospitalization and/or institutionalization.

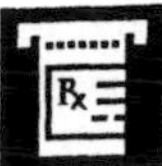

Medications

DRUGS OF CHOICE

The parkinsonian manifestations of DLBD may be managed with anti-parkinsonian agents as outlined on the chapter on idiopathic Parkinson's disease (IPD). While such medications may be helpful, they are complicated by side effects in this disorder, particularly confusion and visual hallucinations. Low doses of combination carbidopa/levodopa medications are best tolerated, with relatively increased toxicity from dopamine agonists and anticholinergic preparations in this patient population.

Carbidopa/levodopa or C/L: (brand name Sinemet, multiple generic formulations) is the preparation that provides the standard of care for people with idiopathic PD. While its use is controversial as a first line agent due to predictable development of motor fluctuations after prolonged exposure to levodopa, it is nevertheless the most efficacious and biologically effective medication available. Doses vary, but patients are usually initiated with 25/100 mg TID and titrating gradually to a total daily dose of dopamine of 300–800 mg. (Note the 25 mg refers to Carbidopa, and the 100 mg refers to L-Dopa).

The **complications of levodopa therapy** are common to all the dopaminergic agents and include confusion, hallucinations, gastrointestinal distress including nausea and vomiting, orthostatic hypotension, and others. The long-term motor complications associated with levodopa usage include dyskinesias (involuntary abnormal movements), dystonias (abnormal involuntary posturing), on/off symptoms in which medication quits working abruptly, and complicated combinations of all of the above.

Cholinesterase inhibitors: are an emerging class of medications for the treatment of dementia. Originally targeted to treat the symptoms of Alzheimer's dementia, the therapeutic benefit of these agents on the cognitive and behavioral features seen in DLBD are being increasingly documented. Except for donepezil, these agents typically need to be taken with food and titrated slowly to their target doses in order to avoid GI side effects.

Tacrine: (Cognex, 80–160 mg/day) was the first cholinesterase inhibitor released. It has largely been replaced by newer agents secondary to frequent dosing requirements, poor GI tolerability and potential hepatotoxicity.

Donepezil: (Aricept, 5–10 mg/day) is given once daily and occasionally causes GI upset. It can cause bradycardia when used concomitantly with beta-blockers.

Rivastigmine: (Exelon, 6–12 mg/day) is given twice daily. It must be given with food in order to avoid nausea and/or vomiting.

Galantamine: (Reminyl, 16–24 mg/day) is also given twice daily and should be administered with food.

Atypical antipsychotics: are used to treat the symptoms of drug-induced hallucinations in PD as well as the spontaneous hallucinations and behavioral disturbances associated with DLBD. These medications are normally given in dosages representing a fraction of that used for patients with schizophrenia.

Clozapine: (Clozaril, 12.5–25 mg/day) is the prototypic atypical antipsychotic. Its use is complicated by the rare, but life-threatening potential side effect of agranulocytosis. Weekly CBC is required during the first 6 months of therapy followed by every two weeks testing thereafter.

Quetiapine: (Seroquel, 25–100 mg/day) is another atypical antipsychotic currently on the market that, like clozapine, shows no dose-dependent extrapyramidal side effects.

ALTERNATIVE DRUGS

N/A

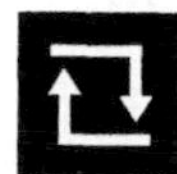

Follow-Up

PATIENT MONITORING

- Some patients with DLBD have a relatively rapid course and will require monitoring every 2–3 months. Psychiatric consultation may assist in the management of DLBD patients.
- By its very nature, DLBD requires steadily increasing doses of medications, for the treatment of dopaminergic deficiency, the side effects of (exogenous) dopaminergic therapy, and especially for the cognitive/behavioral abnormalities.

EXPECTED COURSE AND PROGNOSIS

DLBD is a progressive, neurodegenerative disorder. DLBD is typically more relentless than Parkinson's disease in its progression, some authors suggesting significant disability—emotionally, cognitively, and physically—by 7–10 years after onset of symptoms.

PATIENT EDUCATION

Support groups for parkinsonian disorders are available locally in many areas of the country. There are several large national organizations that provide educational materials to patients and their families. Regular daily exercise has been proven beneficial in alleviating many symptoms of immobility in DLBD, especially when coupled with careful titration and use of proper medications.

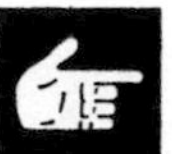

Miscellaneous

SYNONYMS

- Parkinson's with dementia (PDD)
- Dementia with Lewy bodies (DLB)
- Alzheimer's with extrapyramidal features (AD with PD)

ICD-9-CM: 294.10 Dementia conditions classified elsewhere

SEE ALSO: MULTIPLE SYSTEM ATROPHY, PROGRESSIVE SUPRANUCLEAR PALSY

REFERENCES

- Ahlskog JE. Diagnosis and differential diagnosis of Parkinson's disease and parkinsonism. Parkinsonism and Related Disorders, 2001;7:63–70.
- McKeith IG, Burn DJ, Ballard CG, et al., Dementia with Lewy bodies. Semin Clin Neuropsychiatry 2003;8:46–57.
- Sulkava R. Differential diagnosis of parkinsonism. Adv Neurol 2003,91: 383–396.

Author(s): Lawrence W. Elmer, MD, PhD

Distal Myopathies

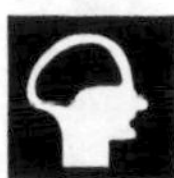

Basics

DESCRIPTION

Myopathic disorders usually produce a pattern of weakness predominantly in proximal muscle groups of the arms and legs. However, occasionally patients with myopathies can present with predominantly distal weakness. Several distinct clinical entities were united under an umbrella of distal myopathy syndrome. They include Welander (late adult type I), Markesbery-Udd (late adult type II), Nonaka or familial inclusion body myopathy (IBM) (early adult onset type I), Miyoshi or limb-girdle muscular dystrophy (early adult onset type II), Laing (early adult onset type III), and myofibrillar (Desmin) myopathy with onset varying from childhood to the seventh decade.

EPIDEMIOLOGY

Distal myopathies are rare. Given clinical and genetic heterogeneity of distal myopathies, no specific data on prevalence and incidence are available.

Some myopathies were discovered among specific ethnic groups, however. For example, myopathy of Welander type was noted in a large cohort of Scandinavian patients; Markesbery-Udd myopathy was described in English, French-English, and Finnish families; Nonaka and Miyoshi were first reported in the Japanese literature, although a lot of non-Japanese cases were described as well.

ETIOLOGY

Distal myopathies are genetically heterogeneous disorders.

Pattern of Inheritance

- Welander, Markesbery-Udd and Laing myopathies demonstrate an autosomal-dominant pattern of inheritance. Nonaka and Miyoshi are inherited in an autosomal-recessive fashion or can be sporadic.
- The pattern of inheritance of desmin myopathy varies from autosomal dominant and sporadic (more common) to autosomal recessive to X-linked.

Gene Localization

Gene localization was determined for Welander (2p13), Markesbery-Udd (2q31), Nonaka (9p1-q1), Miyoshi (2p12-14, 10, and others), Laing (14), desmin (11q21-23—autosomal dominant or sporadic; 2q35—autosomal recessive; 12—X-linked).

Gene Proteins

Several gene proteins were identified. MM (dysferlin) for Miyoshi (located at 2p12-14); HIBM (IBM2) for familial or hereditary IBM; MPD1 for Laing; and TMD for Markesbery-Udd myopathy.

RISK FACTORS

N/A

PREGNANCY

Morbidity during pregnancy might be related to cardiac manifestations (cardiomyopathy and conduction defects) in cases of desmin myopathy. Patients with other forms seem not to be at increased risk for complications during pregnancy.

ASSOCIATED CONDITIONS

Cardiac complications were encountered in numerous patients with desmin myopathy and manifested as conduction defects, syncopal episodes, and cardiomyopathy with associated heart failure. Similar features were described in some cases of Markesbery-Udd and Nonaka myopathies.

Diagnosis

DIFFERENTIAL DIAGNOSIS

Muscle Disorders

- Facioscapulohumeral dystrophy
- Scapuloperoneal myopathy
- Emery-Dreifuss muscular dystrophy (humeroperoneal)
- Myotonic dystrophy
- Oculopharyngeal dystrophy
- Inflammatory myopathies (inclusion body myositis, polymyositis)
- Metabolic myopathies (debrancher and acid-maltase deficiency)
- Congenital myopathies (nemaline, central core, centronuclear)

Peripheral Nerve Disorders

- Charcot-Marie-Tooth disease
- Acquired neuropathies

Motor Neuron Disorders

- Spinal muscular atrophy (distal adult forms)
- Progressive muscular atrophy (distal forms)
- Amyotrophic lateral sclerosis

Disorders Of Neuromuscular Transmission

- Myasthenia gravis (distal form)
- Congenital myasthenic syndrome (slow channel, acetylcholinesterase deficiency)

SIGNS AND SYMPTOMS

Initial site of weakness and the age of onset vary depending on a type of distal myopathy.

- Welander: weakness begins in the distal upper extremities, usually finger and wrist extensors. Later, distal lower limbs become affected. Involvement of proximal muscles is rare, even as the disease progresses. Muscle stretch reflexes and sensory examination are normal as a rule. The onset of first symptoms is after 40 years of age.
- Markesbery-Udd: weakness starts in the anterior compartment of the distal lower extremities (ankle dorsiflexors). Progression is more rapid than in Welander cases. Patients first develop weakness after age of 40.
- Nonaka/familial IBM: weakness begins late in the second or third decade. Initial weakness is in the distal leg anterior compartment (ankle dorsiflexors) and toe extensors. (Patients present with foot drop and steppage gait.) Can progress to generalized weakness.
- Miyoshi: symptoms develop between the ages of 15 and 25. Initial symptoms are in the distal lower extremity posterior compartment. (Patients cannot walk on their toes or climb stairs.)
- Laing: weakness begins in the anterior compartment of the legs and neck flexors, followed by distal finger extensor involvement. Patients develop weakness between 4 and 25 years of age.
- Desmin: it is unclear if desmin myopathy is a distinct entity. Most patients develop weakness between 25 and 45 years of age, although there are reports of onset in infancy and later in life. It can start in either hands or legs, and usually progresses to proximal muscles, sometimes including respiratory musculature. Cardiac involvement is common, and on occasion can precede development of skeletal muscle weakness.

LABORATORY PROCEDURES

Three tests might be helpful in establishing a diagnosis of distal myopathy:

1. Creatine enzymes (CK). It is normal, slightly, or moderately (3–5 × normal) elevated in all conditions, except Miyoshi myopathy, in which it is increased up to 150 × normal.
2. Electrodiagnostic testing (nerve conduction studies/EMG). Usually, consistent with a myopathic process. Normal nerve conduction results or reduced amplitudes of motor responses. Myopathic EMG pattern: early recruitment, and small motor unit potentials (of reduced amplitude and duration).
3. Muscle biopsy. Myopathic dystrophic features, such as fiber size variability, increased amount of central nuclei, fiber splitting present uniformly. A distinctive but not pathognomonic histologic finding; vacuoles are seen in specimens from patients with Markesbery-Udd and Nonaka myopathies. They might be also present in Welander and desmin myopathy cases. The vacuoles are lined with granular material that is basophilic on staining with hematoxylin and eosin and purple-red with Gomori trichrome stain, or so-called rimmed vacuoles. The vacuoles exhibit acid phosphatase activity. On electron microscopy, in addition to autophagic vacuoles, some patients with Nonaka/familial IBM and Welander have nuclear or cytoplasmic 15–18 nm filamentous inclusions.

IMAGING STUDIES

Neuroimaging is not helpful for making a diagnosis.

SPECIAL TESTS

Although localizations for all distal myopathies and gene proteins for some of them are known, no commercially available genetic tests have been introduced so far.

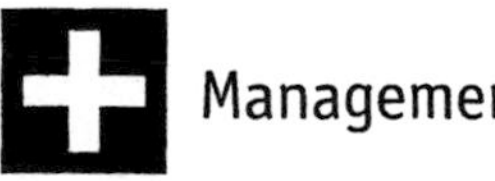

Management

GENERAL MEASURES

- Lower limb weakness usually requires the use of *mobility aids*, such as braces, a cane, or a walker within a decade of the diagnosis. A wheelchair is often needed for mobility several years afterward.
- Associated cardiac problems, such as conduction defect and heart failures are to be managed by a cardiologist and might require implantation of pacemaker.

SURGICAL MEASURES

Surgical correction of contractures is possible.

SYMPTOMATIC TREATMENT

Prophylaxis of contractures includes physical therapy. Occupational therapy is helpful to maximize function as weakness progresses.

ADJUNCTIVE TREATMENT

N/A

ADMISSION/DISCHARGE CRITERIA

Patients with distal myopathies are followed in an outpatient setting. Admissions might be required for treatment of associated conditions or corrective surgeries (see above).

Medications

DRUG(S) OF CHOICE

No medication is currently available for treatment of distal myopathies.

ALTERNATIVE DRUGS

N/A

Follow-Up

PATIENT MONITORING

Patients should be followed by a neurologist, physiatrist, and physical and occupational therapists. If there are signs of cardiac involvement, regular monitoring of a cardiac status by a cardiologist is also required. A Muscular Dystrophy Association (MDA) clinic is ideal for a multidisciplinary approach, longitudinal assessment, and education of patients with distal myopathies.

EXPECTED COURSE AND PROGNOSIS

Gradual worsening of the symptoms is expected. The speed of progression varies from one patient to another and depends on the age of the disease onset. Heart disease has the most significant impact on life span.

PATIENT EDUCATION

Muscular Dystrophy Association can be a source of services and education to patients affected by those disorders: 3300 E. Sunrise Drive, Tucson, AZ 85718; 800-572-1717; *www.mdausa.org.*

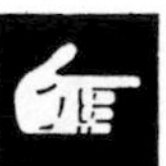

Miscellaneous

SYNONYMS

Distal muscular dystrophies

ICD-9-CM: 359.1 Hereditary progressive muscular dystrophy

SEE ALSO: N/A

REFERENCES

- Barohn RJ. Distal myopathies and dystrophies. Semin Neurol 1993;13: 247–255.
- Gardner-Medwin D, Walton J. The muscular dystrophies. In: Walton J, Karpati G, Hilton-Jones D, eds. Disorders of voluntary muscle, 6th ed. Edinburgh: Churchill Livingston, 1994:580.
- Gowers WA. A lecture on myopathy and a distal form. Br Med J 1902;2:89–92.
- Somer H. Distal myopathies: 25th ENMC international workshop. Neuromusc Disord 1995;5:249–252.

Author(s): Yelena Lindenbaum, MD

Down Syndrome

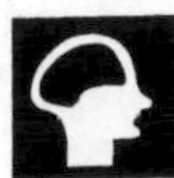

Basics

DESCRIPTION

Down syndrome (DS) is a genetic disorder involving an extra copy of a region (partial translocation trisomy) or the entire chromosome 21. Classic features observed in DS are phenotypically mapped to the 21q22 band of chromosome 21 (Chr21), known as the critical region. These include:

- Mental retardation (MR)
- Bilateral palmar ("simian") crease
- Short digits/extremities
- Midfacial hypoplasia
- Median epicanthal fold
- Oblique palpebral fissures
- Low/flat nasal bridge
- Protruding tongue
- Congenital heart disease

EPIDEMIOLOGY

Incidence/Prevalence

- Incidence: about 1 in 600–1,000 live births
- About 50% of spontaneous abortuses are trisomies (primarily chromosomes: X, 13, 18, or 21). Trisomy 21 has the greatest gestational survival rate (approximately 20%).
- DS is the most common genetically identified type of MR (4–12% of the MR population).

ETIOLOGY

The cause is unknown. Three types of chromosomal abnormalities are observed:

Aneuploidy

- Due to meiotic nondisjunction
- 95% of DS cases
- Results in trisomy 21
- Frequency increases with increasing maternal age
- Nonfamilial

Chromosomal Rearrangement

- Due to unbalanced Robertsonian translocation (partial trisomy 21) between portions of Chr21 and usually Chr14 (t14;21)
- 4% of DS cases
- Sporadic in about two thirds of cases; familial in one third
- Results in triplication of a portion of Chr21
- The classic DS phenotype requires triplication of critical region.

Mosaicism

- Typically occurs during embryogenesis or early cell division results in two cell lines: normal and trisomic in about 1 to 2% of DS cases.

RISK FACTORS

- The incidence of trisomy 21 offspring due to maternal nondisjunction correlates with maternal age:

MATERNAL AGE	*INCIDENCE*
<30 years old	<1/1,000 births
≥45 years	1/54 births

- One third of translocation DS cases are familial involving a balanced carrier parent. The theoretical risk of affected offspring from a balanced carrier parent is (monosomy 21 is lethal):

OFFSPRING	*THEORETICAL RISK*
Female carrier:	
DS	20%
Balanced carrier	40%
Normal	40%
Male carrier:	
DS	5%
Balanced carrier	50%
Normal	50%

PREGNANCY

- About 31% of females are anovulatory; 39% ovulate regularly.
- Approximately 50% are fertile.
- Infertility may exist in males.

ASSOCIATED CONDITIONS

- Additional physical stigmata:
  - —Low-set ears
  - —Hypotonia
  - —Infantile spasms
  - —Brushfield spots (light "speckles" around iris)
- Congenital medical comorbidity:
  - -Cardiac (e.g., atrioventricular defect, tetralogy of Fallot, patent ductus arteriosus, ventricular or atrial septal defects): 40% to 50%
  - -Mitral valve prolapse, aortic regurgitation
  - -Gastrointestinal (duodenal atresia, tracheoesophageal fistula): 12%
  - -Unstable atlantooccipital/atlantoaxial joints: 12% to 20%
  - -Anomalies resulting in sleep apnea
  - —Endocrinopathies: Diabetes mellitus, Hypothyroidism (congenital and acquired type, thyroid antibodies) (By adolescence: 15% In adults: up to 50%).
  - —Immunologic/hematologic abnormalities: Recurrent infections, Aberrant delayed hypersensitivity reaction: 59%, Viral hepatitis, Leukemia: 1% of children, Anemia.
  - —Dermatologic (e.g., eczema, psoriasis)
  - —Ophthalmologic: 77%; Cataracts: congenital, 3%; acquired, 30% to 60%; Myopia; Macular degenerative disease; Strabismus: 49%; Blocked tear duct.
  - —Dental (e.g., gingivitis)
  - —Obesity
  - —Hearing deficits: 15% to 50%
  - —Seizures
  - —Alzheimer's disease (AD): neuropathology: in almost all over 40 years old
    - -Dementia: about 30% of adults over 40 or 50 years old
  - —Psychiatric

Diagnosis

DIFFERENTIAL DIAGNOSIS

- See chapter on Mental Retardation.

SIGNS AND SYMPTOMS

- MR (mild to severe)
- Low-normal intelligence in about 10% of cases
- Aberrant/delayed growth pattern
- Common physical exam findings:
  - —Physical stigmata and comorbid features
  - —Mild bradycardia and hypotension
  - —Heart murmur (congenital or acquired)
  - —Microbrachycephaly
  - —Nystagmus
  - —Hearing/visual deficits
  - —Olfactory deficits
  - —Pyramidal signs secondary to subluxated upper cervical joints

LABORATORY PROCEDURES

- Cytogenetic studies of:
  - —All patients to rule out familial partial translocation type
  - —Parents: if translocation type revealed
  - —Relatives: if carrier parent identified
  - —Several tissue samples may be needed for detecting mosaicism.

IMAGING STUDIES

- X-rays of cervical spine (as early as in 2 year olds)
- Consider
  - —MRI or CT: if suspect coexisting CNS disease (e.g., seizures, dementia, focal deficits)
  - —Gastrointestinal studies: for suspected congenital anomalies

SPECIAL TESTS

- Neuropsychological assessment: typically verbal<nonverbal skills
- Consider:
  - —EEG (suspected seizures)
  - —Evoked potentials (for neurosensory deficits)
  - —Audiometry/ophthalmologic
  - —Electrocardiogram
  - —Echocardiogram: some recommend in all newborns by the age of 2 months

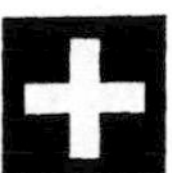

Management

GENERAL MEASURES

- Multidisciplinary approach
- Verbal skills are often inadequate to express symptoms; thorough examination and diagnostic testing are necessary.
- Assess for congenital anomalies and secondary complications.
- Routine vaccinations and consider hepatitis and flu vaccinations.

SURGICAL MEASURES

Sometimes required for:

- Congenital anomalies
- Tubes for middle ear effusion
- Subluxated cervical joints

SYMPTOMATIC TREATMENT

- Failure to thrive in infants:
  —Consider congenital anomalies
  —Consider surgical correction
- Heart failure:
  —Infants/children: consider congenital heart disease
  —Adults: congenital anomalies or acquired valvular insufficiency
  —Pulmonary hypertension: secondary to pulmonary hypoplasia
  —ECG, CXR, ECHO, cardiology consultation
- Dermatologic disorders (e.g., psoriasis, eczema):
  —Topical agents, dermatologic consult
- Bacterial skin infections:
  —Good hygiene, sitz baths, topical antibiotics
- Otitis media: close management/monitoring
  —Decongestants
  —Antibiotics
  —Frequently chronic/recurrent:
  -Long-term antibiotic treatment often beneficial
  -Often associated with hearing loss
  *Affecting language/social development
  *May be prevented by placement of tubes for drainage of effusion
- Hypothyroidism:
  —Thyroid replacement therapy
- Seizures:
  —Work up and treat accordingly
- Psychopathology or functional/cognitive decline:
  —Rule out underlying medical/neurologic disease.
  —Monitor cognitive/adaptive functioning.
  —If underlying treatable disorder is not revealed, then:
  -Diagnostic workup for AD
  -Obtain psychiatric consultation
  —Address psychosocial/competency issues
  —Depressive symptoms
  -Suspect early AD in adults
  -Conduct serial cognitive screenings before and during treatment
  -Consider:
  *Psychiatric consultation
  *Psychosocial needs
  *Low doses of selective serotonin reuptake inhibitors
  *Behavioral or psychotherapeutic modalities

ADJUNCTIVE TREATMENT

- Ophthalmologist
- Audiologist/speech therapist
- Consider
  —Cardiology consult
  —Genetics consultant/counselor for translocation DS subtype
  —ENT specialist for recurrent upper respiratory infections or otitis media

ADMISSION/DISCHARGE CRITERIA

- Severe congenital anomalies requiring inpatient treatment or surgery

Medications

DRUG(S) OF CHOICE

No established drugs.

Contraindications

N/A

Precautions

N/A

ALTERNATIVE DRUGS

N/A

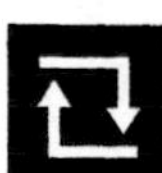

Follow-Up

PATIENT MONITORING

- Thorough annual physical/neurologic examinations monitoring for:
  —Congenital anomalies and secondary or acquired complications
  —Nutritional status, weight, and height
  —In children: signs/symptoms of leukemia (consider annual CBC with differential)
  —Infections
  —Hearing deficits throughout life span (in adults may be premature age-related loss)
  -Consider annual ENT evaluation
  —Geriatric disorders (40 years or older), which can occur prematurely in DS
  —Conduct: ECHO by 2 months of age, annual cardiac assessments
  —Fasting glucose and thyroid function test at least every 2 years throughout life span
- Consider annual:
  —Thyroid panel in adults 35 years and older
  —Fasting glucose in adults with hypothyroidism or with obesity
- Neuropsychological assessments:
  —At regular intervals during childhood
  —In young adults for a baseline measure
  —Recommend annual assessments in adults over 30 years old using:
  -Mini-Mental Status Exam (MMSE) if mild MR to moderate MR
  -Test for severe impairment (easier but similar to the MMSE): if moderate/severe MR
  -Assessment of adaptive functioning, particularly "nontestable" patients with profound MR
- Dental care (every 6 months)

EXPECTED COURSE AND PROGNOSIS

- Shortened life span. Many survive beyond 50 years old with a few surviving into seventies or eighties.
- Leukemia accounts for low survival in about 1% of children with DS.
- Bronchopneumonia is a common cause of death in adults.
- Age-related conditions/disorders occur prematurely in adults (e.g., skin wrinkling, graying of the hair, immunologic aberrancies) and neurodegenerative disorders (e.g., macular degeneration and AD) reported to be more prevalent.

PATIENT EDUCATION

National Down Syndrome Society: 800-221-4602, *www.ndss.org*

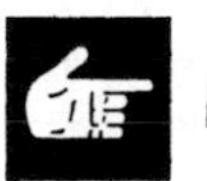

Miscellaneous

SYNONYMS

Trisomy 21 (pertains specifically to nondisjunction type of DS)

ICD-9-CM: 758.0 Down syndrome

SEE ALSO: N/A

REFERENCES

- Albert M, Cohen C. The test for severe impairment: for the assessment of patients with severe cognitive dysfunction. J Am Geriatr Soc 1992:405:449–453.
- Folstein M, Folstein S, McHugh P. "Mini Mental State": a practical method for grading the cognitive state of patients for the clinical. J Psychiatr Res 1975:12: 189–198.
- Peuschel SM. Health concerns in persons with Down syndrome. In: Peuschel SM, Tingey C, Rynders JE, et al., eds. New perspectives on Down syndrome. Baltimore: Paul H. Brooks, 1987:113–134.

Author(s): Karen L. Brugge, MD

Dysmyelinating Disorders

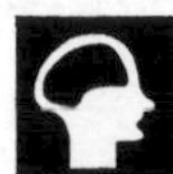

Basics

DESCRIPTION

Dysmyelination of the CNS refers to the production of an abnormal and unstable myelin sheath, often associated with hypomyelination. Frequently of metabolic origin, many dysmyelinating disorders are represented in the sphingolipidoses (see Sphingolipidoses). Four novel disorders are presented: adrenoleukodystrophy (ALD), Pelizaeus-Merzbacher disease (PMD), Canavan disease, and Alexander disease.

EPIDEMIOLOGY

Incidence/Prevalence

ALD: incidence is not known. Estimates range from 1 in 20,000 to 1.1 in 100,000 births.

Race

ALD is panethnic. Canavan disease affects all ethnic groups but is especially prevalent among Ashkenazi Jews and Saudi Arabians.

Age

See Signs and Symptoms, below.

Sex

Because of X-linked inheritance, patients with ALD and PMD are male.

ETIOLOGY

Genetics

ALD and PMD are X-linked. Canavan disease is autosomal recessive. Alexander disease is presumed to be autosomal recessive despite infrequency of involved siblings.
Genes for ALD, PMD and Canavan have been identified. Prenatal diagnosis is available for ALD, PMD, and Canavan disease.

RISK FACTORS

N/A

PREGNANCY

N/A

ASSOCIATED CONDITIONS

N/A

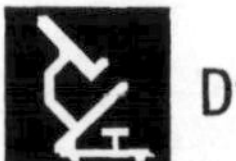

Diagnosis

DIFFERENTIAL DIAGNOSIS

The dysmyelinating diseases presented in this chapter must be differentiated from other inherited metabolic neurodegenerative disorders. Additionally, disorders of dysmyelination, which are characterized by the production of an abnormal and unstable myelin sheath, should be distinguished from disorders of demyelination, which are characterized by destruction of apparently normal myelin. Examples of demyelinating disorders in childhood are multiple sclerosis, Devic disease (neuromyelitis optica), acute disseminated encephalomyelitis (ADEM), acute necrotizing encephalomyelitis, and central pontine myelinosis. Other causes of progressive dementia to consider include encephalitis, chronic infections such as subacute sclerosing panencephalitis (SSPE), exposure to neurotoxins and drugs of abuse, side effects of medications, collagen vascular diseases, and CNS complications of other diseases such as sickle cell anemia and end-stage renal disease.

SIGNS AND SYMPTOMS

- ALD: peroxisomal disorder that can cause damage to the CNS and adrenal cortex. Patients present with a history of normal early development with onset of neurologic/behavioral symptoms, commonly hyperactivity, and school failure, between 4 and 8 years of age. Subsequent onset of adrenal insufficiency is seen in 90% of patients. The course is characterized by progressive dementia, visual loss with optic atrophy, pyramidal tract dysfunction, dysphagia, deafness, and seizures. A second phenotype, which is characterized by progressive paraparesis and sphincter disturbance due to spinal cord disease (adrenomyeloneuropathy), is seen in young men.
- PMD: infantile onset variant is the classic form. A prominent, irregular nystagmus and head tremor or head rolling are noted at birth or during the first few months of life. Progressive dementia, ataxia, spasticity, and choreoathetotic movements ensue. The connatal variant is present at birth and is much more rapidly progressive.
- Canavan disease: onset of symptoms by 3 months of age. Megalencephaly is common but not invariable (also seen in Tay-Sachs disease and Alexander disease). Lack of psychomotor development, progressive spasticity, optic atrophy, seizures, and dysphagia
- Alexander disease: patients with the infantile form present between 6 months and 2 years of age with megalencephaly and/or hydrocephalus (the large head is usually due to an enlarged brain but some do develop hydrocephalus due to obstruction at the aqueduct of Sylvius), psychomotor retardation, spasticity, and seizures. A juvenile-onset form and an adult-onset form characterized by progressive bulbar weakness, spasticity, ataxia, and cognitive deterioration are described.

LABORATORY PROCEDURES

See Special Tests, below.

IMAGING STUDIES

- MRI in patients with ALD shows characteristic symmetric periventricular white matter lesions in the posterior parietal and occipital lobes.
- The MRI in patients with Alexander disease is significant for marked demyelination with frontal predominance.

SPECIAL TESTS

- ALD: abnormally high levels of very long chain fatty acids in plasma and fibroblasts. Mutation is found in the gene for ALD, which encodes for a transport protein in the peroxisomal membrane.
- PMD: tigroid appearance of the white matter on myelin stains because of islands of spared myelin against a nonmyelinated background. Mutation in the gene encoding proteolipid protein.
- Canavan disease: deficient aspartoacylase activity in skin fibroblasts. Detection of mutation in the gene encoding aspartoacylase.
- Alexander disease: Rosenthal fibers, protein inclusions formed in astrocytic footplates, are the characteristic histologic finding.

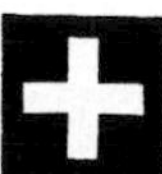

Management

GENERAL MEASURES

Patients with ALD who demonstrate early cerebral involvement by MRI, neuropsychological testing, and/or neurologic exam should be considered candidates for bone marrow transplant. Matched unrelated human umbilical cord blood transplantation may be an option when a suitable bone marrow donor is not available.

SURGICAL MEASURES

N/A

SYMPTOMATIC TREATMENT

Patients with ALD will usually require treatment for adrenal insufficiency.

ADJUNCTIVE TREATMENT

Physical therapy may improve quality of life.

ADMISSION/DISCHARGE CRITERIA

Patients are usually admitted for evaluation and treatment of complications of their disease.

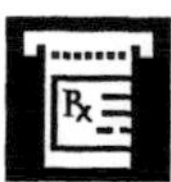

Medications

DRUG(S) OF CHOICE

No specific medication treatment is available to slow or stop the progression of these diseases.

ALTERNATIVE DRUGS

N/A

Follow-Up

PATIENT MONITORING

Patient follow-up is guided by the predicted course and potential complications of the disease.

EXPECTED COURSE AND PROGNOSIS

- ALD: rapid deterioration to a vegetative state once neurologic symptoms become evident.
- PMD: by school age boys are mute and confined to a wheelchair. Patients die of an intercurrent illness in late adolescence or early adulthood.
- Canavan disease: death may occur within the first decade, although survival into the second and third decade is not uncommon.
- Alexander disease: most die in a vegetative state in infancy or during the preschool years. A few children survive to the second decade.

PATIENT EDUCATION

- United Leukodystrophy Foundation, 2304 Highland Dr., Sycamore, IL 60178. Phone: 800-728-5483. *www.ulf.org*
- Canavan Foundation, 600 West 111th Street #8A, New York, NY 10025. Phone: 212-316-6488. *www.canavanfoundation.org*
- National Tay-Sachs and Allied Diseases Association, 2001 Beacon St., Ste. 204, Brighton, MA 02135. Phone: 800-90-NTSAD. *www.ntsad.org*

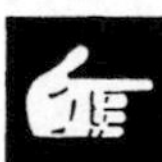

Miscellaneous

SYNONYMS

N/A

ICD-9-CM: 330.0 Leukodystrophy

SEE ALSO: N/A

REFERENCES

- Kapelushnik J, Varadi G, Nagler A. Matched unrelated human umbilical cord blood transplantation for X-linked adrenoleukodystrophy. J Pediatr Hematol Oncol 1998;20(3):257.
- MacCollin M, DeVivo DC. Peroxisomal diseases: Zellweger syndrome, adrenoleukodystrophy, and Refsum disease. In: Rowland LP, ed. Merritt's textbook of neurology. Philadelphia: Williams & Wilkins, 1995:577–581.
- Malm G, Ringden O, Anvret M, et al. Treatment of adrenoleukodystrophy with bone marrow transplantation. Acta Paediatr 1997;86:484.
- Rapin I, Traeger E. Cerebral degenerations of childhood. In: Rowland LP, ed. Merritt's textbook of neurology. Philadelphia: Williams & Wilkins, 1995:597–603.
- Scriver CR, Beaudet AL, Sly WS, et al., eds. The metabolic and molecular bases of inherited disease, 7th ed. New York: McGraw-Hill, 1995.

Author(s): Eveline C. Traeger, MD

Dystonia

Basics

DESCRIPTION

Dystonia is an involuntary movement characterized by sustained muscle contractions, which may cause twisting, repetitive and patterned movements, or abnormal postures.

EPIDEMIOLOGY

Incidence/Prevalence

Incidence

Generalized dystonia: 2 per million/year
Focal dystonia: 24 per million/year

Prevalence

Generalized dystonia: 3.4 per 100,000
Focal dystonia: 30 per 100,000

Race

Dystonia is seen worldwide, though more prevalent among some ethnic groups. The prevalence of generalized dystonia among Ashkenazi Jews is 6.8 per 100,000 population, twice that of the United States population.

Age

Dystonia can occur at any age.

ETIOLOGY

Dystonia can represent a specific disease or be a symptom of an underlying nervous system disorder or insult. Most patients with dystonia have primary dystonia, i.e., idiopathic. Primary dystonias are characterized by a lack of both neurologic findings other than dystonia and distinct neuropathology. Primary dystonia may occur sporadically or be inherited. The inherited primary dystonias follow autosomal-dominant inheritance patterns; three gene loci are currently known: *DYT1* on chromosome 9q, *DYT6* on 8p, and *DYT7* on 18p. These all demonstrate low penetrance (30–40%) and variable expression. Only with *DYT1* is the gene product known (torsinA, an ATP-binding protein). The genetic mutation consists of a 3 base pair (GAG) deletion. This mutation, most prevalent among the Ashkenazi Jews, results in early-onset limb dystonia with subsequent generalization.
Other inherited primary dystonias include dopa-responsive dystonia (DRD), rapid-onset dystonia-parkinsonism, and myoclonic dystonia. Since these conditions are characterized by additional neurologic findings, they are classified among the dystonia-plus syndromes, which include both sporadic and inherited conditions. DRD is caused by mutations within the gene for GTP cyclohydrolase 1 on chromosome 14 (*DYT5* on 14q). This is the rate-limiting enzyme in the formation of tetrahydrobiopterin, a cofactor of tyrosine hydroxylase, the rate-limiting enzyme in dopamine synthesis. These patients respond dramatically to low doses of levodopa. A similar but much less common phenotype has been seen with mutations in the tyrosine hydroxylase (TH) gene, resulting in TH deficiency. This autosomal-recessive disorder also responds to levodopa.
Less commonly, presentations of dystonia are due to insults to the CNS, i.e., secondary dystonia, or the dystonia may be part of an inherited neurodegenerative disease or an inherited disorder of metabolism. Examples of secondary dystonia are numerous and varied; see Associated Conditions, below. The clinical and family history and presence of other neurologic findings set these conditions, as well as the dystonia-plus syndromes, apart from the primary dystonias.

RISK FACTORS

- Family history of dystonia or other neurologic disease
- Exposure to antipsychotic medications
- Perinatal stress
- Toxin exposure

PREGNANCY

No known relationship of dystonia and pregnancy.

ASSOCIATED CONDITIONS

- Dystonia-plus syndromes
  —Sporadic
    -Parkinson's disease
    -Progressive supranuclear palsy
    -Multiple system atrophy
    -Cortical-basal ganglionic degeneration
  —Inherited
    -Dopa-responsive dystonia
    -Rapid-onset dystonia—parkinsonism
    -Myoclonic dystonia
- Secondary causes of dystonia
  —Medications
    -Dopamine receptor antagonists: antipsychotics, antiemetics
    -Anticonvulsants
    -Levodopa, dopamine agonists
  —CNS infections
  —Perinatal CNS insult; kernicterus
  —Toxins
    -Manganese
    -Carbon monoxide
    -Carbon disulfide
    -Cyanide
    -Methanol
  —Head injury
  —Stroke
  —Multiple sclerosis
  —Brainstem or spinal cord lesions
  —Brain tumor
  —Brain surgery, i.e., thalamotomy
  —Arteriovenous malformation
- Inherited neurodegenerative diseases
  —X-linked recessive
    -"Lubag" or X-linked dystonia-parkinsonism of the Philippines
  —Autosomal dominant
    -Huntington's disease
    -Spinocerebellar ataxias
    -Dentatorubropallidoluysian atrophy (DRPLA)
  —Autosomal recessive
    -Wilson's disease
    -Hallervorden-Spatz disease
    -Neuroacanthocytosis
    -Ataxia telangiectasia
  —Maternal (mitochondrial) inheritance
    -Leber's hereditary optic neuropathy
- Inherited disorders of metabolism
  —Lipid storage disorders
    -Metachromatic leukodystrophy
    -Niemann-Pick disease, type C
    -Gangliosidoses
  —Amino acid disorders

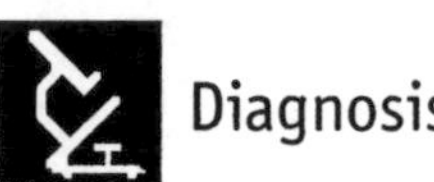

Diagnosis

DIFFERENTIAL DIAGNOSIS

Other hyperkinetic movement disorders may simulate dystonia:

- Chorea—brief movements that occur continuously and randomly among different body parts
- Tics—brief, intermittent movements or sounds; range from jerks (clonic tics) to sustained contractions (tonic or dystonic tics)
- Paroxysmal dystonia—sudden onset of dystonic movements lasting minutes to hours
- Pseudodystonia
  —Atlantoaxial subluxation
  —Syringomyelia
  —Arnold-Chiari malformation
  —Trochlear nerve palsy
  —Posterior fossa mass
  —Soft tissue neck mass
  —Psychogenic

SIGNS AND SYMPTOMS

Dystonia can occur in a wide variety of clinical presentations, e.g., inversion of a foot, excessive blinking, head tilting or turning, a change in speech or handwriting. Dystonia is usually exacerbated by voluntary activity, i.e., action dystonia. This can be a task-specific action dystonia, such as writer's cramp, when only the act of writing results in dystonia. Sometimes activity in one body part results in dystonia in another body part, i.e., overflow dystonia. Eventually, dystonic movements are seen at rest but usually disappear with sleep. Stress and fatigue may result in worsening of the dystonia, while sensory tricks, such as touching the chin in cervical dystonia (the *geste antagoniste* phenomenon) can relieve it. Dystonia may fluctuate, being minimal in the morning and worsening throughout the day. This diurnal dystonia is a characteristic feature of dopa-responsive dystonia. Dystonic movements may also occur suddenly, lasting for short periods; this is paroxysmal dystonia, which may be inherited as an autosomal-dominant trait or be secondary to medications or underlying neurologic disease.

Dystonia can be classified by distribution:

- Focal dystonia: affects a single body part; examples include cervical dystonia (torticollis); blepharospasm; writer's cramp.
- Segmental dystonia: affects one or more contiguous body parts; example is craniocervical dystonia, e.g., blepharospasm and torticollis.
- Multifocal dystonia: involves two or more noncontiguous body parts, for example, foot dystonia and torticollis.
- Generalized dystonia: segmental dystonia affecting one or both legs, the trunk, and one other body part.
- Hemidystonia: affects one half of the body; usually associated with lesion in the contralateral basal ganglia (especially the putamen).

Clinical features of the more common dystonias:

- *Cervical dystonia:* This is the most common focal dystonia, characterized by turning, tilting, flexion, or extension of the head and neck. Shoulder elevation and scoliosis are common.
- *Cranial dystonia:* Blepharospasm is a focal dystonia characterized by involuntary closure of the orbicularis oculi muscles. It usually begins as an increased frequency of blinking and progresses to clonic contractions of the eyelids, which may become more forceful and sustained. It may impair activities dependent on vision, such as driving and reading. It is often associated with dystonic contractions of other facial/cervical muscles.
- *Limb dystonia:* In adults, this manifests as a task-specific action dystonia, occurring with writing, typing, sporting activities, or playing a musical instrument. In children, limb dystonia most commonly presents as inversion of a foot while walking or running.
- *Laryngeal dystonia (spasmodic dysphonia):* This manifests as either excessive closing (adductor type) or prolonged opening of the vocal cords (abductor type). The former is more common and is characterized by an effortful and strained voice. The latter is characterized by a whispering voice.

Clinical features suggestive of a secondary dystonia:

- Abnormal neurologic findings other than dystonia
- Hemidystonia
- Onset at rest
- Rapid progression
- Initial involvement of legs in adults
- Initial involvement of cranial structures in children
- Speech involved early

LABORATORY PROCEDURES

Only needed if there is a suspicion of secondary dystonia

- Serum free copper and ceruloplasmin

IMAGING STUDIES

Only needed if there is a suspicion of secondary dystonia due to a structural lesion

- MRI or CT

SPECIAL TESTS

Only needed if there is a suspicion of secondary dystonia

- Urinalysis for 24-hour copper and amino acids
- CSF—lactate, pyruvate
- Slit-lamp examination—Kayser-Fleischer ring
- Skin biopsy—fibroblasts for lysosomal enzymes
- Genetic testing

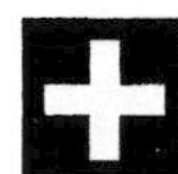

Management

GENERAL MEASURES

The majority of patients with idiopathic dystonia are treated with botulinum toxin injections and medications. A trial of carbidopa/levodopa (25/100 mg PO tid) should be considered in children and young adults with limb-onset dystonia for the possibility of DRD. If a secondary dystonia is identified, treatment for that condition is indicated. Surgical therapy is only rarely performed for intractable generalized dystonia.

SURGICAL MEASURES

Bilateral pallidotomy

SYMPTOMATIC TREATMENT

N/A

ADJUNCTIVE TREATMENT

- Physical/Occupational therapy
- Biofeedback
- Braces that mimic the *geste antagonistique*

ADMISSION/DISCHARGE CRITERIA

Admission is needed only when dystonia is so severe as to cause myoglobinuria, neuromuscular blocking agents are then required with subsequent mechanical ventilation.

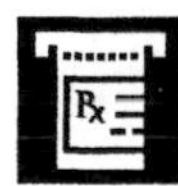

Medications

DRUG(S) OF CHOICE

- Botulinum toxin—type A
  - -Blepharospasm: 10-15 U per eye
  - -Cervical dystonia: 100-300 U
  - -Writer's cramp: 25-100 U
- Anticholinergics
  - —Trihexyphenidyl: initial dose—1 mg; titrate slowly to 6-12 mg qd in divided doses
- Benzodiazepines
  - —Clonazepam: initial dose—0.5 mg; titrate slowly to 1-12 mg qd in divided doses

Contraindications

- Allergies to above medications
- Botulinum toxin contraindicated in:
  - —Myasthenia gravis
  - —Eaton-Lambert myasthenic syndrome
  - —Motor neuron disease
  - —Aminoglycoside antibiotics
  - —Pregnancy

Precautions

Neutralizing antibodies may form to botulinum toxin.

ALTERNATIVE DRUGS

- Intrathecal baclofen
- Carbamazepine and phenytoin for paroxysmal dystonia

Follow-Up

PATIENT MONITORING

Patients should be seen 3 to 4 weeks after the first injection of botulinum toxin to assess for efficacy and complications. Injections should be given no more often than every 3 months to reduce development of antibodies to the toxin.

EXPECTED COURSE AND PROGNOSIS

Dystonia typically starts focally and can remain focal or progress to segmental or generalized. Childhood-onset dystonia is more likely to become generalized, while adult-onset dystonia tends to remain focal or segmental. Dystonia is a lifelong disorder; however, spontaneous remissions can occur occasionally in idiopathic dystonia.

PATIENT EDUCATION

The WEMOVE organization: *www.wemove.org.*

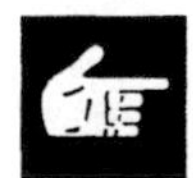

Miscellaneous

SYNONYMS

Torsion dystonia
Torticollis
Dystonia musculorum deformans

ICD-9-CM: 333.6 Dystonia—idiopathic; 333.7 Dystonia—due to drugs; dystonia—symptomatic; 781.0 Dystonic movements

SEE ALSO: CHOREA

REFERENCES

- Fahn S, Bressman S, Marsden CD. Classification of dystonia. Adv Neurol 1998;78:1-10.
- Jankovic J. Medical therapy and Botulinum toxin in dystonia. Adv Neurol 1998;78:169-183.
- Jankovic J, Leder S, Warner D, et al. Cervical dystonia: clinical findings and associated movement disorders. Neurology 1991;41:1088-1091.

Author(s): Paul G. Wasielewski, MD

Dystonic Reactions

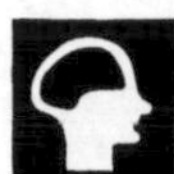

Basics

DESCRIPTION

Dystonia: involuntary muscular contraction leading to sustained postures that may be associated with writhing/twisting (athetoid) movements. A dystonic reaction (DR) implies that the dystonic activity observed is acute and has an identifiable cause, often medication. Movements associated with DR are often repetitive and appear paroxysmal.

EPIDEMIOLOGY

Incidence/Prevalence

DR is commonly seen in psychiatric practice affecting 2% to 12% of patients taking neuroleptics. DR may also occur with other drugs and substances.

Age

Children and young adults are much more vulnerable to this adverse effect of neuroleptics; the elderly rarely develop acute DR to neuroleptics. Predictors of DR for patients receiving neuroleptics, in order of importance: younger patients, male gender, dose, and potency of agent.

Sex

DR from neuroleptic exposure in the context of psychiatric disease favors males (2:1).

ETIOLOGY

- The pathophysiology of DR is not known. DR appears to be mediated by acute dopamine blockade or relative hyperactivity of the cholinergic environment.
- Agents implicated in the production of acute DR:
  - —Dopamine blocking antipsychotic agents: butyrophenones, phenothiazines, benzamides
  - —Dopamine blocking antinausea agents: metoclopramide, prochlorperazine, domperidone
  - —Serotonin agonist anxiolytic agent: buspirone
  - —Serotonin agonist antimigraine agents: sumatriptan
  - —Selective serotonin reuptake inhibitor antidepressants: e.g., fluoxetine
  - —Monamine oxidase inhibitor antidepressants
  - —Diphenhydramine (several patients have been described who developed DR after administration of the antihistamine diphenhydramine; it is of note that diphenhydramine is the drug of choice for most DRs)
  - —Erythromycin (single case report)
  - —Illicit drugs: cocaine (reported to lower threshold for the development of DR when taken in conjunction with neuroleptics; two cases of DR associated independently with cocaine have been reported)
  - —Tricyclic antidepressant (weak neuroleptic potential rarely associated with extrapyramidal reactions)

Genetics

There appears to be a higher incidence of DR among relatives of patients with idiopathic or torsion dystonia.

RISK FACTORS

Patients with a past history of acute dystonic reactions are at higher risk of future reactions upon reexposure to neuroleptics. Risk is also increased by neuroleptic dose and potency.

PREGNANCY

N/A

ASSOCIATED CONDITIONS

Endocrinopathies: hyperthyroidism, hypoparathyroidism, hyperglycemia

Diagnosis

DIFFERENTIAL DIAGNOSIS

Secondary dystonias may begin suddenly, often after some event, such as trauma, and are seen in association with other disorders, such as parkinsonism. Primary dystonias often begin insidiously and are more likely to be related to specific actions (e.g., writer's cramp). Acute dystonia may occur in the context of Parkinson's disease as dystonic cramps, often affecting feet in the morning, reflecting low dopamine levels. The signs of DR are dramatic, often frightening, and may be mistaken for seizure activity. However, unlike seizure, the acute DR is not associated with altered consciousness or postictal confusion. Simple partial seizures that are not associated with loss of consciousness may still pose a problem of differentiation. Paroxysmal dyskinesia, a poorly understood movement disorder associated with sudden involuntary movements, may be associated with dystonia. This group of disorders includes paroxysmal dystonic choreoathetosis, paroxysmal exertion-induced dyskinesia, transient paroxysmal dystonia, or torticollis of infancy.

SIGNS AND SYMPTOMS

Movements associated with DR include forced eye deviation with rotation of head up and back (oculogyric crisis, OGC), blepharospasm, torticollis, trismus, dysarthria, opisthotonus, and rarely laryngeal/pharyngeal spasm that may interfere with breathing and has been implicated in sudden death related to neuroleptic use. The onset of symptoms usually occurs 2 to 24 hours after initiation of first dose of neuroleptic. In the setting of parenteral administration of an antiemetic, such as prochlorperazine, the reaction may be immediate. The duration of the reaction is variable and may last days, waxing and waning. Signs may be more generalized in children and more circumscribed in adults. The region of the body involved may be constant or fluctuate during a DR, and the associated spasms and movements may be painful. Tonic lateral flexion of the trunk with backward rotation may occur 3 to 10 days after initiation of neuroleptic treatment, the Pisa syndrome.

LABORATORY PROCEDURES

Investigation should be appropriate for the setting. If a patient has a DR immediately after receiving a neuroleptic agent, no investigation may be indicated. Where the offending agent is not known but strongly suspected, a drug screen is indicated. If the tonic posture (opisthotonus) or other findings suggest a non-drug related cause (as in the setting of renal dialysis), a search for metabolic or infectious etiologies should be initiated. In the setting of an unexplained movement disorder, especially in a young patient, testing may include ceruloplasmin, serum copper, slit-lamp examination (to rule out Wilson's disease, a treatable entity), creatine kinase, myoglobin, glucose, lactate, pyruvate, uric acid, creatine, liver function studies, erythrocyte sedimentation rate, antinuclear antibody screen (see Dystonia; Torticollis).

IMAGING STUDIES

- If history and physical examination suggest the possibility of a focal underlying process, such as stroke, MRI of the appropriate anatomic area is indicated. However, for DR that is obviously drug induced, imaging is not required.
- If seizure remains a question on a clinical basis, electroencephalography is indicated.

SPECIAL TESTS

N/A

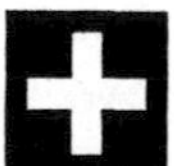

Management

GENERAL MEASURES

Treatment of an acute dystonic reaction includes dose adjustment or discontinuation of the offending agent, administration of medication to abort this reaction, and reassurance of the patient as these reactions are often frightening and painful.

SURGICAL MEASURES

- DR, due to neuroleptic agents, is self-limited and does not require ongoing treatment once the offending agent is removed and DR resolves.
- Late-occurring dystonia, tardive dystonia, in the setting of chronic neuroleptic drug exposure, may respond to chemodenervation with botulinum toxin.

SYMPTOMATIC TREATMENT

N/A

ADJUNCTIVE TREATMENT

N/A

ADMISSION/DISCHARGE CRITERIA

Admission for observation should be considered for severe DRs for observation and monitoring because of the tendency for waxing and waning and the need for repeated administration of anticholinergic agents.

Medications

DRUG(S) OF CHOICE

Many DRs are frightening, dramatic, may be painful, and require parenteral treatment.

- Mild reaction:
  - —Diphenhydramine 50 mg PO tid for several days or
  - —Benztropine 1–4 mg PO qd/bid (maximum dose 6 mg/d)
- Moderate to severe reactions:
  - —Diphenhydramine 50 mg IV, followed by several days of oral treatment
  - —Midazolam 2 mg IV
  - —Benztropine 1 mg IV q15–20 mins up to 3 doses
  - —Biperiden 2 mg IM/IV q 30 min (maximum doses 4 in 24 hours)
- Injectable medications are usually effective within 20 minutes. The effect may occasionally wear off with recrudescence of the dystonic reaction, necessitating a second injection.

Contraindications

- Known hypersensitivity to any of these medications.
- Diphenhydramine should not be used in neonates or nursing mothers.
- Benztropine is contraindicated in patients under 3 year of age.

Precautions

- Antihistamines (diphenhydramine) medications should be used with caution in patients with asthma, increased intraocular glaucoma, cardiovascular disease, hyperthyroidism, benign prostatic hypertrophy, and bladder neck obstruction.
- Acute dystonia related to Parkinson's disease: the acute dystonic cramp associated with Parkinson's disease may respond to adjustment medication if related to "off" time or part of a peak dose phenomenon.

ALTERNATIVE DRUGS

Other agents, such as lorazepam, biperiden, and benztropine, may be effective.
Consider hospitalization for observation as DR may recur and laryngeal/pharyngeal involvement is possible.

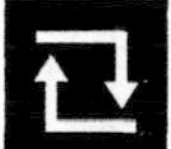

Follow-Up

PATIENT MONITORING

Patients who have experienced acute dystonic reactions are at higher risk for future reactions when taking neuroleptic medications. The use of prophylaxis with medications such as anticholinergics, antihistamines, or amantadine may be considered if long-term neuroleptic use is required and should be decided on an individual basis.

EXPECTED COURSE AND PROGNOSIS

Most DRs resolve rapidly with treatment as above. Failure to respond to several doses of parenteral anticholinergic medication should prompt additional evaluation.

PATIENT EDUCATION

Patients should be educated about the risk of recurrence of DR with neuroleptic medication.

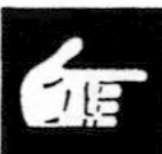

Miscellaneous

SYNONYMS

N/A

ICD-9-CM: 333.7 Dystonia due to drugs; 781.0 Dystonic Movements; 847.0 Dystonia due to trauma

SEE ALSO: PARKINSON'S DISEASE, WILSON'S DISEASE, DYSTONIA, TORTICOLLIS

REFERENCES

- Barach E, Dubin LM, Tomlanovich MC, et al. Dystonia presenting as upper airway obstruction. J Emerg Med 1989;7:237–240.
- Etzel JV. Diphenhydramine-induced acute dystonia. Pharmacotherapy 1994;14: 492–496.
- Garcia G, Kaufman MB, Colucci RD. Dystonic reaction associated with sumatriptan. Ann Pharmacother 1994;28:1199.
- Gerber PE, Lynd LD. Selective serotonin-reuptake inhibitor-induced movement disorders. Ann Pharmacother 1998;32: 692–698.
- Goetz CG, Horn SS. Treatment of tremor and dystonia. Neurol Clin 2001;19: 129–144.
- Jankovic J, Fahn S. Dystonic disorders in Jankovic J, Tolosa E. Parkinson's disease and movement disorders, 2nd ed. 1993; Baltimore: Williams & Wilkins, 337–374.
- Keepers GA, Casey DE. Prediction of neuroleptic-induced dystonia. J Clin Psychopharmacol 1987;8:342–345.
- Spina E, Sturiale V, Ancione M, et al. Prevalence of acute dystonic reactions associated with neuroleptic treatment with and without anticholinergic prophylaxis. Int Clin Psychopharmacol 1993;8:21–24.
- Tolosa E, Alom J, Marti MJ. Drug-induced dyskinesias in Jankovic J, Tolosa E. Parkinson's disease and movement disorders, 2nd ed. 1993; Baltimore: Williams & Wilkins, 375–397

Author(s): Peter J. Barbour, MD

Encephalitis

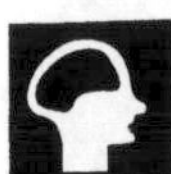

Basics

DESCRIPTION

- Encephalitis is an inflammation of the parenchyma of the brain. CNS function may be affected by direct invasion of the offending organism, vasculitis, hydrocephalus, or demyelination.

EPIDEMIOLOGY

Incidence/Prevalence

- There are approximately 20,000 cases of encephalitis each year in the United States. Herpes simplex virus (HSV) is the most common cause of sporadic focal encephalitis in the United States.

Race

- There is no evidence of any ethnic predominance.

Age

- The disease occurs in all ages.

Sex

- Males and females are equally affected.

ETIOLOGY

- Encephalitis may be caused by viruses, bacteria, amebae, or other parasites, and may be divided into seasonal and nonseasonal infections. Viruses are most common. Nonseasonal viruses are the herpes viruses, particularly herpes simplex type 1 (HSV-1), but also herpes simplex type 2 (HSV-2), varicella-zoster virus, Epstein-Barr virus (EBV), cytomegalovirus (CMV), and human herpesvirus type 6 (HHV-6). Other nonseasonal viruses include adenoviruses, enteroviruses, and rabies virus. One parasite, *Toxoplasma gondii,* may also cause nonseasonal encephalitis. Seasonal viruses include the mosquito-borne viruses (LaCrosse, or California group, St. Louis, Western Equine, Eastern Equine, Japanese, Venezuelan, and West Nile) and the tick-borne viruses (Colorado tick and Powassan). Other seasonal causes of encephalitis are bacterial diseases, including Rocky Mountain spotted fever *(Rickettsia rickettsii)*, ehrlichiosis (both monocytic and granulocytic), Lyme disease *(Borrelia burgdorferi)*, syphilis *(Treponema pallidum)*, tuberculosis *(Mycobacterium tuberculosis)*, Whipple's disease *(Tropheryma whippelii)*, and leptospirosis. Two amebae, *Naegleria* and *Acanthamoeba,* may also be responsible for seasonal encephalitis.
- HSV-1 encephalitis may occur from the primary infection or with reactivation of latent infection in the trigeminal ganglion with spread to the temporal lobe cortex and limbic structures. HSV-1 causes the majority of cases of HSV encephalitis in adults; in newborns most cases are caused by HSV-2.
- Postinfectious encephalitis may occur after influenza, measles, or varicella, or after immunizations. It is generally thought to be an acute inflammatory, demyelinating disease.

Genetics

- There is no known genetic predisposition for encephalitis.

RISK FACTORS

- Cases of encephalitis are generally sporadic, although outbreaks may occur, particularly with the arthropod-borne viruses. Generally, mosquito-borne encephalitis occurs from early summer to early fall, whereas tick-borne encephalitis occurs from spring to early fall. Patients who are immunocompromised, including those with HIV and AIDS, are at increased risk for certain causes of encephalitis, including *Acanthamoeba,* varicella-zoster virus, CMV, EBV, HHV-6, adenovirus, enterovirus, and *Toxoplasmosis.*

PREGNANCY

- Little is known regarding encephalitis in pregnancy. Neonatal HSV-2 infection is acquired during delivery by exposure of the fetus to maternal genital secretions. The risk of transmission is much higher during maternal primary infection compared to reactivation.

ASSOCIATED CONDITIONS

N/A

Diagnosis

DIFFERENTIAL DIAGNOSIS

Infectious Etiologies

- Viral meningitis
- Acute bacterial meningitis
- Brain abscess
- Fungal meningitis
- Mycobacterial meningitis
- Primary HIV infection

Noninfectious Etiologies

- Benign or malignant brain tumor
- Cerebrovascular accident
- Sarcoidosis
- Systemic lupus erythematosus
- Wegener's granulomatosis
- CNS vasculitis
- Arachnoiditis
- Migraine
- Drugs, including nonsteroidal antiinflammatory drugs, trimethoprim/sulfamethoxazole, and OKT3

SIGNS AND SYMPTOMS

- The onset of symptoms is rapid, with fever, nausea and vomiting, headache, and nuchal rigidity all being common. Alterations of consciousness, ranging from confusion and abnormal behavior to coma may be seen, as well as focal or generalized neurologic signs. These may include motor weakness, reflex asymmetry, aphasia, cranial nerve palsies, ataxia, seizures, or cortical blindness. For HSV encephalitis, clinical manifestations may progress over 2–3 weeks.

LABORATORY PROCEDURES

- Baseline blood work should include CBC and differential, blood cultures, serum electrolytes and glucose, liver function tests, and an HIV test. Serum may be sent for specific antiviral IgG antibodies, and determination of the cause of some cases of encephalitis may rely on the demonstration of a fourfold or greater increase in the viral antibody titer between acute and convalescent sera samples for the arthropod-borne viruses, HHV-6, and coxsackieviruses, echoviruses, and enteroviruses 70 and 71.

IMAGING STUDIES

- MRI scans of the brain may be helpful in suggesting the likely etiologic organism of encephalitis. For example, in HSV-1 encephalitis high-signal-intensity lesions on T2-weighted images may be localized to the medial and inferior temporal lobes of the brain, whereas Eastern Equine encephalitis generally localizes to the basal ganglia and thalami. The cranial MRI may be normal early in the course of encephalitis.

SPECIAL TESTS

- Although brain biopsy is the gold standard for diagnosis, it is rarely done. Instead, CSF obtained by lumbar puncture is the most important and accurate diagnostic tool. Opening pressure, Gram stain, CSF culture, protein, glucose, and cell count and differential, and polymerase chain reaction (PCR) for HSV should all be done. Opening pressure typically is mildly to moderately elevated. CSF is generally clear, with up to several hundred white cells/mm^3, mostly mononuclear cells, although polymorphonuclear cells may predominate early in the illness. Protein levels are generally normal to mildly elevated, and CSF glucose is generally normal. A hemorrhagic CSF may be seen with HSV encephalitis. PCR assay for HSV DNA may be falsely negative if collected during the first 48 hours of symptoms. The sensitivity of this test is very high if collected during the first 10 days of symptoms and then drops if collected further into the course of the illness.

- EEG usually is abnormal and shows diffuse bilateral background slowing, sometimes with epileptiform activity. When HSV-1 is the cause of the encephalitis, periodic complexes with sharp-and-slow waves at regular intervals of 2–3 seconds or focal slowing originating from the temporal lobes may be seen.

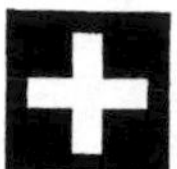

Management

GENERAL MEASURES

- A thorough search for epidemiologic, physical, or historical (e.g., travel, seasonal, zoonotic, or entomologic exposures) clues is imperative. No specific therapy other than supportive care is available for most cases. Empiric therapy for the few treatable organisms may be reasonable. Patients should be covered for HSV with acyclovir. If Lyme disease, Rocky Mountain spotted fever, or ehrlichiosis are suspected, doxycycline should be used. Use of amphotericin B should be limited to patients with exposure to lakes or other bodies of fresh water or immunocompromised hosts, unless amebic encephalitis is clinically suspected.

SURGICAL MEASURES

- There are no surgical measures for encephalitis.

SYMPTOMATIC TREATMENT

- If the patient has increased intracranial pressure, hyperventilation, dexamethasone, and hyperosmolar agents are indicated. Seizures are not uncommon in encephalitis and should be managed with standard anticonvulsant therapy. The usual ICU care for comatose patients includes aggressive pulmonary toilet, hydration and nutrition, and deep venous thrombosis prophylaxis.

ADJUNCTIVE TREATMENT

N/A

ADMISSION/DISCHARGE CRITERIA

- Patients are admitted for supportive care and evaluation of the etiology of the infection.

Medications

DRUG(S) OF CHOICE

- *Herpes encephalitis:* Acyclovir 10 mg/kg IV q8h or foscarnet 60 mg/kg IV q8h for 10–14 days
- *Varicella-zoster virus:* Acyclovir 10 mg/kg IV q8h for 10–14 days
- *Cytomegalovirus:* Ganciclovir 5 mg/kg IV q12h for 14 days
- *Rocky Mountain spotted fever, ehrlichiosis, Lyme disease:* Doxycycline 100 mg IV q12h for 7–10 days; in children under age 8, substitute chloramphenicol 50 mg/kg/day IV divided q6h
- *Leptospirosis:* Penicillin G 4 million units IV q4h for 7–10 days

Contraindications

- Known hypersensitivity to individual agents

Precautions

- Foscarnet, ganciclovir, acyclovir, and penicillin may all require dose adjustment for renal insufficiency.

ALTERNATIVE DRUGS

N/A

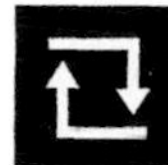

Follow-Up

PATIENT MONITORING

- Once hemodynamically and neurologically stable, close monitoring is not indicated.

EXPECTED COURSE AND PROGNOSIS

- The course and prognosis of the disease is highly variable depending upon the pathogen. The clinical course may range from mild with no sequelae to a rapidly deteriorating course with death or severe neurologic deficits or death. The fatality rate is the highest for Eastern Equine encephalitis with reported rates of 50%–75%.

PATIENT EDUCATION

- Website: *http://www.cdc.gov/epo/mmwr/other/case_def/enceph1.html* or *http://www.kidshealth.org/parent/common/encephalitis.html.*
- National Encephalitis Foundation Inc., 332 North 9th Street, San Jose, CA 95112-3347. Phone: 408-298-2060.

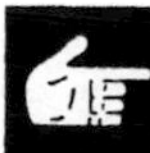

Miscellaneous

SYNONYMS

- Encephalomyelitis

ICD-9-CM: 323 Encephalitis, myelitis, encephalomyelitis; 320.0-320.9 Bacterial meningoencephalitis; 323.0 Encephalitis due to viral diseases; 323.1 Encephalitis due to rickettsial diseases; 323.2 Encephalitis due to protozoal diseases; 323.4 Encephalitis due to infections classified elsewhere; 323.5 Encephalitis following vaccination; 323.6 Postinfectious encephalitis; 323.9 Encephalitis of unspecified cause

SEE ALSO: N/A

REFERENCES

- Pruitt A. Infections of the nervous system. Neurol Clin N Am 1998;16: 419–447.
- Rubeiz H, Roos R. Viral meningitis and encephalitis. Semin in Neurol 1992;12: 165–177.
- Townsend GC, Scheld WM. Infections of the central nervous system. Adv Intern Med 1998;43:403–447.
- Whitley RJ. Viral encephalitis. N Engl J Med 1990;323:242–250.

Author(s): Thomas C. Keeling, MD; Susan L. Koletar, MD

Encephalopathy, Hepatic

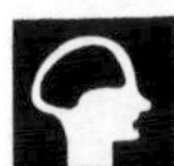

Basics

DESCRIPTION

- Hepatic encephalopathy is classified into acute and chronic varieties according to its associated liver abnormality. Acute hepatic failure is characterized by an encephalopathy and coagulopathy within 6 months of the onset of liver disease. A subcategory is fulminant hepatic failure that develops within 8 weeks of the onset of the hepatic dysfunction. Chronic liver disease evolves over a longer time and is associated with a fluctuating course of cerebral dysfunction, although some patients accumulate progressive motor and cognitive deficits

EPIDEMIOLOGY

Incidence

- Acute hepatic failure affects >2,000 Americans per year. All are encephalopathic, and the mortality is about 80%.
- Conservatively, 1 in 3,000 of the American population is susceptible to chronic hepatic encephalopathy, based on the prevalence of cirrhosis.

Age

- The age range is wide, but most cases with chronic hepatic encephalopathy are middle-aged adults.

Sex

N/A

Race

N/A

ETIOLOGY

- Many cases of acute liver are due to acute viral hepatitis or drug-induced liver injury (especially acetaminophen overdose). Less common causes include ischemia of the liver and toxins (e.g., mushroom poisoning or Wilson's disease).
- Chronic liver disease has a more varied association with encephalopathy, and the incidence is not well defined. Most cases are related to alcoholic cirrhosis. GI bleeding is a common precipitant of the encephalopathy in such patients, as this presents an increased load of nitrogen to the hepatic and then systemic circulation. Electrolyte disturbances, drugs (especially sedative drugs), infection, and surgery are other precipitants.
- The specific cause of the brain dysfunction is not known, but exposure of the brain, via the systemic circulation, to nitrogenous substances (including ammonia and increased aromatic amino acids, which can act as false neurotransmitters) are probable causes. Increased γ-aminobutyric acid (GABA), manganese, and opioids in the brain are also proposed to cause brain dysfunction. The cerebral edema that often accompanies acute hepatic encephalopathy is related to osmotic-induced astrocytic swelling (probably related to ammonia), as well as brain hyperemia.

RISK FACTORS

- The risk for chronic hepatic encephalopathy is increased after portal-systemic shunting procedures used to treat portal hypertension, especially bleeding esophageal varices, including transjugular intrahepatic portal-systemic shunting (TIPS).

PREGNANCY

- Acute fatty liver of pregnancy occurs late in pregnancy. It is associated with jaundice and a small liver. Often, the fetus is male with a deficiency of long-chain 3-hydroxyacyl-COH dehydrogenase.

ASSOCIATED CONDITIONS

- Hypoglycemia, hyponatremia, pulmonary infections, sepsis, coagulopathy (with bleeding complications, including subdural hematoma) are common accompaniments.
- *Hepatorenal syndrome* occurs in some cirrhotic patients and consists of worsening azotemia with sodium retention, oliguria, and hypotension. It probably is related to altered renal hemodynamics. The *hepatopulmonary syndrome* comprises hypoxemia-related right-to-left intrapulmonary shunts associated with increased endothelin-1 and pulmonary nitric oxide.
- *Acquired (non-wilsonian) hepatocerebral degeneration* associated with cognitive changes, extrapyramidal findings, ataxia, and myelopathy with widespread CNS damage may complicate protracted or repeated bouts of portal-systemic encephalopathy.

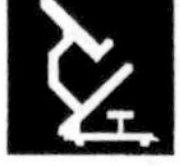

Diagnosis

DIFFERENTIAL DIAGNOSIS

- Intoxications with alcohol and drugs
- Infections, e.g., sepsis, meningitis
- Subdural hematomas, especially if bilateral, may be associated with fluctuating level of consciousness without strong lateralized features
- Alcohol withdrawal syndromes
- Other metabolic disorders, including hypoglycemia

SIGNS AND SYMPTOMS

- Acute hepatic failure is characterized by an initial delirium, often with delusions and hyperkinesis. Chronic hepatic encephalopathy shows greater fluctuation, with relapses and remissions over a long period of time, although acute decompensation also is possible. Even at their best, patients with chronic portal-caval shunting show decreased psychomotor speed and deficits in visual perception, orientation, and constructive ability. Disorders of attention underlie these deficits. Some patients develop extra-pyramidal movement disorders, including chorea or athetosis. Asterixis or flapping tremor is a transient loss of tone of muscles, causing the part of the body that is sustained against gravity to slump. This can include the outstretched arms and wrists, the head on the neck, or the whole body while standing upright.
- There are four stages of hepatic encephalopathy (Table 1).

Table 1 Stages of Hepatic Encephalopathy

STAGE	MENTAL STATUS	ASTERIXIS
I	Euphoria or depression, mild confusion, slurred speech, disturbed sleep	+/−
II	Lethargy, confusion	+
III	Stupor: sleeps but rousable, confused and incoherent	+
IV	Coma	−

LABORATORY PROCEDURES

- EEG shows typical triphasic waves in adult patients who are moderately encephalopathic, succeeded by diffuse delta (frequencies ≤4 Hz) and suppression in coma.
- No diagnostic liver abnormalities on commonly available biochemical testing, but elevated serum ammonia is highly suggestive.
- Respiratory alkalosis is characteristic.
- Elevated glutamine in the CSF is characteristic, but lumbar puncture often is contraindicated.

IMAGING STUDIES

- CT scanning is helpful in gauging the degree of cerebral edema (cortical sulci less visible, increased visibility of white matter, and basal cisterns obliterated) in acute hepatic encephalopathy. With chronic hepatic encephalopathy there is increased T1 signal in the globus pallidus.

SPECIAL TESTS

- In young patients, Wilson's disease is worth excluding. The diagnosis is made by finding any of the following combinations:
  - —Serum ceruloplasmin <20 mg/dL *and* Kayser-Fleischer rings
  - —Serum ceruloplasmin <20 mg/dL *and* a copper concentration >250 μg/g dry weight on a liver biopsy sample
  - —Compatible clinical picture and urinary excretion <100 μg copper/day in the urine

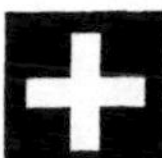

Management

GENERAL MEASURES

- Decrease ammonia production in the gut. Evacuate the bowel with laxatives and lactulose (also helps to convert ammonia to ammonium, which is less well absorbed) and enemas. Use neomycin to kill colonic bacteria.
- Give 20% glucose IV to prevent and correct for hypoglycemia.
- Restrict dietary protein and give carbohydrate supplements to exceed 1,600 calories/day.
- Check for and correct coagulopathy.
- Survey for and treat infections.

SURGICAL MEASURES

- Liver transplantation is appropriate for certain patients with acute hepatic failure (Table 2). Surgery should be done promptly, before the patient develops severe cerebral edema.

ADMISSION/DISCHARGE CRITERIA

- Patients with impaired consciousness require hospital admission, as do patients with acute hepatic failure or disease, in anticipation of encephalopathy. Patients with upper GI bleeding require emergency therapy for the bleeding and careful monitoring for encephalopathy.
- Discharging patients is an individual matter, with due consideration to medical status and support measures being in place.

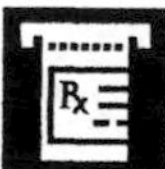

Medications

DRUG(S) OF CHOICE

- *Induction therapy:* Acutely, lactulose syrup 30–60 mL is given every hour until diarrhea occurs. Neomycin 0.5–1.0 g every 6 hours is given orally.

Table 2 Criteria for Consideration of Liver Transplantation in Acute Liver Failure

Acetaminophen toxicity	pH <7.3 (regardless of coma grade) or prothrombin time >100 sec and serum creatinine >3.4 mg/dL (300 μmol/L) in patients with grade III or IV encephalopathy
All other causes	Prothrombin time >100 sec (regardless of coma grade) and any three of the following:
	Age <10 yr or >40 yr
	Liver failure caused by non-A, non-B hepatitis, halothane-induced hepatitis, or idiosyncratic drug reactions
	Duration of jaundice before the onset of encephalopathy >7 d
	Prothrombin time >50 sec
	Serum bilirubin >17.5-mg/dL (300 μmol/L)

From O'Grady JG, Gimson AES, O'Brien CJ, et al. Controlled trials of charcoal hemoperfusion and prognostic factors in fulminant hepatic failure. Gastroenterology 1988;94:1186, with permission.

SYMPTOMATIC TREATMENT

- Patients with impaired consciousness should be cared for in an intensive care setting with the usual supportive measures.
- Mannitol has limited effectiveness in controlling cerebral edema.
- Consider mild hypothermia as a means of preventing brain hyperemia and increased intracranial pressure.
- Patients with bleeding complications may require transfusions of platelets or fresh frozen plasma.

ADJUNCTIVE TREATMENTS

- Branched-chain amino acid infusions, flumazenil (a benzodiazepine receptor blocker), hemoperfusion, and extracorporeal liver assist techniques are unproven, but the latter two occasionally can "bridge" the patient who is to undergo liver transplantation.

- *Maintenance therapy:* Chronic encephalopathy, especially in patients with portal-systemic shunting, can be controlled by regular oral administration of lactulose and reducing dietary protein.

Contraindications

- Avoid sedating drugs, especially benzodiazepines and barbiturates, and any measure that produces a systemic alkalosis, which increases ammonia production from ammonium ion.

Precautions

- Avoid hypocalcemia, which increases ammonia production. Vigorous paracentesis may produce electrolyte imbalance and precipitate or aggravate encephalopathy. Prevention of constipation is important. Any patient who is to undergo surgery should be monitored closely and the anesthesiologist informed well in advance of the surgery.

ALTERNATIVE DRUGS

- Alternative antibiotics such as metronidazole may be worthwhile.

Follow-Up

PATIENT MONITORING

- Acutely, patients need to be checked at least daily for clinical level of consciousness. Serial or continuous EEG monitoring offers a sensitive and objective assessment. The Mini-Mental State Examination is commonly used to track attention and concentration, but the Confusion Assessment Method and the Delirium Symptom Interview are alternatives. After discharge, follow-up with a family physician helps to ensure compliance with the treatment regimen.

EXPECTED COURSE AND PROGNOSIS

- Mortality and morbidity are high in patients with all types of hepatic coma. Survivors may be left with neurologic impairment. Severity of encephalopathy, small liver size and epileptiform activity on EEG are unfavorable prognostic features.

PATIENT EDUCATION

- Regular follow-ups, checks for compliance with diet, prompt recognition and treatment of gastrointestinal bleeding and infections, and care with medications are important measures.

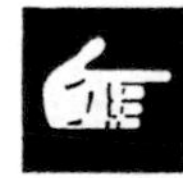

Miscellaneous

SYNONYMS

- Portal-systemic encephalopathy
- Hepatic coma

ICD-9-M: 572.2 Hepatic coma/hepatic encephalopathy

SEE ALSO: N/A

REFERENCES

- Blei AT. Pathophysiology of brain edema in fulminant hepatic failure, revisited. Metab Brain Dis 2001;16:85.
- Chapman RW, Forman D, Peto R, et al. Liver transplantation for acute hepatic failure. Lancet 1990;335:32.
- Lockwood AH. Hepatic encephalopathy. Boston: Butterworth-Heidenhain, 1992.
- Wijdicks EF, Plevak DJ, Rakela J, et al. Clinical and radiological features of cerebral edema in fulminant hepatic failure. Mayo Clin Proc 1995;70:119.

Author(s): G. Bryan Young, MD

Encephalopathy, Hypertensive

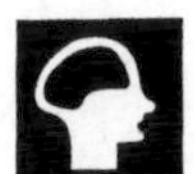

Basics

DESCRIPTION

- Hypertensive encephalopathy (HE) is a complication of malignant or accelerated hypertension and consists of focal and generalized central neurologic features. It is a medical emergency.

EPIDEMIOLOGY

Incidence

- HE is uncommon, but the exact incidence is unknown. Its incidence has lessened since effective antihypertensive therapy has been more available and more widely utilized.

Age

- HE can occur at any age, even young children. Manifestations are similar for different ages.

Sex

N/A

Race

- Given that hypertension is more prevalent in patients of African origin, HE is likely more common in this population. The racial difference is likely increased where there are discrepancies in medical care.

ETIOLOGY

- HE mainly occurs in the context of sudden elevations in blood pressure. This is common in acute or chronic renal failure, especially with volume overload or with the use of erythropoietin. The sudden withdrawal of some antihypertensives, especially clonidine, a centrally acting α-agonist, may precipitate HE. Other causes include the ingestion of tyramine-containing foods in patients taking monoamine oxidase inhibitors, sudden BP elevation in patients with pheochromocytoma, and lower gastrointestinal or urinary tract stimulation in paraplegic patients (autonomic hyperreflexia).
- In HE, the normal autoregulation of blood flow through capillaries is overwhelmed, allowing for engorgement of the capillary beds by high-pressure blood flow. This leads to vasogenic edema, fibrinoid necrosis of the walls of small vessels, and focal or multifocal ischemia, possibly due to vasospasm or occlusion of vascular beds by increased interstitial pressure.

RISK FACTORS

- Renal artery stenosis, renal failure, coarctation of the aorta, pregnancy (especially with a previous history of toxemia)

PREGNANCY

- Eclampsia is HE in the context of pregnancy-induced hypertension. Its manifestations are identical to those of HE. The HELLP (hemolysis, elevated liver enzymes, and low platelets) syndrome may occur as a complex associated with eclampsia. Intracerebral hemorrhages, often in the posterior cerebrum and commonly fatal, are frequent complications of the HELLP syndrome.

ASSOCIATED CONDITIONS

- HE occurs most commonly in patients with chronic renal failure, pregnancy (toxemia or eclampsia), and immunosuppression or interferon therapy.

Diagnosis

DIFFERENTIAL DIAGNOSIS

- Occipital blindness and seizures occur as complications of cancer chemotherapy, transplantation, transfusion, or HIV-1 infection.
- Focal deficits in hypertensive patients require the exclusion of intracerebral hemorrhage or infarction.
- Occipital blindness, in particular, requires the exclusion of infarction in the posterior cerebral artery distribution.
- HE may mimic amphetamine or cocaine overdose, encephalitis, or cortical venous thrombosis.

SIGNS AND SYMPTOMS

- Clinical features include headache, visual disturbance (especially field defects, blurred vision, and cortical blindness), confusion, focal neurologic signs, and focal, multifocal, or generalized seizures.
- Hypertensive changes are found in the fundi, including papilledema. Papilledema is not always present and is commonly absent in the reversible posterior leukoencephalopathy syndrome.
- Many patients show end-organ damage, including renal dysfunction with proteinuria and cardiac left ventricular hypertrophy and strain if the hypertension has been present for a prolonged period of time.

LABORATORY PROCEDURES

NA

IMAGING STUDIES

- MRI studies commonly show occipital-parietal lobe edema bilaterally that classically involves the white matter. However, the adjacent cortex may also be involved in the reversible posterior leukoencephalopathy or occipitoparietal encephalopathy syndrome.
- Altered blood–brain barrier permeability can be demonstrated using gadolinium (or equivalent large molecule markers with other scanning modalities, such as CT) scans.
- Imaging is helpful in excluding some of the conditions mentioned in the Differential Diagnosis.

SPECIAL TESTS

N/A

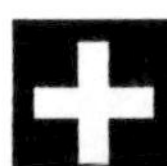

Management

GENERAL MEASURES

- With the clinical picture and exclusion of other processes (mainly by imaging), it should be possible to make a definitive diagnosis of HE. The main therapy is to lower the BP and to stop the ongoing process. Close observation in an intensive care environment, with monitoring of BP, neurologic status, renal output, and airway protection, is indicated.
- The cause of the hypertensive crisis should be sought and removed or treated directly, if possible.

SURGICAL MEASURES

- In severe, recurrent, refractory hypertension, bilateral nephrectomy is sometimes performed. This is a last resort measure because all renal functions (including renal erythropoietin production and vitamin D metabolic activity) will be lost, unless a transplant is performed.

SYMPTOMATIC TREATMENT

- Acute epileptic seizures should be treated. If coma is protracted, EEG monitoring is helpful in detecting and treating nonconvulsive seizures. Antiepileptic drug therapy for ongoing seizures usually begins with lorazepam or diazepam, followed by IV phenytoin (PHT) or fosphenytoin (15–20 mg/kg IV of PHT or PHT equivalents). For refractory cases, endotracheal intubation, assisted ventilation, and anesthesia with midazolam, propofol, isoflurane, or pentobarbital may be necessary.

ADJUNCTIVE TREATMENTS

- Angiotensin-converting enzyme (ACE) inhibitors are slow in action but appear to have a beneficial effect in blocking vascular permeability in the brain, related to angiotensin II. Furosemide helps to maintain sodium diuresis in the face of declining blood pressure. In renal failure, extra fluid can be removed using hemodialysis or peritoneal dialysis.

ADMISSION/DISCHARGE CRITERIA

- All patients with malignant hypertension and HE should be admitted and preferably managed in an ICU setting. Discharge can be considered when BP is controlled and renal function is stable in the absence of significant permanent neurologic sequelae.

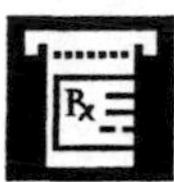

Medications

DRUG(S) OF CHOICE

- Induction therapy
  - —Blood pressure is lowered effectively by sodium nitroprusside 0.25–8.0 μg/kg/minute IV, although other rapidly acting, IV-administered antihypertensives, such as labetalol, may be helpful.
  - —Eclampsia is best treated with magnesium sulfate 4–5 g IV, followed by an infusion of 1 g/hour for 24 hours. Alternatively, 10 g is given IM, followed by 5 g IM every 4 hours for 24 hours. Patients should be monitored for magnesium toxicity by checking for loss of deep tendon reflexes and with serum magnesium concentration determination.
- Maintenance therapy
  - —There are six classes of maintenance antihypertensive therapy: diuretics, antiadrenergic drugs, vasodilators, calcium channel blockers, ACE inhibitors, and angiotensin receptor antagonists. The appropriate class and specific drug should be selected based on the underlying cause of the hypertension, severity of the hypertension, age of the patient, use of other medications, and goals of therapy. Guidelines were developed by the World Health Association in 1999.

Contraindications

- Labetalol should not be used in patients with heart failure, asthma, bradycardia, or heart block. Avoid diazoxide in patients with aortic dissection or myocardial infarction (cardiac stroke volume may increase with diazoxide.)

Precautions

- Care should be taken that the DBP does not fall below 95 mm Hg during the acute treatment phase, because this may compromise cerebral or myocardial perfusion.

ALTERNATIVE DRUGS

- Diazoxide 50–100 mg can be given as an IV bolus. The same dose can be repeated in 5–10 minutes, up to 600-mg total daily dose.

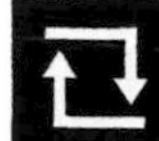

Follow-Up

PATIENT MONITORING

- Patients require regular follow-up for BP checks and neurologic review.

EXPECTED COURSE AND PROGNOSIS

- Neurologic prognosis usually is excellent. Most patients recover without neurologic deficits, but small infarcts may produce some focal signs and symptoms (uncommon in younger individuals). Most with acute symptomatic seizures do not require long-term antiepileptic drug therapy.

PATIENT EDUCATION

- The importance of regular medical checkups and compliance with medications should be stressed. Weekly blood pressure monitoring in the home by the patient, cohabitant, or visiting nurse is ideal.

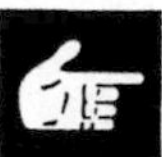

Miscellaneous

SYNONYMS

- Reversible posterior leukoencephalopathy
- Occipitoparietal encephalopathy syndrome

ICD-9-CM: 401.0 Hypertensive encephalopathy; 401.0 Malignant hypertension; 642 Hypertension complicating a pregnancy, childbirth, or puerperium

SEE ALSO: NA

REFERENCES

- Hinchey J, Chaves C, Appignani B, et al. A reversible posterior leukoencephalopathy syndrome. N Engl J Med 1996;334:494.
- Hirschl MM. Guidelines for the treatment of hypertensive crises. Drugs 1995;50:991.
- 1999 World Health Organization. International Society of Hypertension Guidelines for the Management of Hypertension. J Hypertens 1999;17:151.
- The Eclampsia Trial Collaborative Group. Which anticonvulsant for women with eclampsia? Evidence from the Collaborative Eclampsia Trial. Lancet 1995;345:1455.

Author(s): G. Bryan Young, MD

Encephalopathy, Hypoxemic

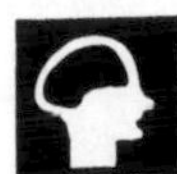

Basics

DESCRIPTION

- Hypoxic-ischemic encephalopathy (HIE) occurs in the setting of cardiovascular arrest. With the advent of cardiopulmonary resuscitation (CPR), large numbers of patients in whom circulation is reestablished are left with injury to the brain. An important duty of physicians in this setting is to establish the prognosis for recovery in a given individual. With cessation of circulation and respiration, an immediate cascade of energy depletion occurs. Lactate elevates, adenosine monophosphate rises, potassium leaks out of cells, and eventually calcium-mediated injury releases enzymes that cause breakdown of cellular fatty acids. Within minutes, neurons sustain irreversible damage that varies with different neuronal populations. Thus, a variety of patterns of neurologic injury occur in the setting of HIE.

EPIDEMIOLOGY

- In an observational cohort study in New York City, of 3,243 consecutive out-of-hospital cardiac arrests in a 6-month period, 1.4% survived. Of the in-hospital arrests, about 30% survive the CPR, and 10% survive to discharge. In one cohort of 1,832 patients with CPR, 1,472 died initially, 235 did not awaken after CPR, and of 124 who awoke after CPR, 61 were normal, 28 had moderate disability, and 36 were severely disabled. HIE occurs predominantly in populations at risk for cardiovascular arrest; therefore, it is seen commonly in elderly patients, usually those with cardiac or respiratory diseases.

Race

- HIE occurs in all races.

Sex

- HIE occurs with equal frequency in male and female populations.

ETIOLOGY

- HIE is due to any lack of oxygen and blood flow to the brain for more than a few minutes, as opposed to focal perfusion problems seen in stroke, and different from toxic exposures (such as carbon monoxide) or hypoglycemia.

RISK FACTORS

- Ischemic heart disease
- Hypertension
- Hyperlipidemia
- Smoking
- Known ventricular dysrhythmias

PREGNANCY

N/A

ASSOCIATED CONDITIONS

- See Risk Factors

Diagnosis

DIFFERENTIAL DIAGNOSIS

- Diagnosis usually is obvious and based on the clinical scenario. Differential includes other encephalopathies. In settings such as after open heart surgery, there may be other etiologies of an encephalopathy, such as sepsis, multifocal embolism, and medication effects.

SIGNS AND SYMPTOMS

- With resumption of circulation, resumption of brain activity occurs at varied rates. The extent of neurologic recovery ranges from complete cerebral inactivity to rapid resumption of normal consciousness in seconds. Various neurologic syndromes are seen between these two extremes. *Amnestic syndrome:* a discrete memory disorder may occur, with reduced recall of events before the arrest (retrograde amnesia) and a more profound impairment in acquiring new memories (anterograde amnesia). Due to injury to bilateral hippocampi. *Cortical blindness:* inability to see despite intact anterior visual pathways. Pupillary light reflexes remain normal. In some cases, patients deny blindness (Anton's syndrome). Due to border zone infarction in distal posterior cerebral arteries. *Action myoclonus:* sudden, rapid, arrhythmic movement of the limbs, face, or trunk may occur, often after severe global ischemic injury. If the patient is aware enough, myoclonic jerks may occur with attempted movement. Due to widespread ischemic change. *Bibrachial paresis (man in the barrel syndrome):* occasionally patients show bilateral arm paralysis with relative sparing of leg and face function. Due to injury in the arm areas of the cortex lying in watershed regions between the anterior and middle cerebral arteries. *Hypoxic-ischemic leukoencephalopathy:* a rare syndrome in which, after apparent recovery, within a few weeks patients show progressive intellectual change, involuntary movements, incoordination, and ultimately a vegetative state and death. Due to widespread white matter demyelination and necrosis. *Parkinsonian syndrome:* patients may develop parkinsonian signs of bradykinesia, rigidity, and gait disorders. Due to injury of basal ganglia. *Choreoathetosis:* writhing or jerking movements of the limbs or trunk. Due to basal ganglia involvement. *Vegetative states:* patients in whom no conscious interactions occur after months of survival. Sleep/wake cycles may occur, but patients do not interact with their environment. Due to severe injury to multiple cortical areas.
- Clinical examination is the key element in assessment of HIE. The neurologic examination is directed primarily toward assessment of the level of responsiveness, pupillary responses, corneal responses, oculocephalic responses (doll's eyes, cold calorics), respiratory pattern, and patterns of motor response (hemiplegic, decorticate, or decerebrate posturing, flaccid).

LABORATORY PROCEDURES

- There are no specific laboratory findings in HIE. Initial respiratory acidosis and lactic acidosis reverse rapidly with resumption of effective respiration and circulatory support.

Pathologic Findings

- On autopsy there are ischemic neurons, loss of neurons, and occasionally generalized edema. Areas most affected include cerebellar Purkinje cells, hippocampal cells, and certain cortical neuronal populations (layers 3 and 5).

IMAGING STUDIES

- CT or MRI show little or no change initially after HIE. Later in the course of disease, either atrophy or white matter demyelination may be seen.

SPECIAL TESTS

- Cortical somatosensory evoked responses may be useful in prognosis of HIE. Bilateral loss of cortical peaks (N20 peaks) is consistent with a 100% chance of mortality. In patients with vegetative states, PET scanning may show reduced cerebral metabolic rates. EEG may be used to judge the level of coma. Patterns on EEG, such as burst suppression, a very low voltage pattern, alpha coma, or electrocerebral inactivity, all have a poor prognosis.

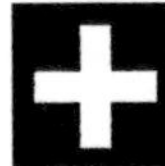

Management

GENERAL MEASURES

- Resumption of circulation and respiration is the key in caring for hypoxic-ischemic encephalopathy. Prevention of recurrent ventricular fibrillation or ventricular tachycardia, or restoration of metabolic status may be necessary. Appropriate nutritional support and fluids per standard ICU care are necessary. Reducing the risk of nosocomial infections, preventing venous thromboembolism, and avoiding stress peptic ulceration are important. Rapid treatment of fever, hypotension, hypoxemia, and metabolic disturbances aids in preventing secondary neuronal damage.

SURGICAL MEASURES

N/A

SYMPTOMATIC TREATMENT

- If patients are agitated, appropriate sedative medications may be helpful as long as respiration is carefully monitored.

ADJUNCTIVE TREATMENT

N/A

ADMISSION/DISCHARGE CRITERIA

- Most patients with a cardiac arrest or other cause of acute hypoxemic encephalopathy will require admission to the hospital. Discharge depends on the extent of injury and speed of recovery. Patients with significant hypoxic encephalopathy may require inpatient rehabilitation to achieve an optimal functional status.

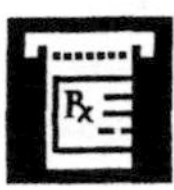

Medications

DRUG(S) OF CHOICE

- Despite multiple studies of various clinical agents, no specific treatments have been shown to be useful in improving the outcome after HIE.

ALTERNATIVE DRUGS

N/A

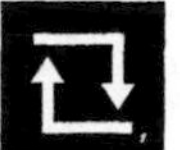

Follow-Up

PATIENT MONITORING

- Patients with significant HIE should be followed for signs of late deterioration. Usual follow-up is via the attending service or cardiology service.

EXPECTED COURSE AND PROGNOSIS

- Clinical outcome from HIE correlates closely with level of responsiveness of the patient. Patients who can be aroused during the first 12 hours after arrest usually do better, although mortality is still about 25%. Patients who are still decorticate, decerebrate, or flaccid and unresponsive at 24 hours have a 7% chance of survival. Absent pupillary response to light or corneal reflex for >6 hours after arrest indicates an extremely poor chance for survival. Any progression of neurologic signs in the first 48 hours denotes a poor prognosis. Other indicators of poor prognosis include the following at day 3 after arrest: abnormal brain stem responses, absent verbal response, absent withdrawal to pain, and age >70 years. Of out-of-hospital arrests, duration of CPR >than 15 minutes is related to a poor prognosis. Burst suppression or an isoelectric EEG in the first week has a 100% mortality in some series.

PATIENT EDUCATION

- Close communication with the patient's family is key to caring for patients with in HIE. Providing information about the patient's level of response, results of testing, and prognosis for recovery are key to allowing families to make important decisions regarding care.

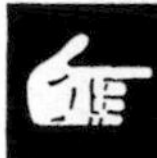

Miscellaneous

SYNONYMS

- Anoxia
- Anoxic brain damage
- Anoxic encephalopathy
- Anoxic ischemic encephalopathy
- Hypoxia

ICD-9-CM: 348.1 Anoxic brain damage

SEE ALSO: N/A

REFERENCES

- Bass E. Cardiopulmonary arrest: pathophysiology and neurologic complications. Ann Intern Med 1985;103:920–927.
- Lombardi G, Gallagher EJ, Gennis P. Outcome of out-of-hospital cardiac arrest in New York City. JAMA 1994;271:678–683.
- Hamel MB, Goldman L, Teno J, et al. Identification of comatose patients at high risk for death and severe disability. JAMA 1995;273:1842–1848.
- Madl C, Kramer L, Yeganehfar W, et al. Detection of nontraumatic comatose patients with no benefit of intensive care treatment by recording of sensory evoked potentials. Arch Neurol 1996;53:512–516.
- Taffet GE, Teasdale TA, Luchi RJ. In-hospital cardiopulmonary resuscitation. JAMA 1988;260:2069–2072.
- Zandbergen EGJ, de Haan RJ, Stoutenbeek CP, et al. Systematic review of early prediction of poor outcome in anoxic-ischaemic coma. Lancet 1998;352;1808–1812.

Author(s): Alexander D. Rae-Grant, MD

Encephalopathy, Metabolic and Toxic

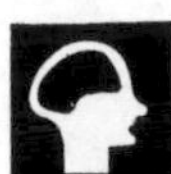

Basics

DESCRIPTION

- Metabolic encephalopathy most commonly is a disorder in which the patient exhibits *global neurologic dysfunction,* such as confusion, lethargy, or coma, as a result of *disruption of a biochemical process or introduction of a toxin.* It is also possible for patients to exhibit a focal neurologic deficit due to exacerbation of a previous underlying lesion (e.g., glucose dysregulation causes worsening hemiparesis in a patient with previous recovery from stroke). Many medical conditions can result in encephalopathy, and key to effective therapy is *diagnosis of the underlying cause.* Encephalopathy may have a single etiology or may be due to multiple metabolic derangements. In multifactorial encephalopathy, the observed cumulative effect often is greater than the individual insults would predict. Patients with preexisting neurologic disease generally have a heightened susceptibility to metabolic or toxic derangements. Some of the potential causes of metabolic and toxic encephalopathy are reviewed in Differential Diagnosis. Several other specific encephalopathies related to disease state are covered in other chapters within this text, including renal dysfunction, hepatic dysfunction, and sepsis.
- The underlying medical problem often is obvious to the clinician. However, some cases of encephalopathy are not readily apparent in origin and require *swift* diagnosis and treatment to prevent irreversible neuropathic changes.

EPIDEMIOLOGY

- The precise frequency of metabolic encephalopathy is known, but neurologists are commonly consulted in such cases. It occurs frequently in elderly populations, particularly in patients with multiple medical problems or polypharmacy.

ETIOLOGY

- See Differential Diagnosis

RISK FACTORS

- Various medications, advanced age, prior neurologic disease, dementia, various medical diseases

PREGNANCY

- Not a specific risk factor

ASSOCIATED CONDITIONS

- See specific conditions

Diagnosis

DIFFERENTIAL DIAGNOSIS

- The following list reviews a variety of causes of metabolic and toxic encephalopathy. For the specifics of each of these disorders, consultation of subspecialty texts is recommended.
  - —Glucose misregulation, e.g., hypoglycemia, nonketotic hyperosmolar state, hyperglycemia, diabetic ketoacidosis
  - —Electrolytes/fluid imbalance, e.g., osmolarity/sodium dysregulation, pontine myelinolysis, calcium disorders, magnesium disorders, phosphate disorders
  - —Endocrine dysfunction, e.g., cortisol abnormalities, thyroid dysfunction, adrenal dysfunction
  - —Toxic exposures, e.g., iatrogenic, accidental, intoxication, environmental exposure, drug withdrawal
  - —Pulmonary disease, e.g., pneumonia, pulmonary embolism
  - —Nutritional deficiency, e.g., vitamin B_{12}, folate, niacin, thiamin (Wernicke's syndrome)
  - —Psychiatric abnormalities, e.g., bipolar disorder, schizophrenia
  - —Renal dysfunction
  - —Sepsis/septic states
  - —Hepatic dysfunction
  - —Primary neurologic disease

SIGNS AND SYMPTOMS

- Patients with metabolic or toxic encephalopathy show various stages of altered mental status: confusion, inattention, lethargy, stupor, or coma. They may be delirious, with signs of agitation, hallucination, increased motor activity, and sympathetic overactivity. Brainstem function usually is intact in such patients. Patients who are encephalopathic often show a *gradual progression* from their normal function to encephalopathy in a variety of degrees from confusion to coma. The patient's mental status may show fluctuation. Early in the development of encephalopathy, the patient may experience minor changes in personality, including mood elevation/depression, mood swings, and inappropriate affect. The patient may proceed to display confusion, inattention, hallucination, delirium, and memory dysfunction. Motor dysfunction is common. including psychomotor retardation, hyperactivity, asterixis, myoclonus, gegenhalten (paratonic rigidity), and tremor.
- Extraocular eye movements usually are normal in encephalopathic patients. Patients may exhibit roving conjugate eye movements. Abnormalities of brainstem reflex (loss of doll's eye response, loss of cold water calorics) can occur in severe metabolic encephalopathies but should suggest other disorders, such as brainstem infarction.
- *Hypersympathetic function* is often observed in metabolic and toxic encephalopathies, with tachycardia, hypertension, diaphoresis, hyperreflexia, and clonus exhibited on examination.
- Abnormalities in breathing patterns are encountered with metabolic and toxic dysfunctions. These include, but are not limited to, apnea, sustained hyperventilation, and Cheyne-Stokes respiration (crescendo-decrescendo breathing with intervening periods of apnea).

LABORATORY PROCEDURES

- Chemistry laboratory examinations: basic metabolic profile and liver function testing, including electrolytes, glucose, calcium, and magnesium; include ammonia level
- Hematologic evaluation: should include CBC, platelets, differential, and peripheral smear
- Arterial blood gas: assists in establishing the acid/base status, as well as oxygenation and ventilation
- Urine or serum toxicology: depending on the patient's history, ethanol, drugs of abuse, expanded toxicology, or specific drugs (or metabolites) should be investigated
- Cultures of blood, urine, sputum, or wounds
- ECG: The clinician should look for baseline rhythm, as well as any signs of focality implying an ischemic event.
- Additional specific tests if ingestion is suspected. Check with local poison control.

IMAGING STUDIES

- Head CT: In patients with metabolic encephalopathy, head CT usually is normal. If clinical examination shows focal signs not explained by previous historical details, then contrast may be needed to assess for focal lesions. Caution must be used with contrast, because it may worsen the underlying condition and metabolic encephalopathy.
- MRI: If the patient has focal deficits, MRI can provide more substantive information on brain parenchyma. MRI also allows better visualization of the brainstem when the clinical examination suggests involvement.

SPECIAL TESTS

- Lumbar puncture: include evaluation of glucose, protein, cell counts, lactic acid, and culture. The opening pressure should be noted to evaluate increased intracranial pressures. Other specific tests should be performed as guided by the patient's history and examination (e.g., Lyme disease, syphilis). Before the patient undergoes a lumbar puncture, a head CT should be obtained to rule out possible sources for herniation, such as large focal mass lesions.
- EEG: useful in ruling out seizure activity (e.g., nonconvulsive status epilepticus). It also is helpful to look for signs of generalized dysfunction. Although the EEG rarely yields the specific cause of encephalopathy, it is useful for categorization and prognostication. Once the etiology has been determined and the treatment initiated, EEG can be a useful tool to determine improvement over time.
- Brainstem auditory evoked responses (BAER): can assist the neurologist in localization of brainstem abnormalities.

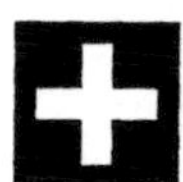

Management

GENERAL MEASURES

- Once the underlying cause of the metabolic or toxic encephalopathy has been determined, the treatment should be directed toward it. Thus, the treatment will be variable depending on cause. In general, avoid, if at all possible, sedating agents while the workup is in progress so as not to confound the clinical examination. If agitation prevents adequate medical or surgical care of the patient, short-acting sedative/anxiolytic agents, such as midazolam, propofol, or fentanyl, are more desirable than agents with prolonged effects.
- If the patient's mental status is so depressed as to prevent adequate protection of the airway, intubation and mechanical ventilation should be used.

SURGICAL MEASURES

- No specific surgical measures are needed.

SYMPTOMATIC TREATMENT

- Specific treatments for septic, renal, and hepatic encephalopathies are discussed elsewhere. In patients with exposure to toxins, antidotes may be available (contact the local poison control center), or the patient may benefit from hemodialysis.

ADJUNCTIVE TREATMENT

- Depends on the underlying cause of encephalopathy

ADMISSION/DISCHARGE CRITERIA

- *Close monitoring of the neurologic examination* is essential in patients with encephalopathy. As the patient becomes more lethargic, obtundation and airway protection may become a crucial consideration. Thus, if a patient is having a progressive decline in mental status, admission to a neurology or medicine critical care unit is highly recommended.

Medications

DRUG(S) OF CHOICE

- Drugs to be used are dependent on the underlying condition.

ALTERNATIVE DRUGS

N/A

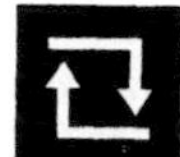

Follow-Up

PATIENT MONITORING

- Patients often exhibit a hypersympathetic state; thus, monitoring of heart rate and BP should be done frequently. The nursing staff should be trained to perform a thorough neurologic evaluation if they are not commonly asked to make this evaluation.

EXPECTED COURSE AND PROGNOSIS

- Although metabolic encephalopathy is one of the most frequently encountered entities in critically ill patients, it is most often *not necessarily fatal.* If the underlying metabolic or toxic origin can be ascertained and treated, the patient has *potential for complete recovery.* The cause of death in patients who are critically ill and suffer from an encephalopathy is often neurologic.

PATIENT EDUCATION

N/A

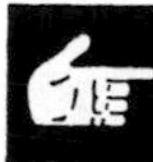

Miscellaneous

SYNONYMS

- Acute confusional state
- Delirium
- Acute organic brain syndrome
- Acute brain disorder
- Clouded sensorium
- Septic syndrome

ICD-9-CM: 348.3 Encephalopathy, unspecified; 349.82 Encephalopathy, toxic

SEE ALSO: ENCEPHALOPATHY, RENAL; ENCEPHALOPATHY, HEPATIC; ENCEPHALOPATHY, SEPTIC

REFERENCES

- Bleck TP. Metabolic encephalopathies. In: Weiner WJ, Shulman LM, eds. Emergent and urgent neurology, 2nd ed. Philadelphia: Lippincott Williams & Wilkins, 1999.
- Hund EF, Böhrer H, Martin E, et al. Disturbances of water and electrolyte balance. In: Hacke W, Hanley DF, Einhäupl KM, et al., eds. Neurocritical care. Heidelberg: Springer-Verlag, 1994: 917–927.
- Riggs JE. Neurological manifestations of electrolyte disturbances. In: Aminoff MJ, ed. Neurology and general medicine. Philadelphia: Churchill Livingstone, 2001:307–316.
- Shaw PJ. Thyroid disease and the nervous system. In: Aminoff MJ, ed. Neurology and general medicine. Philadelphia: Churchill Livingstone, 2001:317–339.
- Windebank AJ, Feldman EL. Diabetes and the nervous system. In: Aminoff MJ, ed. Neurology and general medicine. Philadelphia: Churchill Livingstone, 2001:341–364.
- Young GB. Renal diseases. In: Hacke W, Hanley DF, Einhäupl KM, et al., eds. Neurocritical care. Heidelberg: Springer-Verlag, 1994:928–935.

Author(s): Teresa L. Smith, MD; Bradford Worrall, MD, MSc

Encephalopathy, Progressive Pediatric

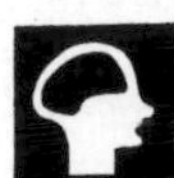

Basics

DESCRIPTION

- Encephalopathy is a generalized cerebral dysfunction that may be static or progressive in nature. Progressive encephalopathies in childhood affect the gray matter (poliodystrophies), white matter (leukodystrophies), or both.

EPIDEMIOLOGY

- Lysosomal storage disorders are seen as often as 1 in 7,000. Total incidence of neurodegenerative disorders approaches 1 in 1,000.

ETIOLOGY

Genetics

Storage Disorders

- *Lipidoses:* Excess lipid forms due to specific lysosomal enzyme deficiencies and is stored in gray matter nuclei.
  - —Hexosaminidase A deficiency (Tay-Sachs disease), hexosaminidase B deficiency (Sandhoff's disease)
  - —Sphingomyelinase deficiency (Niemann-Pick disease)
  - —Glucocerebrosidase deficiency (Gaucher's disease)
  - —Trihexosidase deficiency (Fabry's disease)
  - —Neuronal ceroid lipofuscinoses (NCL). Various forms (Batten disease, Jansky-Bielschowsky, Kufs, etc.).
- *Mucopolysaccaridoses:* Hunter disease (MPS II; Xq2), Hurler-Scheie disease (MPS I; 22q), Sanfilippo disease (MPS III), Morquio (MPS IV; 3p), and Maroteaux-Lamy syndrome (MPS VI; 17q) all have genetic defects resulting in enzymatic derangement. Sly disease (MPS VII) occurs with a deficiency of β-glucuronidase.
- *Leukodystrophies:* Diseases with enzymatic defects that result in dysmyelination due to accumulation of various substances.
  - —Metachromatic leukodystrophy: (autosomal recessive) deficiency of arylsulfatase results in storage of sulfatide in myelin
  - —Krabbe disease or globoid cell leukodystrophy: (autosomal recessive) deficiency of β-galactocerebrosidase
  - —X-linked adrenoleukodystrophy: increased plasma very-long-chain fatty acids
  - —Alexander disease: leukoencephalopathy with megalencephaly, unknown etiology
  - —Canavan's disease: spongy degeneration, deficiency of aspartoacylase
  - —Pelizaeus-Merzbacher leukodystrophy: mutation of gene for proteolipid protein
- *Metabolic encephalopathies*: predominantly autosomal recessive disorders
  - —Aminoacidopathies
  - —Organic acidemias
  - —Urea cycle defects
  - —Defects in glucose metabolism
  - —Wilson's disease, galactosemia, phenylketonuria, and Lesch-Nyhan syndrome
- *Other:*
  - —PEHO (progressive encephalopathy with hypsarrhythmia and optic atrophy): autosomal recessive, with decreased IGF-1 level, increased NO production, and eventual cerebellar degeneration
  - —Alpers' syndrome: autosomal recessive poliodystrophy linked to cytochrome c oxidase (COX) deficiency
  - —Aicardi-Goutieres syndrome (encephalopathy, basal ganglia calcification, and persistent CSF pleocytosis): autosomal recessive
  - —Seitelberger disease (infantile neuroaxonal dystrophy)
  - —Rett syndrome (microcephaly, hand wringing, regression): X-linked dominant (X;3)(p22.1-q13.31), Xp22.11, Xp11.3-Xp21, 18[del(18)(q22.3)]
  - —Hallervorden-Spatz disease: abnormal iron deposition in the brain, recessive gene on chromosome 20p
  - —Menkes disease: X-linked deficiency of copper
  - —Epileptic encephalopathies, includes West disease, Lennox-Gastaut syndrome, progressive myoclonic encephalopathy
  - —Autosomal dominant trinucleotide disorders (Huntington's disease)
  - —Zellweger syndrome (cerebrohepatorenal syndrome): peroxisomal disorder
  - —Refsum's disease: disorder of phytanic acid metabolism
  - —Other leukoencephalopathies: childhood ataxia with central hypomyelination

Mitochondrial Disorders

- Mitochondrial encephalopathies are due to derangements of energy metabolism; may be maternally inherited.
  - —MELAS (mitochondrial encephalopathy with lactic acidosis and strokelike episodes)
  - —Kearns-Sayre syndrome (ophthalmoplegia, hearing loss, encephalopathy)
  - —MERRF (myoclonic epilepsy and red ragged fiber syndrome)
  - —Leigh syndrome (encephalopathy with lactic acidosis)
  - —MNGIE syndrome (myoneurogastrointestinal encephalopathy) mutation coding for thymidine phosphorylase

Acquired

Infectious

- Acquired immunodeficiency disease syndrome (AIDS)-HIV-1 encephalopathy
- Progressive multifocal leukoencephalopathy caused by the JC virus
- Subacute sclerosing panencephalitis (rubeola) and progressive subacute rubella encephalitis
- Chronic enteroviral encephalitis and other retroviral infections
- Prion diseases, such as Creutzfeldt-Jakob disease, cause progressive cerebral dysfunction by transmitted protein particles

Other

- Systemic disorders, such as hepatic dysfunction, uremia, and porphyrias, can cause progressive encephalopathy.
- Hashimoto's encephalopathy with thyroiditis and antithyroid antibodies.

RISK FACTORS

- Genetic predisposition
- Measles, rubella, HIV, and other viral infections/vaccination

PREGNANCY

- Transmission of infectious agents can occur.

ASSOCIATED CONDITIONS

- Seizures
- Visual changes/ophthalmoplegia
- Ataxia
- Hypotonia/spasticity
- Myoclonus
- Dysmorphic features
- Micro/macrocephaly
- Peripheral neuropathies
- Cutaneous or visceral manifestations

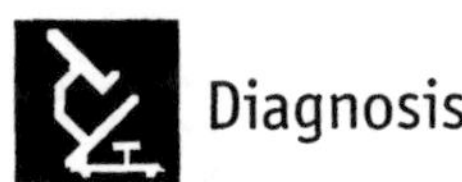

Diagnosis

DIFFERENTIAL DIAGNOSIS

- Static encephalopathies caused by nonprogressive neurologic insult
- Mental retardation of genetic etiology
- Seizure disorders and migraine variants
- Acute encephalopathies (delirium)

SIGNS AND SYMPTOMS

- Cognitive defects
- Deterioration of academic achievement
- Developmental, Language regression
- Behavioral changes and/or psychoses
- Worsening motor, visual, or auditory dysfunction
- Ataxia
- Abnormal movement
- Tremor, Dystonia
- Poor sucking
- Intractable seizures
- Associated motor and sensory peripheral neuropathies
- Hypotonia or spasticity

LABORATORY PROCEDURES

Blood

- Electrolyte panel to check for acidosis
- Serum amino acid levels
- Lactate, Pyruvate
- Ammonia levels
- Lysosomal enzyme assays in white cells

- Very-long-chain fatty acids
- Serum ceruloplasmin levels
- Ultrastructure of lymphocytes reveal membrane-bound inclusions of lysosomal storage, curvilinear, fingerprint, or granular patterns in ceroid lipofuscinoses, and abnormal mitochondria in mitochondrial disorders

Urine

- Urine organic acids
- Excretion of dextran and heparan sulfate
- *N*-acetylaspartic acid

CSF

- Glucose, Protein
- Lactate
- Viral polymerase chain reaction (PCR) and viral antibody levels

IMAGING STUDIES

- MRI usually is necessary:
  - —Poliodystrophies: MRI may show cortical atrophy, widening of sulci and fissures, increased extraaxial fluid and atrophy, and altered signal intensities in deep gray matter.
  - —Leukodystrophies: MRI may show altered signal intensities in white matter (unifocal, multifocal, or confluent).

SPECIAL TESTS

- EEG may demonstrate pathognomonic epileptiform discharges and patterns in various neurodegenerative disorders. West syndrome (an epileptic encephalopathy): hypsarrhythmia. Lennox-Gastaut syndrome: slow spike-and-wave pattern. Periodic spike and/or slow wave complexes are seen in SSPE and CJD.
- Ophthalmologic examination may reveal a retinal cherry-red spot (e.g., Tay-Sachs disease, Niemann-Pick disease), retinal degeneration, ophthalmoplegia (e.g., KSS), and optic atrophy (e.g., Krabbe disease)
- Nerve conduction studies may show peripheral nerve involvement.
- Evoked potentials demonstrate abnormalities depending on the etiology.
- Biopsy of tissue (skin, conjunctiva) will reveal abnormal intracellular inclusions and accumulation of abnormal materials in the various storage diseases. Muscle biopsy will reveal ragged red fibers in mitochondrial disorders.
- Genetic testing, including mitochondrial DNA analysis, is available for the majority of the disorders. Prenatal diagnosis is potentially available for all of the disorders with known genetic defect.
- Neuropsychological testing should be performed to assess the progression of deficits in the various cognitive domains.

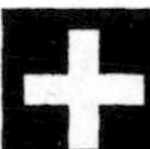

Management

GENERAL MEASURES

- Gene modulation; experimental.
- Enzyme replacement and bone marrow transplantation have been attempted, particularly in the leukodystrophies.
- Vitamin supplementation with coenzyme Q, folate, thiamin, and vitamin C has been tried, particularly in mitochondrial encephalopathies. Sodium selenite and vitamin E have been suggested in Batten disease.
- Dietary modification in cases of defects in glucose metabolism, aminoacidopathies, organic acidemias, and other inborn errors of metabolism is directed toward the specific defect. Glycerol trioleate oil has been tried in adrenoleukopathy.
- Lactic acidosis is managed with oral sodium bicarbonate or sodium citrate.
- Wilson's disease is treated with the copper chelating agent penicillamine.
- HIV encephalopathy is treated with antiretroviral drugs.
- HIV encephalopathy antiretroviral drugs.
- The other viral encephalopathies have no proven therapy, but immunomodulation with agents such as interferon, cimetidine, and inosiplex have been used.

SURGICAL TREATMENT

- Diagnostic biopsies and other supportive measures, such as CSF shunt procedures and tendon release procedures for spasticity

SYMPTOMATIC TREATMENT

- Seizures are treated with anticonvulsants. Valproic acid usually is the first line of antiepileptic drug therapy. Other anticonvulsants, such as lamotrigine, topiramate, and felbamate, are used for difficult-to-control seizures.
- Spasticity can be treated with muscle relaxants, such as baclofen and tizanidine.

ADJUNCTIVE TREATMENT

- Rehabilitation with physical, occupational, and speech therapy

ADMISSION/DISCHARGE CRITERIA

- Patients may be admitted for
  - —Treatment of intractable seizures
  - —Progressive deterioration of mental status
  - —Acute respiratory distress
  - —Infections
- Discharge to home or facility usually requires extensive nursing facilities

Medications

DRUG(S) OF CHOICE

N/A

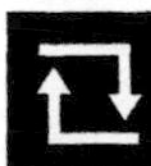

Follow-Up

PATIENT MONITORING

- Serial neuroimaging, cognitive testing, visual examinations, and blood levels can be used to monitor these patients.

EXPECTED COURSE AND PROGNOSIS

- The progressive course of these disorders may be protracted over several years or rapidly deteriorate in a matter of months in the more aggressive types. The infantile forms of most of the neurodegenerative diseases are notoriously relentless with a rapid downhill course. There is usually a progression of worsening of neurologic deficits, intractable seizures, stupor, and coma. Death often occurs as a result of respiratory compromise.

PATIENT EDUCATION

- Most of the individual diseases have support groups and organizations that help disperse knowledge. Examples include
  - —Batten Disease Support and Research Association
  - —National Gaucher Foundation
  - —United Leukodystrophy Foundation
  - —National Organization for Rare Disorders
  - —International Rett Syndrome Association

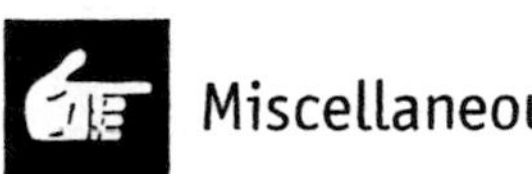

SYNONYMS

- Neurodegenerative disorder
- Childhood dementia

ICD-9-CM: 330.0 Childhood cerebral degenerations, leukopolioencephalopathy; 330.1 Cerebral lipidoses

REFERENCES

- Dyken P, Krawieki N. Neurodegenerative diseases of infancy and childhood. Ann Neurol 1983;13:351–364.
- Menkes JH, Sarnat HB, eds. Child neurology, 6th ed. Philadelphia: Williams & Wilkins, 2000.
- National Institute of Neurological Disorders and Stroke (NINDS). *www.ninds.nih.gov*
Online Mendelian Inheritance in Man. *www.ncbi.nlm.nih.gov/Omim*
- Sato T, DiMauro S, eds. Mitochondrial encephalomyopathies. New York: Raven Press, 1993.
- Swaiman KF, ed. The practice of pediatric neurology, 4th ed. St. Louis: CV Mosby, 1999.

Author(s): Akila Venkataraman, MD; Steven G. Pavlakis, MD

Encephalopathy, Renal

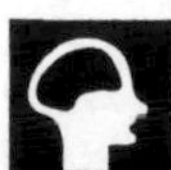

Basics

DESCRIPTION

- Renal encephalopathy is the occurrence of CNS dysfunction associated with either *renal failure itself or the dialysis process.* Renal patients may have other diseases causing encephalopathy.
- *Acute uremic encephalopathy* is suggested by development of daily to hourly fluctuating signs, including lethargy, confusion, irritability, hyperventilation, ataxia, myoclonus, and/or seizure. It appears to correlate with the *rapidity with which renal failure ensues,* rather than any single laboratory abnormality.
- *Dialysis dysequilibrium syndrome (DDS)* consists of headache, muscle cramps, disorientation, asterixis, somnolence, and possibly severe symptoms including frank psychosis, stupor, or generalized seizures that occur *during or after dialysis.*
- *Progressive dialysis encephalopathy (PDE)* or *dialysis dementia* is *related to the use of aluminum* as both a phosphate-binding agent and as a constituent of water used in the dialysis procedure. Its initial presentation is effortful speech with word-finding difficulties (in 93% of patients). Behavioral changes include depression, paranoia, apathy, and somnolence. Myoclonus begins in the upper extremities and then becomes multifocal. Other manifestations may include parkinsonism, ataxia, and seizures.

EPIDEMIOLOGY

- The precise frequency of uremic encephalopathy and dialysis dysequilibrium is not known. The incidence of PDE has decreased in recent years due to modifications of dialysis protocols to prevent aluminum exposure.

ETIOLOGY

- *Acute uremic syndrome:* Several compounds, such as urea itself, purines, guanidine, and phenols, may have toxic effects on the nervous system. Possible methods of action include disturbed energy balance, altered sodium transport, increased blood–brain barrier permeability, increased exposure to aluminum, increased brain calcium, and decreased brain magnesium. These imbalances may alter neuronal transmission.
- *Dysequilibrium syndrome:* There is an increase in water content in the brain parenchyma as a result of changes in osmolarity during dialysis. As the osmolutes are greater in the brain than in the plasma, the net flow of water into the brain occurs over a lag time created by diffusion of osmotically active particles from the brain into the extracellular spaces.
- *Progressive dialysis encephalopathy:* The exact mechanism of PDE remains unclear despite the implication of aluminum. Neurofibrillary degeneration similar to Alzheimer's disease (AD) may occur in PDE. The aluminum deposits in PDE are intracytoplasmic rather than intraneuronal as seen in AD, giving support to the theory that this may be aluminum-mediated neurotoxicity.

RISK FACTORS

- Patients are more likely to suffer dysequilibrium syndrome soon after initiation of dialysis. Aluminum in the dialysate is a risk factor for PDE.

PREGNANCY

N/A

ASSOCIATED CONDITIONS

- Uremic neuropathy
- Restless leg syndrome

Diagnosis

DIFFERENTIAL DIAGNOSIS

Acute Uremic Syndrome

- Hypertensive encephalopathy
- Septic encephalopathy
- Diabetic ketoacidosis
- Thrombocytopenia purpura/hemolytic uremic syndrome
- Anoxia
- Circulatory failure
- Toxin exposure (methanol, salicylates, paraldehyde, formaldehyde, ethylene glycol)

Dysequilibrium Syndrome

- Depression
- Hypotension induced hypoxic-ischemic encephalopathy
- Air embolism
- Subdural hematoma
- Hypernatremia or hyponatremia
- Wernicke's encephalopathy
- Hypoglycemia

Progressive Dialysis Encephalopathy

- Subdural hematoma
- Wernicke's encephalopathy
- Hypercalcemia/hyperparathyroid
- Depressive psychosis
- Alzheimer's dementia
- Creutzfeldt-Jakob disease
- Multifocal ischemic disease

SIGNS AND SYMPTOMS

Acute Uremic Syndrome

- Lethargy followed by inattention and confusion
- Delirium and hallucinations
- Motor manifestations such as myoclonus, carpopedal spasm, and asterixis
- Sleep disturbance
- Catatonia (rare)

Dysequilibrium Syndrome

- General: headache (diffuse, throbbing, or similar to preexisting migraines), nausea, vomiting
- Mental status: irritability, agitation, disorientation, drowsiness
- Ocular findings: exophthalmoses, increased intraocular pressure, papilledema
- Other: seizure, coma, psychosis, death

Progressive Dialysis Encephalopathy

- Speech disturbance: decrease fluency, word-finding difficulty, word substitutions, dysarthria, stammering
- Motor abnormalities: myoclonus (upper extremities affected first), athetoid movements, asterixis, gait disturbance
- Behavioral changes: apathy, depression, paranoia, somnolence, directional disorientation

LABORATORY PROCEDURES

- General chemistry panel: This will enable the clinician to look at electrolyte abnormalities, blood urea nitrogen, and serum creatinine.
- Arterial blood gas: The patient's acid–base status can be evaluated along with any signs of hypoxia and hypercapnia.
- Urinalysis with microscopic examination: The information obtained can assist with determining the cause of renal failure.
- Drugs of abuse screen and toxin screen.
- Serum aluminum level may be of assistance in the patient suspected of having PDE.
- Other rule-out investigations include blood cultures and CSF examination (see below).

IMAGING STUDIES

- In isolated renal encephalopathies, brain imaging often is unrevealing. Given the possibilities within the differential diagnosis, a head CT can point to another source for the physical examination changes (intracranial hemorrhage, stroke, subdural hematoma, subarachnoid hemorrhage). Imaging studies do not show specific changes in renal encephalopathy syndromes.

SPECIAL TESTS

- EEG shows a diffuse nonfocal slowing of background rhythms and superimposed bisynchronous burst of high-voltage slow wave. Generalized epileptiform activity is seen in one fourth of children with acute uremic syndrome but rarely seen in adults. In PDE, the most common reported finding is frontally predominant rhythmic delta. Triphasic waves also are seen in these encephalopathies, although they are more common in hepatic encephalopathy.

- Consider a lumbar puncture (LP) if meningitis is a concern. Because the patient with renal failure may have a bleeding diathesis, caution should be used. Measures such as cryoprecipitate and desmopressin acetate may shorten bleeding times. Once an LP has been established as safe by physical examination and head CT as needed, the results can demonstrate elevated protein (80–100 mg) and pleocytosis in 50% of uremic patients (7–600 cells/mm^3).

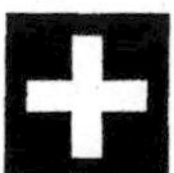

Management

GENERAL MEASURES

Acute Uremic Encephalopathy

- Identify the cause of the acute renal failure. Once the acute cause has been established, treat if reversible (e.g., obstructive uropathy or use of medication such as meperidine, acyclovir, magnesium, chronic NSAID).
- Dialysis if the patient has been exposed to a nephrotoxin or has acidosis, electrolyte imbalance, or fluid overload.
- Establish good urine flow by support of hemodynamic parameters.
- Maintain adequate nutrition to prevent further protein catabolism.
- Treat seizures if they occur. Dilantin is an acceptable choice because it is does not have active metabolites, but free levels must be monitored due to the decreased protein binding of dilantin in uremia. Dilantin should be dosed at q8h in this patient population.

Dysequilibrium Syndrome

- Avoid rapid osmotic shifts from the plasma to the brain.
- Increase the osmolarity of the dialysate by adding urea, sodium, mannitol, or glycerol.
- Decrease the flow rate during dialysis.
- Avoid hypotonic solutions.
- Consider using hemofiltration rather than hemodialysis.

Progressive Dialysis Encephalopathy

- Undertake preventative strategies.
- Monitor aluminum concentrations in dialysates.
- Avoid aluminum-containing antacids.
- Consider treatment with deferoxamine to chelate aluminum.
- Consider renal transplantation.

SURGICAL MEASURES

- If the cause of the patient's acute illness can be treated with dialysis, the clinician must establish a vascular access.

SYMPTOMATIC TREATMENT

- Dialysis or other measures as previously discussed above.

ADJUNCTIVE TREATMENT

N/A

ADMISSION/DISCHARGE CRITERIA

- If a patient is showing signs of encephalopathy that are not reduced by the regular dialysis session, hospital admission is warranted for workup of alternative causes of encephalopathy and to monitor potential progression of the patient's clinical state.

Medications

DRUG(S) OF CHOICE

- *Dilantin:* Although not typically needed, if the patient is having recurrent seizures then loading with dilantin is a reasonable action. Dilantin dosage should be adjusted for the patient's level of liver dysfunction and administered in three doses 8 hours apart. Typical loading dose for seizures is 15–18 mg/kg. May use fosphenytoin to avoid superficial phlebitis. In adults, initial dose is 100 mg PO tid; monitor free levels to achieve a therapeutic dose.
- *Thiamine:* Because thiamine is significantly water soluble, thiamin replacement should be given to patients undergoing dialysis. Wernicke's encephalopathy, although infrequent, has been observed in both children and adults on chronic dialysis.
- *Deferoxamine:* This chelating agent is used in patients who are suspected of having elevated aluminum levels producing a dialysis dementia syndrome. The weekly dose is 4–6 g, with 1–2 g given IV during the last 2 hours of dialysis.

Precautions

- Be aware of various side effects of dilantin or other seizure medications used.

Contraindications

N/A

ALTERNATIVE DRUGS

N/A

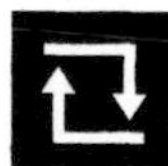

Follow-Up

PATIENT MONITORING

- Although PDE has been described with a wide range of aluminum concentrations (15–>1,000 μg/L), following aluminum levels may still be useful to the clinician.

EXPECTED COURSE AND PROGNOSIS

- The outcome for patients with renal encephalopathies can be excellent, provided there are few other comorbid conditions (such as GI bleed or sepsis). Mortality from acute renal failure without intervening illness is only 10%. Most patients recover from their encephalopathy after dialysis. Issues such as hypotension during dialysis can create additional problems, including ischemic stroke, which may preclude a complete recovery. Reversal of PDE has been reported after renal transplant.

PATIENT EDUCATION

- Diet suggestions and recipes can be found at the following website: *www.rockwellmed.com/links.htm*
- More information can be obtained from a search of the FDA's website: *www.fda.gov/default.htm*

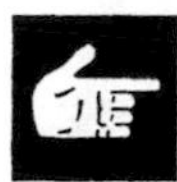

Miscellaneous

SYNONYMS

- Uremic encephalopathy or acute uremic encephalopathy
- Dialysis dysequilibrium syndrome
- Dialysis encephalopathy

ICD-9-CM: 348.3 Unspecified encephalopathy; E879.1 Kidney dialysis as a cause of abnormal reaction of patient; 38.95 Venous catheterization for dialysis

SEE ALSO: N/A

REFERENCES

- Bleck TP. Metabolic encephalopathies. In: Weiner WJ, Shulman LM, eds. Emergent and urgent neurology. Philadelphia: Lippincott Williams & Wilkins, 1999:223–253.
- Raskin NH. Neurological complications of renal failure. In: Aminoff MJ, ed. Neurology and general medicine. Philadelphia: Churchill Livingstone, 2001:293–306.
- Young GB. Renal diseases. In: Hacke W, Hanley DF, Einhäupl KM, et al., eds. Neurocritical care. Heidelberg: Springer-Verlag, 1994:928–935.
- Widjicks E. Neurologic complications of critical illness. New York: Oxford University Press, 2001.

Author(s): Teresa Smith, MD; Bradford Worrall, MD

Encephalopathy, Septic

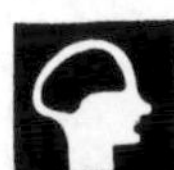

Basics

DESCRIPTION

- Septic encephalopathy refers to the *alteration of brain function* in the *presence of microorganisms or their toxins* in the blood. It is generally a *diagnosis of exclusion,* as a number of conditions may exist in a febrile patient to account for the encephalopathy

EPIDEMIOLOGY

- The incidence of septic encephalopathy is not precisely known, but its occurrence probably is underestimated. It is a common reason for neurologic consultation in the ICU.

ETIOLOGY

- The etiology is multifactorial.
  - —CNS infection: By definition, in order to make a diagnosis, one should rule out any CNS infection. This can generally be done with CSF evaluation. However, some patients with septic encephalopathy (especially those with a protracted course) have been found to have cerebral microabscesses at autopsy despite normal CSF *ante mortem.* This has not been a consistent finding, and septic encephalopathy occurs in noninfectious causes of sepsis such as pancreatitis.
  - —Metabolic dysfunction: In patients with multiorgan failure, secondary metabolic disarray may manifest as altered mental status. However, encephalopathy can be the first manifestation of sepsis prior to significant organ failure. One possible explanation is that hepatic dysfunction that occurs early in sepsis is difficult to recognize with available tests. Electrolyte disturbances are commonly detected in sepsis. Total parenteral nutrition is associated with hypophosphatemia and hyperosmolality. At autopsy, central pontine myelinolysis has been found in some patients. It is critical to recognize that the cumulative impact of metabolic disarray in sepsis may exceed the sum of the individual abnormalities.
  - —Alteration of the blood-brain barrier: Cytokines and other factors such as nitric oxide are released by cells during sepsis and increase the permeability of cerebral endothelial cells. Chemicals, both endogenous and exogenous, normally excluded from the brain may enter and influence brain function. Thus, drugs that normally have limited penetration of the CNS may have effects beyond what is expected during these circumstances. In addition, disruption of the blood-brain barrier may interfere with the diffusion of oxygen despite adequate delivery due to accumulation of edema. The cytokines themselves may have a direct effect on the brain as well.
  - —Alteration of neurotransmitter function: Alterations of neurotransmission have clearly been demonstrated in metabolic encephalopathies. An increase in the ratio of aromatic to branched chain amino acids can be found in the serum of septic patients. This results from altered systemic metabolism and muscle breakdown. In addition, there may be abnormal levels of other endogenous peptides, including benzodiazepine-like substances and hormones that in the setting of abnormal blood-brain barrier function may result in the alteration of neurotransmitter function in sepsis.
  - —Iatrogenic: Sedative drugs are commonly used in the septic patient. Effects of these medications may be enhanced due to increased penetration of the CNS. Clearance of the drugs may be impaired secondary to altered metabolism associated with organ dysfunction.
  - —Dysfunction of vasomotor reactivity: During sepsis, there is a reduction in carbon dioxide-induced vasomotor reactivity that may result in cerebral hypoperfusion. This may be mediated by cytokines and nitric oxide. Thus, ischemia may occur even at BP levels above the lower limit of autoregulation.

RISK FACTORS

- Immunocompromised states increasing risk of infection and sepsis
- Structural brain abnormalities increase susceptibility to all encephalopathies

PREGNANCY

N/A

ASSOCIATED CONDITIONS

N/A

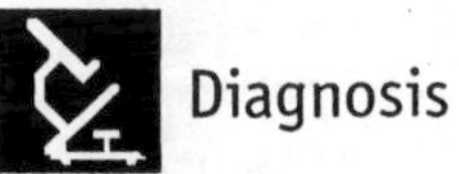

Diagnosis

DIFFERENTIAL DIAGNOSIS

- Septic encephalopathy is a diagnosis of exclusion and entails a workup of alternative causes. The differential diagnosis of septic encephalopathy includes but is not limited to
  - —Systemic infection
  - —Cortical venous thrombosis
  - —Intracranial hemorrhage related to coagulopathy
  - —Heat stroke
  - —Nonconvulsive status epilepticus
  - —Postictal confusion
  - —Endocarditis
  - —Deep vein thrombosis
  - —Intoxication/withdrawal
  - —Fat embolism
  - —Drug fever
  - —Acetylsalicylic acid toxicity
  - —Malignant neuroleptic syndrome
  - —Pulmonary, renal, or hepatic failure
  - —Adrenal failure
  - —Thyroid storm

SIGNS AND SYMPTOMS

- The clinical picture is similar to that of multifocal encephalopathy of other causes. Alteration of mental status is the fundamental neurologic abnormality. The level of consciousness ranges from clouding of consciousness to coma. Patients with only mild symptoms often show fluctuations in their clinical condition. Attention, memory, and concentration are impaired, as is written communication. Paratonic rigidity (increased resistance to movement of a limb throughout the entire range of motion) is characteristic. If the limb is moved very slowly, the rigidity resolves. Tremor, asterixis, and multifocal myoclonus also occur, although less frequently. Generally pupillary reflexes are intact. Seizures and focal findings may occur, especially in those with underlying structural disease that may be microscopic in nature. The presence of peripheral neuropathy is more common in patients with encephalopathy, and the severity of the neuropathy increases with the severity of the encephalopathy.

LABORATORY PROCEDURES

- Sepsis is a systemic inflammatory disorder that generally results from an infection. It is associated with multiorgan dysfunction that may manifest in a wide variety of serologic abnormalities.
- The severity of the encephalopathy is directly correlated with the peripheral white blood cell count, serum creatinine and urea, alkaline phosphatase, and bilirubin. On the other hand, serum albumin and Pao_2 are inversely related to the severity of encephalopathy. However, the patient may show evidence of altered mental status even prior to the onset of organ failure. Thus, serologic evaluations may only reveal evidence of an inflammatory process.
- Coagulation parameters should be monitored, as this system is frequently disturbed in sepsis with potential hemorrhages, including intracranially, as a consequence.

IMAGING STUDIES

- Noncontrast head CT is generally normal, especially in patients without focality on examination or EEG. This is used to exclude alternative causes of encephalopathy (e.g., intracerebral hemorrhage, abscess, infarction, subdural hematoma). There are insufficient data on the use of MRI and septic encephalopathy.

SPECIAL TESTS

- Lumbar puncture is indicated to exclude a CNS inflammatory process such as infection. The most common abnormality on CSF analysis in patients with septic encephalopathy is mild elevations of protein. Cell counts, glucose, stains, and cultures are either normal or negative.
- EEG is considered a more sensitive indicator of CNS dysfunction than is physical examination. It is always abnormal in the encephalopathic patient with bacteremia. Reduction in faster frequencies and a slowing of rhythms with increasing severity are the most common findings. Triphasic waves are common. A burst suppression pattern can be found in advanced cases; however, none of these findings are specific. The EEG is also prognostic. Mortality rises with the degree of EEG abnormality; however, the EEG is not an absolute predictor of poor outcome. Some patients with burst suppression have made full neurologic recoveries.
- Somatosensory evoked potential (SSEP) response testing has demonstrated slowing of the subcortical component of the dorsal column–medial lemniscal pathway that carries information from the periphery to the somatosensory cortex. However, there was no correlation between the subcortical sensory evoked potential and the severity of illness.

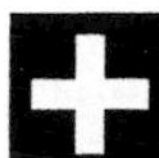

Management

GENERAL MEASURES

- There is no specific treatment for septic encephalopathy. Once secondary causes have been ruled out, the focus of treatment should be directed at the underlying cause.

SURGICAL MEASURES

- No specific surgical measures are indicated.

SYMPTOMATIC TREATMENT

- There are observations that patients may improve with flumazenil, a γ-aminobutyric acid-A antagonist, although the risk of potentiating seizures may limit its use. Infusions of amino acid solutions rich in branched chain amino acids have improved the mental status of patients with hepatic encephalopathy. Neither of these is an accepted treatment for septic encephalopathy but may be areas of future exploration.

ADJUNCTIVE TREATMENT

- Treatment should be directed at the underlying cause and comorbidities. Appropriate antibiotic regimens, as well as supportive care, are indicated and should be aggressively pursued, including respiratory care (mechanical ventilation if indicated, hemodialysis for patients with renal impairment, fluid and electrolyte management, and pressors for those with hemodynamic instability). If seizures are suspected, then antiepileptic medications should be initiated. Many patients require intensive care management.

ADMISSION/DISCHARGE CRITERIA

- Patients with sepsis typically are already admitted into the hospital. The need for critical care becomes important when the patient's encephalopathy significantly clouds his or her mental status such that he or she cannot protect the airway. By definition, encephalopathic patients require close observation and are unstable.

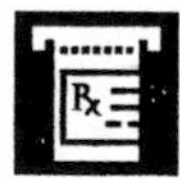

Medications

DRUG(S) OF CHOICE

- As with all patients with encephalopathy, sedation should be minimized and the particular agent chosen carefully. In general, the underlying condition and patient's comorbidities should dictate pharmacologic interventions.

ALTERNATIVE DRUGS

N/A

Follow-Up

PATIENT MONITORING

- The patient's underlying condition will dictate the degree of follow-up. Intensive care may be indicated. Serial neurologic examinations by staff trained in such evaluation to detect changes should be performed.

EXPECTED COURSE AND PROGNOSIS

- Encephalopathy is a common occurrence in sepsis. Whether it is an independent predictor of mortality is unclear, but mortality is higher with more severe degrees of encephalopathy.

PATIENT EDUCATION

N/A

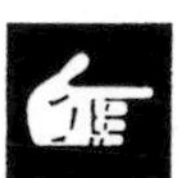

Miscellaneous

SYNONYMS

- Acute confusional state
- Delirium
- Acute organic brain syndrome
- Clouded sensorium
- Septic syndrome

ICD-9-CM: 348.3 Unspecified encephalopathy

SEE ALSO: N/A

REFERENCES

- Bolton CF, Young GB. Neurological complications in critically ill patients. In: Aminoff MJ, ed. Neurology and general medicine. Philadelphia: Churchill Livingstone, 2001:341–364.
- Terborg C, Schummer W, Albrecht M, et al. Dysfunction of vasomotor reactivity in severe sepsis and septic shock. Intensive Care Med 2001;27:1231–1234.
- Young BG. Neurological complications of systemic critical illness. Neurol Clin 1995;13:645–658.
- Young GB, Bolton CF, Archibald YM, et al. The electroencephalogram in sepsis-associated encephalopathy. J Clin Neurophysiol 1992;9:145–152.
- Zauner C, Gendo A, Kramer L, et al. Impaired subcortical and cortical sensory evoked potential pathways in septic patients. Crit Care Med 2002;30: 1136–1139.

Author(s): Robert Cavaliere, MD; Teresa Smith, MD; Bradford Worrall, MD

Epilepsy, Absence Seizures

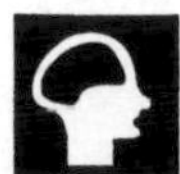

Basics

DESCRIPTION

- Absence seizures are generalized seizures characterized by paroxysmal loss of consciousness and brief discontinuation of activity followed by abrupt recovery with no recollection of the event.

EPIDEMIOLOGY

Incidence/Prevalence

- Absence seizures account for 2%–16% of seizures in all ages and are the seizure type most commonly undiagnosed.

Race

- No known difference

Age

- Absence seizures are seen more often in childhood, but they also occur in about 10%–15% of adults with epilepsies, often combined with other generalized seizures.

Sex

- Some studies showed twofold preponderance in girls.

ETIOLOGY

- There is increasing evidence that genetic factors are involved in the etiology of typical absence seizures. On the other hand, acquired disorders are more common in atypical absence seizures.

Genetics

- A family history of epilepsy is found in 15%–44% of patients with generalized absence seizures. Recent genetic studies have shown a mutation in the gene encoding for γ-aminobutyric acid (GABA) receptors.

RISK FACTORS

- History of febrile seizures

PREGNANCY

- About 25% of pregnant women have an increase in seizure frequency. Antiepileptic drug levels usually decline during pregnancy and should be monitored carefully.

ASSOCIATED CONDITIONS

N/A

Diagnosis

DIFFERENTIAL DIAGNOSIS

- Accurate diagnosis starts with a careful history: description of the seizures, including the duration and frequency, presence or absence of an aura, and postictal events. Primary diagnostic considerations for staring spells include absence seizures, complex partial seizures, and daydreaming. In contrast to absence seizures, complex partial seizures are much less frequent, are often preceded by an aura followed by postictal confusion, and are rarely activated by photic stimulation or hyperventilation. Daydreaming usually is caused by boredom, is of variable duration, can be interrupted by stimulation, and is never associated with clonic components. Absence seizures may frequently be misdiagnosed as nonepileptic disturbances of behavior. In addition, clouding of consciousness with ocular and oromotor automatisms may occur in partial and other generalized epilepsies.
- Absence seizures comprise the primary seizure type in several epilepsy syndromes. The syndromic diagnosis is important to determine optimal treatment and prognosis.
  —Childhood absence epilepsy (CAE): the most common syndrome with typical absence seizures
  —Juvenile absence epilepsy (JAE)
  —Juvenile myoclonic epilepsy (JME)
  —Myoclonic absence epilepsy (MAE)
  —Eyelid myoclonus with absences
  —Perioral myoclonus with absences
  —Stimulus-sensitive absence epilepsies
  —Idiopathic generalized epilepsy with phantom absences
- Atypical absence seizures occur in children with severe symptomatic or cryptogenic epilepsies and usually are associated with other types of seizures (atonic, tonic, and myoclonic).

SIGNS AND SYMPTOMS

- The main characteristic features are abrupt onset of brief staring, cognitive impairment. and change in facial expression. Duration is <20 seconds and is not followed by postictal changes. Many patients have associated minor motor movements, such as eye rolling, eyelid fluttering, head nodding, or subtle oral automatisms. Less frequently, mild sporadic myoclonic jerks of the head or extremities or change in muscle tone accompany absence seizures. Occasionally, autonomic features such as change in skin color, urinary incontinence, or pupillary dilation are present. Hyperventilation for 3 minutes will provoke an absence in nearly all untreated children with CAE.
  —In CAE, absence seizures begin between ages 5 and 10 years. The seizures occur many times per day. About 30% of children with CAE later develop generalized tonic-clonic (GTC) seizures.
  —JAE begins between 10 and 15 years. JAE patients usually have less frequent absences than those with CAE but higher risk for developing GTC seizures.
  —JME usually begins in adolescence with initial manifestations of myoclonic seizures, which predominantly occur on awakenings from sleep. GTC seizures usually develop later.
  —MAE usually is accompanied by severe bilateral rhythmical clonic jerks, often associated with a tonic contraction.
- The neurologic examination usually is normal in patients with typical absence seizures.
- Atypical absence seizures usually occur in children with subnormal mental function and are characterized by a less abrupt clear onset and offset, which usually is progressive. Atypical absence seizures last longer and have a higher incidence of changes in postural tone.

LABORATORY PROCEDURES

Electroencephalography

- Video-EEG is the single most important diagnostic procedure. In CAE, the EEG has a normal background and is characterized by bursts of rhythmic, generalized, high-amplitude 3-Hz spike-and-wave discharges of 4–20 seconds' duration, typically exacerbated by hyperventilation. In JAE, discharges are similar but with faster frequency, mostly 4–5 Hz with frequent polyspikes. JME is characterized by the occurrence of generalized polyspike and slow-wave discharges of 3–6 Hz. Atypical absences usually occur in the context of abnormal background and an ictal EEG of slow <2.5-Hz spike-and-slow wave.

IMAGING STUDIES

- Patients usually have normal neuroimaging. Neuroimaging, preferably MRI, is indicated if the patient has atypical features of the seizures, developmental delay, or abnormal neurologic examination.

SPECIAL TESTS

- Questionable cases could be evaluated with long-term video-EEG monitoring to record and characterize their events.

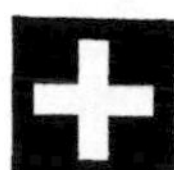

Management

GENERAL MEASURES

- Typical absence seizures often are easy to control with antiepileptic medications.

SURGICAL MEASURES

N/A

SYMPTOMATIC TREATMENT

- Contact sports, unsupervised swimming, driving, and other potentially dangerous activities should be restricted until seizures are well controlled. Bicycle helmets are mandatory.

ADJUNCTIVE TREATMENT

N/A

ADMISSION/DISCHARGE CRITERIA

- Patients who present with prolonged periods of stupor and impaired memory or cognitive functions could be suffering from absence status epilepticus. Inpatient EEG monitoring may be diagnostic by showing prolonged generalized bursts of spike-and-wave discharges. Intravenous or rectal benzodiazepines could be helpful for both treatment and diagnosis.

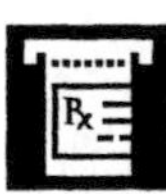

Medications

DRUG(S) OF CHOICE

- Ethosuximide: first drug of choice for isolated typical absences, with 70% rate of control. The initial dosage is 15 mg/kg/day, gradually increased to a daily maintenance dose of 20–mg/kg. Serious but rare side effects include aplastic anemia, Stevens-Johnson syndrome, and hepatic impairment. Common side effects include GI disturbances, anorexia, weight loss, drowsiness, photophobia, and headache.
- Valproic acid: second choice if ethosuximide fails to control absence attacks or the patient develops GTC seizures. Effective for 75% of patients with absence seizures, as well as generalized convulsive and myoclonic seizures. Initial dosage is 10–15 mg/kg/day. Maintenance dose in children is 30–60 mg/kg/day in three divided doses. Serious side effects include acute hepatic failure and acute pancreatitis. Common side effects include nausea, vomiting, dyspepsia, weight gain, polycystic ovaries, tremor, transient hair loss, and thrombocytopenia.
- Lamotrigine: may control absences and generalized seizures in 50%–60% of patients, but may worsen myoclonic jerks. Lamotrigine may have less cognitive side effects. It requires long titration prior to establishing therapeutic efficacy. It is used mainly as an adjunctive therapy and can be used as a monotherapy for children >12 years. For children ages 2–12 years taking valproic acid, lamotrigine could be added at 0.15 mg/kg/day and increased every 2 weeks by 0.15 mg/kg/day to a maximum of 5 mg/kg/day. In adults and children >12 years, lamotrigine can be added to valproic acid at a dose of 25 mg every other day and gradually increased to a maximum of 200 mg/day. Lamotrigine monotherapy can be given to patients >12 years at 25 mg daily and increased to a maximum of 100 mg/day. An allergic rash that could progress to Stevens-Johnson syndrome is the most common and probably most serious adverse effect. Other common side effects include headache, nausea, diplopia, dizziness, tremors, and ataxia. Side effects are more common with rapid titration or when combined with valproic acid.

Contraindications

- Valproic acid is contraindicated for children <2 years and for patients with hepatic disease.
- Vigabatrin, tiagabine, and carbamazepine are contraindicated for treatment of absence seizures, as they tend to exacerbate the seizures and could produce absence status epilepticus.

Precautions

- Neural tube defects occur in 1%–2% of offspring of women who took valproic acid during pregnancy.

ALTERNATIVE DRUGS

- Clonazepam or acetazolamide may be useful adjunctive drugs.

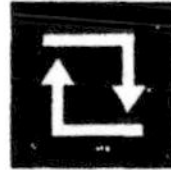

Follow-Up

PATIENT MONITORING

- Patients taking ethosuximide should have blood counts to monitor for aplastic anemia. Those taking valproic acid should be monitored for thrombocytopenia and hepatotoxicity. Therapeutic trough levels range from 40–100 mg/mL for ethosuximide and 50–100 mg/mL for valproic acid.

EXPECTED COURSE AND PROGNOSIS

- Typical absence seizures generally have a favorable prognosis. CAE carries the best prognosis; up to 95% of children with CAE will have complete remission. JAE has a less favorable prognosis than CAE but is better if absence seizures are the only seizure type. JME is usually a lifelong epilepsy.
- Poor prognostic factors include history of associated GTC or myoclonic seizures or absence status, positive family history of epilepsy, abnormal EEG background, or subnormal intelligence.

PATIENT EDUCATION

- Compliance with antiepileptics should be encouraged to avoid breakthrough seizures.
- Epilepsy Foundation of America. Phone: 1-800-EFA-1000; website: *www.epilepsyfoundation.org*
- Freeman J, Vining E, Pillas D, eds. Seizures and epilepsy in childhood: a guide for parents. Baltimore: The Johns Hopkins University Press, 1990.

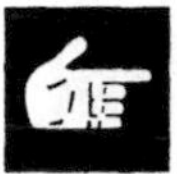

Miscellaneous

SYNONYMS

- Absence seizures (petit mal seizures)
- Childhood absence epilepsy (pyknolepsy)
- Juvenile absence epilepsy (nonpyknoleptic absence epilepsy)
- Juvenile myoclonic epilepsy (Janz disease)

ICD-9-CM: 345.0 Nonconvulsive generalized epilepsy

SEE ALSO: N/A

REFERENCES

- Camfield CS, Camfield PR, Gordon K, et al. Epileptic syndromes in childhood: clinical features, outcomes and treatment. Epilepsia 2002;43[Suppl 3]:27–32.
- Kramer U, Nevo Y, Neufeld MY, et al. Epidemiology of epilepsy in childhood: a cohort of 440 consecutive patients. Pediatr Neurol 1998;18:46–50.
- Ferrie CD, Giannakodimos S, Robinson RO, et al. Symptomatic typical absence seizures. In: Duncan JS, Panayiotopoulos CP, eds. Typical absences and related epileptic syndromes. London: Churchill Communications Europe, 1995:241–252.
- Panayiotopoulos CP. Absence epilepsies. In: Engel JJ, Pedley TA, eds. Epilepsy: a comprehensive textbook. Philadelphia: Lippincott-Raven Publishers, 1997:2327–2346.

Author(s): Khaled Zamel, MD

Epilepsy, Febrile Seizures

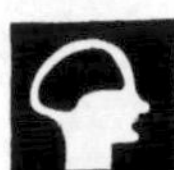

Basics

DESCRIPTION

- Febrile seizures are defined as "an event in infancy or childhood, usually between 3 months and 5 years, associated with fever, but without evidence of intracranial infection or defined cause." Febrile seizures are distinct from epilepsy, which is characterized by recurrent nonfebrile seizures. The febrile illness must have a temperature >38.4°C either before or after the seizure.
- Febrile seizures are simple or complex. Simple febrile seizures occur as solitary events, are generalized, and last <15 minutes. Complex febrile seizures have one or more of the following features: focality, duration >15 minutes, or recurrence in <24 hours. A complex febrile seizure or series of seizures that occur without recovery between events and lasts >30 minutes is termed *febrile status epilepticus.*

EPIDEMIOLOGY

Incidence/Prevalence

- The majority of febrile seizures are simple (65%). The most frequently described complex feature is focality, followed by recurrence and prolonged duration. Febrile status epilepticus accounts for only 5% of all febrile seizures, but accounts for 25% of all childhood status epilepticus and more than two thirds of status epilepticus in the second year of life.

Age

- Febrile seizures occur in 2%–5% of all children <5 years of age. They are most common between 6 months and 3 years, with peak incidence at 18 months. Onset after 7 years is uncommon.

Sex

- Boys are affected slightly more frequently than girls.

ETIOLOGY

Genetics

- No definitive gene or locus for febrile seizures has been identified. However, children with a positive family history of febrile seizures are more likely to experience febrile seizures and to have recurrences. Genetic studies favor a multifactorial or polygenic mode of inheritance, although autosomal dominant, incomplete penetrance modes of inheritance also may occur.

RISK FACTORS

- First- or second-degree relative with a history of febrile seizures
- Neonatal nursing stay ≥1 month
- Presence of developmental delay
- Attendance at day care
- Height of temperature

PREGNANCY

N/A

ASSOCIATED CONDITIONS

- Include upper respiratory infections, otitis media, roseola infantum, tonsillitis, and gastroenteritis. Herpesvirus-6 (roseola or exanthema subitum) is commonly associated with febrile seizures.

Diagnosis

DIFFERENTIAL DIAGNOSIS

- Febrile seizures are distinguished from epilepsy by the absence of previous febrile seizures, CNS infection, and other precipitating causes (e.g., trauma, electrolyte imbalance, toxins). Nonepileptic events that can mimic seizures (e.g., breath-holding spells) can be excluded by a careful history. Shaking rigor (shivering) in a febrile child is frequently misdiagnosed as febrile seizures.

SIGNS AND SYMPTOMS

- Febrile seizures often occur early in the course of a febrile illness. Tonic-clonic seizures are most common, but partial seizures can occur. A typical seizure involves a cry, loss of consciousness, and atonic posture. Breath-holding or circumoral cyanosis may be observed, along with vomiting and incontinence. Focality may be observed during the clonic phase. Postictal lethargy or sleep is common. The majority of events are brief (<15 minutes).

LABORATORY PROCEDURES

- The incidence of meningitis with febrile seizures is 2%–5%. Lumbar puncture should be performed in any child presenting with meningismus, bulging fontanelle, prolonged lethargy, recurrent seizures, or status epilepticus, or in infants <12–18 months (unreliable clinical signs of meningitis in this age group). In children >18 months without clinical suspicion for meningitis, a lumbar puncture is unnecessary. Lumbar puncture is still recommended in children with a first, complex febrile seizure.
- Routine laboratory studies (e.g., CBC, electrolytes) are indicated only as part of the evaluation of febrile illness.

IMAGING STUDIES

- Brain CT scans are of limited benefit in the setting of febrile seizures. Brain MRI scans are only indicated in the evaluation of complex febrile seizures.

SPECIAL TESTS

- EEGs are only likely to be abnormal in the older child and in children with a family history of febrile seizures, with complex febrile seizures, or with preexisting neurodevelopmental abnormalities.

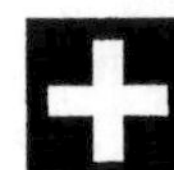

Management

GENERAL MEASURES

- Because most febrile seizures are brief, symptomatic care usually is unnecessary. If seizures persist, are recurrent, or develop into status epilepticus, treatment is mandatory. Because febrile seizures are a benign, self-limited condition that represents an age-dependent response to fever, long-term prophylactic treatment is unwarranted.

SURGICAL MEASURES

N/A

SYMPTOMATIC TREATMENT

- The primary goal of management is treatment of ongoing seizure activity. Treatment of the fever is unnecessary. If the patient is actively seizing upon arrival to the hospital, treatment should be initiated. IV diazepam or lorazepam is effective. Rectal diazepam or diazepam gel can be used if IV access is difficult. If the child continues to seize after an adequate dose of benzodiazepine, a status epilepticus treatment protocol should be initiated.
- For seizures that are prolonged or recurrent, parents can be instructed to administer rectal diazepam.

ADJUNCTIVE TREATMENT

- There is little evidence suggesting that antipyretic therapy has any benefit in febrile seizures. In one study, 50% of children with febrile seizures had previously received antipyretic medication before the febrile seizure. Children whose febrile seizure occurs at the onset of fever have the highest risk of recurrence and the most difficulty initiating therapy prior to the febrile seizure.
- Alternatively, diazepam given orally or rectally (0.5 mg/kg) at onset of a febrile illness reduces the recurrence risk by 50%. The reduction in seizure recurrence must be weighed against the sedative side effects of treatment.

ADMISSION/DISCHARGE CRITERIA

- A child presenting with a first-time febrile seizure warrants medical observation but rarely needs hospital admission. If the child is alert and active, and the etiology of fever is diagnosed and treated, the child can be discharged. Parents should be counseled that 16% of children experience another febrile seizure within 24 hours. Hospital admission is necessary with severe underlying febrile illness, recurrent seizures, prolonged febrile seizure or status epilepticus, and prolonged postictal state.

Medications

DRUG(S) OF CHOICE

Symptomatic

- Rectal diazepam or diazepam gel has been proven to be effective in treating prolonged febrile seizures. Five minutes of continuous seizure activity or repeated seizures within 30 minutes is the criterion for treatment. Dosing is based on age and weight: 0.5 mg/kg for 0–5 years of age, 0.3 mg/kg for 6–11 years, and 0.2 mg/kg for ≥12 years. Alternative drugs include sublingual or rectal lorazepam, which has not been as extensively studied.

Prophylactic

- Recent studies have failed to confirm the efficacy of phenobarbital and suggest the possibility of long-term cognitive and behavioral side effects; therefore, long-term phenobarbital therapy is rarely, if ever, warranted.
- Daily treatment with valproic acid does not consistently reduce febrile seizure recurrence.

Contraindications

- Known hypersensitivity to medications

Precautions

N/A

ALTERNATIVE DRUGS

- Chronic benzodiazepine use has not been well studied as a prophylactic treatment. Carbamazepine and phenytoin are ineffective in febrile seizure recurrence.

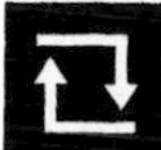

Follow-Up

PATIENT MONITORING

- Children with febrile seizures require only routine pediatric follow-up.

EXPECTED COURSE AND PROGNOSIS

Febrile Seizure Recurrence

- Approximately 33% of children with a first febrile seizure will have a recurrence, and 10% will have ≥3 febrile seizures. Several factors are associated with an increased risk of recurrence, including a family history of febrile seizures and an early age at onset of febrile seizure (before 18 months). The risk of recurrent febrile seizures is 50% when the first seizure occurs before 1 year and 20% when the first seizure occurs after 3 years. The risk appears to be related to the duration for which the child will be in the age group for febrile seizures. Other risk factors include the peak temperature and the duration of the fever before the seizures. Children with multiple risk factors are at higher risk for recurrence. For example, a child with ≥2 factors has a 30% recurrence risk compared to 60% for a child with ≥3 risk factors.
- The presence of a neurodevelopmental abnormality, complex febrile seizures, gender, and ethnicity do not carry an increased risk. If the initial febrile seizure is prolonged, a recurrent febrile seizure is also more likely to be prolonged.

Development of Epilepsy

- Epidemiologic studies have shown that 2%–10% of children with febrile seizures develop subsequent epilepsy. Conversely, 15% of children and adults with epilepsy have a history of prior febrile seizures. In general, the risk of epilepsy after a simple febrile seizure is <1%, similar to the risk in the general population.
- Several studies of adults with intractable temporal lobe epilepsy and mesial temporal sclerosis report that up to 40% had a history of prolonged febrile seizures. Population-based studies have failed to document this association, as have prospective studies on febrile seizure patients.

Intelligence and Neurodevelopment

- Longitudinal, population-based studies have shown no effect of febrile seizures on neurodevelopmental outcome.

PATIENT EDUCATION

- Counseling and reassurance are the most important mainstays of therapy. Instructions on how to respond to subsequent events are important, including the use of symptomatic treatment with benzodiazepines and when to utilize emergency services.

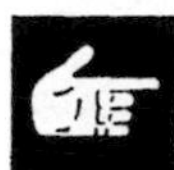

Miscellaneous

SYNONYMS

- Febrile convulsions

ICD-9-CM: 780.31 Febrile seizures

SEE ALSO: EPILEPSY, STATUS EPILEPTICUS

REFERENCES

- Baram T, Shinnar S. Febrile seizures. San Diego: Academic Press, 2002.
- Camfield P, Camfield C, Hirtz D. Treatment of febrile seizures. In: Engel J, Pedley TA, eds. Epilepsy: a comprehensive textbook. Philadelphia: Lippincott-Raven Publishers, 1997:1305.
- Hirtz DG, Camfield CS, Camfield PR. Febrile convulsions. In: Engel J, Pedley TA, eds. Epilepsy: a comprehensive textbook. Philadelphia: Lippincott-Raven Publishers, 1997:2483.
- Nelson KB, Ellenberg JH. Prognosis in children with febrile seizures. Pediatrics 1978;61:720–727.
- Rosman NP, Colton T, Labazzo RNC, et al. A controlled trial of diazepam administered during febrile illnesses to prevent recurrence of febrile seizures. N Engl J Med 1993;329:79–84.
- Shinnar S. Febrile seizures. In: Swaiman KF, Ashwal S, eds. Pediatric neurology principles and practice, vol. I, 3rd ed. St. Louis: Mosby, 1999:676.

Author(s): Julie Paolicchi, MD

Epilepsy, Generalized

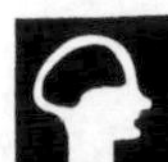

Basics

DESCRIPTION

- Epilepsy syndromes can be divided into two general groups: partial (focal) and generalized (primary). Generalized epilepsies originate from multiple (bilateral) areas of the brain simultaneously. Partial seizures originate from a single focus (although they often secondarily generalize or spread to both hemispheres). The speed of generalization of a focal seizure may be fast, so only close scrutiny of the EEG can determine if the seizure was primarily or secondarily generalized.

Specific Epilepsy Syndromes

- Benign familial neonatal convulsions (BFNC): onset in first week of life, lasting only 3–5 days; generalized usually less frequent than focal seizures
- West syndrome (infantile spasms): onset 1–24 months; idiopathic or symptomatic; infantile spasms, myoclonic seizures; EEG shows hypsarrhythmia pattern; accompanied by mental retardation
- Lennox-Gastaut syndrome (LGS): onset within first 14 years, usually within first 5 years; atonic, tonic, atypical absence seizures most common, also have generalized tonic-clonic (GTC), myoclonic; usually accompanied by psychomotor retardation that may precede or follow onset of seizures; may be idiopathic or symptomatic; ictal EEG shows slow (1.5–2.5 Hz) spike-and-wave discharges; lifelong; notoriously difficult to control
- Benign myoclonic epilepsy of infancy: myoclonic seizures between ages 4 months and 3 years.
- Childhood absence epilepsy: typical absences, with GTC seizures in 40% and rarely myoclonic seizures beginning between ages 3 and puberty; may have dozens of absence seizures per day; EEG shows typical 3-Hz spike-and-wave discharges; up to 80% have complete remission, usually in late adolescence; strong genetic component (75% monozygotic twin concordance)
- Myoclonic-astatic epilepsy (Doose syndrome): myoclonic, astatic, and less commonly absence seizures beginning in first 5 years of life
- Juvenile absence epilepsy: generally same as childhood variant, except onset after puberty; GTC seizures are more common (up to 80%); remission is uncommon
- Juvenile myoclonic epilepsy (JME): myoclonic and GTC seizures (absences in 10%–25%) beginning between ages 7 and 30 years, usually between 10 and 18. Myoclonic jerks of upper extremities as well as GTC seizures upon awakening are characteristic; EEG shows spike and slow waves; tends to be lifelong; positive family history of seizures in 20%–50% of patients
- Progressive myoclonic epilepsies: myoclonic, GTC seizures with gradual neurologic deterioration; causes include a variety of mitochondrial diseases, inborn errors of metabolism, and degenerative diseases

EPIDEMIOLOGY

- Prevalence of generalized epilepsies is 20–30 per 100,000 people. Cumulative incidence of generalized epilepsy from birth through age 80 is approximately 3%. Absence, myoclonic, tonic, clonic, and atonic seizures are much more common in childhood, whereas tonic-clonic seizures have a bimodal incidence in childhood and old age.

ETIOLOGY

- May be idiopathic or symptomatic. Idiopathic generalized epilepsy is often part of an epilepsy syndrome, such as JME or benign rolandic epilepsy. Symptomatic seizures may announce the presence of a myriad of disorders (metabolic, infectious, toxic).

Genetics

- Several genetic disorders that directly result in generalized epilepsy have been described, such as channelopathies. Many diseases that lead to generalized seizures are genetically determined (e.g., inborn errors of metabolism). The gene(s) that causes JME has been localized to 6p.

RISK FACTORS

- Many epilepsies are more common when there is a positive family history.

PREGNANCY

- Pregnancy in epileptic patients is a reason for referral to a neurologist for evaluation of risks to the mother and child. Seizure activity and medication levels may change with pregnancy.

ASSOCIATED CONDITIONS

- Generalized seizures are more common when structural abnormalities of the CNS are present.

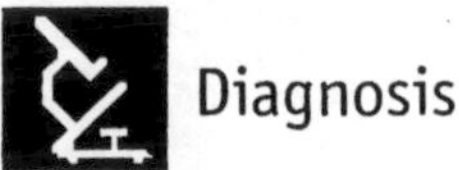

Diagnosis

DIFFERENTIAL DIAGNOSIS

- Psychogenic spells
- Atypical presentations of movement disorders

SIGNS AND SYMPTOMS

- GTC seizures: loss of consciousness followed by tonic stiffening of the body, often accompanied by a loud cry due to respiratory musculature involvement. After a variable period of time, a clonic phase ensues, typified by synchronous muscular contractions. This phase may result in tongue biting or other physical injury. The contractions then slow in frequency until ceasing, often with characteristic slow labored breathing and sometimes loss of bladder control. Patient may have decreased level of consciousness for a variable period of time afterward. The tonic and clonic phases may reoccur in various orders and be accompanied by marked increases in pulse and BP.
- Absence: sudden onset of decreased level of awareness and behavioral arrest without warning, lasting <15 seconds. May be accompanied by automatisms (purposeless motor activity, e.g., lip smacking, picking at clothes) No aura and usually no postictal symptoms. Atypical absences have unusual features, such as significant tonic features, postictal confusion, and atypical EEG findings
- Atonic: sudden loss of postural tone. May be so slight as to result only in brief nodding of head.
- Myoclonic: very brief muscle contractions (<0.5 second), often appearing as twitching or tremors
- Infantile spasms: brief, may be flexor, extensor, or both; resultant gross movement often appears as if the baby is reaching out or posing.
- Special attention should be paid to other signs of neurologic or systemic disease, such as growth curves, mental and motor development, dysmorphic features, and cutaneous findings.

LABORATORY PROCEDURES

- EEG most helpful when diagnosis is uncertain. Abnormalities are often but not always seen between seizures (interictally). Video-EEG monitoring is the gold standard to capture seizures and should be strongly considered in any patient in whom seizure type is unclear or in whom the first antiepileptic drug (AED) is not effective.

IMAGING STUDIES

- MRI with gadolinium contrast is the study of choice.

SPECIAL TESTS

- PET scans and nuclear medicine studies (SPECT imaging, SISCOM evaluation) are specialty tests to rule out focal onset seizures (which may be amenable to surgery).

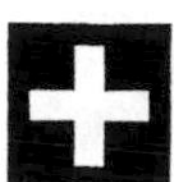

Management

GENERAL MEASURES

- The main focus is educating the patient and family about epilepsy and treatment with AEDs.

SURGICAL MEASURES

- Other than the placement of vagal nerve stimulators, surgery is not indicated in primarily generalized seizures except in refractory cases, in which palliative callosotomy is used for atonic and GTC seizures.

SYMPTOMATIC TREATMENT

- AEDs are initiated as soon as possible. Second-line nonmedication therapies include ketogenic diet (effective in select group of patients, mechanism unknown) and vagal nerve stimulation.

ADJUNCTIVE TREATMENT

N/A

ADMISSION/DISCHARGE CRITERIA

- It is important to keep in mind that seizure patients who usually are well controlled and have a breakthrough seizure may have a new underlying cause, such as infection or metabolic derangement.

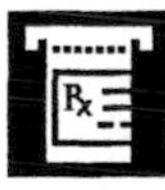

Medications

DRUG(S) OF CHOICE

- With the advent of numerous new AEDs, the drug of choice often is decided on a case-by-case basis. Research has shown that, in general, all of the old drugs and the newer drugs are roughly equally effective in seizure reduction. Side-effect profiles are the main differentiating factor among AEDs. The risks and benefits of each drug to the specific patient must be considered. Probable duration of treatment, treatment goals of the patient, and disability caused by the seizures are all factors.
- Phenytoin (Dilantin) is most often the drug of choice in GTC seizures due to its generic status, long history of proven efficacy, and relatively low side effect profile. Gum hypertrophy, hormonal disturbances, and peripheral neuropathy are possible
- Carbamazepine (Tegretol) is common first-line agent for GTC seizures, but it can exacerbate absence seizures.
- Ethosuximide (Zarontin) is the drug of choice in pure absence seizures. It is ineffective against all other seizure types. It has few significant side effects other than reversible leukopenia.
- Valproate (Depakote, Depakene, Depacon) is the drug of choice in epilepsies in which absence seizures coexist with other seizure types. It is very safe, but there is a small risk for hepatotoxicity. Tremor and weight gain are common.
- Phenobarbital (Luminal) is often the drug of choice in neonates. It also is effective against most other seizure types, but it can worsen absence seizures. Mental slowing and drowsiness are common but often decrease with time.
- Lamotrigine (Lamictal) often is used as a second-line agent. Rash can rarely be a serious side effect.
- Topiramate (Topamax), zonisamide (Zonegran), and levatiracetam (Keppra) are all showing promise for treatment of generalized epilepsies. Keppra has no significant drug-drug interactions and is renally excreted.
- Felbatol is used in LGS and as a third-line agent in other refractory epilepsies.
- Vigabatrin is not available in the United States but has been shown to be effective in LGS.
- Adrenocorticotropin hormone (ACTH) and steroids are proven beneficial in West syndrome.

Contraindications

- AEDs are notorious for drug-drug interactions, especially the older agents (phenytoin, carbamazepine, valproate, phenobarbital). Significant morbidity and even mortality can be caused by the resulting toxic levels of medications, as well as subtherapeutic levels leading to breakthrough seizure activity. Drugs that interact with AEDs include warfarin, antifungals, calcium channel blockers, and rifampin.

Precautions

- Antiepileptic medications tend to have several side effects in common, including effects on cognition, balance, gait, and GI function. As with many medications, allergic reactions can occur and be fatal.

ALTERNATIVE DRUGS

- Switching to a new drug or adding a second drug should be done only after a therapeutic trial of the initial AED.

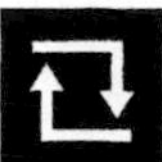

Follow-Up

PATIENT MONITORING

- Follow-up with a neurologist is recommended to determine the future need for AED therapy, as well as to receive specialized counseling regarding the diagnosis of epilepsy.

EXPECTED COURSE AND PROGNOSIS

- After a single unprovoked seizure with a normal EEG and MRI, the chance of a second seizure is only 30%–40%. The prognosis for generalized epilepsies depends to a large extent on the particular epilepsy syndrome and presence or absence of definable causes.

PATIENT EDUCATION

- Activities should not generally be restricted, except driving or flying (which is often dictated by state laws). Patients should get adequate sleep and avoid alcohol and any known stimuli.
- Epilepsy Foundation of America. Website: *www.efa.org*

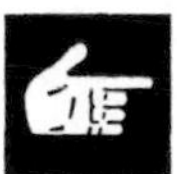

Miscellaneous

SYNONYMS

- Grand mal seizures (antiquated)
- Epilepsy, major (motor)

ICD-9-CM: 345.9 Epilepsy, generalized; 345.1 Epilepsy, generalized, convulsive; 345.0 Epilepsy, generalized, nonconvulsive; 345.4 Epilepsy, secondarily generalized

SEE ALSO: N/A

REFERENCES

• Liprace JD, Sperling MR, Dichter MA. Absence seizures and carbamazepine in adults. Epilepsia 1994;35:1026–1028.

Author(s): Mark R. Gibson, MD; Joseph Sirven, MD

Epilepsy, Infantile Spasms

Basics

DESCRIPTION

- The triad of infantile spasms (IS), a hypsarrhythmic EEG pattern, and mental retardation constitutes West syndrome.

EPIDEMIOLOGY

- 90% of patients with IS present in infancy. The incidence is estimated at 0.24–0.6 per 1,000. IS comprises 1.4%–3.9% of all childhood seizure types.

ETIOLOGY

- In the majority (60%) of patients with IS, a specific etiology can be identified. (symptomatic IS). A second group of infants (termed *cryptogenic*) is assumed to have underlying CNS dysfunction based on abnormal neurologic examination or developmental delay. Idiopathic cases are defined as having normal development, neurologic examination, neuroimaging studies, and unremarkable etiologic evaluations. Family studies support a genetic susceptibility to epilepsy that requires environmental stimuli to precipitate seizures.
- Symptomatic etiologies include
  - —Prenatal causes: cerebral dysgenesis, Sturge-Weber syndrome, Aicardi's syndrome, hydrocephalus, congenital infections, trauma; genetic etiologies include tuberous sclerosis, Down's syndrome, and incontinentia pigmenti.
  - —Perinatal disorders: hypoxic-ischemic encephalopathy, CNS infections, trauma, stroke
  - —Postnatal disorders: metabolic disorders such as pyridoxine dependency, nonketotic hyperglycinemia, maple syrup urine disease, phenylketonuria, mitochondrial encephalopathias

RISK FACTORS

- Any CNS injury to the early developing brain

PREGNANCY

N/A

ASSOCIATED CONDITIONS

- Developmental delay and mental retardation; only 10% of patients are developmentally normal at the time of diagnosis. Patients may also manifest other seizure types, especially focal and tonic seizures.

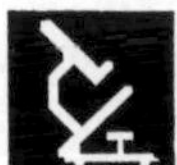

Diagnosis

DIFFERENTIAL DIAGNOSIS

- IS sometimes are misinterpreted as normal infant movements such as hiccuping, posturing, or lack of head control.
  - —Myoclonus in infancy: Differential of myoclonus in infants includes movement disorders such as hyperexplexia (excess startle response), and benign and hereditary essential myoclonus. Benign neonatal sleep myoclonus begins in the first month of life. The movements occur only in sleep, cannot be stopped by gentle restraint, and are eliminated on arousal. Infants are typically neurodevelopmentally normal, and spells usually remit by 6 months of age.
  - —Benign myoclonus of infancy: onset between 3 and 15 months of age with clusters of tonic or myoclonic jerks frequently involving the head and trunk. EEGs are normal, and there is no evolution into epilepsy. The course is self-limited, diminishing within 3 months of onset and ceasing before 2 years of age. The diagnosis is made retrospectively, once serial EEGs and neurologic development remain normal.
  - —Shuddering attacks are uncommon paroxysmal events that may start in infancy, but they also may occur later in childhood. They consist of behavioral arrest but no loss of consciousness, tonic posturing, and flexion or extension of the head and neck. Ictal EEG is normal.
  - —Spasmus nutans is a condition of asymmetric nystagmus, head nodding, and anomalous head position in infants.

SIGNS AND SYMPTOMS

- IS presents as a cluster of spasms of brief, usually bilaterally symmetric contractions of the muscles of the trunk, neck, and extremities. predominantly flexor, extensor, or mixed flexor-extensor. The events are stereotyped in an individual child and vary from a massive abrupt contraction of all flexor muscles to a brief subtle head nod. Clusters predominate on awakening. The number of spasms and clusters/day can be variable. Associated phenomena include nystagmus, eye deviation, autonomic features (flushing, pallor, pupillary dilation), or a cry at the conclusion of the spasm.
- Arrest of neurologic development or a loss of milestones often accompanies the onset of IS. Neurologic examination abnormalities are present in approximately 70% of patients.

LABORATORY PROCEDURES

- Focus on uncovering an etiology for IS, especially metabolic causes (4% of cases). Evaluation includes serum electrolytes, liver function tests, CBC, serum ammonia, lactate, pyruvate amino acid quantification, biotinidase assay, cholesterol profile to screen for peroxisomal disorders, and urine organic acid quantification; chromosome analysis if examination suggests a syndrome. CSF should be tested for lactate for mitochondrial disorders and glycine for nonketotic hyperglycinemia. Ophthalmologic examination is included to evaluate for Aicardi's syndrome, congenital infections, neurodegenerative diseases, and tuberous sclerosis; Wood's lamp skin examination for tuberous sclerosis.

IMAGING STUDIES

- Head MRI is recommended to evaluate for CNS malformation, present in 20% of IS cases, stroke, hypoxic-ischemic encephalopathy, infection, or tuberous sclerosis. Abnormal neuroimaging studies are seen in 70%–80% of cases and are associated with a poor prognosis.

SPECIAL TESTS

- A prolonged EEG that includes sleep is recommended. Ictal video-EEG recording is optimal. The characteristic demonstration of IS, hypsarrhythmia, is a background interictal pattern of disorganized, high-voltage activity with bursts of multifocal and generalized epileptic activity. Hemispheric asymmetry and focal epileptiform abnormalities are not uncommon. Early in IS, hypsarrhythmia may not be present or present only in deep sleep, so serial EEGs may be necessary. The ictal EEG pattern typically consists of an initial slow wave followed by low-amplitude fast activity (14–16 Hz) or diffuse attenuation, referred to as an *electro-decremental response.*
- To evaluate if pyridoxine deficiency is the etiology of IS, pyridoxine 100 mg IV is administered during the EEG. If significant background improvement is noted, chronic pyridoxine treatment is initiated.

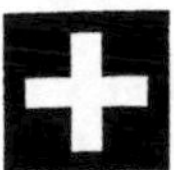

Management

GENERAL MEASURES

- Both adrenocorticotropin hormone (ACTH) and corticosteroids are efficacious in treating IS. Other options include newer antiepileptic drugs.

SURGICAL MEASURES

- Surgical resection of focal cortical regions is reserved for children with persistent IS despite appropriate treatment. Surgical resection of areas of hypometabolism on PET, often located posteriorly in the temporal and occipital lobes, has led to recovery.

SYMPTOMATIC TREATMENT

- Developmental assessments and early intervention programs

ADJUNCTIVE TREATMENT

- H_2-blockers such as ranitidine for steroid-induced gastritis
- Diuretic therapy for steroid-induced hypertension and irritability

ADMISSION/DISCHARGE CRITERIA

- Patients presenting with IS often are hospitalized for video-EEG monitoring to allow etiologic evaluation and initiate therapy.

Medications

DRUG(S) OF CHOICE

- *ACTH:* Intramuscular ACTH is the most frequently used treatment. Treatment success is based on resolution of both the spasms and the hypsarrhythmia, so a follow-up EEG is required and must include sleep. Relapse occurs in up to 47% of patients but often can be successfully treated by a second course of therapy. Proponents of the low-dose regimen (20–40 U/m^2) recommend an increase in dose if spasms continue for 2 weeks. Proponents of the high-dose regimen, which tends to be preferred, recommend 150 U/m^2 of body surface area per day, followed by a rapid taper over 1–2 weeks if spasms are gone and the EEG is not hypsarrhythmic. This approach minimizes side effects but has a high relapse rate, so longer tapers are often used, with every-other-day dosing after the first weeks to minimize side effects.
- *Corticosteroids:* The most common alternative to ACTH therapy is corticosteroids. Oral steroids are easier to administer but have similar side effects. Prednisone is administered at 2 mg/kg/day in 2–4 divided doses for 4 weeks, followed by a taper. Patients who fail to respond to ACTH can respond to steroids, and vice versa. Studies have suggested a lower responder rate and a higher relapse rate with steroid therapy compared to ACTH.
- *Vigabatrin:* For patients who do not respond to or cannot tolerate either ACTH or corticosteroids, vigabatrin has shown effectiveness, especially for children with tuberous sclerosis. Unlike ACTH, response to vigabatrin is dose dependent: increasing doses up to 150 mg/kg/day gradually decreases spasm frequency. Ideal duration of therapy is unknown but is commonly continued for 1 year after cessation of IS, or up to 3 years of age.
- *Antiepileptic drugs:* Other antiepileptic drugs, including high-dose valproate, topiramate, tiagabine, nitrazepam, and zonisamide, have been used in uncontrolled trials.

Precautions

- Side effects of steroids/ACTH include GI irritation, hypertension, irritability, cushingoid weight gain, electrolyte imbalance, hypoglycemia, and acne. The patient should be monitored for BP, Hemoccult in stool, serum electrolytes, and glucose in the urine. During the course of therapy, the immune system is suppressed so that routine immunizations are contraindicated.
  - —Vigabatrin is not approved for use in the United States, nor is it commercially available because of risk for retinal damage resulting in loss of peripheral vision. Regular ophthalmologic or visual evoked response examinations are used to screen for this problem.
  - —Risk of valproate-induced hepatotoxicity is highest in the IS age group.

Contraindications

- Known hypersensitivity to these drugs

ALTERNATIVE TREATMENT

- High-dose vitamin B_6 (pyridoxine) 300–500 mg/kg/day has been used in uncontrolled trials. For refractory IS, the ketogenic diet has been attempted.

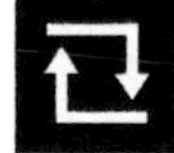

Follow-Up

PATIENT MONITORING

- For patients treated with ACTH or steroids, routine monitoring of BP, urine glucose, and stool Hemoccults are performed at home. Follow-up EEGs are important to assess response.

EXPECTED COURSE OF PROGNOSIS

- IS can spontaneously remit: 89% of patients have been reported to be spasm-free at 5 years. However, the risk of poor neurologic outcome is high: 80%–90% with mental retardation and >50% with epilepsy. Of infants with IS, 30%–40% progress to Lennox-Gastaut syndrome. Prognosis is directly related to etiology: symptomatic cases have significantly worse outcome. Early cessation of the spasms and normalization of the EEG may have good prognostic significance.

PATIENT EDUCATION

- Parents require extensive training in ACTH administration, managing side effects of therapy, and precautions regarding immunosuppression.

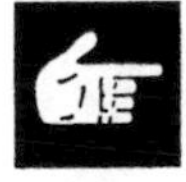

Miscellaneous

SYNONYMS

- West syndrome

ICD-9-CM: 345.60 Infantile spasms

SEE ALSO: EPILEPSY, LENNOX-GASTAUT SYNDROME

REFERENCES

- Baram TZ. Myoclonus and myoclonic seizures. In: Swaiman KF, Ashwal S, eds. Pediatric neurology: principles and practice. St. Louis: Mosby, 1999:668.
- Baram TZ, Mitchell WG, Tournay A, et al. High-dose corticotropin (ACTH) versus prednisone for infantile spasms: a prospective, randomized, blinded study. Pediatrics 1996;97:37.
- Holmes G, Vigevano F. Infantile spasms. In: Engel J, Pedley TA, eds. Epilepsy: a comprehensive textbook, vol I. Philadelphia: Lippincott-Raven Publishers, 1998:627.
- Ohtahara S, Yamatogi Y. Severe encephalopathic epilepsy in infants: West syndrome. In: Pellock JM, et al., eds. Pediatric epilepsy: diagnosis and therapy, 2nd ed. New York: Demos Medical Publishing, 2001:177.
- Snead OC, Benton JW, Hosey LC. Treatment of infantile spasms with high dose ACTH: efficacy and plasma levels of ACTH and cortisol. Neurology 1989;39:1027–1031.

Author(s): Juliann Paolicchi, MD

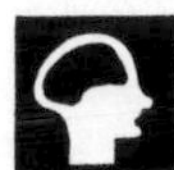

Basics

DESCRIPTION

- Lennox-Gastaut syndrome (LGS) is characterized by multiple seizure types refractory to treatment with antiepileptic drugs (AEDs).

EPIDEMIOLOGY

Incidence/Prevalence

- LGS accounts for 1%–4% of all childhood epilepsy; 10% of epilepsies present in the first 5 years. Prevalence rates are 0.1–0.28 per 1,000. The annual incidence is estimated at 2 per 100,000 children. The prevalence and percentage of LGS are higher in patients with mental retardation (MR; 0.06 per 1,000 and 7%, respectively).

Race

- No racial differences have been identified.

Age

- Although LGS is defined as having onset in children 1–8 years, the mean age at onset is 26–28 months (range 1 day–14 years).

Sex

- Males are affected more than females.

ETIOLOGY

- The syndrome is divided into primary (idiopathic) or secondary (symptomatic). Secondary cases (65%–75% of patients with LGS) are associated with a host of injuries to the developing brain: genetic causes (tuberous sclerosis), cerebral dysgenesis, infectious, hypoxic-ischemic, or traumatic etiologies. No significant genetic factors have been identified except for genetic-associated etiologies.

RISK FACTORS

- 30%–40% of patients with infantile spasms develop LGS.

PREGNANCY

N/A

ASSOCIATED CONDITIONS

- At onset, 20%–60% of patients have MR. The subsequent proportion of patients with MR increases because of cognitive deterioration that occurs with LGS. Behavioral problems and psychological diseases, ranging from hyperactivity to autism, are common.

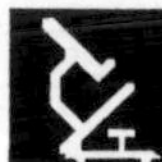

Diagnosis

DIFFERENTIAL DIAGNOSIS

- LGS can be difficult to distinguish from other childhood epilepsy syndromes of multiple seizure types and cognitive dysfunction.
- Myoclonic astatic epilepsy (Doose syndrome) consists of myoclonic, atonic, and atypical absence seizures. Myoclonic astatic epilepsy is predominantly idiopathic, has a better prognosis, and does not develop from West syndrome. Patients with childhood myoclonic epilepsies, such as benign myoclonic epilepsy of infancy, severe myoclonic epilepsy of infancy, and progressive myoclonic epilepsy, tend to have myoclonic seizures as their predominant feature, rarer tonic seizures than LGS, faster EEG (>2.5 Hz) patterns, and more variable cognitive decline.

SIGNS AND SYMPTOMS

- The most frequent seizure types in LGS are tonic, tonic-clonic, myoclonic, atypical absences, and "head drop," which are a form of atonic, tonic, or myoclonic seizures. Tonic seizures are the most prevalent, occurring in 74%–90% of patients. They occur in both awake and sleep states, and can involve the head and trunk, including the arms, or the whole body. Apnea and facial flushing are commonly associated. Events tend to be brief, lasting only a few seconds to a minute. They can occur multiple times per day, sometimes up to hundreds of seizures per day.
- Atypical absences are often subtle with a gradual onset and offset and an incomplete loss of consciousness. They may be accompanied by myoclonic jerks or automatisms.
- Atonic seizures, myoclonic seizures, and myoclonic-atonic seizures can produce sudden "drop attacks" that can be very injurious. Frequency ranges from 10%–56%. Generalized tonic-clonic seizures occur in 15% of patients; complex partial seizures occur in 5%.
- Status epilepticus (54%–75% of patients) can develop from multiple seizure types and tends to be prolonged, resistant to treatment, and recurrent.

LABORATORY PROCEDURES

- The initial evaluation of patients with LGS requires an extensive metabolic and radiologic evaluation to determine the etiology.

IMAGING STUDIES

- Brain MRI is indicated to determine neuroanatomic etiologies of the disorder, such as cerebral dysgenesis, stroke, and hypoxic-ischemic encephalopathy.

SPECIAL STUDIES

- The EEG pattern that characterizes LGS is the generalized spike-and-wave interictal pattern in an otherwise slow background. The slow spike-and-wave or sharp-and-slow-wave complexes occur as generalized bursts with frequencies between 1.5 and 2.5 Hz. The interictal background slowing may be transient or continuous. Continuous slowing is associated with a poor cognitive outcome. The ictal (seizure) EEG patterns depend on the seizure types.

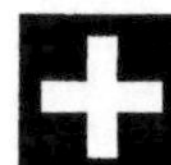

Management

GENERAL MEASURES

- Because freedom from seizure is rarely achievable, the primary goal of treatment is maximizing seizure control and quality of life. Monotherapy is rarely effective. Patients can have periods of relative seizure control, which usually correspond to marked improvements in cognition, alertness, and developmental progress. Unfortunately, cognitive deterioration resumes along with the seizures.

SURGICAL MEASURES

- Two surgical procedures have been used in LGS, but neither has been investigated in case-control studies. In corpus callosotomy, fibers in the anterior corpus callosum are surgically resected. The goal of the procedure is palliation: only 8% of patients are seizure-free, but 61% have improvement in seizures. Drop attacks, atonic seizures, and secondarily generalized seizures are most responsive to this procedure. Benefits are not permanent; seizure frequency can resume over time.
- The vagus nerve stimulator, used to treat medically intractable epilepsy, delivers electrical afferent input to the brainstem via the left vagus nerve. The device is approved for use in refractory partial seizures but also is used for refractory generalized seizures, including LGS. Seizure freedom is rarely achieved. In small studies, 72% of LGS patients experienced a 50% reduction in seizure frequency with up to 5-year follow-up.
- Isolated cases in which resection of localized lesions improved seizure control have been reported.

SYMPTOMATIC TREATMENT

- Intercurrent illness, stress, changes in AED regimen, and use of concomitant mediations can trigger an increase in seizures. Many LGS patients have weekly or monthly periodicity in seizure frequency unrelated to other factors or AEDs, so a long-term approach is often advisable. Parents and caregivers should be instructed on therapy for seizure exacerbation, such as intermittent use of the benzodiazepines.
- Treatment of status epilepticus needs to be individualized. IV phenytoin and benzodiazepines are the mainstays of therapy.

ADJUNCTIVE TREATMENT

- See Medications

ADMISSION/DISCHARGE CRITERIA

- Because children with LGS have multiple daily seizures, admission to the hospital usually is reserved for exacerbations, respiratory compromise, or status epilepticus.

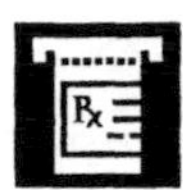

Medications

DRUGS OF CHOICE

- Broad-spectrum AEDs are the mainstay of treatment. Sedating side effects can exacerbate seizure frequency, and tolerance is common.
  - —Valproate has broad-spectrum effectiveness against the seizure types of LGS. Sedative/ cognitive side effects are minimal, except at higher concentrations. Dose-dependent side effects include ataxia, tremor, and platelet dysfunction. Idiosyncratic reactions include weight gain, alopecia, and, of most concern in children <2 years of age, hepatotoxicity, which can be fatal.
  - —Newer AEDs tested for efficacy in double-blind, placebo-control trials include felbamate, lamotrigine, and topiramate. Felbamate is effective in LGS but is associated with dangerous idiosyncratic reactions: aplastic anemia and hepatotoxicity. Although the incidence of both of these reactions is low (1 in 4,000–8,000 and 1 in 18,000–25,000 treated patients, respectively), their severity has limited its use.
  - —Topiramate is an effective adjunctive treatment for most LGS seizure types. Common adverse events are somnolence, anorexia, cognitive or behavioral problems, renal stones, and glaucoma.
  - —Lamotrigine is an effective adjunctive treatment. The most concerning side effects are idiosyncratic skin reactions: rash in 10%–12% of patients treated for LGS, Stevens-Johnson syndrome, and toxic epidermal necrolysis. Risk factors for development of lamotrigine-induced rash include younger age (children > adults), concomitant valproate treatment, a high starting dose, and rapid dose titration.
  - —In the past, long-acting benzodiazepines such as clonazepam and nitrazepam were used for treatment of LGS. Tolerance and sedative side effects tend to limit their long-term effectiveness.
  - —Carbamazepine usually is avoided in LGS because it can exacerbate the slow spike-and-wave pattern causing increased seizures or obtundation, as can phenytoin. Further trials are needed to determine the effectiveness of levetiracetam and zonisamide.

ALTERNATIVE DRUGS

- The ketogenic diet is a treatment alternative for children with medically refractory epilepsy including LGS. The diet consists of a high proportion of fats compared to small amounts of carbohydrate and protein in a ratio of 3:1 or 4:1, which induces ketosis. Overall, one third of patients on the diet experience significant or complete seizure control. Side effects include an inability to tolerate the diet, sedation, GI disturbance, and social limitations. The long-term cardiovascular side effects of a high fat diet are under investigation.

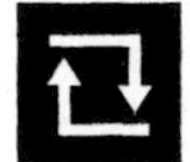

Follow-Up

PATIENT MONITORING

- LGS patients require neurologic care in specialized epilepsy centers to address their multiple neurologic and medical needs.

EXPECTED COURSE AND PROGNOSIS

- Despite the many advances in epilepsy treatments, the outcome of patients with LGS remains poor. By adolescence, the combination of continued seizures, MR, and behavioral difficulties leads to profound social consequences. In a 10-year follow-up study, MR was found in 95% of patients in the primary group and 100% in the secondary group.
- Psychiatric problems can progress from mood instability and personality disturbances in the young child to acute psychotic episodes in older children and adolescents. The main characteristics of mental deterioration include apathy, memory disorders, perseverance, and impaired vision or speech. Poor prognostic factors include secondary or symptomatic LGS, particularly after West syndrome, early onset of seizures, higher frequency of seizures, and continuous slow spike-and-wave EEG background. Mortality rates of 3%–7% is related to intercurrent illness or accidents.

PATIENT EDUCATION

- Patient/caregiver education should address the many social, educational, and medical needs.
- The National Epilepsy Foundation provides information and support. Website: *www.efa.org*
- MRDD services can assist with nursing and respite care needs.

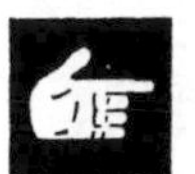

Miscellaneous

SYNONYMS

N/A

ICD-9-CM: 345.91 Epilepsy, unspecified—with mention of intractable epilepsy; 345.11 Generalized convulsive epilepsy—with mention of intractable epilepsy; 780.39 Intractable seizures

SEE ALSO: EPILEPSY, INFANTILE SPASMS

REFERENCES

- Glauser T, Diego M. Encephalopathic epilepsy after infancy. In: Pellock JM, Dodson WE, eds. Pediatric epilepsy: diagnosis and therapy, 2nd ed. Demos Medical Publishing, 2001:201.
- Holmes GL. Generalized seizures. In: Swaiman KF, Ashwal S, eds. Pediatric neurology: principles and practice, vol. 1, 3rd ed. Mosby, 1999:634.
- Genton P, and Dravet C. Lennox-Gastaut syndrome and other childhood epileptic encephalopathies. In: Engel J, Pedley TA, eds. Epilepsy: a comprehensive textbook. Philadelphia: Lippincott-Raven Publishers, 1997:2355.
- Glauser TA, Levisohn PM, Ritter F, et al. Topiramate in Lennox-Gastaut syndrome: open label treatment of patients completing a randomized controlled trial. Topiramate YL Study Group. Epilepsia 2000;41:S86–S90.
- Donaldson JA, Glauser TA, Olberding LS. Lamotrigine adjunctive therapy in childhood epileptic encephalopathy (the Lennox Gastaut Syndrome). Epilepsia 1997;38:68–73.

Author(s): Juliann Paolicchi, MD

Epilepsy, Status Epilepticus

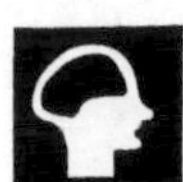

Basics

DESCRIPTION

- Status epilepticus (SE) is a prolonged seizure or multiple seizures without full recovery of consciousness between seizures. The amount of time allowed before beginning abortive therapy varies with the clinical situation and individual preference. In most cases, initial medications should be given after 5 minutes of continuous seizure activity or more than 2 seizures without full recovery. Prolonged seizure activity has been shown to cause irreversible neuronal damage in animals and is associated with significant morbidity and mortality in humans. SE is divided into generalized convulsive status epilepticus (GCSE), nonconvulsive status epilepticus (NCSE), and focal status epilepticus (FSE).

EPIDEMIOLOGY

Incidence/Prevalence

- Approximately 60 per 100,000 per year. Bimodal incidence peaks in early childhood and old age (due to hypoxia and stroke).

Race/Sex

- Affects sexes and races equally.

ETIOLOGY

- Decrease in neuronal electrical inhibition is theorized, but the exact mechanism is unknown.

Genetics

- Predisposition to SE seems to have a heritable component, but the genes and mode of transmission remain unknown with the exception of a few rare genetic diseases.

RISK FACTORS

- Previous episode of SE
- Low antiepileptic drug (AED) levels (poor compliance, drug interactions)
- Metabolic: hyponatremia, hypernatremia, hyperglycemia, hypocalcemia, renal or hepatic insufficiency
- Medications: theophylline, sympathomimetic agents, penicillins, general anesthetics, antipsychotics agents, antidepressants, anticholinergics
- Medication withdrawal: AEDs, sedative-hypnotics
- Structural lesions
- Trauma
- Hypoxia
- Toxic: Carbon monoxide, cocaine, amphetamines
- Infection: meningitis, encephalitis, brain abscess
- Autoimmune: CNS vasculitis
- General (risk factors for seizures): emotional or physical stress, lack of sleep, menstrual cycle, stimulants, individual provoking factors (e.g., flashing lights)
- Roughly one third of SE cases represent the presentation of epilepsy, one third occur in known epileptics, and one third are symptomatic

PREGNANCY

- Eclampsia is the combination of hypertension, edema, and seizures. Most older AEDs are pregnancy class D (can cause harm to fetus), but the risks of prolonged seizures to both the mother and unborn child usually far outweigh the risks of medications. The newer medications are class C (unknown effects).

ASSOCIATED CONDITIONS

- Epilepsy; see Risk Factors

Diagnosis

DIFFERENTIAL DIAGNOSIS

- *Convulsive:* basically limited to psychogenic seizures and unusual presentations of movement disorders (myoclonus, tremors, chorea). Psychogenic spells can be extremely difficult to distinguish from epileptic seizures, and there are many case reports of unnecessary intubation and medication-induced coma. Even experienced epilepsy specialists may need to use video-EEG monitoring. Movement disorders do not affect consciousness (although a number of disease states can cause both movement disorders and seizures, e.g., CJD, hypoxia). The hyperactive reflexes and sustained postures seen in stroke and hypoxia victims can resemble seizures, as can hypocalcemic tetany.
- *Nonconvulsive status:* basically the differential for altered mental status, which includes
  - —Trauma: concussion, intracranial hemorrhage, intracranial hypertension
  - —Infectious: meningoencephalitis
  - —Toxic: drug overdose, poisoning
  - —Metabolic: electrolyte abnormalities (especially hypernatremia), hypoglycemia, hypoxia, hypercarbia, liver failure, renal failure, thyroid and adrenal disorders
  - —Psychiatric: fugue state, psychogenic spells, malingering
  - —Other: cerebral vasculitis

SIGNS AND SYMPTOMS

- *GCSE:* loss of consciousness followed by tonic contraction of various muscle groups, often accompanied by eye deviation and head turning. Usually followed by clonic phase with rhythmic muscle contractions. The contractions often become gradually less frequent and apparent in fewer muscles. Tone may be increased or decreased. Eventually, contractions may cease as the muscles are critically fatigued (and often damaged) with only occasional twitches observed clinically. More subtle signs include hypertension, tachypnea, and pupillary dilation.
- *NCSE (complex partial status, absence status):* impaired alertness and consciousness to a widely varying degree. Can range from mild inattentiveness, word-finding difficulty, and poor memory to deep coma. Can be misinterpreted as drug intoxication, fatigue, or psychiatric illness. Patients may demonstrate automatisms (lip smacking, picking at clothes).
- *FSE:* repetitive clonic contractions of a muscle group, such as the hand and finger flexors.

LABORATORY PROCEDURES

- Investigations of possible causes include urine and serum drug screens, serum AED levels, and electrolytes including calcium, glucose, LFTs, and creatinine. If meningitis or encephalitis is suspected, perform CSF studies. In general, provoking factors should be ruled out, even in known epilepsy patients. SE can cause multiple serum laboratory anomalies, including metabolic acidosis (often marked but usually not requiring correction), elevated creatine kinase, and electrolyte abnormalities. Prolonged convulsive status may result in rhabdomyolysis and resultant renal failure. Serum prolactin usually is elevated with epileptic seizures and normal with psychogenic spells, but the sensitivity and specificity of this test are relatively low.

IMAGING STUDIES

- CT without contrast is the study of choice if intracranial bleeding or tumor is a suspected source of seizures. MRI with gadolinium contrast is the preferred study after the patient is stabilized to determine the presence of any structural lesion that may predispose to seizures.

SPECIAL TESTS

- EEG often is helpful if the diagnosis is uncertain but must be interpreted in the context of the patient's clinical presentation. Interictal EEG (performed between seizures) is helpful when abnormal (may demonstrate subclinical seizure activity or epileptogenic abnormalities), but a negative interictal EEG does *not* rule out seizures. Conversely, psychogenic spells often coexist with epileptic seizures, so an *ab*normal interictal EEG does not diagnose seizures.

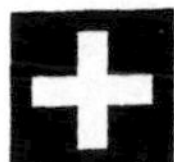

Management

GENERAL MEASURES

- Always begin with the ABCs! Airway protection may become necessary, especially in convulsive status. Intubation should always precede the use of high-dose barbiturates or benzodiazepines. Laboratory tests should be drawn as soon as possible to determine the presence of correctable causes of status (metabolic disturbances, drug overdose).

SURGICAL MEASURES

- Only considered in extremely refractory cases of status with known resectable lesions

SYMPTOMATIC TREATMENT

N/A

ADJUNCTIVE TREATMENT

N/A

ADMISSION/DISCHARGE CRITERIA

- Patients with SE almost always should be admitted for observation (to the unit if respiratory or cardiovascular status is compromised). The exception would be chronic, intractable seizure patients with a known history of status in whom possible causes of breakthrough seizures are ruled out or corrected.

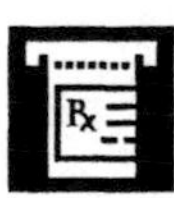

Medications

DRUG(S) OF CHOICE

- Thiamine 100 mg IV followed by glucose 50 g IV should be administered to any patient in status in whom nutritional deficiency and abnormal glucose are possible.
- *GCSE:* Lorazepam (Ativan) is the usual drug of choice, administered at 0.1 mg/kg to a maximum dose of 8 mg at 2 mg/min. Alternatively, diazepam (Valium) 5–10 mg IV q5 min to maximum 30 mg per 8 hours. If seizures continue after 2 minutes, administer fosphenytoin (Cerebyx) 20 mg/kg (1.5 g for a 75-kg person) IV at maximum rate 150 mg/min in adults, 3 mg/kg/min in children.
- Note: Fosphenytoin is measured in "phenytoin equivalents." If "mg" is written, it is universally and automatically converted to phenytoin equivalents by pharmacists. For example, if 1.5 g of fosphenytoin is ordered, the dose administered will be *equivalent* to 1.5 g of phenytoin.
- If IV access not available, diazepam can be given as a rectal gel and fosphenytoin can be given IM. Phenytoin should not be given IM in SE because of slow erratic absorption.
- If fosphenytoin is not available, phenytoin can be dosed at 20 mg/kg IV at maximum rate of 50 mg/min.
- If seizures continue, an additional 5 mg/kg IV dose of fosphenytoin is administered, followed by IV phenobarbital at a dose of 20 mg/kg at maximum rate of 150 mg/min. If these regimens fail (around 15 minutes of status), a neurologist and an EEG team should be urgently consulted. Anticipatory intubation will nearly always be necessary at this point. The next step is inducing electrical shutdown of the CNS (verified with EEG) with one of the following:
  - —IV pentobarbital 5–15 mg/kg loading dose, followed by 5 mg/kg/hour; titrate to EEG
  - —IV midazolam 0.2 mg/kg load, then 0.1 to 0.4 mg/hg/hour; titrate to EEG
  - —IV propofol 2 mg/kg load, then 0.1–0.2 mg/kg/min (6–12 mg/kg/hour); titrate to EEG
- *NCSE:* Begin as for benzodiazepines and fosphenytoin. Further treatment of nonconvulsive status is controversial. Most authorities consider nonconvulsive status as urgent but nonemergent. Some epileptologists believe that some treatments may actually worsen NCSE. Consultation with a neurologist is recommended.

Contraindications

- Known allergies to specific AEDs

Precautions

- Benzodiazepines, barbiturates, and fosphenytoin, especially at higher doses, can cause respiratory and cardiovascular depression necessitating intubation. Phenytoin and fosphenytoin can cause arrhythmias (heart block and prolonged QT interval).

ALTERNATIVE DRUGS

- IV valproate (Depacon) may be helpful, especially in NCSE or as a third-line agent in refractory GCSE. Other anesthetic agents such as lidocaine have been used anecdotally to stop refractory SE.

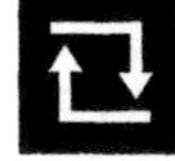

Follow-Up

PATIENT MONITORING

- AEDs should be continued (preferably using the agent that aborted the initial seizure). If only benzodiazepine therapy was required, patient should be loaded with phenytoin or fosphenytoin PO/IV/IM 15–20 mg/kg over 4 hours and then 5 mg/kg/day. Patient should be monitored closely for 24–48 hours while the search for provoking factors is completed. Routine neurology consultation is advisable. Repeat EEG is advisable in cases in which nonconvulsive status or subclinical seizures are suspected (failure of mental status to improve, prolonged focal weakness). Keep in mind that prolonged decreased awareness after GCSE may be due to NCSE instead of drug effect or postictal state.

EXPECTED COURSE AND PROGNOSIS

- Depends primarily on the presence or absence of a provoking factor. Overall mortality is 10%–20%, with the highest mortality in elderly stroke victims. In general, having an episode of SE increases the risk for future seizures, as well as future SE. NCSE and FSE are generally more difficult to treat. Permanent neurologic and psychological deficits may be related to prolonged SE. Most of the mortality of SE is related to the underlying cause (bleed, tumor, infection), but prolonged seizure activity alone is estimated to cause 5% mortality.

PATIENT EDUCATION

- In general, factors that increase seizure risk will increase risk of status: emotional and physical stress, fatigue, sleep deprivation, poor medication compliance, drug-drug interactions, other medications.

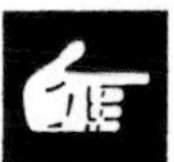

Miscellaneous

SYNONYMS

- Status (rarely may be confused with status migrainosus)

ICD-9-CM: 345.3 Epilepsy, status (grand mal); 345.7 Epilepsy, status focal

SEE ALSO: N/A

REFERENCES

- Corey LA, Pellock JM, Boggs JG, et al. Evidence for a genetic predisposition for status epilepticus. Neurology 1998;50:558–560.
- Treiman DM, et al. A comparison of four treatments for generalized convulsive status epilepticus. N Engl J Med 1998;339:792–798.

Author(s): Mark R. Gibson, MD; Joseph Sirven, MD

Fibromyalgia

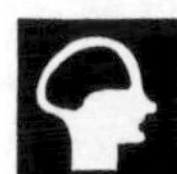

Basics

DESCRIPTION

- Fibromyalgia is a musculoskeletal pain amplification syndrome that includes symptoms of pain, stiffness, and exhaustion; physical findings of specific areas of tenderness; and no evidence of any specific etiology for cause of symptoms. Many terms have been used for similar medical conditions over the years, including tender points with rheumatism, neuralgia, fibrositis, psychogenic rheumatism, myofascial pain syndrome, shell shock, posttraumatic stress disorder, Gulf War syndrome, chemical sensitivity syndrome, chronic fatigue syndrome, and variant reflex dystrophy.

EPIDEMIOLOGY

Incidence/Prevalence

- Clinically detectable fibromyalgia as defined by strict American College of Rheumatology criteria is present in approximately 3%–7% of the US population. The actual number of affected individuals who seek medical help is smaller and based on multiple factors, including an individual's ability to cope with the condition.

Race

- All races are affected.

Sex

- There is a female predominance of approximately 5:1.

Age

- The typical onset is between ages 9 and 60 years; most commonly presenting between ages 40 and 60. In the pediatric population, early precursors of this condition may include "growing pains" or "early migraines."

ETIOLOGY

- The specific cause of fibromyalgia is unknown; however, a number of inciting events are known to be associated with this condition. They include trauma (particularly head and or neck injury from motor vehicle accident), recent infection, and stress. Families with multiple afflicted members are known to occur. Other disease associations within affected families include depression, obsessive-compulsive disorder, and anxiety disorder. Recently, a link has been found with a functional polymorphism in the serotonin transporter gene in affected individuals. Sleep disturbances also play an important role in the pathology. Fibromyalgia patients lack stage 4, non-REM (or slow-wave) sleep relative to controls. Intrusion of alpha waves on slow delta waves is seen on EEG patterns. Normally during stage 4 sleep, we should see delta waves only. Alpha waves are an indication of a lighter (more easily arousable) sleep. This same EEG pattern can be experimentally induced by sleep depriving healthy subjects. Serotonin may be the neurotransmitter that mediates slow-wave sleep. Tryptophan crosses the blood–brain barrier and is converted to serotonin. Inhibition of serotonin production is associated with a decrease in slow-wave sleep and an increase in somatic symptoms; therefore, theories have been put forth to suggest that fibromyalgia may result from an insufficient concentration of circulating tryptophan.

RISK FACTORS

- Risk factors include preceding trauma (whiplash injury), infection, and/or other inciting events all superimposed on a genetically predisposed individual.

PREGNANCY

- Fibromyalgia has no known untoward effects on the mother or the developing fetus during pregnancy.

ASSOCIATED CONDITIONS

- Neuralgia, fibrositis, myofascial pain syndrome, posttraumatic stress disorder, Gulf War syndrome, chemical sensitivity syndrome, chronic fatigue syndrome, and variant reflex dystrophy are all conditions with considerable overlap with patients with fibromyalgia. Associated conditions may include anxiety disorder, depression, irritable bowel syndrome, restless legs syndrome, temporomandibular joint (TMJ) syndrome, and Premenstrual syndrome.

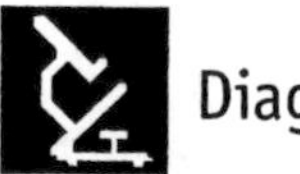

Diagnosis

DIFFERENTIAL DIAGNOSIS

- Early stage of inflammatory connective tissue disorders such as systemic lupus erythematosus or rheumatoid arthritis, Ehlers-Danlos benign hypermobility joint syndrome, hypothyroidism, psychogenic rheumatism, dyskinetic phase of parkinsonism, diffuse idiopathic skeletal hyperostosis (DISH), Paget's disease, multiple myeloma, and cyclic edema are some of the disorders that can mimic fibromyalgia. A number of disorders can cause a secondary fibromyalgia, including cervical/lumbar syndromes, referred pain syndromes, chronic steroid use (tender shins, diffuse fibromyalgia), occult/overt neoplasm, connective tissue diseases, hypokalemia, and diabetes mellitus with neuropathies.

SIGNS AND SYMPTOMS

- In childhood, a common presentation is "growing pains" or "migraines." In young adulthood, "chronic fatigue" eventually may evolve to global pain. Patients will generally describe aches/pains and/or articular pains with possible joint tenderness, although no actual synovitis is detected. Subjective feeling of swelling usually involves the hands, usually worse in the morning and better by midday. Stiffness lasts approximately 1 hour after awakening. An associated sleep disorder characterized by a nonrestorative sleep is common. Barometric weather changes may exacerbate symptoms. Activity may exacerbate some individuals' symptoms, causing them to seek a more sedentary state. Physical examination is characterized by the presence of diffuse tender points (>11 of 18) in all four quadrants of the body. The amount of pressure applied is approximately 4 lb (8.8 kg) at each point. Typically patients will be tender at other sites outside of the 18 tested points. On occasion, testing a tender point might elicit a sudden withdrawal-like response from the subject (jump sign). The term *trigger point* is sometimes used. Trigger points are soft-tissue regions that, either spontaneously or following direct pressure, cause radiating pain, paresthesias, and autonomic symptoms. The diagnosis of fibromyalgia is made once the above noted symptoms have been persistent for >3 months.

LABORATORY PROCEDURES

- Fibrositis is a clinical diagnosis and is confirmed by the presence of normal laboratory data helping to exclude other conditions. Although there are documented laboratory abnormalities in the majority of patients affected by fibromyalgia (threefold elevation in CSF substance P, elevation in CSF nerve growth factor, decrease in CSF angiotensin-converting enzyme level, decrease in 24-hour urine 5-HIAA level), these tests are not routinely obtained as part of the clinical screening profile. Laboratories helpful for excluding other conditions include the presence of normal ESR, TSH, muscle enzyme levels, hemoglobin and hematocrit, rheumatoid factor (RF), and antinuclear antibody (ANA). ANA levels may be positive in 30% of affected individuals; however, these do not indicate an underlying autoimmune condition.

IMAGING STUDIES

- There are no specific imaging abnormalities.

SPECIAL TESTS

- There are no special laboratories needed for diagnostic purposes.

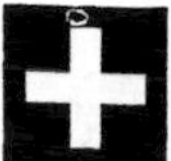

Management

GENERAL MEASURES

- An explanation of the condition is the initial approach. Reassurance; job modification with avoidance of repetitive activities; physical therapy consisting of weight loss, abdominal support exercises, and posture training; and heat therapy consisting of ultrasound and hot packs may all play a role. Exercising to increase heart rate to >150 beats/min is usually more effective than flexibility maneuvers.
- Sleep induction therapy is an important component of treatment of fibromyalgia. Various medications used in this effort are listed in the Drug(s) of Choice section.

SURGICAL MEASURES

N/A

SYMPTOMATIC TREATMENT

- Use of analgesics, acupuncture, biofeedback, and other stress management and relaxation techniques in conjunction with the medications listed below often is beneficial.

ADJUNCTIVE TREATMENT

- *Autonomic dysfunction therapy:* TMJ syndrome is treated with orthodontic bracing/night brace. Irritable bowel syndrome uses agents that decrease GI motility or might benefit from the use of peppermint oil extract. Zinc, magnesium, or manganese supplements might help modulate some symptoms.

ADMISSION/DISCHARGE CRITERIA

- Admission is not required for this condition.

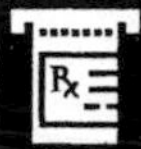

Medications

DRUG(S) OF CHOICE

- Medications include nonsteroidal antiinflammatory drugs and muscle relaxants. On occasion, injection of trigger points with lidocaine steroid is indicated.
- Tricyclic antidepressants at night time (e.g., doxepin [Sinequan] or nortriptyline 10 mg; increase by 10 mg every 3–4 weeks until the patient is able to sleep through the night). Use of selective serotonin reuptake inhibitors (SSRIs; e.g., fluoxetine), usually in the morning, may often provide patients with an energy boost. They probably work by increasing 5-hydroxytryptamine levels in synaptic cleft.

Contraindications

- The medications above should not be prescribed for any patient with a known hypersensitivity to a particular drug. SSRIs should not be used in conjunction with monoamine oxidase inhibitor (MAOI) drugs, and because of its long half-life fluoxetine should be discontinued at least 5 weeks before starting an MAOI antidepressant.

Precautions

- Fluoxetine may be associated with insomnia, changes in weight and appetite, decrease in seizure threshold, and, rarely, activation of mania or hypomania in predisposed individuals.

ALTERNATIVE DRUGS

- Other adjuncts used to modulate pain include sleep aids such as antihistamines or benzodiazepines, and anticonvulsants (γ-aminobutyric acid inhibitors, e.g., gabapentin).

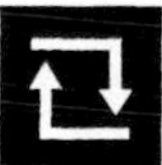

Follow-Up

PATIENT MONITORING

- For many patients, fibromyalgia is a chronic disease. Encouragement and regular follow-up are helpful to ensure compliance with a graded exercise program, identification of contributing stress and depression, and adjustment of symptomatic medications.

EXPECTED COURSE AND PROGNOSIS

- Generally, fibromyalgia has a fluctuating course. Treatment is aimed at empowering the patient to understand the illness and be an active participant in its treatment. Promotion of a positive outlook helps to minimize depression as a result of the chronic pain and helps to reduce disability seeking. On average, 20% of patients obtain complete relief, 60% obtain a 50% decrease in symptoms, and 20% obtain little relief of symptoms.

PATIENT EDUCATION

- There is no definite diet plan for patients with fibromyalgia. A number of diets supported by anecdotal evidence only have been proposed. A normal healthy balanced diet is the best approach. Numerous fibromyalgia support chapters are presently active throughout the United States.

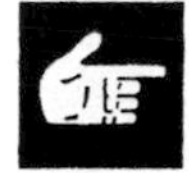

Miscellaneous

SYNONYMS

- Fibrositis

ICD-9-CM: 729.1 Fibromyalgia

SEE ALSO: N/A

REFERENCES

- Bengston A, Ernerudh J, Vrethem M, et al. Absence of autoantibodies in primary fibromyalgia. J Rheumatol 1990;17:1682–1683.
- Goldenberg DL. Fibromyalgia syndrome. JAMA 1987;257:2782–2787.
- Katz W. Pain management in rheumatic diseases. Curr Opin Rheumatol 2002;14:1.
- McCarty GA. Autoantibodies and their relationship to rheumatic diseases. Med Clin North Am 1986;70:237–261.
- Middleton GB, McFarlin JE, Lipsky PE. The prevalence and clinical impact of fibromyalgia in systemic lupus erythematosus. Arthritis Rheum 1994;37:1181–1188.
- Smart P, Waylonis G, Hackshaw KV. The immunologic profile of patients with fibromyalgia. J Am Assoc Phys Med Rehabil 1996;76:231–234.
- Waylonis GW, Perkins RH. Post-traumatic fibromyalgia: a long term follow-up. Am J Phys Med Rehabil 1994;73:403–412.
- Wolfe F, et al. The American College of Rheumatology 1990 criteria for the classification of fibromyalgia. Arthritis Rheum 1990;33:160–172.

Author(s): Kevin V. Hackshaw, MD

Friedreich's Ataxia

Basics

DESCRIPTION

- Friedreich's ataxia (FRDA) is one of the most common forms of autosomal recessive ataxia. In FRDA, the spinocerebellar tracts, dorsal columns, pyramidal tracts, and, to a lesser extent, the cerebellum and medulla are involved.

EPIDEMIOLOGY

Prevalence

- Friedreich's ataxia occurs with a prevalence of approximately 1/50,000 in Caucasian populations.

Race

- It is rare among sub-Saharan Africans and does not exist in the Far East. Particularly high frequency of FRDA was found in Cyprus and among the French-Canadian population.

Sex

- Both sexes are affected with the same frequency as expected given an autosomal recessive pattern of inheritance of the disease.

Age

- Approximately 15% of patients reported with this condition became symptomatic after age 20 years. The only significant differences between these late-onset patients and more typical early-onset patients are a lower occurrence of skeletal deformities in the late-onset groups and normal visual evoked potentials, which were abnormal in 69% of individuals presenting with FRDA before age 20. The disease progresses slower in the late-onset group.

ETIOLOGY

- 98% of cases of FRDA are due to expansion of a GAA trinucleotide repeat intron 1 of the FRDA gene frataxin, whereas 2% are due to point mutations in the frataxin gene located on chromosome 9. Seventeen mutations had been described to date. Larger GAA expansions were correlated with earlier age at onset and shorter times to loss of ambulation. The size of the GAA expansions was associated with the frequency of cardiomyopathy and loss of reflexes in the upper limbs. The GAA repeats were unstable during transmission. Thus, the clinical spectrum of Friedreich's ataxia is broader than previously recognized.

RISK FACTORS

N/A

PREGNANCY

- Morbidity during pregnancy is related to symptomatic manifestations and complications of the disease.

ASSOCIATED CONDITIONS

- Cardiac manifestations are conspicuous in some cases. Approximately half of 82 fatal cases of Friedreich's ataxia died of heart failure, and nearly three fourths had evidence of cardiac dysfunction in life. Abnormalities of the echocardiogram in patients with FRDA were in the form of symmetric, concentric, hypertrophic, or hypokinetic-dilated cardiomyopathy.
- Diabetes was present in 23%. Muscular subaortic stenosis has been described in cases of Friedreich's ataxia.
- Scoliosis is a well-known complication of FRDA. It can cause secondary impairment of pulmonary function.
- Chorea as a rare manifestation of FRDA has been reported.
- Partial deafness and loss of visual acuity occur in a minority of patients with FRDA.

Diagnosis

DIFFERENTIAL DIAGNOSIS

- Spinocerebellar degeneration
- Predominantly cerebellar
  - —Late cortical cerebellar atrophy of Marie-Foix-Alajouanine syndrome
  - —Holmes familial cortical cerebellar atrophy
  - —Alcohol
  - —Drug-induced (phenytoin [Dilantin])
  - —Paraneoplastic
- Cerebellar and brainstem ataxias
  - —OPCA
  - —Dentatorubropallidoluysian atrophy
  - —Machado-Joseph disease

SIGNS AND SYMPTOMS

- Usually begins with gait ataxia; difficulty in standing steadily and running are early symptoms; upper extremity ataxia and dysarthria appear later
- Peripheral neuropathy, mixed sensory and cerebellar ataxia
- Pes cavus, hammertoes, kyphoscoliosis
- Cardiomyopathy in 50% cases; diabetes mellitus in 10%
- Physical examination: decreased or absent deep tendon reflexes, up-going toes, loss of vibratory perception and position sense, positive Romberg, ataxia, dysarthria

LABORATORY PROCEDURES

- Nerve conduction studies: sensory nerve responses absent in lower extremities, slowed in upper extremities. Motor nerve conductions usually are normal or show a mild reduction.

IMAGING STUDIES

- CT scan and MRI are not helpful for making a diagnosis.

SPECIAL TESTS

- DNA testing for GAA repeats of the frataxin gene.

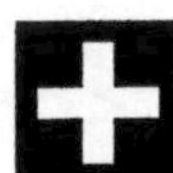

Management

GENERAL MEASURES

- No pathogenetic treatment is currently available; therefore, treatment of FRDA is primarily palliative.

SURGICAL MEASURES

- Surgical correction of foot deformities and contractures is possible.
- Severe cases of scoliosis associated with impairment of pulmonary function and pain can be corrected by surgery.

SYMPTOMATIC TREATMENT

- Loss of balance and coordination usually require using *mobility aids,* such as braces, a cane, or a walker, within a decade of the diagnosis. A wheelchair often is needed for mobility several years afterward. Progressive weakness in the lower limbs can compound the problems caused by loss of coordination.
- *Regular stretching and exercise* as a part of a longitudinal physical therapy program are very important to minimize contractures and maintain strength.
- *Occupational therapy* is needed to determine the appropriate devices and strategies to improve function in the activity of daily living.
- Mild *scoliosis* is sometimes treated with a *brace* fitted around the chest and abdomen.
- *A speech-language pathologist* or speech therapist teaches compensatory techniques for both speech and swallowing. *A dietitian or nutritionist* advises on meals and preparation techniques that make food easier to swallow and increase nutritional content.
- Cardiac problems and diabetes are to be managed by *a cardiologist* and *an endocrinologist,* respectively.

ADJUNCTIVE TREATMENT

N/A

ADMISSION/DISCHARGE CRITERIA

- FRDA, like almost all chronic conditions, is managed primarily on an outpatient basis. Admission might be required for treatment of associated conditions or corrective surgeries (see above).

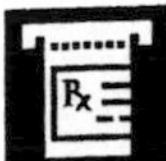

Medications

DRUG(S) OF CHOICE

- Muscle stiffness, spasms, and cramps might be treated with symptomatic medications, such baclofen, diazepam, and gabapentin.
- Baclofen 10 mg 1-3 times per day is titrated up to an effective dose to maximum of 100 mg.
- Diazepam 2–10 mg three times daily.
- Neuropathic pain should be managed with gabapentin 100–900 mg tid, escalating up to a maximal dose of 3,600 mg/day.

Contraindications

- Worsening of gait unsteadiness and excessive sedation are major limitations related to use of these drugs.

Precautions

N/A

ALTERNATIVE DRUGS

- Tizanidine 2–8 mg qd–tid may be used as an alternative antispasticity agent. Gradual titration is required with monitoring for orthostasis, sedation, and LFT abnormalities.

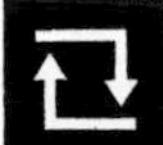

Follow-Up

PATIENT MONITORING

- Careful patient monitoring and multidisciplinary approach with involvement of neurologists, physiatrists, physical and occupational therapists, speech-language pathologists, and, if needed, cardiologists, diabetologists, and orthopedic surgeons can be coordinated through a Muscular Dystrophy Association clinic.

EXPECTED COURSE AND PROGNOSIS

- Gradual worsening of the symptoms is expected. The speed of progression and the effect of FRDA on lifespan vary among patients. On average, people with FRDA live 3–4 decades after the diagnosis. Life expectancy is higher in patients with milder forms of the disease and later age of onset. Heart disease has the most significant impact on lifespan.

PATIENT EDUCATION

- Muscular Dystrophy Association has been a major sponsor of FRDA research and a vital source of services and education to patients affected by this disorder.
- Muscular Dystrophy Association–USA, 3300 East Sunrise Drive, Tucson, AZ 85718. Phone: 800-572-1717, website: *www.mdausa.org*
- National Ataxia Foundation, 2600 Fernbrook Lane, Suite 119, Minneapolis MN 55447-4752. Phone: 763-553-0020, website: *www.ataxia.org*

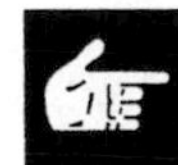

Miscellaneous

SYNONYMS

N/A

ICD-9-CM: 334.0 Friedreich's ataxia

SEE ALSO: SPINOCEREBELLAR ATAXIAS

REFERENCES

- Ackroyd RS, Finnegan JA, Green SH. Friedreich's ataxia: a clinical review with neurophysiological and echocardiographic findings. Arch Dis Child 1984;59:217–221.
- Drake D, Guillory D. Hereditary ataxia. Finding balance. Lancet 2001;358[Suppl]: S36.
- Kaplan J. Spinocerebellar ataxias due to mitochondrial defects. Neurochem Int 2002;40:553–557.
- Koeppen AH. The hereditary ataxias. J Neuropathol Exp Neurol 1998;57: 531–543.
- Lynch DR, Farmer JM, Balcer LJ, et al. Friedreich ataxia: effects of genetic understanding on clinical evaluation and therapy. Arch Neurol 2002;59:743–747.
- Pandolfo M. Molecular basis of Friedreich ataxia. Mov Disord 2001;16:815–821.

Author(s): Lindenbaum Yelena, MD

Gangliosidoses

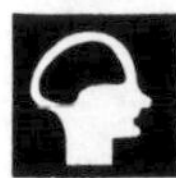

Basics

DESCRIPTION

- Gangliosidoses are a group of diseases that result from enzymatic block and subsequent neuronal ganglioside deposition. Gangliosides are present predominantly in the gray matter. The gangliosidoses include (i) G_{M2} gangliosidoses (deficiency of hexosaminidase A), consisting of infantile G_{M2} gangliosidosis or Tay-Sachs disease, juvenile G_{M2} gangliosidosis, adult G_{M2} gangliosidosis, and normal phenotype with hexosaminidase A deficiency; (ii) Sandhoff disease (deficiency of HEX A and HEX B); and (iii) G_{M1} gangliosidoses, which has infantile, juvenile, and adult variants. All of the gangliosidoses are autosomal recessive disorders.

EPIDEMIOLOGY

- The carrier rate of Tay-Sachs disease is between 1 in 30 and 1 in 40, with a disease incidence of 1 in 4,000 in Ashkenazi Jews; whereas in the non-Jewish population, the carrier rate is 1 in 167, with an incidence of 1 in 112,000. The carrier rate of Sandhoff disease is 1 in 500, with an incidence of 1 in 1,000,000 in the Jewish population. In non-Jewish populations, the carrier rate is 1 in 278, with a disease incidence of 309,000. The incidence of G_{M1} gangliosidoses is 1 in 3,700.

ETIOLOGY

- There are two isoenzymes of βhexosaminidase, HEX A and HEX B. Tay-Sachs disease is caused by gene mutations and complete deficiency of HEX A, with normal HEX B. Patients with juvenile and adult G_{M2} gangliosidoses have partial deficiency of HEX A. Sandhoff disease is induced by mutations of the HEXB gene (encodes β subunit of HEX A and HEX B), with deficiency of HEX A and HEX B. G_{M2} activator deficiency is due to mutations of the G_{M2}A gene and deficiency of the G_{M2} activator protein, with normal HEX A and HEX B.

Genetics

- All forms of G_{M1} gangliosidoses are caused by mutations of the β-galactosidase gene and severe deficiency of acid β-galactosidase.

RISK FACTORS

- Tay-Sachs disease and Sandhoff disease are seen more frequently in the Jewish populations.

PREGNANCY

- The prenatal diagnosis of Tay-Sachs disease, Sandhoff disease, and other G_{M2} gangliosidoses can be made by quantifying HEX A and HEX B in the amniotic fluid (at 16–18 weeks) or the chorionic villi (9–12 weeks) during pregnancy. Prenatal diagnosis of G_{M1} gangliosidoses can be made by measuring acid β-galactosidase activity in amniocytes or chorionic villi.

ASSOCIATED CONDITIONS

- Myoclonic epilepsy, infantile spasms, and a variety of partial or generalized epilepsies are seen in Tay-Sachs disease and other G_{M2} gangliosidoses. Epilepsy is also present in infantile and juvenile G_{M1} gangliosidoses.
- Progressive ataxia and dementia occur often in G_{M2} gangliosidoses. Ataxia is also present in juvenile and adult G_{M1} gangliosidoses.

Diagnosis

DIFFERENTIAL DIAGNOSIS

- Because myoclonic epilepsy, ataxia, loss of milestones, and dementia are all present in the gangliosidoses, the differential diagnosis includes neurodegenerative diseases such as neuronal ceroid lipofuscinosis, progressive myoclonic epilepsy syndrome, aminoacidopathies, organic acidopathies, fatty acid β-oxidation disorders, and mitochondrial cytopathies.
- Because adult and juvenile patients with gangliosidosis can have dystonia, psychosis, spinocerebellar degeneration, corticospinal tract degeneration, or spinal cord anterior horn cell dysfunction, the differential diagnosis includes Kugelberg-Welander disease, spinocerebellar ataxia, Friedreich's ataxia, amyotrophic lateral sclerosis, and other late-onset variants of lysosomal sphingolipidoses.

SIGNS AND SYMPTOMS

- In Tay-Sachs disease, hyperacusis, startle response, and severe irritability occur in the first few months. Developmental retardation, dementia, hypotonia, progressive weakness, poor head control, decrease in attention, visual decline and blindness, cherry-red spot (due to degeneration of ganglion cells around macular fovea centralis), and seizures (myoclonic seizures, infantile spasms, partial and generalized motor seizures) are frequently seen in the first year. Further deterioration in the second year of life results in decerebrate posturing, incoordinate swallowing, and a vegetative state.
- In juvenile G_{M2} gangliosidosis, incoordination and ataxia become apparent between 2 and 6 years. Dementia, loss of speech, spasticity, seizures, and dysfunction of the basal ganglia, cerebellum, corticospinal tracts, and anterior horn cells then are noted over several years. Loss of vision occurs much later than in Tay-Sachs disease; cherry-red spot may not be seen. Optic atrophy and retinitis pigmentosa can occur in the later stages. Decerebrate rigidity and a vegetative state are frequently noted by 10–15 years of life.
- In chronic or adult onset G_{M2} gangliosidosis, the onset is at puberty or early adulthood. Symptoms of spinocerebellar degeneration and lower motor neuron disease are often seen. Psychosis, depression, personality changes, dystonia, and extrapyramidal signs can occur.
- The presentation of infantile Sandhoff disease is similar to Tay-Sachs disease, including the onset and progressive deterioration of neurologic function; however, these patients have organomegaly and occasional bony deformities.
- G_{M2} activator deficiency has a clinical phenotype similar to Tay-Sachs disease and infantile Sandhoff disease.
- In infantile G_{M1} gangliosidosis symptoms are noted early, with severe motor and mental retardation evident in the first year. Feeding difficulty and poor appetite lead to weight loss. Cherry-red spots are seen in 50% of patients. Intractable seizures often occur.
- In juvenile G_{M1} gangliosidosis, the onset is between 6 and 20 months. Psychomotor development is normal in the first year. Ataxia begins at age 1 year, along with strabismus, choreoathetosis, loss of speech, and generalized muscle weakness. Seizures and blindness often occur after age 2 years.
- In adult G_{M1} gangliosidosis, initial symptoms are abnormalities of gait and dysarthria, followed by progressive dystonia of the face and extremities. Mental impairment usually is mild and seizures are rare.

LABORATORY PROCEDURES

- EEG may reveal a variety of epileptiform abnormalities (e.g., hypsarrhythmia). In adult G_{M2} gangliosidosis, electromyograms frequently reveal chronic active denervation and reinnervation, and other changes consistent with anterior horn cell disease. Vacuolated lymphocytes and foam cells in the bone marrow can be detected in infantile and juvenile G_{M1} gangliosidosis.

IMAGING STUDIES

- MRI of Tay-Sachs disease reveals low-signal lesions in areas of abnormal cerebral white matter and the basal ganglia. During later stages, diffuse brain atrophy and compensatory ventriculomegaly may be noted. Severe cerebellar atrophy and mild cerebral atrophy may be noted in juvenile and adult G_{M2} gangliosidoses.
- In all G_{M1} gangliosidoses, diffuse brain atrophy is present on neuroimaging. Low-signal abnormalities of the basal ganglia and high-signal lesions of the white matter may be present in infantile and late-onset G_{M1} gangliosidoses.
- In infantile G_{M1} gangliosidosis, bone x-ray films may detect vertebral deformities, hypoplasia, anterior beaking at the thoracolumbar region, retarded bone age, short long bones, and bilateral dislocation of the hip joints.

SPECIAL TESTS

- Genetic testing of the gangliosidoses requires analysis of either blood or fibroblast samples. The HEXA gene is mapped to chromosome 15q23-24, HEXB gene to chromosome 5q13, and G_{M2A} gene to chromosome 5q32-33. At least 92 mutations in the HEXA gene have been reported in Tay-Sachs disease, and the most frequently seen mutation in Ashkenazi Jews is a four base-pair insertion in exon 11.
- The human β-galactosidase gene is mapped to chromosome 3p21.33. Mutations include missense, nonsense, and insertion varieties.

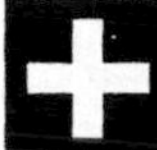

Management

GENERAL MEASURES

- There are no definitive treatment measures for the G_{M1} and G_{M2} gangliosidoses. Only symptomatic and supportive therapies are available.

SURGICAL MEASURES

- Gastrostomy tube placement and Nissen fundoplication may be needed for patients with feeding and swallowing difficulties, and gastroesophageal reflux.

SYMPTOMATIC TREATMENT

- Treatment of epilepsy with a variety of new and old antiepileptic drugs is available. Nutritional support, fluid and electrolyte maintenance, and infectious control with appropriate antibiotics are important. Constipation may be a significant problem and require stool softeners or laxatives.

ADJUNCTIVE TREATMENT

- Physical, occupational, and speech and language therapies are helpful for patients with muscle weakness, coordination difficulty, and language/speech problems.

ADMISSION/DISCHARGE CRITERIA

- Patients with exacerbation of epilepsy often need to be hospitalized for treatment. If severe infections occur (e.g., aspiration pneumonia), patients should be admitted for IV antibiotics and chest physical therapy.

Medications

DRUG(S) OF CHOICE

- Anticonvulsants as required for seizure control. Spasticity of the extremities may benefit from antispasticity drugs such as oral diazepam, dantrolene, baclofen, or tizanidine. Intrathecal baclofen infusions and IM botulinum toxin injections may be effective.

Contraindications

N/A

Precautions

N/A

ALTERNATIVE DRUGS

N/A

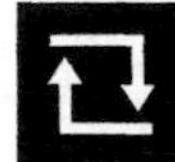

Follow-Up

PATIENT MONITORING

- Patients need to be monitored for seizure control, neurologic function, psychosis or mental decline, and nutritional status.

EXPECTED COURSE AND PROGNOSIS

- The majority of patients with Tay-Sachs disease survive to age 2–4 years. Aspiration pneumonia is often the cause of death. Patients with juvenile G_{M2} gangliosidosis also frequently die of intercurrent infection between 10 and 20 years of age. Adult patients with G_{M2} gangliosidosis may live beyond the third or fourth decade of life. Patients with infantile G_{M1} gangliosidosis typically die of pneumonia by age 2 years. The average lifespan for juvenile G_{M1} gangliosidosis varies between 3 and 10 years. Patients with adult G_{M1} gangliosidosis may survive up to age 60.

PATIENT EDUCATION

- National Tay-Sachs and Allied Diseases Association, 2001 Beacon Street, Suite 204, Brookline, MA 02135. Phone: 617-277-4463; fax: 617-277-0134, website: *http://www.ntsad.org*

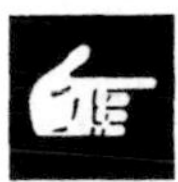

Miscellaneous

SYNONYMS

- Tay-Sachs disease
- Sandhoff disease
- G_{M2} gangliosidosis
- G_{M1} gangliosidosis

ICD-9-CM: 330.1 Tay-Sachs disease; 330.1 Gangliosidosis; 330.1 Sandhoff disease

SEE ALSO: N/A

REFERENCES

- Gravel RA, Kaback MM, Proia RL, et al. The GM2 gangliosidoses. In: Scriver CR, Beaudet AL, Sly WS, et al., eds. The metabolic and molecular bases of inherited disease, 8th ed. New York: McGraw-Hill, 2001:3827–3876.
- Suzuki Y, Oshima A, Nanba E. Beta-galactosidase deficiency (beta-galactosidosis): GM1 gangliosidosis and Morquio B disease. In: Scriver CR, Beaudet AL, Sly WS, et al., eds. The metabolic and molecular bases of inherited disease, 8th ed. New York: McGraw-Hill, 2001:3775–3809.

Author(s): Chang-Yong Tsao, MD

Giant Cell Arteritis

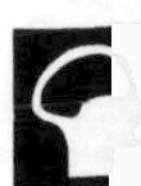

Basics

DESCRIPTION

- Giant cell arteritis (GCA) is a systemic vasculitis characterized by focal granulomatous inflammation of medium and small arteries. Involvement of elastic-containing cranial vessels predominates, including the temporal arteries. Less commonly, vessels of the upper extremities and rarely the aortic arch and great vessels may be involved. Symptoms may include headache, temporal tenderness, jaw claudication, polymyalgia rheumatica, fever, or general malaise. A high degree of suspicion should be maintained for GCA in patients age >60 years because of the risk of acute and severe visual loss. Ocular symptoms complicate 40%–50% of cases.

EPIDEMIOLOGY

Incidence/Prevalence

- Annual incidence rate 50–59 years of age: 2.3/100,000; annual incidence rate 80–89 years of age: 44/100,000

Race

- Rare in African Americans and Asians

Age

- Generally individuals >60 years of age; incidence increases with age; majority will be in their eighth decade

Sex

- Female-to-male ratio of 2–3:1

ETIOLOGY

- The etiology of GCA is unknown, but an immune-mediated process is most widely suspected. A genetic predisposition may exist, as evidenced by an increased prevalence of HLA-DR4 antigen and occasional family clustering.

PREGNANCY

- There is no documented relationship.

ASSOCIATED CONDITIONS

- Polymyalgia rheumatica
- Rheumatoid arthritis

Diagnosis

DIFFERENTIAL DIAGNOSIS

- Nonarteritic anterior ischemic optic neuropathy
- Angle-closure glaucoma
- Migraine
- Temporomandibular joint syndrome
- Trigeminal neuralgia
- Polyarteritis nodosa
- Systemic lupus erythematosus
- Wegener's granulomatosis
- Rheumatoid arthritis
- Takayasu's arteritis
- Churg-Strauss angiitis
- Hypersensitivity reactions

SIGNS AND SYMPTOMS

- GCA is a syndrome that may present with any combination of the following:
  —Headache (initial manifestation in 50%–90% of cases)
  —Pain often gradual onset, diffuse and severe, may be unilateral, usually prominent if not intractable, may be perceived as superficial and may be unresponsive to analgesics
  —Temporal scalp tenderness
  —Point tenderness on palpation over superficial temporal artery
  —Superficial temporal artery may be indurated or have a diminished pulse
  —Abrupt, progressive monocular visual loss with involvement of the fellow eye in 25%–50% of cases
  —Visual loss may be insidious or preceded by episodes of transient monocular loss of vision
  —Partial to complete blindness, largely irreversible
  —Anterior ischemic optic neuropathy (AION) is the most common cause of visual loss as observed in 71%–83% of cases in one series; less frequent causes include central and branch retinal artery occlusion, choroidal infarction, and retrobulbar ischemic optic neuropathy
  —Signs of optic neuropathy may include decreased visual acuity, decreased color vision, afferent pupillary defect, and visual field loss
  —Often altitudinal visual field defect (i.e., respecting the horizontal midline)
  —In cases of AION, the optic disc may show pallid swelling, although hyperemic disc swelling is occasionally seen; peripapillary hemorrhages and cotton wool spots may be noted; as optic disc swelling resolves, optic atrophy occurs
  —Less common ophthalmic presentations are diplopia secondary to cranial neuropathies, amaurosis fugax, orbital inflammation, ocular ischemic syndrome, and Horner's syndrome
  —Polymyalgia rheumatica (>50 years of age, proximal arthralgias and myalgias, morning stiffness, increased ESR >40)
  —Jaw claudication
  —Fever of unknown origin (generally low grade), weight loss, fatigue/malaise
  —Facial pain
  —Neurologic sequelae (ataxia, confusion, hearing loss, ischemic peripheral neuropathy)
  —Hemorrhagic bullae, skin necrosis (over superficial temporal arteries)
  —Extremity claudication
  —Myocardial, renal, visceral, or cerebral infarction
  —Large-vessel involvement (aortic aneurysm or rupture, most commonly thoracic)

LABORATORY PROCEDURES

- There is no specific laboratory test for the diagnosis of GCA, but the Westergren ESR often exceeds 70 mm/hour. A normal ESR does not rule out the diagnosis of GCA, however, as 8%–22% of biopsy-positive GCA cases will have ESR within "normal limits." ESR is a general measure of systemic inflammation, as are C-reactive peptide, fibrinogen, and complement levels, which may also be elevated. Additionally, anemia (hypochromic, microcytic or normochromic, normocytic), polyclonal hypergammaglobulinemia, and a mild leukocytosis may be observed. Liver alkaline phosphatase levels may be elevated in GCA.

IMAGING STUDIES

- Fluorescein angiography (FA) of the fundus may demonstrate a delayed or absent choroidal filling pattern suggesting arteritic ischemic optic neuropathy. FA in cases of nonarteritic ischemic optic neuropathy may show delayed optic disc filling, yet the choroidal circulation is generally not affected. CT or MRI scans are generally not indicated but may be necessary to rule out compressive or infiltrative lesions in atypical cases (e.g., multiple cranial nerve deficits, proptosis, seizure).

SPECIAL TESTS

- Temporal artery biopsy (>2 cm) should be taken from the affected side. A large biopsy is needed because of the commonly observed "skip" lesions in GCA. A positive biopsy is diagnostic and demonstrates granulomatous vasculitis with multinucleated giant cells near a fragmented internal elastic lamina (66% of cases); nonspecific leukocytic infiltration of vessel walls by neutrophils, eosinophils, and T lymphocytes; and intimal fibrosis with narrowing of the lumen. Some authors recommend bilateral temporal artery biopsies; however, biopsy of the symptomatic side usually is adequate. Baseline visual field testing is indicated even without visual symptoms. If large-vessel involvement is suspected, ultrasound and/or angiography should be pursued.

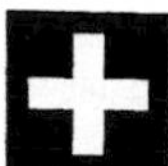

Management

GENERAL MEASURES

- Treatment of GCA focuses on the prevention of serious vascular complications, particularly blindness. Corticosteroids are the mainstay of therapy for GCA and should be instituted when the diagnosis is suspected, even in the face of normal ESR and prior to obtaining temporal artery biopsy. Unfortunately, visual loss often is permanent, and further damage to the affected eye and even in the previously unaffected fellow eye can occur despite high-dose IV methylprednisolone treatment. Therefore, prompt diagnosis and *immediate* corticosteroid intervention is paramount to preventing progressive visual loss. The proper corticosteroid regimen for treatment of GCA has not been established. Initial doses and extended taper schedules should be individualized by the clinical state of each patient. The prominent headache, which is so frequent in GCA, responds rapidly to corticosteroid treatment and typically resolves within 1–2 days. ESR, C-reactive protein, and other acute phase reactants may be used to monitor response to therapy and disease control. Duration of steroid therapy for treatment of GCA may range from 1–3 years.

SURGICAL MEASURES

- Temporal artery biopsy should be performed to confirm the diagnosis of GCA. It is performed under local anesthetic and on an outpatient basis. Biopsy should be completed within 7 days of starting corticosteroids, after which the results of the biopsy may be affected. A negative biopsy does not rule out the diagnosis of GCA.

SYMPTOMATIC TREATMENT

- Analgesics for headache

ADJUNCTIVE TREATMENT

N/A

ADMISSION/DISCHARGE CRITERIA

- Visual symptoms/loss associated with GCA require the patient to see an ophthalmologist on an emergency basis and may involve admission. Admission for GCA is indicated for IV steroid therapy, unstable vitals, large-vessel involvement, ischemic limb, and renal, gastrointestinal, cardiac, or cerebral complication. Alternatively, IV therapy may be given on an outpatient basis.

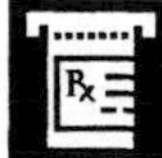

Medications

DRUG(S) OF CHOICE

- The presence and degree of ocular involvement influence the dose and route of corticosteroid therapy. Oral therapy consists of prednisone 20–40 mg/day without ocular involvement and 60–120 mg/day (1–2 mg/kg/day) for cases with ocular involvement. High-dose oral therapy should continue for 8 weeks with gradual taper to achieve the lowest possible maintenance dose. Several authors suggest that IV methylprednisolone 1 g/day (or 250 mg in 6 hours) for 3 days may be beneficial in cases presenting with visual deficit. Patients receiving IV methylprednisolone should be converted to oral prednisone and tapered to maintenance levels. The goal of therapy is to maintain the patient on the lowest dose of corticosteroid that resolves clinical symptoms and maintains ESR >30–40 mm/hour.

Contraindications

- Absolute contraindications to corticosteroid use include hypersensitivity to the drug and systemic fungal infection. Relative contraindications include diabetes, hypertension, tuberculosis, osteoporosis, and congestive heart failure.

Precautions

- From 20%–50% of GCA patients experience steroid-related complications such as progressive osteoporosis, hip and spinal compression fractures, immunosuppression, cushingoid appearance, obesity, peptic ulcer disease, GI bleed, hypertension, diabetes, cataracts, or glaucoma. Gastric prophylaxis may include taking steroids with meals or in divided doses. Additionally, ranitidine (Zantac), sucralfate (Carafate), or omeprazole (Prilosec) may be indicated. Bisphosphonates have been shown to decrease bone loss and may be indicated for some patients.

ALTERNATIVE DRUGS

- In cases where active inflammation is not controlled or intolerable side effects occur, a second immunosuppressive agent (e.g., azathioprine or methotrexate) may be added to spare the steroid dose.

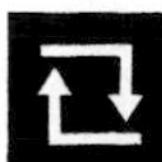

Follow-Up

PATIENT MONITORING

- Patients should be seen every 4–6 weeks to assess the response to therapy. Clinical symptoms and signs, ESR, and other acute phase reactants should be followed as corticosteroids are tapered.

EXPECTED COURSE AND PROGNOSIS

- Relapse most commonly occurs during the initial year of therapy, especially following reduction of steroid dose. Up to 50% of GCA patients may require corticosteroids for greater than 2 years. In general, patients have been reported to have the same life expectancy as age-matched controls. However, profound visual loss in GCA has been found to correlate with decreased quality and duration of life.

PATIENT EDUCATION

- It is necessary to educate each patient regarding the chronic nature of GCA, the spectrum of symptoms, the possibility of relapse, and possible sequelae of long-term steroid therapy

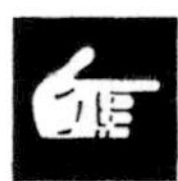

Miscellaneous

SYNONYMS

- Temporal arteritis

ICD-9-CM: 446.5 Giant cell arteritis; 377.41 Ischemic optic neuropathy

SEE ALSO: N/A

REFERENCES

- Dutton GN, Ghanchi FD. Current concepts in giant cell (temporal) arteritis. Surv Ophthalmol 1997;42:99–123.
- Kelman SE. Ischemic optic neuropathies. In: Miller NR, Newman NJ, eds. Walsh and Hoyt's clinical neuro-ophthalmology, vol. 1, 5th ed. Baltimore: Williams and Wilkins, 1998.
- Glaser JS. The ischemic optic neuropathies. In: Albert DM, Jakobiec FA, eds. Principles and practice of ophthalmology: clinical practice. vol. 4. Philadelphia: WB Saunders, 1994.
- Schmidt WA, Kraft HE, Vorpahl K, et al. Color duplex ultrasonography in the diagnosis of temporal arteritis. N Engl J Med 1997;337:1336–1342.

Author(s): James A. McHale, MD; Steven E. Katz, MD

Guillain-Barré Syndrome

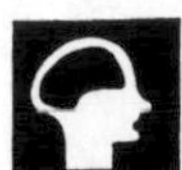

Basics

DESCRIPTION

- An acute, predominantly motor neuropathy of uncertain cause that is the most common cause of acquired generalized paralysis in humans

EPIDEMIOLOGY

Incidence/Prevalence

- Annual incidence 1-2/100,000

Race

- All races affected

Age

- All ages; mean age of onset ~40 years

Sex

- Occurs more frequently in males than females (1.5:1)

ETIOLOGY

- Precise cause is unclear but follows infection in most cases. Infection is thought to produce an immune reaction resulting in cellular and humoral responses that attack unknown myelin components and result in macrophage-induced demyelination.
- Axon may be attacked in severe cases, especially those following *Campylobacter jejuni* infection.

Genetics

- Sporadic disease; some association with HLA types

RISK FACTORS

- Infection precedes disease onset in two thirds/3 of patients. *C. jejuni* infection is the most common precipitating infection occurring in 30%-40%. It causes a gastroenteritis that precedes weakness by 7-14 days. Other infections include influenza viruses, Epstein-Barr virus, cytomegalovirus, human immunodeficiency virus, Coxsackie virus, herpes simplex, hepatitis A virus, and *Mycoplasma pneumonia*. Other possible precipitants include hematologic malignancies, hyperthyroidism, collagen vascular diseases, sarcoidosis, pregnancy, surgical procedures, transplants, immunizations (e.g., swine flu), and certain drugs (e.g., heroin)

PREGNANCY

- Increased incidence

ASSOCIATED CONDITIONS

- See Risk Factors

Diagnosis

DIFFERENTIAL DIAGNOSIS

- Other neuropathies: chronic inflammatory demyelinating polyradiculoneuropathy, vasculitic, toxic, hereditary, porphyria, diptheria, critical illness neuropathy, subacute sensory neuronopathy with cancer, malignant infiltration of nerve roots
- Muscle disorders: periodic paralysis, fulminant polymyositis
- Neuromuscular junction diseases: acute myasthenia gravis, botulism, organophosphate poisoning, prolonged neuromuscular blockade with anesthesia
- Spinal cord disorders: acute compressive lesions, transverse myelitis, multiple sclerosis
- Brainstem disorders: tumor infiltration, encephalitis
- Metabolic disorders: severe hypokalemia, hypophosphatemia
- Psychiatric disorders: conversion disorders, malingering

SIGNS AND SYMPTOMS

- Begins with numbness and tingling in fingers, toes, or trunk that may last 7-10 days.
- Symmetric weakness follows, usually starting in legs and then going to arms (ascending pattern). Facial involvement in approximately 50%.
- Peak weakness reached within 4 weeks of onset.
- Extent of progression variable; approximately 30% require ventilatory assistance
- Tendon reflexes typically absent or depressed.
- Sensory loss variable, particularly when compared to weakness.
- Dull, aching, burning pain involving low back or lower extremities occurs in approximately 90%.
- Autonomic involvement in 70% (blood pressure lability, bowel and bladder involvement, pupillary changes, cardiac arrhythmias). Can be life threatening.
- Variants of typical presentation account for about 15% of all Guillain-Barré syndrome patients.
  - —*Fisher syndrome* (or Miller-Fisher syndrome) may account for 5%; characterized by ophthalmoplegia, ataxia, and areflexia, often without weakness.
  - —*Pharyngeal-cervical-brachial weakness* (3%) weakness in the pharynx, face, neck flexors and arms.
  - —*Paraparetic weakness* (~2%) have only leg weakness and areflexia with variable sensory loss.
  - —*Pure motor variant* (~3%) have no sensory symptoms. Mild sensory abnormalities may be detected on electrophysiologic studies.
  - —*Axonal variant* presents with rapidly progressive weakness and sensory loss with early respiratory insufficiency. Early electrophysiologic studies reveal axonal changes and little to suggest demyelination. Patients with a predominantly axonal picture are more likely to have had preceding *C. jejuni* infection.
  - —*Pure sensory variant* (<1%) present with large fiber, ataxic, areflexic sensory neuropathy with little or no motor involvement, tremor, and autonomic features. Electrophysiologic studies show severe involvement of sensory nerves with relatively few motor findings.
  - —*Acute pandysautonomic variant* (rare) presents with GI disturbances (pain, vomiting, constipation), orthostasis, urinary retention, fatigue, impotence, diminished sweating and salivation, and occasionally pupillary abnormalities.

LABORATORY PROCEDURES

- Spinal fluid analysis: elevated protein without leukocytosis (usually <10 cells/mm^3) in ~90% at time of maximal weakness. Cell count >50 cells/mm^3 indicates alternate diagnosis unless in setting of HIV.
- Anti-G_{M1} antibody testing and serologic testing for *C. jejuni* usually not helpful in diagnosis and do not change therapy, but may indicate poor prognosis if positive.
- Anti-GQ1b antibodies helpful in confirming diagnosis of Fisher syndrome

IMAGING STUDIES

- MRI may show nerve root or cranial nerve enhancement; usually not helpful in confirming diagnosis.

SPECIAL TESTS

- Nerve conduction studies may be normal early in course, becoming abnormal by 2-3 weeks. Changes in the motor nerves usually precede changes in the sensory fibers. Studies show prolonged distal motor latencies, slowed nerve conductions, temporal dispersion of motor response, conduction block, and prolonged F waves. EMG findings depend on extent of axonal involvement. Fibrillations and sharp waves develop if axonal disruption has occurred, usually after the second week. May be severe in some cases with "axonal variant."

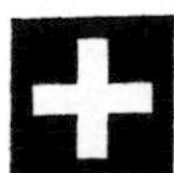

Management

GENERAL MEASURES

- ICU hospitalization for all patients with respiratory compromise, autonomic instability, or complicating medical conditions. IV immunoglobulin *or* plasma exchange for all patients. Monitor ventilatory status closely with serial measurements of forced vital capacity (FVC) and negative inspiratory force (NIF). Consider ventilatory assistance if FVC falls below ~15-20 mL/kg or NIF < −20 to −25 cm H_2O. Neck flexor strength that is not at least antigravity often heralds ventilatory failure.
- Intubation for ventilatory failure or airway protection in patients with severe bulbar weakness.
- Cardiac monitoring for and treatment of arrhythmias or blood pressure instability.
- Aggressive management of neuropathic pain.

SURGICAL MEASURES

- Tracheostomy for patients requiring prolonged intubation

SYMPTOMATIC TREATMENT

- Appropriate supportive care to include physical and occupational therapy, nutritional support, deep vein thrombosis prophylaxis, pulmonary care, and psychological support
- Tube feedings may be required for patients with severe bulbar weakness or those requiring ventilatory support
- Letter boards or electronic devices are important for patients who cannot speak because of intubation or bulbar weakness
- Pharmacologic treatment for depression

ADJUNCTIVE TREATMENT

N/A

ADMISSION/DISCHARGE CRITERIA

- Hospitalization for all but the mildest cases

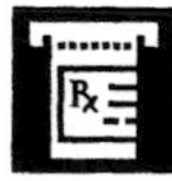

Medications

DRUG(S) OF CHOICE

- Plasma exchange (200-250 cc/kg total exchanged volume divided into 4-6 exchanges over 2-3 weeks) reduces time until initial improvement, return of ambulation, and time on the ventilator; increases percentage of patients improving at 1 and 6 months; and increases percentage of patients showing full recovery at 1 year.
- IV immunoglobulin 0.4 g/kg/day for 5 days is of equal efficacy, increasing the percentage of patients improved at 1 month, and reducing median time to improvement and time to reach independent ambulation.
- Both plasma exchange *and* IV immunoglobulin confers no additional benefits.

Contraindications

- Cardiovascular instability, congestive heart failure, hypotension, renal failure, or severe anemia are relative contraindications to plasma exchange. Theoretical risk of bleeding complications due to depletion of clotting factors, especially fibrinogen. For these patients, IV immunoglobulin probably is a better choice. Sepsis due to chronic indwelling central catheter may be a problem.
- For IV immunoglobulin, congenital IgA deficiency is relative contraindication, because these patients may develop antibodies to IgA that can result in anaphylactic-like reaction.

Precautions

- May need IV fluids if hypotension develops during plasma exchange. Hypocalcemia secondary to anticoagulants used during procedure may need treatment.
- Mild allergic reactions, including chills, aching, fevers, flushing, and tachycardia, usually respond to slowing of infusion rate, but antihistamines, steroids, or both occasionally are needed.

ALTERNATIVE DRUGS

- None. Corticosteroids are not effective and may increase relapse rate.

Follow-Up

PATIENT MONITORING

- Periodic reassessments to ensure that relapse is not occurring

EXPECTED COURSE AND PROGNOSIS

- Degree and extent of progression variable; approximately 75% of patients reach nadir within 7 days of presentation; essentially all by 4 weeks. Some patients progress rapidly to ventilator dependence within days, whereas others have very mild progression for weeks and never lose ambulation.
- Approximately one third of patients eventually require ventilatory assistance. Recovery over weeks to months is usual (~70% of patients).
- 10%–25% will have permanent weakness or other impairments that interfere with activities of daily living.
- 3%–5% die, usually from respiratory distress syndrome, sepsis, or both.
- Poor prognostic factors include advanced age, need for ventilatory support, rapidly progressive weakness, prolonged course of active disease, and axonal involvement, especially reduction of the mean distal compound motor action potential amplitude.
- Approximately 10% of patients have a malignant course with prolonged ventilator dependence and recovery phase extending beyond 2 years.
- 5% of patients may relapse after initial improvement. Relapse best treated like initial episode, although corticosteroids sometimes are effective if fluctuation/worsening of symptoms persists beyond 6 weeks.

PATIENT EDUCATION

- Careful explanation of the natural history of the disease and realistic goals for expected speed and degree of recovery
- Guillain-Barre Syndrome Foundation International, P.O. Box 262, Wynnewood, PA 19096. Website: *www.guillain-barre.com*

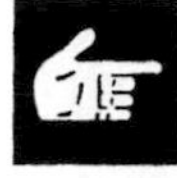

Miscellaneous

SYNONYMS

- Landry-Guillain-Barré-Strohl syndrome
- Acute idiopathic polyneuritis
- Acute ascending paralysis
- Acute inflammatory demyelinating polyradiculoneuropathy

ICD-9-CM: 357.0 Acute infective polyneuritis

SEE ALSO: CHRONIC INFLAMMATORY DEMYELINATING POLYRADICULONEUROPATHY

REFERENCES

- Asbury AK, Cornblath DR. Assessment of current diagnostic criteria for Guillain-Barré syndrome. Ann Neurol 1990;27 [Suppl]:21–24.
- Rees JH, et al. Campylobacter jejuni infection and Guillain-Barré syndrome. N Engl J Med 1995;333:1374–1379.
- Ropper AH. The Guillain-Barré syndrome. N Engl J Med 1992;326:1130–1136.
- van der Meche FGA, Schmitz PIM, Dutch Guillain-Barré Study group. A randomized trial comparing intravenous immune globulin and plasma exchange in Guillain-Barré syndrome. N Engl J Med 1992;326:1123–1129.
- van der Meche FGA, van Doorn PA. Guillain-Barré syndrome and chronic inflammatory demyelinating polyneuropathy: immune mechanisms and update on current therapies. Ann Neurol 1995;37[S1]:S14–S31.

Author(s): John Kissel, MD

Headache, Acute

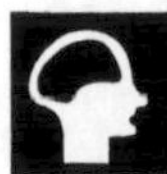

Basics

DESCRIPTION

- Headache is one of the most common symptoms seen in medical practice. Many headaches are chronic or fit readily into the most common patterns of headache. Headaches of new onset that do not fit into the description of migraine, cluster, or tension-type headache need to be analyzed carefully. A single severe headache lasting hours to days in a patient without a history of similar headaches can be classified as acute. Various processes may cause such headaches and may range from benign to life threatening. The acute headache is a particular problem for emergency room physicians, who have only one opportunity to diagnose headaches that require further evaluation and treatment.

EPIDEMIOLOGY

- Approximately 6.6 million office visits are made for headache annually, representing 2% of all primary care visits made in the United States. Over 1.8 million emergency room visits are also made annually. This is 3% of all emergency room visits nationally. Resulting costs are estimated at $15 billion per year. In a single hospital study, of 455 patients screened primarily for headache, 76% were female, mean age 37 years, and 3% had subarachnoid hemorrhage.

ETIOLOGY

- Most acute headache are migraine, tension-type headache, or cluster headache. Each of these entities is dealt with in their respective chapters. A variety of factors are red flags for more significant processes causing headache. The presence of one or more of the following factors is an indication for further evaluation:
  - —Abrupt onset of headache
  - —Anticoagulant use
  - —History of head trauma within the past few months
  - —Fever, immunosuppression, or other symptoms of infection, especially in a parameningeal focus
  - —Prominent neck pain and stiffness, suggesting meningeal irritation
  - —Progressive headache over hours or days
  - —Altered consciousness (including syncope or seizures)
  - —Focal neurologic complaints or findings
  - —Age >40, as the onset of primary headache disorders is rare in this age group and the prevalence of secondary headache disorders is higher
  - —Exposure to products of combustion (or cohabitants/coworkers with similar symptoms) suggesting carbon monoxide exposure
- Acute headache may occur in the following disorders, but is not limited to these conditions:
  - —Brain abscess
  - —Brain tumor
  - —Cerebrovascular disease including venous occlusion
  - —Coital headache
  - —Drug induced, drug withdrawal
  - —Encephalitis
  - —Exertional headache
  - —First migraine
  - —Intracerebral hemorrhage
  - —Low-pressure headache
  - —Meningitis
  - —Pheochromocytoma
  - —Pseudotumor cerebri
  - —Subarachnoid hemorrhage
  - —Temporal arteritis
  - —Tolosa-Hunt syndrome

RISK FACTORS

- Dependent on the primary cause of acute headache. Patients should be asked about medication and drug use, major medical problems, exposures to toxins, recent infections, trauma, and travel.

PREGNANCY

- New headaches in pregnancy may occur due to the onset of migraine. Rarely, cortical vein thrombosis, particularly in the peripartum period, may occur. Headaches may occur with eclampsia. Intracerebral and subarachnoid hemorrhages may occur in patients with berry aneurysms or intracranial malformations.

ASSOCIATED CONDITIONS

- See Etiology; Diagnosis

Diagnosis

DIFFERENTIAL DIAGNOSIS

- Acute glaucoma: eye pain, visual blurring, tender orbit, conjunctival injection
- Brain mass lesion: brain tumor or abscess, usually progresses over days to weeks, and does not usually present as acute headache unless there is superimposed intracranial bleeding
- Carbon monoxide poisoning: exposure setting, others involved in same area, altered mental status, carboxyhemoglobin level
- Encephalitis: hours to days, severe headache, focal neurologic signs (aphasia, hemiparesis), impaired consciousness, seizures, fever, chills
- Exertional headache: minutes, in setting of exercise or straining (Valsalva), sudden, suboccipital, severe, pounding headache lasting minutes; may occasionally be associated with posterior fossa lesions, Arnold-Chiari malformations, or berry aneurysms
- Low-pressure headache: post lumbar puncture or trauma, operation, spontaneous; pancephalic, worse with standing, head shaking; associated with nausea
- Meningitis: hours to days, severe headache with neck stiffness, fever, chills, photophobia, possibly confusion
- Pheochromocytoma: days to weeks, intermittent acute headache, pounding, pancephalic, with acute hypertension
- Pseudotumor cerebri: days to weeks, progressive, pancephalic, worse with recumbency, associated with visual obscurations, occasional sixth nerve palsies, visual field constriction
- Sinusitis: acute sinusitis and other sinonasal problems can be a cause of acute headache and/or facial pain. Less common than perceived by the public. Pain, tenderness over maxillary, ethmoid sinus, with purulent rhinorrhea, respiratory complaints. Vertex pain may occur with sphenoid sinusitis.
- Subarachnoid hemorrhage: immediate, "worst headache of my life," pancephalic, sometimes with loss of consciousness, confusion, mutism, focal neurologic findings, nuchal rigidity
- Temporal arteritis: days to weeks, persistent, aching headache, often temporal, unilateral, associated with malaise, low-grade fever, myalgias, nodular areas temporal arteries, jaw claudication, blindness

SIGNS AND SYMPTOMS

Initial History

- Description of the headache (nature, rapidity of onset, degree and quality of pain, location, relieving/exacerbating factors, prior headache history, change from prior headache)
- Associated symptoms (nausea, vomiting, neurologic symptoms, fever, change in mental status, neck pain or stiffness, dental and sinus symptoms, photophobia, nasal discharge)
- Current medications (including anticoagulants, monoamine oxidase inhibitors, pain medications, other medications)
- Past medical history (major medical or surgical disorders, trauma, infection, drug and alcohol history)

Initial Examination

- Vital signs (temperature, BP, pulse, respirations)
- Dental, sinus evaluation (oral examination, dental percussion, ear examination)
- Check for temporal artery nodularity, tenderness
- Neck examination (rigidity)
- Ophthalmologic examination (for corneal clouding, papilledema, subhyaloid hemorrhages, hypertensive changes)

- General medical examination (including ear, lymph nodes)
- Neurologic examination (level of consciousness, presence of aphasia or neglect, lateralizing signs, up-going toes)

LABORATORY PROCEDURES

- Depends on results of history and physical examination. Considerations include glucose (hypoglycemia or hyperglycemia), electrolytes, CBC (white count elevation in infection, anemia causing headache), PT/PTT (for coagulopathy causing bleeding), drug screen, carboxyhemoglobin (for carbon monoxide exposure), ESR and C-reactive protein (for temporal arteritis).

IMAGING STUDIES

- Any patient with a new headache should be considered for an imaging study. If the headache is suggestive of subarachnoid hemorrhage or intracerebral hemorrhage, a CT scan should be performed as soon. This is positive in subarachnoid hemorrhage in about 90% of patients, but more likely may be negative with a delay of days, with small amounts of blood, or with a low hematocrit. When there is a suspicion of subarachnoid hemorrhage despite negative CT, a lumbar puncture should be performed. MRI is less sensitive acutely in subarachnoid hemorrhage but may show the presence of the aneurysm. Intracerebral hemorrhage is well imaged by CT, and the location and size may determine whether surgical approaches are necessary.
- Imaging studies should be performed for other types of acute headache. MRI may be superior in some types of acute headache conditions. These include intracerebral infections (particularly with the use of gadolinium enhancement), cortical vein thrombosis, CNS inflammatory disorders, and encephalitis. MR angiography of the head and neck may be useful in patients with cerebral aneurysms or dissections of extracranial vessels, or with intracranial vascular anomalies. MR venography may assist in diagnosis of venous sinus thrombosis.

SPECIAL TESTS

- In patients with acute headache in whom there are red flags and initial evaluation is negative, or in which CT is negative and subarachnoid hemorrhage, meningitis, or encephalitis is considered, lumbar puncture is important and may be diagnostic. Lumbar puncture should be avoided in the presence of mass effect or lateralized processes to avoid precipitating cerebral herniation.
- Cerebral arteriography is standard in patients with cerebral aneurysms and should be performed on all intracranial vessels to assess for secondary aneurysms, which occur occasionally.

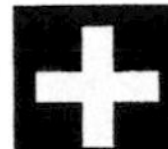

Management

GENERAL MEASURES

- A warm, comfortable, quiet environment may be useful. Photophobic patients may be treated in a dark environment. Reassure the patient that effective analgesia will be provided and that appropriate diagnostic studies will be performed.

SURGICAL MEASURES

- Depends on primary cause of headache

SYMPTOMATIC TREATMENT

- Medications are the primary symptom therapy for acute headache.

ADJUNCTIVE TREATMENT

- See Medications

ADMISSION/DISCHARGE CRITERIA

- Patients considered to have a major cause for acute headache as outlined above should be admitted for definitive treatment. Any patient with a sudden, severe, unexplained headache may be considered for admission unless a rapid outpatient evaluation can be undertaken safely. Patients can be discharged when the primary diagnosis has been made and effective therapy is underway.

Medications

DRUG(S) OF CHOICE

- Analgesics may be used in acute headache. These include over-the-counter analgesics (aspirin, acetaminophen, ibuprofen, naproxen) with or without caffeine. Combination medications (e.g., acetaminophen, butalbital, caffeine) may be used. For more severe headache, opioids may be necessary (codeine and congeners, meperidine, morphine). In the emergency room setting, antiemetics may be useful and at times effective for headache control (chlorpromazine). If the headache is migrainous, specific therapy with various vasoactive agents may be considered (sumatriptan, other "triptan" medications, isometheptene, dihydroergotamine).

Contraindications

- Depend on the individual medication considered. Although symptomatic therapy is important for patient comfort, the primary concern is effective diagnosis and treatment of the underlying cause of headache. Nonsteroidal agents are contraindicated in patients with renal failure or peptic ulcer disease. Vasoactive substances are contraindicated with cardiac disease or intracranial vascular disease.

Precautions

- Antiemetic medications may cause symptomatic hypotension.

ALTERNATIVE DRUGS

N/A

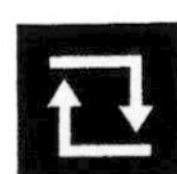

Follow-Up

PATIENT MONITORING

- Patients should be followed carefully until their acute headache has resolved satisfactorily. Specific monitoring parameters depend on the etiology.

EXPECTED COURSE AND PROGNOSIS

- Depends on primary cause

PATIENT EDUCATION

- Depends on primary cause

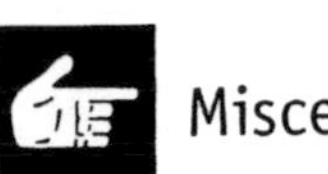

Miscellaneous

SYNONYMS

- See specific diagnosis areas

ICD-9-CM: See specific diagnosis areas

SEE ALSO: SPECIFIC DIAGNOSIS AREAS

REFERENCES

- Cady R, Dodick DW. Diagnosis and treatment of migraine. Mayo Clin Proc 2002;77:255–261.
- Drexler ED. Severe headaches. Postgrad Med 1990;87:164–180.
- Lipton RB, Stewart WF. Migraine in the United States: a review of epidemiology and health care use. Neurology 1993;43:S11–S15.
- Sands GH, Newman L, Lipton R. Cough, exertional, and other miscellaneous headaches. Med Clin North Am 1991;75 [Suppl 3]:733–747.
- Silberstein SD, Marcelis J. Headache associated with changes in intracranial pressure. Headache 1992;32:84–94.

Author(s): Alexander D. Rae-Grant, MD; John Castaldo, MD

Headache, Chronic

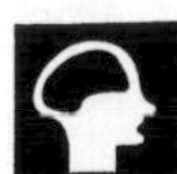

Basics

DESCRIPTION

Headache occurring more than 15 days per month.

- Primary chronic headache
  - —No identifiable cause or
  - —No temporal correlation between the onset of an underlying disorder that causes secondary chronic headache and the headache onset.
- Secondary chronic headache: caused by an underlying disorder

EPIDEMIOLOGY

Incidence/Prevalence

Incidence unknown. Prevalence: 3.2% to 4.7%, versus 12% to 38% for episodic headaches

ETIOLOGY

- Development of chronic headache
  - —75% develop from episodic migraine
  - —8% develop from episodic tension-type headache
  - —16% develop without previous headache history ("new onset daily headache"): should be classified as chronic migraine or tension-type headache
- Medication overuse: frequently causes episodic headache to evolve into chronic headache

Genetics

- Chronic tension-type headache exhibits multifactorial inheritance.
- Chronic cluster headache exhibits autosomal-dominant inheritance.

RISK FACTORS

- Medication overuse
- History of episodic migraine
- Family history of chronic headache
- Coincident major depressive disorder
- Sex
  - —Female predominance in chronic migraine, chronic tension-type headache, hemicrania continua, chronic paroxysmal hemicrania, and idiopathic stabbing headache
  - —Male predominance cluster headache

PREGNANCY

N/A

ASSOCIATED CONDITIONS

- Psychiatric disorders: often remit following successful treatment of chronic headache
  - —Anxiety disorders (23%–70%)
  - —Mood disorders (25%–59%)
  - —Somatoform disorders (6%)
- Medication overuse (30%–40%)
  - —Defined as the use of:
    - -At least three simple analgesic medications (e.g., single-agent, nonbarbiturate, nonsedative) per day at least 5 days per week
    - -Triptans and/or complex analgesics or Opioids and/or ergots at least 3 days per week
  - —Concerns
    - -Short-acting medications cause rebound headaches that are confused with underlying headache.
    - -Medication overuse may make chronic headaches refractory to prophylactic medications.
    - -Medication overuse may reflect attempt to treat undiagnosed psychiatric disturbance.
    - -Systemic toxicities of analgesics

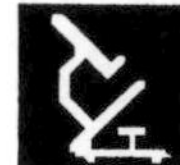

Diagnosis

DIFFERENTIAL DIAGNOSIS

- Primary chronic headache
  - —Chronic migraine
  - —Chronic tension-type headaches
  - —Hemicrania continua
  - —Chronic cluster headache
  - —Chronic paroxysmal hemicrania
  - —Chronic hypnic headache
  - —Idiopathic stabbing headache
- Secondary chronic headache
  - —Posttraumatic headache
  - —Cervical spine disorders
  - —Cranial neuropathies
  - —Ophthalmic disorders
  - —Vascular disorders: arteriovenous malformation, arteritis, arterial dissection, subdural hematoma
  - —Nonvascular disorders: increased or decreased CSF pressure, infection, neoplasm, Chiari malformation
  - —Oromandibular disorders
  - —Sinus and ear disorders

SIGNS AND SYMPTOMS

Chronic Migraine/Transformed Migraine

51% to 78% of chronic headache patients

- Present >1 month
- History of episodic migraine
- Period of increasing headache frequency with decreasing severity of migrainous symptoms (nausea, vomiting, photophobia, phonophobia) over 3 to 4 months
- Chronic tension-type headache with superimposed episodic migraine should be considered chronic migraine
- Triggers generally persist and can induce acute migraine attacks
- Pain is severe but patients attempt to sleep

Chronic Tension-Type Headaches

15% to 46% of chronic headache patients

- Present >6 months
- History of episodic tension-type headaches
- At most one migrainous symptom
- Two of the following pain characteristics:
  - —Compressive quality
  - —Mild to moderate intensity
  - —Bilateral location
  - —Not aggravated by routine physical activity
- Chronic tension-type headache with disorder of pericranial muscles involves:
  - —Tenderness of pericranial muscles

Hemicrania Continua

- Present >1 month
- Unilateral, continuous but fluctuant pain ranging from moderate to severe intensity
- Absence of triggers
- At least one autonomic symptom (conjunctival injection, ptosis, lacrimation, nasal congestion, rhinorrhea, eyelid edema) during periods of severe headache
- Complete symptomatic relief following indomethacin treatment

Chronic Cluster Headache

- One to eight attacks per day lasting 15 to 180 minutes; >5 attacks total
- Cluster of daily attacks lasting >1 year with <14 days of remission
- Pain strictly unilateral, always on the same side, periorbital and temporal region
- Attacks associated with autonomic symptoms: miosis, facial sweating, plus those autonomic symptoms listed for hemicrania continua
- Attacks occur at same time of the day
- Pain is severe, causing agitation
- Pain is boring, throbbing, or compressive
- Migrainous symptoms in <50%; rarely associated with aura
- Usually develops from episodic form of cluster headache; 50% revert spontaneously to episodic form
- Triggers: REM sleep (sleep deprivation shortens REM period; therefore, patients avoid sleep, alcohol, nitrates)

Chronic Paroxysmal Hemicrania

- Four attacks per day during at least half of the headache period
- 50 attacks total
- Attacks last 2 to 45 minutes
- Strictly unilateral, always on the same side
- Located predominantly in periorbital and temporal regions
- Attacks associated with autonomic symptoms ipsilateral to pain
- Indomethacin completely alleviates symptoms
- Pain is boring, throbbing, and severe, causing agitation and restlessness
- Occurs at irregular intervals during day and night
- Absence of migrainous symptoms
- Different from chronic cluster headache in male patients by temporal pattern of attacks, and response to indomethacin
- 10% triggered by head movements or pressure applied to cervical spine

Chronic Hypnic Headache

- Present >1 month
- Headaches last 5 to 60 minutes
- Absence of autonomic symptoms
- One to three attacks per evening, waking patient from sleep

- Headaches develop only during REM sleep, rarely during napping
- Maximum prevalence in 60- to 70-year-olds

Idiopathic Stabbing Headache/Ice-Pick Headache/Jabs-and-Jolts Syndrome/Ophthalmodynia

- Attacks on 24 days per month at irregular intervals
- Pain lasting <1 second, sharp, causing shock-like response ("jolt")
- Pain is typically unilateral, located in the orbit, forehead, and/or temple
- Absence of autonomic symptoms, triggers
- Additional subtype of headache in 58%
- High coincidence of ocular pathology

LABORATORY PROCEDURES

N/A

IMAGING STUDIES

Brain MRI or CT

- Chronic migraine: not indicated if symptomatically stable unless abnormal neurologic examination
- Chronic tension-type headache: identifies treatable abnormality in 0.5% to 2.4% of patients
- Brain MR venogram: venous sinus thrombosis in 10% of chronic migraine and chronic tension-type headache patients

SPECIAL TESTS

- Lumbar puncture: opening pressure may be >20 cm H_2O in 21% of chronic headache patients
- Only half of chronic headache patients with elevated intracranial pressure have papilledema

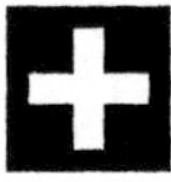

Management

GENERAL MEASURES

- Exclude secondary causes of chronic headache
- Identify comorbid psychiatric factors
- Medication detoxification:
  - —Gradually taper barbiturates, benzodiazepines, and opioids
  - —Gradually switch from short-acting nonsteroidal antiinflammatory drugs (NSAIDs) (regular indomethacin, aspirin) to long-acting NSAIDs (sustained-release indomethacin, naproxen, ketoprofen, tolfenamate, mefenamate, ibuprofen)

SURGICAL MEASURES

Chronic cluster headache: gamma-knife radiosurgery, trigeminal rhizotomy, or trigeminal root transection for medically-refractive cases

SYMPTOMATIC TREATMENT

Limit acute treatments, particularly short-acting NSAIDs, opioids, and ergots

ADJUNCTIVE TREATMENT

- Psychotherapy: stress management, relaxation therapy, and biofeedback proven efficacious
- Physiotherapy: cervical spine manipulation, massage, TENS, and ergonometric review have limited evidence supporting use for chronic tension-type headaches
- Acupuncture proven ineffective

ADMISSION/DISCHARGE CRITERIA

- Emergency admission may be required for:
  - —Complicated migraine
  - —Suspicion of secondary chronic headache
  - —Chronic headache with dehydration from persistent vomiting
  - —Severe comorbid psychiatric disorders
- Nonemergent admission may be required for:
  - —Comorbid medical conditions requiring monitoring
  - —Detoxification from opioids, barbiturates, benzodiazepines, or ergots
  - —Failed outpatient detoxification

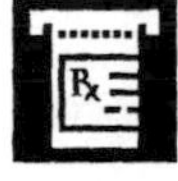

Medications

DRUG(S) OF CHOICE

- Chronic migraine
  - —Acute treatment: triptans
  - —Prophylaxis: amitriptyline
- Chronic tension-type headache
  - —Acute treatment: long-acting NSAIDs
  - —Prophylaxis: amitriptyline
- Hemicrania continua:
  - —Indomethacin PRN for acute treatment, scheduled for prophylaxis
  - —Reconsider diagnosis if no relief following indomethacin
- Chronic cluster headache
  - -Acute treatment: oxygen supplementation, triptans
  - -Prophylaxis: lithium
- Chronic paroxysmal hemicrania: indomethacin
- Chronic hypnic headache: lithium carbonate qPM
- Idiopathic stabbing headache: indomethacin

Contraindications

- Avoid ergots in patients with vascular disease, pregnancy, or coincidence use of oral contraceptives
- Avoid triptans in patients with vascular disease or hypertension

Precautions

- Toxicity with overdosage of lithium and anticonvulsant medications
- Limit use of methysergide to less than 5 months due to retroperitoneal fibrosis

ALTERNATIVE DRUGS

- Chronic migraine
  - —Acute treatment:
    - -Outpatient: long-acting NSAIDs
    - -Inpatient: dihydroergotamine antiemetics
  - —Prophylaxis: fluoxetine, doxepin, tizanidine, β-blockers, anticonvulsants (divalproex, topiramate)
- Chronic tension-type headache: tizanidine; botulinum toxin injection into tender points
- Hemicrania continua: aspirin, long-acting NSAIDs
- Chronic cluster headache
  - —Acute treatment: DHE, intranasal lidocaine
  - —Prophylaxis: verapamil, methysergide, anticonvulsants (valproate, topiramate)
    - -May supplement with steroids
- Chronic paroxysmal hemicrania: aspirin, verapamil
- Chronic hypnic headache: flunarizine, indomethacin
- Idiopathic stabbing headache: verapamil

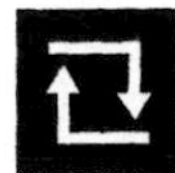

Follow-Up

PATIENT MONITORING

Per routine.

EXPECTED COURSE AND PROGNOSIS

- Response to preventative medications takes up to 10 weeks following detoxification.
- 40% to 80% of patients with medication overuse revert to episodic headaches following detoxification.
- Failure to improve following aggressive management is highly suggestive of psychiatric comorbidity.

PATIENT EDUCATION

- Encourage regular sleep habits and exercise.
- Diet: encourage regular meals.
  - —Dietary supplementation with L-5-hydroxytryptophan (100 mg qd) may reduce analgesic use during detoxification.
- Organizations
  - —International Headache Society. Website: *www.i-h-s.org*.

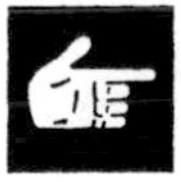

Miscellaneous

SYNONYMS

Chronic daily headache

ICD-9-CM: 784.0 Headache

SEE ALSO: HEADACHE, MIGRAINE

REFERENCES

- International Headache Society. Diagnostic criteria URL: *http://216.25.100.131/ihscommon/guidelines/pdfs/diagnost.pdf.*
- Silberstein SD, Lipton RB, Dalessio DJ, eds. Wolff's headache and other head pain, 7th ed. New York: Oxford University Press, 2001.

Author(s): Monique A. Anawis, MD, JD; Mark K. Borsody, MD, PhD

Headache, Cluster

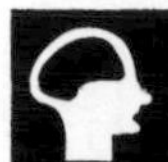

Basics

DESCRIPTION

- Cluster headache is a primary headache disorder characterized by discrete repetitive attacks of unilateral headache with associated ipsilateral autonomic features (including lacrimation, rhinorrhea, ptosis, meiosis). The episodic form is most common and includes periods of attacks (clusters) followed by periods of remission lasting at least 14 days. Chronic cluster headaches occur when attacks occur for 1 year without a remission or when remissions last for <14 days.

EPIDEMIOLOGY

Prevalence

- Estimates vary from 0.1%–0.4% of the population.

Sex

- More common in men than women, with the gender ratio varying from 6–7:1 in the 1960s to 2.1:1 in the 1990s.

Age

- Peak age of onset is 25–50 years, although cluster headaches can occur in teens and children. Men tend to develop their first cluster attack at age 20–30, whereas women have two peaks of cluster onset: late teens/20s and 50–60 years of age.

Race

- Some authors report an increased incidence of cluster HA in African Americans.

ETIOLOGY

Pathophysiology

- Exact cause is unknown.
- One theory suggests involvement of the cavernous sinus portion of the carotid artery. It is here that the trigeminal nociceptive pathways and autonomic fibers are anatomically close together. Activation of these systems would result in the typical features of cluster headache: unilateral orbital pain, lacrimation and rhinorrhea (parasympathetic), ptosis, and meiosis (sympathetic).
- The periodicity of cluster attacks suggests involvement of the hypothalamus, specifically the suprachiasmatic nucleus, which is involved in regulation of circadian rhythms, and the posterior hypothalamus, which contains nuclei involved in autonomic function.
- Recent studies involving PET scans demonstrate activation of various parts of the brain in cluster patients: anterior cingulate gyrus, prefrontal cortex, insula, and contralateral thalamus (each associated with pain); ipsilateral hypothalamic gray (unique to cluster headaches); and extracerebral areas including the cavernous sinus (suggesting activation of the trigeminothalamic system).

Genetics

- Not known to have a genetic component, although recent studies suggest a 14-fold increased risk of cluster headaches in first-degree relatives.

RISK FACTORS

- Include smoking and alcohol use

PREGNANCY

- Women often experience remission while pregnant.
- Menarche, menstruation, menopause, oral contraceptives, and hormone replacement therapy have no known affect on cluster headaches.

ASSOCIATED CONDITIONS

- Leonine facies: sharp facial features, deep nasolabial furrows, telangiectasia, peau d'orange skin
- History of migraines
- Tall stature
- Duodenal ulceration/peptic ulcer disease, secondary to increased gastric acid production
- Psychological conditions (type A personality)

Diagnosis

DIFFERENTIAL DIAGNOSIS

- Migraine headaches
- Trigeminal neuralgia
- Temporal arteritis
- Sinusitis
- Paroxysmal hemicrania
- Hemicrania continua
- SUNCT syndrome (short-lasting unilateral neuralgiform pain with conjunctival injection and tearing)
- Carotid or vertebral artery dissection
- Glaucoma
- Brain tumor
- Cervical cord tumor or infarction
- Arteriovenous malformation
- Intracranial or carotid aneurysms
- Tolosa-Hunt syndrome
- Pheochromocytoma
- Acute angle-closure glaucoma
- Corneal erosion
- Dental problem

SIGNS AND SYMPTOMS

- Cluster headache presents as a rapid-onset headache reaching its peak intensity within minutes.
- The pain often is continuous and is described as deep, boring, or explosive in quality. The phrase "like a hot poker in the eye" has been used to describe the attacks.
- Most patients are unable to remain still during an attack and may bang their heads against walls to relieve the pain.
- Unilateral headache, most often located around the orbit. May radiate to the face, ear, neck, hemicranium, jaw, or teeth.
- Patients have ipsilateral conjunctival injection, lacrimation, rhinorrhea, nasal congestion, sweating, ptosis, meiosis, pallor, or eyelid edema.
- Nausea, vomiting, photophobia, and phonophobia may occur. Auras are rare.
- Individual attacks last approximately 45–90 minutes. Cluster periods last 2–12 weeks, during which patients have 1–3 attacks per day. Remissions may last months to years.
- Patients commonly experience a cluster period at the same time each year, and cluster attacks at the same time each day.
- The attacks remain on the same side of the head during an individual cluster period but switch sides during the next cluster period in 15% of patients.
- Nocturnal attacks are more common, resulting in sleep deprivation, daytime napping, fatigue, and depression.

LABORATORY PROCEDURES

- May help rule out other causes of headache, such as an elevated ESR or C-reactive protein in temporal arteritis or abnormal endocrine studies with a pituitary tumor.

IMAGING STUDIES

- CT and MRI are generally not useful in the diagnosis of cluster headache.

SPECIAL TESTS

N/A

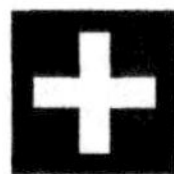

Management

GENERAL MEASURES

- Early and accurate diagnosis is essential.
- Advise patients that cluster attacks are easily managed with fast-acting therapies and may be prevented with a variety of prophylactic medications.
- Prophylactic medications are often tapered near the end of the cluster period and may be restarted if symptoms recur.

SURGICAL MEASURES

- Indicated for patients with unilateral headaches who do not respond to medical therapy or have contraindications to the medications.
- Procedure of choice is radiofrequency thermocoagulation of the trigeminal ganglion (75% effective).
- Alternatives include alcohol injection into the supraorbital/infraorbital nerves or gasserian ganglion, gamma knife radiosurgery, microvascular decompression of the trigeminal nerve, and section of the trigeminal nerve.

SYMPTOMATIC TREATMENT

- Rapid onset and short duration of cluster headaches mandate fast relief of symptoms. Oxygen and subcutaneous sumatriptan achieve this quickly and effectively.

ADJUNCTIVE TREATMENT

- Some individuals may benefit from physical therapy, massage, acupuncture, or other relaxation techniques, although none of these alternative therapies has proven efficacy.

ADMISSION/DISCHARGE CRITERIA

- Patients rarely require hospitalization unless they have suicidal ideation.

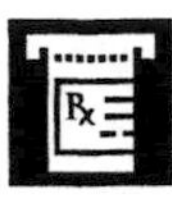

Medications

DRUG(S) OF CHOICE

Abortive Therapy

- Oxygen given as 100% O_2 through a non-rebreather face mask at 7–10 L/min for 15 minutes. Effective in 70% of patients. Portable cylinders are available for patients, although some may find this to be cumbersome. Safe in patients with cardiovascular risk factors.
- Sumatriptan is currently the most rapid and effective treatment (75%–100% of patients achieve relief). May be self-administered as 6-mg SC injection.
- Dihydroergotamine 0.5–1.0 mg IV/IM/SQ; IV is most effective.

Contraindications

- Sumatriptan is contraindicated in patients with uncontrolled hypertension, ischemic heart disease, or vascular disease. Dihydroergotamine should be avoided in patients with cardiovascular disease.

Precautions

- Patients with cardiac risk factors should have a cardiovascular evaluation before receiving sumatriptan or dihydroergotamine. Be cautious of potential drug interactions (including monoamine oxidase inhibitors).

Preventative Therapy

- Verapamil 120–480 mg/day. Agent of choice for episodic and chronic cluster.
- Valproic acid 250-001,000 mg daily.
- Lithium carbonate 300 mg bid. More effective for treatment of chronic cluster than episodic cluster.
- Methysergide is effective but may only be given for 3 months because of potential side effects.
- Prednisone provides more rapid relief than the other preventative agents, which often take 2 weeks to be effective. Therefore, a taper (60 mg/day for 10–14 days) is often started along with one of the above preventative agents.
- Ergotamine derivatives (ergotamine tartrate, DHE-45) also provide more rapid relief of symptoms; may be used for 2–3 weeks without causing rebound headaches.

Contraindications

- Verapamil should not be used in patients with bradycardia and other types of arrhythmias. Ergotamine derivatives are contraindicated in patients with cardiovascular disease and in pregnancy.

Precautions

- Patients using valproic acid should have baseline and routine CBC and LFTs checked; those on lithium must have renal and thyroid function tests monitored. Methysergide, when used for more than 3 months, may cause fibrosis of the pleural and pericardial linings and of the retroperitoneum.

ALTERNATIVE DRUGS

- Zolmitriptan 5–10 mg PO may be used for acute cluster attacks when patients prefer oral medications. Intranasal lidocaine may be useful as an adjunctive therapy in the setting of acute attacks. Other potential medications include topiramate, melatonin, capsaicin, methylphenidate, antispasticity drugs, clonidine, diltiazem, histamine, and somatostatin.

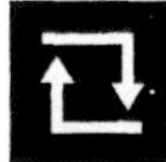

Follow-Up

PATIENT MONITORING

- Patients should be followed closely to ensure that prophylactic medications are effective, to watch for signs of recurrence, and to monitor for potential side effects of medications.
- Patients have at increased risk for suicide and should be monitored for symptoms of depression.

EXPECTED COURSE AND PROGNOSIS

- Natural history not well known
- Most often a lifetime disorder
- Estimated that 13% of episodic cluster patients progress to have chronic clusters, whereas the reverse occurs in 33% of patients
- Complete remissions occur rarely

PATIENT EDUCATION

Activities

- Practice proper sleep hygiene.
- Avoid afternoon naps.
- Avoid volatile substances (e.g., gasoline, paint).
- High altitudes (>5,000 feet) and airplane travel may precipitate attacks.
- Attacks may occur after bursts of anger, rage, anxiety, and excessive physical activity.

Diet

- Alcohol precipitates attacks during cluster periods but not during remissions.

Organizations

- American Headache Society. Website: *www.ahsnet.org*
- American Academy of Craniofacial Pain. Website: *www.aahnfp.org*
- National Headache Foundation. Website: *www.headaches.org*
- American Council for Headache Education. Phone: 800-255-ACHE

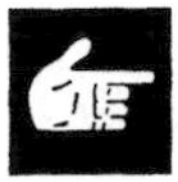

Miscellaneous

SYNONYMS

- Hemicrania angioparalytica
- Migrainous neuralgia
- Histaminic neuralgia
- Autonomic faciocephalalgia
- Suicide headache

ICD-9-CM: 784.0 Headache; 346.2 Cluster headache

SEE ALSO: HEADACHE, MIGRAINE; TRIGEMINAL NEURALGIA AND OTHER FACIAL PAIN SYNDROMES

REFERENCES

- Bahra A, May A, Goadsby PJ. Cluster headache: a prospective clinical study with diagnostic implications. Neurology 2002;58:354–361.
- Bajwa ZH, Sabahat A. Approach to the patient with headache syndromes other than migraine. 2003. Available at *wwbw.uptodate.com.*
- May A, Bahra A, Büchel C, et al. PET and MRA findings in cluster headache and MRA in experimental pain. Neurology 2000;55:1328–1335.
- Newman LC, Goadsby P, Lipton RB. Cluster and related headaches. Med Clin North Am 2001;85:997–1011.
- Silberstein SD, Lipton RB, Dalessio DJ. Wolff's headache and other head pain, 7th ed. New York: Oxford University Press, 2001.
- Silberstein SD, Stiles A, Young WB, et al. An atlas of headache. New York: Parthenon Publishing Group, 2002.

Author(s): Emily T. Klatte, MD

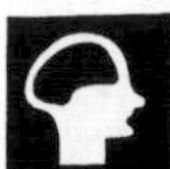

Basics

DESCRIPTION

- The term *migraine* is used to describe a paroxysmal headache with some or all of the following features: unilateral, pulsating, of moderate or severe intensity, aggravated by routine physical activity, duration of 4–72 hours, nausea and/or vomiting, and photophobia and/or phonophobia. These symptoms help to distinguish migraine from tension-type headache, which typically lacks associated features. In practice, most recurrent and disabling headaches are likely to be a form of migraine and responsive to antimigraine therapy. Attacks should be separated by pain-free intervals.
- The most important factor in migraine classification is the presence or absence of aura. The classification system published in 1988 by the International Headache Society also includes several migraine variants.
  —Migraine without aura
  —Migraine with aura
    -Migraine with typical aura
    -Migraine with prolonged aura
    -Familial hemiplegic migraine
    -Basilar migraine
    -Migraine aura without headache
    -Migraine with acute-onset aura
  —Ophthalmoplegic migraine
  —Retinal migraine
  —Childhood periodic syndromes that may be precursors of or associated with migraine
    -Benign paroxysmal vertigo of childhood
    -Alternating hemiplegia of childhood
    -Cyclic vomiting
    -Paroxysmal torticollis
    -Alice in Wonderland syndrome
  —Complications of migraine
    -Status migrainosus
    -Migrainous infarction
  —Unclassifiable migraine-like disorder

EPIDEMIOLOGY

Incidence/Prevalence

- Prevalence is about 13% and peaks in the age range 25–55. Of migraineurs, 64% have migraine without aura, 18% have migraine with aura, 13% have migraine both with and without aura, and 5% have aura without headache.

Sex

- Female-to-male ratio in postpubertal ages is 3:1.

Age

- Migraine is present but less common in pediatric populations.

ETIOLOGY

- Migraine is a form of neurovascular headache that involves dysfunction of brain stem pathways. The pathophysiology is incompletely understood; however, the predominant theory is that certain individuals have a "hyperexcitable" brain. The trigeminovascular system is activated by triggers (stress, chemicals, afferent stimulation) and/or hypothalamic input. During aura, neuroimaging studies have shown an initial period of hyperemia followed by a wave of oligemia across the cortex at a rate of 3 mm/min. This may account for the phenomenon of "spreading depression," which has been found in animals and postulated to cause the slow march of neurologic symptoms during aura. Trigeminovascular input leads to release of vasoactive peptides (including serotonin), resulting in vasodilation of meningeal blood vessels, neurogenic extravasation of plasma protein, and further activation of trigeminal afferents, producing pain. The dorsal midbrain, periaqueductal gray, dorsal raphe nucleus, pons, and locus caeruleus are important modulators of the nociceptive inputs centrally.

Genetics

- Epidemiologic studies suggest a genetic contribution to the disorder; however, specific inheritance patterns have not been elucidated for most migraine types. Familial hemiplegic migraine is associated with a calcium channel abnormality and has been mapped to chromosomes 1 and 19.

RISK FACTORS

N/A

PREGNANCY

- Approximately 70% of pregnant women experience improvement or remission of symptoms, but recurrence in the postpartum period is common. Pregnancy influences treatment options. Triptans are pregnancy category C, and ergots are contraindicated in pregnancy.

ASSOCIATED CONDITIONS

- Stroke, myocardial infarction, Raynaud's phenomenon, fatigue, depression, and anxiety have been associated with migraine.

Diagnosis

DIFFERENTIAL DIAGNOSIS

- Episodic tension-type headache
- Cluster headache
- Sinus headache
- Arteriovenous malformation
- Transient ischemic attack
- Arterial dissection
- Venous sinus thrombosis
- Vasculitis (including giant cell arteritis)
- Infection (meningitis/encephalitis)
- Tumor
- Pseudotumor cerebri
- Simple partial seizure (in the differential diagnosis of aura)

SIGNS AND SYMPTOMS

- Some patients may experience stereotyped premonitory symptoms such as change in mood, change in energy level, or excessive yawning. An aura can be any transient visual, sensory, motor, or other focal neurologic symptom. The symptoms generally develop gradually over 5–20 minutes. Some of the most common auras are scintillating scotoma, photopsia, and paresthesias.
- Headache characteristics and accompanying features:
  —Moderate or severe intensity
  —Unilateral (can be bilateral) throbbing/pulsating pain
  —Aggravated by movement/activity
  —Anorexia/nausea/vomiting
  —Photophobia/phonophobia
  —Osmophobia
  —Diarrhea
  —Blurred vision
  —Lightheadedness

LABORATORY PROCEDURES

- Laboratory tests are not routinely useful or necessary, but they may be performed to exclude secondary causes of headache (e.g., giant cell arteritis).

IMAGING STUDIES

- MRI can show cortical abnormalities during or after attack, but findings are not specific. Appropriate imaging studies are warranted in the setting of a new-onset headache, a change in headache pattern (to rule out a secondary disorder), focal neurologic symptoms/signs, or a suspected seizure.

SPECIAL TESTS

- EEG may show spikes or slowing during an attack, but it is not generally useful for diagnosis or management. Lumbar puncture is not indicated in routine cases.

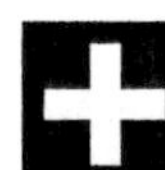

Management

GENERAL MEASURES

- Avoid identifiable triggers.
- Maintain regular sleep and meal schedules.
- Stress-management techniques.
- Avoid analgesic overuse.
- Use headache calendar to monitor disability (e.g., missed work) and effect of therapy.

SURGICAL MEASURES

N/A

SYMPTOMATIC TREATMENT

- Use of analgesic/abortive medication as soon as headache attack is recognized.
- Rest in a dark quiet room.
- Ice pack on forehead may help.
- Caffeine may be effective.
- Control nausea/vomiting with medications.
- Sleep often resolves headache.

ADJUNCTIVE TREATMENT

- Preventive therapy is recommended for patients with frequent attacks, prolonged attacks, and/or attacks that significantly interfere with their daily routine.

ADMISSION/DISCHARGE CRITERIA

- Patients may require admission for symptomatic management of nausea/ vomiting or for treatment of status migrainosus. Admission may be necessary for evaluation of focal neurologic deficits, impaired consciousness, or suspected secondary disorder.

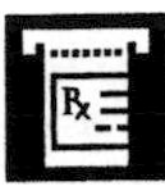

Medications

DRUG(S) OF CHOICE

Acute Therapy

- Many migraines will respond to nonspecific medications. The triptans and DHE are considered "migraine-specific therapies" and have well-established efficacy. Triptans act predominantly as 5-$HT_{1B/D}$ receptor agonists, causing cranial vasoconstriction and decreasing the release of neuropeptides. Ergots act at the same receptor but are not as selective in their binding and, therefore, have more side effects than the triptans.
- Aspirin
- Nonsteroidal antiinflammatory drugs (NSAIDs)
- Combination analgesics
  - —Aspirin and caffeine with or without acetaminophen
  - —APAP/dichloralphenazone/isometheptene (Midrin)
- Triptans
  - —Almotriptan, naratriptan, frovatriptan, sumatriptan, rizatriptan, zolmitriptan
  - —Available in multiple routes of administration (oral, nasal spray, rectal suppository, subcutaneous injection)
- Ergot derivatives
  - —Ergotamine/caffeine (Cafergot)
  - —DHE
- Antiemetics
  - —Prochlorperazine
  - —Metoclopramide
  - —Chlorpromazine

Preventive Therapy

- β-Blockers
  - —Propranolol
  - —Timolol
- Tricyclic antidepressants
  - —Amitriptyline, Nortriptyline
- Calcium channel blockers
  - —Verapamil
- Anticonvulsants
  - —Divalproex sodium; only FDA approved anticonvulsant for migraine prophylaxis
  - —Gabapentin
  - —Topiramate
- Selective serotonin reuptake inhibitors; widely used but poor evidence of efficacy
- Serotonin antagonists: methysergide
- NSAIDs; most useful for menstrual migraine prophylaxis

Contraindications

- *Ergots* are contraindicated in peripheral or coronary artery disease, uncontrolled hypertension, pregnancy, or breast-feeding.
- *Triptans* are contraindicated in coronary artery disease, Prinzmetal angina, uncontrolled hypertension, recent monoamine oxidase inhibitor use, severe liver disease, or presence of severe/prolonged neurologic deficits accompanying headache.
- *β-Blockers* are contraindicated in severe asthma.

Precautions

- *β-Blockers* may cause aggravation of asthma, bradycardia, hypotension, depression, or masking of hypoglycemia symptoms.
- *Tricyclic antidepressants* may cause cardiac arrhythmias, sedation, or aggravation of angle-closure glaucoma.
- *Divalproex sodium* may cause weight gain, hair loss, tremor, liver dysfunction, or neural tube defects in developing embryos. Women of childbearing age should take supplemental folic acid.
- *NSAIDs* can cause renal dysfunction and should be used with extreme caution in patients with a history of GI bleeding.
- *Methysergide* can cause weight gain, vasoconstriction, or fibrosis (pulmonary, cardiac, retroperitoneal).

ALTERNATIVE DRUGS

- *Butalbital-containing products or opioids* have potential for habituation and are generally not recommended.
- *Intranasal lidocaine* is safe but efficacy has been underwhelming
- *Toradol* may be used in acute attacks.
- Recommended treatment of status migrainosus is repeated doses of DHE 0.5–1 mg parenterally every 8 hours, in combination with an antiemetic. Corticosteroids may also be used for refractory attacks.

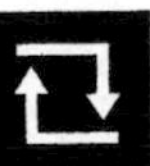

Follow-Up

PATIENT MONITORING

- Patients should keep a headache calendar to document frequency of attacks.

EXPECTED COURSE AND PROGNOSIS

- The goal of therapy is to reduce headache frequency and minimize missed work or activities.

PATIENT EDUCATION

- American Council for Headache Education, 19 Mantua Road, Mount Royal, NJ 08061. Phone: 800-225-ACHE, website: *www.achenet.org*
- World Headache Alliance. Website: *www.w-h-a.org*

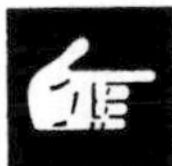

Miscellaneous

SYNONYMS

N/A

ICD-9-CM: 346.0 Classic migraine; 346.1 Common migraine; 346.2 Variant of migraine (includes cluster, basilar, retinal); 346.8 Other forms of migraine (hemiplegic, ophthalmoplegic); 346.9 Migraine, unspecified; Fifth digit subclassification: 0 = without mention of intractable migraine, 1 = with intractable migraine

SEE ALSO: N/A

REFERENCES

- Cady R, Dodick DW. Diagnosis and treatment of migraine. Mayo Clin Proc 2002;77:255–261.
- Goadsby PJ, Lipton RB, Ferrari MD. Migraine: current understanding and treatment. N Engl J Med 2002;346: 257–270.
- Headache Classification Committee of the International Headache Society. Classification and diagnostic criteria for headache disorders, cranial neuralgias, and facial pain. Cephalgia 1988;8[Suppl 7]: 1–96.
- Lipton RB, Stewart WF, Diamond S, et al. Prevalence and burden of migraine in the United States: data from the American Migraine Study II. Headache 2001;41: 646–657.
- Silberstein SD, Lipton RB, Goadsby PJ. Headache in clinical practice, 2nd ed. London: Martin Dunitz; 2002.

Author(s): Roxanne M. Valentino, MD

Headache, Post Lumbar Puncture

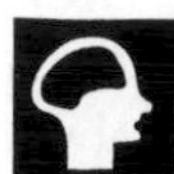

Basics

DESCRIPTION

- Positional, often disabling, headache is a common complication of diagnostic lumbar puncture (LP). The International Headache Society has defined post lumbar puncture headache (PLPHA) by the following essential characteristics. (a) The headache is bilateral and develops in <7 days after LP procedure. (b) The headache occurs or worsens <15 minutes after assumption of the upright position and disappears or improves <30 minutes after resumption of the recumbent position. (c) The headache generally disappears within 14 days of the LP procedure. The pathophysiology of PLPHA is still uncertain. The prevailing theory postulates that leakage of CSF through the LP needle site leads to intracranial CSF hypotension and hypovolemia. This in turn is compensated by dilation of intracranial veins and traction on pain-sensitive meningeal structures with erect posture that can be relieved with recumbency.

EPIDEMIOLOGY

- Most contemporary series studying the incidence of PLPHA consistently found that it occurred in 20%–30% of cases. No specific clinical characteristics reliably predict whether PLPHA will occur.

RISK FACTORS

- Risk factors include young age, female gender, lower body mass index, needle size, and history of headache disorder. Diagnostic LP had a higher but variable risk for the disorder than does spinal anesthesia. Recently the Technology and Therapeutics Subcommittee of the American Academy of Neurology produced a consensus statement on this issue. They noted that factors that did *not* seem to affect the occurrence of PLPHA in review of the current literature included amount of CSF removed, duration of recumbency, sitting or lying position during the procedure, or experience of the procedurist. They also noted that needle size and design (cutting vs. nontraumatic), failure to replace stylet prior to removal from the subarachnoid space, and inattention to maintaining the cutting edge parallel to the dural fibers may be crucial in the evolution of the disorder.

PREGNANCY

- Not a specific risk factor

ASSOCIATED CONDITIONS

N/A

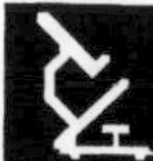

Diagnosis

DIFFERENTIAL DIAGNOSIS

- The diagnosis usually is evident from the clinical circumstances. Consider post-LP meningitis if the patient develops progressively increasing recumbent headache, nausea, vomiting, fever, or severe neck stiffness. The diagnosis of PLPHA is made clinically when a patient within 1 week of LP complains of positional headache that resolves with recumbency. Most commonly the LP is a diagnostic tap, but the syndrome is also seen post LP for radiologic myelographic procedures and occasionally after spinal anesthesia. The differential can become more complex in patients with already previously established headache disorders, such as migraine, pseudotumor cerebri, meningitis, and toxic metabolic states where vascular headache may worsen after LP. In these cases, recumbency may ameliorate the headache, but not completely.

SIGNS AND SYMPTOMS

- The most characteristic symptom of PLPHA is a headache that occurs after LP and worsens with upright posture. Patients who develop this syndrome may have done well for a few days after the LP and may slowly and progressively worsen over ensuing days. Others will develop the symptoms immediately after the tap and complain of positional headache from the moment they leave the procedure room. PLPHA may be severe and associated with nausea, vomiting, vertigo, dizziness, tinnitus, photophobia, teichopsia, diplopia, or neck or scapular pain, and require that patients remain in bed all day. Most often the headache resembles migraine in its disabling severity and throbbing character and associated autonomic symptoms of nausea, vomiting, visual disturbances, and light and sound sensitivity. The presence of positional diplopia or tinnitus is unique for this disorder. Unlike migraine, however, PLPHA is rarely unilateral in location and often is completely, or nearly completely, ameliorated with taking the recumbent position. When the syndrome is prolonged and does not respond to conservative measures, diplopia due to cranial nerve VI palsy may develop and not fully resolve with taking the recumbent position. The headache itself may become ameliorated with recumbency, but in refractory cases may persist to a considerable degree even while in the recumbent position.

LABORATORY PROCEDURES

- No laboratory tests are required to make the diagnosis of post-LP headache. When the diagnosis is in doubt, especially when meningitis or a spontaneous dural CSF leak is suspected, an LP can be performed to assess CSF pressure and cell count. This is to be avoided whenever the diagnosis is clinically certain because it may worsen the syndrome and symptoms.

IMAGING STUDIES

- No diagnostic testing is needed to make a diagnosis of PLPHA. In severe or prolonged cases that fail to resolve with the usual measures in 14 days, a gadolinium-enhanced MRI may be helpful. The typical finding is meningeal enhancement in a diffuse pattern over the convexity. A less common observation is "sagging" of the brain toward the skull base.

SPECIAL TESTS

- When the diagnosis is in doubt, patients should be brought to the outpatient office for physical examination. Funduscopic and neurologic examination findings are normal. The patient is examined in both recumbent and sitting positions, and the time and pattern of headache onset and resolution are noted. Abdominal hand pressure applied at the onset of positional headache in the sitting position nearly always ameliorates or resolves the headache pain. A pragmatic trial of oral or IV triptans may alleviate some of the post-LP vascular headache and should not be used to substantiate a suspected diagnosis of migraine.

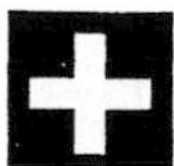

Management

GENERAL MEASURES

- Needle design appears to be a provocative culprit in the occurrence of the disorder. The "pencil point" noncutting, atraumatic needles, such as Whitacre or Sprotte, have a duller tip and an oval opening just proximal to the tip, in contrast to the Quincke needle with sharp edges and an opening at the tip. There is convincing class I evidence in the anesthesiology literature for less PLPHA with noncutting needles compared to cutting needles with bevels parallel to dural fibers. Recently a large randomized trial of Sprotte versus Quincke 20-gauge needle for neurologic diagnostic taps showed considerably less headache in the patients assigned to receive the nontraumatic Sprotte needle for the procedure. Although anesthesiologists use smaller LP needles (usually 22–25 gauge), this size is inappropriate for neurologists who need to collect CSF for diagnostic purposes using larger-bore needle types, usually 20–21 gauge. Many neurologists believe that removing the needle from the CSF space while rolling the patient to the prone position, fluid replenishment, and caffeine use are important to prevent the syndrome, no matter which needle is selected.

SURGICAL MEASURES

- Not usually applicable. Rare case reports of PLPHA refractory to epidural blood patch have required open surgical closure.

SYMPTOMATIC TREATMENT

- The treatment of PLPHA is bed rest, caffeinated fluid and salt replacement, and time. Most often the syndrome resolves in 24–48 hours of bed rest, with bathroom privileges only.

ADJUNCTIVE TREATMENT

- When the problem becomes more prolonged and does not appear to be lessening in response to conservative methods, an epidural blood patch sometimes is warranted. This is performed by anesthesiologists/pain management physicians who take a small amount of blood from the patient's antecubital vein and infuse it in the lumbar epidural space in the region of the tap. Theoretically this provides a "blood patch" to the rent in the dural sac, allowing time for it to seal off, scar, and heal. Oddly, however, this technique of epidural blood patch also has been shown to be effective in spontaneous cervical dural tears, even when the blood is infused into the lumbar region. This raises the question of the true pathophysiology of the PLPHA syndrome and whether elasticity of the dura may be more the problem than strict CSF hypovolemia, as some have suggested. The technique of epidural blood patch is safe and generally painless, and produces rapid "on the table" response in most patients.

ADMISSION/DISCHARGE CRITERIA

- Most patients with PLPHA do not require admission. Patients with refractory headache not responding to outpatient blood patch, with uncontrolled vomiting, or patients who are suspected of having meningitis or other illness should be considered for admission.

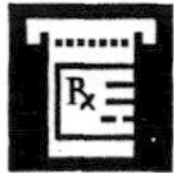

Medications

DRUG(S) OF CHOICE

- There is no specific drug therapy for PLPHA. Caffeinated beverages may be helpful in prevention. Either nonspecific pain medications (acetaminophen, aspirin, ibuprofen) or migraine medications (caffeinated medications, triptans) may be tried.

ALTERNATIVE DRUGS

N/A

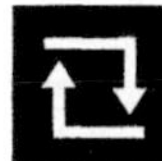

Follow-Up

PATIENT MONITORING

- Patients should be monitored for resolution of headache.

EXPECTED COURSE AND PROGNOSIS

- Most patients can expect a full recovery in 1–2 weeks.

PATIENT EDUCATION

- Patients should be informed of the cause of the PLPHA. They should be educated about consumption of additional fluids, use of the recumbent position, and need to call the office for symptoms of progressive headache, fever, or chills.

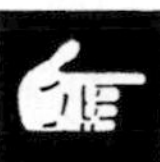

Miscellaneous

SYNONYMS

N/A

ICD-9-CM: 349.0 Post lumbar puncture headache

SEE ALSO: N/A

REFERENCES

- Braune HJ, Huffman GA. A prospective double-blind clinical trial, comparing the sharp Quincke needle (22G) with an "atraumatic" needle (22G) in the induction of post-lumbar puncture headache. Acta Neurol Scand 1992;86:50–54.
- Evans RW. Complications of lumbar puncture. Neurol Clin 1998;16:83–105.
- Evans RW, Armon C, Frohman EM, et al. Assessment: prevention of post-lumbar puncture headaches: report of the Therapeutics and Technology Assessment Subcommittee of the American Academy of Neurology. Neurology 2000;55:909–914.
- Halpern S, Preston R. Postdural puncture headache and spinal needle design. Meta-analyses. Anesthesiology 1994;81:1376–1383.
- Lybecker H, Moller JT, May O, et al. Incidence and prediction of postdural puncture headache. A prospective study of 1021 spinal anesthesias. Anesth Analg 1990;70:389–394.
- Strupp M, Brandt T, Muller A. Incidence of post-lumbar puncture syndrome reduced by reinserting the stylet: a randomized prospective study of 600 patients. J Neurol 1998;245:589–592.
- Tarkkila PJ, Miralles JA, Palomski EA. The subjective complications and efficiency of the epidural blood patch in the treatment of postdural puncture headache. Reg Anesth 1989;14:247–250.

Author(s): John Castaldo, MD

Heavy Metal Poisoning, Neurologic Complications

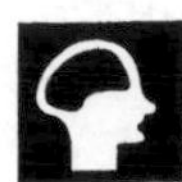

Basics

DESCRIPTION

- Heavy metals associated with adverse neurologic effects include lead, mercury, manganese, arsenic, thallium, organotins (trimethyltin and triethyltin), and aluminum. Although iron and manganese are essential for the activity of certain enzymes, excessive levels can cause disruption of normal neuronal functioning. The toxic effects of heavy metal poisoning can present insidiously or abruptly, depending on the particular metal and the nature of exposure (i.e., acute or chronic; high or low level). Neurotoxicity of metals involves various mechanisms, including generation of free radicals that initiate lipid peroxidation and alter neuronal cell membranes and disruption of cellular respiration, oxidative phosphorylation, and ATP-dependent processes. Recognition of the signs and symptoms of metal poisoning is essential to minimize neuronal damage, remove at-risk persons from further exposure, and reduce accumulated levels of metal in tissue by therapeutic chelation.

EPIDEMIOLOGY

Incidence/Prevalence

N/A

Race

- All races and ethnic groups can be affected.

Age

- Two peaks are present, one in pediatric patients and the other in adults exposed to occupational hazards.

Sex

- Both sexes can be affected; most often diagnosed in males.

ETIOLOGY

- Neurologic dysfunction of the central and/or peripheral nervous system (CNS, PNS) caused by excessive occupational or environmental exposure to one or more heavy metals.

Genetics

N/A

RISK FACTORS

- Include occupation (e.g., welder, iron worker), hobbies (e.g., lead stained glass crafting), water supply (e.g., lead pipes), fish and seafood consumption, age (children at greater risk for lead and mercury encephalopathy), psychosocial factors (e.g., history of pica and object mouthing), nutrition (e.g., iron deficiency anemia susceptibility to lead poisoning), and concurrent medical problems (e.g., diabetes)

PREGNANCY

- Pregnancy has not been shown to affect the course of neurologic complications of heavy metal intoxication. Heavy metal intoxication during pregnancy may adversely affect the fetus.

ASSOCIATED CONDITIONS

N/A

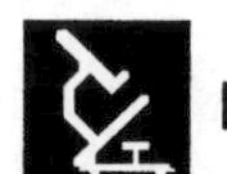

Diagnosis

DIFFERENTIAL DIAGNOSIS

- The differential diagnosis is very extensive because heavy metal poisoning is often clinically nonspecific. Other common non-neurotoxic causes of the presenting symptoms should be evaluated (e.g., metabolic encephalopathy, tumor, stroke, diabetes mellitus, Parkinson's disease, and other idiopathic neurodegenerative disorders).

SIGNS AND SYMPTOMS

- Signs and symptoms are diffuse and nonspecific and may involve the CNS and/or PNS. All of the heavy metals can induce an encephalopathy syndrome; peripheral neuropathy can be noted in poisoning from aluminum, arsenic, lead, mercury, organotins, and thallium. Tremors and movement disorders can occur with poisoning from aluminum, lead, manganese, mercury, and thallium. Other significant symptoms include headache and cerebral edema (lead, organotins), nausea and emesis (thallium, arsenic, organotins), cranial neuropathy (thallium), psychosis (manganese, mercury, thallium, arsenic), loss of memory (lead, aluminum, thallium, arsenic), and seizures (lead, organotins, thallium, arsenic, aluminum).

LABORATORY PROCEDURES

- Screening for recent heavy metal exposure should be performed on blood and urine specimens. Hair or nail samples can be used to determine more remote exposures and may reveal abnormally elevated levels even if blood and urine are normal. Sural nerve biopsies may demonstrate wallerian-type dying back axonal degeneration with secondary demyelination (arsenic, thallium) or segmental demyelination (lead). δ-Aminolevulinic acid (ALA) levels are elevated in blood and urine samples in lead poisoning cases.

IMAGING STUDIES

- MRI or CT, with and without contrast, is appropriate in patients with mental status changes, atypical seizures, or focal neurologic findings to rule out non-neurotoxic intracranial processes (e.g., subdural hematoma, abscess, tumor, stroke). Imaging may reveal atrophy of the cerebellum (mercury), hippocampus (organotin), or cerebral cortex (lead). Edema can be noted in lead poisoning. High-signal lesions in the globus pallidus may occur with manganese poisoning.
- In children, radiographs of long bones may reveal epiphysial bands of increased density (i.e., lead lines) that can document remote exposures to lead.

SPECIAL TESTS

- EMG/nerve conduction testing and EEG can be of benefit to document the presence and pattern of peripheral neuropathy and seizure activity, respectively. Neuropsychological assessment can be helpful to document the extent and pattern of cognitive deficits. Serial neuropsychological testing can follow improvements in performance after cessation of exposure and can assist in determining prognosis.

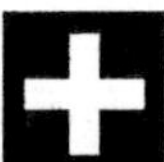

Management

GENERAL MEASURES

- A comprehensive personal, occupational, and medical history is required to document potential past or current chemical exposures. All chemicals that the patient may have come in contact with must be determined. The home water supply and regional environment should be investigated. All further exposures to heavy metals must be avoided. All symptomatic patients should be considered for chelation therapy to reduce the body burden of accumulated metals.

SURGICAL MEASURES

N/A

SYMPTOMATIC TREATMENT

- *Lead poisoning:* Mannitol should be administered to control cerebral edema associated with lead encephalopathy. Immediate chelation therapy is required for encephalopathic patients with serum levels >70 μg/100 mL; IV diazepam can be administered to control seizure activity associated with encephalopathy. Hemodialysis may be necessary in patients with renal failure. Chelation therapy may be helpful for patients with peripheral neuropathy due to chronic lead exposure. Chelation therapy is with BAL (British anti-Lewisite) or $CaNa_2EDTA$ (calcium disodium ethylenediamine tetra-acetic acid).
- *Thallium poisoning:* Gastric lavage and whole bowel irrigation should be used to remove thallium from the GI tract following acute ingestion. Patients with acute poisoning should be monitored in the ICU. Traditional chelating agents are not effective in thallium poisoning. Prussian blue or activated charcoal should be administered instead to enhance fecal elimination. Diuretics can be used to enhance urinary excretion. Hemodialysis may be necessary in patients with thallium-induced acute renal failure.
- *Arsenic poisoning:* Gastric lavage and whole bowel irrigation should be used to remove arsenic from the GI tract following acute ingestion. Chelation therapy should be started immediately after acute ingestion with either BAL, DMSA (2,3-dimercaptosuccinic acid), or penicillamine. The patient should be monitored during initial treatment in the ICU. Activated charcoal can be administered to reduce further GI absorption. Hemodialysis may be necessary in patients with arsenic-induced acute renal failure.
- *Manganese poisoning:* Chelation is helpful to improve clinical symptoms and reduce the body burden in patients with encephalopathy; $CaNa_2EDTA$ is the chelating agent of choice. Chelation therapy may reduce the high signal abnormality in the putamen-globus pallidus but may not improve parkinsonian symptoms. Levo-dopa and dopamine agonists have not been very effective in controlling manganese-induced tremor but are not contraindicated.
- *Mercury poisoning:* Symptomatic patients with serum mercury levels of >15 μg/L should undergo chelation therapy with either BAL, DMSA, or penicillamine. Gastric lavage should be performed on patients who have ingested elemental or inorganic mercury. Hemodialysis with L-cysteine or DMSA infused into the dialyzer may be necessary to reduce body burden in patients with mercury-induced renal dysfunction.

ADJUNCTIVE TREATMENT

- Physical therapy and leg braces should be considered for patients with severe peripheral neuropathy. Nutritional supplements (including B vitamins) may hasten recovery from peripheral neuropathy. Cognitive and vocational retraining may be necessary for patients with permanent cognitive deficits.

ADMISSION/DISCHARGE CRITERIA

- Admission will generally be required for patients with acute neurologic events such as seizure activity, encephalopathy, severe weakness, persistent headache, and psychosis. Heavy metal tissue levels and history of exposure should be determined. Discharge is appropriate once the metal exposure has been determined and the patient has been stabilized with appropriate chelation and supportive therapy.

Medications

DRUG(S) OF CHOICE

- Chelation therapy with agents as listed for lead, thallium, arsenic, manganese, and mercury poisoning. Aluminum poisoning can be chelated with $CaNa_2EDTA$. Organotins can be chelated with BAL, DMSA, or penicillamine.

Contraindications

- None

Precautions

- BAL can frequently cause an elevation in SBP and DBP, accompanied by tachycardia. Penicillamine can induce renal dysfunction and should be used with caution in patients with impaired renal function.

ALTERNATIVE DRUGS

N/A

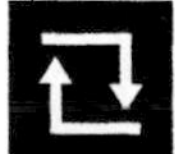

Follow-Up

PATIENT MONITORING

- Neurologic recovery from heavy metal intoxication and serum and/or tissue metal levels should be monitored. Serial testing with neuropsychological and neurophysiologic testing may be of benefit to follow recovery and determine prognosis.

EXPECTED COURSE AND PROGNOSIS

- Most patients improve with chelation therapy and supportive care. Prognosis and potential for permanent neurologic sequelae are variable and depend on the chronicity and severity of exposure. The most common residual deficits are memory loss and impaired cognition following encephalopathy, and persistent motor dysfunction in patients with severe peripheral neuropathy.

PATIENT EDUCATION

- Patients must be educated on strategies to avoid future exposures to heavy metals: protective clothing and masks/respirators, proper ventilation of the workplace, workplace monitoring of air levels of heavy metals, and individual body burdens. Materials Safety Data Sheets (MSDS) for materials used in the workplace should be reviewed. Advise patients on nonoccupational sources of exposure to heavy metals.
- Heavy metal poisoning support groups and resources. Website: *www.medhelp.org/healthtopics/Heavy_Metal_Poisoning.html*
- Heavy metal poisoning information. Website: *www.rxaddict.com/g/conditionpage/Poisoning_Heavy_Metals*

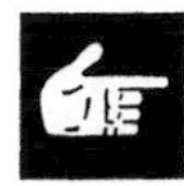

Miscellaneous

SYNONYMS

N/A

ICD-9-CM: 984.9 Unspecified toxic effects of lead; 985.9 Unspecified toxic effects of other heavy metals

SEE ALSO: ENCEPHALOPATHY; NEUROPATHY; PARKINSON'S DISEASE

REFERENCES

- Discalzi G, Pira E, Herrero-Hernandez E, et al. Occupational Mn parkinsonism: magnetic resonance imaging and clinical patterns following $CaNa_2$-EDTA chelation. Neurotoxicology 2000;21:863–866.
- Feldman RG, ed. Occupational and environmental neurotoxicology. Philadelphia: Lippincott-Raven Publishers, 1999.
- Henritig FM. Lead. In: Goldfrank LR, Flomenbaum NE, Lewin NA, et al., eds. Goldfrank's toxicologic emergencies, 6th ed. Stamford, CT: Appleton & Lange, 1998;79:1277–1317.
- Mercurio M, Hoffman RS. Thallium. In: Goldfrank LR, Flomenbaum NE, Lewin NA, et al., eds. Goldfrank's toxicologic emergencies, 6th ed. Stamford, CT: Appleton & Lange, 1998;82:1350–1357.
- Sue YJ. Mercury. In: Goldfrank LR, Flomenbaum NE, Lewin NA, et al., eds. Goldfrank's toxicologic emergencies, 6th ed. Stamford, CT: Appleton & Lange, 1998;80:1319–1331.

Author(s): Robert G. Feldman, MD; Marcia H. Ratner, PhD

Herpes Zoster

Basics

DESCRIPTION

- Herpes zoster (shingles) is a painful vesicular rash that usually occurs in a dermatomal distribution. The infection occurs in individuals who have had chicken pox. The causative agent, varicella-zoster virus, lies dormant in the dorsal root ganglia following chicken pox. If reactivation of the virus occurs, herpes zoster will manifest along the involved ganglion's distribution.

EPIDEMIOLOGY

Incidence/Prevalence

- Occurs in 600,000–1,000,000 persons annually in the United States. Incidence increases with increasing age.

Race

- More common in whites than blacks, with blacks 25% less likely than whites to develop zoster among those exposed to chicken pox.

Sex

- Affects both sexes with equal frequency.

ETIOLOGY

- Herpes zoster is caused by reactivation of the varicella-zoster virus, which lies dormant in the dorsal root ganglia following infection with chicken pox. The reactivation is believed to be in part secondary to an alteration in the patient's immune system; however, the exact etiology of varicella-zoster reactivation is unclear.

RISK FACTORS

- The primary risk factor for herpes zoster is previous chicken pox infection. Other factors that may increase the risk of developing herpes zoster are those involving a depression of the patient's immune system, including advancing age, AIDS, lymphomas, and chemotherapy.

PREGNANCY

- Herpes zoster is rare in pregnancy.

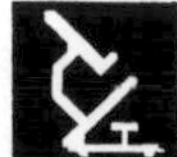

Diagnosis

DIFFERENTIAL DIAGNOSIS

- Appendicitis
- Bell's palsy
- Cholecystitis and biliary colic
- Corneal ulceration
- Ulcerative keratitis
- Conjunctivitis
- Herpes simplex
- Renal calculi
- Trigeminal neuralgia

SIGNS AND SYMPTOMS

- Herpes zoster is preceded by approximately 2 days of pain, tingling, or burning in a dermatomal distribution. This prodromal phase results in a high incidence of misdiagnosis and is the reason herpes zoster is included in the differential diagnosis of many conditions whose symptoms may involve pain or sensory disturbances.
- The prodrome may be followed by symptoms including fatigue, malaise, low-grade fever, and headache. The most characteristic finding is that of a vesicular rash in a unilateral dermatomal pattern. The rash is rarely bilateral. The lesions progress from vesicles to pustules to crusting lesions until the rash resolves. The dermatomes of the thorax are the most commonly involved. The pain may or may not resolve with resolution of the rash. Zoster sine herpete is a form of zoster in which there is no rash, but there are pain and paresthesias in a dermatomal pattern.
- Pain lasting >1 month is described as postherpetic neuralgia.
- Herpes zoster ophthalmicus is defined as zoster involving the distribution of the ophthalmic division of the fifth cranial nerve and may involve the cornea. Herpes zoster oticus or Ramsey-Hunt syndrome is defined as zoster involving the distribution of the facial nerve and can cause severe ear pain as well as paralysis of the facial muscles.

LABORATORY PROCEDURES

- Monoclonal antibody tests
- A Tzanck smear of vesicular lesions can be done but will not distinguish between herpes simplex and varicella-zoster infections.
- Biopsy may be obtained and sent for direct immunofluorescence testing.
- Although laboratory testing may be performed, the diagnosis is most commonly clinical.

IMAGING STUDIES

N/A

SPECIAL TESTS

N/A

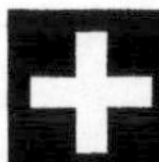

Management

GENERAL MEASURES

- Therapy should be aimed at decreasing pain, shortening the duration of the disease, preventing complications, and minimizing the risk of postherpetic neuralgia. Although analgesics are indicated to treat the pain, antiviral agents also may be used and are most effective if given within the first 72 hours of onset of the patient's symptoms. Studies involving antiviral agents suggest their primary benefit may be reducing the incidence and duration of postherpetic neuralgia. Oral steroids have been used to treat herpes zoster; however, there is conflicting evidence as to their efficacy.

SURGICAL MEASURES

N/A

SYMPTOMATIC TREATMENT

- Herpes zoster usually causes severe pain. Analgesia should include nonsteroidal antiinflammatory drugs and/or narcotics. Dressings may be applied to the rash, including wet dressings with tap water or Burow solution (5% aluminum acetate). Discomfort also may be relieved by using certain lotions, including calamine lotion.

ADJUNCTIVE TREATMENT

N/A

ADMISSION/DISCHARGE CRITERIA

- Herpes zoster is an outpatient disease in most cases; however, admission may be required in some instances, including some cases of herpes zoster ophthalmicus. Ophthalmologic consultation should be obtained in all cases of herpes zoster ophthalmicus. Another indication for admission is in the immunocompromised patient when evidence of dissemination exists. Dissemination should be suspected in the ill-appearing or toxic patient and in patients who have involvement of more than one dermatome.

Medications

DRUG(S) OF CHOICE

- Antiviral agents given within the first 72 hours may reduce the duration and severity of postherpetic neuralgia. Although the most widely studied drug is acyclovir, famciclovir and valacyclovir share similar pharmacotherapeutic properties with acyclovir. Famciclovir and valacyclovir offer dosing regimens that are more convenient and easier to comply with. Whether or not the patient is treated with antiviral agents, a strong analgesic should also be prescribed

Contraindications

- Caution should be used in administering antiviral agents in patients who have renal failure or who are taking nephrotoxic drugs because of the risk of inducing hemolytic uremic syndrome, which has been documented in patients receiving valacyclovir.

Precautions

- As above

Dosages

- Acyclovir 800 mg PO five times per day for 7 days
- Famciclovir 500 mg PO every 12 hours for 7 days
- Valacyclovir 1,000 mg PO every 8 hours for 7 days

ALTERNATIVE DRUGS

- Amitriptyline 25 mg PO qhs has been used for management of postherpetic neuralgia with some success.
- Narcotic analgesics
- Corticosteroids have been proposed by some authors to reduce acute pain, as well as the severity of postherpetic neuralgia. Although the literature suggests that corticosteroids have no effect on postherpetic neuralgia, there is some evidence supporting their use to reduce the acute pain of herpes zoster. There have been no studies examining the theoretical risk of corticosteroid-induced dissemination of localized zoster.

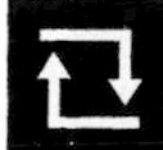

Follow-Up

PATIENT MONITORING

- Patients should be monitored for resolution of rash and cessation of pain. Patients with herpes zoster ophthalmicus should be monitored by ophthalmology for secondary ocular complications (corneal scarring, impaired vision).

EXPECTED COURSE AND PROGNOSIS

- Following the 1- to 3-day prodrome, acute herpes zoster typically resolves after 2 weeks.
- Postherpetic neuralgia presents in about 15% of patients following herpes zoster and is defined as pain that persists for >1 month following resolution of the rash. The incidence of postherpetic neuralgia increases significantly with age, approaching 70% in patients who develop herpes zoster after age 70 years.

PATIENT EDUCATION

- The vesicular lesions of herpes zoster contain the varicella virus; therefore, patients should be advised of that fact and avoid close contact with immunocompromised patients and patients who have not had chicken pox or the varicella vaccine.

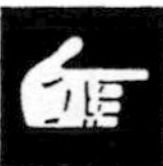

Miscellaneous

SYNONYMS

- Shingles

ICD-9-CM: 053.9 Herpes zoster; 053.2 Herpes zoster with ophthalmic complications; 053.71 Herpes zoster oticus; 053.19 Postherpetic neuralgia

SEE ALSO: N/A

REFERENCES

- Alper BS, Lewis PR. Does treatment of acute herpes zoster prevent or shorten postherpetic neuralgia? A systemic review of the literature. J Fam Pract 2000;49: 255–264.
- Brody MB, Moyer D. Varicella-zoster virus infection. The complex prevention-treatment picture. Postgrad Med 1997;102: 187–190, 192–194.
- Kost RG, Straus SE. Post-herpetic neuralgia–pathogenesis, treatment, and prevention. N Engl J Med 1996;335:32–42.
- Lancaster T, Silagy C, Gray S. Primary care management of acute herpes zoster: systematic review of evidence from randomized controlled trials. Br J Gen Pract 1995;45:39–45.
- Nikkels AF, Pierard GE. Recognition and treatment of shingles. Drugs 1994;48: 528–548.
- Wood MJ. Current experience with antiviral therapy for acute herpes zoster. Ann Neurol 1994;35[Suppl]:S65–S68.

Author(s): Chris Melton, MD

Hemiballismus

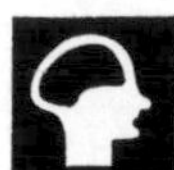

Basics

DESCRIPTION

- Hemiballismus is a hyperkinetic movement disorder characterized by violent flailing movements involving mainly proximal limbs on the same side of the body. Hemiballismus is considered an extreme form of chorea because as ballistic movements subside with time, they have the appearance of classic chorea.

EPIDEMIOLOGY

Incidence

- Uncommon, with an annual incidence of around 1 per 500,000 in the general population. Of 3,084 patients seen at a tertiary care movement disorders clinic, only 21 had hemiballismus.

Age

- Mean age at presentation >60 years of age. It is rare in children; however, Sydenham's chorea can be unilateral and of such large amplitude to resemble hemiballismus.

Sex

- Hemiballismus occurs equally in males and females.

Race

- There is no racial predisposition.

ETIOLOGY

- Hemiballismus typically is caused by a lesion involving the contralateral subthalamic nucleus or its connections with the substantia nigra, putamen, caudate nucleus, globus pallidus or thalamus. The onset usually is acute, over minutes or hours, although evolution over weeks to months has been described depending on the mechanism of injury. Hemorrhagic and ischemic strokes account for about two thirds of all cases of ballismus. Other potential etiologies include head trauma, space-occupying lesions, CNS infections, demyelinating disease, autoimmune diseases (especially systemic lupus erythematosus), hyperglycemia or hypoglycemia, medications (levodopa, oral contraceptives, phenytoin, tardive syndromes of dopamine-blocking agents), complications of surgical procedures for treatment of Parkinson's disease, and calcification of the basal ganglia.

RISK FACTORS

- The list of potential risk factors is extensive. However, vascular risk factors, especially hypertension, are most important because stroke is the main cause of hemiballismus.

PREGNANCY

- There is no specific relationship to pregnancy except that chorea gravidarum occasionally can be severe and unilateral enough to resemble hemiballismus.

ASSOCIATED CONDITIONS

- *Cerebrovascular disease:* ischemic and hemorrhagic stroke, vascular malformations
- *Autoimmune disorders:* systemic lupus erythematosus, scleroderma, antiphospholipid antibody syndrome, Sydenham's chorea
- *Metabolic disorders:* hypoglycemia, hyperglycemia
- *Infectious diseases:* syphilis, tuberculosis, toxoplasmosis, meningoencephalitis, cryptococcosis, AIDS
- *Tumors:* primary CNS malignancies, metastatic tumors, cystic lesions, abscesses
- *Drugs:* levodopa, dopamine agonists, anticonvulsants (e.g., phenytoin), oral contraceptives (hormonal changes, e.g., pregnancy)
- *Surgical procedures:* subthalamic deep brain stimulation, thalamotomy
- *Head trauma*

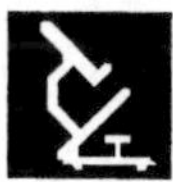

Diagnosis

DIFFERENTIAL DIAGNOSIS

- Ballistic movements are unlikely to be confused with any other hyperkinetic movement disorders or focal seizures.

SIGNS AND SYMPTOMS

- Ballistic movements are large, proximal usually rotatory throwing or kicking movements that often are violent and relentless. The movements may be volitionally suppressed for brief periods of time. They interfere with motor activity and stress makes them worse. In half of patients, the leg and arm of the same side are equally affected. In about two thirds the face also is involved. For reasons that are unclear, the left side is more commonly affected. Other neurologic signs, such as cognitive or affective changes, hemiparesis, sensory impairment, and changes in tone and muscle stretch reflexes, suggest involvement of adjacent motor and sensory pathways.

LABORATORY PROCEDURES

- Laboratory procedures are directed at diagnosing the underlying cause. CBC, routine blood biochemistry, fasting and postprandial blood glucose, sedimentation rate, VDRL, ANA, PT, aPTT, pregnancy test, and urine analysis are first steps in the evaluation. In selected patients, the following tests may be obtained: HIV tests, anticonvulsant blood levels, throat culture, and antistreptolysin antibody titers.

IMAGING STUDIES

- Brain MRI or CT should be performed to search for the cause of hemiballismus. MRI is more sensitive, allows for anatomic localization of the causative brain lesion, and may show changes in the basal ganglia in patients with ballistic movements due to metabolic derangements.

SPECIAL TESTS

N/A

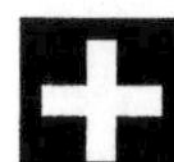

Management

GENERAL MEASURES

- Management requires identification of the cause of hemiballismus, mainly focusing on neuroimaging and identifying and treating risk factors, with special emphasis on vascular risk factors. Once the etiology has been established, the disorder causing the hemiballismus must be treated appropriately depending on its nature. In addition, supportive care directed at preventing self-injury and other complications, such as aspiration pneumonia, pulmonary embolism, and urinary tract infection, should be provided.

SURGICAL MEASURES

- Surgery usually is reserved for patients with refractory hemiballismus. Several surgical targets have been studied, but currently those that have a putative benefit are the globus pallidus, thalamus, and zona incerta. The clinical results of different surgeries with different targets are difficult to compare. However, >90% of patients show significant postoperative improvement.

SYMPTOMATIC TREATMENT

- Medication, primarily dopamine receptor-blocking agents, is method of choice for symptomatic treatment. See Medications.

ADJUNCTIVE TREATMENTS

- Combination therapy is needed in some cases.

ADMISSION/DISCHARGE CRITERIA

- All patients should be admitted for diagnostic evaluation and started on treatment for the ballismus. Discharge criteria and workup depend on the underlying diagnosis.

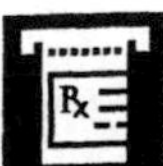

Medications

DRUG(S) OF CHOICE

- *Neuroleptics:* These drugs are the first-line treatment for ballistic movements because of their proven efficacy. Antagonism of the postsynaptic D_2 dopamine receptor seems to be the common feature among agents effective in the treatment of hemiballismus. Chlorpromazine, promethazine, perphenazine, prochlorperazine, haloperidol, pimozide, and tiapride, among other neuroleptics, have been shown to be effective in the treatment of hemiballismus. Clozapine in low doses (50 mg/day) also is useful. Response usually is dramatic and starts within 2 days and almost always within 7 days. If treatment will be prolonged or there are side effects, consider using a benzodiazepine, a dopamine-depleting agent (e.g., reserpine, tetrabenazine), or a GABA-ergic agent such as valproate.
- *Sedative/hypnotics:* A variety of sedative drugs (e.g., barbiturates, chloral hydrate, benzodiazepines) have been used for treatment of hemiballismus. Their efficacy is very modest and related to their tendency to induce sleep.
- *Catecholamine-depleting agents:* Reserpine and tetrabenazine are effective for the treatment of hemiballismus, but the experience with these drugs is more limited than with neuroleptics.
- *GABA-ergic agents:* Valproic acid at various antiepileptic doses have been used with good results. Progabide 900 mg has been reported to be effective in patients who were unresponsive to neuroleptics.

Contraindications

- Neuroleptics should not be used in patients with prior history of hypersensitivity, neuroleptic malignant syndrome, and prolonged QT syndrome.

Precautions

- The main problems with the use of dopamine receptor-blocking agents is the development of extrapyramidal side effects, such as akathisia, drug-induced parkinsonism, neuroleptic malignant syndrome, and tardive dyskinesia. Other side effects include sedation, cardiac conduction abnormalities, weight gain, maculopapular rash, cholestatic jaundice, transient leukopenia, and photosensitivity.

ALTERNATIVE DRUGS

- If pharmacologic measures are ineffective, consider stereotaxic surgical options.

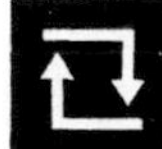

Follow-Up

PATIENT MONITORING

- Dependent on the etiology of the hemiballismus

EXPECTED COURSE AND PROGNOSIS

- The course and prognosis depend on the underlying cause. Overall, good prognosis for survival and recovery is expected, especially when the cause is vascular. In some patients, hemiballismus may evolve into a hemidystonia

PATIENT EDUCATION

- There are no support groups or organizations providing information for patients with hemiballismus. The condition is mentioned briefly at *www.wemove.org.*

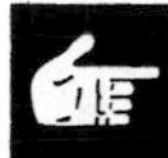

Miscellaneous

SYNONYMS

- Ballism
- Hemichorea

ICD-9-CM: 333.5 Hemichorea

SEE ALSO: N/A

REFERENCES

- Bressman SB, Greene PE. Treatment of hyperkinetic movement disorders. Neurol Clin 1990;8:51–75.
- Dewey RB, Jankovic J. Hemiballismus-hemichorea: clinical and pharmacological findings in 21 patients. Arch Neurol 1989;46:862–867.
- Klawans HL, Hamilton M, Nausieda PA, et al. Treatment and prognosis of hemiballismus. N Engl J Med 1976;99: 222–224.
- Krauss JK, Borremans JJ, Nobbe F, et al. Ballism not related to vascular disease: a report of 16 patients and review of the literature. Park Rel Disord 1996;2:35–45.
- Miyawaki E. The pathophysiology and management of ballism. Neurologist 1998;4:120–130.
- Shannon KM. Hemiballismus. Clin Neuropharmacol 1990;13:413-425.
- Shannon KM. Ballism. In: Jankovic J, Tolosa E, eds. Parkinson's disease and movement disorders. Baltimore: Williams & Wilkins, 1998:365–375.
- Vitek JL. Stereotaxic surgery and deep brain stimulation for Parkinson's disease and movement disorders. In: Watts RL, Koller KC, eds. Movement disorders. Neurologic principles and practice. New York: McGraw-Hill, 1997:237–255.

Author(s): Xabier Beristain, MD; Joanne M. Wojcieszek, MD

Hereditary Spastic Paraparesis

Basics

DESCRIPTION

- Hereditary spastic paraparesis (HSP) represents a group of rare, genetically transmitted, neurodegenerative diseases characterized by the development of progressive weakness and spasticity of the lower extremities. A clinical classification distinguishes pure HSP from "complicated" HSP, in which other neurologic and non-neurologic abnormalities also are present.

EPIDEMIOLOGY

Incidence/Prevalence

- Reported prevalence rates for pure HSP vary from 1.0 to 20.2 per 100,000.

Race

- No ethnic predominance has been reported. Families with HSP have been identified in many parts of the world, with regional clusters.

Age

- Age of symptom onset varies widely (from infancy to >80 years), with a peak from the second through the fourth decades. The distinction between early onset (before 40 years) and late-onset (after 40 years) HSP is debated, because clinical features do not seem to be distinct.

Gender

- No gender difference was reported, except for X-linked forms of HSP.

ETIOLOGY

- Three modes of genetic transmission have been identified:
  - —Autosomal dominant inheritance with complete or nearly complete penetrance is the most common mode of transmission. Linkage analysis identified loci on chromosomes 14q, 2p, 15q, and 8q. CAG repeat expansions were identified in some families.
  - —Autosomal recessive forms were linked to chromosomes 8, 16, and 15q.
  - —X-linked inheritance is rare and has been linked to loci Xq28, Xq21, and Xq11.

RISK FACTORS

- Consanguinity increases the risk of expression of autosomal recessive forms.

PREGNANCY

- Prenatal genetic studies may be used to assess the risk that the fetus inherited HSP, but this testing is useful only in families with a known linkage to HSP loci. Results should be interpreted with caution.

ASSOCIATED CONDITIONS

N/A

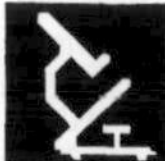

Diagnosis

DIFFERENTIAL DIAGNOSIS

- Clinical diagnosis of HSP requires the presence of progressive spastic paraparesis and a positive family history. However, other possible diagnoses should be ruled out in each patient (particularly in "complicated" forms) through complete neurologic examination and neuroimaging studies. Other causes of spastic paraparesis include
  - —Trauma
  - —Malformations (Arnold-Chiari, tethered cord syndrome)
  - —Acquired structural defects (herniated disc, spondylosis)
  - —Tumors
  - —Vascular disorders (infarcts, hemorrhages, arteriovenous malformations)
  - —Inflammation (transverse myelitis, multiple sclerosis)
  - —Infections (spondylodiscitis, epidural abscess, tertiary syphilis, tropical [HTLV-1 associated] spastic paraparesis, AIDS)
  - —Other neurodegenerative disorders (amyotrophic lateral sclerosis, spinocerebellar ataxias)
  - —Metabolic disorders (B_{12} deficiency, leukodystrophies, mitochondrial diseases)
  - —Familial peripheral neuropathies

SIGNS AND SYMPTOMS

- The main presenting complaint is progressive gait disturbance. Examination shows weakness and spasticity of the lower extremities with hyperreflexia and bilateral Babinski sign.
- In pure HSP, spastic paraparesis may be associated with sensory deficits of the lower extremities, bladder/bowel dysfunction, mild pyramidal involvement of the upper extremities (hyperreflexia, Hoffmann sign, decreased fine movements), and/or slight dysmetria on finger-to-nose testing. Amyotrophy of the lower extremities usually occurs late, in patients with restricted mobility.
- Associated findings, which include ataxia, dysarthria, extrapyramidal signs, cognitive deficits, optic neuropathy, cutaneous abnormalities, ophthalmologic abnormalities, and deafness, lead to the diagnosis of "complicated" HSP, particularly if there is a family history of pure HSP and other diseases have been ruled out.

LABORATORY PROCEDURES

- There is no laboratory diagnostic test for HSP. Genetic linkage studies are increasingly performed, but results must be used with caution for counseling because different mutations may be involved, and all HSP loci have not been identified yet.
- Other laboratory tests aimed at excluding other possible conditions:
  - —VDRL
  - —Serum vitamin B_{12}
  - —HIV and HTLV-1 serologies
  - —Plasma long-chain fatty acids

IMAGING STUDIES

- MRI of the brain and spinal cord is recommended for differential diagnosis. In patients with HSP, MRI is normal or shows atrophy of the spinal cord and/or corpus callosum. Cortical atrophy and foci of increased T2 signal in the cerebral white matter have been reported in some cases.

SPECIAL TESTS

- EMG is useful to rule out peripheral neuropathy. Nerve conduction velocity test are most often normal in HSP.
- Somatosensory evoked potentials obtained after stimulation of the median and tibial posterior nerves may be abnormal with delayed latency and decreased amplitude, even in the absence of clinical sensory deficits.

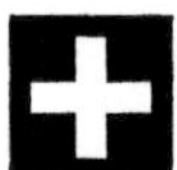

Management

GENERAL MEASURES

- There is no specific treatment for HSP. Management is primarily symptomatic.
- Goals of management:
  - —Preserving function
  - —Limiting handicap
  - —Enhancing quality of life
  - —Preventing medical complications

SURGICAL MEASURES

- Surgery (tenotomies and/r neurotomies) may be useful in the management of severe spasticity with contractures.

SYMPTOMATIC TREATMENT

- Spasticity requires daily stretching exercises and treatment of all potentially irritative factors (urinary tract infections [UTI], pressure sores, ingrown toenail). Multiple medications are available to treat spasticity (see below).

- Bladder dysfunction: The most common complaints are urinary urgency and incontinence. Neurogenic bladder dysfunction is best evaluated by complete urodynamic assessment. It is at least recommended to measure postvoiding residual volumes (PVR), even when the patient does not complain of urinary hesitancy, in order to rule out chronic retention, which might worsen with medications for incontinence. General measures include regular fluid intake and avoidance of irritants (coffee, sodas). Treatments for detrusor hyperactivity include oxybutynin 5 mg qd-tid, tolterodine tartrate (Detrol), and propantheline bromide. If PVR exceeds 100 mL, intermittent self-catheterization is recommended to prevent chronic bladder distention, recurrent UTIs, and vesicorenal reflux. Indwelling bladder catheter is avoided as much as possible because of the risk of chronic infection.
- Sexual dysfunction is a common complaint. Erectile dysfunction can be managed through medications (sildenafil citrate [Viagra]), intracavernous injections, penile prosthesis.
- Bowel dysfunction: Management includes dietary recommendations, adequate fluid intake, regular physical activity, regular bowel schedule (using suppositories to trigger bowel movement or digital rectal evacuation if necessary), daily administration of bulk-forming agents, and cautious use of laxatives.
- Skin care: Prevention of decubiti is a concern mainly for patients with restricted mobility or for those wearing orthoses, particularly if sensation is decreased. Prevention includes frequent change of position, inspection of potential pressure points, use of adequate cushions/mattresses or padding, and avoidance of maceration due to incontinence. Agency for Health Care Policy and Research (AHCPR) guidelines on pressure ulcers for adults can be found on the Internet at *http://text.nlm.nih.gov/ftrs/gateway.*

ADJUNCTIVE TREATMENT

- Physical therapy in the ambulatory patient should be aimed at preserving and optimizing gait through aggressive stretching exercises, neuromuscular stimulation, muscle strengthening, endurance training, and appropriate use of technical aids. In the nonambulatory patient, rehabilitation should be oriented toward preserving range of motion and the ability to transfer. Occupational therapy should focus on upper extremity function, wheelchair assessment, instrumental activities of daily living, and home adaptations. Emphasis is placed on patient education and home exercises. Short periods of intensive rehabilitation may be useful during periods of rapid loss of function or after immobilization due to an intercurrent health problem.

ADMISSION/DISCHARGE CRITERIA

N/A

Medications

DRUG(S) OF CHOICE

- Oral baclofen is commonly used when spasticity is the cause of discomfort or interferes with function. The starting dose is low (10–20 mg qd) and progressively titrated up to 100 mg divided in 3–4 doses daily. Oral tizanidine may be used instead of, or in association with, baclofen at a dose of 2 mg up to 36 mg/day. Intrathecal baclofen pump implantation may be considered in cases of intractable spasticity despite oral treatment at maximum tolerated doses with caution in patients who are still ambulatory, considering the risk of losing function due to increased weakness.

Contraindications

N/A

Precautions

- Tizanidine may cause sedation or orthostatic hypotension and should be titrated up slowly. LFTs should be monitored periodically for chronic tizanidine treatment.

ALTERNATIVE DRUGS

- Other agents used in the treatment of spasticity include dantrolene and diazepam.

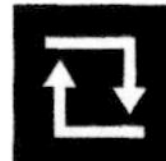

Follow-Up

PATIENT MONITORING

- Monitoring is focused on optimization of symptomatic treatment, preservation of function, and prevention or early treatment of complications, such as UTIs and pressure sores. Development of new neurologic symptoms or abrupt worsening of symptoms must raise the suspicion of misdiagnosis or superimposed condition (e.g., development of cervical spondylosis in a patient with established HSP).

EXPECTED COURSE AND PROGNOSIS

- The rate of progression is highly variable among patients. For a given patient, progression may not be uniform over time. Patients with childhood onset and no or very slow progression have been reported. Many patients remain ambulatory for an extended period of time.

PATIENT EDUCATION

- HSPinfo.org (Hereditary Spastic Paraplegia/ Familial Spastic Paraparesis), 48 W Broadway, Salt Lake City UT 84101. Phone: 801-366-7348, e-mail: info@HSPinfo.org, website: *http://www.HSPinfo.org*

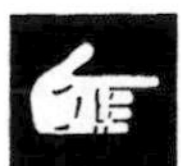

Miscellaneous

SYNONYMS

- Hereditary spastic paraplegia
- Familial spastic paraparesis/paraplegia
- Strümpell-Lorrain disease/syndrome

ICD-9-CM: 334.1 Hereditary spastic paraplegia; 344.1 Paraplegia

SEE ALSO: N/A

REFERENCES

- Bruyn RP, van Dijk JG, Scheltens P, et al. Clinically silent dysfunction of dorsal columns and dorsal spinocerebellar tracts in hereditary spastic paraparesis. J Neurol Sci 1994;125:206–211.
- Coutinho P, Barros J, Zemmouri R, et al. Clinical heterogeneity of autosomal recessive spastic paraplegias: analysis of 106 patients in 46 families. Arch Neurol 1999;56:943–949.
- Fink JK, Heiman-Patterson T, Bird T, et al. Hereditary spastic paraplegia: advances in genetic research. Hereditary Spastic Paraplegia Working Group. Neurology 1996;46:1507–1514.
- Harding AE. Classification of the hereditary ataxias and paraplegias. Lancet 1983;1:1151–1155.
- Jensen LN, Gerstenberg T, Kallestrup EB, et al. Urodynamic evaluation of patients with autosomal dominant pure spastic paraplegia linked to chromosome 2p21-p24. J Neurol Neurosurg Psychiatry 1998;65:693–696.
- Krabbe K, Nielsen JE, Fallentin E, et al. MRI of autosomal dominant pure spastic paraplegia. Neuroradiology 1997;39: 724–727.
- Nielsen JE, Krabbe K, Jennum P, et al. Autosomal dominant pure spastic paraplegia: a clinical, paraclinical, and genetic study. J Neurol Neurosurg Psychiatry 1998;64:61–66.
- Silva MC, Coutinho P, Pinheiro CD, et al. Hereditary ataxias and spastic paraplegias: methodological aspects of a prevalence study in Portugal. J Clin Epidemiol 1997;50:1377–1384.

Author(s): Francois Bethoux, MD

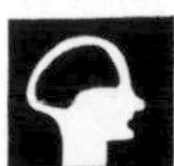

Basics

DESCRIPTION

- In 1869 Johann Frederick Horner, the first professor of ophthalmology in Switzerland, published a case report of eyelid ptosis caused by a neck lesion. Horner's syndrome (HS) is characterized by a lesion of the oculosympathetic pathway. This three-neuron sympathetic pathway runs from the brain to the pupil. The first-order (central) neurons run from the posterior hypothalamus through the brainstem into the spinal cord (via the intermediolateral column) to synapse at the ciliospinal center of Budge at the C8 to T2 level of the spinal cord. Axons of the second-order (preganglionic) neurons then exit the cord via the ventral roots to pass over the apex of the lung to enter the sympathetic cervical chain. This sympathetic chain is associated with the carotid arteries. The second-order neurons synapse at the superior cervical ganglion located at the bifurcation of the cervical carotid artery, which is at the level of the thyroid cartilage. The third-order (postganglionic) neuronal axons leave the superior cervical ganglion to accompany the internal and external carotid arteries. Most third-order axons pass with the internal carotid artery to reach the ipsilateral cavernous sinus and then travel with fibers of the abducens (VI) nerve to pass to the nasociliary branch of the trigeminal nerve and enter the orbit through the superior orbital fissure. These long ciliary nerves pass through the ciliary ganglion (without synapsing) and enter the eye in the suprachoroidal space to innervate the radially oriented iris dilator muscle. Some orbital sympathetic fibers innervate Mueller's muscle, a smooth but minor elevator of the upper eyelid and a rudimentary analogous muscle of the lower eyelid. Both vasomotor (flushing) and sudomotor (sweating) sympathetic fibers of the face travel with branches of the external carotid artery. Therefore, diseases that affect the brain, upper spinal cord, thorax, neck, and orbit can be diagnosed in patients who can present with miosis, partial (1–2 mm) ptosis (upper more than lower lid), and in some cases facial anhidrosis.

EPIDEMIOLOGY

- Nearly 20% of the population has at least 0.4 mm of anisocoria (unequal pupil diameter between the two eyes). The vast majority of such patients, however, have simple (essential, central, or physiologic) anisocoria in that they have equal amounts of anisocoria in bright and dim light. HS is an important diagnostic subset of anisocoric patients. By taking a careful history, one can help localize the part of the three-order neuronal chain that is affected and thereby make an educated differential diagnosis of possible underlying diseases. Ancillary tests include office or bedside pharmacologic pupillary testing and targeted neuroimaging.

ETIOLOGY

- First-order lesions are associated with brainstem or upper spinal cord injury, such as stereotactic thalamotomy, Wallenberg's syndrome, poliomyelitis, multiple sclerosis, syringomyelia, and complicated epidural blocks. Second-order lesions affect the spinal cord and sympathetic chain below the superior cervical ganglion and include apical lung cancer (e.g., bronchogenic carcinoma or so-called Pancoast tumor), birth injury involving the brachial plexus (Klumpke's paralysis), cervical carotid angiography, lymphoma, coronary artery bypass surgery, and radial neck surgery. Third-order lesions involve the superior cervical ganglion and higher and include disorders such as basilar skull fractures, nasopharyngeal carcinoma, cavernous sinus tumors, carotid cavernous fistulas, orbital tumors, and internal carotid artery dissections. In children, congenital cases can be idiopathic or associated with brachial plexus injuries. Acquired cases are presumed to result from a mediastinal tumor (e.g., neuroblastoma) until proven otherwise.

RISK FACTORS

- Risk factors are related to the underlying pathology. For example, smokers are at greater risk for bronchogenic carcinoma.

PREGNANCY

N/A

ASSOCIATED CONDITIONS

- Associated signs and symptoms are dependent on the underlying disease. For example, Wallenberg's syndrome is a lateral medullary infarct with ipsilateral HS, ataxia and facial loss of light touch, contralateral body loss of pain and temperature, dysphasia, hoarseness, nystagmus, and vertigo.

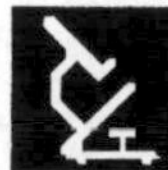

Diagnosis

DIFFERENTIAL DIAGNOSIS

- The differential diagnosis of anisocoria includes those cases of nonphysiologic anisocoria in which the anisocoria is greater in dim-light illumination and the abnormal pupil is the miotic pupil. Examples include pharmacologic causes such as miotic drops to treat glaucoma (e.g., pilocarpine) and intraocular inflammatory disease such as iritis or ocular trauma, both of which can lead to adhesions (posterior synechiae) between the iris and the lens. A careful ocular history and slitlamp examination will rule out the aforementioned examples. It also should be noted that chronic Adie's syndrome (post ciliary ganglionitis with initially large, relatively areflexic pupil that shows denervation hypersensitivity to dilute pilocarpine and is associated with reduced or absent deep tendon reflexes) can develop a small pupil with time, but such cases are unassociated with blepharoptosis. Also, ipsilateral miosis and ptosis can occur in a patient with essential anisocoria and levator aponeurosis dehiscence.

SIGNS AND SYMPTOMS

- The clinical features of HS are (i) anisocoria (the miotic eye being the affected eye as the parasympathetically innervated iris sphincters is unopposed) that is greater in dim light than in bright light; (ii) slower dilation of the affected pupil in dim light (dilation lag that can last up to 15 seconds); and (iii) ptosis of 1–2 mm of the upper lid and occasionally involving the lower lid (upside down ptosis) and apparent (pseudo) enophthalmos that is secondary to blepharoptosis. In some cases, conjunctival injection, reduced intraocular pressure, hemifacial anhidrosis, and lack of blushing are noted. In congenital cases, iris heterochromia (lighter iris color on the affected side) is present because iris melanocyte development depends on sympathetic innervation. Such patients also may have hemifacial and hemicranial straighter hair.

LABORATORY PROCEDURES

- In children suspected of having a neuroblastoma, besides neuroimaging of the thorax and abdomen, a 24-hour urine collection for excessive catecholamine excretion (vanillylmandelic acid and homovanillic acid) is performed in conjunction with an evaluation by a pediatric oncologist.

IMAGING STUDIES

- Targeted CT or MRI scanning is directed by the patient's history, clinical examination, and pharmacologic pupillary testing. Angiography (percutaneous or MR angiography) may be needed in patients with carotid cavernous fistulas or carotid dissections.

SPECIAL TESTS

- Pharmacologic testing is essential because it helps confirm the diagnosis of HS and aids in localizing the order of neuron affected. All pharmacologic pupillary testing should be done before any drops are placed in the patient's eye so that the corneal penetration of the drops is not altered. Oculosympathetic dysfunction is confirmed with topical cocaine (4%–10% in adults). Thereafter, allow 45 minutes before checking each pupil. Cocaine blocks the reuptake of the neurotransmitter norepinephrine at the neuromuscular junction; therefore, any order HS eye does not dilate (or does so minimally, <1 mm) whereas a normal pupil will dilate to cocaine. The Horner's pupil does not dilate because norepinephrine is not being released into the third-order synaptic cleft. Thereafter, one should wait at least 24–48 hours before performing the hydroxyamphetamine (Paredrine 1%) test. Again, one drop is placed in each eye and repeated after several minutes. Hydroxyamphetamine causes release of the presynaptic norepinephrine vesicles. Third-order lesions cause presynaptic terminal degeneration and thereby a lack of norepinephrine vesicles. Unlike eyes that have first- or second-order HS, a third-order HS pupil fails to dilate in response to hydroxyamphetamine. The very good sensitivity and the specificity of pharmacologic testing are not 100%. There is no pharmacologic test to distinguish between first- and second-order HS. One may need to remind the patient that a urine drug screen will remain positive for 24–48 hours after such testing, which could be problematic with a drug toxicity screening for occupational hiring.

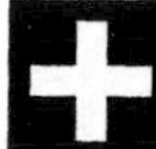

Management

GENERAL MEASURES

- Depend on the underlying pathology

SURGICAL MEASURES

- Depend on the underlying pathology, see below

SYMPTOMATIC TREATMENT

- Ptosis repair (Fasanella-Servat or levator aponeurosis advancement) usually is not required because of its mild (1-2 mm) nature.

ADJUNCTIVE TREATMENT

N/A

ADMISSION/DISCHARGE CRITERIA

- Some patients are diagnosed while they are hospitalized (e.g., for radical neck surgery); for others, the initial neuroimaging typically is done, if needed, as an outpatient. Acquired cases in childhood typically are admitted for a workup to rule out a neuroblastoma.

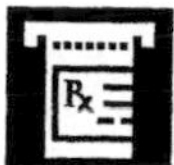

Medications

DRUG(S) OF CHOICE

N/A

ALTERNATIVE DRUGS

N/A

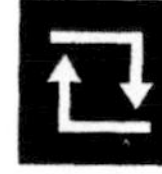

Follow-Up

PATIENT MONITORING

- Once the diagnosis of HS is made, the underlying etiology is monitored on an individual basis.

EXPECTED COURSE AND PROGNOSIS

- HS typically is a permanent condition

PATIENT EDUCATION

- Directed to the underlying condition

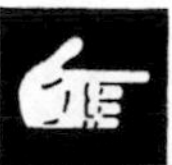

Miscellaneous

SYNONYMS

- Claude Bernard-Horner syndrome

ICD-9-CM: 337.9 Horner's syndrome; 379.41 Anisocoria; 374.43 Ptosis

SEE ALSO: N/A

REFERENCES

- Brazier J, Smith SE. Disorders of the pupil. In: Oxford textbook of ophthalmology, volume 2.Oxford: Oxford University Press, 1999:862–864.
- Horner F. Uber eine Form von Ptosis. Klin Monatsbl Augenheilkd 1869;7:193–198.
- Lee AG, Brazis PW. Clinical pathways in neuro-ophthalmology: an evidence-based approach. New York: Thieme, 1998: 357–388.
- Kardon RH, Denison CE, Brown CK, et al. Critical evaluation of the cocaine test in the diagnosis of Horner's syndrome. Arch Ophthalmol 1990;108:384–387.
- Kardon RH, Thompson HS. The pupil in neuro-ophthalmology. London: Mosby, 1998:13.1–13.9.
- Maloney WF, Younge BR, Moyer NJ. Evaluation of the causes and accuracy of pharmacologic localization in Horner's syndrome. Am J Ophthalmol 1980;90: 394–402.
- Martin TJ, Corbett JJ. Neuro-ophthalmology: the requisiter. St. Louis: Mosby, 2000:191–207.
- Thompson HS, Miller NR. Disorders of pupillary function, accommodation and lacrimation. In: Walsh and Hoyt's clinical neuro-ophthalmology, vol. 1, 5th ed. Baltimore: Williams & Williams, 1998:961–972.

Author(s): Thomas J. Mehelas, MD

Huntington's Disease

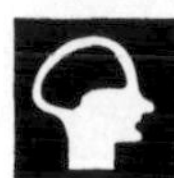

Basics

DESCRIPTION

- Huntington's disease (HD) is a hereditary neurodegenerative disorder characterized by involuntary movements, psychiatric disturbance. and dementia.

EPIDEMIOLOGY

Incidence/Prevalence

- The worldwide prevalence of HD is approximately 5–10 per 100,000. Approximately 25,000 North Americans have manifest HD with an additional 125,000 at risk (parent with HD).

Race

- Reduced prevalence has been reported for certain ethnic backgrounds (Japan, Norway, and individuals of African descent). The disease is endemic in and around Maracaibo, Venezuela.

Age

- The average age of symptom onset is during the third or fourth decade, although onset in childhood and in later life has been reported.

Sex

- No gender predisposition has been identified.

ETIOLOGY

- HD is caused by a mutation on the short arm of chromosome 4 in the first exon of the Huntington gene. Increase in the number of cytosine-adenine-guanine (CAG) triplets beyond 37 produces an expanded polyglutamine sequence that alters the conformation of the polypeptide and engenders a toxic gain of function.

Genetics

- HD is a fully penetrant, autosomal dominant disorder. In adult-onset HD, a CAG expansion of 40–50 is typical. Larger expansions result in juvenile-onset HD. Although the length of the triplet expansion correlates with age of onset, the relationship is imprecise and has limited prognostic value.
- The CAG repeat is unstable, expanding during meiosis. The largest increases occur during spermatogenesis. Meiotic instability provides a mechanism for the phenomenon of anticipation (earlier onset in offspring) and the association of juvenile-onset HD with an affected father.

RISK FACTORS

N/A

PREGNANCY

- Although pregnancy and oral contraceptives can precipitate involuntary movements, the impact of pregnancy on HD is not well characterized.

ASSOCIATED CONDITIONS

N/A

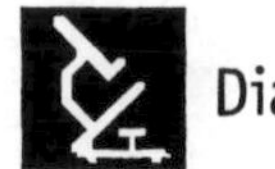

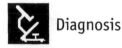

Diagnosis

DIFFERENTIAL DIAGNOSIS

- Hereditary
  - —Benign familial chorea
  - —Neuroacanthocytosis
  - —Wilson's disease
  - —Paroxysmal choreoathetosis
- Metabolic
  - —Hyperthyroidism
  - —Hypoparathyroidism
  - —Electrolyte disturbance
- Infectious/immunologic
  - —Sydenham's chorea (St. Vitus dance)
  - —Viral encephalitis
  - —Multiple sclerosis
  - —Systemic lupus erythematosus
  - —Paraneoplastic
- Cerebrovascular
  - —Hemorrhage/infarct (subthalamic nucleus)
  - —Polycythemia rubra vera

SIGNS AND SYMPTOMS

- Motor disorder
  - —Involuntary movements (may include dystonia, athetosis, tics, as well as chorea).
  - —Impaired pursuit and saccadic eye movements
  - —Motor impersistence (inability to sustain eye closure or tongue protrusion)
  - —Hyperactive tendon reflexes
  - —Incoordination
- Mood disorder
  - —Depression (may precede motor manifestations)
  - —Higher frequency of suicide has been reported in HD
  - —Psychosis
  - —Obsessive/compulsive behaviors
- Cognitive dysfunction
  - —Eludes recognition because of the prominence of motor and psychiatric manifestations and the relative preservation of verbal skills
- The symptoms of HD vary greatly depending upon the age of onset. Onset prior to 20 years of age is associated with prominent rigidity and an increased incidence of seizure (~20%). If symptoms manifest after 50 years of age, chorea may be the only significant symptom and the rate of progression usually is slowed.

LABORATORY PROCEDURES

- Genetic testing: A CAG repeat expansion establishes the diagnosis of HD. The many implications of genetic testing must be carefully considered. Testing of at-risk, presymptomatic individuals must adhere to established guidelines, with participation of a genetic counselor, psychologist, and neurologist. With rare exception, testing is restricted to individuals attaining the age of majority.
- Laboratory evaluation excluding alternative diagnoses
  - —CBC with manual differential (acanthocytes)
  - —Electrolytes
  - —LFTs (Wilson's disease)
  - —Thyroid function studies
  - —Sedimentation rate, antinuclear antibody
  - —Antistreptolysin O (ASO) titers (Sydenham's chorea)
  - —Ceruloplasmin, serum copper, 24-hour urine copper (Wilson's disease)
  - —Pregnancy test (chorea gravidarum)

IMAGING STUDIES

- CT or MRI of the brain demonstrates progressive atrophy of the striatum (caudate nucleus and putamen) that parallels symptom progression. The roles for functional MRI and spectroscopy await definition.
- Functional imaging (PET and SPECT) may improve diagnostic sensitivity and specificity, but current use is restricted to research.

SPECIAL TESTS

- EEG can facilitate the management of seizures in juvenile HD.
- Neuropsychometric evaluation can be performed to assess the extent of cognitive dysfunction.

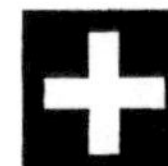

Management

GENERAL MEASURES

- Disease-modifying therapy has yet to be identified.
- Assistance from the social services department is frequently needed because wage-earning years are curtailed.
- Ensure a safe environment because gait disorder and poor balance increase the risk of falls and associated injury.

SURGICAL MEASURES

- Although several trials of fetal tissue transplantation have been reported, its role in surgery for HD awaits further investigation.

SYMPTOMATIC TREATMENT

- Treatment is aimed primarily at controlling involuntary movements and mood disturbance. See Medications.
- Stable environment and well-defined activities can help to control behavioral manifestations.
- Involuntary movements demand caloric intake that can be difficult to sustain, especially when dysphagia and aspiration complicate the management of advanced HD.

ADJUNCTIVE TREATMENT

- Behavioral and supportive psychotherapy can be useful in the management HD.

ADMISSION/DISCHARGE CRITERIA

- Hospitalization does not occur frequently and usually is prompted by exacerbation of psychiatric/behavioral manifestations or to facilitate long-term placement.

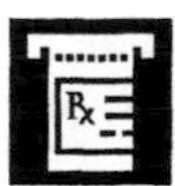

Medications

DRUG(S) OF CHOICE

- Movement disorder: Typical and atypical neuroleptic medications dampen hyperkinetic movements. Dopamine-depleting compounds are used less commonly because of affective side effects. Treatment is deferred until dyskinesia presents an injury risk or interferes with daily activities, and the minimum dose yielding reasonable control is used. As symptoms progress, increasing akinesia and rigidity may respond to dopaminergic therapy. Response to the medicines listed may be enhanced by divided doses.
- Typical neuroleptic
  —Haloperidol (Haldol) 0.5–5 mg qd
- Atypical neuroleptic
  —Risperidone (Risperdal) 0.5–3 mg qd
  —Olanzapine (Zyprexa) 2.5–15 mg qd
- Dopamine-depleting agent
  —Reserpine (Serpasil) 0.5 mg–2 mg qd
- Dopaminergic agent
  —Carbidopa/levodopa (Sinemet) 25/100 mg bid–qid
  —Bromocriptine (Parlodel) 2.5–10 mg qd
- Mood disorder: Selective serotonin reuptake inhibitors and tricyclic antidepressants can moderate the mood disturbance and obsessive-compulsive behaviors. Anticonvulsants are useful in mood stabilization and behavior control and may dampen dyskinetic movements. Neuroleptic medications effectively control psychotic features.
  —Sertraline (Zoloft) 25–200 mg qd
  —Amitriptyline (Elavil) 10–75 mg qd
  —Clomipramine (Anafranil) 25–250 mg qd
- Memory disorder: The efficacy of cognition-enhancing medications in HD awaits characterization.

Contraindications

- Other than known sensitivity or the experience of adverse effects, there are no specific contraindications to available treatments for HD.

Precautions

- When a family history is not readily available, diagnosis of HD often is dismissed. The implications of this diagnosis for the individual and for family members require continued diligence.

ALTERNATIVE DRUGS

- Although a source of great interest, nutritional therapies have not been shown to provide symptomatic benefit or to alter the natural progression of HD. Intriguing results in a recent trial of coenzyme Q_{10} require additional study.

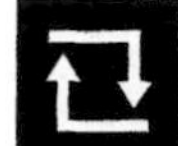

Follow-Up

PATIENT MONITORING

- The frequency of follow-up is dictated by patient need. Semiannual visits provide an opportunity to address questions and obtain information on symptom progression and needed treatment modification.

EXPECTED COURSE AND PROGNOSIS

- Eventually hyperkinetic features are supplanted by increasing rigidity and akinesia. Aspiration pneumonia and other infectious complications are the ultimate cause of death. The interval separating initial symptom recognition and death varies between 15 and 20 years.

PATIENT EDUCATION

- Education is important through the many stages of HD, not only for the individual, but also for the immediate and extended family. Issues surrounding nutrition and the appropriateness of long-term management need to be regularly addressed.
- Huntington's Disease Society of America, 158 West 29th Street, 7th Floor, New York, NY 10001-5300. Phone: 1-800-345-HDSA; website: *www.hdsa.org*

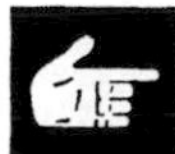

Miscellaneous

SYNONYMS

- Huntington's chorea
- Degenerative chorea
- Woody Guthrie's disease

ICD-9-CM: 333.0 Other extrapyramidal disease and abnormal movement disorders; 333.4 Huntington's chorea; 333.5 Other chorea's (i.e., hemiballism, paroxysmal chorea and rheumatic chorea); 333.9 Unspecified extrapyramidal disease and abnormal movement disorder

SEE ALSO: CHOREA

REFERENCES

- Feigin A, Zgaljardic D. Recent advances in Huntington's disease: implications for experimental therapeutics. Curr Opin Neurol 2002;15:483–489.
- Foroud T, et al. Differences in duration of Huntington's disease based on age at onset. J Neurol Neurosurg Psychiatry 1999;66:52–56.
- Guidelines for the molecular genetic predictive test in Huntington's disease. International Huntington Association and the World Federation of Neurology Research Group on Huntington's Chorea. Neurology 1994;44:1533–1536.
- Harper PS. The epidemiology of Huntington's disease. Hum Genet 1992;89:365–376.
- Higgins DS Jr. Chorea and its disorders. Neurol Clin 2001;19:707–722, vii.
- Kirkwood SC, et al. Progression of symptoms in the early and middle stages of Huntington disease. Arch Neurol 2001;58:273–278.
- Kremer B, et al. A worldwide study of the Huntington's Disease mutation: the sensitivity and specificity of measuring CAG repeats. N Engl J Med 1994;330: 1401–1406.
- Lanska DJ, et al. Huntington's disease mortality in the United States. Neurology 1988;38:769–772.
- Ranen NG, et al. Anticipation and instability of IT-15 (CAG)N repeats in parent offspring pairs with Huntington Disease. Am J Hum Genet 1995;57: 593–602.
- Rosenblatt A, Leroi I. Neuropsychiatry of Huntington's disease and other basal ganglia disorders. Psychosomatics 2000;41:24–30.

Author(s): Donald S. Higgins, Jr., MD

Hydrocephalus

Basics

DESCRIPTION

- Hydrocephalus is a condition that results from an excess of CSF in the brain due to an increase in production of CSF or, more commonly, an obstruction of normal CSF flow or decreased absorption of CSF. The result of this overabundance of CSF is an increase in intracranial pressure (ICP) with corresponding enlargement of the ventricular system of the brain.

EPIDEMIOLOGY

- Congenital hydrocephalus affects approximately 3–4 per 1,000 live births and is commonly associated with any congenital brain malformation. The overall combined incidence of congenital and acquired hydrocephalus in both children and adults is not known.

ETIOLOGY

- Hydrocephalus can be congenital or acquired, and communicating or obstructive (noncommunicating). Acquired hydrocephalus can occur after intracranial hemorrhage, especially intraventricular hemorrhage associated with prematurity, infection, or severe head trauma, or in association with brain tumors. In addition, normal pressure hydrocephalus (NPH) can occur in adults.

Genetics

- A number of genetic disorders are associated with hydrocephalus, such as X-linked hydrocephalus, cytogenetic abnormalities including trisomies 9, 3, and 18, and mendelian conditions such as Hurler syndrome, Walker-Warburg syndrome, and the craniosynostosis syndromes (Crouzon's and Apert).

RISK FACTORS

- Risk factors for hydrocephalus include prematurity (from intraventricular hemorrhage), several first-degree male relatives with congenital hydrocephalus, meningitis, intracranial hemorrhage (especially subarachnoid and intraventricular hemorrhage), and congenital brain malformations (spinal dysraphism, Chiari malformations)

PREGNANCY

- Pregnancy is not contraindicated in women with treated hydrocephalus. Development of hydrocephalus during pregnancy is rare.

ASSOCIATED CONDITIONS

- Myelomeningocele (80%–90% require shunts), Chiari malformations, certain genetic disorders (see Genetics), brain tumors, intracranial hemorrhage, severe head trauma, CNS infections

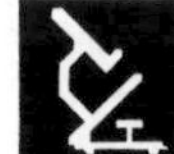

Diagnosis

DIFFERENTIAL DIAGNOSIS

- Brain atrophy (resulting in *ex vacuo* hydrocephalus) secondary to brain ischemia and neurodegenerative disorders, benign intracranial hypertension, hydranencephaly, developmental anomalies (agenesis of the corpus callosum, septo-optic dysplasia).

SIGNS AND SYMPTOMS

- Headache, nausea and vomiting, decreased level of consciousness, confusion or difficulty concentrating, papilledema, abducens and upward gaze palsies, and gait changes. In young children, enlarging head circumference, a bulging and tense fontanelle, splayed sutures, irritability, bradycardia, and sunsetting eyes are commonly seen in hydrocephalus. In NPH, there is a classic triad of dementia, gait abnormalities, and urinary incontinence.

LABORATORY PROCEDURES

- There are no specific laboratory tests that diagnose hydrocephalus. With suspected infection, CSF should be sampled prior to placement of a CSF shunt. Placement of a shunt in the presence of a CSF infection will doom the shunt to failure.

IMAGING STUDIES

- Skull radiographs showing splayed sutures in young children or a "copper beaten" skull may indicate hydrocephalus.
- CT scan shows enlargement of the ventricular system and may provide the underlying cause of the hydrocephalus.
- MRI scan is indicated in cases of suspected aqueductal stenosis and to rule out associated Chiari malformations.

SPECIAL TESTS

- In cases of suspected NPH, a number of ancillary tests to predict responsiveness of NPH to shunting are available. These include a nuclear medicine CSF flow study (using ^{99m}Tc-DPTA) and lumbar puncture (LP). A patient whose symptoms improve after withdrawal of CSF by LP may be more likely to respond to permanent CSF shunting.

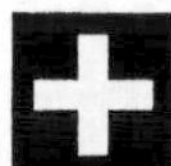

Management

GENERAL MEASURES

- Once the diagnosis is established and the need for treatment confirmed, one should proceed to the specifically indicated surgical option. In cases of acute hydrocephalus where ICP is elevated to a life-threatening level, the usual emergency measures used to lower ICP can be done (elevate the head of the bed, administer 1 g/kg mannitol IV). These measures cannot be a substitute for prompt neurosurgical management of the underlying problem. In cases of neonatal intraventricular hemorrhage, serial LP or ventricular taps can be done until the child has grown large enough that a permanent shunt can be placed.

SURGICAL MEASURES

- Surgical treatment is the mainstay of therapy for hydrocephalus. Several surgical options are available, the goal of which is to bypass the regular CSF pathways.

CSF Shunt

- As a permanent solution to hydrocephalus, closed ventricular draining systems have been in use for >50 years. All CSF shunting systems consist of a proximal ventricular catheter; a one-way valve and reservoir; and a distal catheter terminating in another body compartment. The most common sites for termination of the distal catheter are (in order) the peritoneum, the pleural space, and the venous system (usually the right atrium or superior vena cava).

Endoscopic Third Ventriculostomy

- In selected cases of hydrocephalus, specifically aqueductal stenosis, where the fourth ventricle is normal in size and the lateral and third ventricles enlarged, endoscopic third ventriculostomy (ETV) is a treatment option. In this procedure, a fiberoptic endoscope is passed into the lateral ventricle and then into the third ventricle through the foramen of Munro. A hole is made in the floor of the third ventricle, bypassing the obstruction at the aqueduct. A successful ETV will obviate the need for a permanent CSF shunt. ETV is less successful in cases of hydrocephalus without aqueductal stenosis.

External Ventricular Drainage

- In cases where placement of a permanent shunt is not feasible (e.g., infection or acute hemorrhage) or where drainage of CSF is required temporarily until CSF flow pathways are reestablished (e.g., posterior fossa tumor), placement of an external ventricular drain (EVD) can be a temporizing measure until a permanent shunt can be placed or the indication for CSF diversion is no longer present. The drain is passed into the lateral ventricle and tunneled out through the scalp, draining into an external system. Prolonged use of an EVD is associated with a high CSF infection rate.

SYMPTOMATIC TREATMENT

- The mainstay of symptomatic treatment is surgical therapy.

ADJUNCTIVE TREATMENT

- Supportive care, especially in children, involves monitoring of heart and respiratory rates. Bradycardia and periods of apnea can be ominous signs of increased ICP.

ADMISSION/DISCHARGE CRITERIA

- All patients with symptomatic hydrocephalus should be admitted for management of the condition. In asymptomatic cases where enlargement of the ventricular system is equivocal, it is reasonable to follow a patient both clinically and with serial neuroimaging studies (CT or MRI).
- Patients can be discharged within 1–3 days of surgery provided their symptoms of increased ICP have resolved and the surgeon is satisfied that the shunt is functioning properly. Many neurosurgeons obtain a CT scan of the brain before discharge to ensure that the ventricular catheter is in proper position and the ventricles reduced in size.

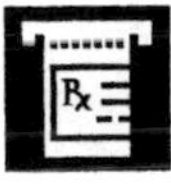

Medications

DRUG(S) OF CHOICE

- Prior to the widespread use of CSF shunts, medical treatment to limit CSF production with acetazolamide (a carbonic anhydrase inhibitor) and furosemide was used as a temporizing measure. These drugs did not provide a permanent solution for hydrocephalus and play no role in the modern management of the condition. Mannitol can be used to acutely lower ICP in an emergency situation.

ALTERNATIVE DRUGS

- No specific alternative drugs are used to treat hydrocephalus.

Follow-Up

PATIENT MONITORING

- CSF shunt devices are associated with a high failure rate (40% at 1 year) and infection rate (5%–10%). As such, patients with shunt devices *in situ* require immediate attention should they develop symptoms of shunt failure. Symptoms of shunt failure or obstruction are similar to those of untreated hydrocephalus and include headache, nausea and vomiting, and a decreased level of consciousness. Evaluation of the patient with a suspected shunt malfunction includes a CT scan of the head and a "shunt series" (a series of plain radiographs tracing the path of the shunt from the skull to the abdomen). In cases where shunt function is equivocal, a radionuclide shunt study can be undertaken to determine if the shunt is patent. Shunt infection can manifest as a shunt obstruction or as fever with no other identifiable source. Shunt infection can be diagnosed by sampling CSF from the shunt reservoir. When shunt malfunction or infection is suspected, immediate referral to a neurosurgeon is indicated. It is not uncommon for a shunted patient to develop subdural fluid collections, which can indicate CSF overdrainage. Many neurosurgeons monitor asymptomatic patients on an annual basis with a CT scan and shunt series.

EXPECTED COURSE AND PROGNOSIS

- CSF shunting devices are associated with a high failure rate. Prior to the development of an adequate surgical treatment of hydrocephalus, the outcome was universally poor. With the use of shunts, mortality for infants with non-tumor-related hydrocephalus has dropped from 64% to 3%–10%. Seventy percent are socially independent and <10% are unemployable.

PATIENT EDUCATION

- Patients and families of those with treated hydrocephalus, either by a CSF shunting device or ETV, should be educated as to the signs and symptoms of shunt failure and to seek prompt medical attention should they develop. Patients with CSF shunts can pursue all regular activities.
- Hydrocephalus Association of America
- Spina Bifida and Hydrocephalus Association of Canada

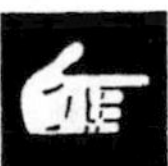

Miscellaneous

SYNONYMS

N/A

ICD-9-CM: 331.30 Communicating hydrocephalus; 331.40 Obstructive hydrocephalus

SEE ALSO: N/A

REFERENCES

- Drake JM, Kestle J, Milner R, et al. Randomized trial of cerebrospinal fluid shunt valve design in pediatric hydrocephalus. Neurosurgery 1998;43:294–305.
- Drake JM, Sainte-Rose C. The shunt book. New York, Blackwell Scientific, 1995.
- Hoppe-Hirsch E, Laroussinie F, Brunet L, et al. Late outcome of the surgical treatment of hydrocephalus. Childs Nerv Syst 1998;14:97–99.
- Laurence K, Coates S. The natural history of hydrocephalus: detailed analysis of 187 unoperated cases. Arch Dis Child 1962;37:345–362.
- Pudenz RH. The surgical treatment of hydrocephalus: an historical review. Surg Neurol 1981;15:15–26.
- Rekate H. Hydrocephalus classification and pathophysiology. In: McClone DG, ed. Pediatric neurosurgery. Philadelphia: WB Saunders, 2001:457–474.
- Schrander-Stumpel C, Fryns JP. Congenital hydrocephalus: nosology and guidelines for clinical approach and genetic counseling. Eur J Pediatr 1998;157:355–362.

Author(s): Patrick J. McDonald MD; Charles C. Matouk, MD

Hyperammonemia

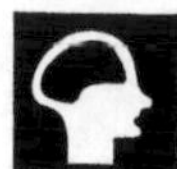

Basics

DESCRIPTION

- Ammonia is present in all body fluids as ammonium ion. Excess ammonia is excreted as urea. Impaired metabolism, from various causes, leads to hyperammonemia, which can cause serious CNS toxicity. This chapter focuses on hyperammonemia due to defects in urea cycle enzymes *N*-acetylglutamate synthetase, carbamyl phosphate synthetase I (CPS I), ornithine transcarbamylase (OTC), argininosuccinate synthetase (citrullinemia), argininosuccinate lyase (argininosuccinic aciduria), and arginase (argininemia).

EPIDEMIOLOGY

Prevalence

- Estimated to be 1 per 30,000 live births.

Age

- Usually seen in neonates; however, can present in childhood.

Sex

- Seen in both sexes.

Race

- Cases have occurred in all races.

ETIOLOGY

- Excess ammonia causes activation of *N*-methyl-D-aspartate (NMDA) receptors, which then activates Na-ATPase leading to ATP depletion and ammonia toxicity. Several other metabolic changes also are involved, such as increased lactate and pyruvate, and decreased glycogen and glutamate.

RISK FACTORS

N/A

PREGNANCY

N/A

ASSOCIATED CONDITIONS

- Urea cycle defects: include deficiencies of *N*-acetylglutamate synthetase, CPS I, OTC, argininosuccinic acid synthetase, argininosuccinic lyase and arginase
- Other metabolic: organic acidemias, congenital lactic acidoses, fatty acid oxidation defects, dibasic amino acid transport defects
- Transient hyperammonemia of the newborn
- Reye syndrome
- Hepatic dysfunction

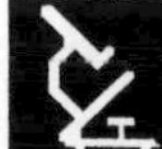

Diagnosis

DIFFERENTIAL DIAGNOSIS

- Because the clinical presentation is nonspecific, differential diagnosis of hyperammonemia depends on laboratory studies.
- Hyperammonemia with respiratory alkalosis is caused by a urea cycle defect or transient hyperammonemia of the newborn. The presence of acidosis, ketosis, and low bicarbonate, along with hyperammonemia, suggests an organic acidemia. Hyperammonemia, in addition to acidosis, ketosis, and increased lactate, indicates congenital lactic acidoses.
- Differential diagnosis for late-onset cases of hyperammonemia also includes liver disease and Reye syndrome. Hepatic transaminases would be elevated in both conditions, but in Reye syndrome bilirubin level would be within normal range.
- Determination of orotic acid and plasma citrulline can help identify the enzyme deficiency. OTC deficiency is associated with elevated urinary orotic acid and trace citrulline level. Plasma citrulline level is very high in AS deficiency ($>1,000$ μmol/L) and moderately high (100–300 μmol/L) in AL deficiency.

SIGNS AND SYMPTOMS

- In neonates, the presentation is nonspecific. Symptoms include poor feeding, lethargy, and vomiting and can lead to coma.
- Patients with partial enzyme deficiencies have a delayed onset and may present with recurrent episodes of vomiting, lethargy, ataxia, and behavioral changes.
- Patients with argininemia present with spastic diplegia.
- Fragile hair (trichorrhexis nodosa) is seen in argininosuccinic aciduria.

LABORATORY PROCEDURES

- Plasma ammonia level (usually >300 μmol/L), arterial blood gas (shows respiratory alkalosis), plasma and urinary amino acid analysis, organic acid and orotic acid determination

IMAGING STUDIES

- CT or MRI of brain may show cerebral edema.

SPECIAL TESTS

- Assay for specific enzymes on liver biopsy specimen. DNA analysis is available for OTC deficiency.

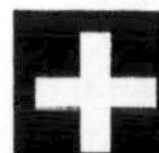

Management

GENERAL MEASURES

- Neonates should be admitted to a neonatal intensive care unit with hemodialysis facilities. No protein intake. Caloric intake in the form of hypertonic glucose and lipids. Monitor ammonia level. Treat any underlying infection.

SURGICAL MEASURES

- Liver transplantation for patients with urea cycle defects

SYMPTOMATIC TREATMENT

- Intravenous sodium benzoate and phenylacetate. Hemodialysis if patient is comatose at presentation or if the ammonia level remains high after several hours of IV treatment.

ADJUNCTIVE TREATMENTS

- Arginine supplementation because it is an essential amino acid for patients with urea cycle defects.

ADMISSION/DISCHARGE CRITERIA

- Admission needed when patients present in hyperammonemic state with an altered mental status, dehydration, or not controlled by oral medications.

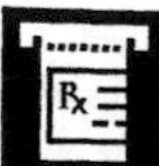

Medications

DRUG(S) OF CHOICE

- Sodium benzoate, sodium phenylacetate, sodium phenylbutyrate. These drugs lower ammonia levels by conjugating with amino acids. Available in IV and oral formulation.

Contraindications

- Hypersensitivity

Precautions

- Due to high sodium content, avoid in congestive heart failure or renal insufficiency. Benzoate may worsen neonatal hyperbilirubinemia by competing with bilirubin for the binding sites on albumin.

ALTERNATIVE DRUGS

N/A

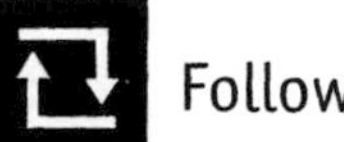

Follow-Up

PATIENT MONITORING

- Growth and development of children. Periodic levels of ammonia, arginine and glutamine.

EXPECTED COURSE AND PROGNOSIS

- Strict adherence to the dietary recommendations and compliance with medications should result in adequate growth and a decrease in episodes of acute hyperammonemia. Overall, there is considerable risk of mortality during acute episodes, and the majority of survivors will have significant cognitive delays.

PATIENT EDUCATION

- Depends on the specific disease entity

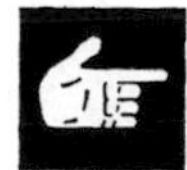

Miscellaneous

SYNONYMS

N/A

ICD-9-CM: 270.6 Hyperammonemia (congenital)

SEE ALSO: ENCEPHALOPATHY, HEPATIC; ENCEPHALOPATHY, PROGRESSIVE PEDIATRIC

REFERENCES

- Albrecht J. Roles of neuroactive amino acids in ammonia neurotoxicity. J Neurosci Res 1998;51:133–138.
- Batshaw ML. Inborn errors of urea synthesis. Ann Neurol 1994;35:133–141.
- Batshaw ML, MacArthur RB, Tuchman M. Alternative pathway therapy for urea cycle disorders: twenty years later. J Pediatr 2001;138[1 Suppl]:546–554.
- Brusilow SW, Horwich AL: Urea cycle disorders. The metabolic and molecular bases of inherited disease. New York: McGraw-Hill 1995;1:1187–1232.
- Consensus statement from a Conference for the Management of Patients with Urea Cycle Disorders. J Pediatr 2001;138:S1–S5.
- Feillet F, Leonard JV. Alternative pathway therapy for urea cycle disorders. J Inherit Metab Dis 1998;21[Suppl 1]:101–111.
- Prasad AN, Breen JC, Ampola MG. Argininemia: a treatable cause of progressive spastic diplegia simulating cerebral palsy: case reports and literature review. J Child Neurol 1997;12:301–309.
- Schaefer F, Straube E, Oh J. Dialysis in neonates with inborn errors of metabolism. Nephrol Dial Transplant 1999;14:910–918.
- Uchino T, Endo F, Matsuda I. Neurodevelopmental outcome of long-term therapy of urea cycle disorders in Japan. J Inherit Metab Dis 1998;21[Suppl 1]:151–159.

Author(s): Kazi Imran Majeed, MD

Hypotonic Infant Syndrome

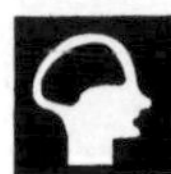

Basics

DESCRIPTION

- The term *hypotonic infant* refers to an infant with hypotonia or decreased muscle tone. Muscle tone is controlled by afferent muscle spindles and α- and γ-motor neurons in the spinal cord, but also is affected by upper motor neurons and corticospinal tract. Hypotonia is characterized by diminished resistance to passive movements and an excessive range of joint mobility. Hypotonic infant syndrome may be seen with severe muscle weakness, but also with only mild weakness or even without obvious weakness.

EPIDEMIOLOGY

Incidence

- Hypotonic infant syndrome is commonly seen in the clinical practice; however, its incidence is not known because it is seen with a large variety of diseases.

Race

- It is seen in all races.

Age

- Occurs more often in the newborn period and the first year of life.

Sex

- Both sexes are affected.

ETIOLOGY

- Lesions at any level of the nervous system, including upper and lower motor units, can cause hypotonia. Hypotonia combined with severe muscle weakness usually is associated with lower motor neuron disorders, including diseases affecting anterior horn cells of the spinal cord, peripheral nerves, neuromuscular junctions, and muscles. Hypotonia without obvious weakness often points to diseases of the central nervous system, connective tissue disorders, and chromosomal diseases, or those involving metabolic, endocrine, or nutritional problems.

RISK FACTORS

N/A

PREGNANCY

N/A

ASSOCIATED CONDITIONS

N/A

Diagnosis

DIFFERENTIAL DIAGNOSIS

- Hypotonia with prominent weakness (lower motor unit disorders): spinal muscular atrophy, congenital myotonic dystrophy, congenital muscular dystrophy, neonatal myasthenia gravis, congenital myasthenic syndrome, congenital myopathies, metabolic myopathies (Pompe's disease, mitochondrial myopathy), hereditary motor and sensory neuropathies, Guillain-Barré syndrome, tick paralysis, infantile botulism
- Hypotonia without prominent weakness:
  - —Cerebral hypotonia: perinatal hypoxia, birth trauma, Down's syndrome, Prader-Willi syndrome, Zellweger syndrome, Riley-Day syndrome, neonatal adrenoleukodystrophy, infantile G_{M1} gangliosidosis
  - —Intrauterine infections (toxoplasmosis, rubella, cytomegalovirus, herpes)
  - —Metabolic, endocrine, nutritional problems: biotinidase deficiency, amino acidosis, organic acidosis, renal tubular acidosis, calcium abnormalities, hypothyroidism, celiac disease, malnutrition
  - —Connective tissue disorders: Ehlers-Danlos syndrome, Marfan syndrome
  - —Acute illness
  - —Benign congenital hypotonia

SIGNS AND SYMPTOMS

- Hypotonia with little or no weakness, normal or increased deep tendon reflexes, craniofacial dysmorphic features, Babinski sign, ankle or knee clonus, or other brain dysfunctions such as language delay, mental retardation, progressive intellectual decline, seizures, aggressive behavior problems, or attention deficit hyperactivity often indicate upper motor unit diseases that affect the cerebrum, cerebellum, brainstem, or spinal cord above anterior horn cells.
- In contrast, hypotonia with significantly severe muscle weakness and atrophy, decreased or absent deep tendon reflexes, and fasciculation, but without Babinski sign or clonus, frequently suggest lower motor unit diseases involving anterior horn cells, peripheral nerves, neuromuscular junction, or muscles. However, there are diseases with both upper and lower motor unit involvements, such as mitochondrial encephalomyopathy, congenital myotonic dystrophy, and metachromatic leukodystrophy.
- Medically treatable hypotonia refers to a condition that can be corrected with specific medical treatment. Hypothyroidism due to thyroid hormone deficiency may present with hypotonia, constipation, failure to thrive, developmental delay, jaundice, and retardation of bone growth. Left untreated, the infant with congenital hypothyroidism may develop mental retardation. Biotinidase deficiency may present with hypotonia, seizures, ataxia, alopecia, skin rash, developmental delay, sensorineural deafness, and lactic acidosis. With early biotin treatment, the clinical features may be reversible. Neonatal myasthenia gravis may present with hypotonia, severe generalized weakness, and respiratory failure, but would be responsive to anticholinesterase treatment. Infantile botulism due to *Clostridium botulinum* toxins occurs in previously healthy infants in the first few months of life, with sudden generalized weakness, hypotonia, poor sucking and swallowing, constipation, ptosis, dilated pupils with sluggish light reflex, lethargy, and respiratory distress. With timely proper ventilatory support, complete recovery is possible; without it, the infant may suffer from respiratory arrest or even sudden death. Infantile Guillain-Barré syndrome is characterized by progressive generalized weakness and areflexia, hypotonia, and respiratory failure. It is immune induced and responsive to intravenous immunoglobulin and plasmapheresis. Tick paralysis is caused by the persistent tick bite with secretion of its toxin, leading to sudden generalized weakness and areflexia, and hypotonia in a formerly normal child. With timely removal of the tick, the child will rapidly and completely become normal.

LABORATORY PROCEDURES

- For lower motor unit diseases:
  - —Serum creatine kinase may be increased in a variety of muscle disorders and some spinal muscular atrophy, and should be done before electromyography and nerve conduction studies.
  - —Blood DNA tests may detect survival motor neuron gene homozygous deletions for spinal muscular atrophy, abnormal CTG trinucleotide repeat expansion for congenital myotonic dystrophy, and mitochondrial DNA mutations of some mitochondrial encephalomyopathies such as mitochondrial encephalomyopathy, lactic acidosis, and strokelike episodes.
  - —Other: stool for culture and exotoxin detection of *C. botulinum* in infantile botulism; CSF for albuminocytologic dissociation in Guillain-Barré syndrome; serum acetylcholine receptor antibodies for myasthenia gravis
- For upper motor unit diseases:
  - —Chromosomal studies for Down's syndrome, Prader-Willi syndrome, and other chromosomal disorders

—Serum studies: very long chain fatty acids for neonatal adrenoleukodystrophy; amino and organic acids, lactate, pyruvate, ammonia, carnitine for disorders of amino acids, organic acids, lactic acids, and urea cycle; lysosomal enzymes for lysosomal disorders; thyroid hormones for hypothyroidism; antibody titers for intrauterine infections (toxoplasmosis, rubella, cytomegalovirus, herpes)

IMAGING STUDIES

- Cranial MRI may detect intracranial ischemia or hemorrhage, increased T2 density of the white matter in the adrenoleukodystrophy or metachromatic leukodystrophy, periventricular calcification for congenital cytomegalovirus infection, diffuse intracranial calcification in congenital toxoplasmosis, and a variety of other brain anomalies. In mitochondrial encephalomyopathy, it may reveal basal ganglia calcification, or cerebral or cerebellar atrophy. Cranial ultrasound study may be necessary at the bedside for neonatal birth asphyxia when MRI is impossible because of the intubation and respiratory support of critically sick and unstable neonates.

SPECIAL TESTS

For Lower Motor Neuron Diseases:

- Electromyography is abnormal in the muscle diseases. Motor and sensory nerve conduction velocity study is useful in the evaluation of peripheral neuropathy.
- Muscle or nerve biopsy may be indicated if there is evidence of myopathy or neuropathy and for more specific diagnosis of the muscle disorders and neuropathy. Muscles may be examined for the specific histochemical staining and special enzymes studies for Pompe's disease, mitochondrial myopathy, specific congenital myopathies, muscular dystrophies, and other studies.
- Repetitive nerve stimulation with low frequency (2–3 Hz) often induces decremental response in myasthenia gravis, whereas stimulation with higher frequency (20–50 Hz often induces incremental response in infantile botulism.
- Edrophonium (Tensilon) IV infusion rapidly and dramatically improves the clinical features of myasthenia gravis, such as ptosis, extraocular ophthalmoplegia, and generalized weakness.

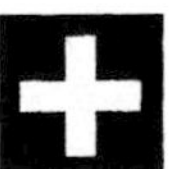

Management

GENERAL MEASURES

- Specific treatment depends on the underlying cause of hypotonia. For example, myasthenia gravis patients will require anticholinesterase such as pyridostigmine or neostigmine. Guillain-Barré syndrome may need plasmapheresis or intravenous immunoglobulin, or even respiratory support. Hypothyroidism requires treatment with thyroid hormone. Biotin replacement is needed for biotinidase deficiency. Tick paralysis requires removal of the tick from the skin of the patient.

SURGICAL MEASURES

- Gastrostomy tube placement and Nissen fundoplication may be required if the patients have severe feeding problems and gastroesophageal reflux. Tenotomy, and tendon transfer or lengthening may be useful for the routine daily care of the patients.

SYMPTOMATIC TREATMENT

- Feeding problems may need special nipples, small and frequent feedings, gavage feedings, or even gastrostomy tube. Postural drainage, suctioning, or vigorous respiratory therapy would be necessary if hypotonia and muscle weakness impair cough reflex or pulmonary functions. Stool softener, laxatives, or dietary control may help constipation. Early infant intervention provides useful stimulation.

ADJUNCTIVE TREATMENT

- Physical, occupational, speech, and language therapy may be helpful when poor fine motor coordination, muscle weakness, and language delay are present.

ADMISSION/DISCHARGE CRITERIA

- Patients may need admission for acute evaluation and treatment of severe weakness associated with hypotonia, such as spinal muscular atrophy, congenital muscular dystrophy, neonatal myasthenia gravis, mitochondrial encephalomyopathy, and infantile botulism. They frequently also require long-term outpatient rehabilitation or follow-up.

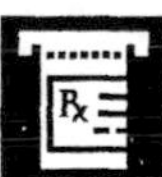

Medications

DRUG(S) OF CHOICE

- Intravenous immunoglobulin is easier for infants with Guillain-Barré syndrome. Intramuscular neostigmine given 30 minutes before feeding is useful for neonatal myasthenia gravis. Biotin is indicated for biotinidase deficiency. Thyroid hormone replacement is necessary for hypothyroidism.

Contraindications

- For intravenous immunoglobulin, congenital IgA deficiency, if complete, is a relative contraindication, because these patients may develop antibodies to IgA that can result in anaphylactic-like reaction.

Precautions

N/A

ALTERNATIVE DRUGS

- Plasma exchange may be useful if intravenous immunoglobulin fails to improve Guillain-Barré syndrome. Pyridostigmine or prednisone may be alternative drugs for myasthenia gravis.

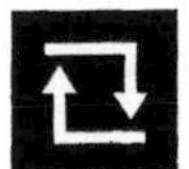

Follow-Up

PATIENT MONITORING

- Patients should be followed regularly after the underlying cause of hypotonia is identified. Patients with hypotonia may have progressive joint contractures or scoliosis and need proper treatment, such as physical therapy or braces. Other problems, such as seizures, may develop and require antiepileptic drug treatment.

EXPECTED COURSE AND PROGNOSIS

- The clinical course and prognosis depend on the underlying diseases of hypotonia.

PATIENT EDUCATION

- Many organizations associated with individual diseases exist to help support patients and their families and research to bring best treatments to the patients.

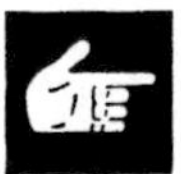

Miscellaneous

SYNONYMS

- Floppy baby syndrome

ICD-9-CM: 781.9 Floppy infant; 781.3 Hypotonia

SEE ALSO: N/A

REFERENCES

- De Vivo DC. The floppy infant syndrome. In: Rowland LP, ed. Merritt's textbook of neurology, 9th ed. Baltimore: Williams & Wilkins, 1995:503–506.
- Dubowitz V. Muscle disorders in childhood. Philadelphia: WB Saunders, 1995.
- Mason TBA II, DeVivo DC. The hypotonic infant. In: Younger DS, ed. Motor disorders. Philadelphia: Lippincott Williams & Wilkins, 1999:103–109.

Author(s): Chang-Yong Tsao, MD

Immunizations, Neurologic Complications

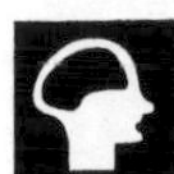

Basics

DESCRIPTION

- Central and peripheral nervous system injuries occur in temporal relationship to immunization in a small number of patients. Nervous system vaccine-related injuries include acute disseminated encephalomyelitis (ADEM), multiple sclerosis (MS), cerebellar ataxia, autism, encephalopathy/encephalitis, seizure disorder, deafness, mononeuropathy/multiplex mononeuropathy, brachial plexopathy, and Guillain-Barré syndrome (GBS). Virtually every vaccine has been reported to be associated with some form of nervous system injury. Although a causal role for vaccination is implied, such an association is rarely established.

EPIDEMIOLOGY

Incidence

- The incidence of vaccine-related neurologic injuries is unknown and varies with the type of injury. The encephalopathy associated with diptheria, pertussis, tetanus (DPT) immunization is reported to be 5 per 100,000 vaccinations in children <age 2, and death related to vaccination in the same age group is reported to be 0 in >29 million immunizations. Epidemiologic studies with prospective case-control designs have been most helpful in establishing or rejecting causality of vaccination to adverse events. In most of these studies, the overwhelming safety of vaccination has become apparent.

Age

- Although generally a disorder of childhood, serious adverse events after vaccination have been reported in adults.

Sex

- A preponderance in one gender has not been reported.

ETIOLOGY

- Injury is considered to be due to the active components of the vaccine or neurotoxicity of adjuvants, preservatives. or contaminants. Generally, the basis of injury is considered to be due to autoimmune "antigenic mimicry" in which the viral/bacterial protein immunogen shares homology with nervous system proteins, usually myelin. In rare instances when the vaccine is inactivated and nonvirulent but live virus/bacteria, injury to the nervous system can result from reactivation of the pathogen as with oral polio virus vaccines.

RISK FACTORS

- Congenital or acquired immunodeficiency states (various congenital immunodeficiency syndromes, cancer chemotherapy using cytotoxic drugs, pregnancy, chronic steroid therapy, HIV infection) can be associated with risk of injury to the nervous system. Most of these states are relative rather than absolute contraindications.

PREGNANCY

- Vaccinations are generally avoided during pregnancy because adverse reactions may occur. Pregnancy is a state of relative immune suppression during which otherwise benign viral infections can become fulminant. Live viral vaccines should be avoided because their virulence during pregnancy can be indeterminate. Live vaccines, such as rubella, can be associated with teratogenic effects in the fetus.

ASSOCIATED CONDITIONS

N/A

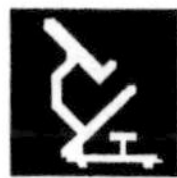

Diagnosis

DIFFERENTIAL DIAGNOSIS

- Includes acute infectious encephalitis, spongiform encephalopathies, metabolic encephalopathies, neoplastic and paraneoplastic disorders

SIGNS AND SYMPTOMS

- The interval from vaccination to injury can range from minutes (anaphylaxis) to 2–3 weeks (ADEM). The more remote the onset, the less likely the symptoms are related to the immunization. Disorders that manifest >6 weeks after immunizations are unlikely to be due to the vaccine, unless the early events after vaccination were clinically silent as is sometimes the case in demyelinating disorders. ADEM typically occurs within days or weeks after immunization. In its most fulminant form, alteration of consciousness can occur, leading to coma. Multifocal neurologic deficits are the rule, and multifocal abnormalities can be seen on MRI studies of the brain and spinal cord. Pathologic evaluation identifies inflammatory lesions in a perivascular distribution in association with primary demyelination. Patients can develop clinical manifestations of meningoencephalitis, optic neuritis, focal solitary lesions that mimic neoplasm, and single or multifocal level myelopathy.

LABORATORY PROCEDURES

- CSF studies: Spinal fluid studies are extremely helpful in diagnosis of ADEM. During the acute phase, CSF most often is normal for protein, cell count, and cultures. In fulminant cases, intracranial hypertension can be reflected in abnormally elevated opening pressures. A modest pleocytosis (50–100 cells) and mild elevation of proteins (always <100 mg/dL) may also be present. In children, predominantly lymphocytic pleocytosis is common, but a polymorphonuclear response can occur in the acute phase as well. In acute fulminant cases with hemorrhagic inflammation, RBCs can be present in the CSF, with xanthochromia as well. Although inflammation is the hallmark of ADEM, evidence of intrathecal IgG synthesis usually is not observed, and oligoclonal IgG bands are distinctly absent. This feature often is helpful in distinguishing ADEM from MS.
- CSF studies also are helpful in the diagnosis of GBS. The typical albuminocytologic dissociation (elevated protein without elevation of the cell count) can be useful for diagnosis.

IMAGING STUDIES

- MRI is the imaging modality of choice. If there are no lesions noted on MRI at the onset of suspected ADEM, imaging should be repeated in 3 weeks. If the MRI is consistently normal at 3 weeks or later, the diagnosis of ADEM should be questioned. Administration of gadolinium is useful in defining acute lesions. The lesions of ADEM can mimic the lesions of MS with a periventricular distribution, including corpus callosum lesions. Although complete resolution can occur clinically, demyelinated lesions can persist for life and result in subsequent confusion regarding diagnosis of MS. CT scan is helpful only if edema or herniation is present.

SPECIAL TESTS

- Immunologic studies: Although generally not the standard of care, patients who experience an adverse event following vaccination should undergo testing for congenital or acquired immune deficiency, including immunoglobulin and complement levels, and T- and B-cell (including CD4 and CD8 subsets) quantitation. Delayed-type hypersensitivity should be examined, with skin tests for common antigens. Preferably, all of these studies should be performed prior to the use of corticosteroids or immunosuppressive agents.
- There is good evidence that patients who develop ADEM have circulating lymphocytes sensitized to myelin basic protein and other myelin proteins.

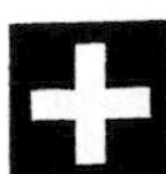

Management

GENERAL MEASURES

- Constitutional symptoms of headache, fever, malaise, and irritability are common in both children and adults with ADEM and should be managed using simple analgesics and antipyretics. Sleep disturbances may occur, particularly in children. Extreme irritability ("inconsolable crying of children"), well known to occur in encephalopathy following DPT, may require the use of sedatives. In general, however, narcotics and sedatives should be minimized because they can cloud assessment of mental status.

SURGICAL MEASURES

- In cases where solitary lesions are present and the diagnosis of a neoplastic process is a primary consideration, biopsy of the lesion may be necessary. In severe cases where increased intracranial pressure due to cerebral edema occurs, intracranial pressure monitoring may be necessary.

SYMPTOMATIC TREATMENT

- As above. Additionally, patients who develop GBS may require ventilator support during the acute phase of their illness.

ADJUNCTIVE TREATMENT

- Extensive rehabilitation with physical, occupational, and speech therapy may be necessary in patients with severe ADEM, GBS, brachial plexopathy, or severe mononeuritis multiplex.

ADMISSION/DISCHARGE CRITERIA

- There are no established criteria for admission or discharge; judgment should be used on an individual basis.

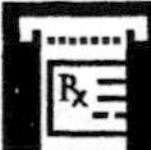

Medications

DRUG(S) OF CHOICE

- Corticosteroids are the mainstay of treatment of ADEM. In particular, severe cases with considerable edema can improve following steroid therapy. Pulse methylprednisolone, 1 gm IV every day or every other day for 5-g total dose is the standard treatment. Considerable improvement can occur in the following 2–4 weeks. Alternate therapies are best considered after a minimum of 3 weeks. In severe cases, where the response is suboptimal at the end of 2 weeks, consideration should be given for plasma exchange because there is good evidence that antibodies mediate the fulminant injury through activation of complement. Plasma exchange is carried out at exchange volumes of 5% of body weight every other day for a total of seven treatments. Oral steroid taper is not necessary except in a few steroid-responsive but steroid-dependent patients.

Contraindications

N/A

Precautions

- Steroids should be administered with caution in patients with hypertension, diabetes, and peptic ulcer disease. Although rare, use of high-dose steroids can be associated with aseptic necrosis of the femur. Psychosis may occur in some patients during administration. In the few patients requiring long-term oral steroids, prophylaxis with trimethoprim/sulfa is indicated for prevention of pneumonia secondary to *Pneumocystis carinii*.

ALTERNATIVE DRUGS

- Nontreatment is an acceptable alternative in any patient, especially patients with intolerance to steroids.

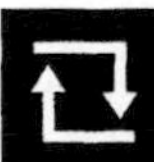

Follow-Up

PATIENT MONITORING

- Following recovery, long-term recurrences are rare. During steroid therapy, especially long-term oral steroid therapy, patients should be monitored regularly for steroid-related complications, including hypertension, glucose intolerance, infections, bone demineralization, GI discomfort, and weight gain.

EXPECTED COURSE AND PROGNOSIS

- Majority of patients make an uneventful recovery; most show complete recovery by 3 months. In the few patients who experience fulminant disease, mortality or severe morbidity can occur. The incidence of such events is unknown.

PATIENT EDUCATION

- The Vaccine Adverse Event Reporting System (VAERS) is a cooperative program for vaccine safety of the Centers for Disease Control and Prevention (CDC) and the Food and Drug Administration (FDA). VAERS is a postmarketing safety surveillance program that collects information on adverse events (possible side effects) occurring after the administration of US licensed vaccines. The VAERS website also provides a vehicle for disseminating vaccine safety-related information. *Website: www.vaers.org*

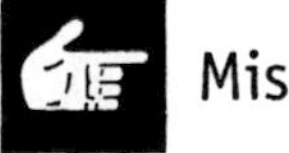

Miscellaneous

SYNONYMS

- Postinfectious encephalomyelitis
- Postimmunization encephalomyelitis

ICD-9-CM: 999.9 Complications, vaccination; 323.5 Encephalitis, encephalomyelitis, or myelitis

SEE ALSO: MULTIPLE SCLEROSIS; TRANSVERSE MYELITIS

REFERENCES

- Stratton KR, Howe CJ, Johnson RB. Adverse events associated with childhood vaccines. Evidence bearing on causality. Washington, DC: Institute Medicine, National Academy Press, 1994.
- DeStefano F, Verstraeten T, Jackson LA, et al. Vaccinations and risk of central nervous system demyelinating diseases in adults. Arch Neurol 2003;60:504.

Author(s): Kottil W. Rammohan, MD

Inclusion Body Myositis

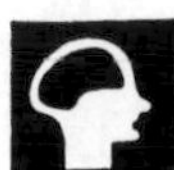

Basics

DESCRIPTION

- Sporadic inclusion body myositis (s-IBM) is an acquired idiopathic inflammatory myositis of insidious onset. It often is characterized by a specific pattern of proximal and distal weakness demonstrating early involvement of forearm flexors and quadriceps muscles. Clinical history, laboratory studies, EMG, and muscle biopsy are used to diagnosis and distinguish s-IBM from polymyositis or dermatomyositis.
- Hereditary inclusion body myopathies (h-IBM) includes a spectrum of hereditary myopathies, often within various ethnic groups, characterized by vacuolated myofibers containing filamentous inclusion, without inflammation. h-IBM may be autosomal dominant (limb-girdle distribution) or autosomal recessive (quadriceps sparing) and have many of the histochemical and ultrastructural changes seen in s-IBM.

EPIDEMIOLOGY

Incidence

- Less than 1 per 100,000 population. s-IBM may account for 15%–28% of all idiopathic inflammatory myopathies. It is considered the most common myopathy in persons $>$50 years of age.
- h-IBM is much rarer than s-IBM in general, although among Iranian Jews the prevalence is estimated at approximately 1 per 1,500.

Age

- s-IBM typically affects persons $>$50 years of age, although some may be as young as 30 years. h-IBM symptoms begin in the second or third decade.

Race

- *s-IBM:* No data are available; most case reports have been of Caucasians.
- *h-IBM:* Most reports include isolated pedigrees within ethnic groups (Iranian Jews, Japanese, and Tunisian kindreds), although one family from India and another Caucasian family from the United States have been reported.

Sex

- *s-IBM:* Male-to-female ratio is 3:1. *h-IBM:* Males and females are affected equally.

ETIOLOGY

- Unknown for both s-IBM and h-IBM. The presence of amyloid deposits within the myofibers of muscle biopsy specimens suggests a degenerative process. Endomysial inflammation in s-IBM, primarily CD8$^+$ T cells, invades non-necrotic myofibers, but it is unclear whether cellular inflammation is primary or secondary. Additional biopsy findings of ragged red fibers and cytochrome *c* oxidase (COX) negative fibers have suggested abnormal mitochondria. Mitochondrial DNA deletions have been detect in approximately 50% of 30 s-IBM patients studied. It is unclear whether these abnormalities are of pathogenic significance or are a secondary phenomenon.

Genetics

- s-IBM is associated with HLADR3, HLA-DR52 and HLA-B8 or HLA-DR3, HLA-DR52, and HLA-DQ2, and specifically (up to 77%) with DR1*0301, DR1*0101 (or DR3*0202), and DQ1*0201 alleles, suggesting an immunogenetic background. Human leukocyte antigen (HLA) testing currently is of no clinical utility.
- s-IBM has been seen among siblings of families and is thought to be related to genetic factors relating to the major histocompatability complex (HLA system).
- Both autosomal dominant and autosomal recessive syndromes have been seen among h-IBM. The autosomal recessive forms seen among Iranian Jews and in Japanese distal myopathy both have been linked to the same locus on chromosome 9p1-q1.

RISK FACTORS

- Other than a possible HLA association, no known risks have been documented in s-IBM. H-IBM often is associated with consanguinity.

PREGNANCY

- No increased risk or associations

ASSOCIATED CONDITIONS

- Other immune-mediated conditions (e.g., Sjögren's syndrome, rheumatoid arthritis) occur in approximately 10% of s-IBM cases. Nonspecific antibodies, such as positive ANA, rheumatoid factor, and SS-A, may be present in 40% of s-IBM cases and do not preclude the diagnosis of s-IBM.

Diagnosis

DIFFERENTIAL DIAGNOSIS

Distal Myopathies

- Welander distal myopathy
- Markesbery distal myopathy
- Nonaka distal myopathy
- Finnish tibial muscular dystrophy

Disorders with Rimmed Vacuoles

- Desmin storage myopathy
- Acid maltase deficiency
- Lysosomal storage disease with normal acid maltase
- McArdle syndrome
- Facioscapulohumeral dystrophy
- Oculopharyngeal muscular dystrophy
- Polymyositis
- Amyotrophic lateral sclerosis (ALS)

SIGNS AND SYMPTOMS

- *s-IBM:* Weakness $>$6 months, with selective involvement of biceps, triceps, flexor digitorum profundus, wrist flexors (greater than wrist extensors), quadriceps, tibialis anterior, iliopsoas, orbicularis oculi muscles, and sparing of deltoid muscles. Amyotrophy may also involve these muscles. Pattern of involvement is quite variable from case to case.
  —Normal, hypoactive, or absent reflexes
  —Dysphagia in up to 40%
  —Transient myalgias (20%)
- *h-IBM:* The hereditary inclusion body myopathies are a spectrum of myopathies whose classification is likely to undergo further revision with time. The two main patterns are an autosomal recessive diffuse weakness with quadriceps sparing and an autosomal dominant limb-girdle weakness with characteristic histologic features on muscle biopsy.

LABORATORY PROCEDURES

- Creatine kinase (CK) may be normal or elevated to 10–12 times normal

IMAGING STUDIES

- MRI or CT demonstrate selective amyotrophy of particular muscle groups but is not necessary for diagnosis.

SPECIAL TESTS

EMG

- Sensory nerve and compound muscle action potentials usually are normal.
- Needle EMG examination may reveal frequent fibrillation potentials and positive sharp waves, and low-amplitude, short-duration motor unit action potentials (MUAPs) or a mixed pattern of both low-amplitude, short-duration and high-amplitude, long-duration MUAPs (chronic myopathic changes).

Muscle Biopsy

Requirements

- Biopsy of involved but not end-stage muscle
- Use of frozen tissue; paraffin-embedded muscle fails to show the characteristic rimmed vacuoles within the myofibers
- Avoid biopsy of a muscle recently examined by EMG

Features of s-IBM

- Vacuolated myofibers (red-rimmed vacuoles on trichrome stain), central or subsarcolemmal 2- to 25-μm diameter, prominent in type I fibers, or evenly distributed between type I and II fibers
- Sparse-to-prominent endomysial inflammation and invasion of non-necrotic myofibers by cytotoxic (CD8$^+$) T cells

- Nuclear or cytoplasmic 15- to 18-nm tubulofilaments (electron microscopy) *or* amyloid deposition in myofibers
- Eosinophilic cytoplasmic inclusions
- Ragged red fibers (often cytochrome *c* oxidase negative)
- Required for muscle biopsy diagnosis of s-IBM

Features of h-IBM

- Muscle biopsy demonstrates many of the same features as in s-IBM, but no mononuclear cell inflammation.
- Ragged red fibers, cytochrome *c* oxidase negative muscle fibers, and mitochondrial abnormalities are seen less often in h-IBM.

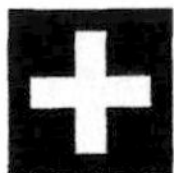

Management

GENERAL MEASURES

- Assistive devices (cane, walker) to prevent falls
- Occupational therapy to prevent contractures of the finger flexors

SURGICAL MEASURES

- Cricopharyngeal myotomy has been reported to relieve dysphagia in s-IBM if pharmacologic interventions fail.

SYMPTOMATIC TREATMENT

N/A

ADJUNCTIVE TREATMENT

N/A

ADMISSION/DISCHARGE CRITERIA

- These myopathies usually are assessed on an outpatient basis, although at end stage, morbidity associated with aspiration pneumonia or falls may necessitate inpatient admission.

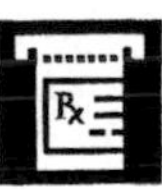

Medications

DRUG(S) OF CHOICE

- Currently, no medications have been shown to be consistently effective for treatment of s-IBM. Several can be tried. Corticosteroids 1–2 mg/kg occasionally stabilize weakness or temporarily prevent progression (in approximately 10% of patients). A 3- to 6-month prednisone trial may be considered and tapered or discontinued if there is no benefit. A previous diagnosis of "polymyositis refractory to corticosteroids" should lead one to consider reevaluation for possible s-IBM.

Contraindications

- Corticosteroids are contraindicated in patients with known hypersensitivity.
- Corticosteroids should not be used in persons with peptic ulcer, except in life-threatening situations.
- Corticosteroids should be used with extreme caution in patients with recent MI, because of an apparent association of corticosteroids and left ventricular free-wall rupture.

Precautions

- Corticosteroids may reduce resistance to and mask clinical signs of infection. Corticosteroids can reactivate tuberculosis, and chemoprophylaxis is used in patients with a history of active tuberculosis undergoing prolonged steroid treatment. Patients should be instructed to notify any surgeon, anesthesiologist, or dentist if a surgical procedure is required and they have recently (within 12 months) been taking glucocorticoids.
- Corticosteroids should be used with caution in persons with diverticulitis, nonspecific ulcerative colitis, cirrhosis, hypothyroidism, hypertension, psychosis, and congestive heart failure.
- Prolonged use of corticosteroids may cause adrenocortical insufficiency, and muscle wasting, pain, or weakness ("steroid myopathy").

ALTERNATIVE DRUGS

- Several double-blind, crossover trials of intravenous immunoglobulin (IVIG) alone or with prednisone failed to demonstrate statistically significant objective improvement in muscle strength, although regional improvements (such as dysphagia) may have been seen. IVIG doses used include 0.4 g/kg/day for 5 days or 1 g/kg/day for 2 days achieve a total dose of 2 g/kg.

Contraindications

- Avoid IVIG in hypoglobulinemia A (risk of anaphylaxis).

Precautions

- Headache, aseptic meningitis, nausea, emesis, irritation at site of infusion

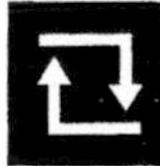

Follow-Up

PATIENT MONITORING

- Patient strength may be monitored at intervals of 6–12 months, with symptomatic treatment for dysphagia or falls as needed.

EXPECTED COURSE AND PROGNOSIS

- In the absence of definitive treatment, weakness progresses slowly and insidiously. There is an increased risk for aspiration pneumonia with dysphagia.

PATIENT EDUCATION

- Patients are told to expect slow and relentless progression of weakness. There is no evidence that a particular diet or dietary supplement is of benefit. Activity is encouraged as tolerated.
- Myositis Association of America, Inc. (MAA), 755 Cantrell Avenue, Suite C, Harrisonburg, VA 22801. Phone: 540-433-7686, web site: *http://www.myositis.org*
- National Organization for Rare Disorders, Inc. (NORD), P.O. Box 8923, New Fairfield, CT 06812-8923. Phone: 203-746-6518, toll-free: 800-999-6673, TDD: 203-746-6927, website: *http://www.rarediseases.org/*

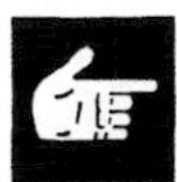

Miscellaneous

SYNONYMS

- IBM, s-IBM, h-IBM
- Familial IBM, f-IBM

ICD-9-CM: 359.8 Inflammatory myopathy for s-IBM; 359.1 Hereditary progressive muscular dystrophy for h-IBM

SEE ALSO: N/A

REFERENCES

- Askanas V, Engel WK. Newest approaches to diagnosis and pathogenesis of sporadic inclusion-body myositis and hereditary inclusion-body myopathies, including molecular–pathologic similarities to Alzheimer disease. In: Askanas V, Serratrice G, Engel WK, eds. Inclusion-body myositis and myopathies. New York: Cambridge University Press, 1998:3–78.
- Dalakas MC, Sonies B, Dambrosia J, et al. Treatment of inclusion-body myositis with IVIg: a double-blind, placebo-controlled study. Neurology 1997;48:712–716.
- Griggs RC, Askanas V, DiMauro S, et al. Inclusion body myositis and myopathies. Ann Neurol 1995;38:705–713.
- Koffman BM, Rugiero M, Dalakas MC. Immune-mediated conditions and antibodies associated with sporadic inclusion body myositis. Muscle Nerve 1997;21:115–117.
- Mendell JR. Sporadic inclusion-body myositis: clinical and laboratory features and diagnostic criteria. In: Askanas V, Serratrice G, Engel WK, eds. Inclusion-body myositis and myopathies. New York: Cambridge University Press, 1998:107–115.

Author(s): Boyd M. Koffman, MD, PhD

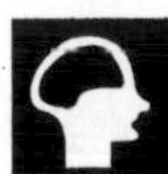

Basics

DESCRIPTION

- Normal bladder function requires the coordinated action of the bladder muscle (detrusor, smooth muscle), internal sphincter (bladder neck, smooth muscle), and external (striated muscle) sphincter. Normal function includes the ability to store urine with limited increase in intraluminal pressure, to initiate voiding voluntarily and to empty the bladder completely. Neural bladder function control occurs primarily in the sacral spinal cord, as well as the pons, diencephalon, and cerebral cortex. Parasympathetic innervation promotes detrusor contraction and sphincter relaxation, whereas sympathetic stimulation results in detrusor relaxation and sphincter contraction.
- Neurogenic urinary incontinence is a symptom resulting from damage to the nerves involved in bladder relaxation or bladder contraction and the coordination of the bladder neck mechanism.
- Common bladder problems associated with neurologic disorders include inability to store (detrusor hyperreflexia), inability to empty (hypotonic bladder/detrusor areflexia) with or without overflow incontinence, or a combination of the two (detrusor sphincter dyssynergia [DSD]).

EPIDEMIOLOGY

- Common occurrence as a result of damage to the integrity of the control mechanisms of the bladder in the central nervous system or to the peripheral nervous system.
- Affects all ages. both genders, and people of all social and economic levels.
- At least 1.5 million individuals have neuropathic bladder.

ETIOLOGY

- Neurologic diseases result in damage to the innervation of the lower urinary tract. If innervation of the lower urinary tract is damaged, it can affect the detrusor, urethra, and sphincter. Often the lesion is combined. Neurologic deficit can occur abruptly or more slowly over time.
- Lesions above the sacral micturition center typically result in loss of inhibition from higher centers, causing detrusor hyperexcitability, with or without sphincter hypertonia and DSD. Lesions at or below the sacral center will result in detrusor areflexia.

RISK FACTORS

- Risk factors are associated with specific conditions known to cause neurogenic bladder.
- Surgery
- Diabetes

PREGNANCY

- History of multiple pregnancies or obstetric trauma can lead to bladder dysfunction.

ASSOCIATED CONDITIONS

- Neurotrauma, brain tumor, meningitis-encephalitis, multiple sclerosis, Parkinson's disease, spinal cord injury, spinocerebellar degeneration, diabetes, stroke

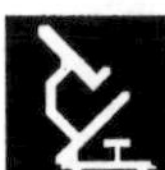

Diagnosis

DIFFERENTIAL DIAGNOSIS

- Unitary tract infection
- Stress incontinence
- Bladder prolapse
- Constipation
- Enlarged prostate
- Surgical complications

SIGNS AND SYMPTOMS

- Neurogenic incontinence presents at any time during the course of an illness. Initial symptoms are urinary urgency, frequency, hesitancy, nocturia, and then leakage of urine.
- Feeling of incomplete emptying, double voiding, nocturia, or a combination symptoms may be indicative of retention or DSD.

LABORATORY PROCEDURES

- Urinalysis/culture and sensitivity test to rule out bladder infection
- Measurement of postvoid residual (bladder ultrasound/intermittent catheterization)
- Urodynamic testing
- Cystoscopy

IMAGING STUDIES

- Ultrasound to identify the integrity of the organs (kidney, bladder, prostate)
- MR scan
- Intravenous pyelogram

SPECIAL TESTS

N/A

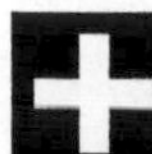

Management

GENERAL MEASURES

- Treatment requires identification of the underlying bladder dysfunction.
- Encouraging patients to keep a voiding diary can help identify symptoms
- Adequate daily fluid intake (48–64 oz/day) is encouraged.
- Avoid caffeinated beverages, aspartame, and alcohol, which are bladder irritants.
- Treat constipation.

SURGICAL MEASURES

- Suprapubic catheter
- Urinary diversion
- Bladder augmentation
- Botulinum toxin injections (detrusor or sphincter)

SYMPTOMATIC TREATMENT

- Quick access to bathroom
- Absorbent products and devices
- Timed voidings
- External catheters
- Intermittent catheterization
- Indwelling urethral catheter

ADJUNCTIVE TREATMENT

- Behavioral therapy/biofeedback to teach special exercises to help strengthen the pelvic floor muscle
- Physical therapy for mobility aids and equipment
- Occupational therapy for assistance with upper extremity function and manageable clothing and equipment (commode chair)

ADMISSION/DISCHARGE CRITERIA

N/A

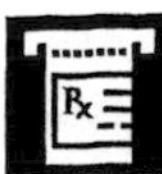

Medications

DRUG(S) OF CHOICE

- Anticholinergic and antimuscarinic agents (oxybutynin and tolterodine)
  - —Oxybutynin: 5–10 mg po bid–qid if cost is an issue
  - —Ditropan XL: begin at 5 mg po qd and increase as needed to 30 mg/day
  - —Detrol LA: 2 mg/day and increase as needed to 4 mg bid
- DDAVP (desmopressin)
  - —This synthetic antidiuretic hormone is useful in treating enuresis
  - —Nasal spray (one puff per nostril qhs) or tablets 0.1–0.2 mg qhs
  - —Caution required when prescribing DDAVP for patients >65. Additional concern about lower extremity edema.
- α-Blockers to relax sphincter
  - —Terazosin (Hytrin): 1 mg qhs and increase as needed to 10 mg/day (reevaluate if no response after 6 weeks)
  - —Quinazoline (Cardura): 1 mg qd, may double dose every 1–2 weeks to maximum 8 mg/day
  - —Tamsulosin HCl (Flomax): initially 0.4 mg/day, then increase to 0.8 mg after 2–4 weeks

Contraindications

- Anticholinergics and antimuscarinics should be avoided if there is suspicion of inability to empty.
- DDAVP should be used with caution in the elderly and in patients with lower extremity edema.

Precautions

- Risk of hypotension with anticholinergics and α-blockers

ALTERNATIVE DRUGS

- Herbal remedies
- Cranberry juice or tablets

Follow-Up

PATIENT MONITORING

- Patients are followed to monitor efficacy of intervention and overall symptom management.

EXPECTED COURSE AND PROGNOSIS

- Incontinence is relatively common and the clinical course may vary.
- There is risk of damage to the upper urinary tract, particularly in SCI.
- Worsening of neurologic symptoms with urinary tract infection usually is reversible after infection is treated.

PATIENT EDUCATION

- Support groups include disease-specific societies (e.g., MS Society, Parkinson's Support Group)
- National Association For Continence (NAFC) (formerly HIP [Help for Incontinent People]), P.O. Box 8310 Spartanburg, SC 29305-8310. Toll-free: 800-BLADDER, phone: 864-579-7900, fax: 864-579-7902, e-mail: memberservices@nafc.org, website: *www.nafc.org*
- National Bladder Foundation, P.O. Box 1095, Ridgefield CT, 06877. Phone 203-431-0005, website: *www.bladder.org*
- Simon Foundation for Continence, Box 835-F, Wilmette, IL 60091. Phone: 800-23SIMON, website: *www.simonfoundation.org*

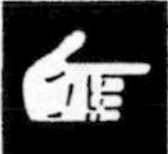

Miscellaneous

SYNONYMS

- Involuntary bladder
- Voiding dysfunction

ICD-9-CM: 596.54 Neurogenic bladder; 596.8 Bladder disorder, NEC; 596.9 Bladder disorder, NOS; 788.3 Incontinence (urinary incontinence); 788.43 Nocturia; 788.9 Bladder (urinary symptoms, NEC)

SEE ALSO: N/A

REFERENCES

- Appel RA. Evaluation and management of urologic disorders in multiple sclerosis. Mult Scler 1995;2:6–9.
- Betts CD, D'Mellow MT, Fowler CJ. Urinary symptoms and neurological features of bladder dysfunction in multiple sclerosis. J Neurol Neurosurg Psychiatry 1993;56: 245–250.
- Blaivas JG. Pathophysiology of lower urinary tract dysfunction. Urol Clin North Am 1985;12:215.
- Namey M. Management of elimination dysfunction. In: Halper J, Holland NJ, eds. Comprehensive nursing care in multiple sclerosis. New York: Demos Vermande, 1997:45–67.
- Schurch B, Stohrer M, Kramer G, et al. Botulinum-A toxin for treating detrusor hyperreflexia in spinal cord injured patients: a new alternative to anticholinergic drugs? Preliminary results. J Urol 2000;164[3 Pt 1]:692–697.
- Stover SL. Epidemiology of neurogenic bladder. Phys Med Rehabil Clin N Am 1994;4:211–220.
- Schmidt RA, Zermann DH, Doggweiler R. Urinary incontinence update: old traditions and new concepts. Adv Intern Med 1999;44:19–57.
- Urinary Dysfunction and Multiple Sclerosis, 1999, Clinical Practice Guidelines. Multiple Sclerosis Council for Clinical Practice Guidelines, Paralyzed Veterans of America, 1999.
- Urinary Incontinence Guideline Panel. Clinical Practice Guidelines. Urinary incontinence in adults: clinical practice guidelines. AHCPR Publication No. 96-0682. Rockville, MD: Agency for Health Care Policy an Research, Public Health Services, US Department of Health and Human Services, 1996.
- Wein AJ. Practical uropharmacology. Urol Clin North Am 1991;18(2):269–281.

Author(s): Marie A. Namey, RN, MSN; Francois Bethoux, MD

Increased Intracranial Pressure

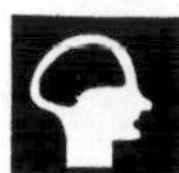

Basics

DESCRIPTION

- Increased intracranial pressure (ICP) is a result of the loss of the ability of the intracranial cavity to accommodate any further changes in the volume of its contents, with a subsequent rise in pressure within the skull. The increased ICP leads to a number of neurologic changes and may result in permanent neurologic injury or death. It is defined as a pressure >20 mm Hg when monitoring ICP.

EPIDEMIOLOGY

Incidence/Prevalence

- Varies significantly depending upon the etiology. Tumors, trauma, infections, and other causes all may impact the incidence and prevalence of increased ICP.

Race

- No predilection

Age

- No predilection

Sex

- No predilection

ETIOLOGY

- The Monro-Kellie doctrine states that the skull is a rigid structure containing three compliant elements: blood, brain, and the spinal fluid. These elements are compressible, and the sum of the pressures of each element contributes to the total ICP. With lesions affecting the brain parenchyma, producing cerebral edema, or other lesions compressing the brain tissue, blood and spinal fluid are forced out of the intracranial cavity. Once the compliance limit has been reached, usually around an ICP of 20 mm Hg, no more fluid is able to be forced out of the skull and the brain tissue begins to become displaced. After this point, any small changes in the volume of the lesion produce significant increases in ICP. Etiologies include
  —Obstruction of CSF pathways
  —Mass lesions, e.g., neoplasms, hematoma
  —Hemorrhages, e.g., subarachnoid hemorrhage, epidural, subdural, intraparenchymal
  —Venous obstruction, e.g., sagittal sinus thrombosis
  —Ischemic strokes
  —Brain injury
  —Infections, e.g., encephalitis, meningitis
  —Generalized seizures and status epilepticus
  —Hepatic encephalopathy
  —Malignant hypertension
  —Idiopathic, e.g., pseudotumor cerebri
  —Eclampsia

RISK FACTORS

N/A

PREGNANCY

- ICP is managed according to management principles outlined below, and the pregnancy is managed according to obstetric principles. Eclamptic states can lead to increased ICP.

ASSOCIATED CONDITIONS

N/A

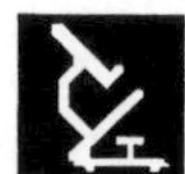

Diagnosis

DIFFERENTIAL DIAGNOSIS

- Increased ICP is a sign of other pathology and does not have differential diagnosis in itself. The inciting etiology will require diagnosis. These etiologies have been outlined above.

SIGNS AND SYMPTOMS

- Headache: common, may be positional, often worse after a period of recumbency. Tends to be generalized and nonfocal.
- Nausea/vomiting: described as "projectile," but this is not reliable. Any persistent vomiting, particularly when headache is present, should prompt a neurologic examination.
- Papilledema
- Blurry vision
- Ataxia
- Cranial nerve palsies, particularly cranial nerves VI and III, with lateral rectus weakness and pupillary dilation
- Diminished level of consciousness, coma
- Hemiparesis
- Cushing's triad: hypertension, bradycardia, and respiratory irregularity. A late finding, when a patient is in extremis. Classic triad seen only a third of the time, but any two of the findings should provoke concern for increased ICP.
- Decerebrate/decorticate posturing

LABORATORY PROCEDURES

- No specific blood work is indicated.
- If any neurosurgical intervention is required or pathology that may require rapid correction of coagulation parameters (such as intracranial hemorrhage) is present, blood should be drawn for a stat platelet count, PT, INR, and PTT, as well as a type and screen or type and cross
- Metabolic screen in cases of suspected metabolic disease.

IMAGING STUDIES

- CT scan
  —Method of choice
  —Performed on an urgent basis
  —Helps rule out surgically decompressible lesions
  —Provides information on the degree and location of cerebral edema, hemorrhage, ventricular size, and any bony abnormalities
  —ICP can only roughly be correlated to CT findings
- MRI
  —Little clinical value in the acute setting
  —Better definition of intraparenchymal lesions
- Angiography
  —Supplements above imaging studies
  —Useful to evaluate vasculitis, aneurysms, arteriovenous malformations, and other underlying vascular causes that may be contributing to increased ICP
- Skull films
  —Not useful

SPECIAL TESTS

- Lumbar puncture is *contraindicated* in cases of suspected increased ICP. The procedure can lead to cerebral herniation and death in a matter of seconds.
- Lumbar puncture may be performed once a CT scan has been obtained and no evidence of impending brain herniation is present.
- Funduscopy to evaluate for papilledema.

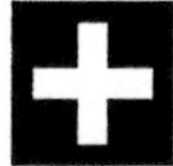

Management

GENERAL MEASURES

- Remembering the Monro-Kellie doctrine assists greatly in medically managing increased ICP, because changing the pressure of any of the three components will decrease the overall ICP. Although the brain contributes 80% of the intracranial volume, the parenchyma is one of the least easily manipulated contributors to ICP. The vascular component, only 10% of the intracranial volume, contributes a significant portion of the ICP that can be manipulated, because regulation of the cerebral vasculature can be easily altered via clinical means.
- To diminish intracranial vascular congestion:
  —Straighten the head
  —Slightly elevate the head to 30 degrees
  —Avoid jugular vein compression, e.g., cervical collars, endotracheal tube tape
  —Reduce positive end-expiratory pressure if the patient is on a ventilator
- To diminish the overall volume of blood and hence extravascular fluid:

- —Mannitol
- —Hyperventilation
  - -Acute early step in managing ICP
  - -Should not be maintained; this maneuver will rapidly diminish the ICP but can lead to ischemia and secondary brain injury
  - -Maintain P_aCO_2 approximately 30 to 35 mm Hg
- —Fluid status
  - -Maintain at two thirds to three fourths of daily maintenance requirements
  - -Avoid hypotonic solutions, e.g., 0.45NS or lactated Ringer solution
  - -Maintain euvolemia, even though using diuretics
- —Avoid hypotension; use pressors as required to keep systolic blood pressure >100
  - -Good evidence that hypotension worsens clinical outcome
- To medically diminish the contribution of cerebral parenchymal pressure to ICP:
  - —Maintain normothermia
    - -Increases of 1°C increases cerebral metabolic rate and, therefore, ICP by 5%–7%
  - —Maintain normal oxygenation
    - -Hypoxia worsens clinical outcome
  - —Barbiturate coma
  - —Antiepileptic medications when required
    - -Seizures increase all cerebral metabolic parameters and adversely affect patient outcome

SURGICAL MEASURES

- Consult neurosurgery early in all cases of increased ICP
- Placement of ICP monitoring devices
- No evidence that placement of ICP monitor changes outcome, but only helps to titrate therapy of increased ICP
- Ventriculostomy for spinal fluid drainage
- Removal of mass lesions, and necrotic or damaged brain tissue

SYMPTOMATIC TREATMENT

- Pain/agitation relief with narcotics, sedatives
  - —Use small doses to alleviate discomfort but not to obscure neurologic examination
- Seizure treatment
  - —Treat aggressively; seizures increase ICP rapidly
  - —May require barbiturate coma if ICP cannot be controlled
- Nausea/vomiting
  - —Antiemetics as required; may sedate patient and confound neurologic examination

ADJUNCTIVE TREATMENT

N/A

ADMISSION/DISCHARGE CRITERIA

- Any patient with increased ICP should be admitted to the hospital for diagnostic procedures, acute intervention, and continuous neurologic assessment.

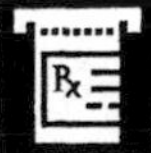

Medications

DRUG(S) OF CHOICE

- *Mannitol* 1 g/kg IV bolus, followed by 0.25–0.5 g/kg IV every 6 hours or more often as needed. Wean as clinical condition improves.
  - —Contraindications: hypotension, renal failure
  - —Precautions: hypotension, renal failure, overshoot of ICP when discontinued, worsening of congestive heart failure due to sudden increase in intravascular volume, hypokalemia, hyperglycemia, subdural hematomas
- *Loop diuretics*, e.g., furosemide, potentiate the effects of mannitol
  - —Contraindications: hypotension, renal failure
  - —Precautions: hypotension, renal failure, overshoot of ICP when discontinued, hypokalemia, hyperglycemia, subdural hematomas
- *Pentobarbital* 5–10 mg/kg IV bolus, followed by 1–2 mg/kg/hour IV, titrated to burst suppression on continuous EEG
  - —Contraindications: hypotension, cardiac compromise
  - —Precautions: hypotension, cardiac and respiratory depression, ileus, infection, loss of neurologic examination
- *Dexamethasone* 6–10 mg IV, only indicated with increased ICP due to neoplasms and encephalitis states; wean according to improvement in patient status
  - —Contraindications: diabetes, significant preexisting infection
  - —Precautions: hyperglycemia, predisposition to infection, electrolyte disturbances, avascular necrosis of hips

ALTERNATIVE DRUGS

N/A

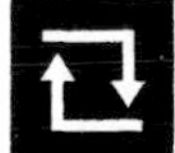

Follow-Up

PATIENT MONITORING

- Patients should be monitored closely with frequent vital signs and neurologic examinations by trained personnel.
- Arterial line, central venous catheter, and Swan-Ganz catheter where required.
- ICP monitor when indicated by neurosurgery.

EXPECTED COURSE AND PROGNOSIS

- Because the etiology of increased ICP may be varied, the overall course and prognosis depend upon correction of the underlying etiology.
- Signs of increased ICP that forebode a grave prognosis include
  - —Progressive increase in ICP despite aggressive medical management
  - —Signs of hypothalamic dysfunction, especially diabetes insipidus
  - —Progressive instability of blood pressure despite treatment and elimination of causes
  - —Worsening or lack of recovery of neurologic function despite aggressive treatment
- Imaging findings consistent with a grave prognosis include
  - —Progressive collapse of the ventricular system
  - —Loss of the basal cisterns
  - —Progressive cerebral edema despite aggressive medical and surgical management

PATIENT EDUCATION

N/A

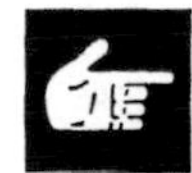

Miscellaneous

SYNONYMS

N/A

ICD-9-CM: 331.3 Communicating hydrocephalus; 331.4 Obstructive hydrocephalus; 348.2 Benign intracranial hypertension (pseudotumor cerebri); 348.4 Compression of brain; 348.5 Cerebral edema

SEE ALSO: N/A

REFERENCES

- Chestnut RM, et al. Medical management of intracranial pressure. In: Cooper PR, ed. Head injury. New York: Williams & Wilkins, 1993:225–246.
- Hughes M, Cohen WA. Radiographic evaluation. In: Cooper PR, ed. Head injury. New York: Williams & Wilkins, 1993:65–91.
- Rengachary SS, Duke DA. Increased intracranial pressure, cerebral edema, and brain herniation. In: Rengachary SS, Wilkins RH, eds. Principles of neurosurgery. London: Wolfe Publishing, 1994:2.0–2.14.
- Ropper AH. Treatment of intracranial hypertension. In: Ropper AH, ed. Neurological and neurosurgical intensive care. New York: Raven Press, 1993:29–53.

Author(s): Scott W. Elton, MD

Lambert-Eaton Myasthenic Syndrome

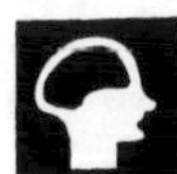

Basics

DESCRIPTION

- Lambert-Eaton syndrome (LES; myasthenic syndrome) is an autoimmune syndrome that results in a defect of neuromuscular transmission. Patients present with symptoms of weakness and autonomic dysfunction.

EPIDEMIOLOGY

Incidence/Prevalence

- Formal epidemiologic studies have not been performed, but LES is a rare neuromuscular disease and is much less common than myasthenia gravis. Although about two thirds of cases have an associated neoplasm (small cell lung carcinoma makes up 90% of these), only 1%–3% of patients with small cell lung carcinoma have LES.

Race

- No study has demonstrated any ethnic predominance.

Age

- LES is primarily a disease that occurs in older individuals. This is especially true for paraneoplastic cases. Cases of LES occurring before age 50 years are less likely to be associated with a tumor. There are case reports of children with LES.

Sex

- Males outnumber females by a 2:1 margin.

ETIOLOGY

- Paraneoplastic LES represents an autoimmune response against the presynaptic terminal of the neuromuscular junction. Antigenic similarity between the tumor (most often small cell lung carcinoma) and the presynaptic terminal results in antibody formation against the presynaptic voltage-gated calcium channels, which are responsible for the release of acetylcholine. The presynaptic terminal reduction in acetylcholine release produces the clinical symptoms. Decreased acetylcholine stimulation of nicotinic receptors on muscle results in weakness, whereas diminished stimulation of muscarinic receptors produces the autonomic symptoms. Cases not associated with a neoplasm (non-paraneoplastic) are less common but also are due to autoimmune dysfunction.

RISK FACTORS

- Smoking, small cell lung carcinoma, and age are the major risk factors. Other lung carcinomas, lymphoma, prostate cancer, cervical cancer, and thymomas are much less commonly associated with LES.

PREGNANCY

N/A

ASSOCIATED CONDITIONS

- Cancer-related LES may have other paraneoplastic syndromes, including encephalomyelitis and cerebellar degeneration. Other autoimmune diseases are associated with LES, such as systemic lupus erythematosus, pernicious anemia, thyroid disease, and myasthenia gravis.

Diagnosis

DIFFERENTIAL DIAGNOSIS

- Myasthenia gravis
- Peripheral neuropathy
- Polyradiculopathy
- Inflammatory myopathy
- Cachexia
- Other paraneoplastic diseases

SIGNS AND SYMPTOMS

- LES presents with slowly progressive weakness and fatigue. Weakness is more prominent in proximal muscles, especially in the lower extremities. After a brief period of muscle activation patients may regain strength, although this is not found in many patients. Muscle stretch reflexes are diminished and typically absent in the lower extremities. It may be possible to enhance reflexes by asking the patient to briefly activate the muscle and then checking the reflex. Muscle pain and paresthesias also can occur, although the sensory examination usually is normal. Autonomic symptoms occur in more than two thirds of all patients and include dry mouth, constipation, impotence, blurred vision, and micturition difficulties. Unlike myasthenia gravis, ocular and bulbar symptoms (ptosis, diplopia, dysphagia) are less prominent and occur in about one third.
- Patients with paraneoplastic LES may have other signs and symptoms due to overlap with other paraneoplastic syndromes. The most common is paraneoplastic cerebellar degeneration and encephalomyelitis.

LABORATORY PROCEDURES

- *Blood work:* A very high voltage-gated calcium channel antibody is strongly supportive of the diagnosis of LES; low titers may be seen in normal patients. High levels do not correlate with disease severity, however. A search for other autoimmune diseases may be performed, including acetylcholine receptor antibody, antinuclear antibody (ANA), and thyroid analysis.

IMAGING STUDIES

- In most cases of LES the symptoms precede the associated neoplasm by <18 months. For this reason, careful monitoring for a lung cancer is necessary, and it is recommended that older patients with a smoking history have a chest x-ray film, CT, or MRI at regular intervals.

SPECIAL TESTS

- There are reports of bronchoscopy detecting a lung carcinoma in the absence of radiologic evidence.

Electrodiagnostic Studies

- EMG is the most helpful test in confirming the diagnosis of LES. Low-amplitude compound muscle action potentials are found at rest, often <10% of normal. This is followed by a >100% increase after a few seconds of exercise. In addition, a decremental response at low rates of stimulation (2–5 Hz) and an incremental response at high rates of stimulation (20–50 Hz) may be found. Needle electrode examination may reveal unstable motor unit action potentials. In mild cases of LES the electrodiagnostic findings may resemble those of myasthenia gravis.

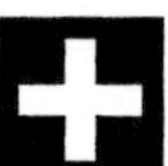

Management

GENERAL MEASURES

- Treatment of LES is geared toward identification and treatment of a potential tumor, medications that enhance neuromuscular transmission, and alteration of autoantibodies. Early and successful treatment of a lung carcinoma usually results in clinical improvement.

SURGICAL MEASURES

- A lung carcinoma may benefit from surgical resection in some cases.

SYMPTOMATIC TREATMENT

N/A

ADJUNCTIVE TREATMENTS

- If a carcinoma is identified, chemotherapy, radiation therapy, and other treatments are geared toward the lung carcinoma.

ADMISSION/DISCHARGE CRITERIA

N/A

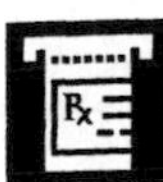

Medications

DRUG(S) OF CHOICE

- Pyridostigmine (Mestinon) inhibits acetylcholinesterase at the neuromuscular junction, resulting in more available acetylcholine for binding to receptors. Strength improvement is seen in some patients with LES, although usually to a mild degree. Dosages of 60 mg q4–6h are typically used. Cholinergic side effects are common and include abdominal cramps, diarrhea, and blurred vision.
- Guanidine hydrochloride increases the release of acetylcholine and may result in symptomatic improvement, especially when given with pyridostigmine. A beginning dose of 5–10 mg/kg/day is given, up to 30 mg/kg/day, divided throughout the day. Side effects include bone marrow suppression, chronic interstitial nephritis, renal tubular acidosis, arrhythmias, paresthesias, encephalopathy, and hepatic toxicity. CBC, LFT, and electrolytes need to be monitored periodically.
- 3,4-Diaminopyridine (DAP) enhances acetylcholine release by blocking potassium channels and results in strength improvement in most patients with LES. A dosage range from 5 mg tid to 25 mg qid is used. Higher dosages are associated with paresthesias, insomnia, and seizures. Cholinergic side effects are similar to those of pyridostigmine. Although DAP is beneficial and is more efficacious than pyridostigmine or guanidine, it is not yet available in the United States, except as on a compassionate-use basis. Pyridostigmine may enhance the effect of DAP. Side effects include paresthesias in the extremities and mouth, and seizures with higher dosages. Cholinergic side effects are common when used with pyridostigmine.
- Immunosuppressants such as prednisone and azathioprine often are used in the treatment of LES and are of benefit in some patients. Azathioprine can minimize the needed dose of prednisone due to its steroid-sparing effects.
- Patients with severe weakness or a rapidly progressive course may benefit from a course of plasmapheresis or intravenous immunoglobulin (IVIG). The effects are short lived, and repeated treatments may be necessary.

Contraindications

- Medications that interfere with neuromuscular transmission can worsen the symptoms of LES. This includes aminoglycoside antibiotics, penicillamine, β-adrenergic blockers, calcium channel blockers, anesthetic neuromuscular blocking agents, quinidine, and iodinated contrast agents.

Precautions

N/A

ALTERNATIVE DRUGS

- Cyclosporine may be beneficial to patients who do not respond to prednisone or cannot tolerate azathioprine.

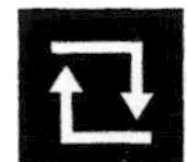

Follow-Up

PATIENT MONITORING

- Careful monitoring for a lung tumor is the most important factor for older individuals with LES. Young patients with other autoimmune diseases in whom a tumor is not found 5 years into the course are very unlikely to develop a lung cancer, and repeated testing is not necessary.

EXPECTED COURSE AND PROGNOSIS

- LES is a chronic disease. Identification of a tumor is the most important prognostic factor in paraneoplastic LES. Symptomatic treatment is less effective if a primary tumor is not identified and treated. Patients with nonneoplastic disease may have a clinical remission after immunosuppressive treatment.

PATIENT EDUCATION

- Information about LES and support groups is available through the Myasthenia Gravis Foundation of America, 123 W. Madison Street, Suite 800, Chicago, IL 60602. Phone: 312-853-0522; website: *www.myasthenia.org/*

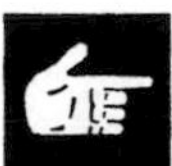

Miscellaneous

SYNONYMS

N/A

ICD-9-CM: 358.1 Myasthenic syndrome

SEE ALSO: N/A

REFERENCES

- O'Neill JH, Murray NMF, Newson-Davis J. The Lambert-Eaton myasthenic syndrome: a review of 50 cases. Brain 1988;111: 577–596.
- Lennon VA, Lambert EH. Autoantibodies bind solubilized calcium channel-omega-conotoxin complexes from small cell lung carcinoma: a diagnostic aid for Lambert-Eaton myasthenic syndrome. Mayo Clin Proc 1989;64:1498.
- Tim RW, Massey JM, Sanders DB. Lambert-Eaton syndrome (LEMS): clinical and electrodiagnostic features and response to therapy in 59 patients. Ann NY Acad Sci 1998;841:823–826.

Author(s): Brad Cole, MD

Leigh's Syndrome

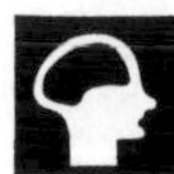

Basics

DESCRIPTION

- Leigh's syndrome (LS) is a subacute necrotizing encephalopathy caused by impaired oxidative energy production.

EPIDEMIOLOGY

Incidence/Prevalence

- Rare

Race

- No ethnic predominance has been reported.

Age

- LS usually affects infants (<2 year old) or young children, although a few cases with adult onset have been reported.

Sex

- Male predominance related to mitochondrial DNA mutations (maternal inheritance)

ETIOLOGY

Biochemistry

- Several isolated or combined defects of the mitochondrial respiratory chain have been associated with LS: pyruvate dehydrogenase deficiency, cytochrome *c* oxidase deficiency, and complex I deficiency and complex II deficiency.

Genetics

- The mutation related to the syndrome can be found in up to two thirds of patients.
- Genomic DNA
  - —Pyruvate dehydrogenase complex, subunit E1α, in chromosome X (X-linked dominant)
  - —Complex I, subunit NADH ubiquinone oxidoreductase, in chromosome 11q13 (autosomal recessive inheritance)
  - —SURF1, in chromosome 9 (autosomal recessive inheritance), is a mitochondrial protein of unknown function; its mutation impairs cytochrome *c* oxidase activity
  - —Nuclear encoded flavoprotein subunit gene of sulfate dehydrogenase (complex II), in chromosome 5 (autosomal recessive inheritance).
- Mitochondrial DNA
  - —Several ATPase 6 subunit mutations and mitochondrial tRNA mutations have been associated with LS (maternal inheritance). The two most common mutations are T8993C and T8993G in the ATPase 6 subunit. Some of the mitochondrial mutations described in LS have been reported in association with other specific phenotypes in older patients: in NARP (neuropathy, ataxia, retinitis pigmentosa), MERFF (myoclonic epilepsy and ragged red fibers), and MELAS (mitochondrial Myopathy encephalopathy, lactic acidosis, strokelike episodes).

RISK FACTORS

N/A

PREGNANCY

- Adult onset of LS is rare. In this event, females should avoid pregnancy due to the morbidity associated with LS.

ASSOCIATED CONDITIONS

- Pearson syndrome

Diagnosis

DIFFERENTIAL DIAGNOSIS

- In children
  - —Pearson syndrome
  - —Infantile beriberi
  - —Lactic acidemia with biotinidase deficiency
- In adults
  - —Multiple sclerosis
  - —Familial spastic paraplegia ("complicated" phenotype)
  - —In sporadic cases, other causes of brainstem dysfunction

SIGNS AND SYMPTOMS

- LS is characterized by a variable combination of retarded motor and intellectual development, seizures, dystonia, swallowing and feeding difficulties, vomiting, ataxia, external ophthalmoplegia, impaired hearing and vision, and peripheral neuropathy. Children may develop acute respiratory distress.
- Differences in clinical presentation have been found associated with specific enzymatic defects:
  - —Cytochrome *c* oxidase associated-LS: Symptoms develop after 6 months and have a milder course. Patients rarely have seizures.
  - —Pyruvate dehydrogenase associated-LS and maternally inherited LS: Symptoms develop in the neonatal or early infantile period. Patients usually have seizures and recurrent apnea.

LABORATORY PROCEDURES

- *Blood work:* Lactic acidosis and high pyruvate blood level are common findings that support the diagnosis of LS in the presence of typical MRI lesions. However, normal lactic acid and pyruvate blood levels do not rule out the diagnosis.
- *CSF:* CSF lactate and pyruvate levels usually are high (>2.2 mmol/L for lactate and 100 μmol/L for pyruvate) and are more sensitive and specific for the diagnosis of LS than blood levels when MRI lesions are typical.

IMAGING STUDIES

- *MRI:* T2 -weighted cranial MRI is more sensitive than CT to detect lesions of subacute necrotizing encephalomyelopathy. Increased signal intensity and edema are commonly found in the substantia nigra, caudate, putamen, and globus pallidus bilaterally and sometimes in tectum, tegmentum, and medullary olive. MRI scan is the most useful tool for premortem diagnosis of the disease.

SPECIAL TESTS

- *Muscle biopsy:* Muscle biopsy does not establish the diagnosis of the disease but may help in the identification of the biochemical defect. Cytochrome *c* oxidase activity and complex II can be investigated by histochemistry; complex I and pyruvate dehydrogenase activity should be assessed biochemically. Characteristically, ragged red fibers are hardly ever found in this disease.
- *Biochemical analysis in other tissues:* Skin fibroblasts, lymphocytes, and liver biopsy can be used for diagnosis of the biochemical defect. Skin biopsy is a less aggressive tool than muscle biopsy; however, the latter is more sensitive for detection of the biochemical deficiency. In addition, liver biopsy seems to be more sensitive than muscle biopsy for the diagnosis of LS, although no extensive data are available.
- *Needle stereotactic brain biopsy:* Only single cases have undergone this procedure, and findings were not useful for the diagnosis.
- *Postmortem evaluation:* Neuropathologic abnormalities include focal, bilaterally symmetric necrotic lesions extending from thalamus to the pons, as well as involving the inferior olives and the posterior columns. The lesions are spongiform and characterized by cystic cavitation, vascular proliferation, neuronal loss, and demyelination. Postmortem neuropathologic findings are especially useful to confirm the diagnosis in affected siblings.
- *DNA studies:* The identification of mutations known to be related to LS in genomic DNA usually is a research laboratory task; however, the study of some of the mitochondrial mutations associated to LS is routinely available, usually under the heading of mitochondrial DNA encephalomyopathy profile or NARP, MERFF, or MELAS profiles.

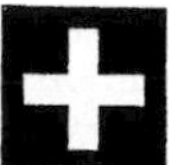

Management

GENERAL MEASURES

- Measures depend on the severity of the phenotype. In severe cases general support measures will be required: gastrostomy or feeding tube, ventilatory support, physical therapy, and symptomatic treatment of seizures and dystonia.

SURGICAL MEASURES

N/A

SYMPTOMATIC TREATMENT

- Same as for General Measures.

ADJUNCTIVE TREATMENT

N/A

ADMISSION/DISCHARGE CRITERIA

- Admission for LS is recommended to treat concurrent complications.

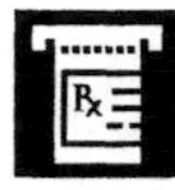

Medications

DRUG(S) OF CHOICE

- In pyruvate dehydrogenase deficiency:
  —Thiamine 100–1,000 mg/day, lipoic acid 100 mg/day, and dichloroacetate 50 mg/kg twice a day
- In complex I deficiency:
  —High-dose riboflavin supplementation (40–300 mg/day) has been attempted with variable success
- For the other biochemical defect no specific treatment is recommended; however it is common practice to try thiamine 100–1,000 mg/day and/or dichloroacetate 50 mg/kg twice a day.

Contraindications

- In the event general anesthesia is needed, volatile anesthetics should be avoided.

Precautions

- If LS is related to mitochondrial mutations, general recommendations for mitochondrial diseases should be followed: vigorous use of antipyretics and avoidance of drugs that are known to inhibit the respiratory chain (phenytoin, barbiturates) or the mitochondrial protein synthesis (tetracyclines).

ALTERNATIVE DRUGS

N/A

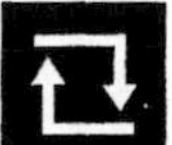

Follow-Up

PATIENT MONITORING

N/A

EXPECTED COURSE AND PROGNOSIS

- Prognosis seems to be related to the biochemical or genetic defect associated with LS:
  —In cytochrome *c* oxidase deficit, patients usually survive until age 5 or 6.
  —In pyruvate dehydrogenase defect, death commonly occurs between 6 and 12 months.
  —In complex I deficiency, prognosis depends on age of clinical presentation and the extent of organ involvement.
- Transient spontaneous remissions have been reported in one fourth of the patients.

PATIENT EDUCATION

- Activities: Avoid exhausting exercise.
- Diet: Ketogenic diet is recommended in pyruvate dehydrogenase deficiency.
- Organizations: Muscular Dystrophy Association. Website: *http://mdausa.org*

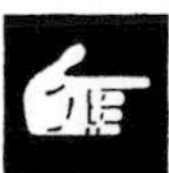

Miscellaneous

SYNONYMS

- Subacute necrotizing encephalomyelopathy

ICD-9-CM: 330.8 Leigh's disease or subacute necrotizing encephalopathy

SEE ALSO: N/A

REFERENCES

- Bourgeron T, Rustin P, Chretien D, et al. Mutation of a nuclear succinate dehydrogenase gene results in mitochondrial respiratory chain deficiency. Nat Genet 1995;11:144–149.
- Brown RM, Dahl HH, Brown GK. X-chromosome localization of the functional gene for the E1 alpha subunit of the human pyruvate dehydrogenase complex. Genomics 1989;4:174–181.
- De Vivo DC. Leigh syndrome: historical perspective and clinical variations. Biofactors 1998;7:269–271.
- DiMauro S, Bonilla E, De Vivo DC. Does the patient have a mitochondrial encephalomyopathy? J Child Neurol 1999;14[Suppl 1]:S23–S35.
- Loeffen J, Smeitink J, Triepels R, et al. The first nuclear-encoded complex I mutation in a patient with Leigh syndrome. Am J Hum Genet 1998;63:1598–1608.
- Morris AA, Leonard JV, Brown GK, et al. Deficiency of respiratory chain complex I is a common cause of Leigh disease. Ann Neurol 1996;40:25–30.
- Rahman S, Blok RB, Dahl HH, et al. Leigh syndrome: clinical features and biochemical and DNA abnormalities. Ann Neurol 1996;39:343–351.
- Swaiman KF. Aminoacidopathies and organic acidemias resulting from deficiency of enzyme activity and transport abnormalities. In: Swaiman KF, Ashwal S, eds. Pediatric neurology. St. Louis: Mosby, 1999:396–397.
- Zhu Z, Yao J, Johns T, et al. SURF1, encoding a factor involved in the biogenesis of cytochrome c oxidase, is mutated in Leigh syndrome. Nat Genet 1998;20:337–343.

Author(s): Carmen Serrrano-Munuera, MD

Leprous Neuropathy

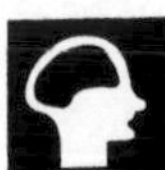

Basics

DESCRIPTION

- Leprosy is an infectious disease that mainly affects the skin, the peripheral nerves, the mucosa of the upper respiratory tract, and the eyes. Leprous neuropathy is the most common type of peripheral neuropathy worldwide. It is caused by direct bacterial infiltration of small-diameter peripheral nerves.

EPIDEMIOLOGY

- Leprosy is indigenous to Hawaii and portions of Florida, Louisiana, and Texas in the United States. It also is seen in immigrants from India, southeast Asia, and central Africa.

Incidence/Prevalence

- Prevalence of 0.9 million cases worldwide in 1996. It has been gradually but steadily declining over several decades.
- Prevalence exceeds 10 per 1,000 in endemic areas such as Asia and Africa.
- One hundred forty-four new cases in the United States in 1995. The majority of leprosy cases diagnosed in the United States are in immigrants from leprosy-endemic countries.

Race

- No racial predilection known

Age

- Leprosy can present at any age but is rare in infancy.

Sex

- Equal in children but 2:1 male preponderance in adults

ETIOLOGY

- The etiologic agent is *Mycobacterium leprae,* an acid-fast bacillus that grows best at 30°C (86°F), which explains its predilection for skin and peripheral nerves. Leprosy is transmitted via transfer of bacteria in nasal discharge of infected individuals to the respiratory tract of susceptible individuals, followed by hematogenous dissemination. The intensity of the cell-mediated immune response to the bacteria correlates with the type of disease expression. Patients with an intense cellular immune response develop disease types toward the tuberculoid end of the spectrum. Little or no cellular immune response is associated with development of lepromatous leprosy.

Genetics

- There is evidence that human leukocyte antigen (HLA)-associated genes influence the type of leprosy an individual develops.

RISK FACTORS

- Exposure to nasal discharge of individuals infected with leprosy

PREGNANCY

N/A

ASSOCIATED CONDITIONS

N/A

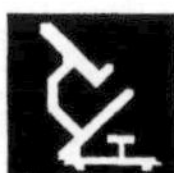

Diagnosis

DIFFERENTIAL DIAGNOSIS

- Leprosy should be considered in presentations with the combination of a skin rash and peripheral neuropathy. The differential also includes the broad differential of peripheral neuropathy.
  —Lupus erythematosus
  —Lupus vulgaris
  —Sarcoidosis
  —Yaws
  —Dermal leishmaniasis other causes of leprosy

SIGNS AND SYMPTOMS

- Indeterminate leprosy (initial infection)
- Solitary hypopigmented macule, which may resolve (about 75%) or persist to progress to one of the other types of leprosy.
- Classification of leprosy types is that of a continuous spectrum based on clinicopathologic features: lepromatous, borderline lepromatous, borderline, borderline tuberculoid, and tuberculoid.

Lepromatous Leprosy

- Multiple symmetric skin lesions affecting face (especially cheeks and nose), limbs, and buttocks, initially macular and evolving into plaques and nodules, typically fairly symmetric. Lesions centers are convex and indurated, and margins are ill defined.
- Nasal congestions and epistaxis
- Ocular: pain, photophobia, loss of vision, glaucoma
- Testicular: sterility, impotence, gynecomastia
- Sensory loss (especially pain, temperature) in distal limbs (palms and soles spared), pinnae of the ears, breasts, buttocks
- Nerve root enlargement, especially superficial nerves such as the greater auricular in the neck, ulnar, peroneal as it passes around the fibula, superficial radial, median
- Motor involvement is late: amyotrophy, clawhand, footdrop
- Reflexes preserved
- Cranial nerve involvement: preferentially V and VII (eye closure and perioral musculature)
- Lucio reaction or phenomenon, a type of necrotizing vasculitis that can occur in lepromatous disease with high mortality

Tuberculoid Leprosy

- Sharply marginated erythematous or hypopigmented macules or plaques that are solitary and asymmetric, occurring in the trunk, buttocks, and face. Tuberculoid leprosy lesions exhibit earlier sensory loss compared with lepromatous lesions.
- Nerve enlargement occurs early and involves nerves contiguous to skin lesions.
- Neuritic pain
- Muscle atrophy, especially in the intrinsic hand muscles
- Resorption of phalanges (late)

Borderline Leprosy

- Skins lesions vary in number and character depending on whether the case is more toward the tuberculoid or lepromatous end of the spectrum.
- Nerve involvement may precede skin lesions in this type, with segmental enlargement and tenderness of nerve trunks.

LABORATORY PROCEDURES

- ELISA to serum antibody to phenolic glycolipid I (PGL-I), a capsular antigen of *M. leprae,* is positive in most patients with multibacillary disease (lepromatous or borderline lepromatous) and often negative in patients with paucibacillary forms of the disease (tuberculous or borderline tuberculous).
- Diagnosis is generally made from demonstration of acid-fast bacteria from smears from affected skin or nasal mucosa.

IMAGING STUDIES

N/A

SPECIAL TESTS

- Dermal scraping or slit-skin biopsy are sent for acid-fast stain or, alternatively, the Ziehl-Neelsen stain to identify *M. leprae.* In tuberculoid leprosy, noncaseating granulomas are present and bacilli often are scant or absent. In lepromatous leprosy, a diffuse granulomatous reaction is present, often with many demonstrable bacilli.
- Nerve biopsy is not usually necessary to make a diagnosis of leprous neuropathy, except in rare cases of isolated nerve involvement.
- Nerve conduction studies/electromyography are helpful to document neuropathy and delineate pattern of involvement.

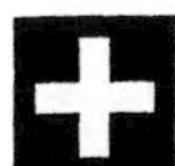

Management

GENERAL MEASURES

- Treatment is given to eradicate the bacteria and to prevent secondary immune reactions that might cause further injury to the nerves. Patients should be evaluated by an ophthalmologist for ophthalmologic manifestations that might threaten vision. Family members should be evaluated for leprosy.

SURGICAL MEASURES

- Occasionally release of contractures and nerve and tendon transplants can improve function. Plastic surgery may be useful to correct or improve facial or other deformities.

SYMPTOMATIC TREATMENT

- Patients should be counseled about the risks of inadvertent injury, such as severe burns to areas rendered insensate by peripheral neuropathy. Insensate limbs should be protected by good footwear, and patients should be warned about the risk of burns.

ADJUNCTIVE TREATMENT

N/A

ADMISSION/DISCHARGE CRITERIA

- Not generally required except in severe reactions to treatment (see Patient Monitoring)

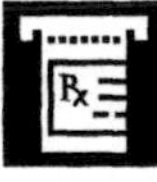

Medications

DRUG(S) OF CHOICE

- Dapsone (diphenylsulfone), a folate antagonist, is the primary therapy.
- The regimen recommended by the US Public Health Service Hospital Long Hansen's Disease Center in Louisiana is given below. These recommendations differ from the World Health Organization (WHO) recommendations, which include a broader regimen because of concerns of dapsone resistance.

US Public Health Service Hospital Long Hansen's Disease Center in Louisiana Regimen

Paucibacillary Disease (Tuberculoid End of Spectrum)

- Dapsone 100 mg PO daily
- Rifampin 600 mg daily
- Duration 1 year

Multibacillary Disease (Lepromatous End of Spectrum)

- Dapsone 100 mg PO daily
- Rifampin 600 mg PO daily
- Clofazimine 50 mg PO daily
- Duration 2 years

WHO-Recommended MDT Regimens

Multibacillary Leprosy

- Rifampicin 600 mg once per month
- Dapsone 100 mg daily
- Clofazimine 300 mg once per month and 50 mg daily
- Duration 12 months

Paucibacillary Leprosy

- Rifampicin 600 mg once per month
- Dapsone 100 mg daily
- Duration 6 months

Single Skin Lesion Paucibacillary Leprosy

- For adults the standard regimens is a single dose of
- Rifampicin 600 mg
- Ofloxacin 400 mg
- Minocycline 100 mg
- Thalidomide is the best therapy for erythema nodosum leprosum.

Contraindications

- All medications are contraindicated in patients with a known history of hypersensitivity reactions.
- Clofazimine and thalidomide are not safe for use during pregnancy.

Precautions

- Adverse effects of dapsone are relatively uncommon but include hemolysis, agranulocytosis, hepatitis, and severe exfoliative dermatitis.
- Clofazimine may cause reddish discoloration of the skin, diarrhea, and abdominal pain.
- Patients may actually have a worsening of their neuropathy or rash when treatment is initiated due to several types of reactions (see Patient Monitoring).

ALTERNATIVE DRUGS

N/A

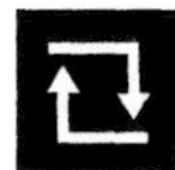

Follow-Up

PATIENT MONITORING

- Patients with leprosy must be followed closely for several types of adverse reactions to treatment.
  - —Leprae type 1 reaction (reversal reaction) is an acute immunologically mediated inflammatory reaction seen in about 50% of patients with borderline leprosy in the first year of therapy. It is manifested as swelling and worsening of skin lesions and of peripheral nerves. Nerve pathology shows inflammation with granulomata and vasculitic changes. Prednisone at initial doses of 60 mg/day is recommended, with treatment required for several months or more and taper guided by clinical response.
  - —Leprae type 2 reaction (erythema nodosum leprosum) is a reaction that occurs in approximately 50% of patients with lepromatous leprosy during the first year of treatment and is attributed to immunologic reaction to massive death of *M. leprae* bacilli (Arthus reaction with deposition of immunoglobulin/complement in skin vessels). This leads to the development of multiple tender skin nodules, as well as fever, arthritis, iridocyclitis, edema, and new peripheral nerve injury in an acute mononeuritis multiplex pattern. Prednisone is also used to treat this reaction. Thalidomide 100–300 mg qhs is useful if prednisone does not quell the reaction.

EXPECTED COURSE AND PROGNOSIS

- In most patients with Lepromatous leprosy (LL), skin lesions typically resolve over months to several years. The peripheral neuropathy may improve, but this depends on the degree of damage present at the time of initiation of treatment. In tuberculoid leprosy, the skin lesions may improve or remain unchanged, and sensory loss often is permanent.

PATIENT EDUCATION

- Centers for Disease Control. Website: *www.cdc.gov/ncidod/dastlr/TB/TB_Hansen.htm*
- World Health Organization information on the eradication of leprosy. Website: *http://www.who.int/lep/disease/disease.htm*

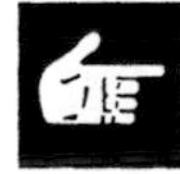

Miscellaneous

SYNONYMS

- Hansen's disease

ICD-9-CM: 030.9 Leprosy; then second diagnosis of 357.4, Polyneuropathy in other diseases classified elsewhere

SEE ALSO: N/A

REFERENCES

- Nations SP, Katz JS, Lyde CB et al. Leprous neuropathy: an American perspective. Semin Neurol 1998:18;113–124.
- Said G. Leprous neuropathy. In: Mendell JR, Kissel JT, Cornblath DR, eds. Diagnosis and management of peripheral nerve disorders. New York: Oxford University Press, 2001:551–564.

Author(s): Joanne Lynn, MD

Lesch-Nyhan Disease

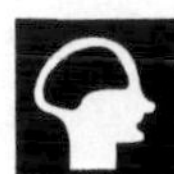

Basics

DESCRIPTION

- Lesch-Nyhan disease (LND) is an inherited metabolic disease characterized by overproduction of uric acid and a characteristic neurobehavioral syndrome. The overproduction of uric acid frequently leads to hyperuricemia, gouty arthritis, and kidney stones composed of uric acid. The neurobehavioral syndrome consists of mental retardation, severe motor handicap, and recurrent self-injurious behavior.

EPIDEMIOLOGY

- LND occurs in all ethnic groups with an estimated incidence of 1 per 380,000 births. Virtually all cases are males.

ETIOLOGY

- LND is caused by inherited mutations in the *HPRT* gene. This gene encodes hypoxanthine guanine phosphoribosyltransferase, an enzyme responsible for recycling the purine bases hypoxanthine and guanine into usable purine nucleotides. In LND, the rate of purine biosynthesis is increased, causing accumulation of uric acid in high concentrations in the blood, spinal fluid, and urine. Gouty deposits may occur in target tissues such as the joints and kidneys.

RISK FACTORS

- Because inheritance is X linked and recessive, female heterozygous carriers are completely asymptomatic, but their male offspring have a 50% risk of contracting the disease.

PREGNANCY

- Because there are no effective treatments for LND, prevention plays an important role in managing the disease. Any female relative of a patient with LND should be counseled regarding her risk of producing an affected child. Genetic tests are available for both carrier testing and prenatal diagnosis.

ASSOCIATED CONDITIONS

- Macrocytic anemia
- Growth retardation

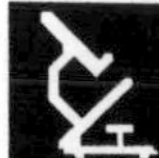

Diagnosis

DIFFERENTIAL DIAGNOSIS

- The differential diagnosis for developmental delay includes a large number of inherited or acquired disorders. The differential diagnosis for self-injurious behavior also is broad and includes severe mental retardation, autism, and several other genetic syndromes. Hyperuricemia is unusual in children, often signifying a metabolic or lymphoproliferative disorder, or the effect of a medication.

SIGNS AND SYMPTOMS

- Developmental delay is followed by an extrapyramidal syndrome resembling cerebral palsy.
- Self-injurious behavior is characteristic, often with mutilation of the lips and fingers. Choreoathetosis starts early in life, and death usually occurs in the teens or 20s from renal failure.
- Renal colic may occur due to stones, and gouty arthritis may occur with joint inflammation.

LABORATORY PROCEDURES

- Serum uric acid
- 24-hour urinary uric acid

IMAGING STUDIES

- Imaging studies of the brain are largely unrevealing. Ultrasound and CT of the kidneys and urogenital system may disclose stones.

SPECIAL TESTS

- Evidence for overproduction of uric acid is a helpful clue but is not sufficient for definitive diagnosis. Diagnosis requires the demonstration of reduced HPRT enzyme activity in blood cells or fibroblasts. Alternatively, a gene test is available to screen for mutations (numerous point mutations mapped to Xq26.1 region). Prenatal testing possible in first trimester (chorionic villus sampling).

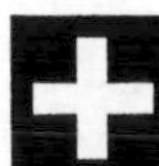

Management

GENERAL MEASURES

- A comfortable and engaging environment is essential for minimizing behavioral problems. Motor dysfunction and behavior problems often worsen with anxiety and stress, such as that associated with hospitalization.

SURGICAL MEASURES

- Patients with LND may undergo most routine surgical procedures with standard anesthetic agents.

SYMPTOMATIC TREATMENT

- Prevention of kidney stones requires generous hydration at all times and allopurinol to reduce the formation of uric acid. There are no consistently effective therapies for the neurobehavioral features. Prevention of self-hitting usually requires physical restraints and sometimes dental extraction to prevent self-biting. Medications sometimes helpful for reducing self-injury include gabapentin, carbamazepine, benzodiazepines, or risperidone.

ADJUNCTIVE TREATMENT

- Wheelchairs must be customized by covering all potentially dangerous parts within reach. Comfortable restraints usually are required in the wheelchair and sleeping environment.
- Behavior therapy can be very helpful to reduce the incidence of self-injurious behaviors.

ADMISSION/DISCHARGE CRITERIA

N/A

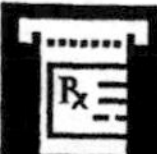

Medications

DRUG(S) OF CHOICE

- Allopurinol

Contraindications

- Impaired renal function is frequent.

Precautions

- Good hydration must be provided.

ALTERNATIVE DRUGS

N/A

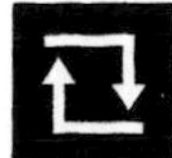

Follow-Up

PATIENT MONITORING

- Regular follow-up is needed to guard against nephrolithiasis and renal failure. Stones may arise even in well-hydrated patients taking allopurinol. The family may require assistance with managing self-injury and other counterproductive behaviors.

EXPECTED COURSE AND PROGNOSIS

- Developmental delay is apparent within the first few months of age. Extrapyramidal signs typically develop between 9 and 18 months of age. Self-injury typically begins between 24 and 36 months of age but may be delayed until late childhood or early adolescence. Although the condition is not progressively degenerative, few patients survive beyond 30 years of age. Most succumb to complications of renal failure or aspiration. A significant proportion experience sudden death of undetermined cause.

PATIENT EDUCATION

- Lesch-Nyhan Syndrome Children's Research Foundation, 210 South Greenbay Road, Lake Forest IL, 60045.
- Emedicine entry for Lesch-Nyhan syndrome. Website: *www.emed.com/neuro/topic630.htm*

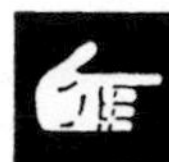

Miscellaneous

SYNONYMS

N/A

ICD-9-CM: 277.2 Lesch-Nyhan syndrome

SEE ALSO: N/A

REFERENCES

- Alford RL, Redman JB, O'Brien WE, et al. Lesch-Nyhan syndrome: carrier and prenatal diagnosis. Prenatal Diagn 1995;15:329–338.
- Jinnah HA, Friedman T. Lesch-Nyhan disease and its variants. In: Scriver CR, Beaudet AL, Sly WS, et al., eds. The molecular and metabolic bases of inherited disease, 8th ed. New York: McGraw-Hill, 2001.

Author(s): H.A. Jinnah, MD, PhD

Leukodystrophies

Basics

DESCRIPTION

- Leukodystrophies are inherited disorders of central myelination resulting in the confluent destruction or abnormal formation of cerebral white matter. Despite substantial progress in our understanding of inherited white matter disorders in recent years, approximately 50% of children with white matter abnormalities do not have a specific diagnosis even after extensive investigations to rule out well-defined leukodystrophies.

EPIDEMIOLOGY

Incidence

- Alexander's disease: rare
- Canavan's disease: rare, 1 in 10,000 in Ashkenazi Jews
- Metachromatic leukodystrophy: 1 in 40,000 to 1 in 100,000
- Krabbe leukodystrophy: 1 in 100,000
- X-linked adrenoleukodystrophy (ALD): 1 in 40,000
- Pelizaeus-Merzbacher disease: 1 in 100,000

ETIOLOGY

- The leukodystrophies are inherited in an autosomal recessive pattern with the exception of Alexander's disease (autosomal dominant) and the X-linked recessive conditions (X-linked ALD and Pelizaeus-Merzbacher), which affect males more severely. Biochemical abnormalities are:
  - —Alexander's disease: *de novo* mutation in glial fibrillary acidic protein gene (GFAP)
  - —Canavan's disease: mutations in aspartoacylase gene
  - —Megalencephalic leukoencephalopathy with subcortical cysts: mutations in the MLC1 gene
  - —Metachromatic leukodystrophy: arylsulfatase A deficiency, multiple sulfatase deficiency, saposin (activator protein) deficiency
  - —Krabbe leukodystrophy: galactocerebrosidase deficiency
  - —X-linked ALD: deficiency of peroxisomal membrane transporter
  - —Pelizaeus-Merzbacher disease: deficient formation of proteolipid protein (PLP) in central nervous system
  - —Vanishing white matter disease: mutations in one of the five subunits of the translation initiation factor eIF2B

RISK FACTORS

- There are no known environmental risk factors.

PREGNANCY

- Prenatal diagnosis available in some cases.

ASSOCIATED CONDITIONS

- In addition to leukodystrophy:
  - —Metachromatic leukodystrophy: peripheral neuropathy, optic atrophy, gallbladder disease
  - —Krabbe leukodystrophy: peripheral neuropathy, visual loss
  - —X-linked ALD: Addison's (adrenal insufficiency)
  - —Pelizaeus-Merzbacher disease: rotatory nystagmus

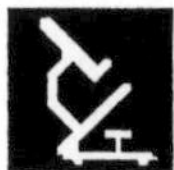

Diagnosis

DIFFERENTIAL DIAGNOSIS

- Multiple sclerosis
- Acute disseminated encephalomyelitis
- CNS vasculitis
- Toxic leukoencephalopathies (e.g. cyclosporine)
- CADASIL (cerebral autosomal dominant arteriopathy with subcortical infarcts and leukoencephalopathy)
- Multiple subcortical infarctions
- Disorders of vitamin B_{12} and folate metabolism
- White matter abnormalities associated with other metabolic conditions, including organic acidurias, aminoacidopathies, and mitochondrial disorders

SIGNS AND SYMPTOMS

Alexander's Disease

- Infantile: macrocephaly, psychomotor regression, seizures, spasticity
- Juvenile: slower development of bulbar signs, ataxia, spasticity with relative preservation of intelligence
- Adult onset: heterogeneous, may mimic relapsing-remitting multiple sclerosis

Canavan's Disease

- Infantile: macrocephaly, hypotonia, developmental delay → seizures and spasticity
- Congenital: marked hypotonia, lethargy, dysphagia, early death
- Juvenile: onset after 5 years of cerebellar dysfunction, cognitive decline → spasticity, optic atrophy

Megalencephalic Leukoencephalopathy with Subcortical Cysts

- Macrocephaly prior to 1 year of age. Early development is normal with eventual development of ataxia, spasticity, and slow deterioration in motor functions. Intelligence remains relatively spared. Seizures may develop.

Metachromatic Leukodystrophy

- Late infantile: initial hypotonia → progressive hypertonia, ataxia, intellectual regression, painful peripheral neuropathy, optic atrophy
- Juvenile: school difficulties, incontinence, and gait clumsiness → extrapyramidal features, hypertonia, intellectual deterioration, pseudobulbar palsy
- Adult onset: initial neuropsychiatric symptoms with progressive frontal dementia → gait disorder, peripheral neuropathy → hypertonia, optic atrophy, spastic tetraparesis, bulbar dysfunction

Krabbe Leukodystrophy

- Infantile: early irritability/hypersensitivity to stimuli → marked hypertonia, loss of vision and hearing, peripheral neuropathy
- Juvenile and adult forms: mental deterioration, pyramidal signs, visual loss, peripheral neuropathy

X-linked ALD

- Six clinical phenotypes have been recognized for this condition:
  - —Childhood cerebral ALD
  - —Adolescent cerebral ALD
  - —Adult-onset cerebral ALD
  - —Amyeloneuropathy
  - —Addison's only
  - —Asymptomatic/presymptomatic
- The childhood cerebral form and amyeloneuropathy are the most common. The childhood cerebral form presents initially with behavioral changes and school difficulties at 2–10 years of age, followed by progressive neurologic dysfunction, visual loss, and adrenal insufficiency. The adolescent and adult-onset cerebral phenotypes have similar features to the childhood cerebral disease but a latter age of onset. Amyeloneuropathy presents in the second to fourth decade of life as progressive spastic paraparesis. Up to half may develop cerebral symptoms, and two thirds develop adrenal insufficiency. Addison's alone may be present in 10%–20% of ALD patients with a high risk of later developing neurologic symptoms. Patients may remain asymptomatic for decades. Different clinical phenotypes can occur within the same family.

Pelizaeus-Merzbacher Disease

- Classic: rotatory eye movements and hypotonia → very slowly progressive involuntary movements and spasticity
- Connatal: onset at birth with severe features and more rapid progression; may have intractable seizures
- X-linked spastic paraparesis

Vanishing White Matter Disease

- Onset from infancy to adulthood
- Chronic progressive cerebellar ataxia, spasticity, optic atrophy, mild mental decline
- Episodes of rapid deterioration following febrile illnesses and minor head trauma

LABORATORY PROCEDURES

- Alexander's disease: mutation analysis of GFAP gene
- Canavan's disease: elevated urinary excretion of *N*-acetylaspartic acid (NAA) decreased aspartoacylase enzyme activity; DNA mutation analysis
- Megalencephalic leukoencephalopathy with subcortical cysts: DNA mutation analysis
- Metachromatic leukodystrophy: arylsulfatase A assay on WBCs or fibroblasts; sulfatides in the urine
- Krabbe leukodystrophy: Galactocerebrosidase assay in WBCs or fibroblasts; mutation analysis
- X-linked ALD: deficiency of peroxisomal membrane transporter (ALDP); accumulation of very-long-chain fatty acids (VLCFA) in blood; DNA mutation analysis
- Pelizaeus-Merzbacher disease: mutations or duplication of the PLP gene
- Vanishing white matter disease: mutation analysis of five subunits of eIF2B

IMAGING STUDIES

- MRI is the study of choice for the evaluation of leukodystrophy:
- Alexander's disease: extensive frontal dominant white matter abnormalities
- Canavan's disease: diffuse hypodensity of white matter and increased NAA peak on magnetic resonance spectroscopy
- Megalencephalic leukoencephalopathy with subcortical cysts: diffusely abnormal; mildly swollen white matter with subcortical cysts in the anterotemporal region and often in the frontotemporal region.
- Metachromatic leukodystrophy: periventricular white matter abnormalities evolve into more extensive, symmetric involvement of the subcortical white matter
- Krabbe leukodystrophy: extensive white matter involvement precedes diffuse cerebral atrophy
- X-linked ALD: symmetric parietooccipital white matter lesions
- Pelizaeus-Merzbacher disease: severe reduction or absence of myelin
- Vanishing white matter disease: diffusely abnormal white matter that vanishes over time and is replaced by CSF

SPECIAL TESTS

- Alexander's disease: histologic finding of Rosenthal fibers on brain biopsy is diagnostic but has been replaced by mutation analysis
- Metachromatic leukodystrophy: nerve conduction studies to assess for peripheral neuropathy; ultrasound to assess for accumulation of sulfatides in gallbladder wall
- Krabbe leukodystrophy: nerve conduction studies to assess for peripheral neuropathy
- X-linked ALD: adrenal function testing in patients with all forms of this disease

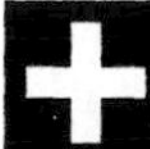

Management

GENERAL MEASURES

- Supportive therapy

SURGICAL MEASURES

N/A

SYMPTOMATIC TREATMENT

- Bone marrow transplantation may result in long-term stabilization and sometimes improvement in clinical symptoms when performed early in cerebral X-linked ALD, the juvenile and adult-onset forms of metachromatic leukodystrophy, and Krabbe's disease. Once neurologic symptoms have progressed beyond the early stages, bone marrow transplantation has not been shown to alter the natural course of these diseases.

ADJUNCTIVE TREATMENT

- Patients with ALD and amyeloneuropathy should be treated for adrenal insufficiency as required.

ADMISSION/DISCHARGE CRITERIA

N/A

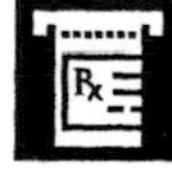

Medications

DRUG(S) OF CHOICE

- No effective drug therapies are currently available.

ALTERNATIVE DRUGS

- Lorenzo's oil has been given to patients with X-linked ALD for more than a decade since it was initially shown to normalize plasma VLCFAs. Recent studies, however, have demonstrated no beneficial effects of Lorenzo's oil on the natural course of the disease. Significant side effects, including elevated liver enzymes and thrombocytopenia, are frequently observed.

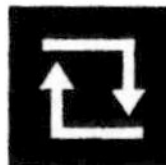

Follow-Up

PATIENT MONITORING

- Presymptomatic boys with X-ALD should be monitored with serial neuropsychological assessments in order to detect early indications of cerebral disease and need for bone marrow transplantation.

EXPECTED COURSE AND PROGNOSIS

- Rate of progression of symptoms is dependent upon the age of onset and characteristics of each individual leukodystrophy.

PATIENT EDUCATION

- Genetic counseling should be provided to patients and their families. Presymptomatic testing of siblings may be offered for some conditions in view of the potential benefit of early bone marrow transplantation.
- United Leukodystrophy Foundation. Website: *www.ulf.org*

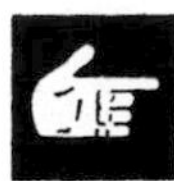

Miscellaneous

SYNONYMS

- Leukoencephalopathies
- Metabolic white matter diseases

ICD-9-CM: 330.0 Leukodystrophy

SEE ALSO: N/A

REFERENCES

- Berger J, Moser HW, et al. Leukodystrophies: recent developments in genetics, molecular biology, pathogenesis and treatment. Curr Opin Neurol 2001;14:305–312.
- Gartner J, Braun A, et al. Clinical and genetic aspects of X-linked adrenoleukodystrophy. Neuropediatrics 1998;29: 3–13.
- Leegwater PA, Boor PK, et al. Identification of novel mutations in MLC1 responsible for megalencephalic leukoencephalopathy with subcortical cysts. Hum Genet 2002;110:279–283.
- Matalon RM, Michals-Matalon K. Spongy degeneration of the brain, Canavan disease: biochemical and molecular findings. Front Biosci 2000;5:D307–D11.
- Rodriguez D, Gauthier F, et al. Infantile Alexander disease: spectrum of GFAP mutations and genotype-phenotype correlation. Am J Hum Genet 2001;69:1134–1140.
- Schiffmann R, Boespflug-Tanguy O. An update on the leukodystrophies. Curr Opin Neurol 2001;14:789–794.
- van der Knaap MS. Magnetic resonance in childhood white-matter disorders. Dev Med Child Neurol 2001;43:705–712.
- van Geel BM, Assies J, et al. X linked adrenoleukodystrophy: clinical presentation, diagnosis, and therapy. J Neurol Neurosurg Psychiatry 1997;63:4–14.

Author(s): Deborah L. Renaud, MD

Lyme Disease, Neurologic Complications (Lyme Neuroborreliosis)

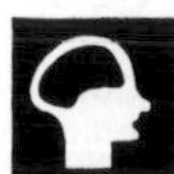

Basics

DESCRIPTION

- Lyme disease is a multisystemic illness associated with both early and late-onset chronic neurologic syndromes.

EPIDEMIOLOGY

Incidence

- The incidence is much higher in the coastal New England, mid-Atlantic, and northern midwestern states.
- 4–5 cases per 100,000 nationally.

Prevalence

- Up to 15% of untreated patients develop early neurologic Lyme disease.
- Chronic Lyme neuroborreliosis is rarer, but the prevalence is unknown.

Race

- Vast majority are white; 2%–3% are black.

Age

- Children <15 years and adults >30 years are at greatest risk

Sex

- Males and females are affected equally.

ETIOLOGY

- Spirochetal infection (*Borrelia burgdorferi* in the United States)
- Transmitted by deer tick (*Ixodes scapularis* in the United States)
- Most patients are infected in spring or summer when the *Ixodes* nymph feeds.
- Initial manifestation is typically the localized, slowly expanding skin rash, erythema migrans (EM).
- If localized disease is untreated, the infection may become disseminated, resulting in early neurologic or cardiac involvement and late manifestations such as oligoarticular arthritis or chronic Lyme neuroborreliosis.

RISK FACTORS

- Residence in, or visitation to, endemic areas during spring and summer

PREGNANCY

N/A

ASSOCIATED CONDITIONS

- Erythema migrans
- Lyme carditis
- Lyme oligoarticular arthritis

Diagnosis

DIFFERENTIAL DIAGNOSIS

Acute Lyme Cranial Neuritis

- Idiopathic (Bell's) facial palsy
- Guillain-Barré syndrome
- Neurosarcoidosis

Acute Lyme Radiculoneuritis

- Herpes zoster
- Cytomegalovirus, Ebstein-Barr virus
- Neurosarcoidosis
- Proximal diabetic neuropathy
- Nonsystemic vasculitic neuropathy

Lyme Meningitis or Meningoencephalitis

- Viral meningitis or meningoencephalitis
- Chronic meningitides

Chronic Lyme Radiculoneuropathy

- Distal sensory diabetic neuropathy
- Other toxic-metabolic neuropathies
- Idiopathic sensory polyneuropathy
- Disc disease
- Fibromyalgia

Chronic Lyme Encephalopathy

- Chronic fatigue/fibromyalgia
- Toxic-metabolic causes
- Depression
- Early Alzheimer's disease
- Neurosyphilis
- Other systemic inflammatory disease

Subacute or Chronic Lyme Encephalomyelitis

- Multiple sclerosis
- Postviral encephalomyelitis

SIGNS AND SYMPTOMS

Acute Lyme Neuropathy: Cranial Neuropathy, Radiculoneuropathy, Meningitis

- In summer/fall, within days to weeks after the onset of infection, cranial neuropathy and/or radiculoneuropathy may develop. A CSF lymphocytic pleocytosis is frequently present; meningeal signs and symptoms may be subtle or absent.
- Other less common syndromes are encephalitis, encephalomyelitis, transverse myelitis, or myositis.
- Any cranial nerve can be affected (most commonly facial palsy in 50%–75% of patients and bilateral in one third). Facial palsy is typically noted within 4 weeks of EM.
- Acute Lyme radiculoneuropathy usually presents with severe sharp, jabbing, or boring pain in the distribution of peripheral nerves or nerve roots. Within days to weeks, neurologic deficits appear, including sensory loss, weakness, or hyporeflexia. Symptoms and signs may be focal or multifocal.

Chronic or Late Lyme Radiculoneuropathy

- Presents months to years after disease onset with sensory symptoms, particularly distal paresthesia or radicular pain. Muscle weakness is slight or absent, and tendon jerks are normal or slightly hypoactive.
- Compared to acute Lyme neuropathy, chronic Lyme radiculoneuropathy is less severe and does not include cranial neuropathy or CSF pleocytosis.
- Patients with distal paresthesia present with symmetric or asymmetric symptoms and signs in a "stocking glove" distribution or truncal paresthesia. The radicular form is less common.

Chronic or Late Lyme CNS Syndromes: Encephalopathy or Encephalomyelitis

- Lyme encephalopathy presents primarily with memory and concentration difficulty.
- Headache, mild depression, irritability, fatigue, or excessive daytime sleepiness may occur.
- Encephalomyelitis usually presents with progressive limb weakness and spasticity, urinary urgency, and occasionally cranial neuropathy.

LABORATORY PROCEDURES

- *Serology:* Within 3–4 weeks, a serum IgM response is detectable and by 6–8 weeks an IgG response develops as the IgM response declines. During early disease (e.g., EM), the patient often is seronegative. Once the disease becomes disseminated and neurologic complications develop, however, the vast majority has a positive IgM or IgG titer.
- *Western blot:* All borderline or positive titers should be confirmed with Western blots to differentiate false- from true-positive titers.
- *CSF analysis:* Lymphocytic pleocytosis typically is found in acute radiculoneuritis, meningitis, encephalitis, encephalomyelitis, transverse myelitis, and sometimes isolated cranial neuritis. Elevated CSF protein without pleocytosis is found in Lyme encephalopathy. Selective concentration of Lyme antibody in CSF is found in most patients with CNS Lyme disease.
- *Neuropsychologic tests:* Typically discloses subtle verbal or visual memory problems
- *EMG/nerve conduction studies:* Patients with acute or chronic Lyme radiculoneuropathy show sensorimotor axon loss, polyradiculo-neuropathy with low-amplitude action potentials (sensory more than motor), and slight slowing of conduction velocities and denervation of distal and proximal muscles. In contrast to the axonal neuropathy in the limbs, patients with acute Lyme facial palsy may show demyelinative physiology with conduction block of facial motor fibers.
- *Electroencephalography:* EEG usually is normal in CNS neuroborreliosis. Seizures, focal sharp activity and focal slowing or dysrhythmia may be seen with encephalomyelitis.

IMAGING STUDIES

- *Brain MRI:* Nonspecific white matter lesions are seen in about 75% of patients with subacute or chronic Lyme encephalomyelitis. Only about 25% of adult or pediatric patients with Lyme encephalopathy have cerebral, nonenhancing, white matter lesions.

SPECIAL TESTS

- *CSF culture:* Culture of *B. burgdorferi* is technically demanding and positive in <10% of patients with known CSF infection.
- *CSF polymerase chain reaction (PCR):* Positive in <50% of patients with CNS or meningeal Lyme disease. Technically demanding, numerous controls required, not standardized.
- *T-cell proliferative response:* A measure of cellular rather than humoral response to *B burgdorferi antigens.* Positive in some seronegative patients. Technically demanding; sensitivity low.
- *Single photon emission computed tomography (SPECT):* Multifocal areas of cortical and subcortical hypoperfusion are often seen in Lyme encephalopathy.

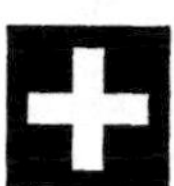

Management

GENERAL MEASURES

- Once the diagnosis of Lyme neuroborreliosis is made, antibiotic therapy should be begun promptly. If there is evidence of CNS invasion (e.g., CSF pleocytosis, selective concentration of antibody in CSF, positive CSF PCR), IV antibiotics (e.g., IV ceftriaxone) should be started. If not, oral antibiotics (e.g., PO amoxicillin) suffice, particularly for isolated cranial neuropathy.

SURGICAL MEASURES

N/A

SYMPTOMATIC TREATMENT

- Neuropathic pain control in patients with acute or chronic radiculoneuritis
- Corneal protection for facial palsy
- Treatment of headache, sleep disorder, depression, spasticity, or seizures if necessary

ADJUNCTIVE TREATMENT

- Physical therapy for limb weakness
- Cognitive rehabilitation for patients with memory disturbance

ADMISSION/DISCHARGE CRITERIA

- Outpatient management is the rule with admission for patients with significant progressive neurologic deficits.

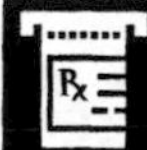

Medications

DRUG(S) OF CHOICE

- For CNS disease, the third-generation cephalosporin, ceftriaxone, is superior to high-dose penicillin because it easily crosses the blood–brain barrier, requires once per day dosing, and has high spirocheticidal activity against *Borrelia.*
- For early neurologic involvement with CSF pleocytosis: 2–4 weeks of IV ceftriaxone 2 g/day in adults (75–100 mg/kg/day in children).
- For isolated facial palsy with normal CSF: 4 weeks of tetracycline 100 mg/PO bid or amoxicillin 500 mg PO tid in adults
- For late central or peripheral neurologic involvement: 4 weeks of IV ceftriaxone 2 g/day in adults (75–100 mg/kg/day in children)
- For encephalomyelitis: 4–6 weeks of IV ceftriaxone therapy

Contraindications

- Known drug allergy
- Patients with penicillin allergy should be skin tested prior to initiating ceftriaxone therapy.

Precautions

- Administer initial dose of IV antibiotic under direct medical supervision.
- Observe for diarrhea (pseudomembranous colitis), right upper quadrant pain (biliary), line sepsis, or phlebitis.
- Treatment duration beyond 4–6 weeks almost never is necessary.
- Symptoms that are unresponsive to prolonged courses of intravenous antibiotics are most likely due to another cause.

ALTERNATIVE DRUGS

- For adults with CNS disease who have penicillin and cephalosporin allergy, consider doxycycline at higher dose (200 mg PO bid). Other alternatives are chloramphenicol, vancomycin, or imipenem.

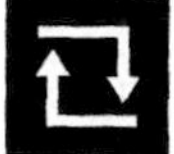

Follow-Up

PATIENT MONITORING

- If elevated initially, expect Lyme antibody titer to remain elevated despite adequate therapy and resolution of symptoms.
- Follow-up CSF studies: pleocytosis resolves, protein declines, CSF PCR reverts to negative.
- Consider follow-up neuropsychologic testing to document improved memory.
- Brain MRI abnormalities may not improve; SPECT abnormalities do improve.

EXPECTED COURSE AND PROGNOSIS

- In acute Lyme radiculoneuropathy, radicular pain often improves over hours to days of IV antibiotic administration, whereas sensory and motor deficits generally resolve completely over weeks to a few months.
- The prognosis for facial and other cranial nerve palsies is excellent.
- In acute or chronic Lyme encephalomyelitis, neurologic function improves, but residual deficits are common.
- In chronic Lyme radiculoneuropathy, symptoms resolve more slowly than in acute Lyme neuropathy over many months, usually with mild residual deficits.
- The outcome is better in Lyme encephalopathy than encephalomyelitis. Improvement in symptoms is slow, beginning 2–3 months after completion of antibiotic therapy and continuing for 6 to 9 months.

PATIENT EDUCATION

- Tick avoidance: beware of high grass, brush, woods in endemic areas in spring/summer

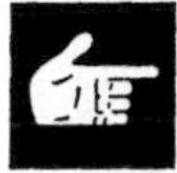

Miscellaneous

SYNONYMS

- Neuroborreliosis
- Bannwarth's syndrome (acute Lyme radiculoneuritis)

ICD 9 CM: 088.81 Lyme disease; 088.81 [320.7] Meningitis-Lyme disease, meningoencephalitis-Lyme disease; 323.9 Encephalitis; 348.3 Encephalopathy; 351.9 Facial neuropathy; 357.0 Polyneuritis, infective (acute); 356.9 Polyneuropathy (peripheral); 723.4 Radiculitis, Arm; 724.4 Radiculitis, leg or thoracic

SEE ALSO: N/A

REFERENCES

- Halperin JJ, Logigian EL, Finkel M, et al. Practice parameters for the diagnosis of patients with nervous system Lyme borreliosis (Lyme disease). Neurology 1996;46:619–627.
- Logigian EL, Kaplan RF, Steere AC. Chronic neurologic manifestations of Lyme disease. N Fngl J Med 1990;323:1438–1444.
- Rahn DW, Malawista SE. Lyme disease: recommendations for diagnosis and treatment. Ann Intern Med 1991;114:472–481.
- Steere AC, Taylor E, McHugh GL, et al. The overdiagnosis of Lyme disease. JAMA 1991;269:1812–1816.

Author(s): Eric L. Logigian, MD

Malignant Hyperthermia

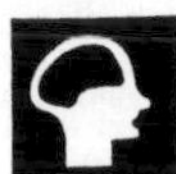

Basics

DESCRIPTION

Malignant hyperthermia (MH) is a condition characterized by elevated calcium concentration in the sarcoplasm after exposure to triggering agents, causing an uncontrolled increase in muscle metabolism.

EPIDEMIOLOGY

Incidence/Prevalence

Incidence of acute MH is approximately 1/15,000 anesthetics in the pediatric population, and 1/50,000 to 1/150,000 in adults.

Sex

Acute MH is more prevalent in males, even prior to puberty.

ETIOLOGY

The ryanodine receptor is the calcium release channel from the sarcoplasmic reticulum. Release of calcium from the sarcoplasmic reticulum normally occurs after depolarization via an action potential. The subsequent calcium release into the myoplasm allows actin-myosin cross-bridge cycling (contraction), which is terminated by calcium reuptake into the sarcoplasmic reticulum (relaxation). Abnormal stimulation of calcium release by triggering agents, possibly combined with abnormal reuptake, causes continuous cross-bridge cycling and consumption of energy stores, both by the contraction apparatus and by sarcoplasmic adenosine triphosphatase (ATPase).

Genetics

The genetics of MH is characterized as autosomal dominant with variable penetrance. Between 20% and 70% of MH susceptible patients have a genetic mutation in the ryanodine receptor. The MH phenotype may be dependent on other proteins that modulate the ryanodine receptor or calcium reuptake.

RISK FACTORS

- Malignant hyperthermia is most commonly caused by exposure to triggering agents including all halogenated inhalation anesthetics, such as sevoflurane and desflurane, and the depolarizing neuromuscular blocker succinylcholine. MH-susceptible patients may not have an episode with their first exposure to a triggering anesthetic; 30% of patients may have had up to three uneventful anesthetics. Triggering and severity of an episode may be ameliorated by mild hypothermia (consistent with the comparatively greater incidence in children as mild hypothermia is less common during pediatric anesthesia).
- Stress has clearly been shown to be a trigger in the porcine model of MH, but evidence for this is weak in humans. Regardless, it has been standard practice to reduce stress in MH-susceptible patients with careful premedication before surgery. There are several case reports of individuals with exercise or heat intolerance who had MH susceptibility demonstrated by halothane-caffeine contracture testing.

PREGNANCY

MH-susceptible women may carry infants to term. There are anecdotal reports of MH episodes occurring during the stress of delivery in hot weather. Epidural analgesia can be given to MH-susceptible patients. Therefore, modern anesthesia techniques can theoretically reduce the risk of MH during delivery.

ASSOCIATED CONDITIONS

- Many physicians suspect an increased incidence of MH susceptibility in patients with myopathies. The King-Denborough syndrome is a dysmorphic complex associated with an increased risk of MH. The majority of patients with central core disease are susceptible to MH.
- Duchenne's and Becker muscular dystrophy have been inconsistently associated with MH episodes. These individuals may have acute hyperkalemic arrests and rhabdomyolysis after the administration of succinylcholine secondary to extrajunctional acetylcholine receptors and dystrophin-poor muscle fragility. In addition, dystrophin-poor muscle may have abnormal resting calcium levels, increased calcium release, and impaired calcium reuptake mechanisms at baseline; the increase of calcium release by inhaled agents may lead to exacerbation of chronic rhabdomyolysis and increased metabolism. The routine use of inhalation anesthetics in these individuals is controversial. If potent inhaled anesthetics are given, careful monitoring of metabolism with end-tidal CO_2 and minute ventilation and muscle injury with serum potassium and urine myoglobin is prudent.
- The evidence for association of MH susceptibility with other myopathies is limited, but is suspected due to the abnormal calcium regulation in these conditions.

Diagnosis

DIFFERENTIAL DIAGNOSIS

Sepsis, thyrotoxic crisis, pheochromocytoma, metastatic carcinoid, serotonin syndrome, neuroleptic malignant syndrome, inadequate ventilation, light anesthesia, cocaine intoxication, iatrogenic overheating, central fever, anaphylactoid reactions.

SIGNS AND SYMPTOMS

- The first sign may be masseter muscle spasm during succinylcholine administration; this may be severe enough to prevent intubation. Approximately 50% of patients with masseter spasm after succinylcholine are found to be MH susceptible. When presented with a patient with masseter spasm after succinylcholine administration, consideration should be given to aborting the anesthetic. If the anesthetic is continued with nontriggering drugs, then consideration should be given to what must be done to facilitate early diagnosis and treatment should MH develop.
- Increased muscle metabolism increases CO_2 production because aerobic metabolism increases in muscle, and lactic acid produced by muscular anaerobic metabolism is neutralized. Metabolic and respiratory acidosis results. Skeletal muscle rigidity may be caused by uncontrolled stimulation of actin-myosin cross-bridge cycling by increased intracellular Ca^{2+} and by muscle temperature above 43.5°C, which causes irreversible contraction. The rigidity of MH is not affected by neuromuscular blockade. In spontaneously breathing patients, tachypnea will be noted; in ventilated patients, increases in end-tidal CO_2 occur despite increasing minute ventilation. Tachycardia and hypertension may be caused directly by hypercarbia, and indirectly by hypercarbic stimulation of catecholamine release. Hyperthermia associated with MH is secondary to muscle hypermetabolism and depends on both the ability to dissipate heat produced and the rapidity of definitive treatment. High concentrations of catecholamines, hypercarbia, and cutaneous vasodilatation lead to flushed, diaphoretic skin.
- Local hyperthermia, acidosis, and depletion of adenosine triphosphate (ATP) cause increased membrane permeability and release of potassium by the hypermetabolic muscle. Hyperkalemia leads to arrhythmias, decreased cardiac output, and cardiac arrest. Continued hypermetabolism, decreased energy stores, local temperature rise, and decreased perfusion lead to rhabdomyolysis. Myoglobinuria can produce renal failure. Pulmonary and cerebral edema and disseminated intravascular coagulation (DIC) are associated with severe or untreated MH.

LABORATORY PROCEDURES

- Arterial and venous blood gases, serum potassium and other electrolytes, urinalysis.
- If urine dipstick is positive for blood, then obtain microscopic analysis for RBCs and quantitative analysis for myoglobin.
- If urine pH is low, consider alkalinization.
- Baseline CK, clotting studies, and creatinine.
- Repeat CK 12 to 24 hours later and until returned to baseline.
- Repeat other abnormal labs at intervals to guide treatment.
- Increased $paco_2$ will be seen, reflected by increased end-tidal CO_2 if this is accurately monitored. A gap between venous po_2 and arterial po_2 will be present, due to increased oxygen extraction by muscle. Increased serum creatine kinase and myoglobinuria reflect muscle damage. The characteristic metabolic and respiratory acidosis secondary to muscle hypermetabolism, along with signs of muscle breakdown and resolution with dantrolene, favor the diagnosis of MH.

IMAGING STUDIES

N/A

SPECIAL TESTS

The halothane-caffeine contracture test is the only approved diagnostic test for susceptibility to MH. It is available in five centers in the U.S. in 2003, and requires 1 g of fresh muscle. Although the test is very sensitive, it lacks specificity. Therefore, the index patient should undergo contracture testing to maximize the predictive value for other family members.

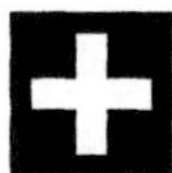

Management

GENERAL MEASURES

The definitive treatment of a known or suspected MH episode is administration of dantrolene as soon as possible and immediate discontinuation of triggering agents. Ventilation with high-flow O_2 through the anesthesia ventilator should be sufficient, as the concentration of inhalational agent in this ventilator will be less than that in the patient.

SURGICAL MEASURES

When an episode occurs during surgery, the procedure should be terminated as soon as possible.

SYMPTOMATIC TREATMENT

Standard treatment of hyperkalemic dysrhythmias should be initiated. Hyperventilation to approach normocarbia, and bicarbonate or tris(hydroxymethyl)-aminomethane (THAM) administration for initial treatment of the metabolic and respiratory acidosis should be titrated. Hyperthermia should be treated with surface cooling, intraperitoneal lavage, ice packs in the axillae and groin, and intravascular administration of cold solution. Aggressive hydration to prevent myoglobin-induced renal failure should be started and monitored by urine output and central venous pressure (CVP).

ADJUNCTIVE TREATMENT

N/A

ADMISSION/DISCHARGE CRITERIA

Patients should be closely monitored until all vital signs and laboratory parameters have been normal for 24 hours. Speed of recovery is dependent on severity of the episode, rapidity of treatment, and development of other sequelae.

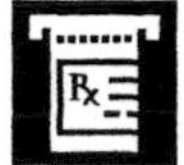

Medications

DRUG(S) OF CHOICE

Dantrolene sodium inhibits Ca^{2+} release from the sarcoplasmic reticulum. The dose is 2.5 mg/kg up to 10 mg/kg in the acute period, then 1 mg/kg every 6 hours for 24 to 36 hours. Intravenous dantrolene may be administered intraoperatively. Side effects include muscle weakness, drowsiness, nausea, and phlebitis. Respiratory compromise is uncommon without preexisting or concurrent causes of muscle weakness

Contraindications

N/A

Precautions

Dantrolene is an antiarrhythmic, increasing atrial and ventricular refractory periods and increasing action potential duration. Administration of dantrolene in the presence of calcium channel blockers may cause hyperkalemia and profound depression of cardiac contractility, but administration for a suspected MH episode should not be held for this reason.

ALTERNATIVE DRUGS

N/A

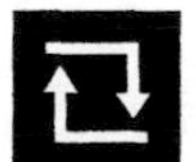

Follow-Up

PATIENT MONITORING

Creatine kinase measurements are recommended 6, 12, and 24 hours after the initial episode, because CK often peaks 24 to 36 hours after treatment of MH. CK values of greater than 20,000 are almost always associated with an MH episode or other severe myopathy.

EXPECTED COURSE AND PROGNOSIS

Administration of dantrolene and cessation of triggering agents halts the syndrome. Hyperkalemia, associated arrhythmias, and respiratory/metabolic acidosis typically resolve. If rhabdomyolysis was extensive, there may be muscle pain and weakness for weeks to months after resolution of acute MH.

PATIENT EDUCATION

Patients who have an MH episode should be counseled regarding the seriousness and heritability of their condition and should wear a "Med-alert" bracelet to inform other health-care professionals. First-degree relatives should be considered susceptible.
The Malignant Hyperthermia Association of the United States. Phone: 203-847-0407, website *www.mhaus.org*, 24-hour hotline 800-MH-HYPER.

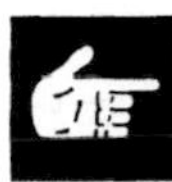

Miscellaneous

SYNONYMS

N/A

ICD-9-CM: 995.86 Malignant hyperthermia

SEE ALSO: N/A

REFERENCES

- Harrison GG. Dantrolene—dynamics and kinetics. Br J Anaesth 1988;60:279–286.
- Kleopa KA, Rosenberg H, Heiman-Patterson T. Malignant hyperthermia-like episode in Becker muscular dystrophy. Anesthesiology 2000;93(6):1535–1537.
- Rosenberg H, Fletcher JE, Brandom BW. Malignant hyperthermia and other pharmacogenetic disorders. In: Barash PG, Cullen BF, Stoelting RK, eds. Clinical anesthesia, 4th ed. Philadelphia: Lippincott Williams & Wilkins, 2001:521–538.
- Sessler DI. Malignant hyperthermia. Acta Anesth Scand 1996;40(suppl):25–30.
- Wappler F. Malignant hyperthermia. Eur J Anesth 2001;18(10):632–652.

Author(s): Miriam Anixter, MD; Barbara W. Brandom, MD

McArdle's Disease (Myophosphorylase Deficiency, Glycogenosis Type V)

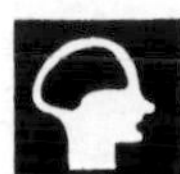

Basics

DESCRIPTION

McArdle's disease is a metabolic muscle disease caused by deficiency of the enzyme myophosphorylase.

EPIDEMIOLOGY

Incidence/Prevalence

McArdle's disease is a rare condition. No data are available about the exact incidence of the disease. In tertiary neuromuscular clinics one or two new cases are diagnosed every year.

Race

No ethnic predominance has been reported.

Age

McArdle's disease can become symptomatic at any age. In most individuals onset of symptoms occurs prior to age 10 years. Rarely the disease affects infants leading to progressive muscle weakness, respiratory insufficiency, and death.

Sex

Male predominance.

ETIOLOGY

- McArdle's disease is caused by the lack of myophosphorylase, the phosphorylase isoenzyme in muscle:
  - —Myophosphorylase activity is undetectable in muscle biopsies (either by immunohistochemistry or direct biochemical analysis) in most patients with McArdle's disease. Up to 10% of residual enzyme activity can be seen in some cases.
  - —Myophosphorylase initiates glycogen breakdown by removing 1,4-glucosyl residues from outer branches of the glycogen molecule, resulting in formation of glucose-1-phosphate. In McArdle's disease the block of this process leads to:
    - -Shortage of glycogen-liberated glucose as a source of adenosine triphosphate (ATP), ultimately impairing the operation of adenosine triphosphatases (ATPases) (sodium-potassium ATPase, calcium ATPase, and myosin ATPase) that couple the hydrolysis of ATP to cell work.
    - -Lack of normal pH fall during exercise with consequent impaired CK reaction equilibrium and exaggerated rise of adenosine diphosphate (ADP), which, among other actions, can also inhibit ATPases.
  - —Exactly how these metabolic changes lead to clinical symptoms is unclear.

Genetics

The disease is in most cases inherited in an autosomal-recessive fashion. The gene for the muscle phosphorylase has been located in chromosome 11q13. Up to 17 different nonsense, missense, and splice junction mutations have been reported. The Arg49Stop mutation is the most common in North America and Europe, accounting for 63% to 81% of the mutations. The incidence of these mutations varies among ethnic groups. Families with apparent autosomal-dominant transmission have been described, although these may in fact represent partial expression of disease in heterozygote carriers.

RISK FACTORS

N/A

PREGNANCY

Labor may constitute an exhausting exercise leading to rhabdomyolysis.

ASSOCIATED CONDITIONS

Rhabdomyolysis
Vitamin B_6 deficiency

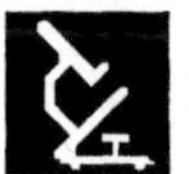

Diagnosis

DIFFERENTIAL DIAGNOSIS

- Inherited metabolic myopathies:
  - —Disorders of carbohydrate metabolism:
    - -Abnormal glycogen metabolism: debrancher enzyme deficiency; phosphorylase b kinase deficiency
    - -Abnormal glycolysis: phosphofructokinase deficiency; phosphoglycerate kinase deficiency; phosphoglycerate mutase deficiency; lactate dehydrogenase deficiency
  - —Disorders of lipid metabolism: carnitine palmitoyltransferase deficiency; muscle carnitine deficiency
  - —Disorders of purine metabolism: myoadenylate deaminase deficiency
- Secondary metabolic myopathies
  - —Endocrine: acromegaly; hypothyroidism; hyperthyroidism; hypoparathyroidism
  - —Electrolyte imbalance: hypo- and hypernatremia; hypo- and hypercalcemia; hypokalemia; hypophosphatemia; hypomagnesemia
- Mitochondrial myopathies
- Vascular insufficiency

SIGNS AND SYMPTOMS

The cardinal symptom of McArdle's disease is exercise intolerance with myalgia, early fatigue, painful cramps (metabolic contractures), and weakness of exercising muscles. Symptoms typically resolve with rest. Although many different physical activities may precipitate this clinical picture, two types of exercise are likely to cause symptoms: brief efforts involving isometric contraction (e.g., lifting weights) or less intense but sustained dynamic exercise (e.g., walking up a long hill). Walking on level ground is usually well tolerated. Most affected individuals function well once they adjust their activities to a level below their individual threshold for symptoms and learn they can exercise longer if they allow a brief rest immediately after the first sensation of muscle pain. This phenomenon is called the "second-wind phenomenon" and is attributed to the combination of increased blood flow stimulated by the activity and the ability to mobilize alternative sources of energy (i.e., fatty acids) for muscle work.

Exercise-induced muscle necrosis and rhabdomyolysis eventually manifest in ~50% of patients; 25% to 50% of these will develop renal failure due to acute tubular necrosis from myoglobinuria. Uncomplicated episodes of myoglobinuria are followed by complete recovery.

There are many variations to this typical presentation. The severity of the symptoms in particular may vary, with some patients complaining only of excessive tiredness and progressive weakness late in life, without cramps or myoglobinuria.

LABORATORY PROCEDURES

- Blood work: There is no specific blood test to diagnose McArdle's disease. However, creatinine kinase (CK) resting level should be obtained since it is moderately increased in 90% of patients. This helps distinguish McArdle's disease from carnitine palmitoyltransferase deficiency, another major metabolic myopathy causing myoglobinuria, where resting CK is usually normal. Serum electrolytes should be checked to rule out electrolyte imbalance as a cause of the symptoms. Endocrine studies such as thyroid function, parathyroid function, and growth hormone levels should be performed only if the systemic clinical picture suggests these diagnoses.
  If rhabdomyolysis is suspected, serum myoglobin, CK, lactate dehydrogenase, electrolytes, and renal function studies should be monitored.
- Urine studies: urine volume, urine sediment, and myoglobin levels are required only if rhabdomyolysis is suspected.

IMAGING STUDIES

No specific imaging studies are useful in the diagnosis of McArdle's disease.

SPECIAL TESTS

- Electromyogram (EMG): EMG is often normal between episodes of myoglobinuria but up to half of the patients may show some nonspecific myopathic abnormalities. The muscle tightness is electrically silent, indicating the presence of true contractures.
- Forearm exercise test: This test is performed by having the patient perform repetitive maximum grip sustained for periods of 1.5 seconds separated by rest periods of 0.5 seconds for a total of 1 minute. Venous blood should be drawn for lactate and ammonia levels prior to exercise, and at 1, 2, 4, 6, and 10 minutes after completion of the exercise. In normal subjects, forearm exercise increases venous lactate to three- to fivefold at the first and third minutes of the test. In patients with muscle disorders affecting the glycolytic or glycogenolytic pathways, lactate cannot be released into the circulation and venous levels do not change. Myophosphorylase deficiency is the most common cause for the lack of production of lactate during this test.
- Muscle biopsy: The diagnosis of McArdle's disease is made by the absence of histochemical staining for myophosphorylase in muscle fibers, while it remains positive in vessel walls. False-positive results can be found in patients with low residual activity or when the fetal phosphorylase isoform is transiently expressed in regenerating fibers after rhabdomyolysis. Additionally, in light microscopy, subsarcolemmal or intermyofibrillar deposits of periodic acid-Schiff (PAS)-stained glycogen can be seen. The muscle can also be sent for direct biochemical assay of myophosphorylase.
- P-31 magnetic resonance spectroscopy: Concentrations of ATP and creatine phosphate are normal at rest but, with exercise, the expected decrease in pH is not seen due to the lack of production of lactate, and the recovery of energy-rich metabolites to baseline is delayed. This tool is essentially used in research protocols.

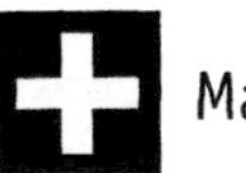

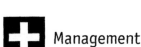

Management

GENERAL MEASURES

There is no specific therapy for McArdle's disease but combined aerobic exercise programs and high-protein diets have had positive effects in some cases.

SURGICAL MEASURES

Not applicable

SYMPTOMATIC TREATMENT

N/A

ADJUNCTIVE TREATMENT

N/A

ADMISSION/DISCHARGE CRITERIA

The diagnosis is usually made in the outpatient setting, and no emergency conditions are associated with the disease except for acute rhabdomyolysis following periods of intense exercise with the consequent risk for acute tubular necrosis.

Medications

DRUG(S) OF CHOICE

Myophosphorylase is the major repository of vitamin B_6 in the body, accounting for 80% of the total body pool. Some patients with McArdle's disease may show signs of subclinical vitamin B_6 deficiency and have reported greater resistance to fatigue with oral vitamin B_6 supplementation.

ALTERNATIVE DRUGS

None

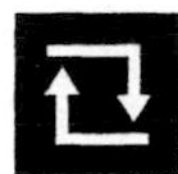

Follow-Up

PATIENT MONITORING

No specific monitoring is required.

EXPECTED COURSE AND PROGNOSIS

Fixed proximal weakness, especially in the shoulder girdle, will appear in up to one third of patients later in life.

PATIENT EDUCATION

Patient should be instructed, especially in childhood, to avoid intense exercise because of the risk of acute rhabdomyolysis. Patients can contact the Muscular Dystrophy Association for educational programs and updates in research and treatment.

Muscular Dystrophy Association, 3300 East Sunrise Drive, Tucson, AZ 85718. Phone: 800-572-1717 or 520-529-2000, website *www.mdausa.org.*

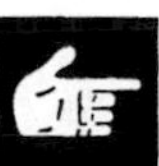

Miscellaneous

SYNONYMS

Myophosphorylase deficiency
Glycogenosis type V

ICD-9-CM: 330.8 Glycogenosis, myophosphorylase deficiency, or McArdle's disease

SEE ALSO: RHABDOMYOLYSIS

REFERENCES

- DiMauro S, Haller RG. Metabolic myopathies: substrate use defects. In: Schapira AHV, Griggs RC, eds. Muscle diseases. Blue books of practical neurology. Boston: Butterworth-Heinemann, 1999: 230–233.
- Jensen KE, Jakobsen J, Thomsen C, et al. Improved energy kinetics following high protein diet in McArdle's syndrome. A 31P magnetic resonance spectroscopy study. Acta Neurol Scand 1990;81(6):499–503.
- Phoenix J, Hopkins P, Bartram C, et al. Effect of vitamin B6 supplementation in McArdle's disease: a strategic case study. Neuromusc Disord 1998;8(3–4):210–212.
- Serratrice G, Pouget J, Azulay JPh. Exercise intolerance: classification and semiology. In: Serratrice G, Pouget J, Azulay JPh, eds. Exercise intolerance and muscle contracture. Paris: Springer, 1999:4–6.
- Slonim AE, Goans PJ. Myopathy in McArdle's syndrome. Improvement with a high-protein diet. N Engl J Med 1985;312(6):355–359.
- Wortmann RL. Metabolic diseases of muscle. In: Wortmann RL, ed. Diseases of skeletal muscle. Philadelphia: Lippincott Williams & Wilkins, 2000:160–162.

Author(s): Carmen Serrano-Munuera, MD

Meniere's Disease and Syndrome

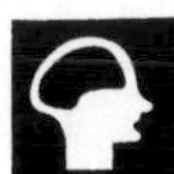

Basics

DESCRIPTION

Meniere's triad of vertigo, hearing loss, and tinnitus is associated with swelling of the endolymphatic space. Meniere's' disease denotes idiopathic endolymphatic hydrops; Meniere's syndrome denotes secondary endolymphatic hydrops.

EPIDEMIOLOGY

Incidence and Prevalence

Incidence estimates vary widely from 15 to 50 per 100,000, with prevalence about 220 cases per 100,000.

Age

Characteristically an affliction of adults, and quite unusual in children.

Sex

It has very modest female preponderance, slight left ear predilection, and often positive family history. Confusion between disease and syndrome confounds the epidemiology.

ETIOLOGY

Typical early endolymphatic distention in the scala media extends to the saccule. Later hydrops occurs in the utricle and vestibular labyrinth. Rupture of the membranous labyrinth admixes periplymph with endolymph. Thereupon a transient improvement of hearing (Lermoyez phenomenon) may occur. Etiopathogenic possibilities include vascular insufficiency, endolymph overproduction, electrolyte or osmotic pressure shifts, impaired endolymphatic flow, or inadequate endolymph resorption. Current consensus favors the latter. The etiology remains controversial.

Genetics

Heterogenetic Meniere's disease families have been described. These rare clusters likely make minor contribution to overall disease burden.

RISK FACTORS

- Trauma (labyrinthine concussion, acoustic trauma; temporal bone fracture; fenestration of the otic capsule)
- Inflammation (autoimmune ear disease; Cogan's syndrome)
- Infection (otosyphilis; viral labyrinthitis)
- Infiltration (leukemia, as in Meniere's original patient; Paget's disease; von Hippel-Lindau–associated neoplasms; histiocytosis)
- Effusion (chronic otitis media; serous labyrinthitis);
- Malformations (Mondini's cochlear dysplasia)
- Endocrine/metabolic (thyroid; diabetes)
- Electrolyte/osmolality shifts

PREGNANCY

Attacks associated with decreased serum osmolality in gravid women and premenstrual attacks associated with fluid retention have been well reported.

ASSOCIATED CONDITIONS

N/A

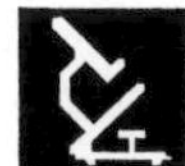

Diagnosis

DIFFERENTIAL DIAGNOSIS

Episodic vertigo occurs with perilymph fistula, migraine, vestibular neuritis, benign paroxysmal positioning vertigo, viral labyrinthitis, and vestibular atelectasis. Vertebrobasilar insufficiency, hyperviscosity syndromes, eighth nerve root entry zone neurovascular compression, vestibular schwannoma, endolymphatic sac tumor, brainstem mass, presyncope, and otosyphilis can masquerade as Meniere's disease. Rarely cerebellar degenerations and familial episodic ataxia must be considered. Astatic seizures mimic otolithic crises.

SIGNS AND SYMPTOMS

Episodes of vertigo lasting from minutes to hours are superimposed on fluctuating hearing loss, aural fullness, and tinnitus. This tetrad varies between patients and over time. Patients often confuse true vertigo with an after-going sense of instability. Cross-coupled accelerations in the semicircular canals (Coriolis effect) may exacerbate vertigo with movement, suggesting other disorders. Hydrops starting in the basal cochlea and leading to rupture of Reissner's membrane at the helicotrema gives the auditory symptoms and Lermoyez phenomenon. Between attacks, some hearing distortion and tinnitus may accompany remitting dysequilibrium and resolving aural fullness. Positive cochlear recruitment may cause painful sensitivity to loud sounds. Cacophonous distortion, muffling, and sometimes diplacusis occur. Abnormal pressure dynamics in the membranous labyrinth may cause the "otolithic crisis of Tumarkin," a sudden drop attack in which the fully conscious patient is thrown to the floor. Pneumatic pressure–induced nystagmus (Hennebert's sign) can be seen. Valsalva- or pressure-induced dizziness (Hennebert's symptom) and sound-induced dizziness (Tullio phenomenon) can also occur. In late stages symptoms become chronic and unremitting. *Atypical Meniere's disease* denotes predominantly vestibular or auditory variants. Presumably strictures in the ductus reuniens or utricular duct result in isolated cochlear or vestibular hydrops. Unilateral onset is typical. Over time bilateral disease features emerge in 10% to 60%. Contralateral fast-phase nystagmus is seen with attacks. Brief ipsilateral "recovery nystagmus" supervenes in attack resolution.

LABORATORY PROCEDURES

No laboratory tests confirm Meniere's disease. Autoimmune disease panel, systemic inflammation markers, RAST, FTA-ABS, thyroid studies, metabolic panel, and CBC evaluate the differential possibilities.

IMAGING STUDIES

MRI and MRA are appropriate for suspected vertebrobasilar insufficiency, neurovascular compression, acoustic neuroma, multiple sclerosis, etc. High-resolution temporal bone CT may show dehiscence of the superior semicircular canal. High-resolution MRI visualized the endolymphatic duct significantly less often in Meniere's patients than in controls. Focused temporal bone MRI detected swelling of the scala media. The primary role of imaging is to exclude other structural pathology.

SPECIAL TESTS

- *Pure tone audiometry* is important. Few causes of low-frequency sensorineural hearing loss give an up-sloping audiogram like early Meniere's disease. With progressive disease, the audiogram becomes peaked around 2000. Thereafter it becomes uniformly depressed or "flat."
- *Speech audiometry* is worse than predicted because of distortion and correlates well with subjective complaints.
- *Electrocochleography* (ECoG) is a very promising short latency evoked response to auditory clicks, in which the summating potential (SP) is sensitive to cochlear basilar membrane distortion. An elevated ratio of SP to action potential (AP) appears to be quite specific but not very sensitive for endolymphatic hydrops.
- *Electronystagmography (ENG)* with bi-thermal caloric testing may show vestibular paresis (>25% decrease in the affected ear), but is not very sensitive and less specific than ECoG. Caloric responses vary with disease stage and the recency of the last attack.
- *Rotational chair testing* may show decreased gain, increased phase lead, and sometimes an asymmetry toward the affected side, as in any peripheral vestibular paresis.
- *Spontaneous nystagmus* can be seen on ENG or with Frenzel goggles. Nystagmus may be elicited by rapid back-and-forth head shaking for 30 seconds, abruptly stopping in the central position and viewing through Frenzel lenses.
- *Marching in place* with eyes closed and arms extended forward will result in a gradual rotation of the patient toward the paretic labyrinth.
- *Osmotic diuresis test* seeks improvement in baseline audiometry 1 to 3 hours after ingestion of a powerful diuretic (typically glycerol), suggesting endolymphatic hydrops.

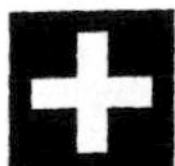

Management

GENERAL MEASURES

A strict low-sodium diet (1.5 to 2 g/d) is universally recommended. Stricter restrictions are arguably more effective. Some advocate avoiding caffeine, chocolate, tobacco, stimulants, stress, and alcohol.

SURGICAL MEASURES

- *Nondestructive surgery* includes endolymphatic sac fistula or shunt procedures. Still quite popular, fibrous overgrowth and success rates indistinguishable from placebo are concerns. Endolymphatic duct stent and cochleosacculotomy have been advocated. Myringotomy and tympanic ventilation tubes have been supplemented by pressure chamber treatments. Recently pressure oscillation through a tympanostomy tube has been used.
- *Destructive (ablative) surgery:* For medically intractable disease, vestibular neurectomy, intratympanic injection of ototoxic drugs (usually gentamicin or streptomycin), and surgical labyrinthectomy (for those without functional hearing in the affected ear) have all been used. Surgical otologic consultation is recommended only after medical therapy has failed. Since Meniere's disease can become bilateral, destructive procedures require appropriate circumspection.

SYMPTOMATIC TREATMENT

During attacks vestibular suppressants (diazepam or meclizine) and antiemetics (prochlorperazine, promethazine, dimenhydrinate, and trimethobenzamide) are useful. Glycopyrrolate is helpful in milder cases.

ADJUNCTIVE TREATMENT

Vestibular rehabilitation may augment central compensation for peripheral vestibular loss in the late chronic stage. Some advocate extension to early disease, although dysequilibrium often substantially remits between attacks.

ADMISSION/DISCHARGE CRITERIA

Medical admission rarely may be indicated to investigate worrisome alternate diagnoses.

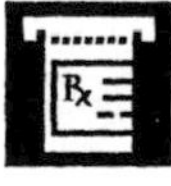

Medications

DRUG(S) OF CHOICE

Diuretics: Mild diuresis with hydrochlorothiazide/triamterene or similar regimen is customary. Acetazolamide should be optimal since dark cells in the labyrinth and the stria vascularis use carbonic anhydrase, but usually it is less clinically useful.

Histamine: Betahistine is a first-line European agent, ostensibly to provide vasodilatation in the labyrinth.

Medical ablation: Historically a selective vestibular toxin was advocated to ablate noisome vertigo.

Contraindications

Anuria or renal failure; elevated serum potassium; avoid combination with multiple potassium sparing diuretics.

Precautions

Gout; lupus; diarrhea; diabetes; hepatic, renal, or chronic pulmonary disease. Pregnancy category D.

ALTERNATIVE DRUGS

Only diuretics and betahistine have controlled randomized trial support. Local and systemic corticosteroids have been used, as well as other immunosuppressives (azathioprine and methotrexate). No controlled trials support frequently used antihistamines. Empirically, vasodilators and calcium channel blockers have been tried.

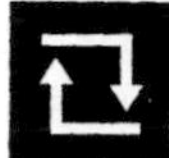

Follow-Up

PATIENT MONITORING

Symptomatic treatment during attacks and regular office visits for dietary and medical management may be combined with periodic audiometry and bithermal caloric ENG.

EXPECTED COURSE AND PROGNOSIS

Unilateral onset of a fluctuating auditory and vestibular decline is punctuated by repeated vertiginous attacks of generally declining frequency. Some contralateral involvement increases from 10% to 15% at 2 years to 30% to 60% at 15 years. Medical treatments do not alter the prognosis for hearing or vestibular loss. Likewise, surgical procedures ablating vertigo do nothing to preserve hearing and may impair it. Some patients have only a few vertiginous spells, mild hearing loss, and a stable course. Others have lifelong relapsing attacks with gradual decline. A minority have an aggressive, unrelenting course with only brief remissions until profound deafness and dysequilibrium ensue. The course of auditory and vestibular symptoms can be independent. Isolated vestibular variants usually, but not always, evolve into more typical forms. Consider other diagnoses if no auditory features emerge after a reasonable time.

PATIENT EDUCATION

Nutritional counseling and repeated encouragement of a low-sodium diet are suggested.

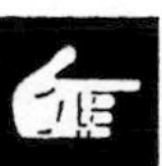

Miscellaneous

SYNONYMS

Endolymphatic hydrops

ICD-9-CM: 386.00 (01 cochleovestibular; 02 cochlear; 03 vestibular; 04 in remission)

SEE ALSO: DIZZINESS/VERTIGO

REFERENCES

- Blakley BW. Update on intratympanic gentamicin for Meniere's disease. Laryngoscope 2000;110(2 pt 1):236–240.
- Claes J, Van de Heyning PH. Medical treatment of Meniere's disease—a review of literature. Acta Otolaryngol Suppl 1997;52:637–642.
- Fitzgerald DC. Perilymphatic fistula and Meniere's disease. Clinical series and literature review. Ann Otol Rhinol Laryngol 2001;110(5 pt 1):430–436.
- Niyazov DM, Andrews JC, Strelioff D, et al. Diagnosis of endolymphatic hydrops in vivo with magnetic resonance imaging. Otol Neurotol 2001;22(6):813–817.
- Paparella MM, Djalilian HR. Etiology, pathophysiology of symptoms, and pathogenesis of Meniere's disease. Otolaryngol Clin North Am 2002;35(3):529–545.

Author(s): Robert W. Jensen, MD, JD

Meningitis, Acute Bacterial

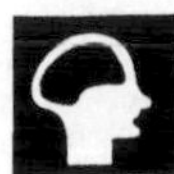

Basics

DESCRIPTION

Acute bacterial meningitis (ABM) is an inflammation of the meninges due to bacterial infection, which, if not treated promptly and appropriately, results in neurologic morbidity and high mortality.

EPIDEMIOLOGY

Incidence/Prevalence

In 1995, a report showed that a total of 5,755 cases of ABM were caused by five major pathogens in the United States: *Streptococcus pneumoniae* (1.1 cases/100,000 persons), *Neisseria meningitidis* (0.6/100,000), group B streptococcus (0.3/100,000), *Listeria monocytogenes* (0.2/100,000), and *Haemophilus influenzae* (0.2/100,000).

Race

There is no evidence of any ethnic predominance.

Age

The disease occurs in all ages.

Sex

Males and females are equally affected.

ETIOLOGY

- The most common pathogens responsible for ABM vary by age group. Among neonates, group B streptococcus (*Streptococcus agalactiae*) is the most common pathogen. While *H. influenzae* type B (HIB) was formerly the most common among children of ages 1 month to 4 years, widespread use of the HIB vaccine has dramatically reduced the incidence of this pathogen, and *S. pneumoniae* (pneumococcus) and *N. meningitidis* (meningococcus) are now the predominant pathogens in this age group. In older children, ages 5 to 18 years, and adults, pneumococcus and meningococcus are most common, while pneumococcus, *L. monocytogenes*, and Gram-negative bacilli are most common in older adults over age 50.
- A subset of patients who have had head trauma, neurosurgery, or CSF shunt are at risk for ABM secondary to *Staphylococcus* spp., Gram-negative bacilli, as well as pneumococcus.
- ABM pathogens generally colonize the nasopharyngeal mucosa of the host, enter the intravascular space, cross the blood–brain barrier, and multiply aggressively in the CSF. There is a paucity of antibody and complement in the CSF, resulting in inefficient phagocytosis of the bacteria. Cytokines contribute to brain edema and elevated intracranial pressure.

Genetics

Complement deficiency is a risk factor for meningococcal disease. Late complement deficiency (C5, C6, C7, C8, or C9) is associated with recurrent meningococcal disease.

RISK FACTORS

Cases of ABM are generally sporadic, though close contact may play a role in some cases. For example, close contacts of patients with meningococcal meningitis may be at risk for developing the disease. One study did suggest that college students residing on campus may be at higher risk of ABM due to *N. meningitidis*. Rifampin, ciprofloxacin, or ceftriaxone may be used to eradicate nasal carriage of this organism. The meningococcal vaccine may also be useful in this population. Children under age 2 who have not been vaccinated with the HIB vaccine are at risk of ABM secondary to this organism. Rifampin or ceftriaxone in children and adults, and ciprofloxacin, rifampin, or ceftriaxone in adults, may be used as prophylaxis if a patient comes into contact with a child with HIB ABM. Other risk factors may include the following:

- Closed head injury with skull fracture or disruption of the cribriform plate
- Parameningeal infections such as sinusitis, chronic otitis, and mastoiditis
- Anatomic defects such as pilonidal sinuses, meningomyeloceles, and meningeal disruption
- Sickle cell anemia and splenectomy may predispose to meningitis due to encapsulated organisms

PREGNANCY

Little is known regarding ABM in pregnancy.

ASSOCIATED CONDITIONS

N/A

Diagnosis

DIFFERENTIAL DIAGNOSIS

- Infectious etiologies:
  - —Viral meningitis
  - —Encephalitis
  - —Brain abscess
  - —Fungal meningitis
  - —Mycobacterial meningitis
  - —Primary HIV infection
- Noninfectious etiologies:
  - —Benign or malignant brain tumor
  - —Cerebrovascular accident
  - —Sarcoidosis
  - —Systemic lupus erythematosus
  - —Wegener's granulomatosis
  - —CNS vasculitis
  - —Arachnoiditis
  - —Migraine
  - —Drugs, including nonsteroidal antiinflammatory drugs (NSAIDs), trimethoprim/sulfamethoxazole, and OKT3

SIGNS AND SYMPTOMS

The classic signs and symptoms of ABM are fever, headache, photophobia, and nuchal rigidity. Less common is vomiting, focal neurologic changes (particularly cranial nerves III, IV, VI, and VII), seizures, and somnolence. Symptoms generally develop rapidly, and ABM should be considered a medical emergency.

LABORATORY PROCEDURES

Baseline blood work should include CBC and differential, blood cultures, serum electrolytes and glucose, liver function tests, and an HIV test.

IMAGING STUDIES

Head CT is useful in patients with coma, papilledema, or focal neurologic signs, but is otherwise not indicated. Obtaining an imaging study should not prevent immediate blood cultures and prompt administration of antibiotics. If no mass effect is seen on imaging, an immediate lumbar puncture should be done.

SPECIAL TESTS

- CSF obtained by lumbar puncture is the most important and accurate diagnostic tool. Opening pressure, Gram stain, CSF culture, protein, glucose, and cell count and differential should be done at a minimum. Latex agglutination for bacterial antigens may be useful if the patient has had prior antibiotic therapy. Opening pressure is typically elevated. In 80% of cases, the organism should be visible on Gram stain. There is usually a neutrophilic pleocytosis ($>$1,000 WBC cells/mm^3), with a predominance of neutrophils. CSF protein is almost always elevated, and hypoglycorrhachia is common. Very rarely, CSF may be normal, particularly in immunocompromised patients, neonates, or in those patients very early in the course of their disease.
- Gram stain is very useful for tailoring antibiotic therapy, although prior antibiotic therapy may make it difficult to interpret.

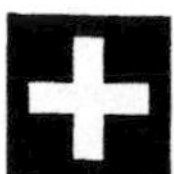

Management

GENERAL MEASURES

- Prompt administration of empiric antibiotics is the most important therapeutic modality. Delay of antibiotic administration has been related to increased neurologic morbidity and mortality. Antibiotic therapy should initially be directed at the most likely pathogens, then tailored specifically to the Gram stain or culture data when available. Infectious disease specialists should be consulted, as antibiotic resistance patterns, particularly of *S. pneumoniae* and HIB, vary widely from region to region.
- Close monitoring is essential, and many of these patients may need endotracheal intubation for airway protection. In patients with elevated intracranial pressure, high-dose dexamethasone, hyperosmolar agents, or hyperventilation may be needed.
- In patients over 2 years of age with ABM due to known or suspected HIB, dexamethasone therapy should be started just prior to antibiotics, because it has been shown to decreases neurologic morbidity. Dexamethasone may also be useful in adults with ABM, but only if there is evidence of elevated intracranial pressure.

SURGICAL MEASURES

N/A

SYMPTOMATIC TREATMENT

Symptomatic treatment includes management of fevers, antiepileptic drugs for secondary seizures, analgesics for headache, and hydration.

ADJUNCTIVE TREATMENT

N/A

ADMISSION/DISCHARGE CRITERIA

Patients are admitted for parenteral antibiotics and careful monitoring. Duration of therapy should be 7 days for HIB and *N. meningitidis*, 10 to 14 days for *S. pneumoniae*, 14 to 21 days for *L. monocytogenes* or group B streptococci, and 21 days for Gram-negative bacilli.

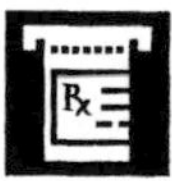

Medications

DRUG(S) OF CHOICE

Empiric Antibiotics

- Age <3 months: ampicillin 100 mg/kg IV q8h plus broad-spectrum cephalosporin such as cefotaxime 50 mg/kg IV q6h or ceftriaxone 50–100 mg/kg IV q12h
- Age 3 months to <18 years: broad-spectrum cephalosporin such as cefotaxime 50 mg/kg IV q6h or ceftriaxone 50–100 mg IV q12h
- Age 18 to <50 years: broad-spectrum cephalosporin such as cefotaxime 2 g IV q6h or ceftriaxone 2 g IV q12h plus vancomycin 1 g IV q12h
- Age 50 and above: ampicillin 2 g IV q4h plus a broad-spectrum cephalosporin such as cefotaxime 2 g IV q6h or ceftriaxone 2 g IV q12h plus vancomycin 1 g IV q12h
- Patients with impaired cellular immunity: ampicillin 2 g IV q4h plus ceftazidime 2 g IV q8h
- Patients who have head trauma, are neurosurgical patients, or who have a CSF shunt: vancomycin 1 g IV q12h plus ceftazidime 2 g IV q8h
- Dexamethasone dosing is 0.15 mg/kg IV q6h for 4 days for both children and adults.

Contraindications

History of allergic reaction to specific antibiotics is a contraindication to their use.

Precautions

None

ALTERNATIVE DRUGS

Space is too limited to list alternative regimens for each suspected pathogen; consultation with an infectious disease specialist is recommended.

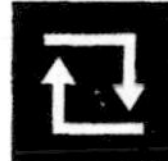

Follow-Up

PATIENT MONITORING

Once hemodynamically and neurologically stable, close monitoring is not indicated. Follow-up lumbar puncture and MRI or CT may be useful in patients who have uncommon pathogens (e.g., Gram-negative bacilli, *Staphylococcus aureus*, etc.) or whose clinical course does not improve as expected. These may aid in evaluation of possible parameningeal focus of infection, and evaluate for complications such as cortical vein thrombosis or subdural empyema.

EXPECTED COURSE AND PROGNOSIS

Overall morbidity in adults in 1995 was 25%. In another recent study, 61% of children had developmental delay and neurologic sequelae after Gram-negative bacillary meningitis. These two reports emphasize the need for the rapid use of antibiotics in patients suspected of having ABM. Despite appropriate therapy, in many of these patients there will be high morbidity and a variety of neurologic sequelae. Many will require physical and occupational therapy after their illness, and some will have massive neurologic deficits.

PATIENT EDUCATION

Information is available on the World Wide Web at *http://www.cdc.gov/ncidod/dbmd/diseaseinfo* or *http://healthlinkusa.com/203.htm*. Also, the Meningitis Foundation of America Inc. may be contacted for information at 7155 Shadeland Station, Suite 190 Indianapolis, Indiana 46256-3922. Phone 800-668-1129.

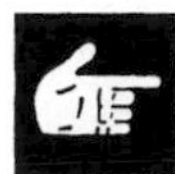

Miscellaneous

SYNONYMS

Bacterial meningitis
Meningitis

ICD-9-CM: 036.0 Meningococcal meningitis; 320 Bacterial meningitis; 320.1 Haemophilus meningitis; 320.2 Pneumococcal meningitis; 320.3 Streptococcal meningitis; 320.4 Staphylococcal meningitis; 320.7 Meningitis in other bacterial diseases classified elsewhere; 320.81 Anaerobic meningitis; 320.82 Meningitis due to Gram-negative bacilli not elsewhere classified; 320.89 Meningitis due to other species of bacteria

SEE ALSO: N/A

REFERENCES

- Fijen CA, Kuijper EJ, et al. Assessment of complement deficiency in patients with meningococcal disease in the Netherlands. Clin Infect Dis 1999;28(1):98–105.
- Harrison LH, Dwyer DM, Maples CT, et al. Risk of meningococcal infection in college students. JAMA 1999;281(20):1906–1910.
- Pruitt A. Infections of the nervous system. Neurol Clin North Am 1998;16(2): 419–447.
- Quagliarello VJ, Scheld WM. Treatment of bacterial meningitis. N Engl J Med 1997; 336:708–716.
- Schuchat A, Robinson K, Wenger JD, et al. Bacterial meningitis in the United States in 1995. N Engl J Med 1997;337(14): 970–976.
- Townsend GC, Scheld WM. Infections of the central nervous system. Adv Intern Med 1998;43:403–447.

Author(s): Thomas C. Keeling, MD; Susan L. Koletar, MD

Meningitis, Aseptic

Basics

DESCRIPTION

Aseptic meningitis is a generic term encompassing a range of conditions that is characterized by an inflammation of the meninges without a readily identifiable bacterial cause after initial stains and culture of the CSF. It is most commonly viral in etiology.

EPIDEMIOLOGY

Incidence/Prevalence

Approximately 10,000 cases of aseptic meningitis are reported in the United States each year. There is summertime predominance, corresponding to enterovirus infections, the primary cause of aseptic meningitis.

Race

There is no evidence of any ethnic predominance.

Age

There is no known age predominance.

Sex

Males and females are equally affected.

ETIOLOGY

- Viruses are the most common etiology for aseptic meningitis. Most common are the enteroviruses (echovirus, coxsackie A and B viruses, polioviruses, and the enteroviruses), which cause up to 80% of aseptic meningitis. Enteroviruses, as well as arboviruses have summertime predominance. Other viruses that can cause aseptic meningitis include lymphocytic choriomeningitis virus in the fall and winter, mumps virus in the winter and spring, and herpesvirus (HSV), Epstein-Barr virus, and cytomegalovirus in any season. HSV accounts for 1% to 3% of all cases of aseptic meningitis. After animal bite, rabies virus should be considered. HIV can cause aseptic meningitis during acute infection, and should always be considered in the differential diagnosis.
- Other potential etiologies for aseptic meningitis includes bacterial (tuberculosis, rocky mountain spotted fever, Q fever, typhus, syphilis, Lyme disease, leptospirosis); fungal (*Candida* sp., *Coccidioides immitis*, *Cryptococcus neoformans*, *Histoplasma capsulatum*); protozoal (toxoplasmosis, malaria, amoebiasis, visceral larval migrans); nematodal (eosinophilic meningitis caused by rat lung worm larvae) and mycoplasmal for infectious etiologies; and malignant etiologies, autoimmune, and collagen-vascular diseases, medications (sulfamethoxazole, trimethoprim, NSAIDs, carbamazepine, isoniazid, penicillin), and vaccinations (mumps and measles) among noninfectious etiologies.

Genetics

There is no known genetic component to aseptic meningitis.

RISK FACTORS

Cases of aseptic meningitis are almost always sporadic. When evaluating the patient, specific features of the history and physical may be helpful. Age, season, lists of medications, potential exposure to HIV, travel history, chronic illnesses, exposure to vectors, herpetic lesions for herpes virus infections, and parotitis with mumps may provide epidemiologic clues.

PREGNANCY

Little is known regarding aseptic meningitis in pregnancy.

ASSOCIATED CONDITIONS

N/A

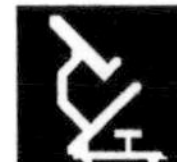

Diagnosis

DIFFERENTIAL DIAGNOSIS

- Infectious etiologies
  - —Viral meningitis
  - —Partially treated bacterial meningitis
  - —Encephalitis
  - —Brain abscess
  - —Fungal meningitis
  - —Mycobacterial meningitis
  - —Primary HIV infection
- Noninfectious etiologies
  - —Benign or malignant brain tumor
  - —Sarcoidosis
  - —Systemic lupus erythematosus
  - —Wegener's granulomatosis
  - —CNS vasculitis
  - —Arachnoiditis
  - —Medications

SIGNS AND SYMPTOMS

The classic signs and symptoms of aseptic meningitis are fever, headache, photophobia, and nuchal rigidity. Also common is vomiting. Focal neurologic deficits, seizures, and significant lethargy are unusual in aseptic meningitis. Usually the symptoms are acute, but occasionally may begin after several days or even weeks of fever or systemic illness.

LABORATORY PROCEDURES

Baseline blood work should include CBC and differential, blood cultures, serum electrolytes and glucose, liver function tests, and an HIV test.

IMAGING STUDIES

Head CT is useful in patients with coma, papilledema, or focal neurologic signs, but is otherwise not indicated. Obtaining an imaging study should not prevent immediate blood cultures and prompt administration of antibiotics if the patient is critically ill. If no mass effect is seen on imaging, an immediate lumbar puncture should be done.

SPECIAL TESTS

- CSF obtained by lumbar puncture is the most important and accurate diagnostic tool. Opening pressure; Gram stain; CSF culture for bacteria, fungus, and virus; and protein, glucose, and cell count and differential should all be done. Opening pressure is typically elevated. CSF WBC is usually less than 500 cells/mm^3, and can be less than 200 WBC/mm^3. Mononuclear cells are the most common leukocyte found in the CSF pleocytosis of aseptic meningitis. CSF glucose is generally normal, and CSF protein is usually normal to slightly elevated.
- Latex agglutination for bacterial antigens may be useful if the patient has had prior antibiotic therapy, and partially treated bacterial meningitis is being considered as the diagnosis. If warranted by the physical exam, other tests that may be useful include CSF cryptococcal antigen, acid-fast stain and culture, serum RPR and CSF VDRL, wet mount for amebic trophozoites, viral culture of CSF, and HSV polymerase chain reaction (PCR). If the patient continues to deteriorate, meningeal or brain biopsy may be necessary.

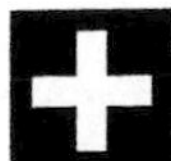

Management

GENERAL MEASURES

Treatment is primarily supportive. Many patients can be treated symptomatically at home, but others may require admission. Criteria for admission may include profound headache, nausea, vomiting, or CSF pleocytosis with a polymorphonuclear leukocytes predominance that may require empiric treatment for acute bacterial meningitis. Oral acyclovir may be useful if herpes meningitis secondary to primary HSV infection is suspected.

SURGICAL MEASURES

There are no surgical measures for aseptic meningitis.

SYMPTOMATIC TREATMENT

Symptomatic treatment addresses pain control, relief of fever, and gentle rehydration.

ADJUNCTIVE TREATMENT

N/A

ADMISSION/DISCHARGE CRITERIA

Patients are admitted if the clinician feels the symptoms are severe enough to warrant admission, or if there is concern about bacterial meningitis with CSF pleocytosis and polymorphonuclear leukocyte predominance. Patients are discharged when their symptoms allow.

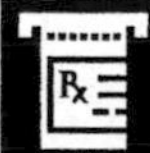

Medications

DRUG(S) OF CHOICE

- Analgesics and antipyretics as necessary
- Herpes: acyclovir 200 mg PO 5×/day for 10 days.
- Partially treated bacterial meningitis: ceftriaxone 2 g IV q12h or cefotaxime 2 g IV q6.
- Other pathogens, if found, should be treated with the appropriate therapy.

Contraindications

Known hypersensitivity to a particular agent.

Precautions

N/A

ALTERNATIVE DRUGS

N/A

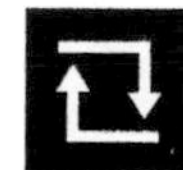

Follow-Up

PATIENT MONITORING

If hemodynamically and neurologically stable, close monitoring is not indicated.

EXPECTED COURSE AND PROGNOSIS

Prognosis is excellent. Most cases of aseptic meningitis are self-limited with no sequelae. In other cases, prognosis is dependent on the underlying etiology.

PATIENT EDUCATION

The Meningitis Foundation of America Inc. may be contacted for information at 7155 Shadeland Station, Suite 190 Indianapolis, Indiana 46256-3922. Phone 800-668-1129, website *http://www.musa.org*. You may also contact your local health department for more information.

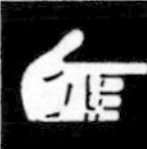

Miscellaneous

SYNONYMS

Viral meningitis
Aseptic meningitis
Meningitis

ICD-9-CM: 047 Meningitis due to enterovirus (includes aseptic meningitis and viral meningitis)
This excludes the following: 049.1 Meningitis due to enterovirus; 060.0-066.9 Meningitis due to arbovirus; 054.72 Meningitis due to herpes simplex virus; 053.0 Meningitis due to varicella zoster virus; 049.0 Meningitis due to lymphocytic choriomeningitis virus; 072.1 Meningitis due to mumps virus; 047.0 Meningitis due to coxsackie virus; 047.1 Meningitis due to ECHO virus; 047.9 Meningitis due to virus not otherwise specified

SEE ALSO: MENINGITIS, ACUTE BACTERIAL; AND MENINGOENCEPHALITIS, CRYPTOCOCCAL

REFERENCES

- Nelson S, Sealy DP, Schneider EF. The aseptic meningitis syndrome. Am Fam Physician 1993;48(5):809–815.
- Pruitt A. Infections of the nervous system. Neurol Clin North Am 1998;16(2):419–447.
- Rubeiz H, Roos RP. Viral meningitis and encephalitis. Semin Neurol 1992;12(3):165–177.
- Townsend GC, Scheld WM. Infections of the central nervous system. Adv Intern Med 1998;43:403–447.

Author(s): Thomas C. Keeling, MD; Susan L. Koletar, MD

Meningoencephalitis, Cryptococcal

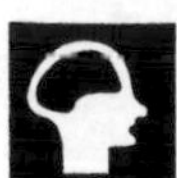

Basics

DESCRIPTION

Cryptococcal meningoencephalitis is caused by fungal infection of both the meninges and underlying brain parenchyma by *Cryptococcus neoformans*. It is the most common cause of fungal meningitis in the United States and an increasingly important opportunistic infection in immunosuppressed patients.

EPIDEMIOLOGY

Incidence/Prevalence

Cryptococcal meningoencephalitis is rare in individuals without impaired cellular immunity. The incidence of cryptococcal meningitis among HIV-infected individuals ranges from 6% to 10%. Cryptococcosis is an AIDS-defining illness in about 40% of these cases. Infection is usually associated with profound immunodeficiency with CD4 count <100 cells/mm^3. It is the third most frequent infection of the CNS seen in patients with AIDS.

Race

No evidence of any ethnic predominance.

Age

Infection affects persons of all ages. The majority, excluding those with AIDS, are between 30 and 60 years of age.

Sex

Males outnumber females 3:1.

ETIOLOGY

Clinical syndromes are due to infection with *Cryptococcal neoformans*, an encapsulated yeast that reproduces by budding. Antigenic specificity of the capsular polysaccharide defines four different serotypes (A, B, C, and D). Serotype A and D are classified as variety *neoformans* and include the large majority of clinical isolates. It is found in soil samples and organic debris such as aged pigeon droppings, in pigeon habitats, and in association with rotting vegetation. Serotypes B and C are listed under the variety *gattii*, which is cultured from several species of eucalyptus trees in tropical and subtropical areas. Var. *gattii* tends to affect patients without predisposing factors, whereas patients infected by var. *neoformans* strains are immunosuppressed, and more frequently have diffusely disseminated lesions and have higher fatality rates. Infection is acquired by inhalation of infectious propagules. Most patients with cryptococcal infection of the CNS have no evidence of concomitant pulmonary involvement, implying they have either asymptomatic, self-limited primary pulmonary disease or reactivation of primary disease. Cell-mediated immunity is the major host defense against infection due to *C. neoformans*.

Genetics

No genetic predisposition established.

RISK FACTORS

Conditions associated with defects in cell-mediated immunity such as HIV infection, organ transplantation, prolonged corticosteroid treatment, malignancy, and sarcoidosis.

PREGNANCY

N/A

ASSOCIATED CONDITIONS

As above.

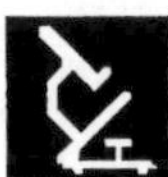

Diagnosis

DIFFERENTIAL DIAGNOSIS

- Infectious
  - —Viral meningitis
  - —Encephalitis
  - —Brain abscess
  - —Fungal meningitis
  - —Mycobacterial meningitis
  - —Toxoplasmosis
  - —Primary HIV infection
  - —Syphilis
  - —Progressive multifocal leukoencephalopathy
- Noninfectious
  - —Carcinomatous meningitis
  - —Lymphomatous meningitis
  - —Cerebrovascular accident
  - —CNS vasculitis
  - —Sarcoidosis
  - —Drugs

SIGNS AND SYMPTOMS

Onset of CNS cryptococcosis may be acute or insidious. Acute manifestations are more common in the immunosuppressed patient. Immune compromise such as in AIDS results in a higher burden of organisms and diminished inflammatory response. Most common symptoms are fever, malaise, and headache. There is typically minimal or no nuchal rigidity. Clinical illness is rarely fulminant, and the subacute onset of symptoms and nonspecific presentation can make it difficult to diagnose. In the immunocompetent host, symptoms may follow a more chronic course over weeks to months. Most present with signs and symptoms of subacute meningitis or meningoencephalitis including confusion, impaired memory, nausea, dizziness, and somnolence. Less common manifestations include visual disturbances, cranial nerve palsies, papilledema, cerebellar signs, and seizures.

LABORATORY PROCEDURES

- CSF examination including examination with India ink. Opening pressure may be markedly elevated (>200 mm H_2O), especially in patients with AIDS, and India ink smears show typical encapsulated yeast forms. Gram stain is usually not sufficient since the organisms can be confused with host cells. Cell counts are characteristically low (<50/μL) in AIDS-associated infection and higher in non-AIDS cases with lymphocyte predominance. Protein and glucose levels are usually only slightly abnormal, with elevated protein and depressed glucose more common in normal hosts. Culture is needed to confirm the diagnosis. Negative cultures do not absolutely rule out infections as only small numbers of organisms are present in some CSF and may be missed. Therefore, large specimens of CSF may be required for diagnosis.
- Extraneural disease is more common in the immunocompromised host. Urine, sputum, and blood cultures should be obtained and any suspicious skin and soft tissue lesions should be cultured and/or biopsied.

IMAGING STUDIES

Any immunocompromised patient with central neurologic dysfunction should undergo CT scan or MRI to exclude possible space-occupying lesions and/or detect hydrocephalus. CT scan of the head is abnormal in up to 30% of AIDS patients with cryptococcal meningitis. Most common abnormalities are cortical atrophy and varying degrees of ventricular enlargement without focal lesions or enhancement. Cryptococcomas can be either single or multiple and occur in up to 25% of patients.

SPECIAL TESTS

Cryptococcal antigen assay is highly sensitive and specific for detection of *C. neoformans* infection. Antigen can be detected in both serum and in CSF, and may be positive before identification of the organism in culture. Antigen presence implies extrapulmonary involvement and necessitates careful evaluation for site of infection. The height of the antigen titer correlates with the burden of organisms. Serial measurement of antigen titers may be useful in following therapy and to predict relapse in immunocompetent patients, but of limited value in AIDS patients.

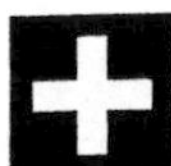

Management

GENERAL MEASURES

Treatment involves initiation of antifungal therapy and supportive care. Treatment options depend on the host immune status. In the non-HIV infected, goal is cure of the infection with CSF sterilization and prevention of long-term neurologic sequelae. In those with coexisting HIV, therapeutic goals are to achieve clinical remission and to prevent relapse with chronic suppressive therapy.

SURGICAL MEASURES

Surgery is rarely required in patients with mass lesions.

SYMPTOMATIC TREATMENT

Supportive care.

ADJUNCTIVE TREATMENT

Systemic corticosteroids may be given for mass lesions with significant edema. Patients with increased intracranial pressure (>200 mm H_2O) may respond to removal of large volumes of CSF with daily lumbar punctures. Lumbar drains or ventricular shunts may be necessary for patients who require more frequent fluid removal for symptom control. Corticosteroids, acetazolamide, and mannitol have no benefit in the management of elevated intracranial pressure.

ADMISSION/DISCHARGE CRITERIA

Patients are admitted for further evaluation, parenteral antibiotics, and careful monitoring.

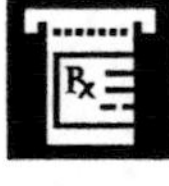

Medications

DRUG(S) OF CHOICE

HIV-negative: induction course of amphotericin B (0.5–1 mg/kg/d) with flucytosine (100 mg/kg/d) for 2 weeks, followed by consolidation therapy with fluconazole (400 mg/d) for an additional 8 to 10 weeks. Optimal duration of consolidation therapy varies from 3 to 6 months.
HIV-positive: induction course of amphotericin B (0.7–1 mg/kg/d) combined with flucytosine (100 mg/kg per in four divided doses) for 2 weeks, followed by consolidation therapy with fluconazole (400 mg/d) for 8 to 10 weeks or until CSF sterile. In conjunction with antiretroviral therapy, lifelong maintenance therapy with fluconazole (200 mg/d) should be administered.

Contraindications

None except systemic allergy.

Precautions

Adverse side effects of amphotericin B include renal injury, nausea, vomiting, chills, fevers, and rigors. Flucytosine dosage must be adjusted on basis of hematologic toxicities. It is necessary to carefully monitor serum electrolytes, renal function, and bone marrow function.

ALTERNATIVE DRUGS

In the setting of significant infusional toxicities or renal failure on conventional amphotericin B, liposomal preparations have been shown to be effective and less toxic. For patients unable to tolerate fluconazole, itraconazole (200 mg twice daily) may be substituted. Salvage therapy with intrathecal or intraventricular amphotericin B may be used in refractory cases.

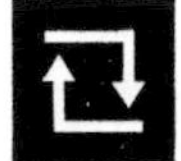

Follow-Up

PATIENT MONITORING

All patients should be monitored for evidence of elevated intracranial pressure. Treatment decisions should not be based routinely or exclusively on CSF or serum cryptococcal antigen titers. In HIV-negative patients, lumbar puncture is recommended after 2 weeks of treatment to assess the status of CSF sterilization. Patients with cryptococcosis involving any site should be evaluated every few months for at least 1 year after therapy. Relapses are more common in chronically immunosuppressed patients, so prolonged therapy is often indicated and close follow-up throughout initial and maintenance therapy is crucial.

EXPECTED COURSE AND PROGNOSIS

Overall mortality has improved with recommended antifungal treatment regimens. However, certain immunosuppressed patients remain at increased risk for more rapid mortality or treatment failure. The most important prognostic factor is the level of immunocompetence. Most patients with no apparent immunosuppression can expect to be cured of the infection with no significant impact on survival. In HIV-negative patients, increased mortality is associated with (a) positive India ink examination of the CSF, (b) CSF WBC count $<20/\mu L$, (c) initial CSF or serum cryptococcal antigen titer >1:32, (d) extraneural sites of infection, and (e) high opening pressure on lumbar puncture. Furthermore, those who relapse after treatment typically have one or more of the following: (a) persistently low CSF glucose concentrations after 4 weeks of therapy, (b) low initial CSF WBC, (c) posttreatment CSF or serum antigen titers of >1:8, and (d) treatment with at least 20 mg of prednisone or its equivalent after completion of therapy. In HIV-positive patients, significant predictors of death during initial therapy are (a) abnormal mental status, (b) CSF antigen titer >1:1024, and (c3) CSF WBC $<20/\mu L$.

PATIENT EDUCATION

The Meningitis Foundation of American Inc., 7155 Shadeland Station, Suite 190, Indianapolis, Indiana 46256-3922. Phone 800-668-1129, website *http://www.musa.org.*

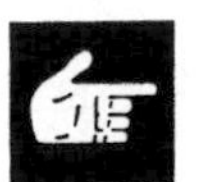

Miscellaneous

SYNONYMS

Cryptococcal meningitis
Cryptococcosis

ICD-9-CM: 117.5, 321.0 Meningitis, cryptococcal

SEE ALSO: N/A

REFERENCES

- Diamond RD. Cryptococcus neoformans. In: Mandell GL, Bennett JE, Dolin R, eds. Mandell, Douglas and Bennett's Principles and practice of infectious diseases, 5th ed. Philadelphia: Churchill Livingstone, 2000: 2707–2718.
- Perfect JR, Casadevall A. Cryptococcosis. Infect Dis Clin North Am 2002;16(4): 837–874.
- Powderly WG. Cryptococcal meningitis and AIDS. Clin Infect Dis 1993;17:837–842.
- Saag MS, Graybill RJ, Larsen RA, et al. Practice guidelines for the management of cryptococcal disease. Infectious Diseases Society of America. Clin Infect Dis 2000; 30:710–718.
- Saag MS, Powderly WG, Cloud GA, et al. Comparison of amphotericin B with fluconazole in the treatment of AIDS-associated cryptococcal meningitis. N Engl J Med 1992;326:83–89.

Author(s): Jennifer L. Klaus, MD

Mental Retardation

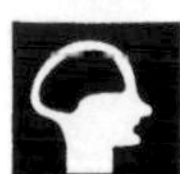

Basics

DESCRIPTION

- Mental retardation (MR) is defined as:
  - —Intelligence quotient (IQ) ≤70.
  - —At least 2 of 10 areas of impaired adaptive functioning such as social, occupational, health/safety skills [see *Diagnostic and Statistical Manual of Mental Disorders,* 4th ed. (DSM-IV), for complete list]. Onset <18 years.
- DSM-IV subclassifies MR by IQ:
  - —Mild MR: 50–55 to 70
  - —Moderate: 50–55 to 35–40
  - —Severe: 35–40 to 20–25
  - —Profound: <20–25
- Note:
  - —Mixed population, etiologically and clinically.
  - —A given IQ score/severity does not imply similar abilities across all cognitive/ functional domains.
  - —MR may not be lifelong/static
- Borderline intellectual functioning (BIF):
  - —IQ of 70 to 90

EPIDEMIOLOGY

Prevalence

For MR (after DSM-IV): 1% or less

Race

Affects all races.

Age

- Grade-school age (97/1,000 MR children)
- Infancy-preschool age (1/1,000)
- Note: Borderline/mild MR may not be detected until school-age years.

Sex

- Male/female ratios:
  - —Severe MR, 1.4–1.8:1
  - —Mild MR, 2–5:1
- Perhaps due to possible greater male predominance in:
  - —Fetal neonatal mortalities
  - —Phenotypic expression of X-linked disorders

ETIOLOGY

Two-group model (may be oversimplified):

- Mild MR (75%–80% of the MR population) is more often familial, cultural or polygenic, idiopathic, and without physical stigmata/ comorbidity
- Severe MR (5%) is most often sporadic, due to identifiable brain injury/cause and associated with physical stigmata/comorbidity

Time and Cause of Injury

- Unknown timing/cause: 12% to 55%
- Prenatal: 23% to 73%
  - —Genetic: 32%
    - -Maldistribution/aneuploidy: most common genetic cause (e.g., trisomy of chromosome 21 most common, then trisomy 18, 13, XO, XXY)
    - -Chromosomal rearrangements: less common
    - -Single gene mutations/deletions/ contiguous gene syndrome: rare (e.g., inborn errors of metabolism, neurocutaneous disorders)
    - -Malformations (genetic, structural, migrational disorders, unknown): 8% (e.g. neural tube defects)
  - —Environmental/Exogenous: 12% (Rubella, HIV, cytomegalovirus, eclampsia, placental abnormalities, teratogens, radiation exposure, malnutrition, etc.)
- Perinatal: 10% to 20%
  - —Environmental/exogenous:
    - -Delivery complications
    - -Infections (e.g., herpes simplex, toxoplasmosis, syphilis, HIV)
  - —Unknown/other
- Postnatal: 2% to 10%
  - —Environmental/exogenous/acquired
    - -Toxins (e.g., lead, pica, carbon monoxide, medications, substance/alcohol abuse)
    - -Infections (e.g., meningitis/encephalitis)
    - -Malnutrition
    - -Other (e.g., psychosocial, trauma)
  - —Unknown/other causes

RISK FACTORS

- Social deprivation/neglect/abuse
- Poverty
- Familial MR
- Gestational folate deficiency (neural tube defects)

PREGNANCY

- Severe/profound MR less likely to reproduce
- Possible congenital/developmental anomalies of the gonads (as in Turner's syndromes)
- Possible neuroendocrinopathies

ASSOCIATED CONDITIONS

Congenital Anomalies

- Cephalic features (shape, size)
- Eyes (hypertelorism, almond shaped, epicanthal folds)
- Lens/retina (subluxated lens, retinal pigmentation)
- Midfacial/oral (cleft palate, high arched palate)
- Ears (malformed, low-set)
- Neck (webbed, short)
- Skin/hair (fibromas, angiomas, pigment, hair texture/whorls)
- Digits (long middle toe, syndactyly, gaps)
- Dermatoglyphic (palmar crease)
- Cardiac anomalies
- Gastrointestinal system (esophageal atresia)
- Renal/ureter anomalies
- Urogenital system
- Musculoskeletal system (subluxated atlantoaxial joint, hip joint dislocation)

Medical comorbidity is common:

- Non-CNS involvement due to congenital anomalies or biochemical/physiologic factors
- Visual/auditory deficits: 10%
- Abnormal body fat distribution (e.g., central)
- Seizures: 9% to 19%
- Cerebral palsy: 20%
- Psychiatric comorbidity: 14% to >70%

Diagnosis

DIFFERENTIAL DIAGNOSIS

It is important to ascertain time of onset of cognitive/functional impairment, any precipitating events, course and any family history (consanguinity, familial pattern of MR/learning disabilities, spontaneous abortions, difficulties with conceiving, neurologic disorders, childhood psychiatric disorders)

- CNS specific causes (e.g., arteriovenous malformation, neoplasia, hydrocephalus)
- Seizures
- Neurosensory deficit
- Sleep disorders
- Endocrinopathies
- Psychiatric illnesses (e.g., depression, eating disorders)
- Childhood psychiatric disorders (see DSM-IV)
  - —Learning disabilities
  - —Pervasive developmental disorders
  - —Autistic and Asperger's disorders

  Rett's and childhood disintegrative disorders (loss of acquired milestones/skills by 5 to 48 months old and by 2 to 10 years old, respectively)

SIGNS AND SYMPTOMS

- Cognitive/developmental/functional deficits
  - —Possible abnormal neonatal sleep/feeding patterns
  - —Delay or loss of milestones
  - —Poor school performance
  - —Impaired social/self-care or other skills
- Aberrant growth pattern
- Physical exam findings such as:
  - —Stigmata/congenital anomalies
  - —Urine odor (musty, maple syrup, etc.)
  - —Cephalofacial features
  - —Soft or focal neurologic signs
  - —Signs of cerebral palsy
  - —Cerebellar signs
  - —Cranial nerve signs
  - —Abnormal higher cortical function
- Syndrome/genetic disorder specific features

LABORATORY PROCEDURES

- No established diagnostic protocol—generally based on clinical presentation
- Some typical blood tests: electrolytes, BUN, Cr, fasting blood sugar (FBS), CBC/ differential, ammonia, uric acid, calcium, magnesium, phosphate, copper, ceruloplasmin, lead, viral titers, RPR

- Endocrine blood/urine tests such as serologic thyroid function test
- Arterial blood gases (ABGs)
- Routine urinalysis

Consider consulting with a geneticist regarding tests for inborn error of metabolism (IBEM) or chromosomal studies

- Results rarely positive unless:
  - —Clinical presentation suggests IBEM
  - —A neonatal presentation with any of the following: hypoglycemia, acidosis, coma, seizures, physical stigmata
- Least helpful if precipitating event is identified/absent physical stigmata
- Some tests for IBEM (see Jones, 1997):
  - —Blood levels of carnitine, pyruvate, lactate, amino acids, organic acids, very long chain fatty acids
  - —ABG and ammonia level
  - —Urine analyses of amino and organic acids, mucopolysaccharides
  - —Fibroblast or white cell culture studies for lysosomal enzyme disease

Consider chromosomal studies, particularly if:

- Prenatal onset
- Familial pattern
- Physical stigmata
- Severe MR
- Idiopathic (according to some experts)

IMAGING STUDIES

- No established protocol, and the cost-to-benefit ratio in idiopathic MR is controversial
- Consider MRI in specific cases such as:
  - —Cephalic abnormalities
  - —Neurofocal deficits
  - —New-onset seizures
  - —Cerebral palsy
  - —Degenerative course
  - —Features of neurocutaneous disorders, neural tube defects, etc.

SPECIAL TESTS

- Neuropsychological assessment
- Also consider:
  - —Electroencephalogram
  - —Evoked potentials (e.g., for neurosensory deficits)
  - —Audiometry/ophthalmologic evaluation
  - —Cerebral fluid spinal studies

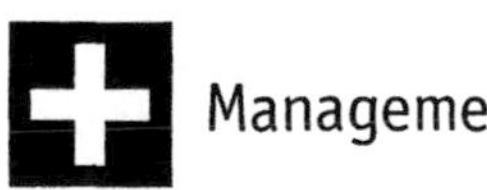

Management

GENERAL MEASURES

If an underlying reversible etiology is identified, appropriate treatment should be implemented accordingly. Management often involves a multidisciplinary approach that addresses educational/training needs and psychosocial issues, provides advocacy, and maximizes level of independence/functioning.

SURGICAL MEASURES

Sometimes for congenital anomalies/medical complications.

SYMPTOMATIC TREATMENT

- Bladder dysfunction:
  - —Consider postvoid residual and cystometric studies.
  - —Anticholinergic agents may be helpful.
  - —Consider imipramine for an enuretic insomniac patient.
- Seizures: anticonvulsant treatment
- Behavioral problems or functional/cognitive decline:
  - —Thorough physical examination by primary physician to rule out underlying medical condition
  - —Thorough neurologic exam to rule neurologic condition (if over 50 years old or an adult with Down syndrome consider dementia)
  - —Treatments to consider: behavioral, cognitive, supportive, group, family psychotherapies, patient/family psychoeducation, pharmacotherapy
- Obesity/overweight (common in MR): dietary consultant, psychologist, psychiatrist

ADJUNCTIVE TREATMENT

Multidisciplinary approach:

- Family and patient counseling
- Psychologist, behaviorist, or psychotherapist
- Psychiatrist (if suspect psychiatric disorder)
- Neurologist (such as for seizures)
- Primary care physician
- Genetics consultant and counselor
- Nutritionist/dietitian
- Speech/physical/occupational therapists

ADMISSION/DISCHARGE CRITERIA

- Patients not previously assessed for MR may require admission for rapidly deteriorating course, unstable conditions, or medical/neurologic complications or surgery
- Most severe cases present at birth/perinatal period and are generally hospitalized for assessment/treatment.
- Children or adults previously diagnosed with MR may require admission for:
  - —New-onset seizures, unstable or treatment resistant seizures
  - —Severe behavioral or psychiatric problems
  - —Other unstable medical conditions

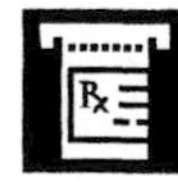

Medications

DRUG(S) OF CHOICE

There are no established medications

Contraindications

N/A

Precautions

N/A

ALTERNATIVE DRUGS

N/A

Follow-Up

PATIENT MONITORING

Generally requires:

- Annual assessments of vocational/educational/functional skills
- Many require annual blood/urine analyses for syndrome specific condition.
- Consider annual neurosensory assessments in patients with deficits.

EXPECTED COURSE AND PROGNOSIS

- Life span is thought to be inversely correlated with severity of MR.
- Adults may be more prone to age-related conditions/disorders.

PATIENT EDUCATION

- Government: Department for MR
- National Down Syndrome Congress, 7000 Peachtree-Dunwoody Rd., Building #5, Suite 100, Atlanta GA 30328. Phone 800-232-6372.
- Special Olympics

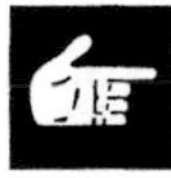

Miscellaneous

SYNONYMS

Developmentally delayed

ICD-9-CM: 319 Mental retardation, unspecified; 317 Mental retardation, mild (IQ 50–70); 318.0 Mental retardation, moderate (IQ 35–49); 318.1 Mental retardation, severe (IQ 20–34); 318.2 Mental retardation, profound (IQ under 20); V62.89 Mental retardation, borderline; 758.0

SEE ALSO: N/A

REFERENCES

- American Psychiatric Association. Diagnostic and statistical manual of mental disorders, 4th ed. Washington, DC: American Psychiatric Association, 1994.
- Jones KL. Smith's recognizable patterns of human malformation, 5th ed. Philadelphia: WB Saunders, 1997.
- Szymanski LS, Wilska M. Mental retardation. In: Tassman A, Key J, Lieberman JA, eds. Psychiatry. Philadelphia: WB Saunders, 1997.

Author(s): Karen Brugge, MD

Mitochondrial Diseases

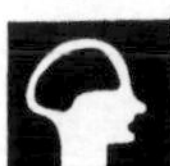

Basics

DESCRIPTION

Mitochondrial diseases are clinically, biochemically, and genetically heterogeneous diseases associated with primary mitochondrial dysfunction. Neurologic, systemic, or both manifestations can be seen in the disorders.

EPIDEMIOLOGY

Incidence/Prevalence

The incidence/prevalence for most mitochondrial diseases is unknown. However, the prevalence of mitochondrial DNA (mtDNA) disease has been estimated to be 1 in 10,000 to 1 in 50,000.

Race

All races are affected.

Age

All ages can be affected.

Sex

Both sexes are affected.

ETIOLOGY

The causes of mitochondrial disorders can be due to nuclear DNA defects, which include defects of substrate transport (such as carnitine palmitoyl transferase deficiency, carnitine deficiency), defects of substrate utilization (such as defects of β-oxidation, pyruvate dehydrogenase complex deficiency), defects of the Krebs cycle (such as fumarase deficiency), defects of oxidation-phosphorylation coupling (such as Luft's disease), and defects of respiratory chain (complex I–V deficiencies). They can also be due to mtDNA defects, which include sporadic large-scale deletions or duplications, point mutations affecting structural genes and synthetic genes, as well as defects of communication between both genomes, which consist of autosomal-dominant multiple mtDNA deletions and autosomal-recessive mtDNA depletion.

Genetics

Genetically inherited mitochondrial diseases may result from defect of mitochondrial or nuclear genome. The former is characterized by maternal inheritance and the latter by mendelian inheritance. Among nuclear DNA defects, most are inherited as autosomal-recessive diseases except pyruvate dehydrogenase deficiency and ornithine transcarbamylase deficiency, which are x-linked diseases. Maternal inheritance is transmitted from the mother to all of her sons and daughters, but only her daughters can pass the mutation to their children. The clinical manifestations are determined by the threshold effect (phenotype occurs when the content of mutated mtDNA reaches certain percentage, for example, the threshold may be 60% to 70% in chronic progressive external ophthalmoplegia) and mitotic segregation (the contents of mutated mtDNA are changed randomly during cell division).

RISK FACTORS

AZT treatment for AIDS may induce mtDNA depletion. Exposure to methyl-phenyl-tetrahydropyridine (MPTP) can cause brain respiratory chain complex I defect and a Parkinsonian syndrome.

PREGNANCY

N/A

ASSOCIATED CONDITIONS

- Reye syndrome: associated with generalized mitochondrial dysfunction, often seen with influenza or varicella and aspirin treatment.
- Aging: associated with an increase in mtDNA mutations and a decrease in mitochondrial respiratory chain function.
- Parkinson's disease: complex I defect in substantia nigra has been shown.
- Huntington's disease: defects of complex II, III, IV in caudate nucleus have been reported.
- Alzheimer's disease: complex IV and pyruvate dehydrogenase defects have been described in the brain.

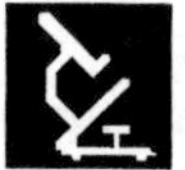

Diagnosis

DIFFERENTIAL DIAGNOSIS

The following mitochondrial disorders need to be differentiated from other diseases.

- Chronic progressive external ophthalmoplegia: myasthenia gravis, oculopharyngeal muscular dystrophy, thyroid oculomyopathy
- Mitochondrial encephalomyopathy, lactic acidosis, stroke-like syndrome (MELAS): viral encephalitis, brain tumor, stroke
- Myoclonic epilepsy and ragged red fibers syndrome: Lafora body disease, progressive myoclonic epilepsy of Unverricht-Lundborg type
- Leber hereditary optic neuropathy: optic neuritis, alcohol-tobacco amblyopia, multiple sclerosis, anterior ischemic optic neuropathy

SIGNS AND SYMPTOMS

The clinical symptoms and signs that may suggest mitochondrial diseases include developmental delay, hypotonia, microcephaly, depression, dementia, mental retardation, central hypoventilation, short stature, seizures, ataxia, migraine headache, sensorineural deafness, ptosis, ophthalmoplegia, optic atrophy, pigmentary retinopathy, cataract, stroke, muscle weakness, exercise intolerance, cardiomyopathy, cardiac arrhythmia, peripheral neuropathy, renal tubulopathy, hepatopathy, pancytopenia, sideroblastic anemia, pancreatic insufficiency, diabetes mellitus or other endocrinopathies, movement disorders, gastrointestinal disorders such as malabsorption, myoglobinuria, multiple lipomas.

LABORATORY PROCEDURES

Elevated serum or CSF lactate, associated with lactate/pyruvate ratio above 20, strongly suggests respiratory chain defects. However, normal serum or CSF lactate with lactate/pyruvate ratio below 20 does not exclude respiratory chain defects. In contrast, increased serum or CSF lactate with lactate/pyruvate ratio below 20 may indicate pyruvate dehydrogenase complex or pyruvate carboxylase deficiencies.

IMAGING STUDIES

Brain MRI or CT may show basal ganglia calcification in mitochondrial diseases. MRI may also reveal multifocal hyperintense T2 signal in the cortex of cerebrum, cerebellum, or subjacent white matter, which is not confined to a single vascular territory, especially in the posterior temporal and occipital areas in MELAS. The increased inorganic phosphate-to-phosphocreatine ratio has been shown in the muscle of mitochondrial myopathy patients. EMG and nerve conduction studies may detect myopathy and neuropathy.

SPECIAL TESTS

Muscle biopsy may reveal ragged red fibers, which represent proliferation of subsarcolemmal mitochondria, and cytochrome c oxidase-negative muscle fibers, which indicate mitochondrial diseases. Muscles also may show respiratory chain defects. Molecular genetic studies may be performed for most common mtDNA point mutations, and most can be done with the blood; however, muscle may be needed to detect mtDNA deletions or depletions. Blood and skin may permit detection of pyruvate enzyme defects. Muscles are needed for the diagnosis of carnitine palmitoyl transferase and carnitine deficiencies.

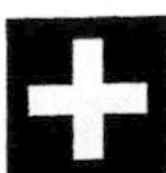

Management

GENERAL MEASURES

- Because mitochondria are virtually present in all organs and systems, mitochondrial diseases often affect multiple organs and systems. Once this disease is suspected, audiograms may detect progressive sensorineural deafness. ECG or echocardiogram may be needed for the diagnosis of cardiomyopathy. Brain MRI may reveal basal ganglia calcification, progressive cerebral or cerebellar atrophy, or other abnormalities.
- During clinical follow-up, other screening for multiorgan involvement in mitochondrial diseases may include muscle weakness, intestinal dysfunction, hepatocellular dysfunction, renal tubulopathy, visual loss or retinitis pigmentosa, pancytopenia, anemia, exocrine pancreatic dysfunction, hyperglycemia, hypocalcemia, growth hormone or sex hormone abnormalities.

SURGICAL MEASURES

- For ptosis due to mitochondrial diseases, surgery to elevate upper eyelids to improve vision may be needed.
- For severe cardiac conduction defects, cardiac pacemaker implantation may be lifesaving.

SYMPTOMATIC TREATMENT

- Seizures may benefit from anticonvulsant treatment; migraine headache requires proper medications.
- Diabetes mellitus or other endocrine abnormalities should be treated if present and sensorineural deafness may require hearing aids.

ADJUNCTIVE TREATMENT

- Moderate aerobic exercise may be useful; prolonged fasting and overexertion should be avoided.
- Optimal nutritional support is also needed.

ADMISSION/DISCHARGE CRITERIA

Patients are sometimes admitted for muscle biopsy when significant sedation is required or for severe complications of these illnesses.

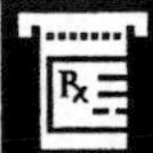

Medications

DRUG(S) OF CHOICE

- Biotin 5–10 mg/d is needed in biotinidase deficiency.
- L-carnitine 50–100 mg/kg/d is lifesaving for carnitine transporter defect and is also prescribed for most patients with secondary carnitine deficiency associated with mitochondrial diseases.
- Coenzyme Q10 is beneficial for coenzyme Q defect and is usually prescribed in respiratory chain defects at 4.3 mg/kg/d but may need much higher dosage with coenzyme Q10 deficiency associated with cerebellar ataxia and other encephalopathy.

Contraindications

Chloramphenicol and tetracycline are inhibitors of mitochondrial protein synthesis; barbiturates can inhibit respiratory chain; valproic acid can sequestrate carnitine. These medications should be avoided.

Precautions

During surgery, halothane or other halogenated anesthetic drugs and succinylcholine should also be avoided to prevent malignant hyperthermia when mitochondrial diseases are suspected.

ALTERNATIVE DRUGS

Dichloroacetate can stimulate pyruvate dehydrogenase complex and has been reported useful in severe lactic acidosis due to pyruvate dehydrogenase complex defects and respiratory chain defects.

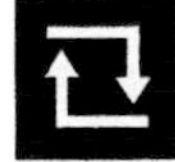

Follow-Up

PATIENT MONITORING

Patients should be monitored regularly for multiple organ/system disorders, which are often seen in mitochondrial diseases, and receive appropriate treatment.

EXPECTED COURSE AND PROGNOSIS

Prognosis of mitochondrial diseases varies tremendously from mild to severe, especially for mtDNA disease because the level of mutant mtDNA in the organs may increase or decrease with time. The clinical course may be static, or rapidly or slowly progressive.

PATIENT EDUCATION

Patients with mitochondrial diseases can be referred to the lay organization, United Mitochondrial Disease Foundation, P.O. Box 1151, Monroeville, PA 15146-1151. Phone/fax 412-856-1297, email: *74743.2705@compuserve.com*; *http://biochemgen.ucsd.edu/umdf*; and another website: *http://www.gen.emory.edu/mitomap.html*.

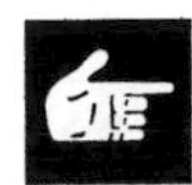

Miscellaneous

SYNONYMS

Mitochondrial cytopathy

ICD-9-CM: 359.9 Mitochondrial disease

SEE ALSO: N/A

REFERENCES

- De Vivo DC. The expanding clinical spectrum of mitochondrial diseases. Brain Dev 1993;15:1–21.
- De Vivo DC, Hirano M, DiMauro S. Mitochondrial disorders. In: Moser HW, ed. Neurodystrophies and neurolipidosis. Amsterdam: Elsevier Science BV, 1997: 389–446.
- Musumecci O, Naini A, Slonim AE, et al. Familial cerebellar ataxia with muscle coenzyme Q10 deficiency. Neurology 2001; 56:849–855.
- Sue CM, Bruno C, Andreu AL, et al. Infantile encephalopathy associated with MELASA3243G mutation. J Pediatr 1999; 19:696–700.
- Tsao CY, Herman G, Boue D, et al. Leigh's syndrome with mtDNA A8344G mutation and a brief review. J Child Neurol 2003; 18(1):62–64.
- Tsao CY, Kien CL. Complete biotinidase deficiency presenting as reversible progressive ataxia and sensorineural deafness. J Child Neurol 2002;17:146.
- Tsao CY, Mendell JR. Combined partial deficiencies of carnitine palmitoyl transferase II and mitochondrial complex I presenting as increased serum creatine kinase level. J Child Neurol 2002;17: 304–306.
- Tsao CY, Mendell JR, Bartholomew D. High mtDNA T8993G (>90%) without typical features of Leigh's syndrome and NARP syndrome. J Child Neurol 2001;16: 533–535.
- Tsao CY, Mendell JR, Lo WD, et al. Mitochondrial respiratory chain defects presenting as nonspecific features in children. J Child Neurol 2000;15:445–448.
- Tsao CY, Mendell JR, Luquette M, et al. Mitochondrial DNA depletion in children. J Child Neurol 2000;15:822–824.

Author(s): Chang-Yong Tsao, MD, FAAN, FAAP

Mucolipidoses

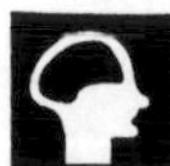

Basics

DESCRIPTION

The term *mucolipidoses* was initially coined to denote a group of lysosomal storage diseases with clinical features common to both the mucopolysaccharidoses and sphingolipidoses but lacking mucopolysacchariduria and sphingolipiduria. These diseases are characterized by variable storage of mucopolysaccharides, glycoproteins, sphingolipids, and/or glycolipids in various tissues, including neurons. A wide spectrum of genetic and metabolic defects, from a mutation in the gene encoding a specific lysosomal hydrolase to defective targeting and endocytosis of multiple hydrolases into lysosomes, underlies this heterogeneous group of disorders.

EPIDEMIOLOGY

Incidence/Prevalence

The mucolipidoses are rare disorders.

Race

The following mucolipidoses have a predilection for a particular subgroup of the population:

- Cherry-red spot myoclonus variant of sialidosis: Italians
- Galactosialidosis: Japanese
- Mucolipidosis IV: Ashkenazi Jews
- Fucosidosis: Italians and the Mexican-Indian population of New Mexico and Colorado.
- Aspartylglucosaminuria: Finnish

Age

See Signs and Symptoms, below.

Sex

Because of autosomal-recessive inheritance, there is an equal number of male and female cases.

ETIOLOGY

Genetics

All the disorders are autosomal recessive. Carrier detection and prenatal testing are available.

RISK FACTORS

N/A

PREGNANCY

N/A

ASSOCIATED CONDITIONS

N/A

Diagnosis

DIFFERENTIAL DIAGNOSIS

Other degenerative disorders.

SIGNS AND SYMPTOMS

- Mucolipidosis I (three types)
  —Sialidosis type 1: cherry-red spot myoclonus variant. Onset in the teen years with progressive visual loss associated with a cherry red spot and nonpigmentary retinal degeneration. Myoclonus and generalized seizures.
  —Sialidosis type 2: congenital and infantile/childhood forms described and characterized by progressive mental retardation, hepatosplenomegaly, and coarsened facial features. A macular cherry red spot, hearing loss, peripheral neuropathy, ataxia, myoclonus, seizures, and dysostosis multiplex may occur.
  Patients with the congenital form may present with hydrops fetalis.
  Patients with kidney involvement have been described.
  —Galactosialidosis: infantile, late infantile, and juvenile/adult onset. Intellectual deterioration, macular cherry red spot, hearing loss, myoclonus, and corneal clouding. Visceromegaly, coarsening of the facial features and skeletal dysplasia.
- Mucolipidosis II or I-cell disease: psychomotor retardation evident by 6 months of age, hepatomegaly, coarse facial features, severe dysostosis multiplex, gingival hyperplasia, and recurrent respiratory infections. [Many features similar to mucopolysaccharidosis (MPS) 1 H/Hurler syndrome, but onset is earlier, course is more rapid, and there is an absence of mucopolysacchariduria.]
- Mucolipidosis III or pseudo-Hurler polydystrophy (a milder form of mucolipidosis II): onset 2 to 4 years of age with a slowly progressive course. Fifty percent of patients have a learning disability or mental retardation. Stiffness of the hands and shoulders with subsequent claw hand deformity, scoliosis, dysostosis multiplex, and coarsening of facial features. Carpal tunnel syndrome. Ophthalmologic triad of corneal clouding, mild retinopathy, and hyperopic astigmatism. (Many features similar to mild to moderately severe MPS I and VI but without mucopolysacchariduria.)
- Mucolipidosis IV: severe psychomotor retardation with peak developmental level of 12 to 15 months by 3 to 4 years of age. Corneal opacification and pigmentary degeneration of the retina leading to visual failure. No storage in the viscera or skeleton.
- Fucosidosis: onset during the first year of life to early childhood with progressive psychomotor retardation. Seizures and deafness. Hepatosplenomegaly, facial coarsening, dysostosis multiplex, recurrent infections, and angiokeratoma.
- α-Mannosidosis: onset during the first year of life to early childhood with progressive mental retardation. Hepatosplenomegaly, facial coarsening, dysostosis multiplex, recurrent infections, deafness, lenticular, and corneal opacities.
- β-Mannosidosis: onset after the first few months of life with progressive mental retardation. Mild facial dysmorphism, hearing loss, and recurrent infections.
- Aspartylglucosaminuria: recurrent infections and diarrhea noted during the first year of life. Mental deterioration starting at about age 5 with IQ below 40 by 15 years of age. Coarsening of facial features and sagging skin folds subtle during the first decade and more obvious afterward. Mild skeletal dysplasia.

LABORATORY PROCEDURES

See Special Tests, below.

IMAGING STUDIES

Bone x-rays to look for skeletal dysplasia.

SPECIAL TESTS

Excessive excretion of oligosaccharides is found in urine. Specific diagnosis is suspected on clinical grounds and confirmed by enzymatic testing.

- Mucolipidosis I: sialidosis type 1 and 2—glycoprotein acid α-neuraminidase
- Galactosialidosis: combined β-galactosidase/α-neuraminidase deficiency due to absence of "protective protein"
- Mucolipidosis II or I-cell disease: multiple lysosomal enzymes due to deficiency of UDP-*N*-acetylglucosamine: lysosomal enzyme *N*-acetylglucosamine phosphotransferase
- Mucolipidosis III or pseudo-Hurler polydystrophy: same as mucolipidosis II
- Mucolipidosis IV: ganglioside sialidase
- Fucosidosis: α-L-fucosidase
- α-Mannosidosis: α-mannosidase
- β-Mannosidosis: β-mannosidase
- Aspartylglucosaminuria: aspartylglucosaminidase

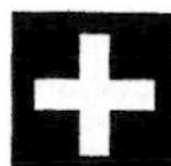

Management

GENERAL MEASURES

Bone marrow transplantation for fucosidosis, α-mannosidosis, and aspartylglucosaminuria is experimental.

SURGICAL MEASURES

N/A

SYMPTOMATIC TREATMENT

Treatment is individualized and aimed at treating complications of the disease.

ADJUNCTIVE TREATMENT

Physical therapy may improve quality of life.

ADMISSION/DISCHARGE CRITERIA

Patients are usually admitted for evaluation and treatment of the complications of their disease.

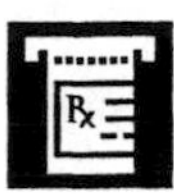

Medications

DRUG(S) OF CHOICE

No specific drug treatment is available.

ALTERNATIVE DRUGS

N/A

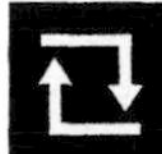

Follow-Up

PATIENT MONITORING

Patient follow-up is guided by the predicted course and potential complications of the disease.

EXPECTED COURSE AND PROGNOSIS

- Mucolipidosis I or sialidosis type 1: survival into middle age without dementia but with a devastating and virtually untreatable myoclonus.
- Type 2: death in infancy in the congenital form, survival to the second decade in milder forms.
- Galactosialidosis: early death to survival into adulthood.
- Mucolipidosis II or I-cell disease: cardiorespiratory complications usually lead to death in early childhood.
- Mucolipidosis III: survival into adulthood is possible.
- Mucolipidosis IV: few patients survive into their teens and beyond. A milder variant has been reported.
- Fucosidosis: severe form with death in the first decade. Survival into the third decade in milder forms.
- α-Mannosidosis: infantile onset with rapid progression and death between 3 and 12 years of age. Later-onset disease more slowly progressive with survival into adulthood.
- β-Mannosidosis: severe form with death by 15 months of age. Milder forms with survival to adulthood.
- Aspartylglucosaminuria: survival to adulthood.

PATIENT EDUCATION

National Tay-Sachs and Allied Diseases Association, 2001 Beacon St., Ste. 204, Brighton, MA 02135; phone 800-90-NTSAD. ML4 Foundation, 714 E. 17th St., Brooklyn, New York 11230. Phone 718-434-5067.

ICD-9-CM: 272.7 Mucolipidosis I, II, III; 271.8 Fucosidosis, mannosidosis

SEE ALSO: N/A

REFERENCES

- Autti T, Santavuori P, Raininko R, et al. Bone-marrow transplantation in aspartylglucosaminuria. Lancet 1997;349:1366.
- Kolodny EH. The mucolipidoses. In: Berg BO, ed. Principles of child neurology. New York: McGraw-Hill, 1996:1115–1140.
- Rapin I. Progressive genetic-metabolic diseases. In: Evans RW, Baskin DS, Yatsu FM, eds. Prognosis in neurological disease. New York: Oxford University Press, in press.
- Scriver CR, Beaudet AL, Sly WS, et al., eds. The metabolic and molecular bases of inherited disease, 7th ed. New York: McGraw-Hill, 1995.
- Vellodi A, Cragg H, Winchester B, et al. Allogenic bone marrow transplantation for fucosidosis. Bone Marrow Transplant 1995;15:153.
- Wall DA, Grange DK, Goulding P, et al. Bone marrow transplantation for the treatment of alpha-mannosidosis. J Pediatr 1998;133:282.

Author(s): Eveline C. Traeger, MD

Mucopolysaccharidoses

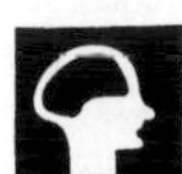

Basics

DESCRIPTION

Mucopolysaccharidoses (MPSs) are chronic and progressive multisystem disorders caused by deficiency of lysosomal enzymes to degrade mucopolysaccharides with resultant marked lysosomal accumulation of one or a combination of the following: dermatan sulfate, heparan sulfate, keratan sulfate, chondroitin sulfate. This accumulation results in cell, tissue, and organ dysfunction. Ten known enzyme deficiencies give rise to six disorders. Residual enzyme activity correlates with clinical course of disease as illustrated by the variable phenotypes due to L-iduronidase deficiency in Hurler syndrome and Scheie syndrome. In contrast, Sanfilippo syndrome can result from four distinct enzyme deficiencies, all of which result in the accumulation of heparan sulfate. Neurologic symptoms are a prominent feature of some MPSs and occur to some degree in all. Profound mental retardation, which is characteristic of MPS I H, severe MPS II, and all subtypes of MPS III, may be absent in other MPS.

EPIDEMIOLOGY

Incidence/Prevalence

A study of MPS in the Netherlands reported an incidence of 1.19 cases per 100,000 births for MPS I; 1.16 cases per 100,000 births for MPS IIIA; 0.67 cases per 100,000 births (1.30 cases per 100,000 male births) for MPS II. Incidence of type IVA is estimated at 1 cases per 200,000 births. Type IVB is rare, as are types VI and VII.

Race

MPS is diagnosed in patients from many ethnic/racial backgrounds.

Age

See Signs and Symptoms, below.

Sex

Because of X-linked inheritance, patients with Hunter syndrome are male.

ETIOLOGY

Genetics

Inheritance is autosomal recessive except for Hunter syndrome (MPS II), which is X-linked. Prenatal diagnosis by enzyme determination following chorionic villus biopsy or amniocentesis is available.

RISK FACTORS

N/A

PREGNANCY

N/A

ASSOCIATED CONDITIONS

N/A

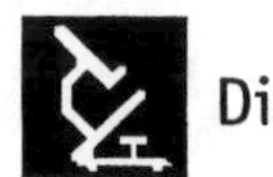

Diagnosis

DIFFERENTIAL DIAGNOSIS

Other degenerative disorders.

SIGNS AND SYMPTOMS

- Hurler syndrome or MPS I H: developmental delay apparent by 12 to 24 months of age. Psychomotor retardation characterized by a maximum functional age of 2 to 4 years followed by progressive deterioration. Corneal clouding, dysostosis multiplex (constellation of radiographic abnormalities), hepatosplenomegaly, and heart disease.
- Scheie syndrome or MPS I S: normal intelligence. Corneal clouding, stiff joints, aortic valve disease.
- Hurler-Scheie compound or MPS I H/S: intermediate between MPS I H and MPS I S.
- Severe Hunter syndrome or severe MPS II: onset of disease occurs between 2 and 4 years of age. Progressive psychomotor retardation, dysostosis multiplex, hepatosplenomegaly, respiratory, and heart disease.
- Mild Hunter syndrome or mild MPS II: normal intelligence. Short stature, heart disease.
- Sanfilippo Syndrome types A, B, C, D or MPS III types A, B, C, D: onset of disease between 2 and 6 years of age. Severe CNS involvement with mild somatic disease. Profound mental retardation, hyperactivity with aggressive behavior. Mild hepatosplenomegaly in young patients.
- Morquio syndrome types A and B or MPS IV types A and B: normal intelligence, spondyloepiphyseal dysplasia (which is specific to this disorder), and corneal clouding.
- Maroteaux-Lamy syndrome or MPS VI: normal intelligence, dysostosis multiplex, corneal opacities, heart disease.
- Sly syndrome or MPS VII: wide spectrum of severity with mental retardation in severe form and normal intelligence in mild form. If present, mental retardation is evident by 3 years of age. Dysostosis multiplex, hepatosplenomegaly.

LABORATORY PROCEDURES

See Special Tests, below.

IMAGING STUDIES

Bone x-rays to look for skeletal dysplasia.

SPECIAL TESTS

MPS may be diagnosed by finding excessive urinary excretion of mucopolysaccharide degradation products. The diagnosis is confirmed by measuring specific enzyme activity in serum, leukocytes, or fibroblasts. Patients with MPS have less than 10% and often less than 1% of residual enzyme activity.

- MPS I H, I S, and I H-S: α-L-iduronidase deficiency
- Severe and mild MPS II: iduronate sulfatase deficiency
- MPS III type A: heparan *N*-sulfatase deficiency
- MPS III type B: α-*N*-acetylglucosaminidase deficiency
- MPS III type C: *N*-acetyl transferase deficiency
- MPS III type D: α-*N*-acetylglucosaminide-6-sulfatase deficiency
- MPS IV type A: galactose 6-sulfatase deficiency
- MPS IV type B: β-galactosidase deficiency
- MPS VI: galactosamine-4-sulfatase (arylsulfatase B) deficiency
- MPS VII: β-glucuronidase deficiency

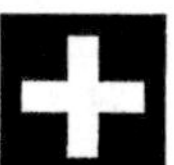

Management

GENERAL MEASURES

- The chronic and progressive course of the MPS warrants periodic evaluation for potential complications, the management of which may improve quality of life. Evaluations should be performed in the following areas: neurologic, cardiovascular, respiratory (including evaluation for obstructive sleep apnea), and joint function.
- Neurologic complications and possible medical and surgical interventions are presented in more detail. It is important to note that patients with MPS I, II, IV, and VI may be at high risk for anesthesia complications because of atlantoaxial instability and presence of a narrowed airway.

SURGICAL MEASURES

Bone marrow transplant (BMT) for patients with MPS I, MPS IV, MPS VI, and MPS VII may lessen visceral and joint symptoms and improve quality of life. BMT can stabilize the CNS in MPS I. BMT performed in patients with MPS 1 H prior to 24 months of age with a Mental Developmental Index >70 can result in continued cognitive development and prolonged survival. Results of BMT for MPS II and MPS III are unsatisfactory.

SYMPTOMATIC TREATMENT

- Progressive communicating hydrocephalus due to failure of reabsorption of CSF in the arachnoid granulations may be seen in MPS I H, MPS II, severe and MPS VI. VP shunt placement may be indicated.
- Corneal clouding leading to significant visual impairment can occur in MPS I, MPS IV, MPS VI, and MPS VII. Consider corneal transplant.
- Glaucoma may develop in patients with MPS I and MPS VI.
- Screening for conductive and sensorineural hearing loss in all patients with MPS. Deafness has been attributed to three causes: frequent middle ear infections, deformity of the ossicles, and probable abnormalities of the inner ear. Hearing aids and myringotomy tubes may improve hearing.
- Development of carpal tunnel syndrome in all MPS patients except those with MPS III and VII. Surgical nerve decompression may be indicated.
- Seizures may develop in patients with severe MPS II and MPS III. Antiepileptic medication should be used to control seizures.
- C1-C2 subluxation/cord compression as a result of a narrowed spinal canal and storage within the meninges (pachymeningitis cervicalis) in patients with MPS IH, MPS IV, MPS VI, and MPS VII. Occipitocervical fusion and laminectomy may be required.

ADJUNCTIVE TREATMENT

Range of motion exercises may help preserve joint function.

ADMISSION/DISCHARGE CRITERIA

Patients are generally admitted for evaluation and treatment of the neurologic, cardiovascular, and respiratory complications of their disorder.

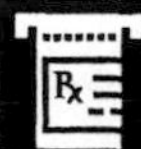

Medications

DRUG(S) OF CHOICE

No specific drug treatment is available.

ALTERNATIVE DRUGS

N/A

Follow-Up

PATIENT MONITORING

Patients should be periodically evaluated for complications of their disorder as described in the management section.

EXPECTED COURSE AND PROGNOSIS

Death is usually due to heart failure but may be secondary to respiratory failure in MPS II or cervical cord compression in patients with MPS IV.

- MPS I H: death by 10 years of age.
- MPS I S: normal life span.
- MPS I H-S: intermediate between I H and I S.
- Severe MPS II: death between 10 and 15 years of age.
- Mild MPS II: survival to adulthood and beyond.
- MPS III: death in teens or early adulthood.
- MPS IV: patients with severe disease may not survive beyond their twenties.
- MPS VI: survival to teens in severe form, adulthood in mild form.
- MPS VII: wide spectrum including hydrops fetalis and survival to adulthood.

PATIENT EDUCATION

National Mucopolysaccharidosis Society, 17 Kraemer St., Hicksville, NY 11801. Phone 516-931-6338.

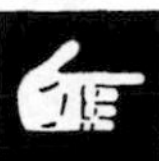

Miscellaneous

SYNONYMS

N/A

ICD-9-CM: 277.5 Mucopolysaccharidosis

SEE ALSO: N/A

REFERENCES

- Kakkis ED, Neufeld EF. The mucopolysaccharidoses. In: Berg BO, ed. Principles of child neurology. New York: McGraw-Hill, 1996:1141–1166.
- McKinnis EJR, Sulzbacher S, Rutledge JC, et al. Bone marrow transplantation in Hunter syndrome. J Pediatr 1996;129:145.
- Moores C, Rogers JG, McKenzie IM, et al. Anaesthesia for children with mucopolysaccharidoses. Anaesth Intensive Care 1996;24:459.
- Neufeld EF, Muenzer J. The mucopolysaccharidoses. In: Scriver CR, Beaudet AL, Sly WS, et al., eds. The metabolic and molecular bases of inherited disease. New York: McGraw-Hill, 1995:2465–2494.
- Peters C, Shapiro EG, Anderson J, et al. Hurler syndrome: II. Outcome of HLA-genotypically identical sibling and HLA-haploidentical related donor bone marrow transplantation in fifty-four children. Blood 1998;91:2601.
- Rapin I. Progressive genetic-metabolic diseases. In: Evans RW, Baskin DS, et al., eds. Prognosis in neurological disease. New York: Oxford University Press, 2000:677–703.

Author(s): Eveline C. Traeger, MD

Multiple Sclerosis

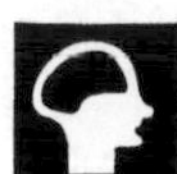

Basics

DESCRIPTION

Multiple sclerosis (MS) is a chronic inflammatory autoimmune disease of unknown etiology that involves demyelination of the CNS with resultant neurologic dysfunction. The manifestations are extremely variable in type and severity.

EPIDEMIOLOGY

Incidence/Prevalence

Approximately 400,000 persons in the U.S. Prevalence varies with latitude: northern U.S. is a high-risk area (prevalence >30 per 100,000); southern U.S is a medium-risk area.

Age

Onset usually between 10 and 59 years (between 20 and 40 years in approximately 70% of patients).

Sex

Female/male ratio of 2:1

Race

Prevalence is higher in Caucasians than blacks or Asians.

ETIOLOGY

- Etiology uncertain but evidence suggests an autoimmune process directed against the protein components of myelin. T lymphocytes are activated against myelin antigens, axons, and/or oligodendrocytes and enter the CNS, triggering an immunologic cascade with recruitment of inflammatory cells and local release of lymphokines and cytokines with resultant injury to myelin and the underlying axon.
- A multitude of environmental factors has been proposed to trigger an autoimmune process. One theory is that an infection triggers the autoimmune response through molecular mimicry. Many infectious agents have been studied; evidence of a link to any particular agent remains inconclusive.

Genetics

Most cases are sporadic; 25% concordance rate in monozygotic twin studies and studies of first-degree relatives (children of patients with MS have 30 to 50× increased risk). Multiple candidate weak MS-susceptibility genes are currently being studied including the gene for CTLA-4 (a molecule expressed on the surface of activated T cells). HLA-DR15, DQ6 haplotype linkage has been demonstrated.

RISK FACTORS

- Female preponderance 2:1
- Caucasian/Northern European
- Temperate latitudes
- Family history of MS

PREGNANCY

The relapse rate decreases significantly during the third trimester. Many studies show an increase in relapse rate in the first 6 months postpartum. Pregnancy does not appear to have a detrimental effect on long-term course or disability.

ASSOCIATED CONDITIONS

- Bell's palsy
- Optic neuritis
- Trigeminal neuralgia
- Uveitis
- Transverse myelitis
- Devic's syndrome

Diagnosis

DIFFERENTIAL DIAGNOSIS

- Acute disseminated encephalomyelitis
- Behçet's disease
- Hereditary ataxias
- Lyme disease
- Metastatic neoplasm
- Migraine
- Neurosyphilis
- Paraneoplastic neurologic syndromes
- Primary CNS lymphoma
- Progressive multifocal leukoencephalopathy
- Sarcoidosis
- Sjögren's syndrome
- Somatization disorders
- Spinal cord compression from tumor or disc
- Strokes in the young
- Syphilis
- Syringomyelia
- Systemic lupus erythematosus
- Transverse myelitis
- Tropical spastic paraparesis/HTLV-1
- Vasculitides
- Vitamin B_{12} deficiency

SIGNS AND SYMPTOMS

- Afferent pupillary defect (Marcus Gunn pupil)
- Ataxia
- Babinski sign
- Bowel dysfunction: constipation, urgency, incontinence
- Cognitive impairment
- Depression
- Diplopia
- Facial palsy or myokymia
- Fatigue
- Gait disorder
- Hyperreflexia
- Incoordination
- Internuclear ophthalmoplegia
- Lhermitte's sign
- Numbness
- Nystagmus
- Pain
- Paralysis
- Paresthesias
- Sexual dysfunction
- Spasticity
- Tonic spasms
- Tremor
- Trigeminal neuralgia
- Urinary frequency, retention, incontinence
- Vertigo
- Visual disturbance or blindness
- Weakness in one or more limbs

LABORATORY PROCEDURES

There is no definitive laboratory test that is conclusive for MS. Blood work (to exclude other disorders):

- ANA (can be positive in low titer in up to 80% of MS patients)
- Anti-SSA antibody (if sicca symptoms)
- HTLV-1 antibody (in myelopathic presentation)
- Vitamin B_{12} level
- FTA-ABS
- Serum Lyme antibody titer

IMAGING STUDIES

- MRI is the most powerful diagnostic tool, abnormal in 90% of patients with clinically definite MS, 60% to 70% probable MS, 30% to 50% possible MS. Cranial MRI: white matter lesions in paraventricular distribution and infratentorial lesions. Acute lesions may enhance with gadolinium.
- The International Panel on the Diagnosis of Multiple Sclerosis convened in 2000 and made recommendations for new diagnostic criteria. The details of these criteria cannot be covered here but may be summarized by maintenance of the traditional requirement to obtain objective evidence of dissemination in time and space of lesions typical of MS. MRI can be useful to demonstrate dissemination in both time and space. Serial MRI scans can be used to demonstrate dissemination in time by the appearance of new T2 or gadolinium-enhancing lesions at least 3 months after an initial scan without a second clinical exacerbation.
- Spinal MRI of cervical and/or thoracic levels is useful to rule out compressive lesions in myelopathic presentation and may demonstrate cord hyperintensities when cranial MRI is not diagnostic. May show cord atrophy in chronic cases.
- Cranial CT is not sensitive enough to detect most MS lesions.

SPECIAL TESTS

- CSF exam may provide additional support for diagnosis if cranial MRI not deemed typical or diagnostic.
  —WBC: normal or modest lymphocytic pleocytosis (<50 cells/mm^3).
  —Total protein should be normal.
  —Protein electrophoresis: presence of oligoclonal bands or elevated IgG index reflect activation of immune cells within CNS, present in 80% with definite MS.
  —CSF Ig abnormalities are not required for the diagnosis of RR MS but are required to meet the new diagnostic criteria for a diagnosis of PP MS (in which MRI abnormalities are often less conspicuous).
- Evoked potentials (visual, somatosensory): less helpful than MRI or CSF but may occasionally be used to demonstrate slowing of conduction through central pathways and presence of second lesion.

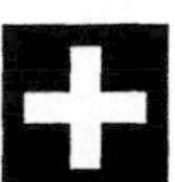

Management

GENERAL MEASURES

- Resist temptation to attribute all symptoms, especially pain, to MS.
- Evaluate for infections when a patient presents with exacerbation and intervene early.
- Aggressively treat fever, which may worsen neurologic function.
- Prescribe stress avoidance/management.
- Prescribe skin care for insensate skin or areas prone to decubiti: seat cushions, frequent position changes, sheepskin, water/foam mattress.
- Prescribe physical therapy, including range of motion (ROM), stretching exercises, strengthening, exercises, gait assessment.
- Prescribe occupational therapy to assist with upper extremity weakness and incoordination, exercise, and assistive devices.
- Prescribe speech therapy to evaluate dysarthria, and problems with deglutition.

SURGICAL MEASURES

- Placement of intrathecal baclofen pump or tenotomy, myotomy, myelotomy for intractible spasticity
- Placement of gastric or jejunal feeding tube for severe swallowing dysfunction
- Urinary diversion procedures for severe voiding problems
- Implantation of deep brain stimulator, gamma knife thalamotomy for intractable tremor

SYMPTOMATIC TREATMENT

- Fatigue—naps, energy conservation, assistive mobility devices, conditioning exercise programs, optimization of sleep, minimization of sedating medications and pharmacotherapy
- Spasticity—rule out conditions that may cause reflex increase in spasticity, such as urinary tract infections, decubiti, cellulitis; physical therapy with emphasis on ROM, daily stretching, exercise, and medications
- Weakness—rest, physical therapy, exercise, energy conservation, cooling vest
- Depression—psychotherapy, antidepressants, exercise
- Dysesthetic pains—medications and TENS units, acupuncture
- Tonic spasms—carbamazepine, phenytoin, gabapentin
- Bladder dysfunction—medications, intermittent self-catheterization, difficult to differentiate several possible patterns of bladder dysfunction based on symptoms alone. Should check postvoid residual to rule out retention or if serious problem with incontinence or frequent UTIs, refer for more detailed urologic evaluation.
- Bowel dysfunction—increased fluid intake to 2 to 2.5 L/day, stool softeners, peristaltic stimulants, increased dietary fiber, enemas, bulking agents, rectal stimulation
- Cognitive dysfunction—cognitive rehabilitation, address fatigue and depression, treat underlying MS
- Tremor—wrist weights, benzodiazepines, primidone, carbamazepine, ondansetron, thalamotomy, or thalamic electrostimulation
- See Medications, below, for appropriate medications

ADJUNCTIVE TREATMENT

- Orthotics—cane and instruction in proper use, walker, ankle-foot orthosis for foot drop, motorized scooter to maintain mobility, conserve energy
- Cooling devices

ADMISSION/DISCHARGE CRITERIA

- MS is managed on an outpatient basis except when abrupt decline prevents the patient from performing normal activities of daily living such as ambulation or transfers, when a serious complication occurs such as urosepsis or deep venous thrombosis/pulmonary embolism, or rehabilitation or chronic long-term care is required. High-dose intravenous corticosteroids generally can be given at home except when close monitoring of hypertension or hyperglycemia due to diabetes mellitus is required.
- Discharge criteria—patients with acute exacerbation should be discharged to home once able to care for self or adequate services are available or to rehabilitation facility if appropriate.

Medications

DRUG(S) OF CHOICE

Acute Exacerbations

- Mild exacerbations, e.g., sensory symptoms, do not require treatment.
- For more severe exacerbations, methylprednisolone 1 g IV qd × 3 to 5 days with or without an oral prednisone taper starting at 60 mg, reduced over approximately 9 to 14 days (restores blood-brain barrier, reduces edema, shortens duration of relapse, and accelerates recovery).
- The Optic Neuritis Treatment Trial results suggest that moderate doses of oral steroids alone may result in higher subsequent relapse rate; therefore, intravenous steroids with or without oral taper are now preferred. Studies of the use of high-dose oral steroids equivalent to IV doses are underway.

Symptomatic Treatment/Medications

- Fatigue
  —Amantadine 100 mg PO bid–tid
  —Modafinil 200–400 mg PO qd; pemoline has been used but less frequently due to concerns about hepatotoxicity,
  —Methylphenidate, and other stimulants.
- Spasticity
  —Baclofen—start 10 mg qd to bid and titrate up to 100 mg or even 200 mg/d if severe in three to four doses per day
  —Tizanidine 4 mg—start with 2 mg qd and gradually increase by 2 mg q3–4d until up to maximum of 32 mg/day. May cause less weakness than baclofen. LFTs must be monitored.
  —Diazepam or clonazepam may relieve spasticity especially at night; use limited by sedation.
  —Baclofen pump, which delivers intrathecal baclofen, may be helpful in severe spasticity not relieved by oral medications.
  —Other approaches to severe refractory spasticity include botulinum toxin injection, intrathecal phenol injection, dorsal root section, myelotomy, or even cordectomy.
- Vertigo
  —Meclizine 12.5–25 mg up to qid; diazepam 2 mg bid to qid PRN
- Bladder dysfunction
  —Hypertonic bladder: avoid caffeine, oxybutynin 2.5 to 5 mg bid to tid, tricyclic antidepressants
  —Hypotonic bladder: bethanechol may improve detrusor contractions; intermittent self-catheterization
  —Bladder-sphincter dyssynergia: anticholinergics and self-catheterization
- Constipation/fecal incontinence
  —Glycerin or Dulcolax suppositories
  —Therevac mini-enemas

- Tremor
  —Often very difficult to treat
  —Weights on the limbs sometimes helpful
  —Propranolol may help action component of tremor (80 mg or more per day)
  —Primidone: start with low doses such as 25 to 50 mg/d and gradually increase to 250 mg bid and further as tolerated. Limited by sedation.
  —Isoniazid 600–1,200 mg/d with pyridoxine may reduce intention tremor
  —Thalamotomy or chronic thalamic stimulation investigational
- Dysesthetic pain
  —Carbamazepine 100 to 200 mg/d to start and gradually increase to 600–1,600 mg/d in 3 to 4 doses for lancinating, sharp pain, e.g., trigeminal neuralgia
  —Gabapentin in doses of 100–1,200 mg tid; other agents that may be helpful include phenytoin, clonazepam, baclofen
  —Tricyclic antidepressants may be helpful for burning, gnawing, aching pains.
- Sexual dysfunction
  —For males, sildenafil, vacuum/tumescence constriction therapy, intracorporeal injections, penile implantation
  —For females, adequate lubrication and stimulation

Disease-Modifying Treatments

Several therapies are available in the U.S. for treatment of MS including three forms of interferon-beta, glatiramer acetate, and mitoxantrone.

- Interferons are natural cytokines that have a wide spectrum of immunomodulating activities. These activities include affects on T-cell activation, alteration of Th1 versus Th2 cytokine production, blood–brain barrier, and antiviral effects. Well-designed studies have been performed with several forms of interferon-beta and have each showed reduction of the exacerbation rate in the range of one third and reduction of new and gadolinium-enhancing lesions on MRI scans. In various trials, the interferons have also demonstrated delayed time of progression in relapsing or secondary progressive disease. The three interferon-beta products are:
  —Interferon-beta 1b (Betaseron)—8 million units (0.25 mg) SC qos
  —Interferon-beta 1a (Avonex)—30 μg IM q week
  —Interferon-beta 1a (Rebif)—22 or 44 μg SC 3 times a week
- Glatiramer acetate (Copaxone) is a synthetic protein that causes inhibition of myelin-reactive T cells and induction of antiinflammatory Th2 cells as well as some bystander suppression of inflammation in the CNS. It is administered as 20 mg SC qd and has been shown to decreases relapse rate by approximately one third and to decrease new MRI lesions.

Treatment of Progressive Disease

- Studies of interferon-beta for the treatment of secondary progressive MS have had mixed results. However, several studies have shown a reduction in acute exacerbations superimposed on a deteriorating baseline and a slowing of progression. Interferon-beta 1b has been FDA approved for secondary progressive MS.
- Slight benefit has been shown with methotrexate 7.5 to 12.5 mg PO q week.
- Mitoxantrone (Novantrone), an anthracenedione antineoplastic agent with immunosuppressive activity, has been shown in one phase III trial to reduce relapse rate and slow progression of neurologic disability. It has been approved for these purposes in SP MS and worsening RR MS. The recommended dose is 5 to 12 mg/m^2 IV infusion every 3 months. Side effects include nausea and alopecia. Lifetime exposure to this medication is limited to 2 to 3 years (cumulative dose of 120–140 mg/m^2) due to dose-related cardiotoxicity. Patients should be monitored with periodic assessments of heart function such as ejection fraction by echocardiogram during their course of mitoxantrone.

Contraindications

- See manufacturer's package insert for each drug. Interferon-beta 1a or 1b should not be used in pregnancy due to abortifacient properties.
- No known drug interactions with other agents.
- Pemoline has been associated with hepatotoxicity.

Precautions

- Interferon-beta side effects: flu-like symptoms (fever, chills, myalgias, headaches) starting 2 to 6 hours and lasting 24 to 48 hours after injection. These gradually lessen over several months. Injection site tenderness, swelling, and occasional skin necrosis as well as LFT abnormalities, leukopenia, anemia, exacerbation of depression. Patients should have a baseline CBC/diff and LFTs and then be monitored approximately 1 and 3 months after initiation of interferon therapy and then every 3 to 6 months. Management of interferon side effects—dose administration before bed so greatest side effects while sleeping; acetaminophen 650 mg q4–6 hrs for 24 hours; nonsteroidal antiinflammatory drugs (NSAIDs) with longer half-life on shot day if acetaminophen not effective; prednisone 10 mg with injection and q6h for 1 to 3 doses on injection day for interferon-beta 1a if above not helpful; pentoxifylline 400 mg bid in addition to acetaminophen; dose reduction and gradual re-escalation; ice or topical anesthetic such as lidocaine 2.5% and prilocaine 2.5% combination for injection site pain.
- Glatiramer acetate is associated with a self-limited postinjection reaction shortly after injection that may include flushing, palpitations, dyspnea, and chest pain or tightness lasting up to 30 minutes. This may be quite alarming to patients unless they are warned about the potential for this reaction ahead of time.
- Tizanidine may cause light-headedness. Many of these medications may cause sedation.

ALTERNATIVE DRUGS

- Other agents used to treat severe relapsing or progressive disease include azathioprine, cyclophosphamide, intermittent intravenous methylprednisolone, intravenous immunoglobulins, plasma exchange, and cladribine. Studies are ongoing on total lymphoid irradiation, bone marrow transplantation, and other agents.
- There is a new emphasis in MS centers to consider trials of treatment with various combinations of therapy such as interferon and methotrexate. However, there is a paucity of phase 3 trials to support efficacy.

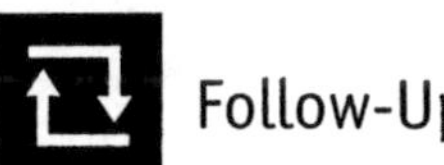

Follow-Up

PATIENT MONITORING

Optimal care with primary care physician sharing care with neurologist with intermittent consultation by urology, psychology, physical medicine and rehabilitation, physical therapy, and occupational therapy as needed. Motor function should be assessed regularly in follow-up visits, and some recommend assessment of time to walk 25 feet as a reliable measure to follow as well as other measures of hand function. Patients should be screened for depression (as depression is very frequent in this population as well as suicide), urinary and sexual dysfunction, fatigue, and cognitive dysfunction at each visit as these problems are not reliably reported as active problems. This condition can also put strains on family relationships, including the primary caregiver, and support should be offered.

EXPECTED COURSE AND PROGNOSIS

- The course is highly variable with several common patterns:
  —Relapsing-remitting—episodes of acute worsening of neurologic symptoms followed by variable recovery and stable period between relapses
  —Secondary progressive—relapsing course that evolves into a gradual course of deterioration with or without superimposed relapses
  —Primary progressive—gradual neurologic deterioration without relapses or remission
- For approximately one third, the disease is relatively benign with minimal disability 10 to 15 years after onset. Approximately one half of MS patients are unable to walk without assistance within 15 years of the initial diagnosis.
- Prognostic factors for severe disease: age of onset >40 years (because older onset patients have higher likelihood of early progressive course), progressive course from disease onset, motor and cerebellar involvement from time of presentation, multiple cranial T2-weighted MRI lesions, poor recovery from relapses, short interval between initial two relapses, and incomplete remissions.
- Approximately 50% of those who present with isolated optic neuritis go on to develop MS.

PATIENT EDUCATION

- National Multiple Sclerosis Society, 205 E. 42nd Street, New York, NY 10017.
  Phone: 800-344-4867 (FIGHTMS), which can also connect patient to nearest local chapter.
  Website: *www.nmss.org*.
- Routine vaccinations are safe and appropriate for MS patients.
- Patients should be warned about potential deleterious effects of heat and fever on neurologic function.

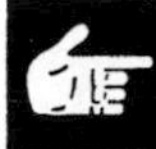

Miscellaneous

SYNONYMS

Disseminated sclerosis

ICD-9-CM: 340 Multiple sclerosis

SEE ALSO: OPTIC NEURITIS, TRANSVERSE MYELITIS

REFERENCES

- Arnold DL, Matthews PM. MRI in the diagnosis and management of multiple sclerosis. Neurology 2002;58(8, suppl 4): S23–31.
- Ghalie RG, Edan G, Laurent M, et al. Cardiac adverse effects associated with mitoxantrone (Novantrone) therapy in patients with MS. Neurology 2002:59: 909–913.
- Goodin DS, Frohman EM, Garmany GP Jr, et al. Disease modifying therapies in multiple sclerosis: report of the Therapeutics and Technology Assessment Subcommittee of the American Academy of Neurology and the MS Council for Clinical Practice Guidelines. Neurology 2002;58: 169–178.
- Jacobs LD, Beck RW, Simon, et al. Intramuscular interferon beta-1a therapy initiated during a first demyelinating event in multiple sclerosis. N Engl J Med 2000; 343:898–904.
- Krupp LB, Rizvi SA. Symptomatic therapy for underrecognized manifestations of multiple sclerosis. Neurology 2002:58 (suppl 4):S32–S39.
- Lublin FD. The diagnosis of multiple sclerosis. Curr Opin Neurol 2002;15(3): 253–256.
- McDonald WI, Compston A, Edan G, et al. Recommended diagnostic criteria for multiple sclerosis: guidelines from the International Panel on the Diagnosis of Multiple Sclerosis. Ann Neurol 2001;50:121–127.
- Noseworthy JH, Lucchinetti C, Rodriguez M, et al. Medical progress—multiple sclerosis. N Engl J Med 2000;343;938–952.
- Paty DW, Ebers GC. Multiple sclerosis. Philadelphia: FA Davis, 1998.
- Rudick RA, Cohen JA, Weinstock-Guttman B, et al. Management of multiple sclerosis. N Engl J Med 1997;337:1604–1611.
- Thompson AJ, Montalban X, Barkhof F, et al. Diagnostic criteria for primary progressive multiple sclerosis: a position paper. Ann Neurol 2000;47:831–835.
- Yong VW. Differential mechanisms of action of interferon-B and glatiramer acetate in MS. Neurology 2002;59: 802–808.

Author(s): D. Joanne Lynn, MD

Multiple System Atrophy

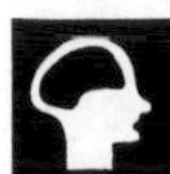

Basics

DESCRIPTION

Multiple system atrophy (MSA) is the prototype of a Parkinson's plus syndrome. Sharing clinical similarities with typical idiopathic Parkinson's disease (IPD), MSA nevertheless presents with a constellation of additional neurologic symptoms. Three major classes of MSA have been described:

- MSA-P (parkinsonism) or striatonigral degeneration (SND): typically presents with parkinsonian features (bradykinesia, rigidity, postural instability, and/or rest tremor), which are virtually resistant to dopaminergic therapy. This syndrome is notoriously difficult to distinguish from IPD at initial evaluation due to transient response to dopaminergic agents.
- MSA-C (cerebellar) or sporadic olivopontocerebellar atrophy (sOPCA): sometimes presenting initially with parkinsonian features, individuals afflicted with this disorder develop concomitant or subsequent cerebellar features, which usually predominate as the disease progresses. Patients usually manifest multiple symptoms of cerebellar dysfunction including ataxia of limb movement, gait and speech, dysrhythmia, dysdiadochokinesis, titubation, impaired check response, nystagmus, and other eye movement abnormalities associated with cerebellar dysfunction. Bulbar symptoms such as dysphagia may develop.
- MSA-A (autonomic) or Shy-Drager syndrome (SDS): typically presents with parkinsonian features and concomitant autonomic dysfunction including orthostatic hypotension without a compensatory tachycardia (defined as a 20 mm Hg drop in systolic BP or a 10 mm Hg drop in diastolic BP from recumbent to standing position without an alternative cause), urinary retention or incontinence, and/or impotence (in males). Other possible features of autonomic insufficiency include anhydrosis, constipation, and reduced/absent pupillary reactivity.

While patients with MSA-C and MSA-A may present without parkinsonian features, once manifest, the parkinsonian features may initially respond significantly to dopaminergic therapy, suggesting at least partial preservation of striatal integrity and primary loss of dopaminergic afferents from the substantia nigra. These benefits from dopaminergic treatment are not typically sustained with time, however, especially as the cerebellar and/or autonomic features advance clinically.

Classical Pathologic Changes in Multiple System Atrophy

Neuropathologic changes in SND include neurodegeneration and glial cytoplasmic inclusions (GCIs) in multiple subcortical structures including globus pallidus, striatum, substantia nigra, inferior olivary nucleus, cerebellum, pons, intermediolateral columns of the spinal cord, and autonomic nuclei of the brainstem. The GCIs are composed of α-synuclein and are common to all varieties of MSA, suggesting a common pathophysiologic process with disorders in which α-synuclein is deposited in the Lewy bodies of IPD and diffuse Lewy body disease (DLBD).

EPIDEMIOLOGY

Incidence/Prevalence

Incidence in individuals past the age of 50 may approach 3/100,000. The prevalence has been estimated at 3 to 5 per 100,000 in the general population.

Race

No known ethnic predilection.

Age

The mean age of onset is the early to mid-fifties, slightly earlier than IPD.

Sex

Some authors suggest a mild male predominance.

ETIOLOGY

There are no clear genetic or environmental causes of MSA. The cerebellar variant must be distinguished from the hereditary multiple system degenerations.

PREGNANCY

N/A

ASSOCIATED CONDITIONS

N/A

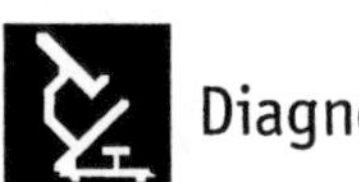

Diagnosis

DIFFERENTIAL DIAGNOSIS

Idiopathic Parkinson's disease
Diffuse Lewy body disease
Corticobasal ganglionic degeneration
Progressive supranuclear palsy
Hereditary ataxias

SIGNS AND SYMPTOMS

Differentiating MSA in its early stages from other akinetic-rigid syndromes such as IPD is difficult, even for specialists. The clinical diagnosis relies on the development of distinct signs and symptoms, none of which is unique to MSA. However, consensus criteria have been developed, which allows for some degree of confidence for antemortem diagnosis (summarized by Gilman, 2002).

The criteria and their corresponding levels of clinical confidence are as follows:

- Possible MSA: one criterion plus two features from other separate domains. If parkinsonism is the criterion, poor levodopa response qualifies as one distinct feature.
- Probable MSA: criterion for autonomic failure/urinary dysfunction plus levodopa-unresponsive parkinsonism or cerebellar dysfunction.
- Definite MSA: pathologic confirmation of pertinent neurodegenerative changes accompanied by the presence of high density of GCIs.

The clinical domains referred to by these criteria include:

- Autonomic and urinary dysfunction
  - —Features
    - -Orthostatic hypotension blood pressure drop of >20 mm Hg systolic or >10 mm Hg diastolic
    - -Occasional urinary incontinence or incomplete bladder emptying
  - —Criteria
    - -Severe orthostatic hypotension—>30 mm Hg systolic or >15 mm Hg diastolic drop in blood pressure or
    - -Persistent urinary incontinence accompanied by impotence in men, or
    - -Both orthostatic changes and urinary incontinence
- Parkinsonism
  - —Features
    - -Bradykinesia
    - -Rigidity
    - -Postural instability
    - -Tremor
  - —Criteria
    - -Bradykinesia, plus
    - -Rigidity, or
    - -Postural instability, or
    - -Tremor
- Cerebellar dysfunction
  - —Features
    - -Gait ataxia
    - -Ataxic dysarthria
    - -Limb ataxia
    - -Sustained gaze-evoked nystagmus
  - —Criteria
    - -Gait ataxia, plus
    - -Ataxic dysarthria, or
    - -Limb ataxia, or
    - -Sustained gaze-evoked nystagmus
- Corticospinal tract dysfunction
  - —Features
    - -Extensor plantar responses with hyperreflexia
  - —No criteria

Other associated clinical features include (a) peripheral neuropathy, especially affecting sphincter musculature; (b) sleep disorders, especially REM sleep behavior disorder and sleep apneas; (c) relative *absence* of cognitive decline; and (d) multiple other motor and sensory symptoms including severe antecollis, spasticity, myoclonus, Raynaud's phenomenon, and pain.

LABORATORY PROCEDURES

There are no specific blood tests to diagnose PSP, but the following tests should be considered to identify potential underlying secondary causes of parkinsonism: serum vitamin B_{12} level, thyroid function tests, serum ceruloplasmin, 24-hour urine copper excretion, and serum α-tocopherol (vitamin E) levels.

IMAGING STUDIES

Functional neuroimaging using PET and SPECT scanning using markers for neuronal activity (fluorodeoxyglucose), dopaminergic terminals, and dopamine receptors may distinguish MSA from IPD, but does not distinguish MSA from other Parkinson's plus syndromes such as PSP. These methods are not being widely implemented.

There is some evidence to suggest that MRI can assist in the diagnosis of MSA. Specifically, brain MRI may reveal hypointensity and/or atrophy in the putamen or, alternatively, hyperintensity and/or atrophy in the cerebellum and brainstem. MRI may also reveal evidence of other causes of parkinsonism such as vascular insults, mass lesions, calcium or iron deposition in the striatum, and cortical atrophy patterns suggestive of other dementing illnesses.

SPECIAL TESTS

Routine studies of autonomic function may help distinguish MSA-A from cases of primary autonomic failure. Cardiac imaging studies visualizing the autonomic innervation of the heart using a SPECT ligand has consistently distinguished MSA-A from IPD with autonomic involvement.

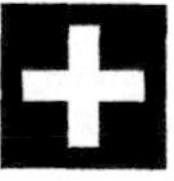

Management

GENERAL MEASURES

There is no effective treatment for MSA. Management is aimed at alleviating the consequences of the motor and autonomic changes associated with MSA.

SURGICAL MEASURES

N/A

SYMPTOMATIC TREATMENT

The extrapyramidal symptoms of bradykinesia and resultant loss of mobility may be overcome by the use of four-wheeled walkers, although the tendency of patients with MSA, especially MSA-C, to fall usually limits the effective duration of this intervention. Dysarthria and dysphagia may benefit from speech pathology intervention. Percutaneous endoscopic gastrostomy (PEG) may be performed to provide life-sustaining nutrition.

ADJUNCTIVE TREATMENT

N/A

ADMISSION/DISCHARGE CRITERIA

MSA is usually managed in an outpatient setting. Rarely, concomitant illnesses, especially aspiration pneumonia, can lead to an acute exacerbation of MSA symptoms, requiring hospitalization for dysphagia, airway management, and issues of decreased mobility.

Medications

DRUG(S) OF CHOICE

Rarely, extrapyramidal symptoms seen in MSA may respond to carbidopa/levodopa administration, sometimes requiring supratherapeutic (i.e., greater than 600–800 mg of levodopa per day) doses. Anticholinergic agents and amantadine may also be of limited usefulness. These responses are usually minimal and short-lived.

Orthostatic hypotension may be treated with increased salt intake, fludrocortisone (0.1–0.4 mg/d in two divided doses), or midodrine (5–10 mg up to three times daily).

Urinary incontinence may be treated with peripheral anticholinergic therapy (oxybutynin 5–10 mg at bedtime, and other formulations).

Constipation is treated with advancing doses of fiber supplements, stool softeners, fruit and vegetable preparations, and/or lactulose.

The ataxia seen in MSA sometimes responds to clonazepam 0.5–1.0 mg at bedtime.

Antidepressants, especially selective serotonin reuptake inhibitors, have helped in cases of depression.

Contraindications

Individuals with a history of congestive heart failure or renal insufficiency should not be prescribed a high-salt diet and should be carefully monitored if given a volume-expanding agent such as fludrocortisone.

Precautions

Severe *hypertension* can result from aggressive treatment with volume expanding or vasoactive therapies. Careful monitoring of blood pressure during titration of these agents is mandatory.

ALTERNATIVE DRUGS

N/A

Follow-Up

PATIENT MONITORING

Like other Parkinson's plus syndromes, the progression of MSA is relentless and refractory to most common treatment modalities, resulting in death within an average of 6 to 9 years after symptom onset. Patients are monitored in the outpatient setting, usually at 4- to 6-month intervals. Judicious use of antidepressant medications and timely discussion of PEG tube placement are recommended to assist patients and their families prepare for future decline.

EXPECTED COURSE AND PROGNOSIS

Due to its progressive nature, the symptoms of MSA always worsen with time. Over time, the limited responsiveness of MSA patients to dopaminergic therapy typically deteriorates. Death usually occurs as a consequence of cardiac arrhythmia or aspiration pneumonia.

PATIENT EDUCATION

The postural instability characteristic of MSA syndromes prevents the use of ambulatory exercise, although stretching and strengthening exercises in a sitting position may be useful. Aqua therapy with close supervision may help forestall some of the immobility issues associated with this illness. Speech therapy is useful for speech and swallowing disturbances. Frequently, patients continue to be classified as IPD patients, confounding their understanding and expectations of treatment options and prognosis.

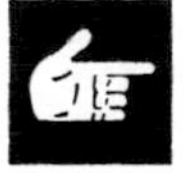

Miscellaneous

SYNONYMS

None

ICD-9-CM: 333.0 Shy-Drager syndrome (orthostatic hypotension with multisystem atrophy)

SEE ALSO: PARKINSON'S DISEASE, DIFFUSE LEWY BODY DISEASE, PROGRESSIVE SUPRANUCLEAR PALSY

REFERENCES

- Gilman S. Multiple system atrophy. In: Jankovic J, Tolosa E, eds. Parkinson's disease and movement disorders, 4th ed. Philadelphia: Lippincott Williams & Wilkins, 2002:170–184.
- Kaufmann, H. Multiple system atrophy. Curr Opin Neurol 1998;11:351–355.
- Tison F, Yekhlef F, Chrysostome V, et al. Parkinsonism in multiple system atrophy: natural history, severity (UPDRS-III), and disability assessment compared to Parkinson's disease. Mov Disord 2002;17:701–709.

Author(s): Lawrence W. Elmer, MD, PhD

Muscular Dystrophy, Congenital

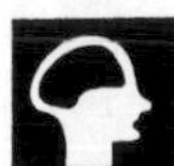

Basics

DESCRIPTION

Congenital muscular dystrophies refer to a group of rare heterogeneous muscle diseases presenting in the neonatal period or early infancy (<6 months) with diffuse muscle weakness and atrophy, hypotonia with or without joint contractures, variable brain abnormalities and mental retardation, and dystrophic changes in the muscle. Included in the congenital muscular dystrophies are Fukuyama congenital muscular dystrophy, Walker-Warburg syndrome, muscle-eye-brain disease, laminin-α_2 (merosin)-deficient and -positive congenital muscular dystrophy, integrin-α_7–deficient congenital muscular dystrophy, rigid spine congenital muscular dystrophy, Ulrich congenital muscular dystrophy, and other unlinked congenital muscular dystrophies.

EPIDEMIOLOGY

Incidence/Prevalence

Merosin-deficient congenital muscular dystrophy consists of 50% of congenital muscular dystrophies. The incidence of Fukuyama congenital muscular dystrophy is 1/18,000 in Japan; that of laminin-α_2–positive congenital muscular dystrophy is 1/60,000. The incidence of other types of congenital muscular dystrophies is unknown.

Race

Fukuyama congenital muscular dystrophy is seen in Japan and Taiwan, and rare in other areas. Muscle-eye-brain disease is described most often in Finland. Other types of congenital muscular dystrophies are reported in all races.

Age

Onset is from birth to first few months of life in all types of congenital muscular dystrophies.

Sex

Males and females are equally affected in all types of congenital muscular dystrophies.

ETIOLOGY

Genetics

All of the above congenital muscular dystrophies are autosomal-recessive diseases. Laminin-α_2 (merosin)-deficient congenital muscular dystrophy is linked to chromosome 6q22-23 (gene product: merosin). Fukuyama congenital muscular dystrophy is linked to chromosome 9q31-q33 (gene product: fukutin). Muscle-eye-brain disease is linked to chromosome 1p32-p34 (gene product: glycosyltransferase). Integrin-α_7–deficient congenital muscular dystrophy is linked to chromosome 12q13 (gene product: α_7 integrin). Rigid spine congenital muscular dystrophy is linked to chromosome 1p35-36 (gene product: selenoprotein N1). Ulrich congenital muscular dystrophy 1-2 is linked to chromosome 21q2 (gene product: collagen VI A1-2); Ulrich congenital muscular dystrophy 3 is linked to chromosome 2q3 (gene product: collagen VI A3). Other congenital muscular dystrophies are unlinked.

RISK FACTORS

N/A

PREGNANCY

N/A

ASSOCIATED CONDITIONS

- Forebrain abnormalities including cobblestone lissencephaly and mental retardation are seen in Fukuyama congenital muscular dystrophy, muscle-eye-brain disease, and Walker-Warburg syndrome.
- Cerebral white matter abnormalities are also frequently seen in Fukuyama congenital muscular dystrophy, muscle-eye-brain disease, Walker-Warburg syndrome, and laminin-α_2 (merosin)-deficient congenital muscular dystrophy.
- Eye abnormalities are present in muscle-eye-brain disease and Walker-Warburg syndrome.
- Seizures and epilepsy may occur in Fukuyama congenital muscular dystrophy, Walker-Warburg syndrome, muscle-eye-brain disease, and laminin-α_2 (merosin)-deficient congenital muscular dystrophy.
- Early spine contractures, rigidity, and scoliosis are seen in rigid spine congenital muscular dystrophy.
- Distal joint laxity is seen in all types of Ulrich congenital muscular dystrophies.
- Severe cardiac involvements are reported in muscle-eye-brain disease and Fukuyama congenital muscular dystrophy.

Diagnosis

DIFFERENTIAL DIAGNOSIS

- Mitochondrial encephalomyopathy
- Congenital myopathies
- Congenital myasthenic syndrome
- Congenital myotonic dystrophy
- Metabolic myopathies

SIGNS AND SYMPTOMS

- In all types of congenital muscular dystrophies, there are generalized hypotonia, diffuse muscle weakness and atrophy, variable early and multiple joint contractures, and onset from birth or the first few months of life.
- In the classical or pure form of congenital muscular dystrophy, which is merosin positive, there are no ophthalmologic abnormalities and the patients are usually mentally normal. Congenital hip dislocation or subluxation is frequently seen. In merosin-deficient congenital muscular dystrophy, no abnormal ophthalmologic findings are demonstrated, but severe weakness with inability to ambulate independently is shown in complete merosin deficiency.
- Fukuyama congenital muscular dystrophy, seen mostly in Japan, typically consists of severe congenital muscular dystrophy, mental retardation, and mild cobblestone lissencephaly. Muscle-eye-brain disease, seen predominantly in the Finnish population, reveals congenital muscular dystrophy, mental retardation, retinal hypoplasia, and cobblestone lissencephaly. In Walker-Warburg syndrome, congenital muscular dystrophy, severe mental retardation, retinal abnormalities, and severe cobblestone lissencephaly are present. Although mental retardation is seen in Fukuyama congenital muscular dystrophy, muscle-eye-brain disease, and Walker-Warburg syndrome, marked eye abnormalities are present in muscle-eye-brain disease and Walker-Warburg syndrome but not in Fukuyama congenital muscular dystrophy. Seizures and epilepsy are also reported in Fukuyama congenital muscular dystrophy, muscle-eye-brain disease, Walker-Warburg syndrome, and laminin-α_2 (merosin)-deficient congenital muscular dystrophy.
- In rigid spine congenital muscular dystrophy, typical clinical features include congenital or infantile hypotonia, stable or slowly progressive weakness, poor head control, early spinal rigidity and scoliosis, and early respiratory insufficiency. Delayed motor milestones and mental retardation have been reported in integrin-α_7–deficient congenital muscular dystrophy. Distal joint laxity is seen in all Ulrich congenital muscular dystrophies, and spine rigidity is also reported in Ulrich congenital syndrome type 1 and 2.

LABORATORY PROCEDURES

- Serum creatine kinase may be mildly to moderately increased in all congenital muscular dystrophies.
- EMG shows myopathic changes in most patients with congenital muscular dystrophies.
- Muscle biopsy reveals dystrophic changes and increased connective tissue in the majority of congenital muscular dystrophies.
- EEG may show epileptiform discharges when seizures or epilepsy occur.

IMAGING STUDIES

Brain MRI demonstrates a variety of congenital brain abnormalities, including polymicrogyria, pachygyria, cobblestone lissencephaly, and diffuse or patchy prolonged T1 and T2 signals in cerebral white matter in Fukuyama congenital muscular dystrophy, Walker-Warburg syndrome, muscle-eye-brain disease, and laminin-α_2 (merosin)-deficient congenital muscular dystrophy. Brain MRI is normal in laminin-α_2 (merosin)-positive congenital muscular dystrophy and all other congenital muscular dystrophies.

SPECIAL TESTS

- Complete or partial muscle and skin laminin-α_2 (merosin) deficiency is detected in laminin-α_2 (merosin)-deficient congenital muscular dystrophy by immunohistological staining. Secondary partial laminin-α_2 deficiency is also shown in Fukuyama congenital muscular dystrophy and muscle-eye-brain disease.
- Normal laminin-α_2 (merosin) is seen in the muscles of classic or pure form of congenital muscular dystrophy, Walker-Warburg syndrome, rigid spine congenital muscular dystrophy, integrin-α_7-deficient congenital muscular dystrophy, and other congenital muscular dystrophies.

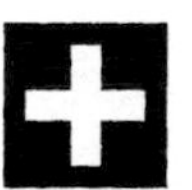

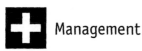

Management

GENERAL MEASURES

Currently, no specific treatment or cure is present for all types of congenital muscular dystrophies.

SURGICAL MEASURES

Tenotomies, tendon transfer, and tendon lengthening may be necessary for some patients to help in standing and ambulation. Progressive scoliosis may require spinal fusion to preserve pulmonary function and respiratory failure. Those with severe cardiac conduction defects may need pacemaker placement to prevent sudden death.

SYMPTOMATIC TREATMENT

Antiepileptic drugs are needed to treat seizures and epilepsy. Physical, occupational, speech and language therapy, braces, and special education are often necessary because muscle weakness, joint contractures, learning problems, and mental retardation are often present in many patients with congenital muscular dystrophies. Special eyeglasses may be needed in patients with visual problems. Antispastic drugs such as baclofen, diazepam, dantrolene, or botulinum toxin injection often reduce spasticity of the extremities.

ADJUNCTIVE TREATMENTS

Passive stretching to improve contractures, night splints, and serial plaster casts may be useful.

ADMISSION/DISCHARGE CRITERIA

Patients are admitted for diagnostic evaluations and treatments such as muscle biopsy, brain MRI, and speech, occupational, and physical therapy.

Medications

DRUG(S) OF CHOICE

N/A

ALTERNATIVE DRUGS

N/A

Follow-Up

PATIENT MONITORING

Patients should be followed regularly for seizure control, joint contractures, nutritional, and other supportive treatments.

EXPECTED COURSE AND PROGNOSIS

- Most patients with laminin-α_2-positive congenital muscular dystrophy are mentally normal but delayed in motor development, and only one third of patients can stand up at age 5 years. Most patients die of respiratory failure during the second decade of life.
- Patients with complete laminin-α_2-deficient congenital muscular dystrophy can sit but never walk, and rarely may die of respiratory failure during infancy; those with partial laminin-α_2-deficiency can walk independently.
- In Fukuyama congenital muscular dystrophy patients, both mental and motor development are severely delayed; only some can stand at age 4 years, and rare patients can walk a few steps. Most die of respiratory failure by age 20 years.
- Patients with Walker-Warburg syndrome have severe mental retardation, generalized weakness, and motor delay, and usually die in the first few months of life.
- Those with muscle-eye-brain disease also have mental retardation and generalized weakness, but usually can sit and walk. Most can live to age 10 to 30 years.
- Those patients with rigid spine congenital muscular dystrophy may develop early life-threatening respiratory insufficiency due to progressive weakness, spinal rigidity, and scoliosis. They require frequent respiratory therapy and may benefit from scoliosis surgical treatment such as timely spinal fusion.
- Ulrich congenital muscular dystrophies and integrin-α_7-deficient congenital muscular dystrophy both have slow clinical course.

PATIENT EDUCATION

In general, all types of congenital muscular dystrophies are rare diseases and the patients need to be referred to muscular dystrophy association clinics or multiple specialty clinics for education and proper care.

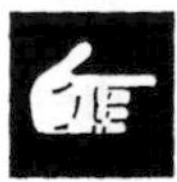

Miscellaneous

SYNONYMS

Muscular dystrophy

ICD-9-CM: 359.0 Congenital muscular dystrophy; 359.1 Hereditary progressive muscular dystrophy

SEE ALSO: N/A

REFERENCES

- Cohn RD, Campbell KP. Molecular basis of muscular dystrophies. Muscle Nerve 2000; 23:1456–1471.
- Emery AE. The muscular dystrophies. Lancet 2002;359:687–695.
- Flanigan KM, Kerr L, Bromberg MB, et al. Congenital muscular dystrophy with rigid spine syndrome: a clinical, pathological, radiological, and genetic study. Ann Neurol 2000;47:152–161.
- Mercuri E, Sewry C, Brown SC, et al. Congenital muscular dystrophies. Semin Pediatr Neurol 2002;9:120–131.
- Muntoni F, Guicheney P. ENMC sponsored workshop on congenital muscular dystrophy held in Naarden, The Netherlands, October 27–28, 2000. Neuromuscul Disord 2002;12:69–78.
- Tsao CY, Mendell JR. The childhood muscular dystrophies: making order out of chaos. Semin Neurol 1999;19:9–23.
- Tsao CY, Mendell JR. Childhood muscular dystrophies sharing a common pathologenesis of membrane instability. In: Younger DS, ed. Motor disorders. Philadelphia: Lippincott Williams & Wilkins, 1999:139–148.
- Tsao CY, Mendell JR. The muscular dystrophies. In: Appel SH, ed. Current neurology, vol 17.IOS Press, 1997:1–46.
- Tsao CY, Mendell JR, Rusin J, Luquette M. Congenital muscular dystrophy with complete laminin α_2-deficiency, cortical dysplasia, and cerebral white matter changes in children. J Child Neurol 1998;13:253–256.

Author(s): Chang-Yong Tsao, MD, FAAN, FAAP

Muscular Dystrophy, Duchenne's and Becker's (Dystrophin-Related Disorders)

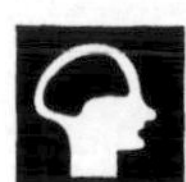

Basics

DESCRIPTION

Muscular dystrophies are progressive neuromuscular diseases that are genetic myopathies, caused by defects in structural proteins resulting in muscle degeneration and weakness. Dystrophinopathies are muscular dystrophies in which the primary abnormality involves dystrophin. Dystrophin is an intracellular protein localized to the subsarcolemmal region of skeletal and cardiac muscle.

Duchenne's and Becker's muscular dystrophies are the most common dystrophinopathies that share the same gene defect but have variable phenotypic expressions.

Less common dystrophinopathies are Duchenne outlier, female Duchenne muscular dystrophy (DMD), and female Duchenne carrier.

EPIDEMIOLOGY

Incidence/Prevalence

- Duchenne's
  —Incidence: 1:3,500 male births
  —Prevalence: 1:25,000
  -30% spontaneous mutation rate
  —Inheritance: x-linked recessive
  —Defect: absent dystrophin (may be up to 3% of normal)
- Becker's
  —Incidence: 1:16,000 to 1:33,000 of male births
  —Inheritance: x-linked recessive
  —Defect: decreased or defective dystrophin (3%–20% of normal)

Race

All races are affected equally.

Age

- Duchenne's
  —Onset by 3 years of age
- Becker's
  —Onset after age 5 to 7 years

ETIOLOGY

Genetics

- Duchenne's and Becker's are x-linked recessive disorders; hence they occur primarily in boys. They are caused by a mutation in the dystrophin gene, which is located on chromosome Xp21.
- An out-of-frame mutation causes Duchenne's. The mutation disrupts dystrophin production.
- No dystrophin, but rarely 3% of normal dystrophin content may be present.
- An in-frame deletion causes Becker's.
  —Shortened but semifunctional dystrophin (20% of normal)
- Reduced expression of normal dystrophin results in outlier DMD.
- *Carrier female*
  —Heterozygotes with normal dystrophin gene on one X chromosome, a mutant gene on the other, and are asymptomatic
- By Lyon hypothesis, when more than half of X chromosome in a muscle fiber express a mutant gene for dystrophin, the muscle fiber is prone to degeneration and can cause clinical symptoms in female carriers.
- 30% to 35% of dystrophinopathies have a point mutation and may not be detectable by routine clinical testing.
- Female Duchenne phenotype presents occasionally in Turner syndrome and has clinical features similar to the male Duchenne.

RISK FACTORS

- Family history of maternal uncles with DMD
- Female carrier donates an X chromosome to a susceptible son and also to carrier daughters.
- Spontaneous mutation—30% to 35%

PREGNANCY

Prenatal diagnosis is possible in the first trimester by chorionic villus sampling to determine deletion and may be more accurate if a family member is known to be involved.

ASSOCIATED CONDITIONS

- Contractures, particular in Achilles' tendon
- Obesity
- Nonprogressive mental retardation with mean IQ = 85
- Kyphoscoliosis (worsens ambulation)
- Impaired pulmonary function
- Cardiomyopathy
- Gastrointestinal tract disorders, including malabsorption, megacolon, volvulus, cramping, and dysmotility
- Emotional disorders, including depression

Diagnosis

DIFFERENTIAL DIAGNOSIS

- Congenital myopathies—group of myopathies with abnormal muscle histology and fiber-type abnormalities presenting mostly as infantile hypotonia
- Congenital muscular dystrophy—present at birth, unpredictable, slow progressive course, with CNS anomalies
- Mitochondrial myopathies—with or without ragged red fibers, multiorgan involvement, and respiratory pathway enzyme deficiencies
- Metabolic myopathies—usually with abnormal muscle lysosomal storage diseases due to enzyme deficiencies, e.g., acid maltase deficiency
- Facioscapulohumeral muscular dystrophy—autosomal dominant face, shoulder, and upper limb involvement; slow progression
- Emery-Dreifuss—X-linked, onset age 5 to 15 years, upper arms and peroneal muscles, slow progression
- Limb girdle—autosomal recessive, onset age 10 to 20 years, shoulder or pelvic girdle

SIGNS AND SYMPTOMS

- Duchenne's
  —Delayed motor development and delayed walking
  —Onset of gait abnormalities evident by 3 to 5 years
  —Calf hypertrophy can be as early as 1 to 2 years
  —Waddling gait
  —Gowers's sign—child "climbs up by his thighs"
  —Toe walking
  —Lordosis and later kyphoscoliosis
  —Proximal, and later distal, limb weakness
  —Difficulty in climbing stairs and frequent falls
  —Contractures later
  —Bulbar weakness may be late
  —Cardiomyopathy
  —Wheelchair-bound by 12 years
  —Death by second or third decade
  —Absent tendon reflexes later
- Becker's
  —More slowly progressive than Duchenne's
  —Muscle weakness usually after 5 years
  —Still ambulatory after 12 years
  —Less severe weakness than Duchenne's
  —Death in adulthood as late as 50 years
- Duchenne outlier
  —Clinically presents like Duchenne's dystrophy with same early symptoms, but with a slower course.
  —Residual dystrophin in 10% of muscle fibers.
  —Still ambulatory by 16 years.
  —Life expectancy may be more than 25 years.
- Female Duchenne muscular dystrophy
  —Normal dystrophin gene on one X chromosome and a mutant gene on the other.
  —According to Lyon hypothesis random inactivation of one X chromosome may leave more than half of mutant X chromosomes to be operant, resulting in various degrees of muscle weakness.
  —Such a scenario leaves these females with clinical signs and symptoms similar to male Duchenne, with laboratory findings of partial absence of dystrophin, elevated creatine phosphokinase (CPK), and Duchenne-type muscle biopsies.

LABORATORY PROCEDURES

- Serum creatinine kinase up to 10,000–30,000 IU early but is lower when disease progresses
- Serum aldolase increases
- Restriction fragment length polymorphic markers for carrier detection

- Muscle biopsy—histology reveals fiber size variation, fiber degeneration and regeneration, endomesial fibrosis
- Absent dystrophin staining for Duchenne's
- Partial dystrophin staining for Becker's
- Chorionic villus sampling in first trimester reveals muscle pathology

IMAGING STUDIES

- Plain x-ray: useful for scoliosis detection
- Chest x-ray: may reveal cardiac enlargement

SPECIAL TESTS

- ECG: Many patients exhibit ECG abnormalities such as tall right precordial R waves with increased R/S amplitude in V_1 and deep Q waves in left precordial leads. ECG is useful to monitor for evidence of conduction system abnormalities including arrhythmias, ectopy, and intraatrial conduction defects.
- EMG can be avoided if clinical features, history, and CPK rule in the diagnosis.

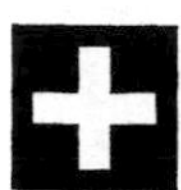

Management

GENERAL MEASURES

- There is no cure, and management is largely symptomatic.
- Early detection and genetic counseling
- Testing of other family members
- Early information to family members/parents
- Multidisciplinary approach involving neurologist, geneticist, cardiologist, orthopedist, pulmonary medicine, psychologist, nutritionist, nursing coordinator, physical therapist, and social worker
- Encouragement of active exercise as much as tolerated

SURGICAL MEASURES

- Scoliosis prevention, detection, and management to keep correct posture
- Achilles' tendon stretching and cord release
- Orthopedic care, e.g., scoliosis and contracture surgery

SYMPTOMATIC TREATMENT

- Physical and occupational therapies may be beneficial. Contractures occur early and emphasis should be placed on aggressive stretching regimens for heel cords, iliotibial bands, and hips. Nighttime ankle/foot orthoses may prevent or lessen development of heel-cord shortening.
- Calcium supplementation to prevent decreased bone density

ADJUNCTIVE TREATMENT

- Cardiac care, eg., arrhythmias, cardiomyopathy, and congestive heart failure
- Pulmonary care, e.g., pneumonia prevention, postural drainage, and pulmonary toileting in end stage
- Psychiatric and psychological care

ADMISSION/DISCHARGE CRITERIA

- Admit patients with pulmonary and cardiac complications.

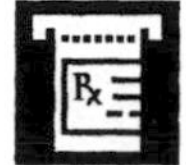

Medications

DRUG(S) OF CHOICE

- Prednisone initiated at 0.75 mg/kg/day improves muscle strength, pulmonary function, and functional ability with maximal improvement attained within 3 months of initiation. Chronic prednisone doses of 0.65 mg/kg/d will maintain these improvements, slow worsening, and may prolong ambulation for up to 2 years. Side effects include weight gain, growth retardation, development of cushingoid features, behavioral changes, and excessive body hair. The weight gain may be enough to secondarily impair ambulation.

Contraindications

- Avoid anticholinergics and ganglion-blocking agents, which can cause decreased muscle tone.
- Avoid cardiotoxic drugs such as halothane.

Precautions

- Proper evaluations prior to general anesthesia to reduce neuromuscular blockade.

ALTERNATIVE DRUGS

- Deflazacort 1.2 mg/kg/d; this is a corticosteroid that has benefits similar to prednisone but with fewer side effects.

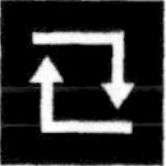

Follow-Up

PATIENT MONITORING

- Early genetic consultation and counseling with multidisciplinary team and evaluations
- 3- to 6-month clinic visits depending on severity and need for services

EXPECTED COURSE AND PROGNOSIS

- Duchenne's
  - —Long leg braces by 9 years
  - —Wheelchair-bound by 12 years
  - —Death in second decade
- Becker's
  - —May reach adult life
- Outlier DMD
  - —May reach 25 years or more

PATIENT EDUCATION

- Muscular Dystrophy Association, 3300 E. Sunrise Drive, Tucson AZ 85718-3208. Phone 800-572-1717, website *www.mdausa.org*.
- Other support groups
- Housing is very important; avoid houses with stairs.
- Educational and school planning
- Special camps
- Modification of educational activities

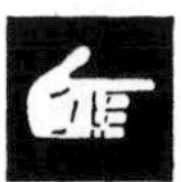

Miscellaneous

SYNONYMS

Aran Duchenne muscular dystrophy
Becker's: Late-onset x-linked muscular dystrophy

ICD-9-CM: 359.4 Hereditary progressive muscular, dystrophy/Duchenne/Becker type; 359.1 Muscular dystrophies/other than Duchenne/Becker type; 359.8 Other myopathies

SEE ALSO: N/A

REFERENCES

- Arahata K, Hoffman EP, Kunkel LM, et al. Dystrophin diagnosis: comparison of dystrophin abnormalities by immunofluorescent and immunoblot analysis. Proc Natl Acad Sci USA 1989;86:7154.
- Bakker E, Goor N, Wrogemann K, et al. Prenatal diagnosis and carrier detection of Duchenne muscular dystrophy with closely linked RFLPs. Lancet 1985;1:655.
- Baumbach LL, Chamberlain JS, Ward PS, et al. Molecular and clinical correlations of deletions leading to Duchenne and Becker muscular dystrophies. Neurology 1989;39:465.
- DeSilva S, Drachman DB, Mellits D, et al. Prednisone treatment in Duchenne muscular dystrophy: long-term benefit. Arch Neurol 1987;44:818.
- Dubowitz V. Muscle disorders in children. Philadelphia: WB Sanders, 1978.
- Heiman-Patterson TD, Natter HM, Rosenberg HR, et al. Malignant hyperthermia susceptibility in x-linked muscular dystrophies. Pediatr Neurol 1986;2:356.
- Malhotra SB, Hart KA, Klamut HJ, et al. Frame-shift deletions in patients with Duchenne and Becker muscular dystrophy. Science 1988;242:755.
- Mendell JR, Province MA, Moxley RT III, et al. Clinical investigation of Duchenne muscular dystrophy: a methodology for therapeutic trials based on natural history controls. Arch Neurol 1987;44:808.

Author(s): Samuel Dzodzomenyo, MD

Muscular Dystrophy, Fascioscapulohumeral

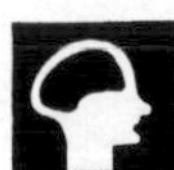

Basics

DESCRIPTION

Facioscapulohumeral muscular dystrophy (FSHD) is a chronic progressive myopathy that is characterized by weakness initially restricted to the facial and shoulder girdle muscles. Though the clinical presentation is typical in the majority of cases, there is considerable heterogeneity both in the pattern and severity of muscular weakness.

EPIDEMIOLOGY

Incidence/Prevalence

The prevalence of FSHD is 1 in 20,000, making it the third most common dystrophy after Duchenne and myotonic dystrophy. It is an autosomal-dominant disorder.

Race

There is no clear evidence of a racial predilection.

Age

Most affected individuals showing signs of FSHD by age 20. The frequency of sporadic mutations is approximately 30%.

Sex

There is high penetrance in both sexes.

Genetics

The FSHD genetic defect consists of deletion of a critical number of a 3.3-kb DNA tandem repeat unit localized to the long arm of chromosome 4 (4q35). Individuals with FSHD have fewer than 10 repeats, whereas normal individuals have 15 or more. The deletion on 4q35 does not contain an expressed sequence of DNA (i.e., a functional gene). Furthermore, chromosomal aberrations that result in loss of the entire 4q35 region do not cause FSHD. The current hypothesis is that expression of nearby genes is influenced by a critical reduction in the number of the 3.3-kb repeats caused by the FSHD-associated deletion, causing a toxic gain of function.

RISK FACTORS

The genetic mutation described above.

PREGNANCY

Approximately 30% may experience a worsening of symptoms during pregnancy. Patients should be cautioned that proximal lower extremity weakness may increase fall risk. There is no clear evidence of increased fetal loss in patients with FSHD.

ASSOCIATED CONDITIONS

As listed below.

Diagnosis

DIFFERENTIAL DIAGNOSIS

- Idiopathic brachial plexopathy: a prominent history of acute onset of severe shoulder and/or neck pain, followed by weakness and atrophy of shoulder girdle muscles, usually separates idiopathic brachial plexopathy from FSHD.
- Atypical presentations of inflammatory myopathies (e.g., polymyositis) are suggested by marked neck flexor weakness. Patients with FSHD usually have relative sparing of the neck flexors while the neck extensors may be quite weak.
- Other dystrophies (e.g., limb-girdle dystrophy): patients with limb-girdle dystrophies may have significant scapular winging resembling FSHD though typically with only minimal facial weakness. Emery-Dreifuss muscular dystrophy, an X-linked condition, has a scapuloperoneal distribution of weakness resembling FSHD. However, unlike FSHD, they also have prominent contractures, minimal facial involvement, and a characteristic cardiac rhythm disturbance (atrial standstill).
- Spinal muscular atrophy syndromes may rarely present with a scapuloperoneal distribution of weakness. These are readily differentiated on electrodiagnostic studies by the finding of neuropathic rather than the myopathic motor unit potentials seen in FSHD.

SIGNS AND SYMPTOMS

In general, close attention to specific features of the history, inheritance pattern, and careful attention to the pattern of muscle weakness is key in accurate diagnosis. The presence of slowly progressive facial weakness, scapular winging, and proximal upper extremity weakness sparing the deltoids is characteristic of FSHD. Most patients present during the first or second decade with slowly progressive proximal upper extremity weakness and are usually unaware of facial weakness. However, on specific inquiry a history of sleeping with eyes open, inability to whistle, or difficulty drinking with a straw is usually elicited. Examination reveals facial weakness in essentially all patients (an inability to bury the eyelashes fully, pout the lips, or whistle, and dimples may be noted at the corners of the mouth with resultant reduction in facial expressivity). Extraocular, bulbar, and respiratory muscles are characteristically spared. The pectoral muscles are often atrophic, leading to axillary creasing; the clavicle angle is flattened. The scapula is prominent and deviates outward and upward on shoulder abduction and elevation. The deltoid is spared, but the biceps and triceps are often affected. This, in combination with relative preservation of the forearm muscles, gives the arm a distinctive "Popeye" appearance. Frequently, there is prominent abdominal muscle weakness with an exaggerated lumbar lordosis, and a deviation of the umbilicus in the vertical direction (usually upward) upon attempting a sit-up (Beevor sign). This is a feature uncommon in other myopathies. Initially, lower extremity involvement is less impressive and is typically confined to the distal muscles, particularly the anterior compartment. However, as the disease progresses, patients usually develop hip-girdle as well as knee extensor and flexor weakness. Side-to-side asymmetry of muscle weakness is characteristic and often striking.

Disease progression is typically descending, starting in the facial and scapular fixator muscles and later involving the upper arm, distal lower extremity, and hip-girdle muscles. Most patients relate a slow, steady progression, although some patients describe a stuttering course with periods of slow or no progression interrupted by periods of more rapid loss of muscle strength.

Extramuscular Manifestations

- Retinal telangiectasias are seen commonly on retinal fluorescein angiography.
- Retinal detachment, usually in the setting of severe exudative retinopathy, occurs only rarely (Coats' disease).
- Atrial conduction abnormalities including atrial tachycardia, and mild conduction delay occur frequently, and there is believed to be a higher susceptibility to inducible atrial arrhythmias. High-grade atrioventricular block requiring a pacemaker is unusual and suggests an alternative diagnosis such as myotonic dystrophy, or rarely, Emery-Dreifuss muscular dystrophy.
- High-frequency deafness appears to be a frequent accompanying feature, and is usually mild.
- Some patients, usually those with severe infantile onset FSHD, may suffer from mental retardation and seizures.

LABORATORY PROCEDURES

Serum creatine kinase (CK) is normal or elevated, and is typically not greater than 3 to 5 times normal. A higher level suggests an alternative diagnosis (e.g., inflammatory myopathy).

IMAGING STUDIES

N/A

SPECIAL TESTS

- Needle EMG typically is abnormal with myopathic motor units in affected muscles, but the findings are nonspecific. Insertional activity is typically increased.
- The availability of a sensitive and specific molecular diagnostic test precludes the need for diagnostic muscle biopsy in most cases of suspected FSHD. Muscle biopsy should only be performed when the molecular diagnostic test is negative. Accurate molecular diagnosis, performed on blood leukocyte DNA, has a sensitivity and specificity of 95% or greater. The test employs a DNA probe that detects, after restriction enzymes digestion, restriction fragments on 4q35 that contain the 3.3-kb repeat units. In a small percentage of patients, interpretation of the molecular diagnosis is complicated by translocations that occur between 4q35 and a similar region on 10q26, and by rare deletions that include the target of the diagnostic probe.
- Muscle biopsy findings are myopathic, with a variable degree of inflammatory infiltrate, but otherwise nonspecific. Muscle biopsy in individuals with negative DNA testing serves to exclude other myopathic conditions.

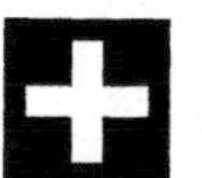

Management

GENERAL MEASURES

Treatment is largely symptomatic.

SURGICAL MEASURES

Surgical fixation of the scapula to the chest wall in an attempt to improve functional strength of proximal shoulder muscles is successful but is associated with a number of complications if not performed by experienced surgeons. Moreover, bilateral surgical fixation of the scapula also reduces overall shoulder mobility. Careful consideration of residual muscle strength, rate of disease progression, and the presence of limitation of the shoulder joint should be made before this surgical procedure.

SYMPTOMATIC TREATMENT

Other beneficial supportive interventions include ankle-foot orthoses for foot drop and various forms of knee bracing. Several bracing techniques have been devised to improve shoulder mobility with variable success. In general, such bracing has to be tightly fitting making it impractical for prolonged daily use.

ADJUNCTIVE TREATMENT

Physical therapy is of benefit to maintain range of motion and prevent joint contractures. The role of exercise in FSHD has not been fully studied. In general, a low- to moderate-intensity exercise program is felt to be safe in FSHD.

ADMISSION/DISCHARGE CRITERIA

Admission is generally not required except for rare cardiac complications.

Medications

DRUGS(S) OF CHOICE

No specific pharmacologic recommendations can be made at present. Albuterol has been suggested as a potential treatment based on its presumed effect in upregulation of muscle protein synthesis. However, a randomized trial failed to show benefit. Corticosteroids and other immunosuppressive agents have not been shown to be helpful.

Contraindications

N/A

Precautions

N/A

ALTERNATIVE DRUGS

N/A

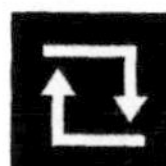

Follow-Up

PATIENT MONITORING

Follow-up at 3-month intervals is a reasonable approach; this should be individualized based on degree of functional disability.

EXPECTED COURSE AND PROGNOSIS

Because of the slow progression of FSHD, most individuals adapt remarkably well to their disabilities and remain relatively functional. However, about 20% of patients become nonambulatory.

PATIENT EDUCATION

MDA; 3300 East Summit Dr., Tucson, AZ 85718-3208. Website *http://www.MDAUSA.org.*
FSH Society Inc.; 3 Westwood Rd., Lexington MA 02420. Website *http://www.fshsociety.org.*

Genetic Testing

- Athena Diagnostics, 377 Plantation St., Worcester, MA 01605. Website *www.AthenaDiagnostics.com.*
- University of Iowa Hospitals and Clinics, Department of Pathology, Microbiology Laboratory, 200 Hawkins Dr., Boyd Tower 6004 GH, Iowa City, IA 52242-1182; contact Beth Alden: *beth-alden@uiowa.edu.*

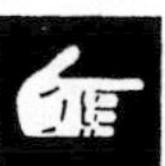

Miscellaneous

SYNONYMS

None

ICD-9-CM: 359.1 Hereditary progressive muscular dystrophy

SEE ALSO: N/A

REFERENCES

- Griggs RC, Mendell JR, Miller RG. The muscular dystrophies. In: Griggs RC, Mendell JR, Miller RG, eds. Evaluation and treatment of myopathies. Philadelphia: F. A. Davis, 1995:122–126.
- Laforet P, de Toma C, Eymard B, et al. Cardiac involvement in genetically confirmed facioscapulohumeral muscular dystrophy. Neurology 1998;51:1454–1456.
- Orrell RW, Tawil R, Forrester J, et al. Definitive molecular diagnosis of facioscapulohumeral dystrophy. Neurology 1999;52:1822–1826.
- Rudnik-Schoneborn S, Glauner B, Rohrig D, et al. Obstetric aspects in women with facioscapulohumeral muscular dystrophy, limb-girdle muscular dystrophy, and congenital myopathies. Arch Neurol 1997;54:888–894.
- Tawil R, Figlewicz DA, Griggs RC, et al. Facioscapulohumeral dystrophy: a distinct regional myopathy with a novel molecular pathogenesis. Ann Neurol 1998;43: 279–282.
- Wijmenga C, Hewitt JE, Sandkuiji LAX, et al. Chromosome 4q DNA rearrangements associated with facioscapulohumeral muscular dystrophy. Nature Genet 1992;2:26–30.

Author(s): James C. Cleland, MBChB; Rabi Tawil, MD

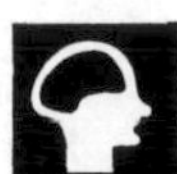

Basics

DESCRIPTION

Myotonic dystrophy (DM) is an autosomal-dominant inherited disorder characterized by progressive skeletal muscle weakness, wasting, myotonia, and other nonmuscular features, such as cardiac conduction defects, cataracts, frontal balding, and intellectual impairment.

EPIDEMIOLOGY

Incidence/Prevalence

Myotonic dystrophy is the most common adult muscular dystrophy with an incidence of 13.5/100,000 living births and a prevalence of 5/100,000 in the Western population.

Race

No data show an ethnic predilection. However, this disease was found to have high incidence in certain regions, such as Quebec, Canada (1:500).

Age

The median age of patients at the onset of symptoms is 20 to 25 years, although a form of congenital myotonic dystrophy can affect neonates. A very mild form of congenital myotonic dystrophy with late onset also occurs.

Sex

Males and females are equally involved.

ETIOLOGY

An expansion of CTG trinucleotide repeats is believed to cause this disease. However, the precise mechanism by which these excessive repeats induce the phenotype of the myotonic dystrophy remains to be clarified.

Genetics

Myotonic dystrophy is an autosomal-dominant disorder. The affected person carries an abnormal gene (myotonic dystrophy protein gene) with an expansion of trinucleotide repeats (CTG), which is located on the 3′ noncoding region of the myotonin protein kinase gene on chromosome region 19q13.2. The number of CTG repeats in the myotonic dystrophy protein gene in normal subjects varies from 4 to 37. The inducing threshold for the myotonic dystrophy is around 50 CTG repeats. The myotonic dystrophy gene codes for a protein termed "myotonin-protein kinase." Like other trinucleotide repeat diseases, the kindreds affected by the myotonic dystrophy often show the phenomenon of anticipation, in which an expanding number of CTG repeats in successive generations is associated with increased severity of the disease.

RISK FACTORS

Positive family history.

PREGNANCY

Congenital DM occurs in 25% of children born to mothers affected by DM. These pregnancies may be complicated by polyhydramnios and poor fetal movements.

ASSOCIATED CONDITIONS

- Sleep apnea; hypersomnia
- Cardiac conduction defects
- Mitral valve prolapse
- Testicular atrophy
- Frontal balding
- Cataracts
- Insulin resistance

Diagnosis

DIFFERENTIAL DIAGNOSIS

- Proximal myotonic myopathy (PROMM)
- Paramyotonia congenita
- Myotonia congenita
- Potassium sensitive periodic paralysis
- Myotonia induced by drugs (clofibrate, diazocholesterol)
- Isaac's syndrome
- Stiff-person syndrome
- Dystonia

SIGNS AND SYMPTOMS

- Classical myotonic dystrophy has its onset from adolescence to the 50s. The majority of DM patients have a slow and progressive course with distal muscles predominantly affected. Weakness and atrophy in the face, tongue, pharynx, masseter, temporalis, and distal limb muscles are characteristic. Myotonia is an impairment of muscle relaxation that occurs in patients with DM but rarely causes significant complaints. It can be elicited by percussion of thenar, wrist extensor, or lingual muscles or by requesting release after sustained handgrip. When this pattern of weakness and atrophy occurs in association with myotonia, the diagnosis of myotonic dystrophy is most likely.
- The recognition of manifestations in nonmuscular systems is very important. These include cardiac conduction disturbances, impaired respiratory drive, personality changes, hypogonadism, posterior subcapsular cataracts, and frontal balding. The impairments in cardiac conduction and respiration are the leading causes of mortality of DM patients.
- Other signs/symptoms
  —Infertility
  —Sleep apnea/hypersomnia
  —Dysphagia/esophageal dysmotility
  —Colonic hypomotility/megacolon
  —Retinal and macular pigmentary degeneration
- Congenital myotonic dystrophy is a severe form of DM affecting children, which is almost always inherited from a DM mother. These patients usually manifest neonatal hypotonia, feeding difficulties, failure of development, mental retardation, and respiratory compromise.

LABORATORY PROCEDURES

- Serum creatine kinase (CK) in DM subjects is normal to threefold elevated. However, this test is nonspecific for the disease. Needle EMG may reveal myotonic discharges with other myopathic features, such as low-amplitude, short-duration, and polyphasic motor unit potentials. This technique is helpful for identifying other affected family members with minimal symptoms. Muscle biopsies are largely avoidable as the DNA test is now available. The typical muscle biopsy would show type 1 fiber atrophy, excessive central nuclei, small angular atrophic fibers, and nuclear clumps.
- The DNA test is the confirmatory test with a sensitivity and specificity approaching 100%. If the CTG trinucleotide repeats exceed 50, the subject is considered to have myotonic dystrophy.

IMAGING STUDIES

N/A

SPECIAL TESTS

N/A

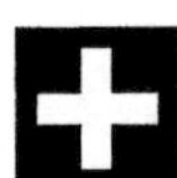

Management

GENERAL MEASURES

There is no specific treatment demonstrated to reverse the progression of DM. Symptomatic treatments are the primary focus of DM management. Optimal care includes a multidisciplinary approach to monitor for and manage manifestations of nonmuscular involvement. Patients with DM often have significantly compromised pulmonary function due to weakness of respiratory muscles and impaired ventilatory drive. Many DM patients have hypersomnia, which is frequently caused by nocturnal sleep apnea. Bilevel positive airway pressure (Bi-Pap) may be effective to reduce these symptoms. Weakened bulbar muscles may cause dysphagia and an increased risk for aspiration pneumonia. A high index of suspicion for these complications is required to detect these problems in their early stage.

SURGICAL MEASURES

- Posterior subcapsular cataracts may require excision.
- Cardiac pacemaker implantation for significant conduction disturbances

SYMPTOMATIC TREATMENT

A footdrop may be benefited by an ankle-foot orthosis.

ADJUNCTIVE TREATMENT

- Weight reduction instruction
- Pulmonary hygiene, cough and deep breathing exercises, postural draining
- Children with congenital myotonic dystrophy require intervention if developmental delay and/or mental retardation exists.

ADMISSION/DISCHARGE CRITERIA

DM patients are usually admitted for ventilation failure and significant disturbances of cardiac conduction.

Medications

DRUG(S) OF CHOICE

The symptom of myotonia usually does not require pharmacologic treatment. Phenytoin does not shorten the P-R interval and is the preferred agent.

Contraindications

Although effective agents to treat myotonia, quinine and procainamide can impair cardiac conduction and should be avoided.

Precautions

Similarly, other antiarrhythmic agents should be used with caution for cardiac ectopy because of the possibility of precipitating heart block. Patients with DM may be more sensitive to sedative medications and have prolonged effects of anesthetics.

ALTERNATIVE DRUGS

N/A

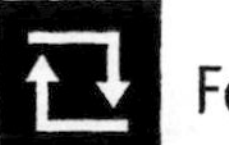

Follow-Up

PATIENT MONITORING

- Periodic cardiac examination is very important. Conventional ECG and/or long-term cardiac monitoring is needed to detect the disturbances of cardiac conduction. Cardiac pacemaker implantation should be considered for patients with unexplained syncope, second-degree heart block, and trifascicular conduction disturbance in conjunction with significant prolongation of the PR interval.
- Patients should be questioned regarding symptoms of hypersomnia and referred for sleep evaluation when appropriate.
- Regular eye examination in DM patients is required to detect cataracts and other ophthalmologic complications.

EXPECTED COURSE AND PROGNOSIS

Although there are exceptions, the number of trinucleotide repeats predicts the severity of DM. For example, patients with congenital myotonic dystrophy may have more than 750 repeats in their leukocytes. The affected children usually have a high risk of death in the neonatal period. The classical DM patients have 100 to 750 repeats in their leukocytes. These patients generally have significantly progressive muscle weakness and other nonmuscular involvement. In contrast, patients with minimal DM have only 50 to 80 repeats. They have very slow progression of muscle weakness without cardiac involvement. In a 10-year longitudinal study in 367 DM patients, the life expectancy was shown to be greatly reduced. The mean age at death was 53.2 years (range, 24–81 years). Death was caused by respiratory problems in 43% of patients. Cardiovascular complications caused death in 20% of patients. The patients with early onset and proximal muscle involvement had greater reduction in their life expectancy.

PATIENT EDUCATION

Genetic counseling should be recommended for all considering reproduction, especially when the affected person is female due to the risk of congenital myotonic dystrophy.
Muscular Dystrophy Association (MDA): 3300 East Sunrise Drive, Tucson, AZ 85718. Phone: 520-529-2000, fax: 520-529-5300, website: *http://www.mdausa.org.*

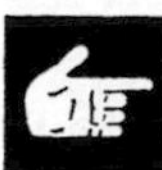

Miscellaneous

SYNONYMS

Steinert's disease

ICD-9-CM: 359.2 Myotonic disorders

SEE ALSO: N/A

REFERENCES

- Broughton R, Stuss D, et al. Neuropsychological deficits and sleep in myotonic dystrophy. Can J Neurol Sci 1990;17(4):410–415.
- Griggs RC, Mendell JR, Miller RG. Evaluation and treatment of myopathies. Philadelphia: F. A. Davis, 1995.
- Harley HG, Brook JD, et al. Expansion of an unstable DNA region and phenotypic variation in myotonic dystrophy. Nature 1992;355:545–546.
- Mathieu J, Allard P, et al. A 10-year study of mortality in a cohort of patients with myotonic dystrophy. Neurology 1999; 52(8):1658–1662.
- Redman JB, Fenwick RGJ, et al. Relationship between parental trinucleotide GCT repeat length and severity of myotonic dystrophy in offspring. JAMA 1993;269:1960–1965.
- Thornton C. The myotonic dystrophies. Semin Neurol 1999;19(1):25–33.

Author(s): Jun Li, MD, PhD

Myasthenia Gravis

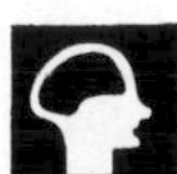

Basics

DESCRIPTION

Myasthenia gravis (MG) is an autoimmune disorder caused by antibodies directed against the acetylcholine receptor of skeletal muscle. Its main feature is muscular weakness, which is made worse by continuing activity, relieved by rest, and improved by the administration of anticholinesterase drugs.

EPIDEMIOLOGY

Incidence/Prevalence

Prevalence is 14 per 100,000 population

Race

No ethnic predominance.

Age and Sex

The most common age at onset is the second and third decade in women and the sixth and seventh decade in men.

ETIOLOGY

MG is an autoimmune disease of the neuromuscular junction with production of antibodies directed against the acetylcholine receptor protein of the skeletal muscle. These antibodies reduce the number of available acetylcholine receptors. Seventy% of patients have thymic hyperplasia, while 20% have thymic tumors. Muscle-like (myoid) cells in the thymus gland bear surface acetylcholine receptors, and a break in immune regulation interferes with tolerance and initiates antibody production.

Genetics

Although MG is not transmitted by mendelian inheritance, family members of patients are 1,000 times more likely to have the disease than the general population, and asymptomatic first-degree relatives show EMG abnormalities. There is a moderate association with human leukocyte antigens (HLAs) B8 and DRw3. This suggests that a genetically determined predisposition to develop MG exists.

RISK FACTORS

There are no specific risk factors for MG.

PREGNANCY

Effects of pregnancy on MG are variable. It can remain unchanged, worsen, or improve. Worsening in the first trimester is more common in primigravidas. Exacerbations in the third trimester and in the postpartum period are more common in subsequent pregnancies.

ASSOCIATED CONDITIONS

- Graves' disease and autoimmune thyroiditis
- Rheumatoid arthritis
- Systemic lupus erythematosus
- Polymyositis
- Aplastic anemia

Diagnosis

DIFFERENTIAL DIAGNOSIS

Patients presenting with ocular or bulbar involvement may be misdiagnosed with stroke, motor neuron disease, multiple sclerosis, or cranial nerve palsies.
Patients with acute generalized weakness can be misdiagnosed with botulism or Guillain-Barré syndrome.
Diseases characterized by excessive fatigability like Lambert-Eaton myasthenic syndrome (LEMS) or fibromyalgia may be diagnosed as MG.

SIGNS AND SYMPTOMS

The ocular muscles are the most commonly involved, with ptosis and diplopia being the initial symptom in 70% of the cases, and present in 90% of cases at some time. Bulbar muscle weakness is the initial symptom in 15% of patients with eventual involvement in 70% to 80% of cases. Presentation as limb weakness is seen in only 15%, and proximal muscles are primarily involved. With severe disease, diaphragm and chest muscles become weak. Weakness is fluctuating, usually mildest in the morning. Testing of muscle strength during maximal effort and after brief periods of rest shows fluctuation. There are two main types of MG: (a) ocular, in which the manifestations are confined to the ocular muscles for 2 years or more; and (b) generalized, in which disease spreads beyond the ocular muscles.

LABORATORY PROCEDURES

Acetylcholine receptor antibodies are measured in the serum. These are seen in 85% of patients with generalized MG and in 50% of patients with ocular myasthenia. Another antibody is the anti-striated muscle antibody, which is thought to have a strong association with thymoma. Thyroid function test should be performed to rule out associated autoimmune thyroid disease, as myasthenic patients respond best to treatment in the euthyroid state.
Systemic infections are a common cause of exacerbations, and chest x-ray as well as urine, sputum, and blood cultures may be needed.

IMAGING STUDIES

CT scan/MRI of the chest are performed to rule out thymic enlargement and thymoma.

SPECIAL TESTS

Edrophonium hydrochloride (Tensilon) test: Tensilon prevents the breakdown of acetylcholine at the neuromuscular junction and improves muscle weakness in myasthenic patients. Tensilon is preferred for diagnostic testing as it can be given intravenously, and has rapid onset (30 seconds) and a short duration of action (about 5 minutes). The test is considered positive when there is unequivocal improvement in an objectively weak muscle. A fractionated test is performed in which 2 mg are given initially, and two further doses of 4 mg are then given at 5-minute intervals if required.
EMG and nerve conduction: repetitive nerve stimulation and single-fiber EMG demonstrate defective neuromuscular transmission.

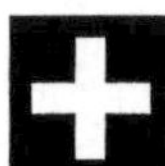

Management

GENERAL MEASURES

In an acute exacerbation, respiratory function should be monitored closely with forced vital capacity (FVC) and negative inspiratory force (NIF) measurements every 4 hours. FVC of less than 1 L and an NIF of less than −20 are indications for elective intubation.
The patient's list of medications should be screened for drugs that can exacerbate myasthenia, and these should be discontinued or changed whenever possible. Such drugs include aminoglycoside antibiotics, beta-blockers, quinidine, d-penicillamine, etc.

SURGICAL MEASURES

Elective thymectomy is performed in patients who have generalized MG and are younger than age 60 and in all patients with thymomas. Patients with disease onset after age 60 rarely show improvement after thymectomy. Thymectomy is not recommended for patients with ocular myasthenia. Prior to thymectomy, effective immunosuppressive treatment must be used to render the patient asymptomatic, as this greatly reduces postoperative morbidity and mortality.

SYMPTOMATIC TREATMENT

Pyridostigmine (Mestinon) may be helpful for the symptoms of weakness of MG (see below).

ADJUNCTIVE TREATMENT

N/A

ADMISSION/DISCHARGE CRITERIA

Most patients with MG can be treated on an outpatient basis. Patients with rapidly progressive weakness or with respiratory insufficiency should be admitted to an intensive care unit setting until they show improvement in weakness and respiratory function.

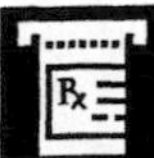

Medications

DRUG(S) OF CHOICE

The drugs used depend on the extent of the disease and on how quickly a therapeutic effect is needed.

- Anticholinesterases: pyridostigmine (Mestinon) is preferred because of its long duration of action (4 to 6 hours). It is available in 60-mg tablets and is started in a dose of 30 mg tid and increased according to response. Mestinon may be the only treatment required for ocular myasthenia, but immunosuppressive drugs must be added in generalized MG.
- Corticosteroids: prednisone is most often used, in a dose of 1.5–2 mg/kg/d. More than 75% of patients show improvement within 2 weeks and are then switched to an alternate-day schedule. The dose is slowly reduced over many months to the lowest dose necessary to maintain improvement; 25% of patients show a transient initial worsening when prednisone is started, and this requires an increase in the dose of Mestinon or, in more severe cases, plasmapheresis.
- Cyclosporine: a useful alternative when steroids are contraindicated or are producing unacceptable side effects. The dose is 5–6 mg/kg/d given in two divided doses 12 hours apart. The dose is adjusted to maintain a trough of serum cyclosporine concentration between 75 and 150 ng/mL. Improvement is seen within 1 to 2 months after starting the drug.
- Azathioprine: can provide relief of symptoms in most patients, but its effect is delayed by 4 to 8 months. It is usually started in a dose of 50 mg/d and increased every week by 50 mg to a total of 150 to 200 mg/d. It is indicated in patients who do not respond to corticosteroids or require large doses that are producing severe side effects.

Contraindications

Cytotoxic agents cannot be used during pregnancy.

Precautions

Major side effects from steroid therapy include weight gain, hypertension, and osteoporosis. Postmenopausal women are especially at risk for osteoporosis, and Fosamax (alendronate sodium) should be given with steroids.
Cyclosporine can be nephrotoxic and patients should have periodic monitoring of urea and creatinine. Blood pressure may rise and need appropriate treatment.
Azathioprine causes leukopenia and liver damage and this requires regular monitoring of CBC and liver function tests. An idiosyncratic reaction with flu-like symptoms can occur in the first 2 weeks of treatment and requires discontinuation of the drug.
Serum IgA should be measured before intravenous immunoglobulin (IVIG) administration, as patients with selective IgA deficiency may develop anaphylaxis to the drug.

Other Therapeutic Measures

- Plasmapheresis provides the most rapid therapeutic benefit and is the treatment of choice in patients with severe generalized disease and respiratory embarrassment. A typical protocol consists of removing 2 to 3 L of plasma three times a week for a total of five to six exchanges. Improvement is usually seen within 48 hours of the first exchange.
- IVIG produces improvement in 50% to 100% of patients. Effects are seen within a week and can last for several weeks or months. The dose is 400 mg/kg/d for 5 days.

ALTERNATIVE DRUGS

N/A

Follow-Up

PATIENT MONITORING

After starting treatment the weak muscles should be evaluated on serial examinations. Once improvement is noted, the dose of steroids can be reduced. Patients younger than 60 years of age with generalized myasthenia should have an elective thymectomy when they are minimally symptomatic.

EXPECTED COURSE AND PROGNOSIS

If MG remains confined to ocular muscles for 2 years or longer, there is little chance it will generalize. Generalized MG responds to immunosuppressive therapy in 80% of patients. Early thymectomy can produce a remission in 35% of nontumor cases and lead to improvement in another 50%. With optimal care most patients lead normal lives.

PATIENT EDUCATION

Patients can obtain information on MG from the Myasthenia Gravis Foundation of America, 123 W. Madison Street, Suite 800, Chicago, IL 60602. Phone: 312-853-0522, website: *www.myasthenia.org.*

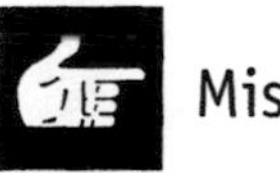

Miscellaneous

SYNONYMS

N/A

ICD-9-CM: 358.0 Myasthenia gravis

SEE ALSO: LAMBERT-EATON SYNDROME

REFERENCES

- Drachmann DB. Medical progress: myasthenia gravis. N Engl J Med 1994;330:1797–1810.
- Sanders DB, Howard JF. Disorders of neuromuscular transmission. In: Bradley WG, Daroff RB, et al., eds. Neurology in clinical practice. Boston: Butterworth-Heinemann, 2000.
- Sanders DB, Scopetta C. The treatment of patients with myasthenia gravis. Neurol Clin 1994:12(2):34.

Author(s): Noor A. Pirzada, MD

Myoadenylate Deaminase Deficiency

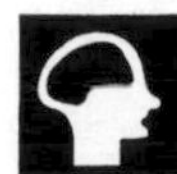

Basics

DESCRIPTION

Myoadenylate deaminase (mAMPD) deficiency is a clinically diverse disorder of skeletal muscle adenosine triphosphate (ATP) catabolism due predominantly to inherited defects in the *AMPD1* gene. Most individuals with this metabolic derangement are asymptomatic, while others are grouped according to clinical, biochemical, and molecular criteria. Exertional myalgia and intolerance without other clinical complications typically characterize symptomatic inherited mAMPD deficiency. Acquired and coincidental mAMPD deficiencies are both secondary to a wide variety of other definable clinical diseases but differ in molecular criteria.

EPIDEMIOLOGY

Incidence/Prevalence

Common, with an incidence of approximately 2% in the entire Caucasian and African-American populations.

Age

Most individuals are asymptomatic. Affected individuals can present as young as 18 months old and up to age 76. Most commonly, clinical features have appeared in over half of all reported cases in the teenage and young-adult years.

Sex

Affects both males and females consistent with the location of the *AMPD1* gene on the short arm of chromosome 1 (p13-p21). The inheritance follows an autosomal-recessive pattern.

Race

Prevalent in Caucasians and African Americans, but rare in Japanese owing to the apparent absence of a common mutation found in the former populations.

ETIOLOGY

All individuals with inherited forms of mAMPD deficiency have identified defects in the *AMPD1* gene. Independent of grouping, the predominant mutant allele in Caucasians and African Americans is defined by double C to T transitions at nucleotide +34 and +143 in the *AMPD1* open reading frame. The former is the dysfunctional mutation and results in a Ql2X nonsense codon and premature termination of mAMPD polypeptide translation. Prevalence of the common *AMPD1* mutant allele in Caucasian sample groups (10%–14%) is sufficient to account for the combined incidence of all forms of mAMPD deficiency in this population. Other rare mutations have also been identified that result in single amino acid substitutions (Q156H in Caucasians and R388W and R425H in Japanese). Individuals with acquired mAMPD deficiency are simple heterozygotes for *AMPD1* mutations in which pathology related to the associated disorder reduces *AMPD1* expression from the normal allele into the deficient range.

RISK FACTORS

Other than inheritance of *AMPD1* mutant alleles, additional risk factors related to symptomatic inherited mAMPD deficiency, although suspected, have not been identified.

PREGNANCY

A normal pregnancy, labor, and delivery without complications have been reported in a woman with symptomatic inherited mAMPD deficiency.

ASSOCIATED CONDITIONS

Coincidental inherited and acquired mAMPD deficiencies have been reported secondary to a wide variety of other definable clinical disorders too numerous to list. The relationship of mAMPD deficiency to clinical involvement in most of these individuals is unknown and may simply reflect the prevalence of *AMPD1* mutations in the general population. Consequently, the number of associated disorders in these two groups of mAMPD-deficient individuals should not be limited to those already described. Notably, clinical symptoms can be more severe than either condition alone when a coincidental inherited mAMPD deficiency is combined with another defect in energy metabolism (termed "double trouble"). In addition, clinical symptoms have been observed in patients with documented multiple partial defects in energy metabolism (including *AMPD1*), a condition referred to as synergistic heterozygosity.

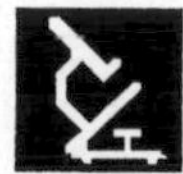

Diagnosis

DIFFERENTIAL DIAGNOSIS

Symptomatic inherited mAMPD deficiency
Exertional myalgia (undefined)
Fibromyalgia

SIGNS AND SYMPTOMS

Symptomatic inherited mAMPD deficiency presents with diffuse symptoms that can include exercise intolerance, fatigue, muscle aches, and pain. This form of the disease is generally not progressive, although some individuals do experience more persistent symptoms over time. Exercise-induced myoglobinuria has been exceptionally reported. Limb muscles, particularly lower ones, are most symptomatic. Cranial, trunk, and respiratory muscles are spared. Even in symptomatic patients, clinical weakness is unusual. Clinical complications of coincidental inherited and acquired mAMPD deficiency are generally defined by the associated disorders that are typically more severe.

LABORATORY PROCEDURES

Serum CK level may be slightly elevated. EMG is often normal, but may reveal small-amplitude, short-duration, motor unit potentials in symptomatic proximal muscles. Serum uric acid elevation has been described. A blunted venous ammonia response during ischemic forearm exercise provides a relatively noninvasive and sensitive diagnostic test for mAMPD deficiency. However, the subject has to perform enough work to prevent a false-negative diagnosis. Adequate effort should produce a concurrent rise in venous lactate of 2.5 to 4 mM (approximately 20 to 35 mg/dL). If mAMPD deficiency is indicated, the diagnosis can be confirmed from muscle biopsy material using enzyme assay or histochemical stain.

IMAGING STUDIES

N/A

SPECIAL TESTS

Polymerase chain reaction (PCR)-based tests are available to identify the C34T mutation in genomic DNA from fresh whole blood.

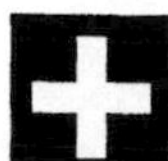

Management

GENERAL MEASURES

Individuals with symptomatic inherited mAMPD deficiency tend to adopt a more sedentary lifestyle in response to their exertional myalgia. However, mild to moderate exercise should be encouraged in these patients since it may promote exercise tolerance. Management of coincidental inherited and acquired mAMPD deficiencies is dictated by treatments appropriate for the associated disorder.

SURGICAL MEASURES

N/A

SYMPTOMATIC TREATMENT

There is no reliable treatment available for individuals with symptomatic inherited mAMPD deficiency. Oral administration of 5-carbon sugars, such as ribose and xylitol, reportedly have minimized exertional myalgia in some individuals with symptomatic mAMPD deficiency, whereas this strategy has been ineffective for others. These sugars are reasonably well tolerated at doses of 15–20 g/d without significant side effects. Treatment of coincidental inherited and acquired mAMPD deficiencies follows courses appropriate for the associated disorder.

ADJUNCTIVE TREATMENT

N/A

ADMISSION/DISCHARGE CRITERIA

N/A

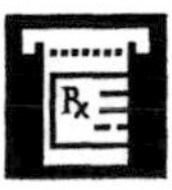

Medications

DRUG(S) OF CHOICE

No medications are currently available for symptomatic inherited mAMPD deficiency.

ALTERNATIVE DRUGS

N/A

Follow-Up

PATIENT MONITORING

Individuals with symptomatic inherited mAMPD deficiency may seek follow-up if they perceive a change in their generally diffuse symptoms or become frustrated with their modified lifestyle. Monitoring of those with coincidental inherited and acquired mAMPD deficiencies will be dictated by the associated disorder.

EXPECTED COURSE AND PROGNOSIS

Although symptomatic inherited mAMPD deficiency is generally not progressive, some individuals experience a worsening of symptoms, such as cramping and pain even at rest. Emotional issues can also develop over time due to patient or physician frustration arising from a lack of reliable treatment. The course and prognosis of coincidental inherited and acquired mAMPD deficiencies should be dictated by the associated disorder.

PATIENT EDUCATION

The Muscular Dystrophy Association maintains a website related to mAMPD deficiency: *http://www.mdausa.orgjdisease/mad.html.*

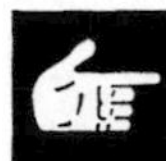

Miscellaneous

SYNONYMS

MDD
MADD
Muscle adenylate deaminase deficiency
Muscle adenylic acid deaminase deficiency
Muscle adenosine monophosphate deaminase deficiency

ICD-9-CM: 359.803 Myoadenylate deaminase deficiency

SEE ALSO: N/A

REFERENCES

- Bruyland M, Ebinger G. Beneficial effects of a treatment with xylitol in a patient with myoadenylate deaminase deficiency. ClinNeuropharmacol 1994;17:492–493.
- Gross M. New method for detection of C34-T mutation in the AMPD1 gene causing myoadenylate deaminase deficiency. Ann Rheum Dis 1994;53:353–354.
- Norman B, Mahnke-Zizelman DK, Vallis A, et al. Genetic and other determinants of AMP deaminase activity in healthy adult skeletal muscle. J Appl Physiol 1998;85: 1273–1278.
- Sabina RL. Myoadenylate deaminase deficiency: a common inherited defect with heterogeneous clinical presentation. Neurol Clin 2000;18:185–194.
- Sabina RL, Holmes EW. Myoadenylate deaminase deficiency. In: Scriver CR, Beaudet AL, Sly WS, et al., eds. The metabolic and molecular bases of inherited disease, 8th ed. New York: McGraw-Hill, 2001:2627–2638.
- Vladutiu GD. Complex phenotypes in metabolic muscle diseases. Muscle Nerve 2000;23:1157–1159.
- Vockley J, Rinaldo P, Bennett MJ, et al. Synergistic heterozygosity: disease resulting from multiple partial defects in one or more metabolic pathways. Mol Gen Metab 2000;71:10–18.

Author(s): Richard L. Sabina, PhD; Safwan S. Jaradeh, MD

Myoclonus

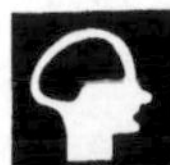

Basics

DESCRIPTION

Myoclonus is a brief sudden muscle jerk. It is caused by either active muscle contractions (positive myoclonus) or a brief interruption of tonic muscle activity (negative myoclonus), as is seen in asterixis. It may involve the face, trunk, or extremities.

EPIDEMIOLOGY

Incidence/Prevalence

Myoclonus is considered a common movement disorder. Myoclonus is not a disease entity in itself, but can be a sign of a wide variety of different illnesses. For this reason, its epidemiology is largely unknown.

Race

No study has demonstrated any ethnic predominance.

Age

Myoclonus may occur at any age, and there is no predisposition for any specific age group.

Sex

Males and females are equally affected.

ETIOLOGY

Myoclonus can occur as a result of a wide variety of disorders. An etiologic classification is summarized as follows:

- Physiologic myoclonus refers to muscle jerks occurring in normal subjects. Examples include hiccups or nocturnal myoclonus.
- Essential myoclonus is usually inherited in an autosomal-dominant fashion and is not associated with any other underlying or progressive illness. As with essential tremor, it is often very responsive to ethanol.
- Epileptic myoclonus is often associated with generalized onset seizures such as juvenile myoclonic epilepsy of Janz.
- Secondary myoclonus refers to a condition in which myoclonus is a manifestation of an underlying neurologic disease. In some of these conditions, myoclonus is the major neurologic manifestation such as in Lance-Adams syndrome (due to cerebral anoxia), bismuth poisoning, or renal failure.
- Hyperexplexia (exaggerated startle syndrome) presents with myoclonus due to an exaggerated startle response to an external stimulus.
- Psychogenic myoclonus represents a voluntary muscle jerk.

RISK FACTORS

Myoclonus is a physiologic manifestation that can be caused by a long list of associated neurologic illnesses. Essential myoclonus is familial (autosomal dominant); thus a positive family history predisposes to the condition. Cortical or spinal cord lesions may produce myoclonus. Degenerative diseases such a Creutzfeldt-Jakob disease, Alzheimer's disease, multiple system atrophy, or corticobasal ganglionic degeneration are associated with myoclonus. Metabolic derangement secondary to liver or renal failure and toxins such as bismuth can cause myoclonic jerks.

PREGNANCY

Pregnancy in itself is not associated with myoclonus.

ASSOCIATED CONDITIONS

- Cortical, brainstem, or spinal cord lesions such as tumors, arteriovenous malformations, encephalitis, ischemia (as in palatal myoclonus), or inflammation
- Progressive myoclonic epilepsies, epilepsia partialis continua, juvenile myoclonic epilepsy, and other childhood myoclonic epilepsies
- Spinocerebellar degeneration
- Basal ganglia degenerations such as multiple system atrophy, corticobasal ganglionic degeneration, and Parkinson's disease
- Dementias such as Creutzfeldt-Jakob disease and Alzheimer's disease
- Encephalitides such as subacute sclerosing panencephalitis, herpes simplex encephalitis, and others
- Metabolic derangements such a hepatic and renal disease, hyponatremia, hypoglycemia, and mitochondrial encephalomyopathies
- Toxic encephalopathies such a bismuth, heavy metal, methyl bromide poisoning, or medications such a levodopa or serotonin reuptake inhibitors
- Posthypoxic encephalopathy (Lance-Adams syndrome).
- Startle syndromes (kyperexplexia).

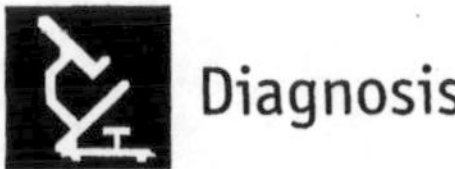

Diagnosis

DIFFERENTIAL DIAGNOSIS

- Tics: in contrast to myoclonus, tics are voluntarily suppressible and are often associated with a premonitory feeling of urgency prior to the tic and a sense of relief afterwards.
- Chorea: consists of quick jerk-like movements, which are in a continuous flow.
- Tremor: tends to be repetitive, whereas myoclonus has a sudden definable onset and end.
- Dystonia: consists of often painful twisting and turning movements that cause abnormal postures.

SIGNS AND SYMPTOMS

Myoclonus may affect one or two adjacent body parts (focal or segmental myoclonus), different noncontiguous body parts (multifocal myoclonus), or the entire body (generalized myoclonus). It may be present at rest, while maintaining a posture, or when a particular movement is performed (action myoclonus). Reflex myoclonus can be triggered by visual, auditory or somesthetic stimuli, such as pinpricking or flicking the fingers or toes. Negative myoclonus consists of a short interruption of tonic muscle activity (asterixis). Asterixis is usually multifocal. When axial muscles are affected, the patient experiences postural lapses that manifest in a bouncy, unsteady gait.

LABORATORY PROCEDURES

N/A

IMAGING STUDIES

N/A

SPECIAL TESTS

Electrodiagnostic Studies

- EMG recordings from involved muscles may sometimes be helpful in characterizing the myoclonus.
- EEG can distinguish cortical from brainstem myoclonus, which has no preceding cortical discharge.
- Somatosensory evoked potentials show an enlarged P25/N33 component in cortical myoclonus, and a cortical correlate may be back-averaged in the simultaneously recording EEG.
- The presence of a Bereitschaftspotential prior to the EMG discharge on the back-averaged EEG suggests the possibility of psychogenic myoclonus.

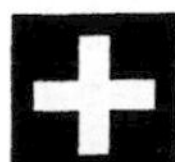

Management

GENERAL MEASURES

The most important measure is to correctly subclassify myoclonus and treat the underlying disease process. Essential myoclonus, like essential tremor, responds very well to small doses of alcohol (e.g., a glass of red wine), a feature that is not found in other types of myoclonus.

SURGICAL MEASURES

Myoclonus is generally treated successfully with medications, and surgical treatment is rarely recommended. However, there are reports of successful surgical management of myoclonus. Spinal myoclonus may respond to removal of a compressive lesion in or adjacent to the spinal cord. A recent study demonstrated alleviation of hereditary essential myoclonus by neurostimulation of the ventral intermediate thalamic nucleus. Older studies show improvement of myoclonus with destructive lesions of the lateral ventral nucleus of the thalamus.

SYMPTOMATIC TREATMENT

Myoclonus secondary to cortical lesions and epileptic myoclonus respond best to valproate, clonazepam, or a combination of these. Piracetam has also been shown to be effective in the treatment of myoclonus; however, it is not readily available in the United States at this time. Primidone has been tried successfully as well. In several cases, combinations of the above medications are needed. Negative myoclonus is much more resistant to treatment than positive myoclonus. The above medications may be tried, but are much less effective. Clonazepam appears to be most effective for brainstem myoclonus. *N*-acetylcysteine has been shown to be beneficial in the symptomatic treatment of myoclonus in the Unverricht-Lundborg disease. Occasionally, serotonin reuptake inhibitors may be helpful. Beta-blockers may be helpful in essential myoclonus. A combination of 5-hydroxytryptophan and carbidopa has been found to be successful in the treatment of Lance-Adams syndrome (postanoxic myoclonus).

ADJUNCTIVE TREATMENT

N/A

ADMISSION/DISCHARGE CRITERIA

The criteria for admission depend, in general, on the underlying disease and not the myoclonus itself. However, rarely, action myoclonus or negative myoclonus of the lower extremities can be so severe as to affect the patient's ability to walk or feed himself, which may necessitate hospitalization.

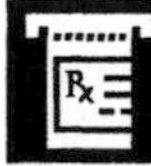

Medications

DRUG(S) OF CHOICE

Aside from the symptomatic medications discussed above, amelioration of myoclonus depends largely on treating the underlying cause for the myoclonic syndrome.

ALTERNATIVE DRUGS

N/A

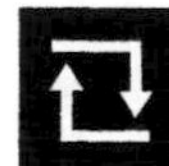

Follow-Up

PATIENT MONITORING

Patients should be followed on an individualized basis, depending on the severity of the myoclonus. Most of the time, the underlying disorder that causes the myoclonic syndrome dictates the frequency of follow-up and the need for hospitalization.

EXPECTED COURSE AND PROGNOSIS

In general, the prognosis depends on the underlying disorder that causes the myoclonic syndrome. Myoclonus itself does not tend to cause complications, unless associated with seizures, which may lead to hypoxia, aspiration, or traumatic injuries.

PATIENT EDUCATION

Support groups for myoclonus:
Moving Forward, 2934 Glenmore Ave., Kettering, OH 45409. Phone 513-293-0409.
Myoclonus Research Foundation (MRF), 200 Old Palisade Rd., Suite 17D, Fort Lee, NJ 07024. Phone: 201-585-8114, website *www.research@myoclonus.com.*

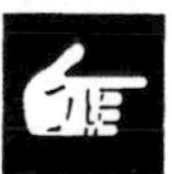

Miscellaneous

SYNONYMS

Jerks
Lightning-fast movements
Involuntary movements

ICD-9-CM: 333.2 Myoclonus

SEE ALSO: TREMOR

REFERENCES

- Daniel DG, Webster DL. Spinal segmental myoclonus. Successful treatment with cervical spinal decompression. Arch Neurol 1984;41:898–899.
- Hurd RW, et al. Treatment of four siblings with progressive myoclonus epilepsy of the Unverricht-Lundborg type with N-acetylcysteine. Neurology 1996;47: 1264–1268.
- Kelly JJ, Sharborough FW, Daube JR. A clinical and electrophysiological evaluation of myoclonus. Neurology 1981;31:581–589.
- Kupsch A, Trottenberg T, Meissner W, et al. Neurostimulation of the ventral intermediate thalamic nucleus alleviates hereditary essential myoclonus. J Neurol Neurosurg Psychiatry 1999;67(3):415–416.
- Lhermitte F, Talairach J, Buser P, et al. Postanoxic-action and intention myoclonus. Stereotactic study and destruction of the lateral ventral nucleus of the thalamus. Rev Neurol 1971;124(1): 5–20.
- Marsden CD. Dystonia, myoclonus, tics & paroxysmal dyskinesias. In: Fahn S, Marsden CD, Jancovic J, eds. 8th annual course: a comprehensive review of movement disorders for the clinical practitioner. New York: Columbia University Press, 1998:597–655.
- Marsden CD, Hallet M, Fahn S. The nosology and pathophysiology of myoclonus. In: Marsden CD, Fahn S, eds. Movement disorders. London: Butterworth, 1982:196–248.
- Obeso JA. Classification, clinical features, and treatment of myoclonus. In: Watts RL, Koller WC, eds. Movement disorders. New York: McGraw-Hill, 1997:541–550.
- Obeso JA, Artieda J, Rothwell JX, et al. The treatment of severe action myoclonus. Brain 1989b;112:765–777.
- Quinn NP, Rothwell JC, Thompson PD, et al. Hereditary myoclonic dystonia, hereditary torsion dystonia and hereditary essential myoclonus: an area of confusion. Adv Neurol 1986;50:391–402.
- Van Woert MH, et al. Fluoxetine in the treatment of intention myoclonus. Clin Neuropharmacol 1983;6:49–54.
- Van Woert MH, Rosenbaum D, Howieson J, et al. Long-term therapy of myoclonus and other neurological disorders with I-5-hydroxytryptophan and carbidopa. N Engl J Med 1977;296:70–75.

Author(s): Dorothee Cole, MD

Myopathy, Congenital

Basics

DESCRIPTION

Congenital myopathies, rare heterogeneous groups of muscle disorders, are characterized by muscle weakness and hypotonia presenting at birth or in the first few months and usually with very slow or lack of progression. However, rare onset in later childhood or even adulthood has been reported. Common congenital myopathies are initially referred to as those with obvious structural abnormalities, including central core disease, nemaline rod myopathy, and myotubular myopathy. There are also uncommon forms of congenital myopathies, including multicore myopathy, fingerprint body myopathy, congenital fiber type disproportion, and protein surplus myopathies due to accumulation of abnormal proteins, such as desmin-related myopathies and actinopathies.

EPIDEMIOLOGY

Incidence/Prevalence

Incidence of nemaline myopathy is 0.02 in 1,000 live births. Incidence of other congenital myopathies is unknown.

Race

No ethnic predilection is noted.

Age

Onset mostly at birth or in the first few months; recently, adult onset has been reported in some patients.

Sex

Both sexes are equally affected.

ETIOLOGY

- Myotubular myopathy is inherited as an X-linked recessive disease in neonatal cases, as autosomal-recessive disease in late infantile and early childhood cases, but as autosomal-dominant diseases in late childhood cases.
- Nemaline rod myopathy is inherited as autosomal-dominant disease, linked to chromosome 1q, but also as sporadic diseases.
- Central core disease is usually inherited as autosomal-dominant disease, linked to chromosome 19, with the mutation of ryanodine receptor gene as the molecular marker of the disease that is associated with susceptibility to malignant hyperthermia. However, it also can be a sporadic disease.
- Multicore disease is inherited as autosomal-dominant disease.
- Congenital fiber type disproportion is usually sporadic.
- Recently recognized desmin-related myopathies are usually autosomal-dominant diseases, rarely as autosomal-recessive or sporadic diseases.
- Also a newly recognized congenital myopathy, actinopathy is due to accumulation of thin filaments of muscle fibers, actin.

RISK FACTORS

N/A

PREGNANCY

N/A

ASSOCIATED CONDITIONS

- Malignant hyperthermia, especially with central core disease and multicore disease
- Skeletal abnormalities including congenital hip dislocation, scoliosis, clubfoot
- Ophthalmoplegia, ptosis, especially with myotubular myopathy
- Respiratory failure, especially with myotubular myopathy, multicore disease, nemaline rod myopathy, and desmin-related myopathies
- Seizures, especially with myotubular myopathy
- Cardiomyopathy, especially with myotubular myopathy, nemaline rod myopathy, and desmin-related myopathies
- Exercise intolerance, especially with desmin-related myopathies
- Mental retardation, especially fingerprint body myopathy
- Gastroesophageal reflux

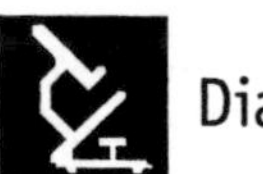

Diagnosis

DIFFERENTIAL DIAGNOSIS

- Spinal muscular atrophy
- Congenital muscular dystrophy
- Congenital myotonic dystrophy
- Pompe's disease
- Debranching enzyme disease
- Mitochondrial myopathy
- Carnitine deficiency
- Congenital peripheral polyneuropathy
- Congenital myasthenic syndrome

SIGNS AND SYMPTOMS

Most patients with congenital myopathies present with generalized hypotonia, delayed motor milestones, and generalized muscle weakness and atrophy. Respiratory failure, ptosis, or ophthalmoplegia may be seen. Slender body habitus, long narrow face, and skeletal abnormalities such as clubfoot, congenital hip dislocation, and kyphoscoliosis are often noted. However, some patients with congenital myopathies can be asymptomatic or only present with mild muscle weakness. Occasionally, cardiomyopathy is seen in the patients with nemaline rod myopathy and myotubular myopathy. Mental impairment is reported in fingerprint myopathy.
Desmin-related myopathies, a newly recognized group of disorders, may present in late adolescence or adulthood, with scapuloperoneal or distal muscle weakness, and some patients may also have respiratory insufficiency, cardiomyopathy, and cardiac arrhythmia.

LABORATORY PROCEDURES

- Serum creatine kinase is usually normal or mildly increased.
- EMG shows either normal or myopathic features.
- Nerve conduction studies are normal; repetitive nerve stimulation is normal.

IMAGING STUDIES

Sonographic, CT, or MRI studies of muscles are not useful to recognize specific congenital myopathy.

SPECIAL TESTS

Muscle biopsy is necessary to diagnose specific congenital myopathy. In central core disease, central cores appear as central or eccentric areas of muscles devoid of oxidative enzyme activity. In nemaline myopathy, nemaline rods are seen as red cytoplasmic or perinuclear clusters on modified trichrome staining. In myotubular myopathy, central nuclei are detected in many muscle fibers. In the multicore disease, multiple small fusiform lesions without mitochondria are present. In the fingerprint myopathy, ovoid inclusions are seen. In congenital fiber type disproportion, type 1 fiber smallness and predominance and type 2 fiber hypertrophy are seen.
Recently, the demonstration of desmin, the intermediate filament protein of the muscle fibers, in the cytoplasmic bodies, and of α-actinin in the intranuclear rods, expands the spectrum of the congenital myopathies to protein surplus myopathies, which include desmin-related myopathies and actinopathy.

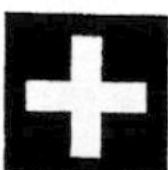

Management

GENERAL MEASURES

In general, only supportive treatment is available for all types of congenital myopathies.

SURGICAL MEASURES

Associated congenital hip dislocation, scoliosis, or clubfeet may require surgical treatment.

SYMPTOMATIC TREATMENT

- Ankle-foot orthoses may be needed for footdrop.
- Back bracing may help scoliosis.
- Respiratory support or gastrostomy feeding may be necessary in respiratory failure or gastroesophageal reflux.

ADJUNCTIVE TREATMENT

- Physical therapy often is needed to prevent joint contractures.
- Wheelchair may be needed.

ADMISSION/DISCHARGE CRITERIA

Patients may be admitted for muscle biopsy for diagnosis and surgical treatment of scoliosis, gastrostomy tube placement, and then discharged to home.

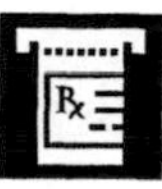

Medications

DRUG(S) OF CHOICE

No specific drugs are available for any type of congenital myopathies.

Contraindications

Because malignant hyperthermia is associated with central core and multicore myopathies, these patients should avoid halothane or other halogenated anesthetic agents and succinylcholine, which may precipitate malignant hyperthermia.

Precautions

Patients should wear medical alert bracelet or necklace indicating their risk of malignant hyperthermia associated with anesthesia.

ALTERNATIVE DRUGS

N/A

Follow-Up

PATIENT MONITORING

Patients should be followed regularly for respiratory insufficiency, cardiomyopathy, or cardiac arrhythmia if present in some congenital myopathies, and the need of braces, physical therapy, nutritional support, or scoliosis treatment.

EXPECTED COURSE AND PROGNOSIS

- Central core disease is usually mild, nonprogressive, but with rare exceptions.
- Nemaline myopathy may run mild to severely progressive course with some fatal outcome, especially those with neonatal onset.
- Myotubular myopathy may also run mild to severely progressive course, even fatal outcome, especially with neonatal onset.
- Congenital fiber-type disproportion usually has mild, nonprogressive course.
- Desmin-related myopathies may be fatal in the infancy or early childhood due to respiratory failure.

PATIENT EDUCATION

Because all types of congenital myopathies are rare, the patients should be referred to the Muscular Dystrophy Association clinics for care, education, and support: Muscular Dystrophy Association, 3300 E. Sunrise Dr., Tucson, AZ 85718-3208. Phone: 1-800-572-1717, website *www.mdausa.org*.

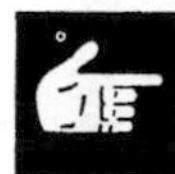

Miscellaneous

SYNONYMS

Myopathy

ICD-9-CM: 359.0 Congenital myopathy; 359.1 Nemaline myopathy; 359.0 Central core myopathy; 359.0 Myotubular myopathy

SEE ALSO: N/A

REFERENCES

- Dubowitz V. Muscle disorders in childhood, 2nd ed. London: Saunders, 1995.
- Engel AG, Franzini-Armstrong C. Myology, 2nd ed. New York: McGraw-Hill, 1994.
- Goebel HH, Borchert A. Protein surplus myopathies and other congenital myopathies. Semin Pediatr Neurol 2002;9(2):160–170.
- Griggs RC, Mendell JR, Miller RG. Evaluation and treatment of myopathies. Philadelphia: F. A. Davis, 1995.

Author(s): Chang-Yong Tsao, MD, FAAN, FAAP

Myopathy, Metabolic

Basics

DESCRIPTION

Metabolic myopathies are a group of muscle disorders stemming from defective energy utilization due to abnormalities in glycogen, lipid, purine, or mitochondrial metabolism.

EPIDEMIOLOGY

Incidence/Prevalence

Rare. Prevalence rates between 1:40,000 and 1:1,000,000 for each individual disorder. However, collectively they are not uncommon.

Race

No known difference.

Age

Age of onset varies from infancy through middle age.

Sex

No known difference except for the two X-linked disorders of carbohydrate metabolism.

ETIOLOGY

Skeletal muscle is highly energy dependent and uses three major sources of adenosine triphosphate (ATP): high-energy phosphate compounds such as phosphocreatine; glycogen; and fatty acids. The intensity and length of exertion determines which energy source is used:

- At rest—fatty acids
- During exercise
  - —First few minutes—high-energy phosphate compounds
  - —Minutes to an hour—glycogen
  - —Hours—fatty acids

Genetics

Inheritance patterns vary by disease. Most disorders are autosomal recessive. Others follow X-linked, mitochondrial, or, rarely, autosomal-dominant modes of transmission.

RISK FACTORS

None

PREGNANCY

No known relationship.

ASSOCIATED CONDITIONS

The following conditions occur with some of the metabolic myopathies:

- Disorders of carbohydrate metabolism: hepatomegaly, cardiomyopathy, *ketotic* hypoglycemia, anemia
- Disorders of lipid metabolism: cardiomyopathy, cirrhosis, *hypoketotic* hypoglycemia
- Disorders of mitochondrial function: deafness, neuropathy, retinopathy, seizures, stroke

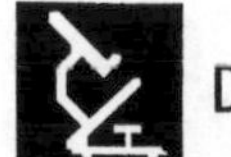

Diagnosis

DIFFERENTIAL DIAGNOSIS

Other myopathies—include endocrine, drug-induced, and inflammatory myopathies
Muscular dystrophies
Fibromyalgia
Polymyalgia rheumatica

SIGNS AND SYMPTOMS

Enzyme deficiencies present with signs and symptoms that are dynamic, static, or both. Most diseases have a usual manner of presentation. They are listed below by their presenting signs and symptoms, energy metabolism pathway, and mode of inheritance.

Dynamic Signs and Symptoms

Cramps/myalgias, fatigue, reversible weakness, myoglobinuria

- Carbohydrate metabolism
  - —Myophosphorylase (MyoP)—autosomal recessive (AR)
  - —Phosphofructokinase (PFK)—AR
  - —Phosphorylase b kinase (PBK)—AR and X-linked recessive (XR)
  - —Phosphoglycerate kinase (PGK)—XR
  - —Phosphoglycerate mutase (PGM)—AR
  - —Lactate dehydrogenase (LDH)—AR
  - —β-Enolase—AR
- Lipid metabolism
  - —Carnitine palmitoyltransferase II (CPT II)—AR
  - —Very-long-chain acyl-CoA dehydrogenase (VLCAD)—AR
  - —Short-chain 3-hydroxyacyl-CoA dehydrogenase (SCHAD)—AR
- Purine metabolism
  - —Myoadenylate deaminase deficiency (MADD)—AR
- Mitochondrial disorders
  - —Multiple—mitochondrial inheritance (Mito)

Static Signs and Symptoms

Progressive, proximal weakness

- Carbohydrate metabolism
  - —Acid maltase (AMD)—AR
  - —Debrancher enzyme—AR
  - —Brancher enzyme—AR
  - —Aldolase A—AR
- Lipid metabolism
  - —Carnitine transporter—AR
  - —Medium-chain acyl-CoA dehydrogenase (MCAD)—AR
  - —Long-chain acyl-CoA dehydrogenase (LCAD)—AR
- Mitochondrial disorders—Mito

Both Dynamic and Static Signs and Symptoms

- Carbohydrate metabolism: MyoP, PFK, PBK, debrancher
- Lipid metabolism: VLCAD, LCAD, SCHAD, TP
- Mitochondrial: mitochondrial DNA depletion myopathy—AR

Clues to Metabolic Pathway Affected

- Carbohydrate metabolism
  - —"Second wind" phenomenon—when muscle symptoms develop, a brief rest results in improved exercise tolerance.
  - —Symptoms are associated with brief, vigorous, isometric exercise such as squatting or lifting a heavy weight, or with short duration, vigorous aerobic activity such as sprinting 100—800 m.
- Lipid metabolism
  - —Symptom onset associated with fasting, illness, cold, or anesthesia
  - —Onset of symptoms with prolonged (4–12 hours) exertion
  - —Episodes mimicking a Reye-like syndrome or coma
  - —Family history of sudden infant death syndrome
- Mitochondrial
  - —Multisystem involvement
  - —Central and/or peripheral nervous system involvement
  - —Ptosis, external ophthalmoplegia

LABORATORY PROCEDURES

- Serum—creatine kinase (CK), lactate, pyruvate, LDH, free and total carnitine, ammonia ($NH3^+$), liver transaminases (including GGT), potassium, phosphate, calcium, creatinine
- Urine—myoglobin, ketones, organic/dicarboxylic acids, and acylglycines
- CSF—lactate, pyruvate, protein, amino acids

IMAGING STUDIES

Phosphorous magnetic resonance spectroscopy is in use at research facilities.

SPECIAL TESTS

- Nerve conduction studies—exclude acquired demyelinating polyneuropathies.
- Repetitive nerve stimulation—excludes neuromuscular junction disorders in cases with ptosis or ophthalmoplegia.
- Needle electromyography (EMG)—confirms myopathy with findings of abnormal spontaneous activity (fibrillation potentials and positive sharp waves) and/or short duration, low amplitude motor units that recruit early seen in some cases. EMG is often normal in metabolic myopathies without permanent weakness.
- ECG and echocardiography—evaluate symptomatic cardiac involvement and exclude presymptomatic disease.
- Forearm exercise test (FET)—a useful screening tool for carbohydrate and purine metabolism disorders. Collect baseline CK, pyruvate, lactate, and ammonia ($NH3^+$) levels.
  - —Have the patient squeeze a ball or hand dynamometer vigorously for 1 minute, intermittently squeezing for 3 seconds and relaxing for 1 second.
  - —Draw blood samples for lactate and $NH3^+$ at 1, 2, 4, 6, and 10 minutes after exercise. All blood samples should be placed on ice.

—Interpretation of FET results
 -In normal subjects, both the lactate and $NH3^+$ levels should rise at least 2½- to 5-fold within 1 to 4 minutes (lactate) and 2 to 6 minutes ($NH3^+$) after exercise.
 -In disorders of carbohydrate metabolism, lactate levels should not rise or be blunted (less than twofold elevation), while $NH3^+$ levels should rise normally, by at least 2½-fold.
 -In disorders of purine metabolism, such as myoadenylate deaminase deficiency, the rise in $NH3^+$ levels is blunted, while the lactate response is normal, at least a 2½-fold rise.
 -If both the lactate and $NH3^+$ levels do not rise by at least 2½-fold, this suggests inadequate effort and the test should be repeated.

- Muscle biopsy—allows sampling of the muscle for histologic review, histochemical analysis, biochemical assays, and genetic analysis. An open biopsy is preferable to needle biopsy.
 —Carbohydrate metabolism
 -Histology—vacuoles and accumulation of glycogen staining positive with periodic acid-Schiff (PAS) stain.
 -Histochemical—diminished or absent staining for the enzyme on the muscle tissue sections in myophosphorylase, phosphofructokinase, or acid maltase deficiencies.
 Biochemical—quantitative enzyme function assays can be performed on muscle tissue.
 -Commercial testing is available for deficiencies of all the glycolytic defects (AMD, debrancher, brancher, MyoP, PFK, PBK, PGK, PGM, LDH) except aldolase A and β-enolase.
 -Mutation analysis—genetic testing is available commercially for the most common mutations causing myophosphorylase deficiency (McArdle's disease).
 —Lipid metabolism
 -Histology—vacuoles and accumulation of glycogen staining positive with oil-red-O (ORO) stain.
 -Biochemical—commercially available assays can be performed on muscle tissue for free and total carnitine levels along with CPT II.
 —Mitochondrial metabolism
 -Histology—"ragged red fibers" and diminished muscle staining for oxidative enzymes (NADH, SDH, and COX).
 -Biochemical—analysis for mitochondrial enzyme deficiencies.
 -Mutation analysis—testing is commercially available for some disorders (MELAS, MERRF, NARP, LHON, KSS/CPEO) via blood and/or muscle tissue. In mitochondrial myopathies, disease-causing mutations may segregate disproportionately with muscle tissue rather than other tissues during embryogenesis. Therefore, mutation analysis on muscle tissue provides a higher diagnostic yield for mitochondrial myopathies.

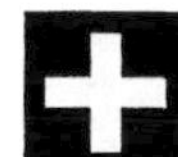

Management

GENERAL MEASURES

The major therapeutic goal in metabolic myopathies is avoidance of provocative factors such as brief bursts of exertion for carbohydrate disorders and fasting for disorders of lipid metabolism. In the future, treatment will consist of enzyme replacement and/or genetic therapy.

SURGICAL MEASURES

None

SYMPTOMATIC TREATMENT

Most patients with a metabolic myopathy derive benefit from a low-intensity, graduated exercise program with emphasis on aerobic exercise. Dietary modification may benefit some patients. A diet high in protein and fats benefits some patients with carbohydrate metabolism disorders. The obverse is true for disorders of lipid metabolism. These patients benefit from frequent meals and a low-fat, high-carbohydrate diet.

ADJUNCTIVE TREATMENT

Co-management of concomitant cardiac, hepatic, and hematologic dysfunction improves quality of life and may be lifesaving. Seizures in mitochondrial disorders usually respond to conventional anticonvulsant drugs. Malignant hyperthermia, especially prevalent in disorders of carnitine processing, responds to dantrolene.

ADMISSION/DISCHARGE CRITERIA

Rhabdomyolysis or episodes of severe weakness warrant admission. Occasionally, patients present with hypoglycemia, seizures, or stroke and require admission.

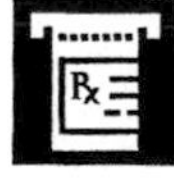

Medications

DRUG(S) OF CHOICE

No medical regimen is yet known.

Contraindications

None

Precautions

None

ALTERNATIVE DRUGS

Some patients with mitochondrial myopathies improve after treatment with coenzyme Q10, 50–100 mg tid, and L-carnitine, 1,000 mg tid, plus an antioxidant vitamin regimen.

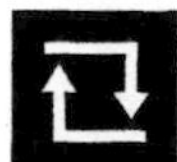

Follow-Up

PATIENT MONITORING

Patients should be seen every 6 to 12 months to monitor disease progression. These visits also facilitate patient education about advances in care.

EXPECTED COURSE AND PROGNOSIS

The clinical course and prognosis are highly variable. Influencing factors include the distinct enzyme involved, the percentage reduction in enzymatic activity, the unique compensatory genetic milieu of each patient, and the environment in which these features play out. Some infantile forms of these disorders cause death due to cardiorespiratory failure prior to the first birthday, while adult-onset forms may present late in life with mild symptoms such as myalgias, cramps, and fatigue.

PATIENT EDUCATION

Muscular Dystrophy Association, 3300 E. Sunrise Drive, Tucson, AZ 85718. Phone: 800-572-1717, website *www.mdausa.org.* Distinct patient organizations exist for many of the individual metabolic myopathies and may be found by searching the Internet.

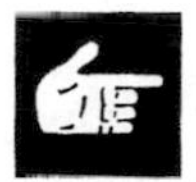

Miscellaneous

SYNONYMS

Myophosphorylase deficiency = McArdle's disease
Phosphofructokinase deficiency = Tarui's disease
Infantile form of acid maltase deficiency = Pompe's disease

ICD-9-CM: 359.89 Other myopathies; 728.89 Rhabdomyolysis (idiopathic); 995.86 Hyperthermia, malignant (due to anesthesia)

SEE ALSO: N/A

ACKNOWLEDGMENT

The views expressed herein are those of the author and do not reflect the official policy of the United States Air Force or the Department of Defense.

REFERENCES

- Darras BT, Friedman NR. Metabolic myopathies: a clinical approach; part I. Pediatr Neurol 2000;22:87–97.
- Pourmand R. Metabolic myopathies. Neurol Clin 2000;18:1–13.
- Vladutiu GD. Laboratory diagnosis of metabolic myopathies. Muscle Nerve 2002;25:649–663.

Author(s): Matthew P. Wicklund, MD

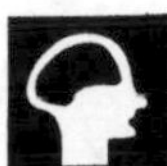

Basics

DESCRIPTION

Toxic myopathies are potentially reversible muscle disorders due to myotoxicity of prescribed or illicit drugs. Suspicion of a toxic myopathy is increased when there is temporal association of drug use prior to the onset of symptoms, absence of preexisting neuromuscular symptoms, and improvement or resolution of symptoms following withdrawal of the suspected toxin. Tentative classification based on the pathogenetic mechanism has been proposed, though knowledge of the mechanism of many toxins is limited. Several authors classify according to whether the myopathy is painful, painless, presence of an associated neuropathy, histopathologic features, drugs of abuse, and focal myopathies.

EPIDEMIOLOGY

Incidence/Prevalence

Incidence is unknown for most toxic myopathies, but appears to be common. For malignant hyperthermia, the incidence is 1 in 15,000 children and 1 in 50,000 adults. Race, age, and sex are not factors.

ETIOLOGY

The mechanism varies depending on the agent. Syndromes include necrotizing myopathy, myoglobinuria, corticosteroid myopathy, hypokalemic myopathy, amphiphilic cationic drug myopathy, impaired protein synthesis, antimicrotubular myopathy, inflammatory myopathy, fasciitis, mitochondrial myopathy, focal myopathies secondary to injections, and unclassified mechanisms. In addition, there are two syndromes constituting emergencies, malignant hyperthermia and neuroleptic malignant syndrome, that should be readily recognized and quickly treated.

Genetics

Malignant hyperthermia is autosomal dominant. Over 50% of families show linkage to the gene encoding the ryanodine receptor. Other candidate genes include the voltage-dependent sodium channel of the skeletal muscle membrane, and the pentameric dihydropyridine receptor.

RISK FACTORS

- Neuroleptic use
- Family history of death following anesthesia
- Autoimmune or other conditions requiring chronic corticosteroid treatment
- High-dose corticosteroids with or without neuromuscular blocking agents or sepsis
- Alcoholism
- Illicit drug use
- Prescribed medications

PREGNANCY

N/A

ASSOCIATED CONDITIONS

Hereditary myopathies associated with malignant hyperthermia
- Evans myopathy
- King-Denborough syndrome
- Central core disease

Potential sequelae of rhabdomyolysis include myoglobinuria and renal failure.

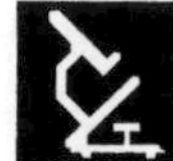

Diagnosis

DIFFERENTIAL DIAGNOSIS

There should be no other identifiable cause of myopathy present. Differential diagnoses are listed by clinical and pathologic findings and may be listed more than once if more than one mechanism of presentation has been described.

Hyperthermia

- Malignant hyperthermia
- Neuroleptic malignant syndrome

Painful Toxic Myopathies

- Myopathic disorders: inflammatory myopathy, mitochondrial myopathy
- Medications: D-penicillamine, procainamide, didanosine, germanium, zidovudine; possibly phenytoin, levodopa, cimetidine, leuprolide, propylthiouracil, streptokinase
- Cholesterol lowering agents:
  —HMG-CoA reductase inhibitors (lovastatin, mevastatin, pravastatin)
  —Fibric acid derivatives (bezafibrate, clofibrate, fenofibrate, gemfibrozil)
  —Nicotinic acid
- Combinations of medications: lovastatin and gemfibrozil may induce a necrotizing myopathy in up to 5%. Lovastatin and cyclosporine may induce a myopathy in up to 30%.
- Fasciitis: the fascia is the connective tissue surrounding the muscle. Inflammation of the fascia is fasciitis, and is listed since symptoms of pain from inflammation of the fascia may be difficult to distinguish clinically from true muscle pain or myalgia. Inflammation may be detected on muscle biopsy when fascia is included with the biopsy for inspection.
- Eosinophilia-myalgia syndrome
- Toxic (rapeseed) oil syndrome
- Ethanol (acute)
- Etretinate
- Hypervitaminosis E
- Ipecac/emetine

Painless Toxic Myopathies

- Corticosteroids (acute high dose, or chronic)
- Myoglobinuria
  —Amphetamines
    -Ethanol (chronic)
    -Heroin
    -Lovastatin
    -Malignant hyperthermia
    -Malignant neuroleptic syndrome
    -Phencyclidine
    -Phenylpropanolamine
    -Succinylcholine
    -Hypokalemic myopathy
      *Amphotericin-B
      *Laxatives
      *Licorice ingestion/carbenoxolone/glycyrrhizate
      *Lithium
      *Mineralocorticoids
      *Thiazide diuretics
      *Toluene abuse
  —Drug-induced lysosomal storage myopathy (amphiphilic cationic drug myopathy)
    -Antianginal: perhexiline
    -Antiarrhythmic: amiodarone
    -Antidepressants: clomipramine, imipramine
    -Antigout (antimicrotubular): colchicine
    -Antimalarials: chloroquine, plasmocid
    -Cholesterol lowering: lovastatin
  —Antimicrotubular myopathy: colchicine, vincristine
- Toxic focal myopathies
  —Ethanol (acute)
  —Intramuscular injections
    -Acute: cephalothin, lidocaine, diazepam
    -Chronic: antibiotics (children), intravenous drug abuse, meperidine, pentazocine, pethidine
- Toxic myopathies associated with drugs of abuse
  —Amphetamines
  —Cocaine
  —Heroin
  —Phencyclidine
  —Volatile inhalation (e.g., toluene, gasoline)

SIGNS AND SYMPTOMS

Myopathic weakness begins after a suitable duration of exposure to a presumed toxin. There is usually no preexisting neuromuscular condition, and symptoms of weakness resolve following removal of the offending agent. Deep tendon reflexes and appreciation of primary sensory modalities are preserved.

LABORATORY PROCEDURES

Laboratory procedures to consider when a toxic myopathy is suspected should be based on suspicions elicited from the history.
- Serum: CPK, potassium, serum toxicology screen
- Urine: 3-methyl-histidine, myoglobin, urine toxicology screen

IMAGING STUDIES

N/A

SPECIAL TESTS

- *In vitro* contracture test (IVCT)—a bioassay that indicates susceptibility to malignant hyperthermia uses increasing concentrations of halothane or caffeine to measure contraction of biopsied skeletal muscle; contraction of muscle at or below the threshold concentration for each agent indicates susceptibility to malignant hyperthermia.

- EMG/NCS—should be considered to exclude an alternate cause of weakness such as demyelinating neuropathy or neuromuscular junction defect. Some agents can cause a neuropathy as well as a myopathy, and nerve conduction studies may also be affected. Such is the case with the antimicrotubular agents colchicine and vinblastine, and possibly with chloroquine and amiodarone. EMG is normal in acute corticosteroid myopathy and demonstrates normal insertional and spontaneous activity with short duration and low-amplitude voluntary motor units in chronic corticosteroid myopathy.
- Muscle biopsy—should be done if there is incomplete or no resolution of weakness following removal of the suspected offending toxin, and may be done sooner to exclude causes of weakness other than toxin-induced myopathy. Knowledge of the pathologic findings and medications that the patient takes can help narrow the differential or confirm a diagnosis.

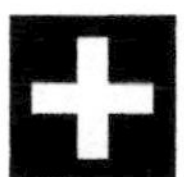

Management

GENERAL MEASURES

Removal of the offending agent—most cases of toxic myopathy require removal of the potentially offending agent. Neuroleptic malignant syndrome can be caused by removal of a dopaminergic agent or use of neuroleptic agents. If discontinuation of a dopaminergic agent is associated with the syndrome, it should be resumed. Malignant hyperthermia and neuroleptic malignant syndrome require additional measures [see Drug(s) of Choice, below] of cooling and hydration.

Hydration for hyperthermia and to prevent renal failure in rhabdomyolysis or myoglobinuria.

SURGICAL MEASURES

N/A

SYMPTOMATIC TREATMENT

N/A

ADJUNCTIVE TREATMENT

N/A

ADMISSION/DISCHARGE CRITERIA

Admission Criteria

- Rhabdomyolysis or myoglobinuria—risk of renal failure
- Hyperthermia following anesthesia or use of neuroleptics
- Impaired ambulation
- Impending respiratory failure

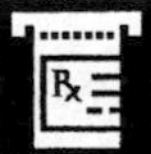

Medications

DRUG(S) OF CHOICE

- Malignant hyperthermia—dantrolene (1 mg/kg) IV as a continuous rapid infusion as needed up to a total dose of 10 mg/kg. The regimen may be repeated if symptoms recur.
- Neuroleptic malignant syndrome—dantrolene (1 mg/kg) IV as needed up to a total dose of 10 mg/kg

Contraindications

None. Only one case of anaphylaxis has been reported through 1999.

Precautions

The intravenous formulation of dantrolene has a high pH and care should be taken to prevent extravasation. If mannitol will be used to prevent or treat late renal complications of malignant hyperthermia, mannitol, 3 g, is required to dissolve each 20 mg vial of dantrolene.

Reporting

The Food and Drug Administration encourages voluntary reporting of adverse events, defined as "any undesirable experience associated with the use of a medical product in a patient." The event should be reported when use of a medication or product causes disability or death, or requires medical intervention or hospitalization. Reports (see the Internet site *http://www.fda.gov/medwatch/report/hcp.htm*) may be submitted by several mechanisms:

- Use the postage-paid MedWatch form (PDF format at *http://www.fda.gov/medwatch/safety/3500.pdf*)
- By Phone: 1-800-FDA-1088
- By Fax: 1-800-FDA-0178
- By Internet at *http://www.accessdata.fda.gov/scripts/medwatch/medwatch-online.cfm*

ALTERNATIVE DRUGS

Neuroleptic malignant syndrome: bromocriptine 2.5–10 mg IV or enterally by NG tube every 4 to 6 hours

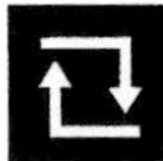

Follow-Up

PATIENT MONITORING

Do not neglect other supportive measures of oxygenation, cooling, and management of metabolic acidosis for malignant hyperthermia or neuroleptic malignant syndrome.

EXPECTED COURSE AND PROGNOSIS

Complete or at least partial resolution of symptoms after treatment.

PATIENT EDUCATION

- Activities—as tolerated
- Diet—N/A
- Organizations
  —Malignant Hyperthermia Association of the U.S., 32 South Main Street, PO Box 1069, Sherburne, NY 13460-4287.
  Phone 800-986-4287, 607-674-7901;
  Fax 607-674-7910;
  Email: *mhaus@norwich.net.*
  —National Organization for Rare Disorders, Inc. (NORD), PO Box 8923, New Fairfield, CT 06812-8923. Phone: 203-746-6518, fax: 203-746-6481,toll free: 800-999-6673, TDD: 203-746-6927,
  email: *orphan@nord-rbd.com*,
  website: *http://www.rarediseases.org/*

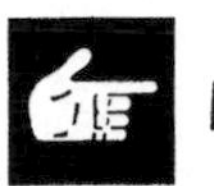

Miscellaneous

SYNONYMS

Drug-induced myopathy
Iatrogenic myopathy
Alcoholic myopathy
Steroid myopathy
Malignant hyperthermia
Neuroleptic malignant syndrome
Fasciitis
Eosinophilic fasciitis
Necrotizing fasciitis

ICD-9-CM: 255.0 Iatrogenic syndrome of excess corticosteroids; use additional E codes to identify the toxic agent; 333.92 Neuroleptic malignant syndrome; use additional E codes to identify the toxic agent; 359.4 Toxic myopathy; use additional E codes to identify the toxic agent; 728.2 Muscle fibrosis; 728.86 Necrotizing fasciitis; 728.89 Eosinophilic fasciitis; 729.4 Fasciitis; 995.86 Malignant hyperthermia; 999.9 Iatrogenic muscle fibrosis (from injection)

SEE ALSO: NEUROLEPTIC MALIGNANT SYNDROME

REFERENCES

- George KK, Pourmand R. Toxic myopathies. Neurol Clin 1997;15:711–730.
- Jurkat-Rott K, McCarthy T, Lehmann-Horn F. Genetics and pathogenesis of malignant hyperthermia. Muscle Nerve 2000;23:4–17.
- Pascuzzi RM. Drugs and toxins associated with myopathies. Curr Opin Rheumatol 1998;10:511–520.
- Victor M, Sieb JP. Myopathies due to drugs, toxins, and nutritional deficiency. In: Engel AG, Franzini-Armstrong C, eds. Myology. New York: McGraw-Hill, 1994:1697–1725.
- Zuckner J. Drug-Induced myopathies. Semin Arthritis Rheum 1990;5:259–268.

Author(s): Boyd M. Koffman, MD, PhD

Narcolepsy

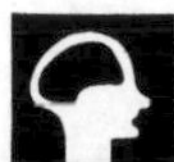

Basics

DESCRIPTION

Narcolepsy is a chronic and disabling neurologic disorder characterized by excessive daytime sleepiness (EDS), cataplexy, sleep paralysis, and hypnagogic hallucinations primarily related to abnormal regulation of rapid eye movement (REM) sleep.

EPIDEMIOLOGY

Incidence

Not determined, because the disorder is chronic. Prevalence has been ascertained in the adult Finnish population (0.026%) and estimated to be 0.05% in the general U.S. population.

Race

No known racial predominance.

Age

Develops around adolescence. Onset may be bimodal (mid-teens and mid-thirties). It then persists lifelong. Excessive daytime sleepiness often develops first with delay in the development of other features; this may lead to a delay in diagnosis.

Sex

Equally common in men and women.

ETIOLOGY

The etiology is uncertain. A strong association with certain human leukocyte antigen (HLA) haplotypes (DR15, DQB1*0602) suggests an autoimmune mechanism. It is likely that narcolepsy results from a deficiency of a neurotransmitter, possibly hypocretin (Orexin). Hypocretins are neurotransmitters whose cell bodies are located in the hypothalamus. Some propose that the pathogenesis likely includes a loss of hypocretin-producing neurons or of hypocretin receptor function, perhaps due to an autoimmune mechanisms.

Genetics

The etiology of narcolepsy is considered to be multifactorial. The 1% to 2% prevalence of narcolepsy within families with an index case does represent a genetic predisposition compared to the 0.05% rate in the general population. Monozygotic twins are concordant for narcolepsy in 25% to 31% of cases. The hypocretin gene was found to be abnormal in narcoleptic dogs in 1999 and a murine narcolepsy model has been produced by knocking out the genes that produce hypocretins.

RISK FACTORS

None are known. Rarely, narcolepsy has been reported after head trauma.

PREGNANCY

There is no known relationship to pregnancy.

ASSOCIATED CONDITIONS

- Obesity
- Type 2 diabetes
- Multiple sclerosis
- Pituitary-hypothalamic pathology (anterior pituitary tumors, craniopharyngiomas, diencephalic sarcoidosis)
- Brainstem lesions

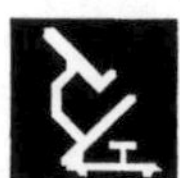

Diagnosis

DIFFERENTIAL DIAGNOSIS

Obstructive sleep apnea
Insufficient sleep syndrome (shift work, jet lag)
Delayed sleep-phase syndrome
Major depression
Chronic fatigue syndrome/fibromyalgia
MS-related fatigue
Familial sleep paralysis
Periodic paralysis
Alcohol or other drug dependence
Restless legs/periodic movements of sleep
Idiopathic hypersomnia

SIGNS AND SYMPTOMS

Narcolepsy is manifested as a classic tetrad of symptoms, most of which may occur in people without narcolepsy. Cataplexy, sleep paralysis, and hypnagogic hallucinations are the result of partial intrusion of REM sleep physiology into wakefulness.

- Excessive daytime somnolence—the most frequent and disabling symptom is an abnormal tendency to fall asleep in the daytime. Narcolepsy often first appears as a tendency to fall asleep or become inattentive in high school classes.
- Cataplexy—usually infrequent and mild, but it is an emotionally induced muscle weakness that is pathognomonic of narcolepsy. Triggered by emotional expressions such as laughter, anger, or excitement, cataplexy is a transient partial or complete muscle weakness of part or the entire body (usually several seconds to several minutes). Its presence may be confirmed by demonstrating transient, simultaneous loss of muscle tone and muscle stretch reflexes in agonist/antagonist muscles. This phenomenon is due to the atonia of disrupted REM sleep—due to inhibition of spinal alpha motor neurons by abnormally activated cells in the medial medulla. Approximately 25% of narcolepsy patients do not seem to exhibit cataplexy.
- Sleep paralysis—a terrifying experience in which the patient becomes transiently unable to move just before sleep onset or just after awakening. This is often associated with a sensation of impending death. These episodes typically last only a few seconds to minutes and terminate spontaneously or by stimulation to hasten full wakefulness. Sleep paralysis is also related to the atonia of REM sleep.
- Hypnagogic hallucinations—vivid dreams, often distressing, that occur at the time of transition from wakefulness to sleep or the reverse. These often involve someone coming into the room or out-of-body experiences.

LABORATORY PROCEDURES

- EDS may be assessed by the Epworth Sleepiness Scale.
- Polysomnography (PSG), an overnight sleep recording (with EEG, EMG, electro-oculography, ECG, pulse oximetry, and respiratory monitoring) should be performed to rule out symptomatic sleep apnea or movement disorders as the cause of EDS. PSG should ideally be performed when the patient has been tapered off of sleeping medications and drugs that might affect sleep onset or REM latency (sedatives, stimulants, or antidepressants).
- Multiple sleep latency test (MSLT) should be performed the next day. REM sleep normally does not occur until 90 minutes after initially falling asleep. However, many patients with narcolepsy exhibit evidence of REM sleep within minutes of falling asleep. Evidence of narcolepsy consists of an abnormal tendency to rapidly fall asleep during an MSLT nap opportunity (within 5 minutes) plus occurrence of two or more episodes of REM sleep during MSLT naps. Such REM-containing naps are especially significant if they take place late in the day, when the propensity for REM sleep is normally low. Approximately 85% of patients with narcolepsy will have a positive MSLT. HLA haplotyping is useful for ruling out narcolepsy in cases of excessive daytime sleepiness attributed to obstructive sleep apnea or other causes.

IMAGING STUDIES

Brainstem MRI abnormalities have been described, but imaging is rarely useful.

SPECIAL TESTS

None

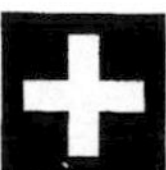

Management

GENERAL MEASURES

Narcolepsy is a lifelong condition that requires treatment with stimulant medication(s) plus self-management of sleep. The latter includes (a) regular, rational periods of bed rest and prevention of sleep deprivation; and (b) planned naps of limited duration (20–30 minutes), especially before activity requiring alertness, such as driving. Shift work should be avoided.

SURGICAL MEASURES

None.

SYMPTOMATIC TREATMENT

EDS can be controlled with a wake-promoting or stimulant medication (modafinil, 200–400 mg/d or methylphenidate 10–40 mg/d) plus planned naps lasting 20 to 40 minutes. Cataplexy can be temporarily suppressed by imipramine 25 mg (or other tricyclic antidepressant drug) taken q4h PRN or a selective serotonin reuptake inhibitor (SSRI)-type antidepressant taken daily. The latter may also control sleep paralysis and hypnagogic hallucinations.

ADJUNCTIVE TREATMENT

Insomnia can occur not infrequently in narcolepsy and may be treated with triazolam with an increase in total sleep time.

ADMISSION/DISCHARGE CRITERIA

Hospital admission is almost never required.

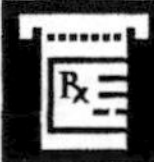

Medications

DRUG(S) OF CHOICE

For treatment of EDS:

- Methylphenidate (Ritalin), 10–20 mg taken 1–2 times a day up to maximum of 100 mg/d.
- Modafinil (Provigil) 200 mg taken 1–2 times a day. It is quite expensive. Modafinil has been shown to stimulate the release of hypocretins in cells present in the anterior hypothalamus.
- Amphetamine (dextro- and mixed dextro- and levoisomers) not to exceed 100 mg/d
- Methamphetamine up to 80 mg/d
- Pemoline up to 150 mg/d

For occasional cataplexy:

- Imipramine 25 mg q4h PRN or other tricyclic antidepressant.
- For cataplexy, sleep paralysis, or hypnagogic hallucinations that occur several times a week or more often, zaleplon (Celexa) 20 mg/d or other SSRI agents may be useful.

Contraindications

Amphetamines are relatively contraindicated for patients with a previous history of chemical dependency.

Precautions

Sympathomimetic adverse effects of amphetamine stimulants include anxiety, tachycardia, palpitations, anorexia, headache, insomnia, and tremor. Patients should be monitored for the development of tolerance and drug dependency, although this is rare in patients without a prior history of chemical dependency. Pemoline has been associated with the risk of acute hepatic failure and manufacturers now recommend that serum transaminases be monitored every 2 weeks during therapy. Modafinil has been associated with adverse side effects of headache, nausea, and nervousness.

ALTERNATIVE DRUGS

Gamma hydroxybutyrate (GHB), an investigational agent, has been helpful for cataplexy during the day for some patients.

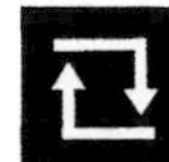

Follow-Up

PATIENT MONITORING

Regular patient visits several times a year.

EXPECTED COURSE AND PROGNOSIS

The severity of narcolepsy may seem to worsen or improve from time to time, but neither complete remission nor relentless progression is known to occur. Symptoms remain lifelong.

PATIENT EDUCATION/ORGANIZATIONS

Narcolepsy Network, Inc., 10921 Reed Hartman Highway, Suite 119, Cincinnati OH 45242. Website *www.narcolepsynetwork.org.*

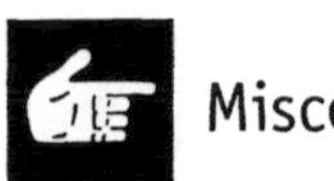

Miscellaneous

SYNONYMS

Narcolepsy-cataplexy syndrome

ICD-9-CM: 347 Narcolepsy

SEE ALSO: N/A

REFERENCES

- Krahn LE, Black JL, Silber MH. Narcolepsy: new understanding of irresistible sleep. Mayo Clin Proc 2001;76:185–194.
- Malik S, Boeve BF, Krahn LE, et al. Narcolepsy associated with other central nervous system disorders. Neurology 2001;57:539–541.
- Overeem S, Mignot E, van Dijk JG, et al. Narcolepsy: clinical features, new pathophysiologic insights, and future perspectives. J Clin Neurophysiol 2001;18:78–105.
- Pollak CP, Wagner DR, Moline ML, et al. Cognitive and motor performance of narcoleptic subjects living in temporal isolation. Sleep 1992;15:202–211.
- Silber MH, Rye DB. Solving the mysteries of narcolepsy: the hypocretin story. Neurology 2001;56:1616–1618.
- U.S. Modafinil in Narcolepsy Multicenter Study Group. Randomized trial of modafinil as a treatment for the excessive daytime somnolence of narcolepsy. Neurology 2000;54:1166–1175.

Author(s): Charles P. Pollak, MD; Joanne Lynn, MD

Neurofibromatosis

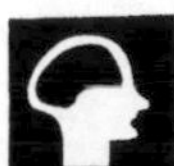

Basics

DESCRIPTION

Neurofibromatosis type 1 (NF-1) is a progressive genetic disease with extreme variability, even within families. NF-1 can be difficult to diagnose in infants, because the appearance of many signs and symptoms is age dependent. The National Institutes of Health (NIH) criteria require that two or more of the following be present: (a) six or more café-au-lait macules greater than 5 mm in diameter in prepubescent individuals or greater than 15 mm in diameter after puberty, (b) two or more neurofibromas of any type (cutaneous, subcutaneous, or plexiform) or one plexiform neurofibroma, (c) freckling in the axilla or groin, (d) a tumor of the optic pathway, (e) two or more Lisch nodules (iris hamartomas), (f) a distinctive osseous lesion such as sphenoid wing dysplasia or thinning of the cortex of the long bones (with or without pseudarthrosis), (g) a first-degree relative (parent, sibling, or child) with NF-1 by the above criteria.
Neurofibromatosis type 2 (NF-2) is an uncommon genetic disorder of tumors affecting the CNS. The diagnostic criteria include individuals with

- bilateral vestibular schwannomas (VS) or
- a family history of NF-2 in a first-degree relative plus
  - —a unilateral VS detected before age 30 or
  - —any two of the following: meningioma, glioma, schwannoma, juvenile posterior subcapsular lenticular opacities.

Most nerve sheath tumors associated with NF-2 are schwannomas and not neurofibromas. The average age of onset of symptoms is 18 to 24 years.

EPIDEMIOLOGY

Incidence/Prevalence

NF-1 affects between 1 in 3,500 to 4,000 individuals worldwide. The incidence of NF-2 is difficult to estimate accurately, because of its rarity. It is estimated to occur in 1 in 40,000 births. There is no racial, ethnic, or gender predilection.

ETIOLOGY

- Both NF-1 and NF-2 are autosomal-dominant diseases, with nearly complete penetrance. Half of cases occur from new mutations.
- The NF-1 gene is on the long arm of chromosome 17. This gene is a tumor suppressor gene that encodes a peptide neurofibromin. Multiple mechanisms cause mutations of this gene, most of which inactivate neurofibromin.
- The NF-2 gene is on chromosome 22 and encodes the protein merlin.

RISK FACTORS

N/A

PREGNANCY

- Healthy women with NF-1 usually have normal pregnancies. Growth of neurofibromas has been reported during pregnancy. Most complications occur from preexisting problems such as pelvic neurofibromas or existing seizures.
- It is not known if NF-2 worsens during pregnancy.

ASSOCIATED CONDITIONS

N/A

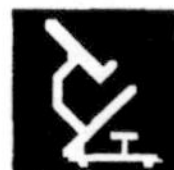

Diagnosis

DIFFERENTIAL DIAGNOSIS

NF-1

- Familial café-au-lait spots
- Schwannomatosis
- Noonan syndrome
- Proteus syndrome
- Watson syndrome

NF-2

- Neurofibromatosis type 1
- Schwannomatosis
- Multiple meningiomas

SIGNS AND SYMPTOMS

NF-1

Pain or weakness can develop from tumor compression of nerves. Associated features include macrocephaly, scoliosis, learning disabilities, seizures, and unidentified bright objects (UBOs) in the basal ganglia, thalamus, cerebellum, and brainstem. UBOs are well-circumscribed, hyperintense lesions without mass effect. Their clinical and pathologic significance is unclear. Rarely, individuals can develop malignant peripheral nerve sheath tumors, pheochromocytomas, juvenile chronic myeloid leukemia, precocious puberty, or renal artery stenosis.

NF-2

- Focal weakness or sensory loss
- Neuropathic pain
- Balance disorder
- Headaches
- Bowel/bladder changes
- Hearing loss/tinnitus
- Visual impairment
- Skin tumors

LABORATORY PROCEDURES

Presymptomatic and prenatal diagnostic testing is available.

IMAGING STUDIES

NF-1

Imaging should be based on the clinical exam.

NF-2

MRI of the head with thin cuts through the internal auditory canals with and without contrast enhancement should be performed to evaluate for VS. Spinal MRI should be performed to evaluate for tumors.

SPECIAL TESTS

NF-1

Clinical findings should dictate any specific testing. Educational testing should be done if there is a possibility of developmental disabilities or learning disabilities. The possibility of a malignant peripheral nerve sheath tumor (MPNST) should be considered in neurofibromas with a change in consistency, rapid change in size, or if persistent unexplained pain is present. Because these tumors are highly aggressive, immediate referral should be made for surgical diagnosis.

NF-2

NF-2 is progressive, and new tumors can develop at any time. Neurologic exams and hearing evaluations should be performed at least annually and when new symptoms occur.

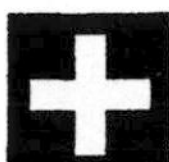

Management

GENERAL MEASURES

- There is no specific treatment or cure for NF-1. Referral to a NF clinic or multidisciplinary treatment team including pediatricians, neurologists, ophthalmologists, surgeons, radiologists, and oncologists should be considered. Seizures can be treated with typical antiseizure medication. Optic pathway tumors should be followed with imaging and ophthalmologic exams. They may require treatment with chemotherapy and less commonly radiation.
- There is no cure or specific treatment for NF-2.

SURGICAL MEASURES

NF-1

Painful or disfiguring neurofibromas can be surgically removed. Plexiform neurofibromas are difficult to completely resect. Dumbbell tumors of spinal nerve roots are difficult to manage. Nerve root and spinal cord compression can occur and surgical removal of the tumors or spinal decompression may be necessary. Patients with tibial dysplasia should be referred to an orthopedic surgeon who is familiar with NF-1. Scoliosis may require spinal fusion.

NF-2

The timing of surgical treatment of VS is critical to preserve hearing and facial nerve function.

SYMPTOMATIC TREATMENT

Pain and itching frequently occur from neurofibromas. The pain can be severe and may require nonsteroidal antiinflammatory drugs (NSAIDs), opiates, or antiseizure medication such as gabapentin.

ADJUNCTIVE TREATMENT

N/A

ADMISSION/DISCHARGE CRITERIA

N/A

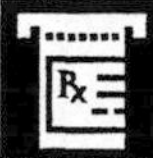

Medications

DRUG(S) OF CHOICE

N/A

ALTERNATIVE DRUGS

N/A

Follow-Up

PATIENT MONITORING

Neurologic exams should be performed at least yearly, as NF-1 is progressive and new manifestations can occur at any time. This exam should always include blood pressure monitoring because of the rare possibility of renal artery stenosis or pheochromocytoma. When optic pathway tumors occur, it is in childhood. Therefore, children should have a yearly exam by an ophthalmologist.
NF-2 patients should have annual neurologic exams, cranial MRI, and hearing evaluations.

EXPECTED COURSE AND PROGNOSIS

- NF-1 is progressive and unpredictable. Patients with more severe disease have increased mortality, but it is difficult to make generalizations because of the extreme variability of the disease.
- The clinical course of NF-2 is variable and dependent on tumor burden. Within families, there is a tendency to similar clinical course. The disease is progressive.

PATIENT EDUCATION

- Genetic counseling should be offered. Because of the progressive nature and unpredictability of the disease many patients benefit from support groups.
- First-degree relatives of patients with NF-2 should be screened for NF-2. All patients with NF-2 should be referred to an audiologist upon diagnosis. Hearing aids, lip reading skills, and sign language may be helpful. Patients with vestibular tumors should be instructed on problems they may develop with balance, including underwater disorientation. Genetic counseling should also be offered. Many patients benefit from support groups.
- National Neurofibromatosis Foundation, 95 Pine St., New York, NY 10005. Phone: 800-323-7938, website: *www.nf.org.*
- The Acoustic Neuroma Association. Phone: 404-237-8023, website: *www.anausa.org.*

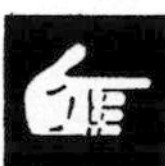

Miscellaneous

SYNONYMS

NF-1

von Recklinghausen's disease

NF-2

Central, bilateral vestibular, or bilateral acoustic neurofibromatosis

ICD-9-CM: 237.71 Neurofibromatosis type 1; 237.72 Neurofibromatosis type 2

SEE ALSO: N/A

REFERENCES

- Friedman JM. Epidemiology of neurofibromatosis type 1. Am J Hum Genet 1999;89: 1–6.
- Friedman JM, Gutmann DH, MacCollin M, et al., eds. Neurofibromatosis—henotype, natural history, and pathogenesis, 3rd ed. Baltimore and London: Johns Hopkins University Press, 1999.
- Gutmann DH, Aylsworth A, Carey JC, et al. The diagnostic evaluation and multidisciplinary management of neurofibromatosis 1 and neurofibromatosis 2. JAMA 1997;278: 51–57.
- National Institutes of Health Consensus Development Conference. Neurofibromatosis conference statement. Arch Neurol 1988;45:575–578.

Author(s): Laura Krietemeyer, MD

Neuroleptic Malignant Syndrome

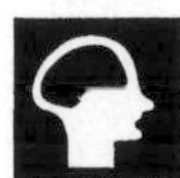

Basics

DESCRIPTION

Neuroleptic malignant syndrome (NMS) is a rare but potentially life-threatening reaction that occurs in patients who are treated with antipsychotic agents (neuroleptics). It appears that the cause of NMS is dopamine blockade, which would explain why this disorder has also been associated with drugs such as:

- Amoxapine (an antidepressant)
- Antiemetics such as prochlorperazine (Compazine), promethazine (Phenergan), and metoclopramide (Reglan)

EPIDEMIOLOGY

Incidence/Prevalence

- Estimated incidence of NMS ranges from 0.02% to 3.2% of patients treated with neuroleptics.
- Reasons for this variability include:
  —Diverse patient populations
  —Different thresholds for diagnosing the disorder
  —Variations in treatment practices
- Incidence of NMS is decreasing due to increased awareness, early detection and treatment, and efforts at prevention.

Race

African Americans may be at higher risk because they have a higher proportion of alleles that code for reduced CYP2D6 enzymatic activity (genetic polymorphisms exist in most of the CYPs).

Age

All ages are affected, although NMS most commonly occurs in adults ages 20 to 50.

Sex

NMS is more commonly seen in men, but this may be attributed to the fact that men are medicated more frequently and more aggressively with neuroleptics than women.

ETIOLOGY

- There is still a fair amount of controversy over the etiology of NMS.
- Dopamine D2 receptor antagonists are associated with this disorder, and it is assumed that NMS is caused by dopamine receptor blockade.
- Studies show that dopamine blockade could lead to hypothalamic dysfunction resulting in:
  —Hyperthermia
  —Labile blood pressure
  —Tachycardia
- Dopamine blockade in the striatum can cause:
  —Tremor
  —Rigidity
  —Rhabdomyolysis (due to prolonged muscular hypertonicity)

RISK FACTORS

- Dehydration
- History of prior episodes of NMS
- High doses of neuroleptics
- Intramuscular administration of neuroleptics
- Rapid rate of neuroleptic loading
- Catatonia
- Iron deficiency
- Use of other medications (especially lithium) in conjunction with neuroleptics
- Prolonged use of seclusion/restraints
- Electrolyte disturbances
- Presence of an organic dysfunction
- Presence of an mood disorder

PREGNANCY

N/A

ASSOCIATED CONDITIONS

N/A

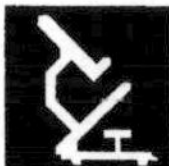

Diagnosis

DIFFERENTIAL DIAGNOSIS

- Catatonia
- Serotonin syndrome
- Heat exhaustion and heat stroke
- Malignant hyperthermia
- Delirium—secondary to anticholinergic toxicity
- Withdrawal of antiparkinsonian agents in a patient with Parkinson's disease
- Thyrotoxicosis
- CNS infections
- Drug toxicity: amphetamines, phencyclidine (PCP), cocaine
- Intermittent acute porphyria
- Pheochromocytoma
- Tetany
- Parkinson's disease and other neurologic disorders

SIGNS AND SYMPTOMS

- Hyperthermia
- Generalized rigidity (lead pipe)
- Autonomic instability
- Mental status changes
- Profuse diaphoresis

Diagnostic Criteria for Neuroleptic Malignant Syndrome

- Recent treatment with neuroleptics (within 7 days before onset)
- Hyperthermia (temperature above 38°C)
- Muscle rigidity
- Exclusion of systemic or neuropsychiatric illness
- And at least three of the following:
  —Change in mental status
  —Change in blood pressure
  —Creatinine phosphokinase (CPK) elevation or myoglobinuria
  —Leukocytosis
  —Metabolic acidosis
  —Tachycardia
  —Diaphoresis or sialorrhea
  —Tremors

LABORATORY PROCEDURES

- CPK
- CBC
- Electrolytes, including calcium and magnesium
- Renal and hepatic function tests
- Urinalysis, including urine myoglobin

Optional Tests to Be Done if Appropriate

- Arterial blood gas
- Toxicology screen
- Coagulation studies
- Blood cultures

IMAGING STUDIES

- CT scan or MRI scan of the head

SPECIAL TESTS

- Lumbar puncture to rule out CNS infection

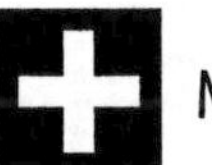

Management

GENERAL MEASURES

- The most critical intervention is to discontinue all neuroleptic agents immediately.
- The discontinuation of other medications such as lithium or anticholinergic agents should be considered.

SURGICAL MEASURES

N/A

SYMPTOMATIC TREATMENT

- IV fluids to correct dehydration, hypotension, and electrolyte imbalance
- A cooling blanket and antipyretics to reduce the temperature
- If rhabdomyolysis occurs, it is important to hydrate patients and alkalinize the urine to prevent renal failure
- Aspiration precautions
- Maintain good nutrition, as this may minimize rhabdomyolysis

ADJUNCTIVE TREATMENT

- Dialysis may be necessary if renal failure develops.
- ECT (electroconvulsive therapy) has been found to be effective both in treating NMS and the underlying psychiatric condition.

ADMISSION/DISCHARGE CRITERIA

- Most patients suspected of having NMS should be treated (at least initially) in the medical intensive care unit.
- Patients may be transferred to a medical or psychiatric inpatient unit once their vital signs are stable, their hydration status and electrolyte imbalance corrected, CPK levels are falling, and there is no evidence of renal failure or cardiorespiratory compromise.

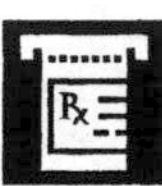

Medications

DRUG(S) OF CHOICE

- In most cases pharmacologic management is instituted if the course of the syndrome fails to improve with supportive measures alone.
- Dopamine agonist agents are the drugs of choice, and some studies have shown that they may decrease mortality and shorten the course of NMS.
- Bromocriptine (Parlodel): a dopamine agonist
  - —Usually the starting doses is 2.5 mg PO tid. The dose can be increased by 2.5 to 7.5 mg daily, up to a daily total of 45 mg in divided doses.
  - —Possible side effects include nausea, vomiting, possible exacerbation of psychotic symptoms.
  - —Caution should be used when administering to children younger than 15 years of age.
- Amantadine (Symmetrel)
  - —Usual adult dose is 200–300 mg PO qd in divided doses
- Sinemet
  - —Usual adult dose is 25/250 mg PO tid or qid
- Dantrolene (Dantrium)
  - —Dantrolene is a muscle relaxant and is specifically recommended for severe hyperthermia. It may be given IV or PO. Initial dose is 1–3 mg/kg IV followed by a total of up to 10 mg/kg/d IV in divided doses or 50–600 mg/d in divided oral doses. Dantrolene may be used in conjunction with bromocriptine if clinically indicated.
  - —Dantrolene may cause hepatitis, and liver function needs to be monitored

Precautions

Complications include:

- Rhabdomyolysis
- Renal failure
- Aspiration pneumonia
- Seizures
- Respiratory or cardiac failure
- Exacerbation of psychiatric illness following discontinuation of antipsychotic agent or treatment with DA agonists

ALTERNATIVE DRUGS

- There are controversial data on the use of benzodiazepines and barbiturates for NMS.
- Nifedipine may be used in hypertension.
- Subcutaneous heparin should be used to prevent pulmonary embolism or deep vein thrombosis.
- Iron deficiency anemia may aggravate NMS. Therefore, iron supplements should be prescribed for patients who are deficient.

Follow-Up

PATIENT MONITORING

Patients with NMS should be off neuroleptics for 2 weeks following resolution of the syndrome. Vital signs and CPK levels need to be monitored.

EXPECTED COURSE AND PROGNOSIS

- The clinical course of NMS usually lasts 2 to 14 days, although in the case of long-acting depot antipsychotic agents it may be prolonged up to 30 days.
- Mortality rate is 10% to 20% from complications listed above. In the absence of these complications the prognosis for full recovery is good.
- Patients who develop NMS are more likely to have a recurrence upon reintroduction of neuroleptic agents. To minimize the risk of a recurrence, several measures may be helpful:
  - —Try a neuroleptic from a different chemical class and with a lower D2 affinity, such as an atypical antipsychotic, (risperidone, olanzapine, quetiapine).
  - —Clozapine is currently recommended for patients who need an antipsychotic and have a history of NMS (but the risk for agranulocytosis needs close monitoring with this agent). In addition, clozapine has also been associated with NMS (but less frequently).
  - —Consider alternative treatments with lithium, valproate, carbamazepine, or ECT.
  - —If an antipsychotic agent is necessary, use the lowest effective dose and increase the dose slowly.
  - —Obtain informed consent from the patient and family and discuss at length risks, benefits, and side effects of treatment. In addition, closely monitor vital signs and CPK levels.

PATIENT EDUCATION

Every patient who has had NMS should be told that he or she is at risk for recurrence if challenged with any dopamine-blocking agent.

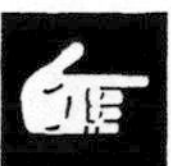

Miscellaneous

SYNONYMS

Neuroleptic midbrain syndrome

ICD-9-CM: 333.92 Neuroleptic malignant syndrome

SEE ALSO: N/A

REFERENCES

- Addonizio G. Neuroleptic malignant syndrome: epidemiology, clinical presentation, diagnosis, and treatment options. Essent Psychopharmacol 1997; 1(4):393–408.
- Caroff SN, Mann SC, Keck PE Jr. Specific treatment of the neuroleptic malignant syndrome. Biol Psychiatry 1998;44(6): 378–381.
- Pelonero A, Levenson JL, Pandurangi AK. Neuroleptic malignant syndrome: a review. Psychiatr Serv 1998;49(9):1163–1172.
- Velamoor VR. Neuroleptic malignant syndrome recognition, prevention and management. Drug Safety 1998;19(1): 73–82.

Author(s): Radu Saveanu, MD

Neuronal Ceroid Lipofuscinoses

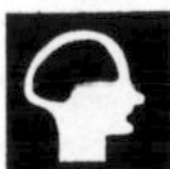

Basics

DESCRIPTION

- Neuronal ceroid lipofuscinoses (NCLs) Group of neurodegenerative disorders characterized by progressive dementia, visual loss, epilepsy and intralysosomal accumulation of a membrane-bound fluorescent lipopigment in neurons and other cells. Although this abnormal lipopigment is widely distributed in the skin, muscle, peripheral nerve, and viscera, signs and symptoms are confined to the central nervous system.
- There are four major subtypes: infantile (NCL1 or Santavuori-Haltia type), late infantile (NCL2 or Jansky-Bielschowsky type), juvenile (NCL3 or Batten type), and an adult recessive form (NCL4 or Kufs type). A dozen atypical variant forms, including Finnish late infantile variant (NCL5), have been described.

EPIDEMIOLOGY

Incidence/Prevalence

- The NCLs are the most common group of neurodegenerative disorders in children.

Race

- NCL2 and NCL3 are the most prevalent subtypes in the United States and Europe. NCL1 and NCL5 are particularly frequent in Finland.

Age

- See Signs and Symptoms

Sex

- Because of autosomal recessive inheritance, there are equal numbers of male and female cases.

ETIOLOGY

Genetics

- Autosomal recessive mode of inheritance except for a rare adult-onset variant that is autosomal dominant. Gene identification has been accomplished for NCL1, NCL2, NCL3, and NCL5. Prenatal diagnosis is available for most subtypes.

RISK FACTORS

N/A

PREGNANCY

N/A

ASSOCIATED CONDITIONS

N/A

Diagnosis

DIFFERENTIAL DIAGNOSIS

- The NCLs are easily distinguished from the other known inherited metabolic neurodegenerative diseases based on physical examination, funduscopic evaluation, and clinical course. It is most important to distinguish between the different forms of the NCLs because they share many clinical features. It also is important to confirm the diagnosis to rule out other neurodegenerative disorders of unknown etiology.

SIGNS AND SYMPTOMS

- Classified according to age of onset, clinical features, ultrastructural morphology, and genetic analysis.
  —NCL1: dramatic onset of psychomotor deterioration, seizures and blindness during the first year of life. The common ocular abnormality is optic atrophy; retinal abnormalities have been reported.
  —NCL2: onset between 2 and 5 years of age, with psychomotor deterioration and intractable seizures. Blindness associated with optic atrophy or retinitis pigmentosa. Vegetative state ensues after symptoms have been present for about 1 year.
  —NCL3: onset between 5 and 15 years of age, with either gradual visual loss resulting in blindness within 3–5 years and/or behavioral symptoms. There is prominent macular degeneration, optic atrophy. or retinitis pigmentosa. Some time after the onset of the visual disturbance, motor dysfunction (apraxia and ataxia), seizures, and slow dementia are noted.
  —NCL4: average onset at 30 years, with a steadily progressive dementia and seizures that ultimately become refractory. Vision usually is not affected.

LABORATORY PROCEDURES

- See Special Tests

IMAGING STUDIES

- Neuroimaging may reveal atrophy.

SPECIAL TESTS

- Diagnosis is suspected based on physical examination, which must include a funduscopic evaluation, and clinical course. EEG, electroretinogram, visual evoked potentials, and somatosensory evoked potentials may add supportive evidence. Confirmation is made by histologic identification of characteristic ultrastructural abnormalities noted on skin or conjunctival biopsy and/or genetic analysis when available.
- Histologic inclusions:
  —NCL1: granular osmiophilic deposits
  —NCL2: curvilinear inclusion bodies
  —NCL3: fingerprint inclusions
  —NCL4: curvilinear inclusion bodies, fingerprint inclusions, granular osmiophilic deposits

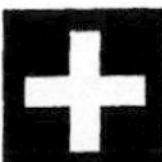

Management

GENERAL MEASURES

- Patients and their families require emotional support.

SURGICAL MEASURES

N/A

SYMPTOMATIC TREATMENT

- Correction of associated visual refractive errors
- Valproate and clonazepam for seizure control
- Psychotropic drugs for treatment of behavior problems

ADJUNCTIVE TREATMENT

- Braille training and visual impairment education

ADMISSION/DISCHARGE CRITERIA

- Patients usually are admitted for evaluation and treatment of the complications of their disease

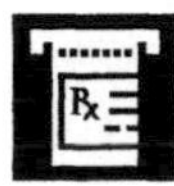

Medications

DRUG(S) OF CHOICE

- No medications are available to reverse the symptoms of these disorders. Antioxidants may temporarily improve mentation.

ALTERNATIVE DRUGS

N/A

Follow-Up

PATIENT MONITORING

- Patient follow-up is guided by the predicted course and potential complications of the particular disease.

EXPECTED COURSE AND PROGNOSIS

- NCL1: rapid and severe neuronal devastation. Usually fatal before the end of the first decade.
- NCL2: rapidly progressive. Usually fatal before the end of the first decade.
- NCL3: may remain ambulatory and able to attend school until the late teens, although 25% of patients die in their teens after a more rapidly dementing course with prominent seizures.
- NCL4: slow progression. Duration of illness 20–30 years.

PATIENT EDUCATION

- Batten Disease Support and Research Association, 2600 Parsons Avenue, Columbus, OH 43207. Phone: 800-448-4570.
- Children's Brain Diseases Foundation, 350 Parnassus Avenue, Suite 900, San Francisco, CA 94117. Phone: 415-565-5402.
- National Batten Disease Registry, 1050 Forest Hill Road, Staten Island, NY 10314-6399. Phone: 800-952-9628.

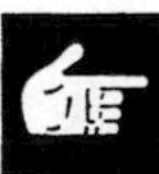

Miscellaneous

SYNONYMS

N/A

ICD-9-CM: 272.7 Ceroid storage disease

SEE ALSO: N/A

REFERENCES

- Dyken PR. The neuronal ceroid lipofuscinoses. In: Berg BO, ed. Principles of child neurology. New York: McGraw-Hill, 1996:1495–1512.
- Goebel HH, Sharp JD. The neuronal ceroid-lipofuscinoses: recent advances. Brain Pathol 1998;8:151.
- National Center for Biotechnology Information. http://www3.ncbi.nlm.nih.gov.
- Wisniewski KE, Kida E, Patxot OF, et al. Variability in the clinical and pathological findings in the neuronal ceroid lipofuscinoses: review of the data and observations. Am J Med Genet 1992;42:525.

Author(s): Eveline C. Traeger, MD

Neuropathy, Diabetic

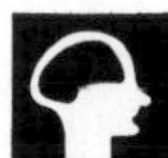

Basics

DESCRIPTION

- Diabetes mellitus (DM) is the most frequent cause of peripheral neuropathy in the developed world. The most common peripheral neuropathic syndrome associated with diabetes is diabetic polyneuropathy, an insidiously progressive, length-dependent peripheral neuropathy. Patients with diabetic polyneuropathy may exhibit distal sensory loss and dysesthesias, autonomic dysfunction, and distal weakness. Morbidity related to diabetic polyneuropathy is significant and includes neuropathic pain, sensory loss leading to limb infections and amputations, and reduced proprioception with unsteady walking and falls.

EPIDEMIOLOGY

- DM is an increasingly common disorder affecting nearly 7% of the US population. Late complications, which include retinopathy, nephropathy, and peripheral neuropathy, are more common with prolonged and severe hyperglycemia.
- More than half of diabetics eventually develop clinically evident peripheral neuropathy. At the time of diagnosis, 8% of diabetics have clinically overt peripheral neuropathy. Fifty percent have overt peripheral neuropathic findings within 10 years of diagnosis.

ETIOLOGY

- Diabetic polyneuropathy results from chronic hyperglycemia, but the precise pathophysiology has not been established. Microangiopathy and metabolic abnormalities are the two major proposed causes. Endoneurial microvascular changes with basement membrane thickening and pericyte degeneration progress to vessel and nerve ischemic injury. Proposed metabolic abnormalities include accumulation of advanced glycosylation end products leading to smooth muscle proliferation and capillary atherogenesis. Accumulation of polyol constituents, such as sorbitol and fructose, ultimately may lead to nerve demyelination and axonal injury. Oxidative stress with excessive free radical production may lead to lipid peroxidation of nerve membranes. Circulating nerve growth factors are also reduced, suggesting a role in pathogenesis.

RISK FACTORS

- Diagnosis of DM with chronically poor glycemic control is the most important risk factor for the development of diabetic polyneuropathy. Older diabetic patients and men are at greater risk. The risk for developing diabetic polyneuropathy can be significantly reduced with a regimen of strict glycemic control. Once axonal injury becomes well established, there are no known effective interventions for reversing diabetic polyneuropathy.

PREGNANCY

- Pregnant women who develop gestational diabetes are not at increased risk for developing diabetic polyneuropathy, unless their hyperglycemia persists beyond 6 weeks postpartum.

ASSOCIATED CONDITIONS

- Several other peripheral neuropathic syndromes occur in diabetics and are distinct from, and often coexist with, diabetic polyneuropathy.
  - —*Cranial neuropathies* related to diabetes include oculomotor, abducens, and trochlear neuropathies presenting with subacute external ophthalmoplegia, frequently preceded by pain. The most common is diabetic oculomotor neuropathy, which presents with ocular or hemicranial pain, ptosis, and diplopia. Sparing of pupil constrictor function may help to differentiate diabetic from compressive causes of oculomotor neuropathy, but pupil function may be spared initially in compressive lesions. The prognosis is favorable in these patients with functional recovery occurring over 1–3 months.
  - —*Compressive mononeuropathies:* Diabetics have increased susceptibility to compression neuropathies, including median neuropathies at the wrists (carpal tunnel syndrome), ulnar neuropathies at the elbows, peroneal neuropathies at the fibular heads, and lateral femoral cutaneous neuropathies (meralgia paresthetica).
  - —*Truncal radiculoneuropathy:* Diabetics may develop subacute thoracic paraspinal, flank, chest wall, or upper abdominal pain, which is generally unilateral, intense, and independent of position or inspiratory movement. Examination may demonstrate abnormal sensation in a radicular or segmental pattern in the thoracic region, occasionally with focal abdominal wall weakness. Recovery occurs over several weeks.
  - —*Lumbosacral radiculoplexus neuropathy:* This syndrome of painful, asymmetric lower extremity weakness (also called Bruns-Garland syndrome or diabetic amyotrophy) is most often observed in older men with type 2 DM. Severe pain involving the back, hip, buttock, or anterior thigh precedes the development of muscle weakness and atrophy affecting both proximal and distal muscles. Weakness may progress over weeks or months, with later involvement of the contralateral lower extremity. Recovery occurs over months, with the degree of recovery directly related to the severity and distribution of weakness.

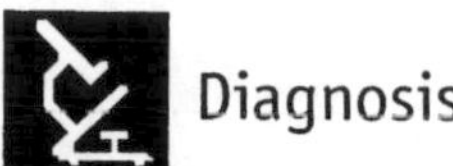

Diagnosis

DIFFERENTIAL DIAGNOSIS

- Differential diagnosis includes peripheral neuropathy due to peripheral neurotoxins, uremia, nutritional deficiency, hypothyroidism, and paraproteinemia, along with hereditary, idiopathic sensory, and chronic immune-mediated peripheral neuropathies.
- The clinical diagnosis of diabetic polyneuropathy can be made in patients with DM and a history of prolonged hyperglycemia. Diagnosis of DM requires a random serum glucose measurement $\geq$200 mg/dL, fasting plasma glucose $\geq$126 mg/dL, or plasma glucose $\geq$200 mg/dL during a 2-hour oral glucose tolerance test. In this setting, a diagnosis of diabetic polyneuropathy is supported by findings of a distal, symmetric, peripheral neuropathy in the absence of other causes of polyneuropathy.

SIGNS AND SYMPTOMS

- The initial symptoms of diabetic polyneuropathy are related to dysfunction of the longest sensory nerve fibers with early impairment of small-fiber sensory function. This may present as tingling or burning paraesthesias in the toes and distal feet with abnormal pain and temperature sensation. Achilles tendon reflexes and vibratory sensation in the toes are often reduced early.
- Hand numbness and sensory loss may develop later as a consequence of the progression of length-dependent neuropathy or from compressive median or ulnar neuropathies. As diabetic polyneuropathy progresses, abnormal sensation may be perceived on the anterior abdomen due to distal involvement of thoracic nerves.
- Autonomic neuropathy may produce postural hypotension with an increased and invariant pulse and reduced sweating in the distal limbs. Gastrointestinal manifestations include delayed gastric emptying, gastroparesis, postprandial sweating, and nocturnal diarrhea. Genitourinary manifestations include bladder atony with difficulty initiating micturition, incomplete bladder emptying, and postvoid dribbling. Most men are aware of erectile impotence, although ejaculation initially is unaffected.
- Large-fiber sensory deficits develop later, with distal proprioceptive loss and sensory ataxia. Patients may complain of gait unsteadiness, with difficulty walking in a dark environment or loss of balance with eyes closed. Romberg's sign is often present. Neurogenic foot arthropathy (Charcot joint) may develop at the instep.
- Distal weakness with reduced strength and bulk for great toe extension, foot dorsiflexion, and intrinsic hand musculature may develop with advanced disease.

LABORATORY PROCEDURES

- *Electrodiagnostic studies:* Nerve conduction studies may demonstrate reduced conduction velocity and amplitudes of sensory nerve action potentials and of compound muscle action potentials in a length-dependent fashion. Needle electromyography may demonstrate denervation and reinnervation in distal muscles with more advanced disease. Electrodiagnostic studies are particularly useful when a superimposed compression neuropathy is being considered.
- *Quantitative sensory testing:* Quantitative sensory testing demonstrates increased vibratory, touch pressure, and thermal sensory thresholds.
- *Autonomic studies* are utilized to assess autonomic function. Heart rate variability to deep breathing (R-R interval testing) may demonstrate loss of the normal sinus arrhythmia with slow deep breathing at six times per minute.
- *Nerve biopsy* is not normally indicated to evaluate diabetic polyneuropathy.

IMAGING STUDIES

N/A

SPECIAL TESTS

See above

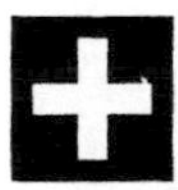

Management

GENERAL MEASURES

- Strict glycemic control can prevent or slow progression of diabetic polyneuropathy. Meticulous foot care is essential to prevent the development of foot infections, which are difficult to treat and may lead to amputation.

SURGICAL MEASURES

N/A

SYMPTOMATIC TREATMENT

- Symptomatic treatment of neuropathic foot pain is frequently required; see Medications.

ADJUNCTIVE TREATMENT

- Podiatric referral for foot hygiene, including nail care and callus removal, should be promoted. Physical therapy may be indicated for patients with sensory ataxia.

ADMISSION/DISCHARGE CRITERIA

- Hospital admission is not generally required.

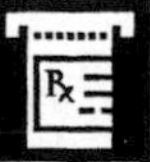

Medications

DRUG(S) OF CHOICE

- Neuropathic pain involving the distal extremities may require treatment. For mild symptoms, ibuprofen 400 mg twice a day may be given in the setting of normal renal function.
- For more severe and continuous neuropathic pain, tricyclic antidepressant agents such as amitriptyline beginning at a low dosage of 10–25 mg at bedtime may be effective over 10 days. If pain relief is inadequate, the dosage may be increased slowly to 100–150 mg at bedtime. Sedation is a prominent side effect of amitriptyline and may be desirable in patients with insomnia related to neuropathic pain. Desipramine and nortriptyline offer less sedation. Tricyclic agents should be used with great caution in patients with heart disease or prostatism.

Contraindications

- Known hypersensitivity, glaucoma, serious cardiac conduction delays, benign prostatic hypertrophy

Precautions

N/A

ALTERNATIVE DRUGS

- Selected anticonvulsants (gabapentin, carbamazepine, phenytoin) are helpful in neuropathic pain.

Follow-Up

PATIENT MONITORING

- Glycemic control should be closely monitored by the primary physician or endocrinologist. Neurologic reexamination at long intervals can document sensory, motor, and autonomic function.

EXPECTED COURSE AND PROGNOSIS

- Progression of polyneuropathy occurs with chronic hyperglycemia and is not inevitable if glycemia is well controlled.

PATIENT EDUCATION

- Exercise, weight loss in obesity, appropriate diet, optimal foot care, and compliance with insulin and/or oral hypoglycemic medications are important for best outcomes.
- National Institute for Neurological Disorders and Stroke Diabetic Neuropathy Information Page. Website: *www.ninds.nih.gov/health_and_medical/disorders/diabetic_doc.htm*
- National Diabetes Information Clearinghouse, 1 Information Way, Bethesda, MD 20892-3560. Website:*ndic@info.niddk.nih.gov*

Miscellaneous

SYNONYMS

N/A

ICD-9-CM: 357.2 Diabetic polyneuropathy; 250.60 for Type 2, controlled; 250.61 for Type 1, controlled; 250.02 for Type 2, uncontrolled; 250.03 for Type 1, uncontrolled

SEE ALSO: N/A

REFERENCES

- Dyck PJ, Thomas PK, eds. Diabetic neuropathy. Philadelphia: WB Saunders, 1999.
- Mokdad AH, Ford ES, Bowman BA, et al. Diabetes trends in the U.S.: 1990–1998. Diabetes Care 2000;23:1278–1283.
- Pirart J. Diabetes mellitus and its degenerative complications: a prospective study of 4400 patients observed between 1947 and 1973. Diabetes Care 1978;1: 166–188, 252–263.
- The Diabetes Control and Complications Trial Research Group. Factors in development of diabetic neuropathy: baseline analysis of neuropathy in feasibility phase of diabetes control and complications trial (DCCT). Diabetes 1988;37:476–481.
- Diabetes Control and Complications Trial Research Group. The effect of intensive treatment of diabetes on the development and progression of long-term complications in insulin-dependent diabetes mellitus. N Engl J Med 1993;329:977–986.

Author(s): Vern C. Juel, MD

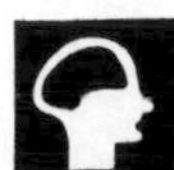

Basics

DESCRIPTION

- Hereditary neuropathies probably account for a majority of the cases referred to large neuromuscular centers. Most common sensory motor hereditary neuropathies fall under the category of Charcot-Marie-Tooth (CMT) neuropathy or disease, which encompasses disorders resulting from different genetic defects involving either the ensheathing Schwann cell or the nerve cell itself. Other less common hereditary neuropathies include sensory and autonomic neuropathies, familial amyloid polyneuropathy, disorders of lipid metabolism, ataxia with neuropathy syndromes, and rare miscellaneous conditions. The subclassification of different categories of CMT is done according to the principal pathology (demyelinating [CMT1, CMT3, CMT4] or axonal [CMT2]), mode of inheritance (autosomal dominant, autosomal recessive, X linked), age at onset (infancy, childhood, adulthood), and the specific gene mutation. CMT1, the most common form, refers to an autosomal dominant demyelinating form (sporadic in 20%). CMT2 refers to an autosomal dominant or recessive axonal form. CMT3 begins in infancy and is associated with severe hypomyelination, inherited in an autosomal recessive or dominant form. CMT4 subgroup includes cases resembling CMT1 or CMT3 phenotype but is inherited only in an autosomal recessive fashion. Although this classification offers some practical considerations, it is far from complete or accurate in considering the variability in phenotype (axonal vs. demyelinating) that could result from different mutations in the same gene. An expected influence of molecular genetics on clinical neurology is now resulting in the currently evolving classification of CMT neuropathies.

EPIDEMIOLOGY

- Estimates suggest a prevalence rate of 1 in 2,500, but exact numbers are difficult to ascertain because of the heterogeneity of the syndromes. Duplication of CMT1A locus is the most prevalent mutation found in CMT1. Female carriers for the X-linked form of CMT caused by connexin 32 (Cx32) mutations have mild signs, but 10% of patients have obvious changes on examination with mild functional impairment.

ETIOLOGY

- It is now well established that mutations in myelin-making Schwann cells, particularly in CMT1, have a profound influence on their axonal counterpart. This results in alterations in the cytoskeletal components and impaired axonal transport leading to preferential distal axonal atrophy and degeneration giving rise to a clinical presentation of a length-dependent axonal neuropathy. In CMT2, the primary axonal form, mutations affecting components of axonal cytoskeleton, their regulators, and axonal transport motors result in primary axonal pathology.

Genetics

- New mutations responsible for different forms of CMT are being discovered at a rapid pace (recent information available at *htpp:/molgen-www.uia.ac.be/CMT mutations/*). Most common CMT mutations are as follows.
  —CMT1A has 1.5-Mb duplication at chromosome 17p11.2-12 encompassing the peripheral myelin protein 22 (PMP22) gene in the majority; others have point mutations.
  —Deletion of the same gene causes the reciprocal disorder hereditary neuropathy with pressure palsies (HNPP).
  —CMT1B has point mutations and small deletions/duplications in myelin protein zero (P0) on chromosome 1q22-23.
  —CMT1C has point mutations in LITAF/ SIMPLE (a putative protein degradation) gene on chromosome 16p13.1-p12.3.
  —CMTX has point mutations, small deletions, or insertions in the Cx32 gene encoding a gap junction protein on chromosome Xq13.1.
  —CMT2A has point mutation in KIF1B (kinesin family member for axoplasmic motor) gene on chromosome 1p35-p36.
  —CMT2B has point mutations in RAB7 (member of RAS oncogene) gene on chromosome 3q27.
  —CMT2E has point mutations in NEFL (neurofilament light chain) gene on chromosome 8p21.
  —CMT4A has point mutations, small insertions, or deletions in GDAP1 (ganglioside-induced differentiation-associated protein 1) gene on chromosome 8p21.1.
  —CMT4B has point mutations, small insertions, or deletions in MTMR2 (myotubularin-related protein 2) gene on chromosome 11q22.
  —CMT4E has point mutations in EGR2 (early growth response 2) gene on chromosome 10q21.1-q22.1.
  —CMT4F has point mutations and deletions in PRX (periaxin) gene on chromosome 19q13.13-q13.2.

RISK FACTORS

N/A

PREGNANCY

- The rate of obstetric complications in CMT patients is in accordance with that of the normal population. Exacerbation of CMT (increasing weakness) was reported as a temporary worsening (35%) or persistent disability (65%) during at least one pregnancy in one third of patients.

ASSOCIATED CONDITIONS

- Essential tremor is present in one third of CMT1 cases but is less common in CMT2 cases. Palpable nerve enlargement is seen in 50% of CMT1 cases. Pes cavus and hammertoes are common (not invariable). Associated deafness has been reported in rare families with demyelinating phenotype.

Diagnosis

DIFFERENTIAL DIAGNOSIS

- In sporadic cases or when a reliable family history is unavailable, a broad differential of peripheral neuropathy with an insidious onset and slowly progressive course, as in toxic metabolic and deficiency states, should be ruled out.

SIGNS AND SYMPTOMS

- CMT1: type 1A (70%), 1B (20%), 1C (10%)
- Most common form of hereditary motor and sensory neuropathy manifesting in the first or second decade with distal muscle weakness and atrophy, more prominent in the lower than upper extremities. Latter occurs in about two thirds of cases.
- Loss of distal muscle stretch reflexes (majority areflexic throughout).
- Early age at onset of motor impairment is predictive of a more severe course.
- Sensory complaints are minimal, usually not modality specific. Decreased vibration with preservation of position sense is common.
- CMT2: incidence is about half that of CMT1. For types A, B, and D, onset is in the first or second decade (maybe later). Findings on neurologic examination are similar to CMT1. CMT2C may have an onset in infancy or later, with associated vocal cord paralysis and respiratory muscle weakness from diaphragm, intercostal and laryngeal involvement, and minimal sensory loss.
- CMT3 (Dejerine-Sottas syndrome [DDS]): should be considered a severe phenotypic variant of CMT1. Onset is in infancy or early childhood and includes cases with hypotonia at birth with delayed motor milestones. Generalized limb and trunk weakness with prominent large-fiber sensory loss resulting in ataxia and palpable peripheral nerves is common. Muscle stretch reflexes are absent. Skeletal abnormalities, including kyphoscoliosis, pes cavus, and hammertoes, may be prominent. Cases with recessive inheritance and severe hypomyelination at infancy are now being classified as CMT4 to include EGR2 and PRX gene defects.

LABORATORY PROCEDURES

Electrodiagnosis

- CMT1: uniform slowing (by 25% or more of normal, <40 m/s in arms and <30 m/s in legs)
- CMT2: motor normal or mildly slow (not demyelinating range); sensory nerve action potentials reduced or absent
- CMT3: uniform slowing (<20 m/s in arms, <10 m/s in legs)
- HNPP: focal slowing of conduction velocities and loss in amplitude in relation to compression; may have features of mild generalized demyelinating sensory motor neuropathy
- CMTX: uniform slowing with loss of compound muscle action potentials

Pathology

- CMT1: loss of myelinated nerve fibers; many thinly myelinated fibers; prominent onion bulbs
- CMT2: loss of myelinated nerve fibers; axonal atrophy; clusters of regenerating fibers
- CMT3: severe loss of myelinated nerve fibers; many thinly myelinated fibers; prominent onion bulbs
- HNPP: loss of myelinated nerve fibers; occasionally clustered thinly myelinated fibers; tomaculi (focal sausagelike myelin thickening)
- CMTX: loss of myelinated nerve fibers; axonal atrophy; regeneration-associated onion bulbs

IMAGING STUDIES

- White matter abnormalities in brains are seen rarely in patients with X-linked CMT and HNPP.
- In CMTX cases, nonenhancing and symmetric white matter abnormalities were transient, corresponding to acute transient ataxia, dysarthria, and weakness.

SPECIAL TESTS

- Genetic testing is commercially available for some CMT subclasses. The mode of inheritance, age at onset, and clinical features with electrophysiology should guide the clinician in selecting a candidate gene defect for testing.

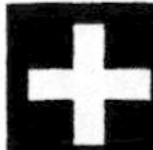

Management

GENERAL MEASURES

- Many patients benefit from ankle-foot orthoses. Appliances may be useful for patients with hand weakness. Patients with DDS phenotype may require knee-ankle-foot orthosis. Patients should be tested to ensure an early diagnosis of possible superimposed diabetes, thyroid dysfunction, or vitamin B_{12} deficiency.

SURGICAL MEASURES

- Corrective surgical procedures for foot deformities may help selected patients, depending on their needs.

SYMPTOMATIC TREATMENT

- A significant number of patients with CMT neuropathies have pain. When neuropathic pain is present, as in the case of idiopathic painful neuropathies, the pain must be treated aggressively with anticonvulsants, tricyclic antidepressants, or antiarrhythmic agents. A monotherapy approach is desirable, but combination therapy might be beneficial in failed cases. Cramping pain can be treated with quinine sulfate.

ADJUNCTIVE TREATMENT

N/A

ADMISSION/DISCHARGE CRITERIA

N/A

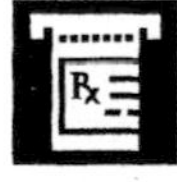

Medications

DRUG(S) OF CHOICE

- There currently is no medical therapy to reverse or slow down the disease process.

Contraindications

N/A

Precautions

- Drugs with neurotoxic side effects, such as cancer chemotherapeutic agents, and particularly those with well-known neurotoxicity, such as vincristine, paclitaxel (Taxol), or doxorubicin (Adriamycin), can result in severe and rapid progression of CMT neuropathy. Patients should be monitored closely while taking such medications or, if possible, switched to less toxic alternatives.

ALTERNATIVE DRUGS

N/A

Follow-Up

PATIENT MONITORING

N/A

EXPECTED COURSE AND PROGNOSIS

- CMT neuropathies usually have an insidious-onset, slowly progressive course with age. Patients with a recent history of notable worsening of their disease should be evaluated for the possibility of superimposed acquired autoimmune neuropathies or metabolic disorders.

PATIENT EDUCATION

- Charcot-Marie-Tooth Association. Website: *www.charcot-marie-tooth.org*
- The Neuropathy Association. Website: *www.neuropathy.org*

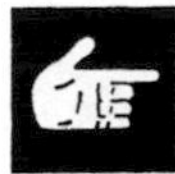

Miscellaneous

SYNONYMS

- Hereditary motor and sensory neuropathies (HMSN, 1975 classification; type I synonymous with CMT1; type II with CMT2 also called neuronal form of peroneal muscular atrophy; type III refers to DDS)

ICD-9-CM: 356.0 Hereditary peripheral neuropathy

SEE ALSO: N/A

REFERENCES

- Berger P, Young P, Suter U. Molecular cell biology of Charcot-Marie-Tooth disease. Neurogenetics 2002;4:1–15.
- Mendell JR, Sahenk Z. Hereditary motor and sensory neuropathies and giant axonal neuropathy. In: Mendell JR, Kissel JT, Cornblath DR, eds. Diagnosis and management of peripheral nerve disorders. New York: Oxford University Press, 2001:429–449.

Author(s): Zarife Sahenk, MD, PhD

Neuropathy, Peripheral

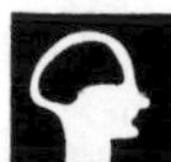

Basics

DESCRIPTION

- Acquired or hereditary disorder of multiple peripheral nerves, with primary injury to sensory and/or motor axons, myelin sheaths, and/or neurons; occasional autonomic involvement. Mononeuropathies are beyond the scope of this chapter.

EPIDEMIOLOGY

Incidence/Prevalence

- Population-based data are sparse, especially by cause. Population prevalence is 2,400 per 100,000 (2.4%), increasing in the elderly to 8,000 per 100,000 (8%). The Neuropathy Association estimates 5%–10% of the US population (about 30 million people) has a polyneuropathy. In the western world, the most common acquired polyneuropathy is diabetes mellitus; worldwide it is leprosy.

Age

- Occurs at all ages.

ETIOLOGY

- Hereditary motor and sensory neuropathies (HMSN), known as Charcot-Marie-Tooth (CMT) or peroneal muscular atrophy. Among many subtypes, the most common are demyelinating type I with secondary axon loss (HMSN I, CMT1) and "axonal" type II (HMSN II, CMT2). Multiple genotypes produce similar phenotypes of different severities, generally with high arched feet, hammertoes, distal weakness (predilection for peroneal muscles causing footdrop), and numbness. Hereditary pattern usually is autosomal dominant (e.g., type Ia, peripheral myelin protein 22 [PMP22] gene duplication on chromosome 17; Ib, myelin protein zero gene on chromosome 1), but occasionally recessive or X linked (e.g., CMTX, connexin 32). Wide range of onset, age, and severity.
- Hereditary neuropathy with liability to pressure palsies (HNPP): autosomal dominant. Deletion in PMP22 on chromosome 17 (converse of HMSN Ia)
- Other hereditary polyneuropathies:
  —Defective DNA repair (Cockayne's syndrome, ataxia telangiectasia)
  —Familial amyloid polyneuropathy
  —Hereditary sensory and autonomic neuropathies (HSAN)
  —Hereditary sensory neuropathies (HSN)
  —Leukodystrophies (metachromatic, globoid cell/Krabbe's), lipoprotein disorders (HDL deficiency/Tangier, abetalipoproteinemia), lysosomal enzyme deficiency (Fabry disease)
  —Peroxisomal disorders (X-linked adrenomyeloneuropathy, Refsum's),
  —Porphyrias (acute intermittent, variegate, others)
  —Miscellaneous: giant axonal neuropathy, myotonic dystrophy, spinocerebellar degenerations, Friedreich's ataxia

RISK FACTORS

- Any genetic predisposition or associated condition listed elsewhere
- Environmental hazards: excessive cold, vibration
- Habits: smoking, alcohol, HIV risks, drugs (cocaine, IV drugs, nitrous oxide)
- Medication toxicity (partial list): amiodarone, chloramphenicol, chloroquine, cisplatin, colchicines, cytarabine, dapsone, disulfiram, ergots, ethambutol, FK-506, gold salts, hydralazine, imipramine, indomethacin, isoniazid, metronidazole, misonidazole, nitrofurantoin, paclitaxel, penicillamine, perhexiline, phenytoin, procainamide, procarbazine, pyridoxine, "statins", sulfonamides, suramin, docetaxel (Taxotere), thalidomide, vincristine
- Occupational toxicity: acrylamide, allyl chloride, arsenic, biphenyls (polychlorinated), cadmium, carbon disulfide, dimethylaminopropionitrile, dichlorodiphenyltrichloroethane (DDT), ethylene oxide, hexacarbons (methyl *n*-butyl ketone, *n*-hexane), lead, mercury, methyl bromide, nitrous oxide, organophosphates, thallium, trichloroethylene, triorthocresyl phosphate, vacor

PREGNANCY

- Generally, heightened risk is associated with specific underlying causes of polyneuropathy (e.g., diabetes, HIV, alcohol), not the polyneuropathy *per se*.

ASSOCIATED CONDITIONS

Immune Mediated

- Collagen vascular diseases
  —Behçet's disease
  —Mixed connective tissue syndrome
  —Relapsing polychondritis
  —Rheumatoid arthritis
  —Scleroderma
  —Sjögren's syndrome
  —Systemic lupus erythematosus
- Demyelinating diseases
  —Acute inflammatory demyelinating polyneuropathy (AIDP; Guillain-Barré [GBS])
  —Chronic inflammatory demyelinating polyneuropathy (CIDP)
  —Multifocal motor neuropathy (MMN)
- Gastrointestinal (celiac disease, inflammatory bowel, primary biliary cirrhosis)
- Granulomatosis
  —Sarcoidosis
  —Wegener's granulomatosis
- Vasculitis
  —Associated with connective tissue syndromes
  —Hypersensitivity
  —Systemic necrotizing vasculitis (polyarteritis nodosa, Churg-Strauss)

Infectious

- Critical-illness polyneuropathy (?mediators of sepsis, ?metabolic)
- Diphtheria
- HIV
- Leprosy
- Lyme disease
- Neurosyphilis (tabes)

Metabolic

- Acromegaly
- Diabetes mellitus
- Hyperlipidemia
- Hypothyroidism, myxedema
- Malabsorption, malnutrition
- Organ system failure (renal, hepatic, pulmonary)
- Porphyria (acute intermittent, variegate)
- Vitamin deficiencies (B_1, cobalamin/B_{12}, E, folate)

Malignancy

- Infiltrating tumor
- Lymphoma, myeloma
- Paraneoplastic (sensory neuropathy or neuronopathy, sensorimotor)

Paraproteins

- Castleman syndrome
- Cryoglobulinemia
- MGUS
- Myeloma
- POEMS syndrome (polyneuropathy, organomegaly, endocrinopathy, M-protein, skin changes), associated with osteosclerotic myeloma
- Primary systemic amyloidosis
- Wäldenstrom's macroglobulinemia

Cryptogenic

- Sensory, sensorimotor

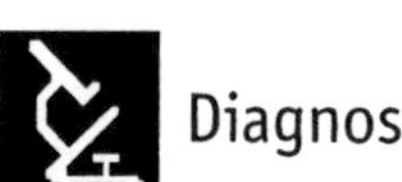

Diagnosis

DIFFERENTIAL DIAGNOSIS

- When confronted with suspected polyneuropathy, the goal is to determine the predominant pathologic process (axon loss vs. demyelination) and likely cause, if possible, to guide specific treatment. An orderly approach is as follows:
  —*Consider whether polyneuropathy is truly present.* Although most patients with polyneuropathy report foot numbness and tingling—usually progressing insidiously from the toes to the balls of feet, then more proximally over plantar and dorsal pedal surfaces—this is not absolutely diagnostic. Occasional patients with CNS disorders (e.g., multiple sclerosis) report "pseudo-neuropathic" distal symptoms but show upper motor neuron (UMN) signs such as hyperreflexia and Babinski signs not observed in polyneuropathy.

—*Consider the time course* (acute over days in AIDP and some toxic neuropathies; subacute over several months in some inflammatory and vasculitic neuropathies; or chronic over many months to many years in most axonal polyneuropathies). Often, polyneuropathies in childhood have a hereditary or inflammatory basis.

—*Consider predisposing medical conditions* (e.g., diabetes), *family history* (e.g., amyloidosis, HMSN), *habits* (see above), and *occupational exposures* (e.g., painters and lead; smelters and arsenic, plastics, and acrylamide; farmers and organophosphate).

—*Consider the anatomic distribution.* At least three fourths of polyneuropathies have a *"fiber-length-dependent" pattern,* commonly known as "stocking glove." Sensory and motor involvement is symmetric, legs > arms and distal > proximal. Predominant pathology is axon loss, mimicked by some chronic inflammatory demyelinating polyneuropathies (CIDP) or confluent mononeuropathy multiplex. Other polyneuropathies show a *proximal ≥ distal pattern,* usually symmetric, such as many demyelinating polyneuropathies (AIDP/GBS, some CIDP). Uncommon polyneuropathies show an *asymmetric or "multifocal" pattern,* such as mononeuropathy multiplex (random lesions, usually vasculitic nerve infarcts, rarely inflammatory or infiltrative). Other multifocal polyneuropathies include MMN and HNPP (formerly known as "tomaculous neuropathy").

—*Consider whether paraesthesias are present and whether sensory symptoms are predominant. "Positive" sensory symptoms* (e.g., tingling, burning, lancinating pain, cutaneous hypersensitivity) are "extra" sensations from abnormal nerves and generally indicate the polyneuropathy is *acquired* (e.g., alcoholic, diabetic). Most acquired axonal polyneuropathies are predominantly sensory or sensory = motor symptomatically, whereas many acquired demyelinating (e.g., AIDP, CIDP, MMN) and most hereditary polyneuropathies (e.g., HMSN I and HMSN II) are motor predominant. The particular quality of the neuropathic pain is not helpful in etiologic diagnosis, beyond the nonspecific but commonplace burning quality of selective small-fiber sensory polyneuropathies. Certain neuropathies are often painful (e.g., alcohol, amyloid, arsenic, cryptogenic, diabetic, neoplastic, porphyric, vasculitic, uremic). Most patients with hereditary polyneuropathies report "negative" symptoms of numbness and weakness without paresthesias (e.g., HMSN); however, many of these patients report nociceptive pain due to tissue stress.

—*Consider whether deep tendon reflexes are reduced out of proportion to muscle weakness, especially proximal areflexia with distal weakness and numbness.* When present, consider demyelinating polyneuropathy (AIDP, CIDP, HMSN I).

—*Consider other informative physical findings.* Palpably enlarged nerves in HMSN I, amyloid, leprosy, occasionally CIDP. Autonomic signs, such as orthostatic hypotension, sweating abnormalities, cold dry extremities, dry eyes and mouth, bowel and bladder dysfunction, and erectile dysfunction, may be seen together or individually in AIDP, porphyria, amyloidosis, and uremia. Other physical findings, including skin changes, are beyond the scope here.

—*Determine if there is selective fiber-type involvement,* which, if present, is etiologically suggestive. Most polyneuropathies are "mixed" in that there is involvement of *large sensory neurons* and their axons (proprioception, vibration, two-point discrimination), *small sensory neurons* and their axons (perception of heat and cold, nonspecific nociception), *motor* neurons and *axons, and* to variable degrees autonomic nerves (postganglionic sympathetic efferents supply arms and legs). Important differential diagnosis of fiber-selective neuropathies includes the following:

- Large sensory neurons and axons (sensory ataxia): paraneoplastic (SCLC), Sjögren's, idiopathic, toxic (excess B_6 >200 mg daily for many months), *cis*-platinum, docetaxel, vincristine), and vitamin deficiency states (B_{12} and E).
- Small sensory neurons and axons (often painful): cryptogenic sensory neuropathy of elderly, diabetes, vasculitis, amyloid, arsenic, Fabry, HIV
- Motor neurons and axons: motor neuron diseases, HMSN II, demyelinating (MMN, AIDP, CIDP), porphyria, lead, dapsone, imipramine
- Autonomic: diabetes, amyloid, AIDP, HIV, vincristine, paclitaxel (Taxol), amiodarone, porphyria, HSAN, idiopathic and paraneoplastic pandysautonomias

SIGNS AND SYMPTOMS

- Numbness (subjective "deadness," loss of vibration, joint position sense)
- Tingling (paresthesias)
- Burning, jabbing (dysesthesias)
- Lancinating pain
- Heat, cold, and/or touch intolerance
- Gait ataxia
- Pseudo-athetosis
- Muscle weakness and fatigability
- Muscle atrophy, sometimes with deformities (e.g., pes cavus)
- Cramping
- Fasciculations
- Myokymia (quivering muscles under skin)
- Hyperhidrosis and anhydrosis
- Sicca complex (dry eyes and mouth)
- Orthostasis
- Sphincter and erectile dysfunction
- Cranial nerve symptoms

LABORATORY PROCEDURES

- A clinically directed approach to laboratory testing of unknown polyneuropathy is more revealing and cost effective than a "shotgun" approach. Rational laboratory testing follows logically from knowing whether the polyneuropathy is acute or subacute/chronic, symmetric or multifocal, predominantly axonal or demyelinating, and fiber-type specific or mixed sensory and motor. Such knowledge requires a *detail-oriented history and neurologic examination, followed by a problem-focused nerve conduction and EMG study designed and performed by a physician well-trained in clinical neurophysiology and neuromuscular diagnosis.*
- Among identifiable polyneuropathies, the most likely cause usually is a known or clinically discernible condition, predisposing genetic disorder, or toxic-metabolic state (e.g., metabolic, medication toxicity, alcoholism, illicit drugs, occupational, environmental). About half of unknown polyneuropathies, especially chronic predominantly axonal polyneuropathies, remain "cryptogenic" after thorough workup, which stands to reason as laboratory tests seek harmful factors extrinsic to nerves, although intracellular causes that cannot be assayed play a role. Commercial "diagnostic panels" for polyneuropathy seldom justify their expense in clinical practice, without clinically driven selection of particular laboratory assays. Until evidence-based and consensus guidelines for polyneuropathy testing are available, the following stepwise testing approach is offered for consideration:
  —*Primary tests* (all patients; need not be repeated if normal within 3–6 months): EMG and nerve conduction studies (NCS). CBC with differential, complete metabolic profile (CMP), fasting blood sugar (FBS), TSH, ESR, RPR, vitamin B_{12}, ANA, rheumatoid factor (RF), serum immunoelectrophoresis (SIEP), UIEP (urine immunoelectrophoresis; note: serum protein electrophoresis [SPEP] may miss a small monoclonal band or a monoclonal present in urine only).
  —*Secondary tests* (often, specific clinical suspicion and/or abnormality above): glucose tolerance test, $HgbA_{Ic}$, methylmalonic acid (especially elderly with serum B_{12} low normal), vitamins B_1 and E, γ-glutamyl transferase (GGT), hepatitis B and C, thyroxine, FTA-ABS, ANA profile (including ds-DNA, SS-A, SS-B), complement (C3, C4, CH50), Lyme titer, HIV, lead and mercury (if motor), arsenic and thallium (if sensory). Chest x-ray film in many for malignancy.

—*Tertiary tests* (uncommon, specific clinical suspicion and/or abnormality above): cryoglobulins, c-ANCA and p-ANCA (especially mononeuropathy multiplex), porphyria (especially motor), angiotensin-converting enzyme, antigliadin Ab (small fiber), lipids (cholesterol, triglycerides, HDL, lipoproteins).
—*Quaternary tests* (rarely, very specific signs, symptoms, and/or family history):
-Acquired polyneuropathies
*G_{M1} ganglioside Ab: MMN; seen in about half of cases; most helpful if NCS does not show conduction block
*Anti-MAG antibody: seen in about half of CIDP cases with IgM MGUS; indicator of refractoriness to conventional immunotherapies.
*Anti-Hu Ab (ANNA-1): paraneoplastic sensory neuropathy; in conjunction with chest x-ray film or CT (identify small-cell lung cancer)
*G_{Q1B} ganglioside: Miller-Fisher variant of AIDP
*Antisulfatide antibody: sensory neuropathies; little practical value
-Hereditary polyneuropathies (selected entities; see Hereditary list)
*HMSN panels (for Charcot-Marie-Tooth): HMSN Ia and Ib, CMT-X
*HNPP: deletion in PMP22 gene locus on chromosome 17
*Transthyretin: suspect amyloid (small-fiber sensory-autonomic neuropathy; other internal organs, often autosomal dominant)

IMAGING STUDIES

- Chest x-ray film (possibly followed by chest CT or other malignancy workup depending on results and clinical suspicion): ?tumor, ?adenopathy
- MRI and CT of spinal cord, occasionally brain: occasionally helps to exclude CNS causes of "pseudo-neuropathic" limb paresthesias and weakness; gadolinium may show root enhancement in demyelinating, infectious, and autoimmune polyradiculoneuropathies or in carcinomatous meningitis
- MRI of brachial or lumbosacral plexus, with gadolinium: very occasional yield for compressive, inflammatory, hypertrophic, infiltrating lesions
- Skeletal survey: paraprotein evaluation for marrow abnormality (plasmacytoma)

SPECIAL TESTS

- Nerve conductions and EMG: essential test to characterize polyneuropathy as likely predominantly axonal or demyelinating, acuteness, and severity.
- Sensory nerve biopsy (usually sural nerve; occasionally superficial peroneal sensory fascicle with peroneus tertius muscle): occasionally performed. Best candidate when suspect "diagnostic" material in nerve, especially epineurial vasculitis (sometimes biopsy peroneus tertius muscle); amyloid; mononuclear cells or edema (inflammation); active myelin breakdown
- CSF: albuminocytologic dissociation in demyelinating polyneuropathies (few or no WBC, elevated protein), such as AIDP and CIDP. HIV-related AIDP has lymphocytic pleocytosis (>50 WBC). CIDP may be associated with very high protein (>125–150 mg/dL). Serologic abnormalities in Lyme polyradiculoneuropathy and neurosyphilis.
- Quantitative sensory testing (QST): measure cold and heat perception, and cold and heat pain, detection thresholds. Quite valuable for small-fiber neuropathy and longitudinal follow-up, pending or during treatment.
- Autonomic testing: quantitative sudomotor axon reflex test (QSART), thermoregulatory sweat test (TST), tilt table (orthostasis), Schirmer's (sicca).
- Cutaneous nerve punch biopsy: verify small-fiber dying-back neuropathy. Specialized technique, with limited availability in few neuromuscular centers.
- Other biopsies: minor salivary gland (Sjögren's), rectal mucosa/fat pad (amyloid).

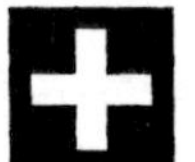

Management

GENERAL MEASURES

- Rational, pattern-recognition, cost-effective approach to diagnostic testing. If unexpected progression occurs during follow-up (clinically, NCS, QST), reopen and widen diagnostic evaluation, including possible nerve biopsy.
- Low threshold for consulting neuromuscular diseases specialized neurologist regarding unexplained polyneuropathy, particularly if progressive in a young patient.
- Treatment of cause—if known—may limit progression or improve neuropathy (e.g., tight glucose control in diabetes, abstinence in alcoholic neuropathy, replete vitamin B_{12} or thyroid if deficient, eliminate neurotoxic exposure).
- Effective immunotherapy for treatable, proven immune-mediated neuropathy.
- Vigorous treatment for neuropathic pain and secondary nociceptive pains.
- Monitor cognitive and psychosocial function on analgesic medications.
- Proactive mitigation of complications of steroids and immunosuppressants (e.g., calcium and biphosphonate therapy with steroids; monitor LFTs, CBC; track cumulative doses of specific immunosuppressants).
- Encourage exercise, as tolerated, and well-balanced diet.
- Discourage megadoses of "alternative" medications, particularly those taken regularly.
- Limit vitamin B_6 to <50 mg/day in polyneuropathy (avoid in sensory neuronopathy).
- Protect limbs with loss of protective sensation from physical and thermal trauma.
- Excellent professional foot and nail care, in appropriate cases (e.g., diabetic).
- Effective pedal arch supports; special shoes as needed (e.g., HMSN).
- Ankle-foot orthoses for footdrop; high shoes for ankle instability.
- Ambulation aids appropriate to sensory ataxia and/or weakness (cane, ideally four-prong; walker, including wheeled walker; wheelchair; electric scooter).
- For severe hypersensitivity, bed cradle over feet to prevent blanket contact.
- Reassure patients with "cryptogenic" sensory/sensorimotor polyneuropathy and elderly patients with "cryptogenic" painful small-fiber neuropathy—after adequate diagnostic evaluation—that recent literature supports usually good prognosis for indolent progression. Follow for unexpected change.
- Medical professionalism. Commitment to ongoing care. Sensitivity to patient's inner experience of disease. Goal is to support capability for a full life.

SURGICAL MEASURES

- Nerve biopsy: selective, recognizing possible persisting pain at biopsy site.
- Other biopsies: skin, minor salivary gland, abdominal fat pad, rectal mucosa, marrow. Conservative approach to surgery of incidental spinal stenoses, unless severe.

SYMPTOMATIC TREATMENT

- Pain management: Neuropathic pain may respond to empirically applied single agents or combinations of low-dose tricyclics, antiepileptic drugs (gabapentin, topiramate, carbamazepine, others), topical analgesics (lidocaine crème or patch, capsaicin), mexiletine, clonidine, opioids (selected). Nociceptive pain may respond to nonsteroidal antiinflammatory drugs (NSAIDs) and cyclooxygenase 2 (COX2) inhibitors. Associated chronic myofascial pain may respond to selective serotonin reuptake inhibitor and tricyclics. Control of secondary nociceptive pain (joints, ligaments): NSAIDs. Nonpharmacologic approaches (e.g., biofeedback, exercise, meditation).
- Autonomic dysfunction: artificial tears, pharmacologic and nonpharmacologic approaches to orthostatic hypotension, support hose, caffeine, midodrine.

ADJUNCTIVE TREATMENT

- Depression: judicious antidepressants; counseling (individual and family), support groups, psychiatrist or psychologist; exercise (important)
- Physical therapy: strengthening, flexibility, endurance range-of-motion
- Occupational therapy: upper extremity adaptive aids; thickened utensil handles; custom splints; work-hardening occupational assessment
- Durable goods; ankle-foot orthoses, cane, walker, wheelchair, scooter

ADMISSION/DISCHARGE CRITERIA

- AIDP: initial monitored setting (telemetry, q shift forced vital capacity until trend clear).
- Elective intravenous immunoglobulin (IVIG) and PLEX (selected cases)
- Immunosuppression complications

Medications

DRUG(S) OF CHOICE

- AIDP/GBS: PLEX and IVIG equivalent efficacy; avoid corticosteroids
- CIDP: corticosteroids, PLEX, IVIG, azathioprine, cyclosporine
- Connective tissue syndromes: treat primary condition, vasculitis if present
- Deficiency states: replete deficient vitamins, nutritional factors
- Familial amyloid polyneuropathy: liver transplantation
- MMN: IVIG, cyclophosphamide, rituximab
- Osteosclerotic myeloma and POEMS syndrome: radiation and/or surgery
- Paraproteinemias (including MGUS): PLEX, IVIG, immunosuppression
- Vasculitis: corticosteroids, cytotoxic agents

ALTERNATIVE DRUGS

- α-Lipoic acid (omega-3)

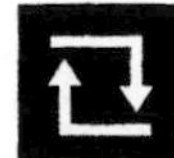

Follow-Up

PATIENT MONITORING

- Variable, depending on cause

EXPECTED COURSE AND PROGNOSIS

- Variable, depending on cause

PATIENT EDUCATION

- Charcot-Marie-Tooth Association (CMTA), 2700 Chestnut Street, Chester, PA 19013-4867. Phone: 800-606-CMTA, website: *www.charcot-marie-tooth.org*
- Guillain-Barre Syndrome Foundation International (GBSFI), P.O. Box 262, Wynnewood, PA 19096. Phone: 610-667-7036, website: *www.guillain-barre.com*
- Muscular Dystrophy Association-USA (MDA; support and advocacy for 43 neuromuscular diseases, including CMT and Friedreich's ataxia). National Headquarters, 3300 East Sunrise Drive, Tucson, AZ 85718. Phone: 800-572-1717, website: *www:mdausa.org*
- The Neuropathy Association (public, nonprofit organization established by people with neuropathy and their families or friends to help those who suffer from disorders that affect the peripheral nerves), 60 East 42nd Street, New York, NY 10165-0999. Phone: 212-692-0662, website: *www.neuropathy.org*

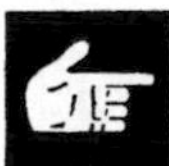

Miscellaneous

SYNONYMS

- Neuropathy polyradiculoneuropathy

ICD-9-CM: 277.3 Autonomic amyloidosis; 337.0 Autonomic idiopathic; 357.2 Diabetic neuropathy; 357.6 Drug-induced neuropathy; 357.7 Toxic induced (arsenic, lead, organophosphates); 356.0 Hereditary; 356.2 Hereditary sensory; 356.4 Idiopathic progressive; 356.8 Idiopathic other specified; 356.9 Idiopathic neuropathy

SEE ALSO: N/A

REFERENCES

- Anonymous. Appropriate number of plasma exchanges in Guillain-Barre syndrome. The French Cooperative Group on Plasma Exchange in Guillain Barre Syndrome. Ann Neurol 1997;41:298–306.
- Barohn RJ. Approach to peripheral neuropathy and neuronopathy. Semin Neurol 1998;18:7–18.
- Bromberg MB, Smith AG. Toward an efficient method to evaluate peripheral neuropathies. J Clin Neuromusc Dis 2002;3:172–182.
- Hughes RAC. Peripheral neuropathy. BMJ 2002;324:466–469.
- Katirji B, Kaminski HJ, Preston DC, et al. Neuromuscular disorders in clinical practice. Boston: Butterworth-Heinemann, 2002.
- Lacomis D. Small-fiber neuropathy. Muscle Nerve 2002;26:173–188.
- Mendell JR, Kissel JT, Cornblath DR. Diagnosis and management of peripheral nerve disorders. New York: Oxford, 2001.
- Wolfe G, Baker NS, Amato AA, et al. Chronic cryptogenic sensory polyneuropathy: clinical and laboratory characteristics. Arch Neurol 1999;56: 540–547.
- Wolfe GI, Kaminski HJ. Autoantibody testing in neuromuscular disorders, part I: peripheral neuropathies. J Clin Neuromusc Dis 2000;2:84–95.

Author(s): Glenn A. Mackin, MD

Neuropathy, Vasculitic

Basics

DESCRIPTION

- Vasculitis is a term that covers a diverse group of disorders in which inflammatory changes destroy blood vessel walls, resulting in ischemia and thrombosis. Inflammatory changes typically result from dysfunctional immunologic mechanisms, but they also occur as a direct consequence of infections. Peripheral nerve damage occurs when inflammation affects the vasa nervorum supplying individual nerves. This most commonly is part of a systemic illness, although peripheral neuropathy may be the sole manifestation of vasculitis. The vasculitides are commonly distinguished by their organ system involvement and the size of the blood vessels pathologically affected.

EPIDEMIOLOGY

Incidence

- The exact incidence of vasculitic neuropathy is unknown. In polyarteritis nodosa, which is considered the most common systemic necrotizing vasculitis, approximately 60% of individuals have peripheral nerve involvement, equating to roughly 5 cases per million people.

Age

- More common at older ages (mean age of onset 60 years)

Sex/Gender

- There is no clear sex or racial predominance.

ETIOLOGY

- Autoimmune disease is the presumed pathologic mechanism, although this remains largely unproven. An inciting antigen is thought to trigger a cascade involving humoral or cellular responses, resulting in leukocyte adherence to the endothelial surface of blood vessel walls. Inflammatory changes then damage the endothelial surface, and the blood vessel may undergo necrosis. The immunologic hypothesis stems from the fact that vasculitides occur with connective tissue diseases, malignancies, and hypersensitivity drug reactions, or in association with infections including syphilis, Lyme disease, rickettsia, human immunodeficiency virus, cytomegalovirus, and *Cryptococcus*.

Genetics

N/A

RISK FACTORS

- Vasculitis occurs in the setting of connective tissue disease, drugs, infections, and malignancy.

PREGNANCY

- There is no known relationship with pregnancy.

ASSOCIATED CONDITIONS

- Peripheral nerve vasculitis is often part of a wider systemic illness. Other organ manifestations that may occur with peripheral nerve involvement include coronary artery disease (Kawasaki disease), necrotizing glomerulonephritis (Wegener's granulomatosus, microscopic polyangiitis), respiratory tract inflammation and eosinophilia (Churg-Strauss), skin disorders (HSP, cryoglobulinemia, leukocytoclastic vasculitis), arthritides (rheumatoid arthritis), and polymyalgia rheumatica (temporal arteritis).

Diagnosis

DIFFERENTIAL DIAGNOSIS

- The differential diagnosis includes diabetic mononeuropathy multiplex, and infectious or carcinomatous causes of polyradiculopathy. Autoimmune conditions, such as multifocal acquired demyelinating sensory and motor neuropathy, may also mimic vasculitic mononeuropathy multiplex. Guillain-Barré syndrome should be considered in cases with more acute onset and symmetric neuropathic involvement. Other conditions with a clinical presentation resembling vasculitic neuropathy include Sjögren's-related sensory neuronopathy, amyloidosis neuropathy, sarcoidosis, and toxic neuropathies related to heavy metal exposure (e.g., arsenic, thallium).

SIGNS AND SYMPTOMS

- Vasculitic neuropathy typically presents as asymmetric weakness and sensory loss in the distribution of multiple individual nerves. Clinical involvement most commonly occurs in the peroneal and ulnar distributions. Symptoms occur acutely or subacutely, and progress in a stepwise pattern to involve one nerve after another. Pain and dysesthesia are common (50%–80%), usually noted at the onset of peripheral nerve damage. Sensory loss and weakness conform to individual peripheral nerves and typically are apparent on neurologic examination. Constitutional symptoms of fever, myalgias/arthralgias, and weight loss are common, and their presence, along with skin, lung, kidney, or joint involvement, should help point to a systemic illness. Besides mononeuritis multiplex, other clinical presentations may occur, including a rapidly progressive, areflexic paralysis resembling Guillain-Barré syndrome, and a slowly progressive, symmetric, distal sensorimotor polyneuropathy. Gradual overlapping involvement of multiple individual peripheral nerves may lead to the appearance of a symmetric distal or generalized sensorimotor polyneuropathy.

LABORATORY PROCEDURES

- Laboratory studies, including complete blood cell count, erythrocyte sedimentation rate, coagulation panel, serum chemistries, liver function tests, urinalysis, serum protein electrophoresis, rheumatoid factor, antinuclear antibody, extractable nuclear antigen antibodies, serum complements, and cryoglobulins, help to identify more widespread systemic disease. Additional testing, aimed at identifying a vasculitis-related illness, include HIV, Lyme titer, syphilis serologies, serum angiotensin-converting enzymes, chest x-ray film, cytoplasmic (c) ANCA (Wegener's granulomatosus), and perinuclear (p) ANCA (Churg-Strauss, microvascular polyangiitis). Cerebrospinal fluid analysis is of limited utility.

IMAGING STUDIES

- There are no specific imaging abnormalities.

SPECIAL TESTS

- *Nerve conduction studies* reveal a multifocal sensorimotor axonopathy with reduced amplitude compound motor and sensory nerve action potentials. Sensory changes tend to be more prominent, and the lower extremities are affected more than the upper extremities. Distal latencies and conduction velocities typically are normal. A few reports describe primarily demyelinating features and motor conduction block, which may be apparent if testing is performed within 1 week of symptom onset. Subclinical abnormalities in asymptomatic nerves may help with diagnosis in difficult cases.
- *Needle electromyography (EMG)* typically demonstrates active denervation (fibrillations, positive sharp waves) and decreased recruitment patterns most severely affecting the distributions of individual peripheral nerves where weakness is present.
- *Nerve biopsy* provides pathologic confirmation of vasculitic neuropathy. The sural, superficial peroneal, or superficial radial nerves are most commonly biopsied. Biopsy features of vasculitis include lymphocytic inflammatory cell infiltration within the blood vessel wall, endothelial cell destruction, fibrinoid necrosis, intimal hyperplasia, vascular sclerosis, and perivascular inflammation. Simultaneous muscle biopsy, looking for inflammatory changes in blood vessels supplying small nerve twigs entering muscle, may increase the diagnostic yield compared to nerve biopsy alone. Overall, the need for diagnostic confirmation by muscle or nerve biopsy is greatest in cases of isolated peripheral nerve vasculitis when there is often no evidence of systemic involvement; it has the least value in cases where systemic disease is obvious.

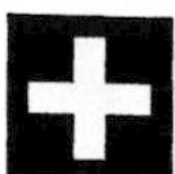

Management

GENERAL MEASURES

- The four basic principles of vasculitic neuropathy management are (i) removal of the inciting antigen (drug reaction, infections, malignancy); (ii) immunosuppressive therapy, (iii) treatment of vaso-occlusion, and (iv) supportive/adjunctive care.

SURGICAL MEASURES

N/A

SYMPTOMATIC TREATMENT

- Neuropathic pain is common. Effective medications include tricyclic antidepressants (amitriptyline, nortriptyline); antiepileptic medications (gabapentin, phenytoin [Dilantin], carbamazepine [Tegretol]); mexiletine; topical creams (capsaicin, lidocaine); transdermal medications (lidocaine patch, fentanyl patch); and scheduled opioid therapy (methadone). Trials of these various medications can be managed through routine clinic visits, but recalcitrant pain may require management by a pain specialist.

ADJUNCTIVE TREATMENT

- Physical and occupational therapy assist in maintenance of strength, flexibility, and functional ability in the setting of neurologic impairment from vasculitic neuropathy. Ankle-foot orthoses may be required for footdrop, and splints may be required to stabilize and protect weakened extremities. Once the underlying vasculitis is under control, aggressive physical therapy may be required to hasten strength recovery.

ADMISSION/DISCHARGE CRITERIA

- Hospital admission is not commonly required, unless the neuropathy is particularly severe and rapidly progressive.

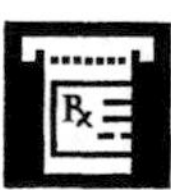

Medications

DRUG(S) OF CHOICE

- *Immunosuppression:* In vasculitic neuropathy associated with systemic necrotizing vasculitis, a *combination* of prednisone (1.5 mg/kg daily) and a cytotoxic agent (cyclophosphamide 2 mg/kg PO daily, or 500–600 mg/m^2 IV pulse every 4 weeks) is recommended. Mesna can be administered intravenously with pulse IV cyclophosphamide to reduce the risk of hemorrhagic cystitis. If clinical improvement is noted, prednisone is then tapered by 5–10 mg every 2–4 weeks. The cytotoxic agent usually is discontinued after 6–12 months. In cases where there is no clinical response, alternative cytotoxic medications, including azathioprine, methotrexate, or cyclosporine, may be considered. Prednisone alone may be sufficient if the neuropathy is slowly progressive, if there is no systemic involvement, or in the setting of temporal arteritis or hypersensitivity reaction. High-dose steroid induction with methyl prednisone (15 mg/kg qd for 3–5 days) may be necessary if the neuropathy is severe or rapidly progressing.
- *Vaso-occlusion:* Antiplatelet therapy with aspirin (81–325 mg daily) may help reduce thromboxane-induced vasoconstriction and platelet activation that is not covered by glucocorticoid administration. Calcium channel blockers may also be helpful.

Contraindications

- Prednisone should be used under supervision in poorly controlled diabetes mellitus or hypertension. Cyclophosphamide may impair renal or liver function and may lead to bone marrow suppression or opportunistic infection. Both prednisone and cyclophosphamide should be used cautiously during pregnancy.

Precautions

- Side effects of long-term prednisone use include weight gain, glucose intolerance, osteoporosis, cataracts, hypertension, acne, and myopathy. Cyclophosphamide may cause hemorrhagic cystitis, bladder and hematologic malignancies, gastrointestinal symptoms, and alopecia.

ALTERNATIVE DRUGS

- Both intravenous immunoglobulin and plasmapheresis have been considered as possible therapies, but no reports demonstrate specific improvement in vasculitic neuropathies.

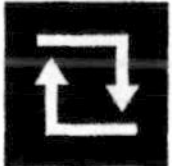

Follow-Up

PATIENT MONITORING

- Patients should be seen frequently when there is active vasculitis and when immunosuppressive therapy is initiated. Follow-up should focus on clinical change, adjustment of medications, and monitoring of adverse effects. Blood testing for patients on cyclophosphamide should include a monthly complete blood count, electrolytes, liver function tests, and urinalysis. Patients on prednisone should be monitored for symptoms of diabetes. Dietary consultation and TB skin testing may be considered before initiating prednisone therapy.

EXPECTED COURSE AND PROGNOSIS

- There are no long-term, prospective studies specific to vasculitic neuropathy. However, 25%–50% of patients with systemic vasculitis fail to respond to therapy or may relapse during treatment. In addition, 40% experience drug-related side effects and up to 85% experience disease-related morbidity primarily involving other organ systems. As in most neuropathies associated with significant axonal damage, clinical stabilization and improvement can be expected, although recovery often is protracted and incomplete.

PATIENT EDUCATION

- There are no specific therapies, activities, or dietary restrictions related to vasculitis. Nutritional therapists may instruct patients regarding appropriate dietary changes while taking prednisone. Information about peripheral nerve vasculitis is available from the following:
  —American Autoimmune Related Diseases Association, Inc. Website: *www.aarda.org*
  —Neuropathy Association. Website: *www.neuropathy.org*

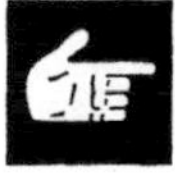

Miscellaneous

SYNONYMS

- Peripheral nerve vasculitis
- Mononeuritis multiplex

ICD-9-CM: 447.6 Vasculitis; 354.5 Mononeuritis multiplex

SEE ALSO: N/A

REFERENCES

- Barohn RJ. Approach to peripheral neuropathy and neuronopathy. Semin Neurol 1998;18:7–18.
- Collins MP, Kissel JT, Mendell JR. Vasculitic neuropathies. In: Antel JP, Birnbaum G, Hartung HP, eds. Clinical neuroimmunology. Boston: Blackwell Science, 1998:316–339.
- Collins MP, Mendell JR, Periquet MI, et al. Superficial peroneal nerve/peroneus brevis muscle biopsy in vasculitic neuropathy. Neurology 2000;55:636–643.

Author(s): Patrick M. Grogan, MD; Jonathon S. Katz, MD

Nonepileptic Seizures

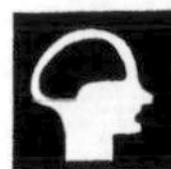

Basics

DESCRIPTION

- Nonepileptic seizures (pseudoseizures) are spells of paroxysmal behavior that resemble epileptic seizures without electroencephalographic evidence of abnormal brain electrical activity during the event. They are most often characterized by convulsive activity but also may present with periods of stiffening, unresponsiveness, staring, or a variety of abnormal behaviors. Almost any type of abnormal behavior may be called a seizure and present for evaluation. Nonepileptic seizures usually are not stereotyped (vary from occurrence to occurrence) and remain refractory to antiepileptic drugs (AEDs). Unlike epileptic seizures, which almost always are $\leq$2 minutes in duration, nonepileptic seizures may go on for many minutes or even hours, frequently waxing and waning.
- Usually all previous evaluations have been normal, including EEGs, neuroimaging (MRI, CT head), and neurologic examination. The best diagnostic data come from a well-performed EEG during an episode of pseudoseizure activity that shows a normal background and no electrographic seizure activity.

EPIDEMIOLOGY

Incidence/Prevalence

- The overall incidence is unknown, but approximately 25%–30% of patients who are monitored at a tertiary epilepsy center are diagnosed with pseudoseizures.

Age

- Usually presents in adulthood

Race

- No apparent predisposition for race

Sex

- From 50%–80% of patients are women. (Note: Gates study quotes 80% female, but other studies reported equal male and female [Gulick TA, Spinks IP, King DW. Pseudoseizures: ictal phenomena. Neurology 1982;32:24–30].)

ETIOLOGY

- The etiology of nonepileptic seizures is not well understood. Most nonepileptic seizures are believed to be conversion symptoms and result from psychological factors. The cause of conversion symptoms in general is controversial. One hypothesis is that conversion symptoms represent an expression of an unconscious psychological need or conflict that has been repressed. Another hypothesis is that conversion symptoms are an unconscious means for patients to obtain secondary gain in the form of support or services.

Genetics

- There are no genetic studies.

RISK FACTORS

- Patients with lower levels of education are at higher risk. In addition, patients with a number of psychiatric diagnoses, including dissociative identity disorder, hypochondriasis, and somatization disorder, are at greater risk. Victims of physical, sexual, or emotional abuse are at significantly increased risk. Some patients with nonepileptic seizures also have true epilepsy (10%–34%), so epilepsy may be a risk factor. Note that because psychiatric diagnoses are common in the epilepsy population, just the presence of psychopathology may not help in the diagnosis.

PREGNANCY

- There is no association with pregnancy.

ASSOCIATED CONDITIONS

- Dissociative disorder, somatization disorder, hypochondriasis, conversion disorder, history of physical or sexual abuse

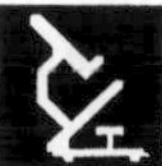

Diagnosis

DIFFERENTIAL DIAGNOSIS

- Epilepsy including frontal lobe epilepsy (which may be very hard to detect with EEG)
- Syncope
- Malingering
- Nonepileptic myoclonus
- Sleep disorders, including narcolepsy and cataplexy, periodic limb movements, night terrors
- Paroxysmal movement disorders
- Panic disorder

SIGNS AND SYMPTOMS

- The manifestations may be extremely varied but usually involve some shaking or unresponsiveness. Symptoms occur often but certainly not always during times of stress. Features that may suggest pseudoseizures rather than true seizures include gradual onset, waxing and waning of symptoms, a long duration, conspicuous absence of postictal confusion, crying during the spell, out-of-phase clonic movements of the limbs, and suggestibility.

LABORATORY PROCEDURES

- CBC, chemistries, AED levels

IMAGING STUDIES

- MRI is the preferred form of neuroimaging. As with epilepsy patients, it is important to rule out a structural pathology in this population.

SPECIAL TESTS

- EEG is indicated; if EEG is normal and an episode is not captured, prolonged EEG recording may be needed. Inpatient video-EEG is the preferred test. This test lasts from 1 to several days as needed. Outpatient ambulatory EEG may be adequate but is prone to artifact that is confounding. Use of suggestion may needed at the time of the EEG to assist patients in having one of their typical spells. Patients with pseudoseizures commonly will respond to suggestion during recording, whereas patients with epilepsy will rarely have a seizure with suggestion.
- If syncope is suspected, Holter ECG monitoring may be indicated, as may be carotid noninvasive testing and neuroimaging (MRI usually is preferable to CT). If disorders of sleep or arousal are suspected, a polysomnogram or multiple sleep latency test may be indicated.

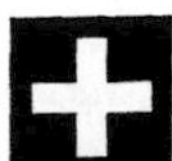

Management

GENERAL MEASURES

- Presenting the patient and his/her family with the diagnosis is the first step to management. It may be the most difficult step. This must be done in a nonconfrontational style. The patient or family may not initially accept the diagnosis. If the patient and/or family are alienated, they may go to other physicians and be treated for the wrong diagnosis or have to repeat the previous evaluations. The neurologist should follow-up with the patient, and AEDs (if any) should be gradually tapered off on an outpatient basis as long as there is no evidence that the patient also has epileptic seizures. *Most* patients are not aware that the events are psychologically mediated. Patients should not be viewed as "crazy" but rather as having inappropriate reaction to some unconscious conflict. They need to be referred to a psychiatrist or psychologist. Treatment by the psychologist/social worker/psychiatrist may include insight-oriented psychotherapy, behavioral therapy, family therapy, hypnosis, and drug therapy.

SURGICAL MEASURES

N/A

SYMPTOMATIC TREATMENT

- Psychotherapy, including psychodynamic therapy, behavioral therapy, family therapy, and hypnosis

ADJUNCTIVE TREATMENT

- Some patients require antidepressant medications during their outpatient treatment.

ADMISSION/DISCHARGE CRITERIA

- In-patient video-EEG monitoring is warranted in patients for whom the diagnosis of pseudoseizures is suspected but not proven. Inpatient monitoring is also indicated if the patient is suspected of having both epileptic and nonepileptic seizures. Sometimes it is important to know which type of seizures (if there is more than one type) is epileptic and which is not. The patient should be discharged when the diagnosis is no longer in doubt.

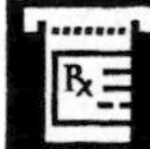

Medications

DRUG(S) OF CHOICE

- There are no recommended medications, but antidepressants and/or anxiolytics are often used. Patients may often be taking multiple AEDs prior to diagnosis; such polypharmacy should be reduced to a minimum.

Contraindications

N/A

Precautions

N/A

ALTERNATIVE DRUGS

N/A

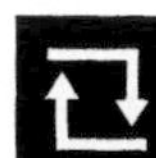

Follow-Up

PATIENT MONITORING

- The patient ideally should be followed by both mental health professionals and a neurologist initially. Taper of AEDs is best handled by the neurologist, if necessary. As the patient improves, the follow-up with neurology can be gradually extended and then terminated when both parties are comfortable.

EXPECTED COURSE AND PROGNOSIS

- Prognosis is better when the diagnosis is made and treatment is commenced closer to the start of the pseudoseizures. A small but significant percentage of patients will improve after learning that the seizures are not epileptic. The rest will need a multidisciplinary approach that may take many months of therapy.

PATIENT EDUCATION

- The only reading materials widely available are books and journal articles, some of which are listed below. There is no organization that acts as an advocate for these patients.

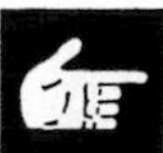

Miscellaneous

SYNONYMS

- Hysterical pseudoseizures
- Pseudoepileptic seizures
- Hysteroepilepsy
- Psychogenic seizures

ICD-9-CM: 300.11 Conversion; 300.14 Dissociative identity disorder; 300.81 Somatization disorder (Briquet's syndrome); 300.70 Somatoform disorder; 301.51 Factitious disorder with physical symptoms

SEE ALSO: N/A

REFERENCES

- Chabolla DR, Krahn LE, So EL, et al. Psychogenic nonepileptic seizures. Mayo Clin Proc 1996;71:493–500.
- Lempert T, Schmidt D. Natural history and outcome of psychogenic seizures: a clinical study in 50 patients. J Neurol 1990;237: 35–38.
- Shen W, Bowman ES, Markand ON. Presenting the diagnosis of pseudoseizure. Neurology 1990;40:756–759.

Author(s): J. Layne Moore, MD

Opsoclonus

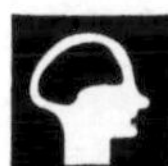

Basics

DESCRIPTION

Opsoclonus affects both eyes and consists of back-to-back saccades (rapid eye movements) in the horizontal, vertical, and torsional planes. It can be continuous, or intermittent, and represents the most dramatic acquired eye movement disorder when the saccades are of large amplitude. The descriptive term saccadomania has been used to describe its striking manifestations. Opsoclonus, however, can also be of very small amplitude, and may require careful observation of the eyes for detection. Other neurologic signs such as ataxia, myoclonus, and an encephalopathic state are commonly associated with opsoclonus.

EPIDEMIOLOGY

Incidence/Prevalence

Opsoclonus is a relatively rare disorder.

Race

Opsoclonus shows no ethnic preference.

Age

Age at presentation depends on the etiology and ranges from infancy to old age.

Sex

Opsoclonus shows no gender preference.

ETIOLOGY

- Opsoclonus has multiple etiologies but in a considerable number of cases the underlying disease process remains undetermined. It is most commonly seen in the context of cancer, and as a parainfectious disorder. In both circumstances the pathophysiology is presumed to be autoimmune with antibodies damaging neurons involved in ocular motor control. Pathologically, damage to pontine structures, possibly including saccade-suppressing omnipause neurons, has been described. Loss of inhibitory input to cerebellar nuclei has also been theorized to produce opsoclonus.
- Opsoclonus occurring in infants and young children is associated with neural crest tumors (neuroblastoma, ganglioneuroma) in more than 50% of the cases. However, only 2% to 3% of children with these tumors develop opsoclonus. Of these patients, 62% also have myoclonus and ataxia. In adults the most common cancers causing opsoclonus as a paraneoplastic syndrome include small cell lung and breast cancers. Numerous other neoplasms have also been implicated (ovarian, bladder, renal, thyroid, pancreatic, transitional cell carcinomas, malignant melanoma, and T-cell lymphoma). It has been estimated that 20% of all adult opsoclonus cases are of paraneoplastic origin.
- Opsoclonus as a parainfectious disorder may be preceded by a viral prodrome, usually on the order of a few days. Coxsackie, parainfluenza, Epstein-Barr virus, and enterovirus are most commonly implicated. Other infections include AIDS, salmonellosis, psittacosis, syphilis, Lyme, and rickettsial diseases.
- Among the rarer etiologies of opsoclonus are the following:
  - —Drug toxicity: phenytoin, amitriptyline, lithium, cocaine, diazepam
  - —Inborn errors of metabolism: biotin responsive carboxylase deficiency
  - —Toxic metabolic states: hyperosmolar nonketotic coma, hyperphosphatasemia, thallium, organophosphates, toluene, strychnine, chlordecone
  - —Demyelinating disorders: multiple sclerosis, acute disseminated encephalomyelitis

RISK FACTORS

N/A

PREGNANCY

N/A

ASSOCIATED CONDITIONS

N/A

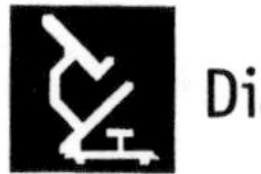

Diagnosis

DIFFERENTIAL DIAGNOSIS

Ocular flutter also consists of back-to-back saccadic oscillations of both eyes. In contrast to opsoclonus, however, ocular flutter occurs only intermittently, and the oscillations are restricted to the horizontal plane. Etiologies of both disorders overlap and they likely represent a pathophysiologic continuum. However, several disease processes have been reported to cause only ocular flutter. These include cyclosporine toxicity, malaria, and carbohydrate-deficient glycoprotein syndrome type Ia.

SIGNS AND SYMPTOMS

Onset of opsoclonus is usually subacute. Visual complaints are nonspecific and range from mild blurring to frank oscillopsia (the visual illusion of movement of stationary objects). Myoclonus, dysarthria, and variable degrees of truncal and appendicular ataxia often coexist, and patients may complain of vertigo and nausea. Encephalopathic states are more commonly associated with paraneoplastic opsoclonus and may be severe. Opsoclonus can be elicited by fixation and gaze shifting and persists during sleep. The frequency of oscillations ranges from 6 to 15 Hz. Very small amplitude opsoclonus may be detectable only during direct ophthalmoscopy.

LABORATORY PROCEDURES

- Obtain urine catecholamines and homovanillic acid in suspected neuroblastoma, and anti-Ri (breast, ovarian cancer) and anti-Hu autoantibodies (small cell lung cancer, neuroblastoma) in suspected paraneoplastic opsoclonus. Note that the presence of these autoantibodies indicates a very high likelihood of cancer, even if the oncologic workup is negative. Repeat testing after several months is mandatory, as delays between the emergence of opsoclonus and tumor detection of up to 1 year have been reported. Even in the absence of autoantibodies, a workup for cancer is required in all adults presenting with opsoclonus.
- Antiviral antibodies and other screens for infectious disorders are indicated when an underlying infectious process is suspected. The sensitivity for detecting a viral CNS infection can be increased by performing polymerase chain reaction (PCR) on the cerebrospinal fluid.

IMAGING STUDIES

MRI of the brain is unrevealing in the majority of cases. Imaging studies of the lungs, breasts, abdomen, and pelvis are elements of the oncologic workup. Octreotide scanning is a sensitive screen for the detection of neural crest tumors.

SPECIAL TESTS

N/A

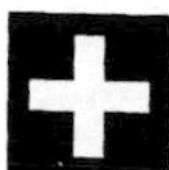

Management

GENERAL MEASURES

- New-onset opsoclonus warrants hospital admission, particularly if other symptoms such as ataxia, myoclonus, and encephalopathy coexist.
- The multitude of etiologies requires diagnostic and therapeutic approaches tailored to each patient. In paraneoplastic opsoclonus two main management strategies need to be applied: treatment of the underlying malignancy and suppression of the immune response against nervous system targets. In adults, the latter is usually attempted with corticosteroids, intravenous immunoglobulin (IVIG), plasma exchange, or immunoabsorption, with the latter being preferred by some. In select cases, several immunomodulatory measures may need to be tried sequentially before a treatment response is achieved.
- Children with neuroblastoma-related opsoclonus respond acutely to adreno-corticotropic hormone (ACTH) or prednisone. Early treatment success, however, needs to be followed up with long immunosuppressant measures (see below), as untreated patients often show a progressive course of developmental and behavioral abnormalities.
- Postinfectious opsoclonus generally has a benign, but sometimes protracted, course. Corticosteroids are commonly applied in this situation. However, concern about potentiating an underlying infection, particularly in children, may make IVIG a better choice. In view of the high rate of spontaneous improvement and unpredictable disease course, it has not been possible to define the value of immunomodulatory treatment in this situation.

SURGICAL MEASURES

N/A

SYMPTOMATIC TREATMENT

Aside from immunomodulatory therapies, benzodiazepines, Mysoline, gabapentin, and thiamine have been tried in the symptomatic treatment of opsoclonus and myoclonus. Unfortunately, no well-designed treatment trials exist to guide the clinician.

ADJUNCTIVE TREATMENT

N/A

ADMISSION/DISCHARGE CRITERIA

N/A

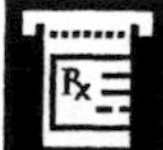

Medications

DRUG(S) OF CHOICE

N/A

ALTERNATIVE DRUGS

N/A

Follow-Up

PATIENT MONITORING

N/A

EXPECTED COURSE AND PROGNOSIS

- Opsoclonus that is not related to neoplastic disease has a much more favorable prognosis than the paraneoplastic variant. Postinfectious opsoclonus, nonetheless, may require weeks or months to resolve and relapses can occur. Complete recovery is common, but mild deficits, such as truncal ataxia, may remain.
- Children with neural crest tumors show a high initial response rate to ACTH or prednisone, but ongoing immunosuppression is often required. A significant proportion of children show signs of permanent CNS injury and of a possibly progressive encephalopathy presenting with expressive language disturbances, attentional deficits, irritability, and delayed motor and cognitive development. Intercurrent illnesses may precipitate recurrences of ataxia and myoclonus. Such patients require long-term treatment with prednisone or other immunosuppressants (methotrexate).
- The least favorable prognosis is encountered in adults with paraneoplastic opsoclonus, especially when an encephalopathic state coexists. Immunoabsorption, and other immune therapies do not show consistent benefit and even responders may be left with permanent cerebellar dysfunction such as truncal ataxia. Occasionally, however, patients may show resolution of opsoclonus after successful tumor removal, and rare patients have improved spontaneously without cancer treatment. Compared to other adult paraneoplastic syndromes, opsoclonus appears to have a somewhat more favorable prognosis.

PATIENT EDUCATION

N/A

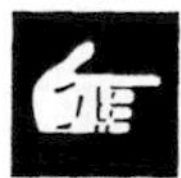

Miscellaneous

SYNONYMS

Opsoclonus-myoclonus syndrome (OMS), opsoclonus-myoclonus-ataxia syndrome, opsoclonus myoclonus ataxic encephalopathy (OMAE), dancing eyes and dancing feet (childhood opsoclonus, myoclonus), saccadomania.

ICD-9-CM: 379.59 Irregular eye movements not elsewhere classified

SEE ALSO: N/A

REFERENCES

- Antunes NL, Khakoo Y, Matthay KK, et al. Anti-neuronal antibodies in patients with neuroblastoma and paraneoplastic opsoclonus-myoclonus. J Pediatr Hematol Oncol 2000;22:315–320.
- Averbuch-Heller L, Remler B. Opsoclonus. Semin Neurol 1996;16:21–26.
- Bataller L, Graus F, Saiz A, et al. , for the Spanish Opsoclonus-Myoclonus Study Group. Clinical outcome in adult onset idiopathic or paraneoplastic opsoclonus-myoclonus. Brain 2001;124:437–443.
- Hasaerts DE, Gorus FK, DeMeirleir LJ. Dancing eye syndrome and hyperphos-phataemia. Pediatr Neurol 1998;18: 432–434.
- Hayward K, Jeremy RJ, Jenkins S, et al. Long-term neurobehavioral outcomes in children with neuroblastoma and opsoclonus-myoclonus-ataxia syndrome: relationship to MRI findings and anti-neuronal antibodies. J Pediatr 2001;139:552–559.
- Mitchell WG, Davalos-Gonzalez Y, Brumm VL, et al. Opsoclonus-ataxia caused by childhood neuroblastoma: developmental and neurologic sequelae. Pediatrics 2002;109:86–98.
- Moretti R, Torre P, Antonello RM, et al. Opsoclonus-myoclonus syndrome: gabapentin as a new therapeutic proposal. Eur J Neurol 2000;7:455–456.
- Rudnick E, Khakoo Y, Antunes NL, et al. Opsoclonus-myoclonus-ataxia syndrome in neuroblastoma: clinical outcome and anti-neuronal antibodies—a report from the Children's Cancer Group Study. Med Pediatr Oncol 2001;36:612–622.

Author(s): Bernd F. Remler, MD

Optic Neuritis

Basics

DESCRIPTION

Optic neuritis refers to inflammation of the optic nerve with variable demyelination. Optic neuritis may be acute, chronic, or subclinical. Acute optic neuritis is most common and is characterized by sudden, usually unilateral vision loss, which progresses over hours to days. The central visual disturbance may be mild or severe. Many patients notice color desaturation and difficulty seeing in dim illumination. Ninety percent of patients have mild to moderate pain in or around the eye, usually worse with eye movement.

EPIDEMIOLOGY

Incidence

Approximately 6 per 100,000. Peak incidence is in the third and fourth decades.

Sex

The female to male ratio is approximately 2:1.

ETIOLOGY

Optic neuritis occurs as the initial symptom of MS in 35% to 62% and is likely a forme fruste of MS in its isolated form.

Causes of Optic Neuritis Other Than MS

- Viral and parainfectious causes—adenovirus, Coxsackie, cytomegalovirus, HIV, hepatitis A, Epstein-Barr virus, measles, mumps, rubella, varicella zoster, herpes zoster
- Postvaccination
- Syphilis
- Lyme disease
- Tuberculosis
- *Mycobacterium pneumoniae*
- Sarcoidosis
- Vasculitides (systemic lupus erythematosus, Wegener's)
- Autoimmune
- Sinus infection
- Bee venom
- Toxoplasmosis
- Cat scratch disease

RISK FACTORS

Patients with known MS are at significant risk of optic neuritis.

PREGNANCY

Little is known concerning the relationship between pregnancy and optic neuritis. In patients with MS, there is a diminished risk of new exacerbations including optic neuritis, especially during the third trimester.

ASSOCIATED CONDITIONS

In patients presenting with isolated optic neuritis, the risk of developing MS is approximately 30% after 5 to 7 years. In long-term follow-up studies (up to 30 years), 75% of women and 34% of men developed clinically definite MS.

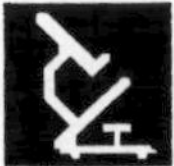

Diagnosis

DIFFERENTIAL DIAGNOSIS

Numerous infectious or inflammatory disorders other than demyelinating disease may cause optic neuritis. Acute optic neuritis can usually be distinguished from other conditions on clinical grounds. History is usually suggestive with compressive optic neuropathy from intracranial tumors, anterior ischemic optic neuropathy, sinus disease, and radiation-induced optic neuropathy. Patients presenting with bilateral anterior optic neuritis should be evaluated for papilledema. Leber's hereditary optic neuropathy (LHON), a mitochondrial disorder usually causing bilateral central visual loss, may mimic optic neuritis, especially in young men in early stages before the fellow eye is involved.

Optic Neuropathies and Ophthalmic Conditions Mimicking Optic Neuritis

- Neuro-retinitis
- Big blind spot syndrome
- Leber's hereditary optic neuropathy
- Diabetic papillitis
- Ischemic optic neuropathy
- Central retinal vein occlusion
- Venous stasis retinopathy
- Optic disc drusen
- Central serous retinopathy
- Carcinomatous meningitis
- Infiltrating neoplasm (lymphoma)
- Radiation-induced optic neuropathy
- Paraneoplastic disorder

SIGNS AND SYMPTOMS

- The diagnosis is a clinical one. Examination should confirm optic nerve dysfunction. Central acuity is usually reduced, but 10% of patients have preserved central vision of at least 20/20. Patients who retain normal or near-normal acuity often have reduced color vision and contrast sensitivity out of proportion to central visual disturbance.
- Virtually all patients with unilateral optic neuritis have a relative afferent pupillary defect (RAPD or Marcus Gunn pupil) in the affected eye. A RAPD may be demonstrated objectively by the swinging flashlight test, or subjectively by asking the patient to compare brightness of a light source in the affected and unaffected eyes.
- Central visual field loss (central scotoma) is the hallmark of optic neuritis, accounting for over 90% of the visual field defects. However, virtually any visual field defect can occur, including cecocentral, paracentral, arcuate, hemialtitudinal, hemianopic, peripheral constriction, and diffuse suppression. The optic disc may appear normal in retrobulbar optic neuritis (approximately two thirds of patients), inspiring the adage "the patient sees nothing and the physician sees nothing." In anterior optic neuritis (or papillitis), the disc may be swollen. Hemorrhage at the disc margin occurs in less than 6% of patients.
- The optic disc may become pale weeks after the initial episode. Transient reversible neurologic dysfunction in response to exercise or exposure to heat is referred to as Uhthoff's symptom (after the German ophthalmologist). Uhthoff's symptom should raise suspicion of, but is not pathognomonic for, MS.

LABORATORY PROCEDURES

Blood Work

The following tests should be considered: CBC/differential, thyroid function tests, vitamin B_{12} and folate levels, RPR, ANA, RF, anti-SSA, anti-SSB, p & c ANCA, HIV, serum and/or CSF angiotensin-converting enzyme level, lyme titer, immunofixation, CSF studies including IgG index and synthesis rate, oligoclonal bands, cryptococcal antigen, AFB smear and culture, cytology, and hypercoagulable studies in selected patients (including anticardiolipin antibodies, protein C & S, antithrombin III, activated protein C resistance, factor V Leiden, plasma viscosity, homocysteine, fibrinogen).

IMAGING STUDIES

Lesions in the optic nerve may be difficult to detect with conventional MRI. Gadolinium enhancement on MRI is demonstrated in the optic nerves of the majority of patients with acute optic neuritis with newer techniques of fat suppression. In most patients, enhancement is no longer observed 1 month after the onset of optic neuritis and correlates with recovery of visual acuity and improvement of visual evoked potential (VEP) amplitudes.

Abnormalities on MRI in the periventricular and other white matter areas are seen in 30% to 70% of patients with isolated optic neuritis and in 90% to 98% of patients with clinically definite MS. The presence of lesions on MRI is a strong predictor of the risk of developing clinically definite MS. Cranial MRI should be considered in an attempt to establish a diagnosis, facilitate counseling of the individual regarding risk of MS, and to guide decisions for treatment.

SPECIAL TESTS

Visual Field Testing

Confrontational visual field techniques may be used for screening, but are insensitive compared to Goldmann perimeter or automated threshold perimetry.

Neurophysiologic Studies

Visual evoked potentials (VEPs) record electrical activity of the occipital lobe in response to visual stimuli. Optic neuritis typically causes prolongation of the latency and decreased amplitude of the P100, the first large positive peak occurring approximately 100 msec after stimulus. Pattern reversal stimulus presentation yields more reproducible results. However, flash VEP can be used to confirm visual pathway integrity when the P100 is not seen with pattern VEPs. Abnormalities of the VEP indicate dysfunction at any point along the visual pathways from the retina to the striate cortex, and are not pathognomonic for demyelinating optic neuropathy. Other disorders can cause VEP disturbance (e.g., compressive lesions, congenital optic nerve anomalies, glaucoma, hereditary and toxic optic neuropathy, and papilledema).

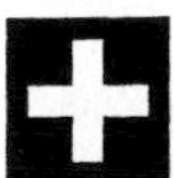

Management

GENERAL MEASURES

The disparity of visual functioning between the two eyes is often sufficient to provoke headache and ocular discomfort. Analgesic agents should be used as necessary. Patching the involved eye for a few days may be helpful if the interocular visual functioning is highly disparate.

SURGICAL MEASURES

N/A

SYMPTOMATIC TREATMENT

There are currently no approved therapies for the symptomatic complaints associated with optic neuritis. In those who experience Uhthoff's phenomenon, high temperatures should be avoided. Ingestion of ice-cold liquids or the use of cooling devices may also be helpful.

ADJUNCTIVE TREATMENT

Formal evaluation by an ophthalmologist is suggested to maximize visual function with refractive techniques and to exclude potentially treatable ophthalmic conditions.

ADMISSION/DISCHARGE CRITERIA

Patients with optic neuritis can be treated with IV corticosteroids in the hospital or at home. Diabetes mellitus and uncontrolled hypertension are comorbidities that may warrant hospitalization.

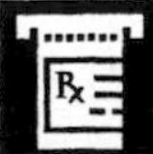

Medications

DRUG(S) OF CHOICE

- Corticosteroids have long been the cornerstone of therapy for optic neuritis despite conflicting studies of effectiveness.
- In most patients 1,000 mg/d of methylprednisolone may be administered as a single daily intravenous infusion for 3 to 5 days, followed by a tapering dose of oral prednisone (starting at 100 mg for 4 days and then tapering by 10 mg every other day) over 2 to 4 weeks.
- Oral prednisone, at least in conventional doses of 1 mg/kg/d, is contraindicated as the sole treatment, although some practitioners are exploring the use of higher doses (2–5 mg/kg/d or more).

Contraindications

In patients with a suspected infectious etiology, corticosteroids should be withheld until appropriate antibiotic therapy is instituted.

Precautions

Common adverse events related to high-dose corticosteroid treatment include gastric irritation, insomnia, euphoria, depression, and occasionally psychosis, tachycardia, hypertension, hypokalemia, hyperglycemia, increased appetite and fluid retention. Pretreatment with an H2 blocker for GI prophylaxis and potassium supplementation should be considered.
A single morning dose of corticosteroids may reduce the risk of insomnia. Blood pressure, potassium, and glucose levels should be monitored. Those with diabetes or hypertension require more careful monitoring that often includes the use of sliding-scale insulin. Mild tranquilizers are effective for insomnia.

ALTERNATIVE DRUGS

While controlled studies are lacking, some consider treating steroid recalcitrant visual loss with either intravenous immunoglobulin (IVIG) or plasma exchange.

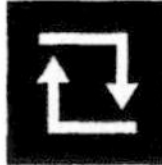

Follow-Up

PATIENT MONITORING

Patients should be reexamined after steroid therapy to exclude a further decline in visual function.

EXPECTED COURSE AND PROGNOSIS

The natural course of acute optic neuritis is variable. Visual deficits typically worsen over a few days to 2 weeks. Most patients then recover rapidly, achieving most of their improvement by 5 weeks. Some continue to recover for up to a year. The mean visual acuity 12 months after the onset is 20/15. Fewer than 10% have visual acuity less than 20/40 at 1 year. Despite recovery of vision to "near normal," most patients are aware of residual visual dysfunction due to deficits in contrast sensitivity, color vision, and depth perception.

PATIENT EDUCATION

See Multiple Sclerosis.

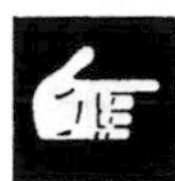

Miscellaneous

SYNONYMS

Inflammatory optic neuropathy
Retrobulbar optic neuritis
Optic papillitis

ICD-9-CM: 377.3 Optic neuritis; 377.30 Optic neuritis, unspecified; 377.31 Optic papillitis; 377.32 Retrobulbar neuritis

SEE ALSO: N/A

REFERENCES

- Beck RW. Optic neuritis. In: Miller NR, ed. Walsh and Hoyt's clinical neuro-ophthalmology, 5th ed. Baltimore: Williams & Wilkins, 1998.
- Beck RW, Cleary PA, Anderson MM, et al. A randomized, controlled trial of corticosteroids in the treatment of acute optic neuritis. N Engl J Med 1992;326:581–588.
- Newman NJ, ed. Walsh and Hoyt's clinical neuro-ophthalmology, 5th ed. Baltimore: Williams & Wilkins, 1998:599–647.
- Optic Neuritis Study Group. The clinical profile of optic neuritis: experience of the optic neuritis treatment trial. Arch Ophthalmol 1991;109:1673–1678.
- Optic Neuritis Study Group. The five-year risk of multiple sclerosis after optic neuritis; experience of the Optic Neuritis Treatment Trial. Neurology 1997;49: 1404–1413.
- Sedwick LA. Optic neuritis. Neurol Clin 1991;9:97–114.

Author(s): Elliot M. Frohman, MD, PhD

Orthostatic Hypotension

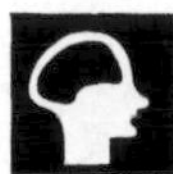

Basics

DESCRIPTION

Clinically, it is important to recognize mild degrees of autonomic failure that present as orthostatic intolerance (OI), postural tachycardia syndrome (POTS) or syncope. Orthostatic hypotension (OH) is a dominant feature of severe autonomic failure. For example, autonomic neuropathy in amyloidosis or diabetes is widespread, progressive, and hallmarks an unfavorable prognosis. OI is defined as (a) symptoms triggered by standing and relieved in supine position, (b) heart rate increase >30 bpm or >120 bpm, and (c) blood pressure is normal or increased. Orthostatic hypotension is defined as (a) blood pressure fall >20/10 mm Hg for 3 minutes, (b) with or without symptoms of cerebral hypoperfusion, and (c) loss of heart rate increase indicates severe autonomic failure. Neurogenic syncope is triggered by reflex mechanism and may occur with both conditions.

EPIDEMIOLOGY

Incidence/Prevalence

In the U.S. 500,000 patients have orthostatic intolerance.

Race

N/A

Age

Orthostatic intolerance may affect all ages. Orthostatic hypotension is more common in the middle aged and the elderly.

Sex

Female > male; multiple system atrophy (MSA) male > female.

ETIOLOGY

Genetics

Unknown, except for familial dysautonomia [Riley-Day syndrome in Ashkenazi Jews on chromosome 9 (q31)].

RISK FACTORS

Falls, injury.

PREGNANCY

- OI—generally improvement during pregnancy
- OH—determined by primary diagnosis

ASSOCIATED CONDITIONS

- Orthostatic intolerance
  - —Small fiber neuropathy
  - —Excessive venous pooling/deconditioning/ prolonged bed rest/weightlessness
  - —Hypovolemia
  - —β-receptor supersensitivity
  - —Brainstem dysregulation, Arnold-Chiari malformation
- Orthostatic hypotension
- Primary autonomic failure
  - —Pure autonomic failure (PAF)
  - —MSA with parkinsonian, cerebellar, and pyramidal features
  - —Acute and subacute pandysautonomia
- Secondary autonomic failure
  - —Peripheral autonomic neuropathy (diabetes, amyloidosis)
  - —Dopamine-β-hydroxylase deficiency (DBH)
  - —Guillain-Barré syndrome
  - —Paraneoplastic (Lambert-Eaton syndrome—small cell lung carcinoma)
  - —Brain tumors—posterior fossa
  - —Autoimmune and collagen disorders (Sjögren syndrome)
  - —Tabes dorsalis
  - —HIV infection
  - —Familial dysautonomia (Riley-Day)

Diagnosis

DIFFERENTIAL DIAGNOSIS

- Non-neurogenic orthostatic intolerance
  - —Anxiety
  - —Cardiogenic syncope
  - —Tachyarrhythmias/bradyarrhythmias
  - —Seizures, pseudoseizures
  - —Porphyria
  - —Pheochromocytoma
  - —Anemia
- Non-neurogenic orthostatic hypotension
  - —Cardiac impairment (myocardial infarction, myocarditis)
  - —Impaired cardiac filling/output (e.g., aortic stenosis, cardiomyopathy, heart failure)
  - —Nephrogenic (nephropathy, hemodialysis)
  - —Blood/plasma loss—hemorrhage, burns, sepsis
  - —Fluid/electrolyte loss—vomiting, diarrhea, fluid loss
  - —Increased intracranial pressure
  - —Drug-induced—centrally acting agents that reduce sympathetic activity (clonidine, methyldopa, reserpine, barbiturates, anesthetics)
    - -Peripheral—guanethidine, bethanidine
    - -α-blockers—prazosin, phenoxybenzamine
    - -β-blockers—propranolol, pindolol, timolol, etc.
    - -Vasodilators—nitrates, alcohol
    - -Diuretics

SIGNS AND SYMPTOMS

- Light-headedness
- Dizziness
- Blurred vision
- Fatigue
- Nausea
- Gastrointestinal symptoms
- Palpitations
- Shortness of breath, hyperventilation, dyspnea
- Headache
- Memory loss (OH in elderly)

LABORATORY PROCEDURES

- ECG normal; Holter monitoring shows episodes of sinus tachycardia.
- Standing plasma catecholamines are increased in some OI patients, but reduced in OH.
- Reduced ACTH and β-endorphin can distinguish OH due to MSA vs. PAF (normal).
- Reduced growth hormone and melatonin in dopamine-β-hydroxylase deficiency.

IMAGING STUDIES

- OI—MRI typically normal; Arnold-Chiari malformation, cervical stenosis (rare)
- OH—MSA—T2-weighted images show putamen hypointensity, olivo-ponto-cerebellar atrophy. Positron emission tomography shows reduced reuptake of F-dopa in MSA.

SPECIAL TESTS

Diagnosis of autonomic failure is made using a battery of autonomic tests:

- Tilt table testing is done at 60 to 80 degrees for 5 to 45 minutes without medications. OI shows sinus tachycardia (>100 bpm) for at least 5 minutes with normal or increased blood pressure. POTS is severe form of OI with orthostatic heart rate >120 bpm. OH shows sustained blood pressure drop >20/10 mm Hg for 3 minutes. Loss of heart rate increment indicates severe autonomic failure. Isoproterenol/nitroprusside infusions are used for evaluation of syncope.
- Heart rate variation to deep breathing and bradycardia/tachycardia ratio during Valsalva maneuver is typically reduced.
- Quantitative sudomotor axon reflex test (QSART)—stimulation of postganglionic sudomotor fibers using iontophoresis of 10% acetylcholine chloride. QSART may be normal in OI but is typically reduced with OH due to peripheral neuropathy.
- Thermoregulatory sweat test—body is covered by alizarin powder and temperature is raised by 1°C. Sweating is indicated by red coloration. Typically, in diabetic neuropathy, sweating is lost in stocking/gloves distribution.

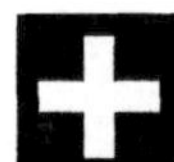

Management

GENERAL MEASURES

Treatment of orthostatic hypotension includes a combination of volume expansion, pressor agents, and supportive measures.

SURGICAL MEASURES

Tumor removal
Brainstem decompression in Arnold-Chiari malformation

SYMPTOMATIC TREATMENT

- Liberalize fluid and salt intake.
- Review all medications to determine if any that might be contributing to orthostasis may be discontinued, especially diuretics, antihypertensive agents, antianginal agents, and antidepressants.
- Have patient move from supine to sitting and standing positions in gradual stages.
- Head-up tilt bed—elevation of bed to 20-degree angle activates the renin-angiotensin-aldosterone system and decreases nocturnal diuresis.
- Elastic body garments (custom-fitted stockings with graded pressure, abdominal binder inflatable, or Easy-wraps)

ADJUNCTIVE TREATMENT

N/A

ADMISSION/DISCHARGE CRITERIA

Frequent loss of consciousness (LOC)/ improvement of orthostatic tolerance.

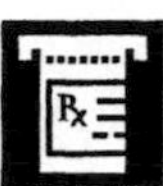

Medications

DRUG(S) OF CHOICE

Orthostatic Intolerance

- Fludrocortisone 0.05 mg PO bid; weekly increase to 0.1–0.3 mg PO bid
  - —3- to 6-lb weight gain is desirable.
  - —Side effects: 50% hypokalemia, 50% hypomagnesemia, peripheral edema
- Sodium chloride (salt tablets): 50 mEq or 1,200 mg PO tid
  - —Side effects: peripheral edema
- Propranolol (Inderal) 10–40 mg PO qid
- Pindolol (Visken) 2.5–5.0 mg bid to tid

Orthostatic Hypotension

- Fludrocortisone (Florinef) 0.05 mg PO bid; weekly increase to 0.1–0.3 mg PO
  - —Side effects: see above
- Sodium chloride: see above
- ProAmatine (Midodrine): starting dose 5 mg tid up to 40 mg/d, last dose before supper.
  - —Side effects: sensation of goose flesh (chills), scalp pruritus; urinary retention; supine hypertension; may increase urinary Na^+ loss.
- Caffeine 250 mg (2 cups) in the morning and 1 cup with meals (postprandial hypotension)
- Erythropoietin (Epoetin alfa) 25–75 mg U/kg IV or SC three times weekly (only for severe autonomic failure)
- Octreotide (Somatostatin) 25 μg SC bid with increase to 100–200 μg tid
- Clonidine (Catapres—α_2-agonists) 0.1–0.3 mg given as 0.2–0.8 mg bid to tid
  - —Indications: autonomic failure due to efferent sympathetic lesion. Note that patients with peripheral lesion become hypotensive.

Contraindications

- Fludrocortisone, ProAmatine—CHF
- Erythropoietin—hypersensitivity to human albumin
- Clonidine—caution with β-blockers; tricyclic antidepressants may cause rebound hypertension

Precautions

Monitor supine hypertension, peripheral edema, and congestive heart failure.

ALTERNATIVE DRUGS

- Orthostatic intolerance: disopyramide 150 mg qid or 300 mg bid
- Orthostatic hypotension: ephedrine sulfate 12.5–25 mg, PO tid

Follow-Up

PATIENT MONITORING

If no improvement of symptoms, repeat tilt study on medications.
Monitor supine hypertension (24-hour BP monitoring might be useful).

EXPECTED COURSE AND PROGNOSIS

Orthostatic Intolerance

Good prognosis—majority of patients improve over time.

Orthostatic Hypotension

- Knowing precise diagnosis is important for prognosis.
- Diabetic neuropathy—increased risk for death/arrhythmias
- MSA survival 5 years from diagnosis
- PAF survival >10 years

PATIENT EDUCATION

Activities

Countermaneuvers (squatting, leg crossing, toe raising, marching, bending forward, abdominal contraction); supine exercise (leg lifting, weight pressing), swimming; relaxation. Avoid overheating and straining maneuvers. Schedule activities for the afternoon since the symptoms are typically worse in the morning.

Diet

High sodium and 2–2.5 L of fluids; small, more frequent, low-carbohydrate meals.

Organizations

The National Dysautonomia Research Foundation, contact person: Linda J. Smith (Email: *ndrf@ndrf.org,* phone: 715-594-3140; fax: 715-594-3140; website: *http://www.ndf.org*)

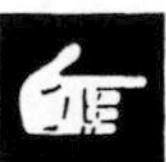

Miscellaneous

SYNONYMS

Orthostatic Intolerance

Postural orthostatic tachycardia syndrome, orthostatic tachycardia, Da Costa syndrome, soldier's heart, effort syndrome, mitral valve prolapse syndrome, neurocirculatory asthenia, idiopathic hypovolemia, chronic fatigue syndrome, vasoregulatory asthenia, partial dysautonomia, irritable heart

Neurally Mediated Syncope

Neurocardiogenic, vasovagal, vasodepressor

Orthostatic Hypotension

- Multiple system atrophy: Shy-Drager syndrome, olivopontocerebellar degeneration (OPCA), striatonigral degeneration
- Pure autonomic failure: Bradbury-Eggleston syndrome

ICD-9-CM: 780.4 Dizziness; 780.02, 780.4 Near syncope; 780.2 Syncope; 780.39 Convulsive disorder—nonepileptic seizure; 458.0 Orthostatic hypotension; 337.9 Autonomic disorder—nonspecified; 333.0 MSA, Shy-Drager Syndrome; 337.1 Autonomic neuropathy

SEE ALSO: N/A

REFERENCES

- Kaufmann H. Syncope. A neurologist's viewpoint [review]. Cardiol Clin 1997;15: 177–194.
- Low PA. Autonomic nervous system function [review]. J Clin Neurophysiol 1993;10:14–27.
- Low PA, Opfer-Gehrking TL, Textor SC, et al. Postural tachycardia syndrome (POTS) [review]. Neurology 1995;45:S19–25.
- Mathias CJ. Orthostatic hypotension: causes, mechanisms, and influencing factors. Neurology 1995;45(suppl 5): S6–S11.
- Morillo CA, Ellenbogen KA, Fernando Pava L. Pathophysiologic basis for vasodepressor syncope [review]. Cardiol Clin 1997;15: 233–249.
- Novak V, Novak P, Opfer-Gehrking TL, et al. Clinical and laboratory indices that enhance the diagnosis of postural tachycardia syndrome (POTS). Mayo Clin Proc 1998;73:1141–1150.
- Robertson D, Davis TL. Recent advances in the treatment of orthostatic hypotension. Neurology 1997;45(suppl 5): S26–S32. 1997.
- Schondorf R, Low PA. Idiopathic postural orthostatic tachycardia syndrome: an attenuated form of acute pandysautonomia? Neurology 1993;43:132–137.

Author(s): V. Novak, MD, PhD

Paraneoplastic Neurologic Syndromes

Basics

DESCRIPTION

Paraneoplastic neurologic syndromes are disorders of the nervous system pathogenetically related to an underlying systemic malignancy, but not due to direct tumor invasion or other indirect effects of cancer.

EPIDEMIOLOGY

Incidence/Prevalence

These disorders are extremely rare and occur in <1% of patients with cancer. Small cell lung cancer has the highest incidence, followed by breast cancer, ovarian cancer, and Hodgkin's disease

Race

No known racial or ethnic predisposition.

Age

Most patients are older than 40. Paraneoplastic opsoclonus-myoclonus (POM) may occur in very young children and infants with neuroblastoma.

Sex

Reflects the sex distribution of the underlying cancer.

ETIOLOGY

- The etiology is unknown, although an inflammatory, immune-mediated mechanism is suspected. Specific serum and CSF onco-neuronal antibodies are detectable in a large percentage of patients. While these antibodies do not appear to be pathogenic, their presence confirms the diagnosis of paraneoplastic disease. Moreover, they are useful markers to prompt search for underlying malignancy, which is occult at the time of neurologic diagnosis in over 50% of patients. Many of these antibodies share specificity to antigens expressed by cells of the CNS and antigens expressed by systemic tumors. These syndromes may result from intrathecal synthesis of some as yet undiscovered antineuronal antibody or from cell-mediated immunity directed against the underlying cancer. The absence of serum or CSF onco-neuronal antibodies does not exclude the diagnosis of paraneoplastic disease.
- A specific area of the nervous system is targeted in each of these syndromes. In patients with paraneoplastic cerebellar degeneration (PCD), the focus of the injury is the cerebellar Purkinje cells. In POM, the pathology is most commonly limited to the brainstem and cerebellum. Patients with paraneoplastic encephalomyelitis/paraneoplastic sensory neuronopathy (PEM/PSN) suffer symptoms related to injury to the limbic structure, cerebellum, and dorsal root ganglia. There is a good deal of clinical overlap been theses syndromes.

Genetics

No known genetic predisposition.

RISK FACTORS

N/A

PREGNANCY

There is no known association between paraneoplastic disorders and pregnancy.

ASSOCIATED CONDITIONS

Systemic malignancy

Diagnosis

DIFFERENTIAL DIAGNOSIS

PCD/POM/PEM

- Primary or metastatic tumor of the cerebellum
- Toxic/metabolic disorders causing ataxia (5-FU, ARA-C, anticonvulsant medications, lithium, alcohol, vitamin B_{12} or B_1 deficiency, heavy metal poisoning, Wilson's disease, etc.)
- Brainstem or cerebellar infarct/hemorrhage
- Infection (bacterial, fungal, or parasitic abscess, encephalitis, PML)
- Demyelinating disease
- Heritable ataxias
- Toxic or metabolic encephalopathy (diabetic hyperosmolar nonketotic coma, lithium, thallium, amitriptyline overdose, toluene, strychnine)
- Hydrocephalus
- Brain metastases
- Cerebral vasculitis
- Multiple cerebral infarcts

PSN

- Acute or chronic inflammatory demyelinating polyradioneuropathy (AIDP/CIDP)
- Monoclonal gammopathy associated polyneuropathy
- Diabetic polyneuropathy
- Vasculitic neuropathy (particularly Sjögren's syndrome)
- B_{12} deficiency
- Toxic neuropathies (vitamin B_6 overdose, chlorobiphenyl, thalidomide)
- Idiopathic subacute sensory neuronopathy

SIGNS AND SYMPTOMS

PCD

- Subacute, progressive pancerebellar dysfunction (may be asymmetrical)
- Gait and limb ataxia
- Dysarthria
- Dysphagia
- Diplopia/nystagmus/oscillopsia
- Vertigo

POM

- Involuntary, arrhythmic, conjugate vertical and horizontal eye movements
- Opsoclonus persists during sleep
- Diffuse or focal myoclonus of virtually any voluntary muscle
- Truncal or head titubation
- Cerebellar ataxia
- Nausea/vomiting
- Vertigo/oscillopsia
- Cognitive abnormalities

PEM/PSN

- Subacute dementia or delirium
- Focal or generalized seizures
- Psychosis
- Spastic hemiparesis/quadriparesis
- Cerebellar ataxia
- Parkinsonism
- Limb anesthesia/paresthesia
- Neuropathic pain
- Sensory ataxia
- Lower motor neuron weakness, fasciculation, and muscle wasting
- Dysautonomia

LABORATORY PROCEDURES

- Blood work: a subset of patients have serum autoantibodies that react with CNS cell antigens and sometimes the underlying tumor.
  —PCD: anti-Yo or APCA; anti-Hu or ANNA-1; Anti-Ri or ANNA-2
  —POM: A subset of adult patients will have circulating serum and CSF antibodies to neural antigens. When opsoclonus occurs as a component of PCD, APCA (anti-Yo) and ANNA-1 (Anti-Hu) antibodies have been noted. ANNA-2 (Anti-Ri) antibody has been found in some female patients with POM and breast or pelvic cancers.
  —PEM/PSN: anti-Hu or ANNA-1
- While not pathogenic, these antibodies point to the causal malignancy. Anti-Yo (APCA) is associated with breast, ovarian, and uterine cancer. Anti-Hu (ANNA-1) is associated with small cell cancers and Anti-Ri (ANNA-2) is seen in association with breast cancer. These antibodies are specific but not sensitive. A patient may harbor a paraneoplastic nervous system disease but be seronegative for antibodies.
- Testing for all three of the above-mentioned antibodies is appropriate in an adult patient with opsoclonus-myoclonus, an otherwise unexplained diffuse encephalopathy or a severe, predominantly sensory polyneuropathy.
- PEM/PSN: Serologic testing to rule out underlying infection (CBC and differential, ESR, and blood cultures if febrile), toxic-metabolic disorders (sodium, calcium, magnesium, liver and renal function tests), and vasculitis (ESR, ANA, RF, ENA, and ANCA) should be performed. Serum and urine immunoelectrophoresis, fasting glucose, serum B_{12} level, and urine heavy metals may also be appropriate.

IMAGING STUDIES

- Neuroimaging is important to rule out alternative causes. Early in the evolution of PCD, POM, and PEM, CT and MRI of the head may be normal. After several months, marked diffuse cerebellar atrophy is usually noted in PCD. Nonspecific areas of abnormal T2 signal abnormalities have been described in some patients with POM and PEM. After several months, brainstem, cerebral, and cerebellar atrophy is often noted.
- An aggressive search for an underlying malignancy should be undertaken. This may include total body CT, mammogram, liver function tests, bone scan, or other tests deemed appropriate by the oncologist. Some have advocated an exploratory laparotomy in patients with APCA (Anti-Yo), if pelvic imaging and mammography are negative, to search for an occult tumor. Pediatric patients should have testing to detect a thoracic or abdominal neuroblastoma. In patients seropositive for ANNA-1 (Anti-Hu), bronchoscopy is indicated even if chest CT or MRI is normal.

SPECIAL TESTS

- Lumbar puncture: after neuroimaging has excluded a mass, CSF should be examined to exclude hemorrhage and infection. Approximately 50% of patients with PCD, POM, and PEM/PSN will have nonspecific inflammatory changes of CSF including a modest increase in protein, CSF lymphocytic pleocytosis, increased IgG index, and the presence of oligoclonal bands.
- PEM/PSN
  - —Electroencephalography may demonstrate diffuse or asymmetric cerebral slowing and focal or multifocal epileptiform activity.
  - —Nerve conduction studies typically show reduced/absent sensory nerve action potentials with relatively preserved compound muscle action potential amplitudes and conduction velocities. EMG may show evidence of muscle denervation.

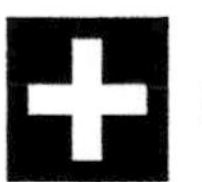

Management

GENERAL MEASURES

Supportive care is paramount to avoid secondary complications like aspiration pneumonia, decubiti, urinary tract infection, deep venous thrombosis, and injury from falls.

SURGICAL MEASURES

N/A

SYMPTOMATIC TREATMENT

Physical therapy may assist with gait and avoidance of joint contractures.

ADJUNCTIVE TREATMENT

N/A

ADMISSION/DISCHARGE CRITERIA

Admission may be required for hydration and evaluation for oncologic workup and exclusion of other neurologic disorders.

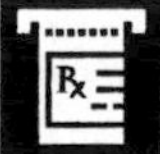

Medications

Unfortunately, there is no specific therapy for these disorders. There are reports of spontaneous remission or improvement with treatment of the underlying cancer. Treatment with thiamine and clonazepam has produced neurologic improvement in anecdotal cases of POM. Pediatric POM associated with neuroblastoma often responds to treatment with corticosteroids, although most patients will be left with residual neurologic deficits. Immunosuppressant medications, intravenous immunoglobulin (IVIG), and plasmapheresis are often tried without significant improvement, although there have been occasional reports of response.

DRUG(S) OF CHOICE

N/A

ALTERNATIVE DRUGS

N/A

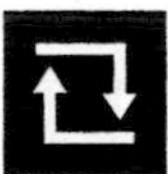

Follow-Up

PATIENT MONITORING

If malignancies are not found on the initial evaluation, periodic reevaluations for malignancy should be conducted.

EXPECTED COURSE AND PROGNOSIS

- In most patients, PCD is permanent and disabling. The disease progresses rapidly over a period of weeks or months and then stabilizes. Most patients will be wheelchair- or bed-bound from their disease.
- The prognosis of adult-onset POM is highly variable. Spontaneous remissions or improvement after treatment of the underlying cancer are frequently noted. Many patients suffer residual disability from cerebellar ataxia. Although childhood cases associated with neuroblastoma do remit with corticosteroid therapy, most children are left with permanent neurologic deficits.
- The onset and course of PEM/PSN is usually subacute and progressive. Most patients stabilize with very severe neurologic deficits. Remission is extremely rare.
- Interestingly, prolonged survivals even without cancer treatment have been seen in all of these syndromes in patients with pelvic and lung cancers. This suggests that heightened immunity may have a beneficial effect on host defenses to cancer. Although patients may die from progression of their underlying cancers, many die from complications of their neurologic disease.

PATIENT EDUCATION

N/A

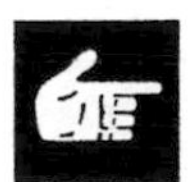

Miscellaneous

SYNONYMS

PCD: Anti-Yo syndrome
POM: "Dancing eyes and dancing feet," infantile polymyoclonia
PEM: Anti-Hu syndrome, paraneoplastic limbic encephalitis
PSN: Anti-Hu syndrome, subacute sensory neuronopathy

ICD-9-CM: PCD/POM: 334.4 Cerebellar ataxia in diseases classified elsewhere: neoplastic disease (140.0–239.9); POM: 333.2 Myoclonus; PEM: 323.8 Other causes of encephalitis; PSN: 357.3 Polyneuropathy in malignant disease

SEE ALSO: N/A

REFERENCES

- Dalmau J, Graus F, Rosenblum MK, et al. Anti-Hu-associated paraneoplastic encephalomyelitis/sensory neuronopathy. A clinical study of 71 patients. Medicine 1992;71:59–72.
- Lucchinetti CF, Kimmel DW, Lennon VA. Paraneoplastic and oncologic profiles of patients seropositive for type I antineuronal nuclear autoantibodies. Neurology 1998;50:652–657.
- Luque FA, Furneaux H, Ferziger R, et al. Anti-Ri: an antibody associated with paraneoplastic opsoclonus and breast cancer. Ann Neurol 1991;29:241–251.
- Marshall PC, Brett EM, Wilson J. Myoclonic encephalopathy of childhood (the dancing eye syndrome): a long-term follow-up study. Neurology 1978;28:348.
- Moll JWB, Vecht CJ. Paraneoplastic syndromes of the central nervous system. In: Vecht CJ, ed. Handbook of clinical neurology, Vinken and Bruyn, vol 69. New York: Elsevier, 1997:349–371.
- Peterson K, Rosenblum MK, Kotanides H, et al. Paraneoplastic cerebellar degeneration. I. A clinical analysis of 55 anti-Yo antibody-positive patients. Neurology 1992;42:1931–1937.
- Posner JB. Paraneoplastic syndromes. In: Posner JB, ed. Neurologic complications of cancer. Contemporary neurologic series. Philadelphia: F. A. Davis, 1995:353–385.

Author(s): Julie E. Hammack, MD

Parkinson's Disease

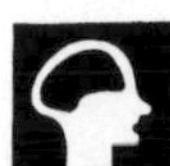

Basics

DESCRIPTION

Parkinson's disease (PD) is a common, progressive neurodegenerative disorder of the extrapyramidal system. PD has a classic pathology, the eosinophilic, cytoplasmic intraneuronal inclusion bodies known as Lewy bodies, which appear in the substantia nigra, locus ceruleus, nucleus basalis of Meynert, and dorsal motor nucleus of the vagus. PD is characterized by a slowly progressive movement disorder with tremor, rigidity, bradykinesia, and gait disorders. It responds to therapies that alter dopaminergic and cholinergic neurotransmission.

EPIDEMIOLOGY

Incidence/Prevalence

PD is a common disorder of the elderly affecting 1-3/1,000 adults in the U.S. It is the second most common neurodegenerative disorder in the U.S. after Alzheimer's disease. Incidence may approach 5 to 20 new cases per 100,000 annually (U.S.).

Race

Highest prevalence in East Indian > Caucasian > African American > Chinese.

Age

The prevalence increases with age, averaging 1% or greater after the age of 65.

Sex

Males are slightly more frequently affected than females.

ETIOLOGY

The cause of PD is unknown. The two most likely contributing factors are genetics and environmental or endogenous toxins.

Genetics

Twin studies have shown that young-adult PD (onset typically before age 40) has a high concordance rate among monozygotic twins. The typical older adult-onset PD in twins had a concordance rate that was similar between monozygotic and dizygotic twins. The risk of developing PD is approximately two to three times above average when a first-degree relative is affected. Rare cases of familial PD are scattered throughout the world, but examination of the gene affected in familial PD (coding for the protein α-synuclein) has not shown similar mutations in the sporadic form of PD. Another gene product, referred to as *parkin*, has also been associated with a hereditary, early adult onset form of PD.

Environment

The greatest risk factor for developing PD is advanced age. Rural residence with exposure to well water and herbicide and pesticide preparations is an additional risk factor, as is exposure to industrial chemicals, especially metals (manganese, iron, and steel alloys).

RISK FACTORS

See above

PREGNANCY

N/A

ASSOCIATED CONDITIONS

N/A

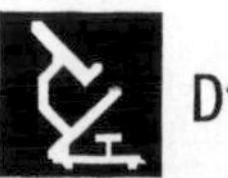

Diagnosis

DIFFERENTIAL DIAGNOSIS

- Essential or familial tremor (10 times higher prevalence than PD and commonly misdiagnosed as PD)
- Diffuse Lewy body disease (DLBD)
- Drug-induced parkinsonism (e.g., antipsychotics, antiemetics, and other dopamine blocking agents)
- Multiple system atrophy (MSA)
- Progressive supranuclear palsy (PSP)
- Vascular parkinsonism
- Posttraumatic parkinsonism
- Wilson's disease
- Frontotemporal dementia with parkinsonism
- Alzheimer's with extrapyramidal features (possibly a DLBD variant)
- Creutzfeldt-Jakob disease

SIGNS AND SYMPTOMS

Primary Motor Symptoms

The early cardinal signs and symptoms of idiopathic PD (tremor, rigidity, and bradykinesia) are essentially *always* asymmetric at onset, progressing slowly (months to years) to involve the contralateral side. The initial symptoms develop insidiously over months to years. Patients may be undiagnosed or misdiagnosed for months (or years) until an experienced clinician performs a careful history and neurologic examination.
The classic tetrad of PD includes:

- Tremor at rest
- Rigidity (with cog-wheeling)
- Bradykinesia (masked facies, decreased blink rate, decreased spontaneous arm swing while walking, slowness in initiating and maintaining movements, slow shuffling gait)
- Postural instability (late manifestation)
- Diagnosis is made from the patient's clinical history, two of three cardinal signs (rest tremor, rigidity, bradykinesia) on exam, and exclusion of secondary causes of parkinsonism.

Other Signs and Symptoms

- Cognitive dysfunction
  - —Bradyphrenia, a slowing of response time
  - —Visuospatial disturbances (typically in late PD)
- Ocular dysfunction
  - —Limitations of upgaze, but not downgaze,
  - —Saccadic eye movements with pursuit
  - —Persistent eye blinking when the forehead is repeatedly tapped (glabellar reflex or Myerson's sign)
- Speech and swallowing disturbances
  - —Monotonous, hypophonia
  - —Palilalia (repetition of the first syllable)
  - —Pooling of saliva with drooling
  - —Dysphagia (late in disease)
- Musculoskeletal abnormalities
  - —Dystonias (fixed postures of hands or feet)
  - —Muscle cramping
  - —Kyphoscoliosis
- Autonomic disturbances
  - —Constipation
  - —Urinary frequency, urgency, and, rarely, incontinence
- Sleep disturbances
  - —Sleep fragmentation
  - —REM sleep behavior disorder
- Symptoms more characteristic of DLBD
  - —Dramatic fluctuations in motor function and mentation
  - —Syncope like spells
  - —Visual hallucinations (sometimes prior to dopaminergic medication)
  - —Exquisite sensitivity to conventional neuroleptics

LABORATORY PROCEDURES

There are no specific blood tests to diagnose PD, but the following tests should be considered to identify potential underlying secondary causes of parkinsonism: serum vitamin B_{12} level, thyroid function tests, serum ceruloplasmin, 24-hour urine copper excretion.

IMAGING STUDIES

There is no evidence to suggest that structural imaging studies (CT, MRI) can assist in the diagnosis of either PD. MRI may reveal evidence of other causes of parkinsonism such as vascular insults, mass lesions, calcium or iron deposition in the striatum, atrophy in the posterior fossa suggestive of multiple system atrophies, and cortical atrophy patterns suggestive of other dementing illnesses.

SPECIAL TESTS

A therapeutic trial of Sinemet, a combination of carbidopa and levodopa, at doses of up to 600–800 mg of levodopa equivalents in 24 hours, is sometimes considered diagnostic of true idiopathic PD when the patient responds with dramatic symptomatic improvement (see Management, below).

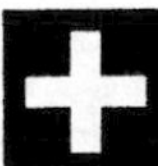

Management

GENERAL MEASURES

See Medications, below.

SURGICAL MEASURES

Stereotactically placed deep brain stimulation (DBS) electrodes for the management of PD are FDA approved. This procedure can be performed bilaterally with few long-term side effects. Electrodes have been placed in either the globus pallidum or subthalamic nucleus with significant improvement in PD symptoms. Ablative pallidotomy is used less now due to side effects.

SYMPTOMATIC TREATMENT

See Medications, below.

ADJUNCTIVE TREATMENT

See Medications, below.

ADMISSION/DISCHARGE CRITERIA

PD is usually managed in an outpatient setting. Rarely, concomitant illnesses (e.g., pneumonia, UTI) can lead to an acute exacerbation of PD symptoms, requiring hospitalization for dysphagia, airway management, and issues of decreased mobility. Psychosis in the setting of idiopathic PD with excessive dopaminergic medication may precipitate hospitalization and/or institutionalization.

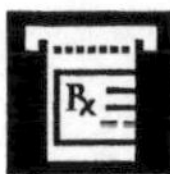

Medications

DRUG(S) OF CHOICE

- Levodopa therapy
  - —Carbidopa/levodopa (C/L) (brand name Sinemet, multiple generic formulations) is the preparation that provides the standard of care for people with idiopathic PD. While its use is controversial as a first-line agent due to predictable development of motor fluctuations after prolonged exposure to levodopa, it is the most efficacious and biologically effective medication available.
  - —Controlled-release form of C/L (Sinemet CR or C/L ER) is only 70% bioavailable on average compared to immediate release C/L, and thus there is a tendency to underdose patients when using this formulation.
  - —The complications of levodopa therapy are common to all the dopaminergic agents and include confusion, hallucinations, gastrointestinal distress including nausea and vomiting, orthostatic hypotension, and others. The long-term motor complications associated with levodopa usage include dyskinesias (involuntary abnormal movements), dystonias (abnormal involuntary posturing), on/off symptoms in which medication quits working abruptly, and complicated combinations of all of the above. As the disease progresses, most patients require additional levodopa doses, with or without the use of adjunctive therapy, in order to avoid "off" periods, defined as a hypokinetic state associated with minimal or no pharmacologic benefit from their medications.
- COMT inhibitors
  - —These molecules block residual breakdown of levodopa in the GI tract by inhibiting catechol-o-methyl transferase (COMT) activity, increasing the bioavailability and effective half-life of C/L. These agents appear to decrease off time in patients with motor fluctuations by approximately 20% to 30%, with some patients concomitantly able to decrease their total daily levodopa intake by 20% to 30%. The most common side effects from these medications are the result of the increased dopaminergic tone induced by the increased bioavailability of levodopa, including onset or exacerbation of nausea, dyskinesias, and/or hallucinations. Other side effects include urine discoloration and diarrhea.
  - —Tolcapone (Tasmar, 100–200 mg tid) had the adverse side effect of lethal hepatic damage in several patients worldwide, resulting in a black-box warning on the PDR insert. There is an absolute requirement for liver function monitoring every 2 weeks for the first year, followed by every 4 weeks for 6 months after that, and then every 8 weeks indefinitely when using this medication. This medication should be prescribed only by specialists familiar with its use and contraindications.
  - —Entacapone (Comtan, 200 mg with every dose of C/L) has not shown any evidence of hepatic toxicity. A new combination pill incorporating carbidopa/levodopa/entacapone—Stalevo—will be newly introduced worldwide in the summer of 2003.
- Dopamine agonists
  - —Dopamine agonists (DAs) have been routinely used since the 1970s as adjunctive therapy to supplement C/L when daily levodopa doses approached or exceeded 600 mg/d. While dopamine agonists, especially the two newer derivatives, are purported as ideal initial treatment for PD, the incidence of adverse events, especially confusion, hallucinations, and orthostatic hypotension increase dramatically as the patient ages. Other potential side effects include nausea, sleepiness (including possibly sleep attacks), and peripheral edema. The frequency of these side effects in clinical practice depends largely on individual patient differences, including age, premorbid conditions (especially dementia), concomitant medications, etc.
  - —Bromocriptine (Parlodel, 15–40 mg/d) and pergolide (Permax, 0.75–3.0 mg/d) are ergot derivatives that are useful as adjunctive therapy. In general, patients placed on adjunctive DA therapy experience 20% to 30% improvement in their overall daily mobility, and some patients concomitantly decrease their total daily dose of C/L by 20% to 30%. Due to cost and side effect profile, bromocriptine is rarely, if ever, used.
- Ropinerole (Requip 9–24 mg/d) and pramipexole (Mirapex, 1.5–4.5 mg/d) are newer, non-ergot derivatives. They were released late in the 1990s with dual indications as monotherapy agents in patients newly diagnosed with PD and as adjunctive agents for patients currently on levodopa therapy.

- Trihexyphenidyl (Artane) 6–15 mg/d and benztropine (Cogentin 1.5–6 mg/d) are anticholinergic agents commonly used in the early treatment of PD. Both have a slightly greater propensity for treating the symptom of tremor. The risk of cognitive effects in the elderly as well as multiple other anticholinergic side effects in all populations limits their usefulness.
- Amantadine (Symmetrel 200–400 mg/d) is an antiinfluenza agent that works through a variety of different mechanisms, including decreasing dopamine reuptake, glutamatergic blockade, and possibly mild anticholinergic effects. It also may be especially useful for the treatment of tremor. Recent data suggest that amantadine at 300–400 mg/d may significantly alleviate the dyskinesias in patients with associated motor fluctuations.
- Selegiline (Eldepryl 5–10 mg/d) is a selective MAO-B inhibitor that delays or decreases the breakdown of dopamine in the brain, resulting in a mild symptomatic benefit. Initial studies suggested that it may be neuroprotective; however, follow-up analysis of the data has failed to show any statistically significant evidence of neuroprotection. Its use in the elderly as well as prolonged use greater than 5 to 10 years is controversial.
- Atypical antipsychotics
  —Atypical antipsychotics are used to treat the symptoms of drug-induced hallucinations in PD. These medications are normally given in dosages representing a fraction of that used for patients with schizophrenia.
  —Clozapine (Clozaril, 12.5–25 mg/d) is the prototypic atypical antipsychotic. Its use is complicated by the rare, but life-threatening potential side effect of agranulocytosis. Weekly CBC is required during the first 6 months of therapy followed by every 2 weeks thereafter.
  —Quetiapine (Seroquel, 25–100 mg/d) is the only other atypical antipsychotic currently on the market that, like clozapine, shows no dose-dependent extrapyramidal side effects.

ALTERNATIVE DRUGS

In patients with dementia, cholinesterase-inhibiting medications may be used.

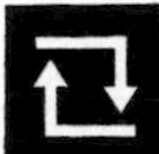

Follow-Up

PATIENT MONITORING

- Patients with idiopathic PD (IPD) are seen usually two to three times per year in an outpatient setting. These visits are typically more frequent when medications are adjusted.
- By its very nature, IPD requires steadily increasing doses of medications, for the treatment of dopaminergic deficiency or the side effects of (exogenous) dopaminergic therapy.

EXPECTED COURSE AND PROGNOSIS

PD is a progressive, neurodegenerative disorder. Progression varies, but most patients are able to maintain productive lives for at least 5 to 7 years after the time of diagnosis. After 10 to 15 years, most patients with PD will experience significant motor fluctuations as their medication improves the symptoms of PD on an intermittent basis throughout the day. After 20 to 30 years of treatment for PD, most patients require at least some assistance with ambulation during the day. Dysphagia with resultant aspiration pneumonia and falling are two common causes of morbidity and mortality in PD.

PATIENT EDUCATION

Support groups for PD are available locally in many areas of the country. There are several large national organizations that provide educational materials to patients and their families. Regular daily exercise has been proven beneficial in alleviating many symptoms of immobility in PD, especially when coupled with careful titration and use of proper medications.

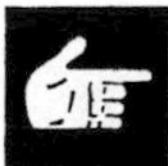

Miscellaneous

SYNONYMS

Shaking palsy (PD)

ICD-9-CM: 332.0 Idiopathic Parkinson's disease

SEE ALSO: DIFFUSE LEWY BODY DISEASE; MULTIPLE SYSTEM ATROPHY; PROGRESSIVE SUPRANUCLEAR PALSY; DEMENTIA, ALZHEIMER'S

REFERENCES

- Ahlskog JE. Diagnosis and differential diagnosis of Parkinson's disease and parkinsonism. Parkinsonism Rel Disord 2001;7:63–70.
- Hauser R, Zesiewicz T. Parkinson's disease: questions and answers, 3rd ed. Coral Springs, FL: Merit Publishing International 2000.
- Waters C. Diagnosis and management of Parkinson's disease, 2nd ed. Laddo, OK: Professional Communications, 1999.

Author(s): Lawrence W. Elmer, MD, PhD

Pituitary Apoplexy

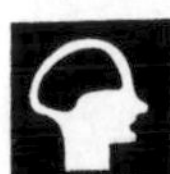

Basics

DESCRIPTION

Pituitary apoplexy is characterized by a hemorrhage, infarction, necrosis, or a hemorrhagic infarction of a pituitary tumor (mostly adenoma), which usually presents suddenly. This is accompanied by an expanding space-occupying sellar lesion, which compresses the sellar and/or para- or suprasellar anatomic structures. Subclinical or silent courses may occur. Histologic findings include hemorrhaged pituitary adenoma tissue, occasionally infarctions, necrosis, cysts, or calcifications. There may be infiltration of adjacent structures (e.g., sphenoid sinus, cavernous sinus, hypothalamus, chiasm).

EPIDEMIOLOGY

Incidence

General incidence of pituitary adenomas is about 10/1,000,000/year.
Incidence of all types of pituitary apoplexy is about 10% to 15% (range 0.6% to 27.7%) of all pituitary adenomas
Symptomatic: acute 6.8%, subacute 2.3%, asymptomatic 7.5%
Tumor type: most frequent nonfunctioning adenoma (null-cell adenoma), followed by prolactinomas and (usually silent) gonadotropinomas. Acromegaly and Cushing's disease rare.

Age

Mean age ranges from 35.3 to 56.6 years. Children are affected extremely rarely.

Sex

Male > female.

ETIOLOGY

- Spontaneous
- External causes (see Risk Factors, below)
- Pathophysiologic and pathoanatomic aspects: hemorrhage and necrosis are frequently the result of increased intratumoral pressure, edema, and pathologic alterations of the microarchitecture of the tumor vessels, which are supported by the regular vascularization of the pituitary originating from branches of the internal carotid artery (meningohypophyseal trunk, superior and inferior hypophyseal arteries)

RISK FACTORS

- (Minor) trauma
- Pregnancy (e.g. Sheehan syndrome)
- Cerebral angiography
- Endocrine stimulation tests
- Radiation therapy
- Dopamine agonist therapy
- Estrogen therapy
- Anticoagulation therapy (also due to dialysis or cardiac/vascular surgery)
- Increased abdominal pressure (also during surgery)
- Chronic coughing and sneezing
- Postoperative tumor remnants in case of incomplete resection

ASSOCIATED CONDITIONS

Pituitary adenoma, sella tumors, and other space-occupying lesions, empty sella, (subarachnoid) hemorrhage, ischemia, necrosis, vascular insults

PREGNANCY

Sheehan syndrome is the occurrence of pituitary apoplexy during or after pregnancy.

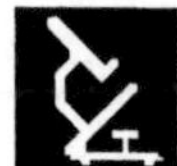

Diagnosis

DIFFERENTIAL DIAGNOSIS

- Subarachnoid hemorrhage (caused by ruptured aneurysm or AV malformation)
- Cavernous-sinus thrombosis
- Venous sinus thrombosis
- Meningitis
- Hemorrhage of another (unknown) intrasellar or intracranial mass lesion
- Acute optic neuritis
- Migraine with aura

SIGNS AND SYMPTOMS

- Usually acute symptoms
- Sudden headache
- Meningism
- Visual disturbances/amaurosis
- Impaired consciousness
- Nausea/vomiting
- Oculomotoric palsies/cranial nerve deficits (nerves III, IV, V, VI)
- Hemiparesis
- Diabetes insipidus
- Signs of (partial or pan-) hypopituitarism
- Signs of anterior lobe hormonal excess (e.g., acromegaly, Cushing's disease)
- Hypothalamic dysregulation (temperature imbalance, disturbance of water/electrolyte balance)
- (Extremely rare) unexpected death

LABORATORY PROCEDURES

- Electrolytes
- Urinary concentration
- Osmolarity of serum and urine
- Serum prolactin level
- Anterior pituitary hormone concentrations (basal)
- Anterior pituitary hormone function tests

IMAGING STUDIES

Head CT (axial and coronal projection) and/or MRI confirms pituitary apoplexy. Additionally, angiography or helical CT angiography to exclude vascular malformations may be required. MRI and CT scan can also identify subclinical or silent lesions (cysts, hemorrhages, necrosis, etc.).

SPECIAL TESTS

- Lumbar CSF puncture (usually bloody or xanthochrome) should be avoided (possible risk of transtentorial brain herniation)
- Doppler ultrasound examination in case of extended subarachnoid hemorrhage (diagnosis/treatment control for vasospasm)
- Ophthalmologic examination (visual fields, visual acuity)

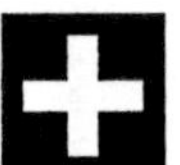

Management

GENERAL MEASURES

Most important measurements: endocrinologic and general stabilization

- Corticosteroids (initially minimum 200 mg hydrocortisone)
- In case of diabetes insipidus: DDAVP (desmopressin)
- Balance of electrolytes
- If necessary: intensive care treatment/ artificial respiratory treatment/brain edema treatment (e.g., mannitol)

SURGICAL MEASURES

Treatment of choice in case of progressive visual disturbances or neurologic deficits, if the patient is in stable condition (e.g., endocrinologic or anesthesiologic parameters)

- (Usually) transsphenoidal surgery with removal of tumor and hematoma (decompression of chiasm)
- (Rarely) craniotomy necessary
- In case of extended subarachnoid hemorrhage, hydro-/hematocephalus or coma, supplemental ventricular drainage

SYMPTOMATIC TREATMENT

Appropriate pain medication may be given for headache.

ADJUNCTIVE TREATMENT

- Generally: conventional radiation therapy, gamma knife/Linac therapy
- Additional pharmacotherapy: in prolactinomas—dopamine agonists; in acromegaly—dopamine agonists, somatostatin analogues; in Cushing's disease—ketoconazole, metapyrone, etomidate, mitotane; here also palliative surgery: bilateral adrenalectomy.
- Hormonal substitution (mentioned above)

ADMISSION/DISCHARGE CRITERIA

Admission

In all cases of acute symptoms listed above for diagnoses and treatment, especially surgical therapy. In case of subacute or silent symptoms, ambulant (conservative) management can be considered.

Discharge

Following recovery, rehabilitation facility or outpatient management

Medications

DRUG(S) OF CHOICE

Endocrinologic substitution with hydrocortisone, T_4, testosterone/estrogens, possibly growth hormone and DDAVP are necessary depending to the individual deficits. Furthermore, for tumor treatment, if necessary, dopamine agonists, somatostatin analogues, etc.

Contraindications

No specific contraindications unless specific hypersensitivity reactions are present.

Precautions

Avoid sudden withdrawal of any of these medications, which are substituted for naturally occurring hormones. Adrenal insufficiency may be precipitated by sudden steroid withdrawal.

ALTERNATIVE DRUGS

N/A

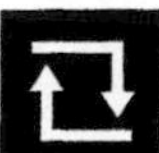

Follow-Up

PATIENT MONITORING

- Regular endocrinologic controls (basal and function tests) for adaption of hormonal substitution. In case of functioning tumors, control of the specific tumor hormones.
- Regular ophthalmologic examinations (visual fields, visual acuity)
- Regular MRI controls (mandatory in nonfunctioning tumors, in endocrine active tumors depending on the endocrinologic parameters)

EXPECTED COURSE AND PROGNOSIS

Usually recovery following a critical clinical course in the acute cases, if hormonal replacement and surgery have been done in time. Lethal courses are rare. In the subclinical or silent cases, the prognosis is generally favorable.

PATIENT EDUCATION

- Information and management of the follow-up examinations listed above.
- Information about the need for endocrine substitution (especially hydrocortisone) in case of stress and emergency situations (e.g., accident, infections, surgery, different diseases, etc.)

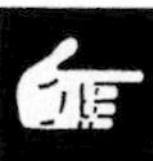

Miscellaneous

SYNONYMS

Pituitary hemorrhage
Pituitary necrosis
Hemorrhagic pituitary adenoma

ICD-9-CM: 253.2 Pituitary necrosis postpartum

SEE ALSO: PITUITARY ADENOMA, SUBARACHNOID HEMORRHAGE

REFERENCES

- Bills DC, Meyer FB, Laws ER, et al. A retrospective analysis of pituitary apoplexy. Neurosurgery 1993;33:602–609.
- Bonicki W, Kasperlik-Zaluska A, Koszewski W, et al. Pituitary apoplexy: endocrine, surgical and oncological emergency. Incidence, clinical course and treatment with reference to 799 cases of pituitary adenomas. Acta Neurochir (Wien) 1993;120:118–122
- Brisman MH, Katz G, Post KD. Symptoms of pituitary apoplexy rapidly reversed with bromocriptine. J Neurosurg 1996;85: 1153–1155.
- Lange M, Woenckhaus M, Segiet W, et al. A rare fatal course of a patient with a spontaneous pituitary apoplexy: Case report and literature review. Neurosurg Rev 1999;22:163–169.
- Onesti ST, Wisniewski T, Post KD. Clinical versus subclinical pituitary apoplexy: presentation, surgical management, and outcome in 21 patients. Neurosurgery 1990;26:980–986.
- Parent AD. Visual recovery after blindness from pituitary apoplexy. Can J Neurol Sci 1990;17:88–91.
- Wakai S, Fukushima T, Teramoto A, et al. Pituitary apoplexy: its incidence and clinical significance. J Neurosurg 1981;55: 187–193.

Author(s): Manfred Lange, MD

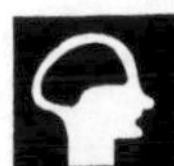

Basics

DESCRIPTION

Atraumatic brachial plexopathy is characterized by acute pain and weakness around the shoulder girdle and arm with variable findings of sensory loss, reflex change, and atrophy developing over the next several weeks. The pattern of weakness depends on whether a portion or the whole plexus is involved.

Epidemiology

Incidence/Prevalence

This is an uncommon disorder occurring at approximately 1.6 per 100,000.

Race

There seems to be no racial predominance in this disorder.

Age

Most cases occur between the ages of 20 and 55 years, although cases have been reported at all ages.

Sex

Brachial plexopathy is more common in males, with a male-to-female ratio of 2:1 to 10.5:1 in various studies.

ETIOLOGY

Many precipitating factors have been suggested as the etiologic factor for brachial plexopathy. Antecedent factors associated with development of brachial plexopathy frequently include viral infection, immunization, invasive medical procedures in the axilla, or trauma at childbirth. Based on the timing of onset after viral illnesses many have postulated an immune-mediated mechanism. Multifocal mononuclear cell infiltrates have been found in some patients after biopsy.

Genetics

A familial form of recurrent brachial neuritis is inherited in an autosomal-dominant manner. The gene defect localizes to chromosome 17.

RISK FACTORS

Traumatic lesions of the plexus are often seen after penetrating wounds or after severe traction on the upper limb with motorcycle or snowmobile accidents.

PREGNANCY

Pregnancy and childbirth can be precipitating factors, especially in cases that are familial.

ASSOCIATED CONDITIONS

- Autoimmune diseases: systemic lupus erythematosus, giant cell arteritis, polyarteritis nodosa, inflammatory bowel disease
- Infectious diseases: HIV infection, CMV infection, Coxsackie-virus infection, parvovirus, *Mycoplasma pneumoniae,* bacterial pneumonia, typhoid, syphilis
- Postimmunization: tetanus toxoid, immune sera, diphtheria, swine flu, hepatitis B vaccination
- Neoplasia: Hodgkin's disease, neuroblastoma, postradiation
- Hereditary neuropathies: hereditary neuropathy with liability to pressure palsies (HNPP)

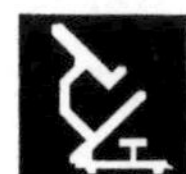

Diagnosis

DIFFERENTIAL DIAGNOSIS

Poliomyelitis
Entrapment neuropathy
Cervical root syndromes
Vertebral artery dissection
Rotator cuff injuries
Subacromial bursitis

SIGNS AND SYMPTOMS

- The onset of brachial neuritis is often dramatic, with acute pain in the shoulder radiating into the neck and into the arm to the level of the elbow. The arm is often held flexed at the elbow and adducted at the shoulder. The pain may be constant for several weeks and may be intermittently painful for long periods. After several weeks, weakness develops in the limb and the distribution varies depending on what portion or portions of the plexus is involved. Lesions that involve the entire plexus affect muscles innervated by C5 through T1, and often the arm hangs limp at the patient's side. Sensory loss involves almost the entire arm.
- Lesions involving the upper trunk produce weakness in the C5 and C6 distribution, causing weakness in abduction of the shoulder and flexion of the elbow, and the shoulder internally rotates. This has been called the "waiter's-tip" posture. Sensory loss is over the lateral arm, forearm, and thumb. Involvement of the lower trunk causes weakness in muscles innervated by C8 and T1 roots. Weakness is present in both median nerve and ulnar nerve innervated intrinsic hand muscles and medial wrist flexors. Sensory loss occurs in the medial two fingers, medial hand, and forearm.
- Lesions at the level of the cords are most often traumatic. Posterior cord lesions cause weakness in muscles innervated by the axillary and radial nerves. This results in loss of shoulder abduction and elbow and wrist extension. Sensory loss occurs in the posterior lateral aspect of the arm, forearm, and dorsal lateral aspect of the hand. Lateral cord lesions cause weakness in muscles innervated by the musculocutaneous nerve and median nerve muscle supplied by roots C6 and C7. This results in weak pronation of the forearm and flexion of the wrist. In medial cord lesions, muscles innervated by the ulnar nerve and those muscles that receive C8 and T1 via the median nerve are affected. Isolated nerves can be affected as they branch off the plexus (e.g., phrenic nerve involvement causing diaphragmatic weakness or isolated suprascapular nerve involvement causing weakness in the supraspinatous and infraspinatous).

LABORATORY PROCEDURES

EMG is very helpful in making the diagnosis and defining the degree of plexus injury. Denervative changes in muscles innervated by two cervical roots and involving at least two peripheral nerves point to the plexus as the site of the lesion. By definition, the lesion must be distal to the roots. Examination of the cervical paraspinal muscles by EMG is normal. Traumatic lesions may cause both plexus lesions as well as cervical nerve root lesions if the root is avulsed. Occasionally neoplastic lesions may also affect the plexus as well as the cervical roots.

IMAGING STUDIES

Plain x-rays of the chest and neck are often very helpful. A lesion at the pulmonary apex with erosion of the first or second rib may be the cause of a lower plexus lesion. Similarly the presence of a cervical rib or elongated C7 transverse process may explain thoracic outlet syndrome symptoms. MRI and CT with contrast are helpful in finding mass lesions compressing or infiltrating the plexus.

SPECIAL TESTS

N/A

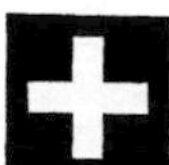

Management

GENERAL MEASURES

Management is largely supportive with efforts focused on pain control and passive and active range of motion exercises for the limb. Corticosteroids do not alter the course of the disease but may be helpful in the acute stage with pain not relieved by narcotics. Prednisone 60 mg/d for a few days with a rapid taper may be useful.

SURGICAL MEASURES

Surgery may occasionally be needed to define the lesion's full extent. Intraoperative electrical monitoring of evoked responses may help determine motor root damage. Occasional nerve grafting along with tendon transfers may allow return of function for some patients.

SYMPTOMATIC MANAGEMENT

Extensive physiotherapy is often needed for many months to maintain range of motion and avoid a frozen shoulder syndrome.

ADJUNCTIVE TREATMENT

N/A

ADMISSION/DISCHARGE CRITERIA

N/A

Medications

DRUG(S) OF CHOICE

Narcotics are often used for pain control in the acute stages.

Contraindications

Known hypersensitivity to narcotic drugs.

Precautions

The clearance of various narcotic agents or their metabolites may be decreased in patients with hepatic or renal dysfunction.

ALTERNATIVE DRUGS

N/A

Follow-Up

PATIENT MONITORING

Regular visits to ensure full range of motion in the joints are recommended.

EXPECTED COURSE AND PROGNOSIS

About one third of nontraumatic plexus injuries return to normal function in 1 year.
Seventy-five percent have full recover at 2 years and almost all by 4 years. Upper brachial plexus lesions recover more quickly. Weakness in the diaphragm and serratus anterior are associated with persistent weakness.

PATIENT EDUCATION

N/A

Miscellaneous

SYNONYMS

Parsonage-Turner syndrome
Brachial neuritis
Neuralgic amyotrophy
Brachial plexus neuropathy

ICD-9-CM: 723.4 Brachial neuritis NOS

SEE ALSO: N/A

REFERENCES

- Beghi E, Kurland LT, Mulder DW, et al. Brachial plexus neuropathy in the population of Rochester Minnesota, 1970–1981. Ann Neurol 1985;18:320–323.
- Botella MS, Garcia M, Cuadrado JM, et al. Parsonage-Turner syndrome in positive HIV patients. Rev Neurol 1997;25:143.
- Chance PF, Windebank AJ. Hereditary neuralgic amyotrophy. Curr Opin Neurol 1996;9:343–347.
- Parsonage MJ, Turner JW. Neuralgic amyotrophy, the shoulder girdle syndrome. Lancet 1948;1:973–978.
- Stratton KR, Howe CJ, Johnston RB Jr. Adverse events associated with childhood vaccines other than pertussis and rubella. Summary of a report from the Institute of Medicine. JAMA 1994;271:1602–1605.
- Suarez GA, Giannini c, Bosch EP, et al. Immune rachial plexus neuropathy: suggestive evidence for inflammatory-immune pathogenesis. Neurology 1996;46:559–561.
- Tsairis P, Dyck PJ, Mulder DW. Natural history of brachial plexus neuropathy. Arch Neurol 1972;27:109–117.

Author(s): J. Ned Pruitt II, MD

Plexopathy, Lumbosacral

Basics

DESCRIPTION

Lesions involving the lumbosacral plexus produce symptoms of weakness, numbness, and pain in the affected lower extremity. Neoplastic infiltration and radiation necrosis are common etiologies and can usually be distinguished based on clinical, radiographic, and electrodiagnostic differences.

EPIDEMIOLOGY

Incidence/Prevalence

Lumbosacral plexopathies are less common than brachial plexopathies, in part because the lumbar plexus is less likely to be involved in trauma.

Race

No demonstrated ethnic predominance.

Age

Many etiologies for lumbosacral plexopathy occur in older individuals.

Sex

Lumbosacral plexopathies due to cancer infiltration are more common in women. Radiation-induced lumbosacral plexopathy occurs in women, but is also seen in young men after treatment for testicular cancer.

ETIOLOGY

- Neoplastic infiltration is a relatively common cause of lumbosacral plexopathy and produces symptoms by mass effect. This can occur by direct extension from pelvic tumors or due to distant metastasis.
- Radiation treatment for pelvic tumors produces a delayed plexopathy, with symptom onset occurring 3 to 5 years after treatment, although the range is broad and may occur from 3 months to 30 years after radiotherapy. The mechanism is not clear, although vascular injury appears to play an important role, as obliterated blood vessels have been found on histologic studies. Radiation plexopathies become more likely with a higher total dose given (3,000–8,000 cGy), increased size of the individual treatment fractions, a higher frequency of treatments, and increased radiation field size.
- A hemorrhage into the retroperitoneum can involve the lumbar plexus, which is formed in the psoas muscle. The hemorrhage can also extend to involve the sacral plexus. The cause is usually heparin therapy, and roughly 5% of patients on intravenous heparin may develop a spontaneous hemorrhage into the psoas muscle. Patients with hemophilia and disseminated intravascular coagulopathy (DIC) are also at increased risk.
- Patients with diabetes may develop subacute painful leg weakness, termed diabetic amyotrophy, or Bruns-Garland syndrome. Diabetic amyotrophy is due to ischemic injury to the nerve roots or lumbosacral plexus. Paraspinal muscle abnormalities on EMG studies suggest that the lesion may be at the nerve root level rather than plexus, although this is debatable.
- Idiopathic lumbosacral plexitis (neuralgic amyotrophy of the lumbosacral plexus) presents with severe hip, anterior thigh, and inguinal pain, and later with progressive weakness and atrophy of the leg.
- Injury to the lumbar plexus and/or the femoral nerve can occur during complicated delivery.
- Inadvertent intraarterial injection into the iliac artery or one of its branches can result in injury to the lumbar plexus in particular. This typically occurs with needle injections into the deep midline buttocks area, as opposed to the outer gluteal quadrant. Vasospasm results in ischemic injury to the lumbar plexus.
- Internal or external iliac artery chemotherapy with cisplatin for local pelvic tumors can induce small vessel injury with subsequent lumbosacral plexus infarction. There may also be a direct toxic effect of the cisplatin on the plexus. Local infusion of Adriamycin, 5-fluorouracil, and other chemotherapeutic agents has also been reported to result in a lumbosacral plexopathy.
- Trauma probably accounts for only 5% of all lumbosacral plexopathies and are often associated with a pelvic fracture.

RISK FACTORS

Pelvic tumors, radiation treatment, diabetes, complicated childbirth, heparin therapy, and trauma.

PREGNANCY

Delivery can result in a lumbar plexopathy. The incidence of obstetrics-related nerve injuries is estimated to occur between 1/2,600 and 1/6,400 of all deliveries.

ASSOCIATED CONDITIONS

Cancer, whether local in the pelvis (colorectal, uterine, cervical, ovarian, prostate and testicular cancers) or from distant sites (breast and thyroid carcinoma, sarcoma, and lymphoma), and diabetes are the major associated diseases.

Diagnosis

DIFFERENTIAL DIAGNOSIS

- Lumbosacral radiculopathy, including cauda equina syndrome; this can be difficult to distinguish clinically and often requires neuroradiologic and EMG studies.
- Sciatic neuropathy—strength of the gluteus medius (thigh abduction) and gluteus maximus (hip extension) are important to assess in this differential. If these muscles are weak, the lesion must be above the sciatic nerve at least as proximal as the plexus or nerve root level.
- Polyneuropathy is a diagnostic consideration in patients who have received chemotherapeutic agents, especially since polyneuropathies affect the lower extremities to a greater degree. To distinguish from plexopathy it is important to look for evidence of polyneuropathy involving the upper extremities.

SIGNS AND SYMPTOMS

In general, lumbosacral plexopathy presents with weakness, sensory loss, paresthesias, pain, loss of reflexes, and atrophy in the affected lower extremity. Many of the etiologies mentioned above may result in bilateral lumbosacral plexopathies resulting in signs and symptoms in both legs. Preferential involvement of the sacral plexus results in more prominent weakness below the knee, and involvement of the gluteus medius and maximus, with a diminished Achilles reflex. Preferential involvement of the lumbar plexus results primarily in weakness of proximal muscles, such as the quadriceps and thigh adductors and patellar reflex loss.

- Patients with cancer infiltration present with back and leg pain in at least 75% of cases. Leg edema and a rectal mass are found in some patients. Bowel and bladder involvement can be seen uncommonly.
- As opposed to neoplastic infiltration, radiation plexopathy presents with paresthesias and indolent leg weakness. Pain may eventually occur, but is less common and not as severe as in cancer infiltration.
- Patients with retroperitoneal hemorrhage due to heparin therapy present with acute-onset low back and leg pain, leg weakness, and paresthesias. The lumbar plexus is involved to a greater degree in retroperitoneal hemorrhage.
- In diabetic amyotrophy, intense pain begins in the anterior thigh, and inguinal region. Over the following weeks, the patient has progressive weakness, primarily in the distribution of the lumbar plexus, although the more distal sacral plexus innervated muscles may also be involved. The opposite leg may be involved to a milder degree. Some patients have a significant degree of weight loss.
- Neuralgic amyotrophy of the lumbosacral plexus presents similarly to diabetic amyotrophy with severe pain and preferential involvement of the lumbar plexus.

LABORATORY PROCEDURES

Blood work: an urgent CBC and PT/PTT are important when a lumbosacral plexopathy is suspected due to retroperitoneal hemorrhage from heparin therapy.

IMAGING STUDIES

MRI with gadolinium is the best test for identifying neoplastic infiltration of the lumbosacral plexus and is more sensitive than CT, although CT can often identify cancer infiltration. A CT of the pelvis should urgently be performed if a patient is suspected of having a retroperitoneal hemorrhage due to heparin therapy. A radionucleotide bone scan may show abnormal uptake in the pelvic, sacrum, and lumbosacral vertebrae in cases of lumbosacral metastasis.

SPECIAL TESTS

Electrodiagnostic Studies

EMG is useful to confirm the diagnosis of lumbosacral plexopathy and to distinguish between neoplastic and radiation etiologies. By nerve conduction study, low-amplitude compound muscle action potentials (CMAPs) and sensory nerve action potentials (SNAPs) are found. The low-amplitude SNAPs distinguish the lesion from a radiculopathy, in which the SNAPs are normal. Needle electrode examination reveals widespread active and chronic denervation involving muscles innervated by the lumbosacral plexus, including the proximal gluteus medius and maximus muscles. The finding of spontaneous, semirhythmic bursts of potentials, called myokymic discharges, is a most useful finding that makes radiation plexopathy a more likely cause than neoplastic infiltration (seen in roughly two thirds of patients with radiation-induced lumbosacral plexopathy).

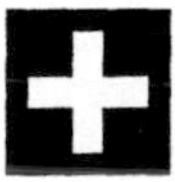

Management

GENERAL MEASURES

If a tumor is identified, radiation treatment may be indicated depending on the tumor type. If the patient is on heparin, this should be discontinued immediately.

SURGICAL MEASURES

A pelvic tumor may in some cases benefit from surgical resection. Surgical evacuation for retroperitoneal hemorrhage is controversial and most patients are treated conservatively.

SYMPTOMATIC TREATMENT

Pain management is an important concern in most causes of lumbosacral plexopathy. Physical therapy may be beneficial.

ADJUNCTIVE TREATMENT

If a neoplasm is identified, chemotherapy, radiation therapy, and other treatments are indicated. Patients with retroperitoneal hemorrhage may require blood transfusion and correction of the bleeding disorder.

ADMISSION/DISCHARGE CRITERIA

N/A

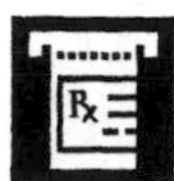

Medications

DRUG(S) OF CHOICE

No specific therapy. Pain management includes nonsteroidal antiinflammatory drugs, tricyclic antidepressants, and narcotic medications.

Contraindications

N/A

Precautions

N/A

ALTERNATIVE DRUGS

N/A

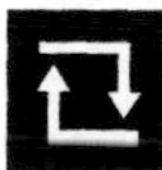

Follow-Up

PATIENT MONITORING

N/A

EXPECTED COURSE AND PROGNOSIS

Prognosis varies widely depending on the etiology. Patients with retroperitoneal hemorrhage, diabetic amyotrophy, neuralgic amyotrophy of the lumbosacral plexus, and postobstetrical plexopathy tend to improve over time. While patients with diabetic amyotrophy have a good recovery, only 40% make a full functional recovery. Patients with radiation plexopathies usually have slow progression of symptoms, although some patients have spontaneously improved. Neoplastic infiltration is typically associated with a poor prognosis, although early treatment results in a better outcome. One study of 30 patients with neoplastic infiltration of the lumbosacral plexus showed that 86% had died 3½ years after the onset of symptoms.

PATIENT EDUCATION

Due to the wide variety of disorders that can cause lumbosacral plexopathy, the patient can be referred to support groups for the underlying disease (e.g., cancer, diabetes, etc.).

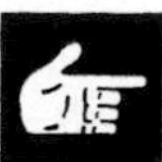

Miscellaneous

SYNONYMS

None

ICD-9-CM: 353.1 Lumbosacral plexopathy

SEE ALSO: N/A

REFERENCES

- Aho K, Sainio K. Late irradiation-induced lesions of the lumbosacral plexus. Neurology 1983;33:953–955.
- Emery S, Ochoa J. Lumbar plexus neuropathy resulting from retroperitoneal hemorrhage. Muscle Nerve 1978;1:330–334.
- Pettigrew LC, Glass JP, Maor M, et al. Diagnosis and treatment of lumbosacral plexopathies in patients with cancer. Arch Neurol 1984;41:1282–1285.
- Subramony SH, Wilbourn AJ. Diabetic proximal neuropathy: clinical and electromyographic studies. J Neurol Sci 1982;53:501–509.
- Taylor BV, Kimmel DW, Krecke KN, et al. Magnetic resonance imaging in cancer-related lumbosacral plexopathy. Mayo Clin Proc 1997;72:823–829.
- Thomas JE, Cascino TL, Earle JD. Differential diagnosis between radiation and tumor plexopathy of the pelvis. Neurology 1985;35:1–7.

Author(s): Brad Cole, MD

Poliomyelitis

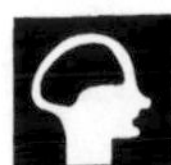

Basics

DESCRIPTION

Polio is a generalized viral infection of humans that can involve the anterior horn cells of spinal cord and motor nuclei of cranial nerves with resultant paralysis.

EPIDEMIOLOGY

Incidence/Prevalence

Today the disease has already been eradicated from large parts of world except Asia and West and Central Africa. In the U.S. and other countries where the wild virus has been eradicated, paralytic polio is still seen due to live attenuated virus vaccine. In 1998, 6,349 confirmed paralytic polio cases were reported worldwide, and 2,289 of these were due to wild virus.

Age

Any age can be affected; however, in 50% of cases children under the age of 3 are affected.

Sex

No sex difference is present.

Season

The disease is most frequent in summer and fall (July through September).

ETIOLOGY

Poliovirus is a single-stranded RNA enterovirus belonging to the Picornaviridae family. It has three serologically distinct types (polio 1, 2, and 3). Polio spreads through food or drink contaminated by feces. Also flies can passively transfer the virus from feces to food.

RISK FACTORS

- Several factors increase the likelihood of paralytic form of the disease:
- Tonsillectomy
- Intramuscular injections
- Immune deficiency
- Hypogammaglobulinemia
- Pregnancy
- Exercise
- Adult age (>18 years)

PREGNANCY

Pregnancy is associated with increased risk of paralytic disease.

ASSOCIATED CONDITIONS

- Vaccine-associated paralytic polio
- Postpolio syndrome

Diagnosis

DIFFERENTIAL DIAGNOSIS

- Acute causes of peripheral neuropathy
- Guillain-Barré syndrome
- Acute intermittent porphyria
- Lyme disease
- Diphtheria
- Transverse myelitis
- Heavy metal poisoning
- Acute spinal cord compressive lesions
- Other viral infections (Coxsackie virus, echovirus)

SIGNS AND SYMPTOMS

- The incubation period varies between 5 and 35 days, and oral and fecal shedding of the virus starts within 24 hours of the exposure.
- About 90% polio infections are asymptomatic.
- Minor illness (abortive polio): 5% to 10% of infected people develop nonspecific influenza-like syndrome characterized by fever, malaise, anorexia, headache, sore throat, and myalgia. Symptoms last 2 to 3 days.
- Nonparalytic poliomyelitis (aseptic meningitis): in about 1% of patients 7 to 10 days after the minor illness, aseptic meningitis is characterized by fever, headache, neck stiffness, and back pain develops. Symptoms resolve completely in most patients.
- Paralytic poliomyelitis: 1% of people infected develop the paralytic form of the disease. Paralysis develops 2 to 5 days after abortive polio when patient starts to recover. Symptoms start with fever, headache, and muscle pain. Asymmetrical weakness develops over several hours to days, affects legs more than arms. Neurologic examination reveals neck stiffness, decreased or absent deep tendon reflexes, and flaccid paralysis. A single muscle or groups of muscles of one or more extremities can be involved. While monoparesis is common in children, quadriparesis is more frequent in adults. Sensory examination is normal. Dysautonomia (cardiac arrhythmias, blood pressure instability, bladder and bowel dysfunction) can be seen. Involvement of cervical or thoracic cord may lead to intercostal and diaphragmatic weakness. Bulbar involvement is seen in 10% to 15% of cases. Symptoms include dysphagia, dysphonia, facial paralysis, diplopia, stridor, and respiratory weakness. Death may result from respiratory insufficiency and autonomic disturbances. Long-term sequelae include weakness, atrophy of limb, and growth failure especially in young children.

LABORATORY PROCEDURES

Blood Work

- Routine blood tests are normal except for lymphocytic pleocytosis.
- CSF examination: typically pleocytosis with increased protein is seen. Cell count does not usually exceed 500 cells/mm^3, initially polymorphonuclear leukocytes shifting to lymphocytic predominance after 72 hours. Protein content increases up to 200 mg/dL in the first few weeks. Virus isolation from CSF is rare.
- Virus can be isolated from feces and throat swabs 2 weeks before paralysis and several weeks after the onset of symptoms.
- A fourfold or greater increase in neutralizing antibody titers between acute phase and convalescent (3 to 6 weeks later) serology is diagnostic.

IMAGING STUDIES

Hyperintense signal of the ventral horns of the spinal cord has been demonstrated on spinal MRI in patients with poliomyelitis. These findings are nonspecific but may be helpful to differentiate acute lower motor neuron syndromes from Guillain-Barré syndrome.

SPECIAL TESTS

Electrodiagnostic Studies

Nerve conduction velocities are usually normal; compound muscle action potentials may have low amplitudes. Needle EMG shows a reduced number of voluntary motor unit potentials; and fibrillation potentials appear at about 3 weeks. As improvement occurs, giant motor units indicating reinnervation appear.

Management

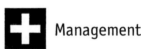

GENERAL MEASURES

Intensive care with respiratory support may be lifesaving. When forced vital capacity decreases below 12 mL/kg (less than 1 to 1.5 L for adults) or significant subjective dyspnea appears, intubation and mechanical ventilation should be considered. Cardiac function should be monitored. Bulbar functions should be followed and aspirations precautions observed.

SURGICAL MEASURES

There are no surgical procedures for the acute illness. For chronic phase correction of scoliosis, tendon lengthening and transfers are examples of rehabilitative surgeries. As improvement may continue up to 2 years, surgical procedures should be postponed until this time.

SYMPTOMATIC TREATMENT

Bed rest, analgesics, and hot wet packs relieve the muscle pain during acute illness.

ADJUNCTIVE TREATMENT

In the acute phase, respiratory exercises, hot packs to relieve pain, and passive exercises to prevent contractures should be performed. Active exercises and occupational therapy can be started at the subacute phase.

ADMISSION/DISCHARGE CRITERIA

For acute paralytic disease, hospitalization and bed rest are mandatory.

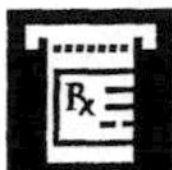

Medications

DRUGS(S) OF CHOICE

There is no specific antiviral agent proven effective against polio infection. Vaccination is the most effective measure for prevention.

Prophylaxis

There are two kinds of polio vaccine, both providing immunity against three types of poliovirus.

- Inactivated polio vaccine (IPV) (Salk)
  - —Administered subcutaneously
  - —Provides only serum humoral immunity; therefore, cannot prevent the multiplication of virus in gastrointestinal system and shedding in stool
  - —Safe for immunizing people with immune system problems

Contraindications

Does not cause vaccine-associated polio. Contraindicated in children allergic to neomycin, streptomycin, or polymyxin B.

- Oral polio vaccine (OPV) (Sabin)
  - —Live attenuated vaccine
  - —Easy to administer
  - —In addition to serum humoral immunity, provides secretory immunity in mucous membranes; therefore, limits the multiplication of virus in gastrointestinal system and prevents person-to-person transmission. Therefore, preferred in areas where the wild virus is still present.
  - —Carries vaccine-associated polio paralysis risk 1 in 2.4 million doses, more common with the first dose.

Contraindications

Contraindicated in children with immunodeficiency, hypogammaglobulinemia, leukemia, lymphoma, malignancy, and lowered resistance due to corticosteroid treatment, chemotherapy, or radiation and close contacts of such patients.

Precautions

Four doses of polio vaccine are enough to protect from polio. Committee on Infectious Diseases of the American Academy of Pediatrics recommends OPV for routine immunization. OPV is administered at ages 2, 4, and 15 months and 4 to 6 years. An additional dose can be administered at 6 months of age in areas with high risk of disease.

Immunization programs in countries where polio has been eradicated may employ combined immunization schedules with both OPV and IPV. The Centers for Disease Control and Prevention recommends first and second doses as IVP in the U.S. This decreases the risk of vaccine-associated poliomyelitis by 50% to 75% and provides the advantages of both vaccines.

For people traveling to areas where polio is common: if vaccinated previously, they should receive an additional dose of the vaccine they previously had. If they have not been previously vaccinated, they should be immunized with IPV. People younger than 18 years of age who have not been vaccinated in infancy can get two doses of OPV separated by 2 months and a third dose 6 to 12 months later.

People over 18 years of age should not be given OPV as the risk of paralysis with OPV is higher in adults.

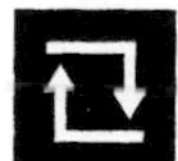

Follow-Up

PATIENT MONITORING

Patients in the convalescent phase of poliomyelitis may require physical therapy, bracing, and other orthoses.

EXPECTED COURSE AND PROGNOSIS

- Recovery from polio infection is complete except paralytic disease.
- CNS involvement determines the outcome of paralytic poliomyelitis. Ten percent of paralytic cases die due to respiratory and bulbar involvement. In bulbar poliomyelitis cases mortality goes up to 60%. Fifty percent of cases recover completely. The rest are left with neurologic sequelae.
- Paralysis is evident by 2 to 3 days of onset of symptoms. Improvement begins in weeks and plateaus by 6 months.
- Postpolio syndrome: in a group of patients, two to three decades after the paralysis, slowly progressive weakness and atrophy of previously affected or unaffected muscles may develop. This condition is called "postpolio syndrome." Fatigue and pain accompany the picture. This is an extremely slowly progressive condition and the patients should be reassured about this.

PATIENT EDUCATION

Polio is a rare disease now and is already eradicated from a large part of the world. However, there is a risk of spread of polio by travelers in areas where polio still exists. Improvement of hygiene and sanitation, and immunization are important to prevent and eradicate polio infections. Immunization programs should be continued until the disease is eradicated all over the world even in areas free of polio.

Centers for Disease Control and Prevention: *http://www.cdc.gov/nip.*

World Health Organization: *http://www.who.int/gpv-polio.*

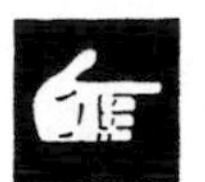

Miscellaneous

SYNONYMS

Heine-Medin disease

ICD-9-CM: 045 Acute poliomyelitis; 045.0 Acute paralytic poliomyelitis specified as bulbar; 045.1 Acute poliomyelitis with other paralysis; 045.2 Acute nonparalytic poliomyelitis; 045.9 Acute poliomyelitis, unspecified

SEE ALSO: N/A

REFERENCES

- Dalakas M, Illa I. Post-polio syndrome: concepts in clinical diagnosis, pathogenesis and etiology. Adv Neurol 1991;56: 495–511.
- Pascuzzi RM. Poliomyelitis and postpolio syndrome. In: Roos KL, ed. Central nervous system infectious diseases and therapy. New York: Marcel Decker, 1997:429–441.
- Simoes EAF. Poliomyelitis. In: Hoeprich PD, Jordan MC, Ronald AR, eds. Infectious diseases. Philadelphia: JB Lippincott, 1994:1141–1149.
- Update on adult immunization. Recommendations of the Immunization Practices Advisory Committee (ACIP). MMWR 1997;46:35–39.

Author(s): Ersin Tan, MD

Polymyositis

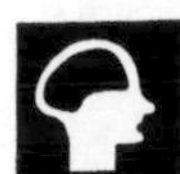

Basics

DESCRIPTION

Polymyositis (PM) is an idiopathic inflammatory myopathy. The syndrome is characterized by primary inflammation of skeletal muscle with myofiber necrosis; other organs may be involved. The history, pattern of weakness, and muscle pathology distinguish polymyositis from the other idiopathic inflammatory myopathies (dermatomyositis and inclusion body myositis).

EPIDEMIOLOGY

Incidence/Prevalence

Most studies have grouped polymyositis and dermatomyositis (DM) together. The annual incidence ranges from 0.1 to 0.93 per 100,000 population.

Race

The incidence among white Americans is 0.32 per 100,000 population. The incidence among black Americans is 0.77 per 100,000.

Sex

Females have PM more frequently in all age groups.

ETIOLOGY

The cause of PM is unknown. A viral etiology has been speculated but not demonstrated. Speculation has included viral infection triggering an altered immune response directed against self-antigens, possibly from cross-reactivity with specific muscle antigens. PM may occur alone or in association with a number of connective tissue diseases, autoimmune, or infectious conditions (see Associated Conditions, below). PM is sporadic, without family history of weakness.

Genetics

PM is associated with human leukocyte antigen (HLA) DR3 in 48% of white patients and also with HLA-B7 and HLA-DRw6 in black patients.

RISK FACTORS

None identified.

PREGNANCY

PM is a rare event in pregnancy. Perinatal mortality approaches 60% in the few cases (less than two dozen) reported.

ASSOCIATED CONDITIONS

- Autoimmune conditions: Crohn's disease, Hashimoto's disease, primary biliary cirrhosis, vasculitis, myasthenia gravis, adult celiac disease, chronic graft-versus-host disease, discoid lupus, ankylosing spondylitis, Behçet's disease, acne fulminans, dermatitis herpetiformis, psoriasis, agammaglobulinemia, autoimmune thrombocytopenia.
- Infections: HIV, human T-cell lymphotrophic virus type I (HTLV-I), *Borrelia burgdorferi* (Lyme disease), *Legionella pneumophila* (Legionnaires' disease).
- Overlap syndromes: PM may be associated with connective tissue diseases, and overlap syndromes are diagnosed when criteria for two diseases are present. PM may occur with scleroderma myositis, Sjögren's syndrome, systemic lupus erythematosus, rheumatoid arthritis, antisynthetase syndrome, and mixed connective tissue disease.
- Malignancy: many authors report an increased association (0%–28%) between PM and malignancy, though the evidence is less strong than that between DM and malignancy.

Diagnosis

DIFFERENTIAL DIAGNOSIS

- Inflammatory myopathies
  - —Dermatomyositis
  - —Inclusion body myositis (especially previously diagnosed PM unresponsive to corticosteroids)
- Toxin-induced inflammatory myopathies
  - —D-penicillamine
  - —Zidovudine
  - —Procainamide
  - —Remote effect of *ciguatera* poisoning
- Sarcoid myopathy
- Infections
  - —Bacterial (tropical pyomyositis)
    - *-Staphylococcus aureus*
    - *-Streptococcus*
  - —Parasitic
    - -Trichinosis
    - -Cysticercosis
    - -Toxoplasmosis
- Sporadic limb-girdle muscular dystrophy
- Metabolic myopathy
- Endocrinopathy
- Progressive muscular atrophy (neurogenic muscular atrophies)

SIGNS AND SYMPTOMS

- Insidious onset of weakness of proximal greater than distal muscles
- Usually symmetric, occasionally asymmetric or focal on presentation
- Neck flexor weakness
- Muscle pain/tenderness may occur
- Dysphagia
- Arthritis in 25% to 65% of PM patients
- Cardiac abnormalities: bundle branch block, atrioventricular conduction defects, atrial dysrhythmias
- Dyspnea, suggesting diaphragm involvement, interstitial lung disease, or aspiration

LABORATORY PROCEDURES

Serum Studies

- Muscle enzymes (elevated up to 50-fold)—creatine kinase. Aldolase, glutamic oxaloacetic transaminase (SGOT) may also be elevated in the serum.
- Erythrocyte sedimentation rate (ESR)—normal in more than half of patients, and not useful in diagnosis, determining treatment efficacy, or prognosis.
- Antibodies—patterns of antibody production may provide additional support for clinical diagnosis of some inflammatory muscle diseases but are usually not clinically useful. Antibodies against MI-2 and Mas antigens are associated with relatively mild muscle disease. Anticytoplasmic antibodies against translational components (antisynthetase and anti-SRP, or signal recognition particle antibodies) are associated with severe muscle and systemic illness. The anti-Jo1 antibody is associated with interstitial lung disease.

IMAGING STUDIES

MRI detects muscle and subcutaneous edema and inflammation, but is rarely helpful in making the diagnosis. Use of MRI may be no better than clinical exam, is expensive, and has been limited to research.

SPECIAL TESTS

- EMG/NCS—sensory action potentials, late responses (F-waves and H-reflexes), conduction velocities, and repetitive nerve stimulation, are normal. The compound muscle action potential (CMAP) is normal in latency and amplitude early in disease; the CMAP amplitude may decrease with disease progression, reflecting loss of myofibers. Needle EMG studies demonstrate increased insertional activity (>500 msec), increased spontaneous activity (fibrillations, occasional complex repetitive discharges, and, rarely, myotonic discharges), and reduced amplitude and duration of voluntary motor unit action potentials (MUAPs). Voluntary MUAPs are often polyphasic with increased recruitment patterns. Chronic PM may demonstrate long duration motor unit action potentials.
- Muscle biopsy is the preferred diagnostic test for PM. Histologic features include myofiber size variation, regeneration, necrosis, an increase in connective tissue, an increase in central nuclei, and inflammation. Inflammation is perivascular, perimysial, and endomysial. Endomysial inflammation consists primarily of activated $CD8^+$ cells, macrophages, very few natural killer cells, and few or no B cells. $CD8^+$ cells focally invade non-necrotic muscle fibers.

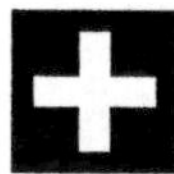

Management

GENERAL MEASURES

Once PM is suspected, the main focus should be exclusion of alternative causes of myopathic weakness and treatment of the disease;

respiratory function should be monitored with vital capacity and negative inspiratory force if presentation includes respiratory distress.

SURGICAL MEASURES

Rarely, cricopharyngeal myotomy may be considered for dysphagia refractory to pharmacologic treatment.

SYMPTOMATIC TREATMENT

Speech pathology evaluation and swallow study should be considered for dysphagia.

ADJUNCTIVE TREATMENT

Physical therapy and occupational therapy should be considered to preserve range of motion.

ADMISSION/DISCHARGE CRITERIA

- Evaluation and treatment of weakness affecting speech, respiration, or ambulation.
- Transfer or admission to a rehabilitation facility should be considered when there is significant weakness.
- Some patients may come to the attention of the neurology service during evaluation by pulmonology for interstitial lung disease and myopathy is detected.

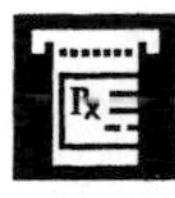

Medications

DRUG(S) OF CHOICE

Prednisone (at least 1 mg/kg/d, typically 60–80 mg) is administered in a single oral daily dose for 3 to 4 weeks, followed by a slow taper over 10 weeks to 1 mg/kg on alternate days. In severe cases, intravenous methylprednisolone 1 g qd or qod for five to six doses can be used to initiate therapy. If prednisone demonstrates efficacy, the dose may be reduced by 5 or 10 mg every 3 to 4 weeks until the least necessary dose is determined. If prednisone is ineffective, another immunosuppressive medication may be initiated and prednisone more rapidly tapered.

Contraindications

Corticosteroids are contraindicated in patients with a known hypersensitivity to any of the corticosteroids.

Corticosteroids should not be used in persons with peptic ulcer (except life-threatening situations).

An apparent association of corticosteroids and left ventricular free-wall rupture after recent myocardial infarction (MI) has been suggested, and corticosteroids should be used with extreme caution in patients with recent MI.

Precautions

- Corticosteroids may reduce resistance to and aid in bacterial, viral, or fungal infections and mask clinical signs of infection. Corticosteroids can reactivate tuberculosis, and chemoprophylaxis is used in patients with a history of active tuberculosis undergoing prolonged steroid treatment. Patients should be instructed to notify any surgeon, anesthesiologist, or dentist if a surgical procedure is required and they have recently (within 12 months) been on glucocorticoids.
- Anaphylactoid reactions are seen in some patients given parenteral glucocorticoids, and may represent hypersensitivity to paraben preservatives.
- Corticosteroids should be used with caution in persons with diverticulitis, nonspecific ulcerative colitis, cirrhosis, hypothyroidism (who may demonstrate an exaggerated response to the drugs), hypertension, psychosis, and congestive heart failure.
- Prolonged use of corticosteroids may cause adrenocortical insufficiency (in supraphysiologic doses), and muscle wasting, pain, or weakness ("steroid myopathy").
- Corticosteroid use is associated with hyperglycemia and hypokalemia.

ALTERNATIVE DRUGS

Considered if prednisone is ineffective or if relief for steroid complications is sought. Consider azathioprine 2 to 3 mg/kg daily orally for approximately 4 to 6 months. If azathioprine is ineffective, consider methotrexate 15 to 25 mg/week orally.

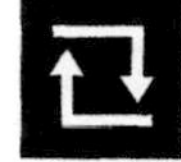

Follow-Up

PATIENT MONITORING

- Recommendations about following creatine kinase vary, depending on the author. Clinical examination is the best measure of progress and treatment efficacy.
- Patients on steroids should have weight, blood pressure, serum glucose, and potassium, and eyes (for cataract formation) monitored.
- For patients on azathioprine or methotrexate, blood count and liver function tests should be monitored every 1 to 2 months.
- Consider supplementing patients on methotrexate (a folic acid analog inhibiting dihydrofolate reductase) with folic acid 5 mg once weekly after the methotrexate dose.

EXPECTED COURSE AND PROGNOSIS

The prognosis in PM without malignancy is relatively favorable, but may require lifelong treatment. Five-year survival rates range from 70% to 93%. Poor prognostic features include older age, malignancy, interstitial lung disease, cardiac disease, respiratory muscle weakness, dysphagia, acute onset, fever, presence of Jo-1 or SRP antibodies, and a delay in, or inadequate, treatment.

PATIENT EDUCATION

Patients who will be on long-term corticosteroids should be told of potential complications such as electrolyte disturbances, osteoporosis, peptic ulcer, weight gain, bruising, insomnia, hyperglycemia, and cataract formation. Such potential complications form the basis for monitoring (see above) and consideration for treatment with potassium and calcium supplementation, a no-added-salt diet, antacids, and exercise program. Physical therapy should also be considered early in the disease to prevent atrophy and preserve muscle function. The Myositis Association of America serves as a source of information for patients as well as patient advocate and support group. Myositis Association of America, Inc. (MAA), 755 Cantrell Avenue, Suite C, Harrisonburg, VA 22801. Phone: 540-433-7686, fax: 540-432-0206, email: *maa@myositis.org*, website: *http://www.myositis.org*.

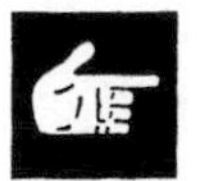

Miscellaneous

SYNONYMS

N/A

ICD-9-CM: 710.4 Polymyositis

SEE ALSO: N/A

REFERENCES

- Amato AA, Barohn RJ. Idiopathic inflammatory myopathies. Neurol Clin 1997;15:615–648.
- Corticosteroids: general statement. In: McEvoy GK, ed. American Hospital Formulary Service. Bethesda, MD: American Society of Health-System Pharmacists, 1995:2094–2102.
- Dalakas MC. Polymyositis, dermatomyositis, and inclusion-body myositis. N Engl J Med 1991;325:1487–1498.
- Litchy WJ. Polymyositis and dermatomyositis. In: Vinken PJ, Bruyn GW, Klawans HL, et al., eds. Handbook of clinical neurology, vol 27: systemic diseases, part III. New York: Elsevier Science, 1998:129–147.
- Love LA, Leff RL, Fraser DD, et al. A new approach to the classification of idiopathic inflammatory myopathy: myositis-specific autoantibodies define useful homogeneous patient groups. Medicine 1991;70: 360–374.
- Mikol J, Engel AG. Inclusion body myositis. In: Engel AG, Franzini-Armstrong C, eds. Myology. New York: McGraw-Hill, 1994:1384–1398.
- Rosenzweig BA, Siegfried R, Binette SP, et al. Primary idiopathic polymyositis and dermatomyositis complicating pregnancy: diagnosis and management. Obstet Gynecol Surv 1998;44:162–170.

Author(s): Boyd M. Koffman MD, PhD

Porphyria

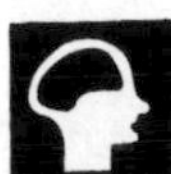

Basics

DESCRIPTION

Porphyria is an autosomal-dominant condition with highly variable expression. It results from a relative deficiency of porphobilinogen deaminase (known as uroporphyrinogen 1) of the heme biosynthesis pathway. Acute intermittent porphyria is the most common porphyria associated with neurologic manifestations and is classified as a hepatic porphyria due to the overproduction and accumulation of porphyrin precursors in the liver.

EPIDEMIOLOGY

Incidence

Porphyria has an incidence of approximately 1 in 50,000. It is much more common in Sweden with an incidence of approximately 1 in 1,000.

Age/Sex

Manifestations usually occur in adult women. Attacks of acute intermittent porphyria are rare before puberty.

ETIOLOGY

The deficiency of porphobilinogen deaminase results in higher levels of aminolevulinic acid and porphobilinogen in both the blood and urine during attacks. How accumulation of these metabolites contributes to the clinical symptoms is not well understood.

Genetics

Many deletions and point mutation in the porphobilinogen-deaminase gene on chromosome 11 have been described.

RISK FACTORS

Many drugs and hormones may precipitate attacks. Drugs that are contraindicated are typically inducers of the P-450 system and include barbiturates, carbamazepine, ergots, synthetic estrogens and progesterones, griseofulvin, valproate, and sulfonamide antibiotics. Attacks in women are often in the luteal phase of their menstrual cycle.

PREGNANCY

As many as 75% of patients experience an exacerbation of porphyria during pregnancy with some series showing up to 20% mortality. During an attack there is a high risk for spontaneous abortions. There are no known effects on the fetus, although there is passive transfer of porphyrins through the placenta.

ASSOCIATED CONDITIONS

N/A

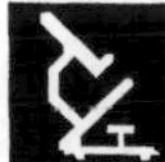

Diagnosis

DIFFERENTIAL DIAGNOSIS

- Acute abdominal pain associated with common conditions such as appendicitis, ectopic pregnancy, or subacute bacterial peritonitis
- Paralytic ileus
- Guillain-Barré syndrome
- Arsenic poisoning
- Thallium poisoning

SIGNS AND SYMPTOMS

Attacks of acute intermittent porphyria manifest themselves as acute attacks of abdominal pain, which is poorly localized and may be associated with abdominal cramping and nausea and vomiting. Neuropsychiatric manifestations also can occur, ranging from restlessness and agitation to delirium with psychosis. Two to 3 days after the onset of abdominal pain the patients often develop a predominantly motor axonal neuropathy. Weakness develops rapidly and is predominantly proximal, although the extensors of the fingers and wrists seem to be usually affected. Reflexes are diminished but are not usually lost in the early course of the illness, unlike in acute demyelinating neuropathies such as Guillain-Barré syndrome. An autonomic neuropathy is frequently encountered and may result in unexplained arrhythmias and wide fluctuations in blood pressure. Rarely seizures may occur.

LABORATORY PROCEDURES

Porphyria is easily diagnosed once the disease is suspected. During an acute attack high levels of porphobilinogen and alanine are present in the blood. Definite diagnosis depends on demonstrating a porphobilinogen deficiency in erythrocytes. Nerve conduction studies and electromyography confirm the axonal nature of the neuropathy and help distinguish it from an acute demyelinating neuropathy or rhabdomyolysis.

IMAGING STUDIES

N/A

SPECIAL TESTS

N/A

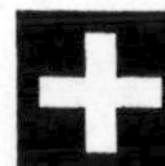

Management

GENERAL MEASURES

Long-term management focuses on avoiding precipitating factors and recognizing the possibility of acute intermittent porphyria in the setting of an acute attack of abdominal pain.

SURGICAL MEASURES

N/A

SYMPTOMATIC MANAGEMENT

Specific treatment of an acute porphyric attack involves intravenous administration of glucose or heme. Both agents inhibit the heme biosynthetic pathway. Glucose is given in doses of 300 g per day and heme in the form of hematin, heme albumin, or heme arginate at doses of 3 to 4 mg per day for 4 days. Narcotics can be used safely to treat the abdominal pain, and phenothiazines are safe for the treatment of nausea and vomiting. Seizures may be difficult to treat since many of the typical anticonvulsants are contraindicated. Benzodiazepines can be used safely.

ADJUNCTIVE TREATMENT

N/A

ADMISSION/DISCHARGE CRITERIA

N/A

Medications

DRUG(S) OF CHOICE

No medications are available to prevent acute attacks. Avoidance of contraindicated drugs is recommended.

Contraindications

Barbiturates, carbamazepine, ergots, danazol, estrogens and progesterones, griseofulvin, valproate, sulfonamide antibiotics, meprobamate, phenytoin

Precautions

N/A

ALTERNATIVE DRUGS

N/A

Follow-Up

PATIENT MONITORING

The acute axonal neuropathy may also affect cranial nerves, causing bulbar weakness and increasing the risk for aspiration. Respiratory weakness can also occur due to involvement of the phrenic and intercostal nerves.

EXPECTED COURSE AND PROGNOSIS

The recoveries from the attacks of acute abdominal pain are often quite rapid. Recovery of strength is dependent on the degree of axonal injury.

PATIENT EDUCATION

Patients should be aware of potential precipitating medications and wear a medical identification bracelet. Family members of patients identified as having porphyria should also be screened for the genetic defect.

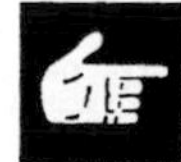

Miscellaneous

SYNONYMS

Acute intermittent porphyria

ICD-9-CM: 277.1 Dis porphyrin metabolism

SEE ALSO: N/A

REFERENCES

- Albers J, Robertson WJ, Daube J. Electrodiagnostic findings in acute porphyric neuropathy. Muscle Nerve 1978;1:292–6.
- Anderson K, Spitz I, Sassa S, et al. Prevention of cyclical attacks of acute intermittent porphyria with a long acting agonist of luteinizing hormone-releasing hormone. N Engl J Med 1984;311:643–645.
- Becker D, Kramer S. The neurological manifestations of porphyria: a review. Medicine 1977;56:411–423.
- Goldberg A. Molecular genetics of acute intermittent porphyria. Br Med J 1985;291: 499–500.
- Tschudy D, Valamis M, Magnussen C. Acute intermittent porphyria: clinical and selected research aspects. Ann Intern Med 1975;83:851–864.

Author(s): J. Ned Pruitt II, MD

Primary Lateral Sclerosis

Basics

DESCRIPTION

Primary lateral sclerosis (PLS) is a clinical term applied to a disorder that in life remains restricted to the corticospinal tracts (CSTs) and is proven only at autopsy. The definition of PLS mandates the exclusion of other likely causes of progressive spastic paraparesis (PSP) such as demyelinating disease, hereditary conditions, structural disorders, malformations, and infection of the CNS.

EPIDEMIOLOGY

Incidence/Prevalence

PLS is a rare disorder, and as a result the incidence and prevalence have not been established. There is no known predilection for race, age, or sex.

ETIOLOGY

PLS is a neurodegenerative disorder with predominant degeneration of the upper motor neurons. Autopsy studies demonstrate loss of large pyramidal Betz cells in layer V with secondary degeneration of the pyramidal tract. There is no known genetic predisposition.

RISK FACTORS

There is a paraneoplastic association of PLS with cancer of the lung and breast and lymphoma; however, a discrete autoantibody has not been isolated.

PREGNANCY

There is no association with pregnancy.

ASSOCIATED CONDITIONS

PSL may be a forme fruste of amyotrophic lateral sclerosis (ALS).

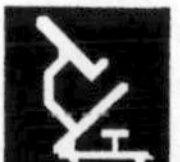

Diagnosis

DIFFERENTIAL DIAGNOSIS

The differential diagnosis includes primarily progressive spinal multiple sclerosis (MS), hereditary spastic paraplegia (HSP), cervical spondylotic myelopathy (CSM), tumors of the foramen magnum, syringomyelia, spinal arteriovenous malformations, human T lymphotrophic virus and HIV infections, and stroke.

SIGNS AND SYMPTOMS

Spasticity in PLS results from the underlying upper motor neuron (UMN) lesion and the disinhibition of velocity-dependent increase in muscle tone during passive stretch. The associated positive clinical signs of this disinhibition are hyperreflexia, Babinski signs, and painful extensor and flexor spasms. The negative signs of spasticity are UMN weakness, fatigability, and incoordination.

LABORATORY PROCEDURES

Electromyography and nerve conduction studies (EMG-NCS) should be performed in all patients for the possibility of ALS, because fibrillation, positive sharp waves, and widespread fasciculation should not be seen in PLS.

IMAGING STUDIES

MRI of the brain and cord excludes structural disorders of the CNS, and in conjunction with sensory evoked responses (SERs) of the arms and legs, auditory evoked responses (AERs), and visual evoked responses (VERs), and lumbar CSF analysis excludes MS and chronic infection.

SPECIAL TESTS

Transcranial magnetic stimulation (TMS) complements EMG-NCS because it quantitates central conduction time, which should be reduced in isolated disease of the CST.

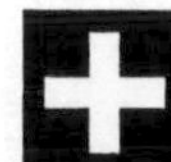

Management

GENERAL MEASURES

The goal of treatment is to prevent or reduce the undesirable consequences of spasticity that include decreased mobility, disabling pain, contractures, dependency for activities of daily living (ADL), sexual dysfunction, and sleep disturbances. Untreated, these consequences lead to low self-esteem and mood disorders. The management of spasticity should ideally be based on ongoing clinical assessment leading to an appropriate therapeutic plan

SURGICAL MEASURES

Selective dorsal rhizotomy (SDR) can be performed in selected patients who do not benefit from other measures to manage spasticity. Physiologically, this procedure reduces spasticity by removing the stimulating afferent input of muscle stretch receptors on motor neurons. However, SDR invariably leaves the patient with some undesirable sensory deficits.

SYMPTOMATIC TREATMENT

Physiotherapy should be prescribed to prevent contractures, improve overall active function, and provide comfort, but it is rarely sufficient therapy alone. Occupational therapy is needed periodically to optimize ability to perform ADLs.

ADJUNCTIVE TREATMENT

N/A

ADMISSION/DISCHARGE CRITERIA

Admission is not generally required except for management of complications such as aspiration pneumonia.

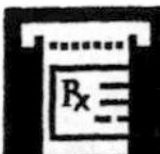

Medications

DRUG(S) OF CHOICE

Oral antispasticity agents should be tried in all patients. Baclofen, a γ-aminobutyric acid analogue, is the drug of choice for the treatment of spasticity associated with PLS. It is given in doses of 10 to 40 mg PO tid to qid (and often higher doses, although the PDR recommended limit is 100 mg per day). It penetrates the blood-brain barrier poorly; thus to obtain significant therapeutic benefit, high doses need to be taken that may induce unacceptable weakness, lethargy, somnolence, and other side effects.

Contraindications

Known hypersensitivity to baclofen.

Precautions

Oral antispasticity agents may cause increased weakness, sedation, and nausea. These agents should be started at low doses and titrated up gradually.

ALTERNATIVE DRUGS

- Alternative oral agents for spasticity include tizanidine, diazepam, clonidine, dantrolene, and cyproheptadine.
- Botulinum toxin can be injected into affected muscles in selected individuals with focal sever spasticity, but there may be bruising, focal weakness, flu-like symptoms, and antibody development with chronic use.
- Baclofen can be delivered intrathecally via a surgically implanted programmable pump with the advantage of easier penetration of the drug into the CNS and higher drug levels. However, the disadvantages include an operative procedure and potential malfunction of the pump system.

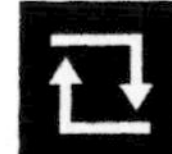

Follow-Up

PATIENT MONITORING

A thorough clinical assessment is crucial in formulating a local management program that requires a multidisciplinary approach. The Ashworth Scale is an objective bedside rating system of spasticity that can be easily applied to patients with PLS, both in initial assessment and in determining treatment benefit.

EXPECTED COURSE AND PROGNOSIS

The course is usually slowly progressive, leading to a bed-bound state over decades. Oropharyngeal involvement can predispose to aspiration pneumonia.

PATIENT EDUCATION

- National Institute of Neurologic Disorders and Stroke information page: *http://www.ninds.nih.gov/health_and_medical/disorders/primary_lateral_sclerosis.htm.*
- Spastic Paraplegia Foundation, P.O. Box 1208, Forston, GA 31808. Phone: 978-256-2673, email: *info@sp-foundation.org*, website: *http://www.sp-foundation.org.*
- Primary Lateral Sclerosis Newsletter, 101 Pinta Court, Los Gatos, CA 95032, *73112.611@compuserve.com.*

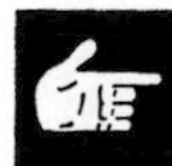

Miscellaneous

SYNONYMS

N/A

ICD-9-CM: 335.24 Primary lateral sclerosis

SEE ALSO: N/A

REFERENCES

- Lassman AB, Sadiq SA. Management of spasticity. In: Younger DS, ed. Motor disorders. Philadelphia: Lippincott Williams & Wilkins, 1999:505–514.
- Younger DS, Chou S, Hays AP, et al. Primary lateral sclerosis: a clinical diagnosis re-emerges. Arch Neurol 1988;45:1304–1307.
- Zhai P, Pagan F, Statland J, et al. Primary lateral sclerosis—a heterogeneous disorder composed of different subtypes? Neurology 2003;60:1258–1265.

Author(s): David S. Younger, MD

Progressive Multifocal Leukoencephalopathy

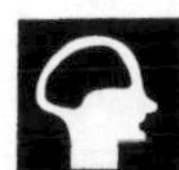

Basics

DESCRIPTION

Progressive multifocal leukoencephalopathy (PML) is a subacute demyelinating disease of the CNS secondary to activation of latent JC virus, usually occurring in immunoincompetent individuals.

EPIDEMIOLOGY

Incidence/Prevalence

PML is a rare disease in the general population. It occurs most commonly in HIV-infected patients, and occurs in approximately 5% of that population. The age-adjusted death rate increased from 0.2 per million persons before 1984 to 3.3 per million persons in 1994, attributable to HIV. During the 16-year period from 1979 through 1994 3,894 PML deaths were reported.

Race

No study has demonstrated an ethnic predominance.

Age

Range 5 to 84 years.

Sex

Males > females.

ETIOLOGY

It is estimated that 70% to 80% of the adult population harbors latent JC virus (a human polyomavirus). An immunocompromised state secondary most commonly to HIV, lymphoproliferative disorders, and iatrogenic immune suppression allows reactivation of the JC virus in oligodendrocytes. PML has been described in immunocompetent individuals.

Genetics

PML appears to be sporadic and genetic factors are not identified.

RISK FACTORS

Immunocompromised state.

PREGNANCY

Little is known about any relationship of PML to pregnancy.

ASSOCIATED CONDITIONS

PML has been described in association with AIDS, chronic neoplastic disease, Hodgkin's disease, lymphoma, myeloproliferative diseases, tuberculosis, sarcoidosis, and multiple immunosuppressive drugs.

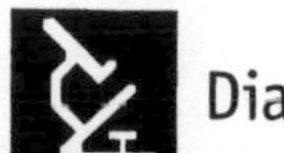

Diagnosis

DIFFERENTIAL DIAGNOSIS

- HIV demyelination
- Multiple sclerosis
- Hypertensive leukoencephalopathy
- Vasculitis
- Lymphoma
- Toxoplasmosis
- Glioma
- Central pontine myelinolysis
- Radiation-related leukoencephalopathy
- Stroke
- Acute disseminated encephalomyelitis
- CMV

SIGNS AND SYMPTOMS

Patients present with focal neurologic deficit including hemiparesis, visual loss, aphasia, ataxia, dysarthria, sensory changes, and cognitive impairment. Headache, seizures, and extrapyramidal syndromes are more rare.

LABORATORY PROCEDURES

Blood Work

There are no specific blood tests to diagnose PML, but the following tests should be considered to rule out other possible etiologies: ESR, CBC, coagulation profile, HIV, RPR, vitamin B_{12}, BUN, creatinine, Na, ammonia level, and toxoplasmosis titer.

IMAGING STUDIES

- CT demonstrates hypodense lesions in the white matter. These lesions are commonly seen in the frontal and parieto-occipital regions, but may occur in any white matter distribution including the posterior fossa. Scattered lesions may enlarge and become confluent. These lesions are usually bilateral, but may be unilateral.
- MRI is much more sensitive in evaluating white matter involvement. MRI often shows T2 hyperintense lesions in the periventricular and subcortical white matter. Lesions are often seen to progress from focal to extensive and confluent areas of T2 hyperintensity. Contrast enhancement is typically absent.
- MR spectroscopy can be used to further evaluate PML, and MR magnetization transfer can help in distinguishing PML from HIV encephalitis.

SPECIAL TESTS

CSF cell count, glucose, and protein are usually normal. Polymerase chain reaction (PCR) for JC virus DNA is specific but not sensitive for PML and should be done to aid in diagnosis. Cytology, cell count, glucose, protein, Gram stain, bacterial culture, fungal culture, AFB, VDRL, and viral screen should be done to rule out other possible causes of white matter lesions. Biopsy remains the standard for diagnosis demonstrating characteristic histopathology; however, clinical and radiographic evidence accompanied by positive PCR for JC virus DNA suffices in most situations.

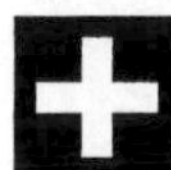

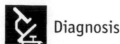

Management

GENERAL MEASURES

PML, with few exceptions, is the result of immunosuppression, and the underlying cause of immunosuppression should be determined if unknown as part of the initial evaluation. Iatrogenic immunosuppressive agents should be discontinued when plausible. When PML is the initial presenting feature of HIV infection (~5%), patients should be offered optimal antiretroviral therapy (HAART). Antiviral therapy directed at the JC virus is of unproven benefit. Cytosine arabinose has been the most commonly used agent, but in a controlled trial in HIV+ patients was ineffective. Other agents under investigation include Cidofovir and interferon.

SURGICAL MEASURES

There are no surgical procedures for the treatment of PML.

SYMPTOMATIC TREATMENT

- Antiseizure medication should be initiated when seizures occur.
- Pain may be present as part of a central pain syndrome and should be treated appropriately. Tricyclic antidepressants and selective serotonin reuptake inhibitor antidepressants, gabapentin, and narcotics may be of benefit.
- Spasticity may occur and can be treated with baclofen or tizanidine.

ADJUNCTIVE TREATMENT

- Physical therapy and occupational therapy may be of benefit when hemiparesis or paralysis occur.
- Intrathecal cytarabine and interferon alpha are of unproven benefit.

ADMISSION/DISCHARGE CRITERIA

Patients should be admitted for initial evaluation, treatment, and stabilization, if rapidly progressive neurologic deficits, fever, or recurrent seizures occur. If a neoplasm or acute infection is strongly suspected, admission for diagnostic evaluation including possible brain biopsy may be necessary. Inpatient rehabilitation should be considered at discharge when deficits dictate.

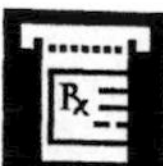

Medications

DRUG(S) OF CHOICE

No specific anti-JC viral treatment is known to be effective. Treatment of the underlying immune disorder may help.

ALTERNATIVE DRUGS

N/A

Follow-Up

PATIENT MONITORING

Patient should be followed every 4 to 6 weeks to observe progression.

EXPECTED COURSE AND PROGNOSIS

Most patients die within 9 months of diagnosis. Spontaneous remission have been reported to occur in as much as 8% of the HIV population. When the underlying cause of immunosuppression can be reversed, survival is improved.

PATIENT EDUCATION

N/A

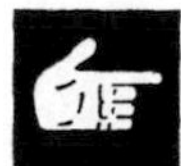

Miscellaneous

SYNONYMS

N/A

ICD-9-CM: 046.3 Progressive multifocal leukoencephalopathy

SEE ALSO: N/A

REFERENCES

- Albrecht H, Hoffman C, Degen O, et al. HAART therapy significantly improves the prognosis of patients with HIV-associated progressive multifocal leukoencephalopathy. AIDS 1998;12(10):1149–1154.
- Bradley WG, Daroff RB, Fenichel GM, et al. Neurology in clinical practice. Boston: Butterworth-Heinemann, 2000:1369–1370.
- DeLuca A, Giancola ML, Cingolani A, et al. Clinical and virological monitoring during treatment with intrathecal cytarabine in patients with AIDS-associated PML. Clin Infect Dis 1999;28(3):624–628.
- Ernst T, Chang L, Witt M, et al. PML and HIV-associated white matter lesions in AIDS: magnetization transfer MR imaging. Radiology 1999;210(2):539–543.
- Hall CD, Dafni U, Simpson D, et al. Failure of cytarabine in PML associated with HIV infection. AIDS Clinical Trials Group 243 Team. N Engl J Med 1998;338(19): 1345–1351.
- Holman RC, Torok TJ, Belay ED, et al. Progressive multifocal leukoencephalopathy in the United States, 1979–1994: increased mortality associated with HIV infection. Neuroepidemiology 1998;17(6): 303–309.
- Yiannoutsos CT, Major EO, Curfman B, et al. Relation of JC virus DNA in the cerebrospinal fluid to survival in acquired immunodeficiency syndrome patients with biopsy-proven progressive multifocal leukoencephalopathy. Ann Neurol 1999;45(6):816–821.

Author(s): Stephen J. Gomez, MD; Paul L. Moots, MD

Progressive Supranuclear Palsy

Basics

DESCRIPTION

Progressive supranuclear palsy (PSP) is one of the Parkinson's plus syndromes. Despite clinical similarities, however, the basic neuropathologic processes are significantly different from idiopathic Parkinson's disease (IPD). Clinically, PSP is regarded as one of the akinetic-rigid syndromes. Pathologically, however, it falls more in the class of tauopathies, which include, but are not limited to, Alzheimer's disease, frontotemporal dementias including Pick's disease, corticobasal ganglionic degeneration (CBGD), and others.

Characterized by early gait disturbance, bradykinesia, rigidity, and occasionally tremor, it is most commonly misdiagnosed as IPD early in its onset. Relentlessly progressive, PSP usually leads to significant motor and cognitive decline in 5 to 7 years, resulting in institutionalization and death.

Like many of the Parkinson's plus syndromes, PSP shares the clinical characteristic of being poorly responsive or totally unresponsive to dopaminergic stimulation.

Classical Pathologic Changes in Progressive Supranuclear Palsy

- Prominent neurofibrillary tangles (NFTs) in multiple subcortical regions as well as cortex, including hippocampus
- Granulovacuolar degeneration in:
  - —Basal ganglia
  - —Brainstem, especially the red nucleus, locus ceruleus, and superior olivary nucleus
  - —Cerebellum

EPIDEMIOLOGY

Incidence/Prevalence

Incidence rates of PSP have been estimated at 0.3 to 1.1 new cases per year per 100,000 individuals. Prevalence rates in the United Kingdom may approach 6 to 7 cases per 100,000 population.

PSP represents approximately 3% to 5% of all cases of parkinsonism, while idiopathic PD represents at least 85%.

Race

No known ethnic predilection.

Age

The median age of diagnosis is mid- to late 50s to early 60s, slightly earlier than idiopathic PD.

Sex

Some authors suggest a male/female ratio of 2:1, while other studies have found no gender differences.

ETIOLOGY

The cause of PSP is unknown. The possibility of infection has been raised due to similarities between PSP and postencephalitic parkinsonism. Rare cases of autosomal-dominant, familial clusterings have been reported, but the gene has not been identified yet. Recent evidence suggests that homozygous carriers of the A0/A0 genotype with mutations of the tau gene may be at increased risk of developing PSP.

PREGNANCY

N/A

ASSOCIATED CONDITIONS

N/A

Diagnosis

DIFFERENTIAL DIAGNOSIS

- Corticobasal ganglionic degeneration
- Diffuse Lewy body disease
- Drug-induced parkinsonism (e.g., antipsychotics, antiemetics, and other dopamine blocking agents)
- Multiple system atrophy (MSA)
  - —Shy-Drager syndrome (SDS)—PD plus autonomic insufficiency
  - —Striatonigral degeneration (SND)—PD plus levodopa unresponsiveness
  - —Olivopontocerebellar atrophy (OPCA)—PD plus ataxia
- Vascular parkinsonism
- Postencephalitic parkinsonism
- Posttraumatic parkinsonism
- Wilson's disease
- Frontotemporal dementia with parkinsonism
- Alzheimer's with extrapyramidal features (probably a DLBD variant)
- Creutzfeldt-Jakob disease

SIGNS AND SYMPTOMS

The earliest symptoms of PSP include frequent falling with profound postural instability (usually affecting >95% of patients at time of diagnosis), usually accompanied by bilateral bradykinesia, i.e., masked facies, paucity of spontaneous limb movement, slowness and shuffling of the gait. On exam, patients occasionally have a resting tremor, but may have complicating postural and intention tremors. The distribution of increased resistance to passive manipulation is predominantly axial, affecting neck and trunk movements more than the limbs. This pattern is the opposite of that seen in IPD. Tremor and rigidity are also typically more symmetric at onset in PSP, differentiating it from the largely asymmetric onset of signs and symptoms in IPD.

The classic neuro-ophthalmologic features of PSP include loss of voluntary vertical gaze, followed by loss of voluntary horizontal gaze. This "supranuclear" ophthalmoplegia can be overcome by doll's-eyes maneuvers, confirming the intact nature of the brainstem nuclei and their connections. Patients may have a neck dystonia with retrocollis and eyelid retraction, resulting in a prominent "staring" appearance. Other neuro-ophthalmologic hallmarks include gaze impersistence, loss of optokinetic nystagmus (first in vertical, then in horizontal planes), and square wave jerks with ocular fixation.

Other frequent symptoms include dysarthria, dysphagia, disinhibition, and frontal lobe symptoms such as perseveration, grasping, apathy, and/or depression.

LABORATORY PROCEDURES

Blood Work

There are no specific blood tests to diagnose PSP, but the following tests should be considered to identify potential underlying secondary causes of parkinsonism: serum vitamin B_{12} level, thyroid function tests, serum ceruloplasmin, 24-hour urine copper excretion.

IMAGING STUDIES

Functional neuroimaging using PET and SPECT scanning with markers for neuronal activity (fluorodeoxyglucose), dopaminergic terminals (beta-CIT, DTBZ, and others) and dopamine receptors (IBZD) may distinguish PSP from idiopathic PD, but does not distinguish from other Parkinson's plus syndromes. These methods are not being widely implemented.

There is no evidence to suggest that structural imaging studies (CT, MRI) can assist in the diagnosis of PSP. MRI may reveal evidence of other causes of parkinsonism such as vascular insults, mass lesions, calcium or iron deposition in the striatum, atrophy in the posterior fossa suggestive of multiple system atrophies, and cortical atrophy patterns suggestive of other dementing illnesses.

SPECIAL TESTS

N/A

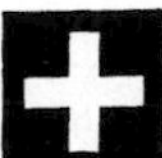

Management

GENERAL MEASURES

There is no effective treatment for PSP. Management is aimed at alleviating the consequences of the motor and cognitive changes associated with PSP.

SURGICAL MEASURES

N/A

SYMPTOMATIC TREATMENT

The primary symptom of gait instability may be overcome by the use of four-wheel walkers, although the predominant tendency of patients with PSP to fall backward usually limits the effective duration of this intervention. Patients with dysarthria or dysphagia may benefit from speech pathology intervention. Percutaneous endoscopic gastrostomy (PEG) may be performed to provide life-sustaining nutrition. Exposure keratitis may be prevented by frequent administration of artificial tears.

ADJUNCTIVE TREATMENT

N/A

ADMISSION/DISCHARGE CRITERIA

PSP is usually managed in an outpatient setting. Rarely, concomitant illnesses, especially aspiration pneumonia, can lead to an acute exacerbation of PSP symptoms, requiring hospitalization for dysphagia, airway management, and issues of decreased mobility. Symptoms of psychosis may precipitate hospitalization and/or institutionalization.

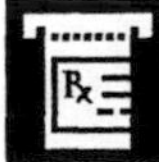

Medications

DRUG(S) OF CHOICE

Rarely, patients with PSP will transiently respond to carbidopa/levodopa (C/L) therapy at the beginning of the disease process. This response is usually minimal and short-lived. Antidepressants, especially amitriptyline and trazodone have helped ameliorate some of the symptoms of rigidity, bradykinesia, and gait disturbance. Botulinum toxin injections have been useful for severe dystonias.

Contraindications

Individuals with a history of cardiac arrhythmias or orthostatic hypotension may have adverse effects when prescribed tricyclic antidepressants.

Precautions

The use of high doses of carbidopa/levodopa and other dopaminergic therapies may be associated with confusion, hallucinations, and agitation, especially in individuals with advanced symptoms of PSP.

ALTERNATIVE DRUGS

N/A

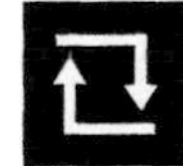

Follow-Up

PATIENT MONITORING

PSP is a relentlessly progressive illness, typically leading to death within 6 to 10 years. Patients are monitored in the outpatient setting, usually at 4 to 6 month intervals. Judicious use of antidepressant medications and timely discussion of PEG tube placement are recommended to assist patients and their families prepare for future decline.

EXPECTED COURSE AND PROGNOSIS

Due to its progressive nature, the symptoms of PSP always worsen with time. Death usually occurs as a consequence of pulmonary embolism or aspiration pneumonia.

PATIENT EDUCATION

The severe gait instability in PSP prevents the use of ambulatory exercise, although stretching and strengthening exercises in a sitting position may be useful. Aqua therapy with close supervision may help forestall some of the immobility issues associated with this illness. Speech therapy is useful for speech and swallowing disturbances. National organizations provide information to patients and their families.

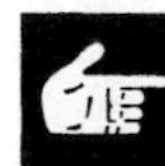

Miscellaneous

SYNONYMS

Steele-Richardson-Olszewski syndrome

ICD-9-CM: 333.0 Progressive supranuclear palsy; Other disorders of the basal ganglia

SEE ALSO: MULTIPLE SYSTEM ATROPHY, PARKINSON'S DISEASE, DIFFUSE LEWY BODY DISEASE

REFERENCES

- Albers DS, Augood SJ. New insights into progressive supranuclear palsy. Trends Neursci 2001;24:347.
- Litvan I. Diagnosis and management of progressive supranuclear palsy. Semin Neurol 2001;21:41.
- Vanacore N, et al. Epidemiology of progressive supranuclear palsy. Neurol Sci 2001;22:101.

Author(s): Lawrence W. Elmer, MD, PhD

Pseudotumor Cerebri

Basics

DESCRIPTION

Pseudotumor cerebi (PTC) is a condition that mainly affects obese women and is associated with significant morbidity due to increased intracranial pressure (ICP). Headaches, transient visual obscurations (TVOs), and progressive visual loss are the most common presenting symptoms. The elevated ICP is transmitted through the optic nerve sheaths to the optic discs, causing papilledema, which is generally considered a medical emergency. CT scan demonstrates no evidence of a mass lesion, while lumbar puncture reveals an elevated opening CSF pressure. This process unchecked can lead to irreversible blindness.

EPIDEMIOLOGY

Incidence/Prevalence

- Obese women of childbearing age are most commonly affected.
- Incidence in the general population (1:100,000):
  - —In women age 20–44, >10% over ideal body weight (13:100,000)
  - —In women age 20–44, >20% over ideal body weight (19.3:100,000)
  - —In men age 20–44, >20% over ideal body weight (1.5:100,000)

Race

No known association with race.

Sex

Female/male ratio of 8:1 in the adult population.

Age

Peak incidence is in the third decade, but can occur from infancy to old age.

ETIOLOGY

The etiology remains elusive; however, the leading theory proposes low conductance to CSF outflow at the arachnoid villi leading to increased CSF volume and increased ICP. The majority of cases are *idiopathic*; but resistance to CSF egress may be *secondary* to venous occlusive disease, meningeal carcinomatosis or other infiltrative processes. A variety of medications including tetracycline, doxycycline, minocycline, fluoroquinolones, nalidixic acid, exogenous growth hormone, birth control pills and hypervitaminosis A are well-documented secondary causes. PTC has also been associated with steroid withdrawal, Addison's disease, hypo- and hyperthyroidism, hypopara-thyroidism, menarche, and menstrual irregularities and pregnancy, betraying a possible underlying endocrine etiology.

Genetics

No known genetic syndrome.

PREGNANCY

No evidence of an increased risk of PTC onset or exacerbation during pregnancy.

ASSOCIATED CONDITIONS

- Obesity/recent weight gain
- Empty sella syndrome
- Systemic lupus erythematosus
- Behçet's disease

Diagnosis

DIFFERENTIAL DIAGNOSIS

The diagnosis of idiopathic PTC is largely one of exclusion. Therefore, it is necessary to rule out other causes of papilledema and increased ICP as well as secondary PTC. Focal neurologic signs other than cranial nerve VI palsy should suggest a diagnosis other than PTC.

- Intracranial mass lesion with obstructive hydrocephalus
- Pseudopapilledema (i.e., optic disc drusen)
- Meningitis (i.e., bacterial, viral, neurosyphilis)
- Venous sinus thrombosis
- Medication related (e.g., tetracycline, growth hormone therapy)
- Endocrine related (e.g., systemic lupus erythematosus, acromegaly)

SIGNS AND SYMPTOMS

- Headache (most frequent symptom)
  - —Generally holocranial or retrobulbar
  - —Relatively constant, "aching" or "throbbing" quality, variable intensity
  - —May be associated with nausea or light-headedness
- Transient visual obscurations
  - —Unilateral or bilateral blurring, dimming, or loss of vision lasting for 2 to 3 seconds
  - —Secondary to optic disc swelling
- Visual loss (optic disc related)
  - —Causes of permanent loss of vision: compressive optic nerve damage, optic disc infarction, choroidal folds, and subretinal hemorrhage
  - —Visual field loss
  - —Enlarged blind spot and generalized constriction are most common.
  - —Nasal step, arcuate defects, and cecocentral scotomas may also be encountered.
  - —Relative afferent pupillary defect with asymmetric optic nerve involvement
  - —Bilateral optic disc swelling secondary to increased ICP (i.e., papilledema) is generally noted; patients with unilateral optic disc swelling or no optic disc edema are rare.
  - —Diplopia, secondary to cranial nerve VI palsy, which may be unilateral or bilateral
  - —Photopsia (seeing "sparkles" or "flashes")

LABORATORY PROCEDURES

Blood work is generally unnecessary in the typical idiopathic PTC patient. In an atypical patient (e.g., thin male) or in a patient with uncharacteristic symptoms or signs (e.g., arthralgias, malar rash, tetanic muscle spasms, cranial nerve III palsy), other laboratory tests may prove diagnostic for secondary forms of PTC: VDRL, FT-ABS, antinuclear antibody, anti-dsDNA, or serum Ca^{2+} determinations.

IMAGING STUDIES

CT and MRI are the main imaging techniques used in PTC. Normal to small-sized ventricles are seen with no evidence of mass lesion. Up to 70% of PTC patients have evidence of an empty sella. Clear differentiation between the optic nerve and sheath, with an enlarged, elongated subarachnoid space, and flattening of the posterior aspect of the globe may also be seen. MRI is better than CT to rule out infiltrative diseases and venous sinus thrombosis.

SPECIAL TESTS

- Lumbar puncture (LP) is necessary to obtain the opening pressure and to rule out infection or inflammation. Opening pressures greater than 200 mm H_2O are considered elevated. Falsely low pressures may occur when the LP requires multiple attempts with reinsertion and redirection of the needle. LP under radiologic guidance should be considered in obese patients, especially when normal landmarks cannot be palpated. CSF analysis should include cell counts, differential, cytology, protein and glucose levels, Gram stain, and routine cultures and sensitivities. These are all within normal limits in idiopathic PTC.
- Visual acuity testing, pupillary responses, slit lamp and dilated funduscopic evaluation, and visual fields are necessary to assess baseline visual function. Stereoscopic optic disc photographs taken on initial evaluation can be used to monitor disease progression. Fluorescein angiography of the fundus may help to differentiate optic disc drusen (i.e., pseudopapilledema) from true papilledema.

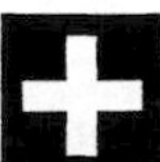

Management

GENERAL MEASURES

Weight loss is the most effective treatment for PTC and may reduce the need for medications or surgery. Suspect exogenous agents should be discontinued. Lumbar puncture initially done for diagnostic purposes may also be therapeutic.

SURGICAL MEASURES

Surgical intervention is necessary to control intractable headaches and to preserve visual function when weight loss and medical therapies are not successful. Serial lumbar puncture can be used to lower ICP; however, the effects are often temporary, and repeat procedures may be poorly tolerated. The main surgical considerations for PTC are lumboperitoneal shunting (LPS) and optic nerve sheath fenestration (ONSF). In a retrospective study of 30 PTC patients who underwent LP shunting, headache improved in 82%, papilledema resolved completely or nearly completely in 96%, and visual acuity or field improved in 68% of patients. Unfortunately, reoperation is the general rule, most commonly due to shunt malfunction. In the previously mentioned PTC study, the mean follow-up duration was 34.9 months and the mean shunt revision rate was 4.2 per patient. In ONSF, multiple incisions are made in the anterior dural covering of the optic nerve. ONSF is useful to decompress the optic nerve in cases with severe papilledema. It is less likely to relieve high ICP in the long run; however, it does reduce the risk of visual loss with recurrent elevation of ICP. In this regard, ONSF is also helpful in cases of PTC with recurrent LPS failure to prevent them from "picking off" vision each time. Gastric bypass surgery may be indicated to improve weight loss in morbidly obese patients.

SYMPTOMATIC TREATMENT

Symptomatic treatment includes judicious use of analgesics for relief of headache.

ADJUNCTIVE TREATMENT

Weight loss is an important component of treatment and may require consultation with a dietitian.

ADMISSION/DISCHARGE CRITERIA

Hospital admission may be indicated (a) for radiologic-guided lumbar puncture and initiation of medical therapy, or (b) for urgent surgical intervention to preserve vision.

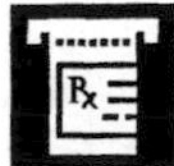

Medications

DRUG(S) OF CHOICE

Carbonic anhydrase inhibitors are the mainstay of medical therapy for PTC, and work by reducing CSF production. Neptazane 50 mg bid to qid and acetazolamide 250 mg bid to 500 mg qid are generally well tolerated.

Contraindications

Carbonic anhydrase inhibitors should not be used in patients with sulfa allergy. They have a relative contraindication during pregnancy (class B) and should definitely not be used during the first 4 months' gestation.

Precautions

Common adverse effects at higher doses include tingling and numbness in the fingers and toes, fatigue, nausea, and metallic taste, K+ wasting. Aplastic anemia is a rare idiosyncratic reaction.

ALTERNATIVE DRUGS

Furosemide in doses of 20 mg bid to 40 mg qid is also effective; however, it is important to monitor serum potassium. Corticosteroids are a controversial alternative that are most useful in patients with an underlying inflammatory condition such as systemic lupus. Prolonged corticosteroid use may be counterproductive by leading to further weight gain and fluid retention. Octreotide, a somatostatin analog has been found in several small case series to lower intracranial pressure, relieve headache, reduce papilledema, and improve vision in PTC patients, although the mechanism of action is unknown. Octreotide is an option in patients with sulfa allergy.

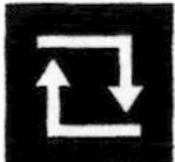

Follow-Up

PATIENT MONITORING

The goal of treatment is to eradicate intolerable headaches and to preserve visual function. It is necessary to monitor the degree of papilledema and formal visual field testing over time. Papilledema may not resolve completely with appropriate treatment and may not recur significantly with ICP once it becomes chronic in nature. Optic disc appearance alone is not adequate to assess for recurrent elevation in ICP; subjective symptoms and visual field progression may be more reliable.

EXPECTED COURSE AND PROGNOSIS

PTC appears to be a self-limited disease. Once the condition is controlled on medication for 6 months to a year, attempts to wean off the medication should be made periodically, especially when weight loss has been achieved. Systemic hypertension is a risk factor for increased visual loss.

PATIENT EDUCATION

Patients should be educated that PTC is self-limited, but that visual loss secondary to the disease may be permanent or progressive.

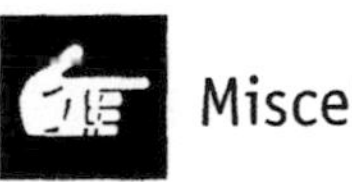

Miscellaneous

SYNONYMS

Idiopathic intracranial hypertension

ICD-9-CM: 348.2 Pseudotumor cerebri; 377.01 Papilledema

SEE ALSO: N/A

REFERENCES

- Burgett RA, Purvin VA, Kawasaki A. Lumboperitoneal shunting for pseudotumor cerebri. Neurology 1997;49:734–739.
- Corbett JJ. Idiopathic intracranial hypertension (pseudotumor cerebri). In: Albert DM, Jakobiec FA, eds. Principles and practice of ophthalmology: clinical practice, vol 4, 2nd ed. Philadelphia: WB Saunders, 2000; Chapter 305.
- Friedman DI, Jacobson DM. Diagnostic criteria for idiopathic intracranial hypertension. Neurology 2002;59:1492–1495.
- Goh KY, Schatz NJ, Glaser JS. Optic nerve sheath fenestration for pseudotumor cerebri. J Neuroophthalmol 1997;17:86–91.
- Miller NR. Papilledema. In: Walsh & Hoyt's clinical neuro-ophthalmology, vol 1, 5th ed. Baltimore: Williams & Wilkins, 1998; Chapter 10.

Author(s): James A. McHale, MD; Steven E. Katz, MD

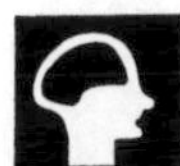

Basics

DESCRIPTION

Rabies ("rage" or "madness" in Latin) is a viral infection that causes rapidly progressive and almost always fatal encephalomyelitis. It is transmitted to humans primarily through close contact with saliva (bites, scratches, licks on broken skin and mucous membranes) of infected animals (dog, bat, raccoon, fox, skunk), rarely through laboratory exposure, inhalation (caves that harbor bats), and iatrogenic (corneal transplant) tissue exposure.

EPIDEMIOLOGY

Incidence/Prevalence

Rabies causes more than 40,000 deaths each year worldwide, primarily in Asia, Africa, and Latin America. About 10 million people receive postexposure prophylaxis each year. In the U.S., 32 cases were reported between 1980 to 1996.

Race

No race difference was reported.

Age

Although rabies can occur at any age, about half of the cases reported occur in children.

Sex

No sex difference was present.

ETIOLOGY

Rabies virus is a single-stranded RNA rhabdovirus. The infection spreads to the human through an infected animal bite. The principal reservoir is the domestic dog in Africa, Asia, and Latin America, while wild animals are the main hosts in developed countries. Among the wild animals, bats are the most common source of rabies. Seventeen out of 20 cases infected by indigenous strains between 1980 and 1996 in the U.S. were attributed to bats. However, a significant proportion of human rabies cases lack an identified route of transmission.

Genetics

No definite genetic factors are identified.

RISK FACTORS

The risk of an unimmunized person to develop rabies after a bite of a rabid animal is 5% to 15%. Modifying factors include the site and the severity of bite and the virus concentration of saliva. Bites on the head and face result in the highest incidence of disease with the shortest incubation period.

PREGNANCY

Transplacental transmission of rabies has rarely been reported, and the possibility of transmission through lactation has not been excluded. Postexposure prophylaxis of pregnant women has been reported as safe in several case reports.

ASSOCIATED CONDITIONS

None

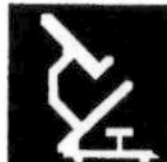

Diagnosis

DIFFERENTIAL DIAGNOSIS

- Other causes of viral encephalitis
  —Herpes simplex virus encephalitis
  —Arbovirus encephalitis
- Nonviral causes of encephalitis
  —Mycoplasma pneumonia
  —Legionnaire disease
  —Central nervous system toxoplasmosis
  —Guillain-Barré syndrome (GBS) (paralytic or dumb rabies cases)
  —Poliomyelitis
  —Tetanus
- Allergic encephalitis due to nerve tissue-derived rabies vaccine
- Acute hepatic porphyria with neuropsychiatric disturbances
- Alcohol withdrawal (delirium tremens)

SIGNS AND SYMPTOMS

The incubation period for human rabies is usually 1 to 3 months after contact with a rabid animal, although varies extremely up to a year. After prodromal phase, patients enter into either excitatory or paralytic phase followed by coma and death.

- Prodromal phase: lasts 2 to 10 days, consisting of fever, malaise, headache, nausea, and sore throat. Abnormal sensations like pain, itching, tingling, and paresthesias at the site of inoculation are important symptoms seen in up to 80% of patients.
- Excitatory (encephalitic, furious) phase: seen in 80% of cases and may last up to a week. There is anxiety, agitation, confusion, and hallucinations. Increased sensitivity to bright light and loud noise and autonomic dysfunction (increased salivation, lacrimation, perspiration, mydriasis, tachycardia, bradycardia, cyclic respiration, urinary retention and constipation) are seen. Hydrophobia resulting from intense spasms of pharyngeal and laryngeal muscles when patients attempt to swallow liquids is the classic manifestation. Aerophobia also induces spasms. Once coma develops, inspiratory spasms replace them. Muscle tone is increased. Cranial nerve dysfunctions (ocular palsies, facial weakness, hoarseness, hippus, nystagmus) are seen. Seizures, although rare, can be seen. Death can result in this phase due to respiratory arrest. If not, patients lapse into coma.
- Paralytic phase: about 20% of patients experience paralytic or dumb rabies which lasts 1 to 4 weeks before coma develops. A progressive, flaccid paralysis develops simulating GBS. Consciousness is spared and there is no agitation. Phobic spasms, inspiratory spasms, and autonomic signs are present.

LABORATORY PROCEDURES

Routine blood work is nonspecific except leukocytosis. CSF examination is normal until late in the disease.

IMAGING STUDIES

Neuroimaging may show nonspecific signs of encephalitis and is not particularly helpful for diagnosis.

SPECIAL TESTS

- Antibody detection in the serum and CSF: serum antibodies may not be present until several days after the onset of symptoms. Rapid fluorescent focus inhibition test measures the neutralizing antibodies, while indirect immunofluorescence assay detects antibody reactive to rabies antigen in infected cell cultures.
- Virus isolation from saliva, nuchal skin, CSF, oral or nasal mucosa, brain
- Antigen detection by direct immunofluorescence from nuchal skin biopsy, corneal, and salivary impressions
- Detection of viral RNA in saliva

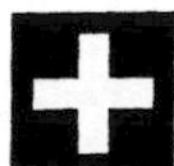

Management

GENERAL MEASURES

Rabies is almost always fatal after the onset of symptoms. Pulmonary and cardiac functions should be monitored. Dysautonomia, seizures, and increased intracranial pressure should be managed aggressively. Sedation with barbiturates, benzodiazepines, and phenothiazines may be necessary.

SURGICAL MEASURES

There is no surgical procedure for rabies. Brain biopsy for diagnosis is debatable because of the risks of the procedure and the inaccessibility of tissues with greatest involvement. If done, eosinophilic viral inclusions (Negri bodies) will be seen.

SYMPTOMATIC TREATMENT

Prophylaxis

- Preexposure prophylaxis
  - —Should be applied to high-risk individuals (veterinarians, certain laboratory workers, animal control workers, travelers to countries where rabies is endemic). Cell or tissue culture vaccines [human diploid cell vaccine (HDCV), purified duck embryo vaccine, purified chick embryo cell vaccine] should be used if possible. Vaccine should be administered IM or ID in the deltoid area on days 0, 7, and 21 or 28 (according to package instructions). Two to 3 weeks after the last injection, the antibody titer should be checked and if inadequate, a booster dose should be given. Follow-up of the antibody titer every 6 months for persons who work with live rabies virus and every year for those under continuous risk (veterinarians, travelers to endemic areas) is recommended.
- Postexposure prophylaxis
  - —Local wound cleaning
    - -The wounds or scratches should be washed with water and soap or detergent immediately followed by ethanol, tincture, or aqueous iodine. Deep wounds should be irrigated by syringe and these solutions applied by cotton-tipped applicators.
    - -An antibacterial agent can be applied to prevent secondary infections. Provide tetanus prophylaxis.
    - -Do not suture the wound. If suturing is unavoidable, do it after immune globulin infiltration.
- Vaccination
  - —Five doses of cell or tissue culture vaccine, 1 mL each is enough. First dose should be given as soon as possible, subsequent doses on days 3, 7, 14, and 28 after the first dose. (WHO recommends a sixth dose on day 90.)
  - —Vaccine should be given IM in the deltoid muscle in adults and anterior thigh in infants.
- Postexposure prophylaxis for those previously immunized: two doses of vaccine on days 0 and 3 IM in the deltoid area should be given. Human rabies immune globulin (HRIG) is contraindicated.

ADJUNCTIVE TREATMENT

N/A

ADMISSION/DISCHARGE CRITERIA

All suspected cases should be followed in the intensive care units.

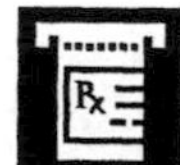

Medications

DRUG(S) OF CHOICE

- HRIG
  - —Infiltrate 20 IU/kg HRIG in the tissues around the wound. As much HRIG as anatomically possible should be given to the wound and rest intramuscularly to the anterior thigh. HRIG should be given as early as possible, but can be given up to 8 days after the first dose of the vaccine. Doses given in and after the 8th day will compromise patient's response to vaccine.

Contraindications

N/A

Precautions

Never draw HRIG with the same syringe with the vaccine and do not administer in the same site.

ALTERNATIVE DRUGS

N/A

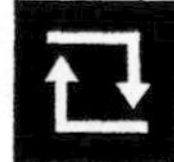

Follow-Up

PATIENT MONITORING

For rare cases of survival, follow-up focuses on the patient's neurologic complications.

EXPECTED COURSE AND PROGNOSIS

Once clinical signs of encephalitis have begun, rabies is almost always fatal. However, both complete recovery of rabies and survival with severe sequelae have been reported.

PATIENT EDUCATION

Unfortunately, many people die from rabies when efficacious preventive measures are available.

Websites

World Health Organization: *http://www.who.int/emc/diseases/zoo*
Centers for Disease Control and Prevention: *http://www.cdc.gov/ncidod/dvrd/rabies*

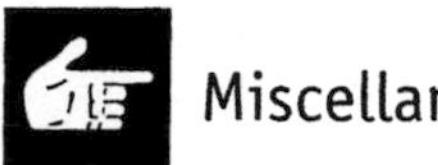

Miscellaneous

ICD-9-CM: 071 Rabies

SEE ALSO: N/A

REFERENCES

- Dreesen DW, Hanlon CA. Current recommendations for the prophylaxis and treatment of rabies. Drugs 1998;56:801.
- Hemachudha T. Rabies. In: Roos KL, ed. Central nervous system infectious diseases and therapy. New York: Marcel Decker, 1997:573–600.
- Noah DL, Drenzek CL, Smith JS, et al. Epidemiology of human rabies in the United States, 1980 to 1996. Ann Intern Med 1998;128:922.
- World Health Organization Expert Committee on Rabies. WHO technical report series No. 824, 8th report. Geneva: World Health Organization, 1992:i–vii, 1–84.

Author(s): Sevim Erdem, MD

Radiculopathy, Cervical

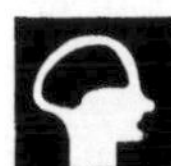

Basics

DESCRIPTION

Cervical radiculopathy (CR) refers to dysfunction of a cervical nerve root, usually due to compression and usually caused by degenerative spine disease or acute disc herniation. Typical clinical picture includes neck and arm pain with or without alterations in strength, sensation, and reflexes.

EPIDEMIOLOGY

Incidence/Prevalence

Annual incidence rate 83.2/100,000 population.

Age

For CR due to herniation of the nucleus pulposus (HNP), incidence highest at ages 50 to 54, mean age 47. CR in older patients more often due to cervical spondylosis and spinal stenosis with root compression due to osteophytes rather than disc material, or to both. Approximation: 50% of compressive CR affects the C7 root, 30% C6, 10% C5, and 10% C8. Isolated T1 radiculopathy is rare.

Sex

Male predominance.

ETIOLOGY

Degenerative spine disease (spondylosis) has two elements: degenerative disc disease (DDD) and degenerative joint disease (DJD). Primarily due to aging; superimposed macro- or micro trauma may aggravate the process. DDD predisposes to HNP ("soft disc"). DJD causes osteophytic narrowing of the neural foramina ("hard disc"). Either process may cause compressive radiculopathy. More advanced spondylosis may also lead to spinal stenosis and cord compression.

RISK FACTORS

The only major risk factor is trauma.

PREGNANCY

N/A

ASSOCIATED CONDITIONS

Osteoarthritis

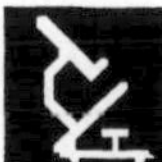

Diagnosis

DIFFERENTIAL DIAGNOSIS

- Brachial plexopathy
- Entrapment neuropathy
- Nerve root tumors (neurofibroma, schwannoma)
- Infection [herpes zoster, Lyme disease, cytomegalovirus (CMV), epidural abscess]
- Meningeal carcinomatosis/lymphomatosis
- Multiple sclerosis (causing radiculopathy)
- Giant cell arteritis
- Non-neuropathic mimickers
  —Cervical myofascial pain
  —Shoulder pathology (bursitis, tendinitis, impingement syndrome)
  —Lateral epicondylitis
  —DeQuervain's tenosynovitis
  —Facet arthropathy
  —Referred pain from heart, lungs, esophagus, or upper abdomen.

SIGNS AND SYMPTOMS

- Features favoring CR as opposed to other etiologies of neck and/or arm pain are
  —Age 35 to 60
  —Acute/subacute onset
  —Past history of cervical or lumbosacral radiculopathy
  —Cervicobrachial pain radiating to shoulder, periscapular region, pectoral region, or arm
  —Paresthesias in arm or hand
  —Pain on neck movement—especially extension or ipsilateral bending
  —Positive root compression signs
  —Radiating pain with cough, sneeze, or bowel movement
  —Myotomal weakness
  —Decreased reflex(es)
  —Dermatomal sensory loss
  —Pain relief with hand on top of head
  —Pain relief with manual upward traction
- Onset acute in half, subacute in a quarter, insidious in a quarter; many patients awake with pain in neck and rhomboid region. Majority of patients symptomatic for about 2 weeks prior to diagnosis. Pain in pectoral region occurs in about 20%. Neck, periscapular, and pectoral region pain may be referred from disc itself; arm pain more likely due to nerve root compression. Only 56% of the patients have neck or shoulder pain, but 99% have pain in the upper arm, often poorly localized. Pain in forearm in 88%, usually poorly localized.
- Cervical range-of-motion (ROM) maneuvers affect size of intervertebral foramen. Pain produced by movements that close the foramen suggest CR. Pain on symptomatic side on putting ipsilateral ear to shoulder suggests radiculopathy; increased pain on leaning or turning away from the symptomatic side suggests myofascial pain. Radiating pain with neck extended and tilted slightly to the symptomatic side suggests CR; brief breath holding in this position sometimes elicits radicular pain. Axial compression (Spurling's maneuver) adds little. Light digital compression of the external jugular veins until the face is flushed sometimes elicits radicular symptoms: unilateral shoulder, arm, pectoral or periscapular pain, or radiating paresthesias into the arm or hand (Naffziger sign), a highly specific but insensitive finding.
- Findings that suggest a lesion at a given level as follows:
  —C5—pain only in neck and shoulder, no pain below elbow, depressed biceps and brachioradialis reflexes, weakness of spinati or deltoid
  —C6—weakness of deltoid or biceps, paresthesias limited to the thumb, sensory loss over thumb only, depressed biceps and brachioradialis reflexes
  —C7—presence of scapular/interscapular pain, pain involving the posterior upper arm, pain involving the medial upper arm, paresthesias limited to index and middle fingers, whole hand paresthesias, depressed triceps reflex, weakness of triceps, sensory loss involving middle finger
  —C8—presence of scapular/interscapular pain, pain involving the medial upper arm, depressed triceps reflex, paresthesias limited to ring and small fingers, weakness of hand intrinsics, sensory loss involving small finger.
  —T1—disproportionate weakness of abductor pollicis brevis (APB).

LABORATORY PROCEDURES

None helpful.

IMAGING STUDIES

Plain cervical spine films with obliques to assess for osteoarthritic changes and osteophytes. MRI to assess for disc herniation and evidence of root compression. Abnormalities on MRI common in asymptomatic individuals. CT myelogram is the most sensitive test.

SPECIAL TESTS

EMG and MRI are complementary studies. Each has about 55% to 70% sensitivity; studies agree in 60% of patients but in 40% only one is abnormal and it may be either one. Agreement higher with abnormal neurologic examination. Mild radiculopathy is difficult to diagnose with either study. Denervation changes on EMG require time to develop, then resolve over time. EMG done less than 3 weeks after onset may be false-negative. EMG done too late in the course is less helpful because of reinnervation.

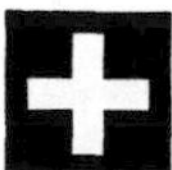

Management

GENERAL MEASURES

- Treatment relies on three approaches: mechanical, medicinal, and surgical. Nerve roots lying in the foramen normally enjoy freedom of movement through a small range. The size of the intervertebral foramen and the lateral recess changes dynamically with neck movement. When neck is extended or tilted or turned ipsilaterally, foramen is narrowest; with flexion or contraversive movement, foramen is wider. When caliber of foramen or lateral recess is narrowed because of osteophyte or HNP, neck movement may cause microtrauma, which induces inflammation and edema. With HNP, intradiscal inflammatory mediators may spill onto the root, exacerbating the process. Mainstay of treatment is to reduce neck movement and increase the size of the foramen.
- Soft cervical collar is usually helpful. For compressive CR, collar should be worn "backward," with high side posterior, to maintain neck in slight flexion and open foramina. Hard collars cannot be turned around in this fashion and are not as useful for a radiculopathy syndrome. Soft collar should be worn at night if tolerated; if not, use cervical pillow. Prolonged use of collar may weaken neck muscles.
- Cervical traction for 15 to 30 minutes tid often very helpful—distracts spine, opens foramina, gives involved root respite. Over-the-door home traction unit adequate; referral to a physical therapist unnecessary. Start with low weight (5–8 lb), advance as tolerated to 12–15 lb. Too rapid weight increase may cause neck or jaw soreness, and limit compliance. Best for patient to face door with neck slightly flexed; combination of flexion and distraction more effective in opening the foramen. However, it is difficult to do anything but stare at the door during treatment, and if facing away from the door appears equally efficacious for the individual patient, it is permissible and may improve compliance.

SURGICAL MEASURES

Consider referral to a spine surgeon in patients with medical research council (MRC) strength of grade 4/5 or worse in any muscle, evidence of myelopathy, or excruciating pain unresponsive to conservative treatment. In a population-based study, 26% required surgery. Newer surgical techniques are much less invasive.

SYMPTOMATIC TREATMENT

Modality physical therapy, or local heat or ice, may provide some relief of axial pain component, but the effects seldom persist much beyond the individual treatment session. Cervical ROM exercises are of no benefit and possibly harmful.

ADJUNCTIVE TREATMENT

Cervical epidural steroids, acupuncture used rarely; spinal manipulation imprudent.

ADMISSION/DISCHARGE CRITERIA

Hospital admission not required for medically treated patients.

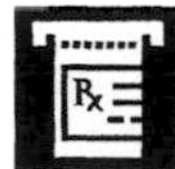

Medications

DRUG(S) OF CHOICE

Nonsteroidal antiinflammatory drugs (NSAIDs) may decrease radicular inflammatory component and relieve pain. Other analgesics are often necessary, including occasional narcotics. When neurologic deficit is moderate (MRC grade 4+/5 in the most involved muscles), a course of oral steroids is reasonable, e.g., prednisone 60–100 mg/day for 7 to 10 days, tapering over the next 7 to 10 days. Caution about short-term steroid side effects. Intensive conservative therapy usually continued for 3 to 6 weeks.

Contraindications

Known hypersensitivity for mediations.

Precautions

Standard precautions for the drug employed.

ALTERNATIVE DRUGS

Muscle relaxants add little; side effects of sedation and depression.

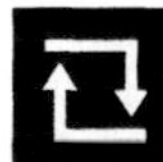

Follow-Up

PATIENT MONITORING

Follow especially strength and reflexes of involved segment; worsening strength or loss of reflex may prompt more aggressive treatment.

EXPECTED COURSE AND PROGNOSIS

The typical patient is significantly improved by 2 to 3 months. Generally favorable long-term prognosis; 90% have minimal to no symptoms on prolonged follow-up. When due to HNP, CR has a tendency to recur: 31% have previous history of CR, 32% have recurrence during follow-up.

PATIENT EDUCATION

Neck owner's manual (Krames 800-333-3032).

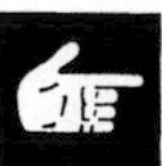

Miscellaneous

SYNONYMS

N/A

ICD-9-CM: 721.0 Cervical spondylosis; 722.0 Cervical disc herniation; 722.4 Cervical disc degeneration; 723.1 Cervicalgia; 723.4 Cervical HNP; 722.6 Degenerative disc disease, NOS; 722.91 Cervical disc disorder, other; 723.3 Cervicobrachial pain; 847.0 Cervical strain; 353.2 Cervical root lesion, NEC

SEE ALSO: N/A

REFERENCES

- Braakman R. Management of cervical spondylotic myelopathy and radiculopathy. J Neurol Neurosurg Psychiatry 1994;57: 257–263.
- Levin KH, et al. Cervical radiculopathies: comparison of surgical and EMG localization of single root lesions. Neurology 1996;46:1022–1025.
- Nardin RA, et al. Electromyography and magnetic resonance imaging in the evaluation of radiculopathy. Muscle Nerve 1999;22:151–155.
- Radhakrishnan K, et al. Epidemiology of cervical radiculopathy. A population-based study from Rochester, Minnesota, 1976 through 1990. Brain 1994;117:325–335.
- Yoss RE, et al. Significance of symptoms and signs in localization of involved root in cervical disc protrusion. Neurology 1957;7:673–683.

Author(s): William W. Campbell, MD, MSHA

Radiculopathy, Lumbosacral

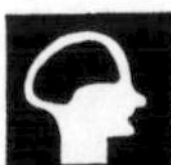

Basics

DESCRIPTION

Lumbosacral radiculopathy (LSR) refers to dysfunction of a lumbar or sacral nerve root often presenting as low back pain with radiating leg pain/paresthesias with or without neurologic deficits of weakness, sensory disturbance, and reduced or absent reflexes.

EPIDEMIOLOGY

Incidence/Prevalence

Multiple studies of incidence and prevalence show disparate numbers but the cumulative lifetime prevalence for low back pain may range from 14% to 65%. Providing an accurate number for LSR is even more difficult but may be around 12% of patients, with low back pain having symptoms that may indicate radiculopathy.

- Majority of herniated discs occur at L4-5 and L5-S1 (>90%), much less frequently at L3-4, and rarely at L1-2 and L2-3.
- Male to female ratio 1.5:1 in one series of surgically proven cases.
- The incidence of degenerative disc disease (DDD) is highest in the fourth and fifth decades, whereas compression from degenerative joint disease (DJD) is at an older age.

ETIOLOGY

LSR is most commonly caused by extrinsic processes such as compression by disc material (DDD) or bone/synovium/ligaments (DJD) and infrequently by intrinsic processes such as infiltration from tumor or infection.

Genetics

N/A

RISK FACTORS

Trauma is a major risk factor; other possible risk factors include cigarette smoking, greater number of hours spent in a motor vehicle, and occupations requiring lifting while twisting the body. Advancing age is a risk factor for DJD.

PREGNANCY

N/A

ASSOCIATED CONDITIONS

Osteoarthritis

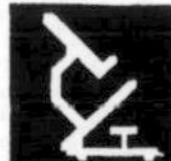

Diagnosis

DIFFERENTIAL DIAGNOSIS

- Tumor
  —Primary, metastatic, carcinomatous meningitis
- Infection
  —Herpes zoster, Lyme, HIV, CMV
- Osteomyelitis (*Staphylococcus aureus* most common, TB)
- Epidural abscess *(S. aureus)*
- Diabetic polyradiculopathy
- Paraneoplastic polyradiculopathy
- Non-neuropathic mimickers
- Facet arthropathy
- Discitis
- Referred pain from abdominal and pelvic organs, aorta

SIGNS AND SYMPTOMS

Features favoring LSR over other etiologies of back pain with radiating leg pain:

- Age over 30
- Acute/subacute back pain, recurrent back pain with radiating symptoms down one or both legs
- Past history of cervical or lumbosacral radiculopathy
- Paresthesias or pain in posterior leg, lateral aspect and sole of foot or lateral leg and top of foot
- Radiating pain with cough, sneeze, or bowel movement
- Positive root compression signs
  —Straight leg raise (Lasegue's sign). With the patient supine, the affected leg is raised by the ankle until pain is elicited. Reproducing the pain or paresthesias under 60 degrees is a positive sign of root compression.
  —Crossed straight leg raise. With the patient supine, the asymptomatic leg is lifted. A positive root compression sign is elicited if there is reproduction of pain or paresthesias in the symptomatic leg on lifting the asymptomatic leg. More specific but less sensitive than the straight leg raise.
  —Femoral stretch test (reverse straight leg raise). With the patient prone, the hip of the symptomatic leg is maximally extended. Reproducing the symptoms is a positive test; most useful in upper level herniated discs (L2, L3, L4).
- Myotomal weakness
- Dermatomal sensory loss
- Decreased reflexes
- Bowel or bladder dysfunction (polyradiculopathy/cauda equina syndrome from canal stenosis)
- No systemic illness
- Findings that suggest a lesion at a given level as follows:
  —High lumbar (L1-3)—sensory signs (altered sensation) in the inguinal region, anterior thigh, and medial aspect of knee. May have weakness in iliopsoas (hip flexion), quadriceps (knee extension), and thigh adductors. Cremasteric reflex (L2) and patellar reflex (L3) may be depressed. Positive femoral stretch test.
  —L4—sensory signs over the knee and medial leg, may have weakness in the quadriceps and tibialis anterior (foot dorsiflexion and inversion). Patellar reflex may be depressed.
  —L5—sensory signs over the lateral leg, dorsomedial foot, and large toe. May have weakness in gluteal muscles (hip extension, hip abduction), tensor fascia latae (abduction and internal rotation of thigh), hamstring muscles (knee flexion), tibialis posterior (plantar flexion and inversion of foot), tibialis anterior, peronei (foot plantar flexion and eversion), extensor hallucis longus (extension of great toe and foot dorsiflexion). No reflex changes.
  —S1—sensory signs over the little toe, lateral foot, and sole of foot. May have weakness in the gluteus maximus (hip extension), hamstring muscles, gastrocnemius (foot plantar flexion), flexor hallucis longus (foot plantar and great toe flexion), and flexor digitorum longus (plantar flexion of the foot and toes except for great toe). Achilles reflex may be depressed.
  —S2-5—sensory abnormalities involving the perianal region, buttocks, posterior thigh, and calf. May have bowel or bladder disturbance. Anal reflex may be absent.

LABORATORY PROCEDURES

N/A

IMAGING STUDIES

- MRI is the imaging procedure of choice in suspected LSR. It has the benefits of imaging in the sagittal view, giving excellent soft tissue resolution, and does not involve radiation. Contraindicated for patients with implanted magnetic sensitive devices, difficult to perform on patients with claustrophobia or obesity.
- CT has a lower sensitivity, but acceptable if there is a need, such as in patients unable to undergo MRI or when more bony detail required. Using intrathecal contrast (CT myelogram) increases the sensitivity, but makes it an invasive procedure with potential for the same adverse reactions as conventional myelography.

- Myelography has a role in some selected cases such as in patients with metallic fixation in place or are morbidly obese. It is capable of evaluating patients in a full weight-bearing position. It has the advantage over CT of imaging in the sagittal plain and better evaluates the cauda equina. Myelography is an invasive procedure and can result in headache, nausea/vomiting, seizures, arachnoiditis, infection, and allergic reaction to the contrast.
- Plain lumbosacral spine films are generally not helpful except in the setting of acute trauma, suspected infection, or malignancy, and then is often only the starting point of the evaluation.
- Of note, there is a high incidence of lumbosacral abnormalities on neuroimaging in asymptomatic individuals. CT and MRI potentially demonstrate abnormalities in 36% and 30%, respectively, of asymptomatic individuals. Therefore, imaging should be done only when clinically indicated, for example, if the patient is a surgical candidate.

SPECIAL TESTS

EMG is complementary to MRI and has the advantage of providing information about nerve function, severity of the lesion, and the prognosis for recovery. Should be done between 3 weeks and 6 months for the highest yield.

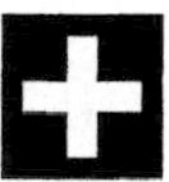

Management

GENERAL MEASURES

Conservative treatments shown to have potential benefit outweighing potential harm include certain medications, gradual return to normal activities, patient education, and low-stress aerobic exercise. Treatment options with weak or equivocal evidence of benefit include manipulation, self-application of heat or ice, epidural steroid injections, wearing a corset, and bed rest of 2 to 4 days.

SURGICAL MEASURES

Referral to surgeon if pain is severe or neurologic deficit persists after 1 month of conservative treatment. May need to refer earlier for suspicion of cauda equina syndrome, infection, malignancy, recent trauma, or severe weakness.

SYMPTOMATIC TREATMENT

See General Measures, above.

ADJUNCTIVE TREATMENT

See General Measures, above.

ADMISSION/DISCHARGE CRITERIA

Not required unless rapidly progressing neurologic deficits, as might be seen in cauda equina syndrome.

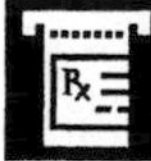

Medications

DRUG(S) OF CHOICE

- Nonsteroidal antiinflammatory drugs (NSAIDs) such as ibuprofen, naproxen, or from the newer class of nonsteroidals, the cyclooxygenase-2 (COX-2) inhibitors like celecoxib and rofecoxib.
- Acetaminophen

Contraindications

Previous hypersensitivity reaction to NSAIDs, history of asthma, and nasal polyps. Also, celecoxib should not be given to patients who have a history of allergic reactions to sulfonamides.

Precautions

Use with caution if there is a history of renal, hepatic, or hematologic disease. May cause gastrointestinal distress (much less common with the COX-2 inhibitors; however, these are currently more expensive).

ALTERNATIVE DRUGS

- Narcotics—rarely indicated, especially in chronic pain, helpful for a brief period during acute symptoms.
- Muscle relaxants—short course may be helpful, limited due to sedation and depression.

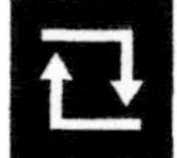

Follow-Up

PATIENT MONITORING

Follow neurologic exam, especially strength and reflexes of involved segment. Worsening or persistent signs and symptoms should prompt more aggressive evaluation and possibly a surgical referral.

EXPECTED COURSE AND PROGNOSIS

Prognosis is favorable, with 80% to 90% of patients recovering from back pain in about 6 weeks regardless of type of treatment.

PATIENT EDUCATION

Weight loss if obese, smoking cessation, avoiding prolonged hours in a motor vehicle, and avoiding excess lifting especially with a twisting motion can help prevent low back pain.

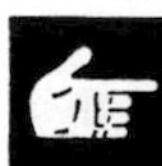

Miscellaneous

SYNONYMS

Sciatica; herniated nucleus pulposus (HNP)

ICD-9-CM: 722.32 Lumbar/lumbosacral disc degeneration; 953.2 Lumbar root injury; 953.3 Sacral root injury; 722.10 Lumbar/lumbosacral disc displacement; 722.2 Intervertebral disc (with neuritis, radiculitis, sciatica, or other pain)

SEE ALSO: N/A

REFERENCES

- Bigos SJ. Perils, pitfalls, and accomplishments of guidelines for treatment of back problems. Neurol Clin 1999;17:179–192.
- Boden SD, Davis DO, Patronas NJ, et al. Abnormal magnetic resonance scans of the lumbar spine in asymptomatic subjects. A prospective investigation. J Bone Joint Surg 1990;72A:403–408.
- Deyo RA, Tsui-Wu Y. Descriptive epidemiology of low-back pain and its related medical care in the United States. Spine 1987;12:264–268.
- Lomen-Hoerth C, Aminoff MJ. Clinical neurophysiologic studies.Which test is useful and when? Neurol Clin 1999;17: 65–74.
- Waddell G. A new clinical model for the treatment of low-back pain. Spine 1987;12:632–644.
- Weisel SW, Tsourmas N, Feffer HL, et al. A study of computer-assisted tomography. I. The incidence of positive CAT scans in an asymptomatic group of patients. Spine 1984;9:549–551.

Author(s): Kristen C. Barner, MD; William W. Campbell, MD, MSHA

Reflex Sympathetic Dystrophy

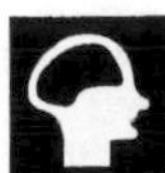

Basics

DESCRIPTION

Reflex sympathetic dystrophy (RSD) usually involves a limb, and combines extreme pain, hyperalgesia and other sensory abnormalities, vasomotor and sweating disturbances, motor disturbances such as spasm, dystonia or loss of mobility, and, later in the course, trophic changes involving hair, nails, skin, and thinning of bone. RSD commonly develops after limb trauma, without (complex regional pain syndrome type 1; CRPS-1) or with (CRPS-2) an obvious nerve lesion. The pain arises from three sources: peripheral, central, and abnormal sympathetic-somatosensory coupling.

EPIDEMIOLOGY

Incidence/Prevalence

The incidence of RSD remains uncertain. Although upper extremity RSD is more commonly reported, a large pain center usually finds cases equally distributed between the upper and lower extremities. RSD occurs with fractures of the radius in 1% to 16% of cases and 15% to 25% after major hemispheric stroke. There is no age, race, or sex predilection.

ETIOLOGY

The exact etiology of RSD is unknown. Useful clinical observations include (a) local and neurogenic inflammation in the limb, (b) α-adrenergic sensitivity at the nociceptor and dorsal root ganglion levels, (c) architectural reorganization of the dorsal horn, and (d) changes in thalamic and anterior cingulate function.

RISK FACTORS

Phenobarbital and isoniazid are drugs associated with the production of RSD, refractory to any standard treatment until the offending agent is removed. Immobilization is the most common major risk factor, followed by trauma or operation, fracture, nerve injury (defining type 2), and stroke with significant paresis. Prior occurrence of RSD increases the probability of the disorder's recurrence, or occurrence in another limb.

PREGNANCY

Pregnancy has been associated with pelvis and lower extremity RSD.

ASSOCIATED CONDITIONS

Any disease associated with a small fiber neuropathy, such as diabetes and collagen-vascular disorders.

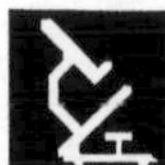

Diagnosis

DIFFERENTIAL DIAGNOSIS

RSD is usually a complication of tissue injury rather than a primary disorder. All of the conditions that could mimic RSD could also underlie RSD, and should be considered. Such diseases include vascular disorders such as deep venous thrombosis, arterial occlusion, and stenosis; inflammatory disorders such as cellulitis and osteomyelitis; anterior compartment syndrome; and occult stress fracture.

SIGNS AND SYMPTOMS

- The diagnosis is established on clinical grounds, based on four symptom groups: sensory abnormalities (spontaneous pain, allodynia, reduced sensation); motor abnormalities (spasm, dystonia, reduced range of motion); autonomic abnormalities (vasomotor, sudomotor, and interstitial fluid disturbances); and trophic changes in hair, skin, nails, and bone. The presence of symptoms in all four groups—definite RSD; three groups—high probability of RSD; two groups—possible RSD; and one group—probably not RSD.
- The syndrome is divided into three stages: early (weeks-6 months) when the limb is dry and warm, middle (3 months-years) when the limb becomes wet and cool, and late (6 months-years). Atrophy sets in while pain and autonomic signs wane. Autonomic symptoms include swelling, temperature changes, erythematous or cyanotic color, and sweating asymmetry. Motor disturbances include severe spasm, various dystonias, postural and action tremors, and progressively limited range of motion. Sensory symptoms include hypesthesia, paresthesia, and severe allodynia. Pain increases when the limb is dependent and with activity, and in severe cases, even with passive range of motion. Trophic changes occur later in the course of the disease, including periarticular osteoporosis, glossy skin, nail and hair growth abnormalities, and contractures.

LABORATORY PROCEDURES

Diffusely increased technetium pyrophosphate uptake by bone scan occurs in RSD, especially in the lower limb, and this study can also exclude a focal inflammatory or infectious process. Autonomic testing of the affected limbs can also be useful to diagnose RSD.

IMAGING STUDIES

Comparative x-ray examinations of the limbs can demonstrate diffuse or local bone demineralization, and exclude a stress fracture. MRI of the limb can show deep tissue swelling and exclude other structural processes.

SPECIAL TESTS

Increased resting sweat output on the affected side is very specific for the diagnosis of RSD. Skin temperature measurements are useful to predict response to a sympathetic block.

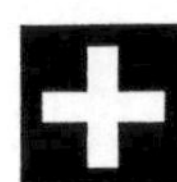

Management

GENERAL MEASURES

Management is most successful when carried out early, in the first 5 months of the disorder. Since presentations are quite diverse, management must be tailored to the main obstacles preventing return to normal function. A rehabilitation program with training and education at its core is the cornerstone of successful management. The program should include psychological intervention to address pacing strategies, coping issues, and approaches to chronic pain. Physical therapy and occupational therapy can address physical and postural issues.

SURGICAL MEASURES

Spinal cord and deep brain stimulation can be of benefit in selected patients.

SYMPTOMATIC TREATMENT

Transcutaneous electrical nerve stimulation (TENS) units and nerve stimulation may be of benefit in selected patients. Lumbar sympathetic blocks as well as stellate ganglion blocks, though never proven effective, are still widely used for relief of pain in RSD. The greatest benefit is derived when they are used in the context of a pain management program.

ADJUNCTIVE TREATMENT

Acupuncture can be of benefit in selected cases.

ADMISSION DISCHARGE CRITERIA

N/A

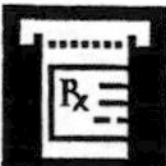

Medications

DRUG(S) OF CHOICE

- *Corticosteroids:* a short trial of prednisone 60 mg for 5 to 7 days is often helpful and should be extended to 3 to 4 weeks if effective. It is most effective for early disease of the lower extremity. Patients with systemic fungal infections, allergy to glucocorticoids, and recent live virus vaccination should not be placed on chronic steroids.
- *Tricyclic antidepressants:* most of the tricyclic antidepressants have some impact on RSD pain. Typically a nonsedating tricyclic is administered during the day such as imipramine or desipramine (in the elderly), with a sedating tricyclic agent such as amitriptyline or nortriptyline at night to aid sleep. The total tricyclic dosage usually begins at 20 to 30 mg and becomes maximally effective between 75 and 150 mg. Patients should not receive these medications if they have cardiac conduction defects (especially prolonged QT interval) or active suicidal ideation. Patients with tachy- or bradycardia, conduction block, Q-T interval prolongation, hypertension or hypotension, agitation, disorientation, hallucinations, dystonia, seizures, decreased secretions, urinary retention, mydriasis, and hyperthermia should be treated with caution.
- *Selective serotonin reuptake inhibitors:* generally not used to treat pain directly, with the possible exception of venlafaxine, but can be very helpful in high doses to manage concomitant depression. May be used in double the usual dose to treat depression, to achieve the desired pain control.
- *Antiepileptic agents:* nearly all agents have been tried, with intermittent success. Gabapentin, carbamazepine, topiramate, Gabitril, clonazepam, keppra, oxcarbazepine, and mexiletine have been beneficial in individual patients. Drugs should be started at the lowest available dose and advanced slowly. The only contraindication is allergy to the drug. All these agents can be associated with various types of cognitive deficits, tremors, ataxia, and other neurologic side effects.
- *Nonsteroidal antiinflammatory drugs:* marginally helpful. When combined with other agents they can produce some added pain relief. They are seldom helpful in isolation. Maximal doses are usually necessary and the antigastrointestinal precautions are always imperative.
- *Adrenergic agents:* clonidine decreases adrenergic transmission by activating presynaptic α_2-receptors. A dosage of 0.1–0.3 mg bid may be effective; higher doses may be needed for improved control. Clonidine can be particularly effective when applied as a patch over an area of scar suspected to harbor an underlying neuroma. Side effects include dry mouth, nausea, dizziness, impotence, nightmares, anxiety, and depression. Phenoxybenzamine, another adrenergic agent, blocks both α_1- and α_2-adrenergic receptors, producing systemic sympathetic blockade through the oral route. Dosage must be advanced until the patient experiences mild symptoms of orthostasis (light-headedness), usually about 80 to 220 mg per day. This drug is most often effective when sympathetic blocks have produced pain relief. It can be used to prolong the effect of sympathetic blocks.
- *Calcitonin:* the only other agent with significant support for efficacy in the literature. It is typically administered in high doses intravenously. It is also available as an intranasal formulation.
- *Antispastic agents:* baclofen, methocarbamol, tizanidine, Artane, and Sinemet can all be helpful for particular movement disturbances.

ALTERNATIVE DRUGS

N/A

Follow-Up

PATIENT MONITORING

Once patients are taught self-management and are on a stable drug regimen (which may take approximately 6 months), they may continue regular follow-up with their primary care physician, with support from the pain specialist as needed.

EXPECTED COURSE AND PROGNOSIS

Patients with RSD may develop complications including infection (cellulitis), ulcers, chronic edema, dystonia, atrophy of muscles in the affected area, and deep venous thrombosis (if immobile). The longer the symptoms and duration of RSD, the poorer the prognosis.

PATIENT EDUCATION

Proper education for the patient and caregiver is essential. Continued passivity on the part of the patient and shopping for health professionals can prove extremely detrimental to long-term control of RSD symptoms.
Web-based information sources:

- International RSD Foundation: *www.rsdinfo.com*
- RSD Syndrome of America: *www.rsds.org*
- International Research Foundation for RSD/CRPS: *www.rsdfoundation.usf.edu*

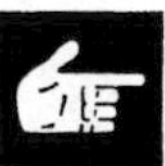

Miscellaneous

SYNONYMS

Complex regional pain syndromes (CRPS) type 1 or type 2

ICD-9-CM: 337.20 RSD; 337.22 RSD lower limb; 337.21 RSD upper limb

SEE ALSO: N/A

REFERENCES

- Kemler MA, Barendse GAM, van Kleef M, et al. Spinal cord stimulation in patients with chronic reflex sympathetic dystrophy. N Engl J Med 2000;343:618–624.
- van Hilten BJ, van de Beek WJT, Hoff JI, et al. Intrathecal baclofen for the treatment of dystonia in patients with reflex sympathetic dystrophy. N Engl J Med 2000;343:625–630.
- Wasner G, Backonja MM, Baron R. Traumatic neuralgias: complex regional pain syndromes (reflex sympathetic dystrophy and causalgia): clinical characteristics, pathophysiological mechanisms and therapy. Neurol Clin 1998;16:851–868.

Author(s): Thomas Chelimsky, MD

Refsum's Disease

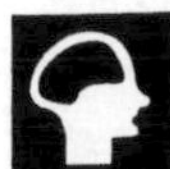

Basics

DESCRIPTION

Sigvald Refsum initially described Refsum's disease in 1945. It is caused by defective metabolism of phytanic acid with subsequent accumulation. This can lead to impairment of function of a wide variety of bodily systems.

EPIDEMIOLOGY

Incidence/Prevalence

Refsum's disease is very rare. Exact incidence and prevalence rates are unknown but United Kingdom figures suggest a prevalence rate of 1/1,000,000. There may be a number of patients particularly with retinitis pigmentosa who are undiagnosed.

Race

The disease may be slightly more common in Scandinavian races and other racial groups with Nordic or Viking ancestry.

Age

The onset of symptoms is usually in late childhood.

Sex

Males and females are equally affected.

ETIOLOGY

Inheritance is autosomal recessive. The defective genes *(PAHX)* are on chromosome 10. Point mutations and deletions have been described. The single enzymatic deficiency in Refsum's disease affects phytanoyl CoA hydroxylase, which normally catalyzes the second step in the breakdown of phytanic to pristanic acid. This results in accumulation of phytanic acid with elevated levels in blood and other tissues including fat and neurons. The mechanism of phytanic acid toxicity is unclear.

RISK FACTORS

N/A

PREGNANCY

Pregnancy may be associated with acute and subacute presentations.

ASSOCIATED CONDITIONS

N/A

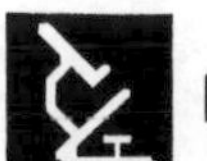

Diagnosis

DIFFERENTIAL DIAGNOSIS

Phytanic acid accumulates in other conditions including Zellweger disease, neonatal adrenoleukodystrophy, infantile Refsum's, and rhizomelic chondrodysplasia punctata. However, these conditions have a different phenotype. Other enzymatic defects in the metabolic pathway of phytanic acid have also been described. Patients with a deficiency of α-methylacyl-CoA racemase have a Refsum's phenotype, but in that condition pristanate levels are also elevated, whereas in classical Refsum's the pristanate to phytanate ratio is <0.0007. Friedreich's ataxia, mitochondrial disease, other hereditary neuropathies, and vitamin E deficiency can usually be differentiated on clinical grounds.

SIGNS AND SYMPTOMS

The cardinal neurologic manifestations include a demyelinating neuropathy, pes cavus, sensorineural deafness, cerebellar ataxia, anosmia, and cranial nerve involvement. There may be marked nerve hypertrophy. Night blindness secondary to retinitis pigmentosa (RP) is common. RP and anosmia occur most frequently. Cataracts, photophobia, and miosis occur less frequently. Cardiac involvement may cause premature death usually secondary to arrhythmias. The skin is thickened and dry, and epiphyseal dysplasia and syndactyly may lead to a characteristic shortening of the fourth toe, which can be diagnostically useful. However, this latter feature is present in only 30% of patients.

LABORATORY PROCEDURES

Nerve conduction studies show evidence of a demyelinating neuropathy. CSF protein levels are often elevated. Plasma levels of phytanic acid are consistently elevated (normal range $<19\mu$mol/L), sometimes >800 μmol/L. Nerve biopsy is no longer particularly useful, but onion bulb formation and targetoid inclusions have been described.

IMAGING STUDIES

N/A

SPECIAL TESTS

N/A

Management

GENERAL MEASURES

Phytanic acid is almost exclusively of exogenous origin, and dietary restriction reduces plasma and tissue levels. Fish, beef, lamb, and dairy products should be avoided. Poultry, pork, fruit, and vegetables are freely allowed. The diet should contain enough calories to prevent weight loss and consequent mobilization of phytanic acid from fat. Dietary treatment needs to be lifelong.

SURGICAL MEASURES

Cataract surgery and orthopedic correction of foot deformities may be necessary in some patients.

SYMPTOMATIC TREATMENT

N/A

ADJUNCTIVE TREATMENT

Occasionally, where phytanic acid levels are extremely high or where the presentation is acute (mimicking Guillain-Barré syndrome) the level can be rapidly reduced by plasma exchange (PEX). PEX should also be considered where dietary control is inadequate. Dialysis is ineffective.

ADMISSION/DISCHARGE CRITERIA

N/A

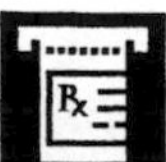

Medications

DRUG(S) OF CHOICE

N/A

ALTERNATIVE DRUGS

N/A

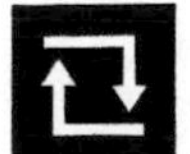

Follow-Up

PATIENT MONITORING

Patient should be assessed at regular intervals by a neurologist. Ophthalmologic, audiologic, and dietary advice is often helpful.

EXPECTED COURSE AND PROGNOSIS

The neurologic, cardiac, and dermatologic sequelae usually can be reversed to some extent by lowering plasma phytanic acid levels. The visual and hearing deficits and anosmia are less responsive to treatment. Pregnancy, rapid weight loss, and fever may be associated with rapid deterioration. Life expectancy is not significantly reduced.

PATIENT EDUCATION

Dietary surveillance needs to be lifelong. There is a Refsum's clinic at the Chelsea and Westminster Hospital, London, UK (phone: 0-044-2082372730).

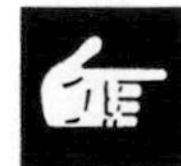

Miscellaneous

SYNONYMS

Heredoataxia hemeralopica polyneuritiformis
Heredopathia atactica polyneuritiformis
HMSN IV.

ICD-9-CM: 356.3 Refsum's disease

SEE ALSO: PEROXISOMAL DISORDERS

REFERENCES

- Gibberd FB, Billimoria JD, Goldman JM, et al. Heredopathia atactica polyneuritiformis: Refsum's disease. Acta Neurol Scand 1985;72(1):1–17.
- Harari D, Gibberd FB, Dick JP, et al. Plasma exchange in the treatment of Refsum's disease. J Neurol Neurosurg Psychiatry 1991;54(7):614–617.
- Jansen JA, Ofman R, Ferdinandusse S, et al. Refsum disease is caused by mutations in the phytanoyl-CoA hydroxylase gene. Nature Genet 1997;17:190–193.
- Jansen GA, Wanders RJ, Watkins PA, et al. Phytanoyl-coenzyme A hydroxylase deficiency—the enzyme defect in Refsum's disease. N Engl J Med 1997;337(2): 133–134.
- Mihalik SJ, Morrell JC, Kim D, et al. Identification of PAHX, a Refsum disease gene. Nature Genet 1997;17:185–189.
- Refsum S. Heredoataxia hemeralopica polyneuritiformis. Nord Med 1945;28: 2682–2685.
- Skjeldal OH, Stokke O, Refsum S, et al. Clinical and biochemical heterogeneity in conditions with phytanic acid accumulation. J Neurol Sci 1987;77:87–96.
- Steinberg D. Refsum disease. In: Scriver CR, Beaudet AL, Sly WS, et al., eds. The metabolic basis of inherited disease, 6th ed. New York: McGraw-Hill, 1989: 2351–2369.
- Verhoeven NM, Wanders RJ, Poll BT, et al. The metabolism of phytanic and pristanic acid in man: a review. J Inherit Metab Dis 1998;21(7):697–728.
- Wills AJ, Manning NJ, Reilly MM. Refsum's disease. Q J Med 2001;94:403–406.

Author(s): Adrian J. Wills, MD

Restless Leg Syndrome

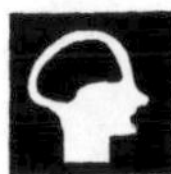

Basics

DESCRIPTION

Restless leg syndrome (RLS) is a disorder characterized by uncomfortable sensations in the calves or feet and, rarely, the upper extremities. The sensations are variously described as painful, tingling, crawling, or "pins and needles." Typically, the sensations begin late in the evening around bedtime and may present as insomnia. However, patients may be awakened by the sensations or they may occur earlier in the day and may interfere with sedentary work or driving. The uncomfortable sensation is immediately quenched by movement of the extremity but frequently returns when movement ceases.

EPIDEMIOLOGY

Incidence/Prevalence

RLS is thought to affect 2% to 5% of the population.

Race

There appears to be no racial preference.

Age

Although the syndrome tends to appear in middle age, symptoms are frequently present for many years prior to presentation.

Sex

Men and women are affected equally.

ETIOLOGY

Etiology is unknown. RLS occurs as an idiopathic form without evidence of any other disease process and as secondary or symptomatic disease in association with several other medical conditions. Some researchers theorize that some of the manifestations of RLS result from disinhibition of descending inhibitory spinal pathways. In addition, the response of many patients to dopaminergic medications suggests that there may be a dysregulation of dopaminergic pathways in the brainstem or spinal cord.

Genetics

Approximately 50% of patients with RLS describe relatives with similar symptoms, suggesting a genetic factor, although the high prevalence of this condition in the general population may make this simply a chance happening. In contrast, families have been described with multiple members clearly affected in a pattern suggestive of autosomal-dominant inheritance. A French-Canadian family was reported with apparent autosomal-recessive mode of inheritance and several candidate locations on chromosome 12.

RISK FACTORS

No known risk factors.

PREGNANCY

Symptoms of RLS have been reported in 10% to 20% of pregnant women and usually resolve after delivery.

ASSOCIATED CONDITIONS

In addition to pregnancy, RLS has also been shown to be associated with iron deficiency with or without anemia and chronic renal failure (especially patients on dialysis). There also appears to be a higher frequency in patients with Parkinson's disease, peripheral neuropathy, and radiculopathy. Tricyclic antidepressants as well as fluoxetine, caffeine, and verapamil have all been demonstrated to increase symptoms of RLS. Other conditions with less well-established associations include:

- Magnesium deficiency
- Folate deficiency
- Rheumatoid arthritis
- Diabetes

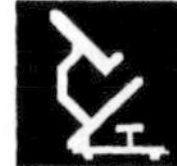

Diagnosis

DIFFERENTIAL DIAGNOSIS

- Nocturnal leg cramps: tend to have an abrupt onset at night and may awaken the patient from sleep. They are painful, tend to be located in the calf or foot, and are accompanied by visible and palpable muscle cramps.
- Fibromyalgia: symptoms tend to occur throughout the day, are not improved by movement, and usually involve more widespread areas of the body (neck, shoulders, and hips).
- Radiculopathy
- Neurogenic claudication
- Akathisia (neuroleptic induced): this syndrome of restlessness with a compulsion to move is seen most commonly with phenothiazine use or in association with Parkinson's disease. In contrast to RLS, the sensory features are less and are more likely to affect the entire body as opposed to the extremities. Symptoms are less prominent at night, and consequently there is less sleep disturbance.
- Small-fiber polyneuropathies: in contrast to RLS, small-fiber polyneuropathies are usually associated with distal sensory loss or abnormal reflexes.
- Painful legs and moving toes syndrome: usually described as aching pain in the feet or toes associated with involuntary writhing movements. The movements are not increased during the evening and night and therefore are not associated with a sleep disturbance.
- Vesper's curse: this is the sudden awakening from sleep with painful calf cramps and fasciculations, frequently with the urge to move. An increase in right atrial filling pressures with subsequent increase in paraspinal venous volume associated with lumbar stenosis has been cited as the cause.

SIGNS AND SYMPTOMS

Diagnostic criteria put forth by the International Restless Legs Syndrome Study Group in 1995 include:

- Desire to move the extremities in association with unpleasant sensations in the calves or feet (and occasionally the upper extremities). These unpleasant sensations are variable and described as a deep burning, tingling, cramping, aching, crawling, or itching.
- Motor restlessness: people with RLS feel a compelling urge to move a limb but do have some choice of which type of movement to perform. The spectrum of movements includes walking, pacing, rocking, shaking, stretching, etc.
- Symptoms are worse at rest with partial and temporary relief with movement, but recur as soon as the patient stops moving and rests.
- Symptoms are worse in the evening or at night, worsening to a peak around midnight and then improving in the morning. These movements may prevent or fragment sleep.
- Although the syndrome is chronic, there is tremendous fluctuation in the intensity of symptoms. Patients may go weeks or months without symptoms followed by nightly occurrences. There is some evidence that stress may play a role as symptoms tend to be more severe at the end of the work week.

LABORATORY PROCEDURES

CBC, electrolytes, BUN and creatinine, vitamin B_{12}, folate, iron, and ferritin.

IMAGING STUDIES

None

SPECIAL TESTS

- Although 80% to 90% of patients with RLS have frequent periodic limb movements (PLMs) during sleep, polysomnography is of little diagnostic value because of the frequency of PLMs in patients without RLS. Thus the diagnosis of RLS is clinical, based on the presence of dysesthesias of the limbs with the desire to move the extremity, motor restlessness, and worsening of the symptoms at rest or at night.
- NCV/EMG should be considered if there is any evidence of distal sensory loss or diminution of reflexes.

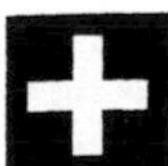

Management

GENERAL MEASURES

The mainstay of treatment is the use of various medications that reduce the uncomfortable symptoms of RLS (see below). There is some evidence that daily vigorous exercise may improve the symptoms of RLS. Also, reduction or the elimination of caffeine may be of benefit.

SURGICAL MEASURES

None

SYMPTOMATIC TREATMENT

- Avoid tobacco products, alcohol, antinausea medications, neuroleptics.
- Avoid sleep deprivation.
- Some patients find a massage or stretching helpful before sleep.
- Hot baths or cold or hot compresses to the limbs.

ADJUNCTIVE TREATMENT

None

ADMISSION/DISCHARGE CRITERIA

N/A

Medications

DRUG(S) OF CHOICE

- Levodopa/carbidopa: historically, levodopa/carbidopa has been the treatment of choice for RLS. The starting dose is 100 mg levodopa and 25 mg carbidopa. Most patients can be controlled with doses of 200 mg of levodopa. Unfortunately, two major problems can occur with this drug. First, many patients will suffer a recurrence of symptoms during the night. In this setting, a second dose can be taken or consideration given to using a sustained release form of L-dopa. However, this preparation tends to be less efficacious. A second problem that may occur with L-dopa, particularly when a second dose is taken, is the onset of paresthesias and restlessness during the day. In this setting, a prolonged trial of a benzodiazepine (clonazepam) may be beneficial. Tardive dyskinesia, a possible long-term side effect of L-dopa, does not usually appear in patients with RLS. However, tolerance to the beneficial effects of the drug also may develop.
- Dopamine agonists: if levodopa/carbidopa becomes ineffective, changing to a dopamine agonist such as pergolide (0.05 mg at bedtime with increase by 0.1 mg every third day) or bromocriptine (2.5 or 5 mg at bedtime) may prove effective. It appears that the daytime occurrence of RLS symptoms is less with the dopamine agonists.
- Other agents that have proven to be effective in the treatment of RLS include the anticonvulsants gabapentin and carbamazepine. Of these, gabapentin has probably been most effective in doses of 300 to 1,000 mg at bedtime.

Contraindications

- Hypersensitivity to levodopa/carbidopa products
- History of melanoma, undiagnosed skin lesions
- Narrow-angle glaucoma
- Nonselective MAO inhibitors

Precautions

There is a 10% incidence of orthostatic hypotension with use of the dopamine agonists.

ALTERNATIVE DRUGS

Benzodiazepines, and specifically clonazepam (0.5 to 2 mg at bedtime), have been shown to be effective at reducing the symptoms of RLS and improving subjective sleep quality, but the major drawback to these drugs is daytime sedation, particularly in the elderly. Finally, opioids (propoxyphene 65 mg, hydrocodone 5 mg, codeine 30 mg) have long been recognized to reduce the symptoms of RLS and improve sleep quality, but the risks of these medications need to be considered.

Follow-Up

PATIENT MONITORING

Polysomnography is of little use in RLS. Therefore, clinical assessment with questioning both the patient and bed partner about the quality of sleep as well as the presence of daytime sleepiness is indicated on a regular basis.

EXPECTED COURSE AND PROGNOSIS

In general the prognosis is good. However, RLS is a lifelong condition, although the intensity of symptoms tends to fluctuate greatly.

PATIENT EDUCATION

Because of the relatively high prevalence of this disorder, numerous support groups are available, such as WEMOVE, website: *www.wemove.org*.

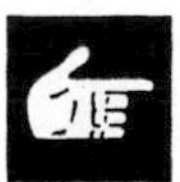

Miscellaneous

SYNONYMS

None

ICD-9-CM: 333.99 Extrapyramidal disease NEC

SEE ALSO: N/A

REFERENCES

- Aldrich MS. Sleep medicine. New York: Oxford University Press, 1999.
- Foreman BH, Chambliss L, Does gabapentin improve restless legs syndrome? J Fam Pract 2003;52(4): 276–279.
- Krieger J, Schroeder C. Iron, brain and restless legs syndrome. Sleep Med Rev 2001;5(4):277–286.
- Stiasny K, Oertel WH, Trenkwalder C. Clinical symptomatology and treatment of restless legs syndrome and periodic limb movement disorder. Sleep Med Rev 2002;6(4):253–65.
- Walters AS, et al., the International Restless Legs Syndrome Study Group. Towards a better definition of the restless legs syndrome. Mov Disord 1995;10:634.

Author(s): Jeffrey Weiland, MD

Rhabdomyolysis

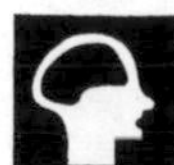

Basics

DESCRIPTION

Rhabdomyolysis is the acute lysis of skeletal muscle. This often causes the release of myoglobin into the circulation and then into the urine, resulting in myoglobinuria.

EPIDEMIOLOGY

Incidence/Prevalence

Because of the many causes of rhabdomyolysis, the exact incidence is unknown.

ETIOLOGY

Many hereditary and acquired diseases may cause rhabdomyolysis, but the most frequent cause is crush injuries. Malignant hyperthermia is a rare cause of rhabdomyolysis associated with certain types of inhaled anesthetics. Although traumatic injury is the most frequent cause of a single episode of rhabdomyolysis, many toxins, drugs, infections, and metabolic derangements may induce the syndrome.

Genetics

The main hereditary disorders that cause rhabdomyolysis are due to inborn errors of metabolism affecting carbohydrate and lipid metabolism within the muscle. The glycolytic defects include deficiencies in muscle phosphorylase (McArdle's disease), phosphorylase b kinase, phosphofructokinase, phosphoglycerate mutase, phosphoglycerate kinase, and lactate dehydrogenase. Lipid metabolism defects may also cause recurrent rhabdomyolysis, with the most common being carnitine palmitoyltransferase deficiency. Defects in long, medium, and short chain fatty acids oxidation may also cause recurrent rhabdomyolysis. More recently, rhabdomyolysis with mitochondrial and respiratory chain disorders have been described. Other biochemical defects can cause recurrent episodes including deficiencies of glucose-6-phosphate dehydrogenase and myoadenylate deaminase. Dystrophinopathies such as Duchenne's muscular dystrophy and Becker's muscular dystrophy are sometimes associated with rhabdomyolysis.

RISK FACTORS

Hereditary causes of rhabdomyolysis are often precipitated by brief, intense exercise or fasting. Malignant hyperthermia is precipitated by the inhaled anesthetic halothane.
Traumatic crush injury may damage the muscle directly, but may also cause ischemia to the muscle, resulting in muscle infarctions. Extreme muscle exertion, even in well-conditioned individuals, may cause rhabdomyolysis. Drugs associated with rhabdomyolysis include alcohol, cocaine, heroin, phencyclidine, amphetamines, phenylpropanolamine, and toluene. Lipid-lowering agents, especially in combination with fibrates, may cause rhabdomyolysis. Snake and insect venoms often cause rhabdomyolysis. Rapid withdrawal of dopaminergic agents may induce a neuroleptic malignant syndrome with rhabdomyolysis.

PREGNANCY

Pregnant women with carnitine palmitoyltransferase deficiency or myophosphorylase deficiency may benefit from intravenous glucose at the time of delivery.

ASSOCIATED CONDITIONS

- Acute renal failure
- Renal tubular acidosis
- Hyperkalemia
- Hypocalcemia
- Compartment syndromes

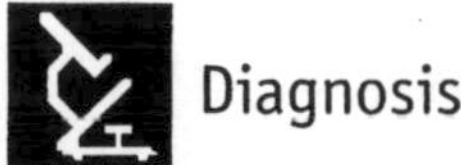

Diagnosis

DIFFERENTIAL DIAGNOSIS

Other causes of pigmenturia such as hematuria, hemoglobinuria and porphyria. A history of recurrent pigmenturia suggests an inborn error in metabolism.

SIGNS AND SYMPTOMS

Rhabdomyolysis that causes myoglobinuria often causes severe myalgias and muscle swelling. Often the patient is unable or unwilling to move due to the severe myalgias. Nausea and vomiting are often present. If an injury has occurred to a well-localized area, a compartment syndrome may develop, causing further damage to the muscle secondary to ischemic as the internal pressures within the muscle compartment rise. Compartment syndrome may lead to arterial and nerve compression with near irreversible damage to the limb. A drop in urine output is a warning of impending renal failure. With rhabdomyolysis, large releases of potassium from the muscle may cause cardiac arrhythmias. Disseminated intravascular coagulation is a rare complication.

LABORATORY PROCEDURES

Pigmenturia is present when concentrations of urine myoglobin are greater than 100 μg/mL. Serum levels of creatine kinase (CK) peak within the first 2 days after the onset of the illness. Hyperkalemia and hyperphosphatemia with hypocalcemia are often present.

IMAGING STUDIES

N/A

SPECIAL TESTS

If the history suggests recurrent episodes of rhabdomyolysis, a muscle biopsy with routine histochemistry and quantitation of enzymes associated with rhabdomyolysis should be done. This can be done after the acute episode has resolved.

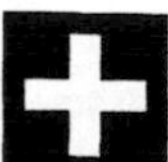

Management

GENERAL MEASURES

The patient should be put to bed rest during the acute phase. The major complications of rhabdomyolysis include renal failure, hyperkalemia, and hypocalcemia. Renal failure can often be prevented with fluid replacement to avoid hypotension and intravenous mannitol or furosemide to maintain urine output. Alkalinization of the urine with intravenous sodium bicarbonate promotes the excretion of myoglobin. Hemodialysis is needed if urine output falls despite these efforts. Hyperkalemia needs to be managed with electrocardiogram monitoring and intravenous glucose and insulin.

SURGICAL MANAGEMENT

Compartment syndrome requires emergent fasciotomy to prevent further ischemia to the muscle and nerve injury.

SYMPTOMATIC TREATMENT

Myalgias often respond to intravenous fluid replacement, but narcotic analgesics may be helpful.

ADJUNCTIVE TREATMENT

N/A

ADMISSION/DISCHARGE CRITERIA

Patients should be admitted for observation and monitoring of renal function until the severity of the episode is determined.

Medications

DRUG(S) OF CHOICE

N/A

ALTERNATIVE DRUGS

N/A

Follow-Up

PATIENT MONITORING

Maintenance of urine output and management of hyperkalemia are key features for the first several days after the onset of the illness.

EXPECTED COURSE AND PROGNOSIS

Most patients recover fully with no lasting effects on their muscle strength if renal failure is avoided. Patients with inborn errors of metabolism or a dystrophinopathy may develop muscle weakness late in life due to recurrent muscle injury.

PATIENT EDUCATION

Precipitating factors need to be avoided.

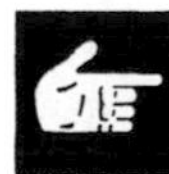

Miscellaneous

SYNONYMS

Myoglobinuria

ICD-9-CM: 791.3 Myoglobinuria

SEE ALSO: N/A

REFERENCES

- DiMauro S, Lamperti C. Muscle glycogenoses. Muscle Nerve 2001;24:984–999.
- Karadimas CL, Greenstein P, Sue CM, et al. Recurrent myoglobinuria due to a nonsense mutation in a COX 1 gene of mitochondrial DNA. Neurology 2000;55:644–649.
- Knochel JP. Pigment nephropathy. In: Greenberg A, ed. Primer on kidney diseases. National Kidney Foundation. San Diego, CA: Academic Press, 1994:149–152.
- Meltzer A, Cola PA, Parsa M. Marked elevations of serum creatine kinase activity associated with antipsychotic drug treatment. Neuropsychopharmacology 1996;15:395–405.
- Penn AS. Myoglobinuria. In: Engel AG, Franzini-Armstrong C, eds. Myology, 2nd ed. New York: McGraw-Hill, 1994: 1679–1696.
- Pierce LR, Wysowik DK, Gross TP. Myopathy and rhabdomyolysis associated with lovastatin-gemfibrozil combination therapy. JAMA 1999;264:71–75.
- Warren JD, Blumberg PC, Thompson PD. Rhabdomyolysis. Muscle Nerve 2002;25: 332–347.

Author(s): J. Ned Pruitt II, MD

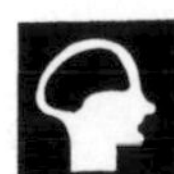

Basics

DESCRIPTION

Rheumatoid arthritis (RA) is a chronic multisystem immune complex disease. Extraarticular manifestations occur in 10% to 20% of patients. Neurologic complications usually occur in patients with moderate to severe RA and can involve the CNS and PNS, including the spine. Chronic synovitis of the spine typically occurs in the cervical region, with damage to the atlantoaxial complex. Complications affecting the PNS are frequent, with carpal tunnel syndrome (CTS; compression neuropathy of the median nerve) being most common.

EPIDEMIOLOGY

Incidence/Prevalence

RA affects 1% to 2% of the population. Cervical spine involvement occurs in 30% to 50% of all RA patients. CTS occurs in 20% to 65% of RA patients. Vasculitis is noted in 5% to 15% of all patients. CNS vasculitis and RA nodules are uncommon.

Race

All races and ethnic groups affected.

Age

Onset is usually between 35 and 50 years of age, but can occur at any age.

Sex

There is a female predilection, accounting for 75% of cases of RA.

ETIOLOGY

RA is mediated by interaction of autoantibodies, such as rheumatoid factor (IgM or IgG class), with circulating immunoglobulins. The immune complexes are composed of IgG combined with IgM or IgG anti-IgG antibodies. Deposition of the immune complexes into the joints and soft tissues induces activation of complement and other inflammatory pathways. Atlantoaxial subluxation (AAS) results from rheumatoid synovial tissue–induced laxity or destruction of the transverse ligament in combination with odontoid erosion. Subaxial subluxation can occur with rheumatoid involvement of the longitudinal ligaments, vertebral endplates, apophyseal joints, and intervertebral discs. Peripheral neuropathy results from entrapment, segmental demyelination, or rheumatoid vasculitis of the small-to-medium size vessels. Nerve entrapment syndromes arise from inflamed synovial sacs and can affect the median, ulnar, and posterior tibial nerves.

Genetics

There can be a genetic predisposition for RA; first-degree relatives of seropositive patients are four times more likely to develop RA than controls.

RISK FACTORS

AAS is more likely in patients with RA of 10 years' duration or longer, seropositivity, erosive and deforming peripheral joint disease, and male gender. Compression neuropathies correlate with the severity of local synovitis. Vasculitis is more likely to occur in patients with long-standing RA; the incidence is higher in males.

PREGNANCY

A hormonal role is suspected in disease expression, because there is an increased risk of RA in nulliparous women and a possible protective effect in women who use oral contraceptives.

ASSOCIATED CONDITIONS

There is a higher incidence of vasculitic complications in RA patients with Felty's syndrome (i.e., RA, splenomegaly, neutropenia, anemia, and thrombocytopenia).

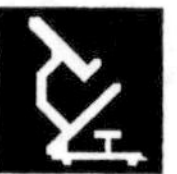

Diagnosis

DIFFERENTIAL DIAGNOSIS

The differential diagnosis is broad and includes other causes of myelopathy, cervical subluxation disorders, CNS and PNS vasculitis, entrapment neuropathies, and peripheral neuropathy. RA must be distinguished from degenerative osteoarthritis and from deforming inflammatory arthritis associated with other connective tissue disorders.

SIGNS AND SYMPTOMS

Spine Involvement

In most cases AAS is asymptomatic, despite the radiologic appearance. Cord and nerve compression is more likely to occur if there is an atlanto-dens interval of greater than 9 mm. Compression of the second spinal nerve roots often causes localized neck pain with radiation to the occiput and scalp. Early signs of cervical radiculopathy are numbness and paresthesias in the glove-stocking distribution. Later signs of progression to cord compromise include myelopathy, lower motor neuron injury at the level of compression, and gait difficulty. Lhermitte's sign (sudden tingling paresthesias that radiate down the spine after cervical flexion) can occur at any stage. Intradural spinal nodules can cause nerve root compression, spinal stenosis, and cord compression.

CNS Involvement

Intraparenchymal rheumatoid nodules can cause encephalopathy, seizures, and obtundation. Cerebral vasculitis can present with seizures, stroke syndromes, encephalopathy, cranial neuropathies, ataxia, and hemorrhage (intracerebral or subarachnoid).

PNS Involvement

CTS typically presents with night numbness, paresthesias, and pain in the thumb, index, and middle fingers of the affected hand. In severe cases, atrophy of the thenar muscles may be present, along with thumb weakness, and retrograde pain up the forearm. Tinel's sign is often positive—reproduction of symptoms elicited by percussion of the median nerve on the volar aspect of the wrist. Phalen's sign may also be present—flexion of the wrist for at least 1 minute, eliciting numbness, tingling, or pain in the median nerve distribution. Tarsal tunnel syndrome presents as paresthesias, pain, and burning in the toes and soles of the feet. Weakness and atrophy of the intrinsic toe muscles may occur.

Other PNS manifestations of RA include mild and severe forms of sensorimotor polyneuropathy, as well as a mononeuritis multiplex.

LABORATORY PROCEDURES

Serologic testing for rheumatoid factor and other autoantibodies is necessary.

IMAGING STUDIES

- To evaluate spinal involvement, lateral radiographs of the cervical spine (flexion and extension views) are required to demonstrate subluxation. Lateral AAS can be demonstrated on open-mouthed, anteroposterior views. MRI can further evaluate bony spinal degeneration and screen for spinal cord compression. MRI is also indicated for patients with suspected basilar invagination for whom standard radiographs are inconclusive. A dynamic flexion-extension MRI may be able to reveal subtle instability patterns (e.g., atlantoaxial instability) of the spinal column.
- MRI (with or without MR angiography) can be helpful for the diagnosis of CNS vasculitis.

SPECIAL TESTS

Somatosensory evoked potentials can evaluate the functional integrity of central sensory pathways. Disease processes affecting the cervical spinal cord may produce prolongation of wave and interwave latencies recorded along these pathways. EMG and sensory nerve conduction studies are the most accurate method to diagnose compression neuropathies and peripheral neuropathies. Sural nerve biopsies can be helpful if the diagnosis of vasculitis is unclear.

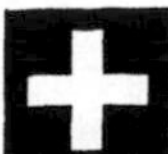

Management

GENERAL MEASURES

- For patients with cervical spine disease, neck pain without neurologic features tends to be self-limited and usually improves. In the absence of cord compression, conservative management is appropriate with antiinflammatory or disease modifying antirheumatic medications, physical therapy, and soft cervical collars.
- Rheumatoid vasculitis is a potentially life-threatening problem that requires high-dose corticosteroids in combination with a cytotoxic drug such as oral cyclophosphamide or methotrexate.

SURGICAL MEASURES

- For patients with AAS, surgical intervention with C1-2 arthrodesis stabilizes the atlantoaxial complex and usually eliminates occipital pain. The indications for surgery include basilar invagination, neurologic abnormality with spinal instability, intractable neck and head pain, vertebral artery compromise, and asymptomatic spinal cord compression on MRI.
- Surgical release of compression neuropathy may be indicated when there is a significant motor or sensory abnormality and evidence of denervation on neurophysiologic testing.

SYMPTOMATIC TREATMENT

Soft cervical collars can stabilize the spine and reduce neck pain in patients with severe AAS. Local corticosteroid injections and splints may be of benefit for compression neuropathies.

ADJUNCTIVE TREATMENT

Simple neck traction may be helpful in patients with severe AAS or subaxial subluxation. Physical and occupational therapy should be considered for patients with myelopathy, peripheral neuropathy, and other forms of weakness.

ADMISSION/DISCHARGE CRITERIA

Admission is uncommon except in cases of acute neurologic deterioration, where the diagnosis is indeterminate or therapeutic intervention is necessary. Patients with CNS or PNS vasculitis are the most likely subgroup to require admission, usually for weakness, seizures, encephalopathy, gait dysfunction, or other acute complications.

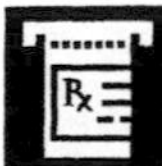

Medications

DRUG(S) OF CHOICE

Pharmacotherapy of neurologic manifestations of RA consists of a combination of corticosteroids and a cytotoxic agent, such as oral cyclophosphamide or methotrexate. The corticosteroid is started at 60 to 100 mg per day and then tapered over several weeks. Monotherapy with one of the cytotoxic agents is then continued for long-term maintenance therapy. The efficacy of other immunosuppressive therapies such as plasmapheresis and intravenous immunoglobulin (IVIG) is unknown.

ALTERNATIVE DRUGS

N/A

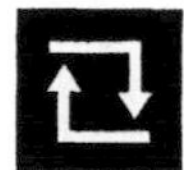

Follow-Up

PATIENT MONITORING

RA patients who should be screened for AAS with radiographic evaluation include those with posterior skull and/or neck pain and stiffness, and patients with long-standing erosive RA in whom radiographs have not been done within the previous 2 or 3 years. Serial neurologic examinations and appropriate follow-up testing (e.g., MRI of the brain or spine, EMG, and nerve conduction testing) is necessary.

EXPECTED COURSE AND PROGNOSIS

The best course of management is to prevent significant morbidity in RA. Aggressive immunosuppressant therapy reduces the neurologic complications of RA. The overall 5-year mortality rate of RA patients with radiographic evidence of cervical subluxation (with or without neurologic symptoms) is similar to that of severe RA patients without cervical involvement. The risk of developing upper cervical spinal cord compression secondary to anterior AAS is increased by male sex, anterior subluxation >9 mm, and coexistent atlantoaxial impaction. There is a higher incidence of fatality with basilar invagination. The prognosis of rheumatoid vasculitis is poor. Independent variables that best predict mortality include cutaneous vasculitis, multifocal neuropathy, and depressed C4 level.

PATIENT EDUCATION

- National Institute of Arthritis and Musculoskeletal Disorders: *www.niams.nih.gov*
- Arthritis Foundation Home Page: *www.arthritis.org*

Miscellaneous

SYNONYMS

N/A

ICD-9-CM: 714.0 Rheumatoid arthritis; 354.0 Carpal tunnel syndrome; 336.9 Myelopathy—spinal cord; 454.1 Vasculitis—cerebral; 447.6 Vasculitis—disseminated

SEE ALSO: VASCULITIS, MYELOPATHY, PERIPHERAL NEUROPATHY

REFERENCES

- Cats A. Rheumatoid arthritis: instability of the cervical spine. In: Klippel JH, Dieppe PA, eds. Rheumatology. 5;4:London: Mosby 1998;4-6.
- Chang DJ, Paget SA. Neurologic complications of rheumatoid arthritis. Rheum Dis Clin North Am 1993;19: 955-973.
- Gurley JP, Bell GR. The surgical management of patients with rheumatoid cervical spine disease. Rheum Dis Clin North Am 1997;23:317-332.
- Matteson EL, Cohen MD, Conn DL. Rheumatoid arthritis: clinical features and systemic involvement. In: Klippel JH, Dieppe PA, eds. Rheumatology. 5;4:London: Mosby, 1998;1-8.
- Paget SA, Erkan D. Case studies: neurologic complications of rheumatoid arthritis. Adv Immunother 2000;7(3): 12-16.
- Rawlins BA, Girardi FP, Boache-Adjei O. Rheumatoid arthritis of the cervical spine. Rheum Dis Clin North Am 1998;24:55-65.

Author(s): Doruk Erkan, MD; Stephen A. Paget, MD; Herbert B. Newton, MD

Sarcoidosis, Neurologic Complications

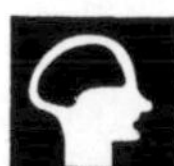

Basics

DESCRIPTION

Sarcoidosis is a chronic disorder of unknown etiology characterized by multisystem dissemination of noncaseating granulomas. Approximately one third of patients with involvement of the CNS have no other known systemic involvement. Sarcoidosis can affect all parts of the nervous system including the brain, spinal cord, and peripheral nerves, as well as muscle.

EPIDEMIOLOGY

Incidence/Prevalence

Worldwide incidence ranges from 1 to 64 per 100,000. The disorder is thought to be more frequent in the southeastern part of the United States.

Race

There appears to be significantly more involvement of African Americans, with a tenfold increase compared to Caucasians in the southeastern part of the United States.

Age

Occurs in all ages.

Sex

A slight preponderance is reported in females.

ETIOLOGY

The cause of this disorder is unknown. Abnormalities of immune regulation in the genetically susceptible individual induced by an as yet unidentified environmental agent is the prevailing hypothesis.

Genetics

A genetic basis for this disease is speculated, but no specific gene has been identified.

RISK FACTORS

There are no known risk factors for this disorder. However, for reasons that are unclear, the disorder favors the nonsmoker.

PREGNANCY

Specific information regarding pregnancy is lacking. Anecdotal reports of remissions as well as flare-ups during pregnancy have been reported.

ASSOCIATED CONDITIONS

None. However, patients with sarcoidosis can have increased susceptibility to mycobacterial infections.

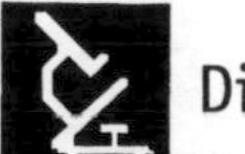

Diagnosis

DIFFERENTIAL DIAGNOSIS

Neurologic dysfunction in sarcoidosis is due to granulomas that act as space-occupying lesions. The granulomas themselves are nontoxic and do not usually elicit any inflammatory response in the adjoining brain. Entities to be considered include infectious disorders such as cryptococcosis, histoplasmosis, coccidioidomycosis, tuberculosis, syphilis, and Lyme disease; inflammatory disorders including vasculitis and berylliosis; and malignancies such as meningeal carcinomatosis, primary lymphoma of the CNS, metastatic disease, and gliomatosis cerebri.

SIGNS AND SYMPTOMS

- In the CNS sarcoidosis affects the basal meninges and the area around the third ventricle, including the thalamus, hypothalamus, and hypophysis. Patients may present with features of meningitis. Multiple cranial nerve palsies are common, especially unilateral or bilateral Bell's palsy. Recurrent seventh nerve palsy of the lower motor neuron type, especially when bilateral, should suggest sarcoidosis. Optic neuritis occurs, especially in the form of papillitis. Hypothalamic and hypophysial involvements are especially common, and can manifest as the syndrome of inappropriate secretion of vasopressin or diabetes insipidus. Almost half of patients with CNS sarcoidosis develop hyperprolactinemia with secondary galactorrhea in either sex. When involved, the spinal cord is usually enlarged with evidence of an intramedullary mass and resultant compressive myelopathy and its clinical manifestations.
- Rarely, sarcoidosis can affect the peripheral nervous system in isolation. The symptoms of peripheral nerve involvement are due to the space-occupying nature of the granulomas that result in expansion of the nerves and sometimes compression. Muscle involvement in systemic sarcoidosis is common. Often, the muscle can be a useful site for biopsy for demonstration of the sarcoid granuloma.

LABORATORY PROCEDURES

- Since meningeal involvement is common, CSF evaluation is particularly helpful. CSF pressure is usually normal. Fluid is colorless unless associated with elevated spinal fluid protein, which causes xanthochromia. Moderate to severe pleocytosis is common, causing some concern of an infectious process. Total WBC counts can be around $100/mm^3$. Most cells are mononuclear and of the T-cell type, mostly of the CD4 phenotype. Some B cells are evident as well. Increased production of intrathecal IgG is common with abnormally elevated IgG index and the presence of oligoclonal bands. Measurement of angiotensin-converting enzyme (ACE) levels in the CSF is of limited value since this enzyme can be transported from serum into CSF across an intact blood–brain barrier. Accordingly when serum ACE levels are elevated, CSF levels may go up as well, although there may not be any evidence of CNS involvement by other studies. Conversely, CSF ACE levels can be normal in patients with isolated spinal cord or brain sarcoid granulomas.
- In every patient with suspected sarcoidosis of the CNS, evaluation should be done to identify multisystemic involvement. This may include measurement of serum ACE levels, liver enzyme levels, bronchoalveolar lavage with phenotyping of the washed cells, and liver or lung biopsy or biopsy of enlarged lymph nodes.

IMAGING STUDIES

Granulomatous involvement of the meninges and parenchyma of the brain and spinal cord can be readily detected by MRI. Detection can be improved with the use of gadolinium, which can show enhancement of the meninges affected by the sarcoid granulomata as well as parenchymal lesions with disruption of the blood–brain barrier. CT of the brain does not have any role in diagnosis of this disorder because of low sensitivity to detect sarcoid lesions.

SPECIAL TESTS

There are no special tests for diagnosis of sarcoidosis of the CNS. In the absence of systemic sarcoidosis, biopsy is the only method of diagnosis. In a third of patients with CNS, sarcoidosis such methods may be necessary.

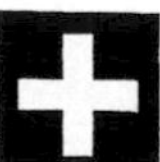

Management

GENERAL MEASURES

The focus of treatment is corticosteroid therapy as well as supportive measures necessary and appropriate to the mode of presentation. Accordingly, encephalopathic patients may require correction of electrolyte imbalance if the problem was related to alteration of electrolytes secondary to diabetes insipidus or syndrome of inappropriate antidiuretic hormone (SIADH). A patient presenting with seventh nerve paresis may require attention to prevent exposure keratitis. Patients with myelopathy may require attention to bowel and bladder function and emergent treatment with steroids to treat compressive myelopathy.

SURGICAL MEASURES

Surgery is not necessary for diagnosis unless the clinical presentation is confusing and the sarcoidosis is confined to the nervous system. In such instances biopsy of the lesion or basal meninges may be necessary to make the diagnosis. When the granuloma is located in the spinal cord, often masquerading as a tumor, excision of the lesion may be necessary.

SYMPTOMATIC TREATMENT

None specific for neurosarcoidosis.

ADJUNCTIVE TREATMENT

Adjunctive therapy to reduce steroid complications is necessary. Diphosphonate therapy to reduce loss of bone mass, H2 blockers for prevention of peptic acid disease, and when appropriate, use of trimethoprim with sulfa for chemoprophylaxis against *Pneumocystis carinii* should be considered.

ADMISSION/DISCHARGE CRITERIA

Admission is necessitated by clinical status of the patient, often dictated by the nature of involvement, such as altered mental status from encephalopathy, spinal cord involvement with paresis, etc.

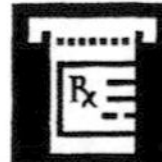

Medications

DRUG(S) OF CHOICE

Corticosteroids are the mainstay of treatment of sarcoidosis, and neurosarcoidosis is no exception. Acutely, patients may be treated with intravenous steroids for disorders that require immediate resolution, such as optic neuritis, transverse myelitis, encephalopathy secondary to diabetes insipidus, or SIADH. Methylprednisolone is administered in doses of 500 to 1,000 mg in D5/0.45 N saline daily for 3 to 5 days. Oral prednisone may be necessary in severe cases and is used in doses of 1 mg/kg daily or every other day, best administered as a single oral dose in the morning. There are no good controlled studies that have examined the dose, route of administration, or duration of treatment necessary for neurosarcoidosis. The duration of treatment can vary from 3 to 18 months, depending on the response and steroid dependence exhibited by these patients.

Contraindications

Corticosteroids are contraindicated in cases of known hypersensitivity or allergy. Steroids should be used with caution in patients with hypertension, diabetes, or known history of gastroduodenal ulceration. However, these conditions are not absolute contraindications for treatment with glucocorticoids since additional therapeutic measures can be instituted to permit their use.

Precautions

Corticosteroid treatment can be associated with glucose intolerance and steroid-induced diabetes. In rare individuals, aseptic necrosis of the femur can occur with need for surgical replacement of the femoral head with prosthesis. Daily treatment for prolonged periods can result in adrenal insufficiency, which can be minimized with alternate day regimen.

ALTERNATIVE DRUGS

A number of drugs have been used as adjunctive therapy with steroids to reduce the granuloma load and to reduce the doses of steroids required. These include methotrexate, cyclosporine, cyclophosphamide and, less often, indomethacin, chloroquine, allopurinol, and levamisole. There are no good studies that have documented the usefulness of any of these agents.

Follow-Up

PATIENT MONITORING

Patients should be monitored for corticosteroid-induced complications as well as response to treatment. Cushingoid side effects can be minimized by reduction of oral salt intake. Patients should be instructed on a low-carbohydrate diet to minimize weight gain as well as glucose intolerance. ACE levels are often not elevated, and therefore seldom helpful in monitoring treatment. The best guide to effective treatment is the clinical response of the individual patient. Imaging with gadolinium-enhanced MRI can be helpful.

EXPECTED COURSE AND PROGNOSIS

Excellent resolution of the symptoms can be expected in the short term with corticosteroid therapy. Patients with extensive basal meningeal disease, endocrinopathy, or spinal cord granulomas often require more chronic therapy. With long-term therapy prognosis for complete resolution is often excellent.

PATIENT EDUCATION

Patients on chronic steroid therapy should be instructed to maintain a 1-g sodium and 1,500- to 2,000-calorie low-carbohydrate diet to minimize weight gain and cushingoid side effects.

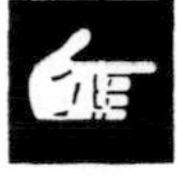

Miscellaneous

SYNONYMS

Hutchinson's disease
Boeck's disease
Uveoparotid fever
Heerfordt's disease

ICD-9-CM: 135 Sarcoidosis; additional codes may apply according to areas of involvement such as meningitis (322.9), encephalitis (323.9), transverse myelitis (323.9), cranial neuropathy (facial paresis 351.8, ocular paresis 378.52, 378.53, and 378.54), optic neuritis/papillitis (377.3), endocrinopathy, myopathy (359.9), neuropathy (355.9)

SEE ALSO: N/A

REFERENCES

- Gullapalli D, Phillips II LH. Neurologic manifestations of sarcoidosis. Neurol Clin 2002:20(1):59–83.
- Nowak DA, Widenka DC. Neurosarcoidosis: a review of its intracranial manifestation. J Neurol 2001;248(5):363–372.
- Zajicek JP. Neurosarcoidosis. Curr Opin Neurol 2000;13(3):323–325.

Author(s): Kottil W. Rammohan, MD

Sleep Apnea

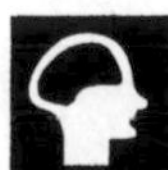

Basics

DESCRIPTION

Obstructive sleep apnea (OSA) is a severely underdiagnosed disorder characterized by intermittent nocturnal upper airway occlusion. This occlusion causes loud, irregular snoring, hemoglobin desaturation, and recurrent arousals from sleep. In addition to its impact on patient well-being, there is a growing body of evidence that untreated OSA has serious long-term cardiovascular effects. OSA also has public health ramifications, largely due to its effects on driving and workplace performance.

EPIDEMIOLOGY

Incidence/Prevalence

OSA is estimated to affect 2% of women and 4% of men over the age of 50. The prevalence is somewhat lower in younger populations, though it has been reported to affect even very young children, largely due to congenital upper airway abnormalities. At least one series suggests that a significant minority of OSA occurs in patients without the "typical" body habitus.

Race

OSA has no well-established racial predilection.

ETIOLOGY

- Partial or complete upper airway obstruction during sleep is the crucial event in the genesis of OSA. The physiologic decrease in pharyngeal muscle tone seen in all sleeping persons is a major contributor, though this effect alone is generally inadequate to cause symptomatic obstruction. Sedative drugs and alcohol accentuate the decrease in muscle tone and can worsen the occlusion. Most patients also have anatomic upper airway narrowing, usually related to the peripharyngeal infiltration of fat seen in obesity. Retrognathia, macroglossia, and abnormally large tonsils, soft palate or uvula are other abnormalities that are sometimes seen. Additionally, posterior movement of the tongue in the supine sleeper narrows the airway further.
- Obstruction of the airway causes apnea or hypopnea in the face of repeated respiratory efforts, oxyhemoglobin desaturation, and ultimately, arousal. Arousal then increases muscle tone in the upper airway, relieving the obstruction. Arousal is usually partial, and may occur more than a hundred times per hour, leading to fragmented sleep.

Genetics

Although familial clustering of OSA has been widely noted, a definitive genetic basis for the disease has not yet been identified.

RISK FACTORS

Risk factors include obesity, increased neck circumference (>16 inches in females, >17 inches in males), retrognathia, macroglossia, other craniofacial abnormalities, acromegaly, hypothyroidism, neuromuscular disorders, and use of alcohol or sedative medications. While some authors believe that chronic nasal obstruction is a risk factor, this subject remains controversial.

PREGNANCY

Several case reports have suggested an association between untreated obstructive sleep apnea and preeclampsia.

ASSOCIATED CONDITIONS

- Multiple large series have demonstrated a relationship between OSA and systemic hypertension; the relative risk of hypertension is greater with more severe degrees of OSA. Whether treatment of OSA improves hypertension is less clear, although this effect has been seen anecdotally.
- There is no definitive evidence that OSA causes pulmonary hypertension or congestive heart failure, though numerous series suggest that these conditions can improve if coexisting OSA is treated.
- Untreated OSA has a well-documented correlation with automobile accidents; one series from Canada demonstrated an accident rate in untreated OSA three times that of non-OSA controls. In another study, patient-reported near-miss rates decreased almost eightfold after treatment with continuous positive airway pressure (CPAP).

Diagnosis

DIFFERENTIAL DIAGNOSIS

The differential diagnosis of OSA includes simple snoring, central sleep apnea, narcolepsy, insufficient sleep, idiopathic CNS hypersomnia, periodic limb movement disorder, psychiatric disorders, and alcohol or sedative drug use.

SIGNS AND SYMPTOMS

Loud, irregular snoring and daytime hypersomnolence are the hallmarks of OSA. Patients commonly awaken in the morning unrefreshed, and often describe falling asleep during quiet activities, such as reading, watching TV, or driving. A history from the patient's bed partner is crucial, and often reveals witnessed episodes of apnea during sleep. Other symptoms include nocturnal choking, sore throat, morning headache, difficulty concentrating, memory impairment, irritability, and depression.

LABORATORY PROCEDURES

A thyroid-stimulating hormone (TSH) level should be measured to assess for hypothyroidism; CBC may reveal polycythemia if nocturnal desaturations are significant.

IMAGING STUDIES

Radiologic studies are generally not useful in OSA.

SPECIAL TESTS

- Polysomnography (PSG) performed in a sleep lab is the test of choice for diagnosing OSA. PSG consists of EEG, electrooculography, EMG, electrocardiography, pulse oximetry, nasal and oral airflow measurements, and measurement of chest and abdominal wall movement, all done during a night of sleep. PSG in a patient with obstructive sleep apnea typically demonstrates repeated apneas and hypopneas with EEG-documented arousal and varying degrees of oxyhemoglobin desaturation.
- The number of apneas and hypopneas per hour of sleep is referred to as the respiratory disturbance index (RDI); an RDI of greater than 5 is usually considered abnormal.
- The high cost of polysomnography has given rise to various portable monitors for home diagnosis of OSA; however, none of these monitors have been well validated, and they should still be considered experimental.

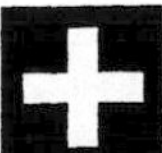

Management

GENERAL MEASURES

- CPAP is the primary nonsurgical treatment for OSA. CPAP acts as a pneumatic splint for the upper airway, preventing obstruction during sleep, and is quite effective in most cases. It can be delivered either via nasal mask or full-face mask, and is titrated to a normal RDI during polysomnography. Compliance data are mixed, although adherence to therapy tends to be greater in those with more severe OSA.
- Mandibular advancement devices are oral appliances custom fit to the patient's mouth, and designed to direct the mandible anteriorly, preventing obstruction at the level of the hypopharynx. Though well tolerated, these devices are not as effective as CPAP, and are only useful in those with mild-moderate OSA.

SURGICAL MEASURES

- Uvulopalatopharyngoplasty (UPPP) is the most commonly performed surgical procedure for OSA. It consists of removal of the uvula, posterior soft palate, and redundant peripharyngeal tissue. Long-term cure rates with this procedure are less than 50%, and many patients ultimately require CPAP or repeat surgery. UPPP is probably most effective in those with mild OSA.
- More invasive base-of-tongue and mandibular advancement procedures can be effective in carefully selected patients; these procedures require an experienced ENT surgeon and carry a higher risk of complications.
- Tracheostomy is curative for OSA, but is reserved for patients with very severe OSA who are noncompliant or unresponsive to maximal CPAP.

SYMPTOMATIC TREATMENT

There is no symptomatic treatment for OSA other than those listed above.

ADJUNCTIVE TREATMENT

Weight loss can decrease the severity of OSA, and can occasionally be curative, but is usually difficult to maintain. Avoidance of the supine sleeping position can also be helpful, and the use of alcohol and sedative medications should be limited if possible.

ADMISSION/DISCHARGE CRITERIA

N/A

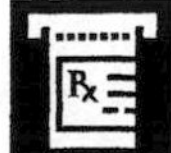

Medications

DRUG(S) OF CHOICE

Although a number of medications have been used to treat OSA in the past, none are effective, and pharmacotherapy is not currently indicated for this disorder.

ALTERNATIVE DRUGS

N/A

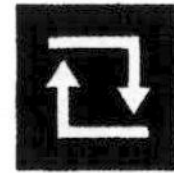

Follow-Up

PATIENT MONITORING

Periodic reassessment of the patient's sleep quality by interview is important to assure sustained response to therapy. If symptoms such as daytime hypersomnolence or snoring recur, repeat PSG is sometimes needed to titrate CPAP or evaluate the need for further therapy.

EXPECTED COURSE AND PROGNOSIS

The prognosis for treated OSA is generally good. While surgery or significant weight loss can sometimes lead to a permanent cure, OSA usually requires lifelong therapy.

PATIENT EDUCATION

- Patients should be advised that weight gain could decrease the effectiveness of most therapies for OSA
- For those patients using CPAP, an experienced respiratory therapist is an invaluable educational resource, and can often provide advice regarding the technical aspects of CPAP use that the physician cannot.
- There is an extensive body of information on OSA available via the Internet, including professional societies, nonprofit organizations, and support groups. Links to many of these groups can be found at *www.sleepapnea.org*.

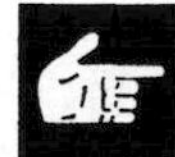

Miscellaneous

SYNONYMS

None

ICD-9-CM: 780.51 Insomnia with sleep apnea; 780.53 Hypersomnia with sleep apnea; 780.57 Other unspecified sleep apnea

SEE ALSO: N/A

REFERENCES

- Engleman HM. Self-reported use of CPAP and benefits of CPAP therapy: a patient survey. Chest 1996;109(6):1470–1476.
- Flemons WW. Obstructive sleep apnea. N Engl J Med 2002;347(7):498–504.
- George CF. Reduction in motor vehicle collisions following treatment of sleep apnoea with nasal CPAP. Thorax 2001;56(7):508–512.
- Peppard PE. Prospective study of the association between sleep-disordered breathing and hypertension. N Engl J Med 2000;342(19):1378–1384.
- Victor LD. Obstructive sleep apnea. Am Fam Physician 1999;60(8):2279–2286.
- Young T. Predictors of sleep-disordered breathing in community-dwelling adults: the Sleep Heart Health Study. Arch Intern Med 2002;162(8):893–900.

Author(s): LeRoy Essig, MD

Sphingolipidoses

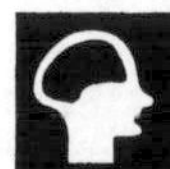

Basics

DESCRIPTION

Degenerative storage disorders are caused by deficiency of an enzyme that is required for the catabolism of lipids that contain ceramide.* The lipids that accumulate in tissues and organs of affected individuals are from the normal turnover of cells and cell components. Differences in properties of the accumulating substances as well as the type of tissue in which a particular lipid component is rapidly turning over account for the diverse clinical manifestation of the disorders.

There are ten diseases, most of which have variable phenotypes that correlate with the level of residual enzyme activity. Central and/or peripheral nervous system involvement is true of all except type 1 Gaucher and Niemann-Pick type B. The clinical features described in this chapter are for the most common phenotype with neurologic manifestations. Less common phenotypes that may be characterized by delayed onset during adolescence or adulthood and associated with variable neurologic and systemic manifestations are described in more extensive reviews.

EPIDEMIOLOGY

Incidence/Prevalence

Tay Sachs: Disease incidence of 1 in 4,000 Ashkenazi Jewish births. Among non-Jews, the disease incidence is 100 times less. Five geographic isolates do exist: Switzerland, Japan, the Pennsylvania Dutch group in Pennsylvania, French-Canadians in Quebec, and Cajuns in southern Louisiana.

Sandhoff: Incidence of 1 in 309,000 non-Jewish infants; 1 in 1,000,000 Jewish births. Several populations have an increased incidence: Creole population in Argentina, Metis Indians in northern Saskatchewan, Lebanese-Canadians, as well as in Lebanon.

Fabry: Estimated incidence of 1 in 40,000.

Niemann-Pick type A: Panethnic but with an increased incidence in Ashkenazi Jews of 1 in 40,000.

Niemann-Pick type C: Panethnic, but with an increased incidence in Spanish-Americans in southern Colorado.

Niemann-Pick type D: All patients share a common ancestry in Nova Scotia. Incidence of 1% in this population.

Gaucher type I: most commonly diagnosed in Ashkenazi Jews. Type 2 is panethnic and Type 3 has a predilection for the population of Northern Sweden.

Krabbe: Incidence estimated at 1 in 100,000 to 1 in 200,000 births. Incidence of 6 in 1,000 births in a large Druze kindred in Israel.

* Niemann-Pick types C/D do not share this common metabolic defect. They are grouped with the sphingolipidoses because of their historical association.

Incidence also increased in the Scandinavian countries.

Metachromatic leukodystrophy: incidence estimated at 1 in 100,000 births. A particularly high incidence in the Habbanite Jewish community in Israel.

Race

See Incidence/Prevalence, above.

Age

See Signs and Symptoms, below.

Sex

Because of X-linked inheritance, patients with Fabry are male. Female heterozygotes may manifest symptoms of the disease but symptoms are less severe and of later onset.

ETIOLOGY

Genetics

The sphingolipidoses are inherited in an autosomal-recessive manner except for Fabry, which is X-linked. Determination of carrier status is possible for some. Prenatal testing is available.

RISK FACTORS

N/A

PREGNANCY

N/A

ASSOCIATED CONDITIONS

N/A

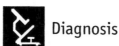

Diagnosis

DIFFERENTIAL DIAGNOSIS

The sphingolipidoses must be differentiated from other inherited neurodegenerative diseases.

SIGNS AND SYMPTOMS

- GM_2 gangliosidosis (Tay-Sachs) and Sandhoff: onset at 3 to 5 months with exaggerated startle response to sound and decreased visual attentiveness. By 6 to 10 months of age, there is progressive weakness and loss of previously attained milestones. Thereafter progression is rapid. A cherry red spot is present in almost all patients. Seizures usually develop by the end of the first year. Macrocephaly from reactive cerebral gliosis is common.
- GM_1 gangliosidosis: onset of developmental arrest before 6 months of age followed by progressive CNS deterioration. Fifty percent of patients have a cherry red spot. Hepatosplenomegaly is almost always present. Skeletal dysplasia seen. Patients become vegetative with generalized spasticity, contractures and generalized seizures.
- Fabry disease: onset in preteen and adolescent boys. Two pain syndromes are described:
  - —Episodic painful, burning sensations in the hands and feet, which may last minutes to several days (Fabry crises)
  - —Constant discomfort of burning paresthesias in the hands and feet. Progressive CNS damage, such as transient ischemic attacks and cerebral hemorrhage, from multifocal small vessel involvement. Reddish-purplish angiokeratoma on the skin, which may be limited to the umbilical and scrotal areas. Hypohidrosis and characteristic corneal and lenticular opacities. Progressive cardiac and renal disease.
- Niemann-Pick type A: onset prior to 6 months of age with psychomotor retardation. A cherry red spot is present in 50% of patients. Progressive spasticity, rigidity, and vegetative state. Hepatosplenomegaly, foam cells in bone marrow.
- Niemann-Pick type C: history of neonatal jaundice. Presents in late childhood with inattention/school difficulties progressing to dementia. Down gaze ophthalmoplegia, ataxia, dystonia, dysarthria, and dysphagia are common. Seizures do occur. Some patients have hepatosplenomegaly.
- Niemann-Pick type D: similar to Niemann-Pick type C but with a slower neurodegenerative course. All patients share a common ancestry in Nova Scotia.
- Gaucher disease type 2: onset from infancy to 6 months of age with progressive CNS damage including marked mental retardation, seizures, hypertonicity with hyperactive reflexes, cranial nerve involvement with strabismus, facial weakness, and dysphagia. Hepatosplenomegaly and bone lesions.
- Farber lipogranulomatosis: onset from infancy to 4 months of age. Swollen, painful joints with subcutaneous nodules over affected joints and pressure points. Progressive aphonia, swallowing, and feeding difficulties due to laryngeal involvement. Lower motor neuron involvement, which manifests as hypotonia and muscular atrophy. Psychomotor development variable from severe involvement to normal intelligence. Some patients exhibit hepatomegaly.
- Krabbe or globoid cell leukodystrophy: onset 3 to 6 months of age with psychomotor delay, tonic seizures, progressive motor impairment with hypertonicity. Deafness and blindness are common. Peripheral neuropathy detected. CSF protein increased. Clinical symptoms restricted to nervous system.
- Metachromatic leukodystrophy (MLD): late infantile form with onset at age 1 to 2 years, with progressive ataxia, hypotonia, and diminished deep tendon reflexes. Progressive optic atrophy and spastic quadriparesis. Slowing of conduction velocities of peripheral nerve. CSF protein increased.

LABORATORY PROCEDURES

See Special Tests, below.

IMAGING STUDIES

Neuroimaging studies may reveal nonspecific changes such as atrophy.

SPECIAL TESTS

Diagnosis is made by enzymatic assay of the specific enzyme in leukocytes, skin fibroblasts, and in some cases, serum.

- GM_2: hexosaminidase A deficiency
- Sandhoff: hexosaminidase A and B deficiency
- GM_1: β-galactosidase deficiency
- Fabry: α-galactosidase A (ceramide trihexosidase) deficiency
- Niemann-Pick type A: sphingomyelinase deficiency
- Niemann-Pick type C/D: defective cellular esterification of exogenously derived cholesterol
- Gaucher: glucocerebrosidase deficiency
- Farber: ceramidase deficiency
- Krabbe: galactocerebrosidase deficiency
- Metachromatic leukodystrophy: arylsulfatase A deficiency

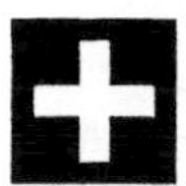

Management

GENERAL MEASURES

N/A

SURGICAL MEASURES

N/A

SYMPTOMATIC TREATMENT

- Carbamazepine or phenytoin, occasionally in combination with amitriptyline, is used to treat the painful neuropathy in patients with Fabry disease.
- Kidney transplant in patients with Fabry disease is successful in most cases.
- Joint replacement and splenectomy in patients with Gaucher type 1 may improve quality of life.
- Bone marrow transplant for treatment of Niemann-Pick type C and Gaucher type 3 may decrease visceral storage.

ADJUNCTIVE TREATMENT

The indication for physical therapy should be assessed on an individual basis.

ADMISSION/DISCHARGE CRITERIA

Patients are usually admitted for evaluation and treatment of the neurologic and respiratory complications of their disorder.

Medications

DRUG(S) OF CHOICE

Enzyme replacement therapy (ERT) with macrophage-targeted glucocerebrosidase (Ceredase) for patients with Gaucher type 1 and type 3 effectively reverses the systemic manifestations of the disease. ERT in patients with Gaucher type 3 can stabilize or slightly improve CNS disease. There are no specific treatments for the other disorders.

ALTERNATIVE DRUGS

N/A

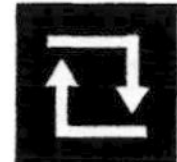

Follow-Up

PATIENT MONITORING

Patient follow-up is guided by the predicted course and potential complications of the disease.

EXPECTED COURSE AND PROGNOSIS

- GM_2 and Sandhoff: vegetative state rapidly ensues with death by 2 to 4 years of age.
- GM_1: death ensues a few years after onset of the disease.
- Fabry: death usually occurs from renal failure, cardiovascular involvement, or cerebrovascular disease. Average age at death is 41 years.
- Niemann-Pick type A: death occurs by 2 to 3 years of age.
- Niemann-Pick type C: indolent downhill course with death in adolescence.
- Niemann-Pick type D: death in adolescence to more prolonged survival.
- Gaucher (infantile): death in infancy.
- Farber: death in late infancy or early childhood.
- Krabbe: death in infancy or early childhood.
- Metachromatic leukodystrophy: death 1 to 7 years after onset.

PATIENT EDUCATION

United Leukodystrophy Foundation, 2304 Highland Dr., Sycamore, IL 60178. Phone: 800-728-5483.
National Tay-Sachs and Allied Diseases Association, 2001 Beacon St., Ste. 204, Brighton, MA 02135. Phone: 800-90-NTSAD.
National Gaucher Foundation, 11140 Rockville Pike, Ste. 350, Rockville, MD 20852-3106. Phone: 800-925-8885.

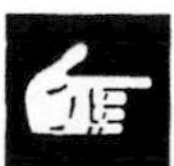

Miscellaneous

SYNONYMS

N/A

ICD-9-CM: 272.7 Sphingolipidosis (Fabry, Niemann-Pick, Gaucher); 272.8 Farber lipogranulomatosis; 330.1 Gangliosidosis (Tay-Sachs, Krabbe, MLD)

SEE ALSO: N/A

REFERENCES

- Brady RO, Patterson MC. Disorders of lipid metabolism. In: Berg BO, ed. Principles of child neurology. New York: 1996: 1091–1114.
- Greer WL, Riddell DC, Gillan TL, et al. The Nova Scotia (type D) form of Niemann-Pick disease is caused by a $G_{3097} \rightarrow T$ transversion in NPC1. Am J Hum Genet 1998;63:52.
- Peces R. Is there true recurrence of Fabry's disease in the transplanted kidney? Nephrol Dial Transplant 1996;11(3):561.
- Rapin I. Progressive genetic-metabolic diseases. In: Evans RW, Baskin DS, Yatsu FM, eds. Prognosis in neurological disease. New York: Oxford University Press, 1992;32: 677–703.
- Schiffman R, Heyes MP, Aerts JM, et al. Prospective study of neurological responses to treatment with macrophage targeted glucocerebrosidase in patients with type 3 Gaucher's disease. Ann Neurol 1997;42:613.
- Scriver CR, Beaudet AL, Sly WS, et al., eds. The metabolic and molecular bases of inherited disease, 7th ed. New York: McGraw-Hill, 1995.

Author(s): Eveline C. Traeger, MD

Spinal Cord, Neoplastic Cord Compression

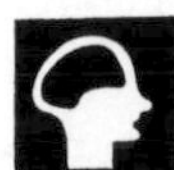

Basics

DESCRIPTION

Neoplastic epidural spinal cord compression (ESCC) is a common neurologic complication of systemic cancer that is associated with severe neurologic morbidity. ESCC develops after growth of metastatic deposits to the vertebral column (85%; usually vertebral bodies), paravertebral space (10% to 12%), or epidural space (1% to 3%). The most common primary tumors include cancers of the prostate, breast, kidney, and lung, as well as melanoma, myeloma, and lymphoma. In children, ESCC can arise from sarcoma, neuroblastoma, and lymphoma. ESCC develops most often in the thoracic spine (70%), but is also noted in the lumbar spine (20%) and cervical spine (10%). Approximately 90% of ESCC occurs in patients with an established diagnosis of cancer. In 10% of cases, ESCC is the first manifestation of the malignancy. After the onset of back pain, neurologic deterioration can occur quickly in patients with ESCC.

EPIDEMIOLOGY

Incidence/Prevalence

The estimated incidence of ESCC is 5% to 14% of all cancer patients in the U.S. This corresponds to more than 25,000 patients each year who are at risk. ESCC occurs most often in adults, with a secondary peak in children.

Race

All races and ethnic groups are equally affected.

Age

Typical presentation is between 45 and 65 years of age.

Sex

The incidence of ESCC is equal between males and females.

ETIOLOGY

- Systemic tumor cells gain access to the vertebral column and spinal bones through hematogenous spread in the majority of cases. The concentration of growth factors found in bone marrow stroma and the wide distribution of drainage of the vertebral venous plexus predispose the thoracic spine to ESCC. Other routes of access include tumors located in paravertebral and epidural sites (e.g., lymph nodes) and the Batson's vertebral venous plexus.
- Neurologic function is disrupted by ESCC through several mechanisms including an increase in the regional venous pressure, microhemorrhages within the spinal cord parenchyma, elevation of serotonin and prostaglandin E_2 levels, increased vascular permeability and secondary edema formation, elevated concentrations of glutamate and calcium, spinal cord ischemia and infarction, and regional demyelination of long tracts.
- Tumor cells most likely to metastasize to the vertebral column have a more aggressive and motile phenotype; these changes are mediated by scatter factor, autocrine motility factor, amplification of oncogenes, and mutation of metastasis-suppressor genes (e.g., *nm23*).

Genetics

ESCC is a sporadic process without any specific genetic influence.

RISK FACTORS

The only risk factor for ESCC is widespread aggressive disease from a systemic malignancy, especially from primaries of the lung, breast, and prostate.

PREGNANCY

Pregnancy does not affect the clinical behavior of ESCC.

ASSOCIATED CONDITIONS

Include other common general and neurologic complications of cancer patients such as infection and sepsis, metabolic encephalopathy, carcinomatous meningitis, and brain metastasis.

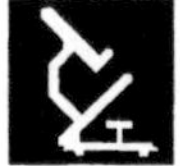

Diagnosis

DIFFERENTIAL DIAGNOSIS

Includes other diseases that can involve the vertebral column and spinal cord, such as herniated disc, degenerative joint disease, epidural abscess, spinal osteomyelitis, primary spinal cord tumor, intramedullary metastasis, leptomeningeal tumor, spondylolisthesis, spinal stenosis, and facet syndrome.

SIGNS AND SYMPTOMS

- Back pain is a common symptom with an annual incidence of 5% and a lifetime prevalence of 60% to 90% in the general population. Most back pain is benign and self-limited; in cancer patients, the presenting symptoms of ESCC are mild at first, then progressively worse. The initial symptom is always pain (95%), which can develop anywhere, but usually in the thoracic spine. The pain is regional and often associated with a radicular component (e.g., down an arm, around the ribs). Several weeks after the onset of pain other symptoms develop, including extremity weakness (75%; usually the legs), autonomic dysfunction (60%; urinary retention, urinary and/or bowel incontinence), sensory alterations (50%) of the lower extremities such as ascending numbness and paresthesias, and gait disturbance.
- The general physical examination often reveals localized pain to percussion over the involved vertebral bodies (usually thoracic). The neurologic examination usually demonstrates leg weakness; early on, the weakness is mild and may involve only the iliopsoas and hamstring muscle groups. Later in the course a myelopathy develops, with upper motor neuron pattern weakness, spasticity, Babinski's sign, and exaggerated reflexes. ESCC of the lumbar region affects the cauda equina and produces a lower motor neuron syndrome (hypotonia, areflexia, muscle atrophy, fasciculations). Sensory loss is mild initially, with distal decrement to vibration and proprioception; with advanced disease, a level develops below the ESCC, characterized by loss of light touch and pinprick sensation.

LABORATORY PROCEDURES

Patients with a history of fever require a white blood cell count, blood cultures, and sedimentation rate to rule out epidural abscess, discitis, and osteomyelitis.

IMAGING STUDIES

Spine x-rays can identify an abnormality of the involved region in 85% to 90% of cases. The most common lesions are vertebral body erosion and collapse, subluxation, and pedicle erosion. MRI of the spine, with and without gadolinium contrast, is the most sensitive imaging test ($\geq$90%). Axial, coronal, and midsagittal enhanced images should be obtained. MRI can easily demonstrate epidural or paravertebral masses and any associated ESCC. The degree of cord displacement is clearly revealed, along with cord damage, as shown by high signal within the parenchyma. Nonmalignant lesions are clearly delineated (e.g., herniated disc, degenerative spine disease). CT and myelography are not as sensitive as MRI and are not required if MRI is available.

SPECIAL TESTS

N/A

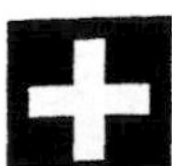

Management

GENERAL MEASURES

Should include symptomatic treatment and consultation by radiation oncology and neurosurgery for treatment evaluation. ESCC is a medical emergency and requires rapid treatment.

SURGICAL MEASURES

Surgical intervention is appropriate for carefully selected patients with ESCC. It should be considered for patients with acute deterioration of neurologic function at presentation, if there is progressive neurologic dysfunction during radiotherapy (RT), an unknown primary tumor, evidence for spinal instability, bone involvement with ESCC, and if the involved tumor is known to be radioresistant (e.g., renal). The anterior surgical approach is preferred (i.e., vertebral body resection) in most patients, since it removes the bulk of the tumor and directly decompresses the spinal cord. Spinal stability is better following the anterior approach than the posterior approach (i.e., laminectomy).

SYMPTOMATIC TREATMENT

Consists of high-dose intravenous dexamethasone and pain control. Pain is often severe and may need treatment before imaging can be performed. Definitive treatment (surgery and/or RT) should begin within 24 hours after the initiation of dexamethasone.

ADJUNCTIVE TREATMENT

- Conventional RT is the mainstay of treatment of ESCC in most patients. The recommended dose is 30 Gy in 10 daily fractions over 2 weeks. The radiation port should include two vertebral bodies above and below the region of compression. RT is also usually necessary after surgical decompression of ESCC. Many patients improve during RT (30% to 50% with increase in leg strength and/or ambulation).
- Chemotherapy has a limited role in most patients with ESCC. In some cases, it can be used as adjunctive therapy in addition to surgical resection or RT. Chemotherapy should be considered first-line treatment for ESCC only from Hodgkin's lymphoma, germ cell tumors, or neuroblastoma, which are very chemosensitive tumors and respond rapidly.

ADMISSION/DISCHARGE CRITERIA

Admission is for initial diagnosis and treatment of ESCC. Readmission may occur for patients with recurrent or progressive spinal disease.

Medications

DRUG(S) OF CHOICE

Intravenous dexamethasone is always necessary as initial treatment of ESCC, to reduce edema and swelling of the spinal cord. Recommended initial dosing consists of a load of 20 to 100 mg, followed by maintenance doses of 2 to 24 mg q6h. Dexamethasone often improves pain and neurologic function. Narcotic analgesics are usually necessary for adequate amelioration of pain.

Contraindications

Patients on chemotherapy must meet appropriate hematologic parameters before proceeding with the next cycle; WBC >2.0, hemoglobin >10.0, and platelets >100,000.

Precautions

All patients should be on an H2 blocking drug while receiving chronic dexamethasone.

ALTERNATIVE DRUGS

N/A

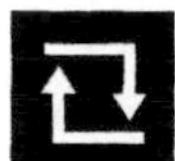

Follow-Up

PATIENT MONITORING

Patients are followed with assessment of neurologic function and spinal MRI every 3 to 6 months.

EXPECTED COURSE AND PROGNOSIS

- ESCC is a severe complication of cancer that requires emergent treatment. In ESCC patients who are ambulatory at the start of treatment, 80% remain so after therapy; only 45% of paraparetic patients and 5% to 10% of paraplegic patients are ambulatory after treatment. Nonambulatory patients have reduced survival due to medical complications such as pneumonia, decubitus ulcers, urinary infections, and septic episodes.
- The most important factor for improved prognosis is preservation of gait and neurologic function at the onset of treatment. Factors related to poor prognosis include very rapid onset of compression and neurologic deficit, duration of paraplegia of greater than 24 hours, and presence of autonomic dysfunction at the time of diagnosis.

PATIENT EDUCATION

University of Washington-ESCC: *www.stat.washington.edu/TALARIA/LS2.3.2.html*
ESCC Patient/Family Resources: *uasom-dl.slis.ua.edu/patientinfo/orthopedics/back/spinal-cord-compression*
University of Michigan-ESCC: *www.cancer.med.umich.edu/learn/bonespinalcord.htm*

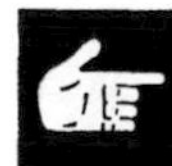

Miscellaneous

SYNONYMS

Epidural spinal cord compression, metastatic spinal cord compression

ICD-9-CM: 198.4 Secondary malignant neoplasm of other parts of CNS; 336.3 Myelopathy-other diseases classified elsewhere; 336.9 Unspecified disease of the spinal cord

SEE ALSO: N/A

REFERENCES

- Byrne TN. Spinal cord compression from epidural metastases. N Engl J Med 1992;327:614–619.
- Lada R, Kaminski H, Ruff RL. Metastatic spinal cord compression. In: Vecht CJ, ed. Handbook of clinical neurology, vol 25 (69): neuro-oncology, part III. Amsterdam: Elsevier Science, 1997:167–189.
- Loblaw DA, Laperriere NJ. Emergency treatment of malignant extradural spinal cord compression: an evidence-based guideline. J Clin Oncol 1998;16: 1613–1624.
- Newton HB: Brain tumors and other neuro-oncological emergencies. In: Shah SM, Kelly KM, eds. Emergency neurology: principles and practice. Cambridge: Cambridge University Press, 1999:326–341.
- Newton HB Neurologic complications of systemic cancer. Am Fam Physician 1999; 59:878–886.

Author(s): Herbert B. Newton, MD

Spinal Cord Syndromes, Acute

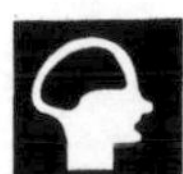

Basics

DESCRIPTION

Acute spinal cord syndromes are neurologic emergencies and may result in permanent loss of function. Examples include complete or incomplete transection of the spinal cord from trauma, injury due to infarction, hemorrhage or disc herniation, and acute spinal cord injury secondary to hyperflexion or hyperextension of the spine in the elderly. Spinal cord compression due to tumor may present acutely. Acute spinal cord syndromes are important to recognize early because prognosis is directly related to the speed and accuracy of diagnosis and subsequent treatment.

EPIDEMIOLOGY

Incidence/Prevalence

The precise incidence is unknown, but this entity is frequently seen in trauma centers and in those that deal with cancer patients.

ETIOLOGY

- Compression due to various mass lesions
- Ischemia due to atherosclerosis, embolic disease, hypercoagulable states or vasculitis

RISK FACTORS

Recent trauma, underlying cancer, coagulopathies, drug abuse, cervical spondylosis, and infection.

PREGNANCY

N/A

ASSOCIATED CONDITIONS

Include cancer and cervical spondylosis.

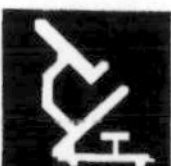

Diagnosis

DIFFERENTIAL DIAGNOSIS

Diagnosis must be made early through a combination of accurate history, directed physical and neurologic exam, and imaging studies. The differential diagnosis to consider when collecting the history and physical exam data can be lengthy, but the mnemonic VIBRATED SPASMS (adapted from Wagner and Jagoda, 1997) is helpful for both acute (A) and chronic (C) spinal cord syndromes:

- **V**ascular (A/C)
- **I**nfectious, idiopathic (A/C)
- **B**$_{12}$ deficiency (C)
- **R**adiation (C)
- **A**myotrophic lateral sclerosis (C)
- **T**umor (A/C), trauma (A), toxic-metabolic (A)
- **E**pidural abscess, electricity (A)
- **D**evelopmental, hereditary (C)
- **S**pondylosis (A/C)
- **P**araneoplastic (C)
- **A**rachnoiditis (A/C)
- **S**yringomyelia (C)
- **M**yelitis (A), multiple sclerosis (A/C)
- **S**ystemic disorders (A/C)

SIGNS AND SYMPTOMS

Symptoms

Patients may give "red flags" in the history that raise the suspicion of acute spinal cord dysfunction. Examples include numbness below a certain level, back pain, hesitancy or incontinence of bladder and bowel functions, and weakness in the lower extremities, especially in such activities as climbing stairs and walking.

Signs

Physical exam findings that raise suspicion and assist in the diagnosis of acute spinal cord syndrome include objective muscle weakness in upper and/or lower extremities, loss of reflexes in affected limbs, sensory level to pin and light touch, loss of vibration and position sense below a certain level, limited range of motion of the spine, change in gait, and loss of sphincter tone. Obvious signs of spasticity (hyperreflexia, clonus, increased tone) usually develop late, and cannot be depended on to make a diagnosis of an acute spinal cord syndrome.

LABORATORY PROCEDURES

Laboratory studies are important especially if cancer is suspected and should include serum CBC, calcium, and PSA; serum protein electrophoresis (SPEP) and urine protein electrophoresis (UPEP) are helpful for a suspected gammopathy.

IMAGING STUDIES

The most helpful imaging study is MRI, which noninvasively images spinal cord tumors, disc protrusions, epidural abscess and hematoma, and intrinsic cord lesions. In patients with epidural metastases plain x-ray films show bony abnormalities approximately 80% of the time. Myelography is usually reserved for cases where more precise imaging of nerve root elements is needed, or where MRI cannot be used (e.g., patients with pacemakers, etc.).

SPECIAL TESTS

Special tests may include bone scan if cancer is suspected. Lumbar puncture is usually not helpful in acute spinal cord dysfunction, but may be very useful in chronic syndromes. Lumbar puncture usually shows a lymphocytic pleocytosis in patients with transverse myelitis, aiding in diagnosis.

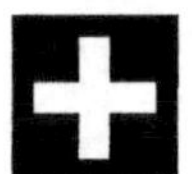

Management

GENERAL MEASURES

- Management depends on etiology. An etiology of tumor is treated with radiation therapy if the tumor is radiosensitive and with decompression if it is not. Blood dyscrasias are treated with coagulation factor replacement or platelet transfusions. Patients at bed rest require prophylactic anticoagulation to reduce the risk of venous thrombosis or pulmonary embolism.
- Medications may be required for acute pain management and spasticity. Careful attention to bladder function is important. Patients frequently require an indwelling catheter due to acute urinary retention. Bowel function is also frequently impaired, and may require laxatives, enemas, and monitoring.

SURGICAL MEASURES

Epidural spinal cord compression due to hematoma is treated with surgical decompression as soon as possible. Epidural abscesses or infections are treated with surgical drainage and IV antibiotics as appropriate. Occasionally acute disc herniations require decompression. Surgical instability of the spine requires stabilization.

SYMPTOMATIC TREATMENT

As above.

ADJUNCTIVE TREATMENT

As above.

ADMISSION/DISCHARGE CRITERIA

Suspicion of spinal cord dysfunction is reason for the immediate admission of the patient. Following treatment, discharge to a rehabilitation facility is common.

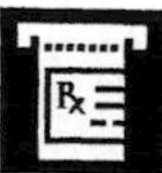

Medications

DRUG(S) OF CHOICE

The common use of high-dose IV methylprednisolone in acute spinal cord injury is now controversial. Antibiotics are used in cases of infection or abscess and cancers are treated appropriately with chemotherapy. Deep venous thrombosis prophylaxis should be instituted in all appropriate patients. Medications for pain management, bowel function, and relief of anxiety are all useful.

Contraindications

Known acute hypersensitivity to medications.

Precautions

Glucose monitoring if corticosteroids are used in spinal cord injury especially for diabetics.

ALTERNATIVE DRUGS

N/A

Follow-Up

PATIENT MONITORING

Careful follow-up of these patients is indicated and depends on the diagnosis. For example, a patient whose tumor was the cause of spinal cord compression is at risk for other metastases at other locations.

EXPECTED COURSE AND PROGNOSIS

This depends on the etiology and severity of neurologic injury. In general, patients with milder deficits, shorter time to decompression of cord compression, younger age, and better general medical status have a better prognosis.

PATIENT EDUCATION

Patients should understand the nature of spinal cord injury, the relationship between their clinical symptoms and the cord injury, the nature of treatments and rehabilitation, and options for care. In rehabilitation they should become acquainted with assistive devices, bowel and bladder regimens, vocational opportunities, etc.

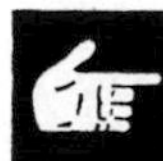

Miscellaneous

SYNONYMS

N/A

ICD-9-CM: 336.9 Spinal cord compression

SEE ALSO: N/A

REFERENCES

- Arce D, Sass P. Recognizing spinal cord emergencies. Am Fam Physician 2001;64:4.
- Daw HA, Markman M. Epidural spinal cord compression in cancer patients: diagnosis and management. Cleve Clin J Med 2000;67:7.
- Hurlbert RJ. Methylprednisolone for acute spinal cord injury; an inappropriate standard of care. J Neurosurg 2000;93:1.
- Schiff D, Batchelor T, Wen P. Neurologic emergencies in cancer patients. Neurol Clin North Am 1998;16:2.
- Wagner R, Jagoda A. Spinal cord syndromes. Emerg Med Clin North Am 1997;15:3.
- Weiner H, Levitt L, Rae-Grant A. Spinal cord compression. In: Neurology for the house officer. Baltimore: Lippincott Williams & Wilkins, 1999:43–48.

Author(s): Lawrence P. Levitt, MD; Stacy Statler, PA-C

Spinal Cord Syndromes, Chronic

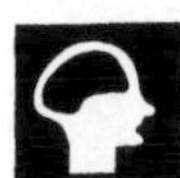

Basics

DESCRIPTION

Chronic spinal cord syndromes are common, particularly in the elderly. They are characterized by progressive spasticity, gait disorders, paresthesias, and bowel and bladder dysfunction. Chronic spinal cord syndromes are recognized by a basic understanding of spinal cord anatomy combined with how a careful history, examination, and laboratory studies fit with various disease processes that affect the cord. A basic understanding of primary motor and sensory tracts is necessary. Thus, for example, amyotrophic lateral sclerosis (ALS) affects motor tracts but spares sensation. Combined system disease due to vitamin B_{12} deficiency affects both the posterior and lateral tracts producing characteristic symptoms and signs.

EPIDEMIOLOGY

Incidence/Prevalence

Precise incidence is not known.

ETIOLOGY

See Risk Factors.

RISK FACTORS

Include cervical spinal degeneration, HIV infection (AIDS myelopathy), malnutrition (B_{12} deficiency), cervical spondylosis (causing myelopathy), trauma (causing syringomyelia), toxin exposure, systemic infection (epidural abscess), radiation (myelopathy), and multiple sclerosis (MS). There are various familial syndromes of chronic spinal cord disease (familial spastic paraparesis, spinocerebellar degenerations, adrenomyeloneuropathy, etc.).

PREGNANCY

N/A

ASSOCIATED CONDITIONS

Include underlying cancer, cervical spondylosis, vasculitis, systemic infections, toxins (e.g., nitrous oxide, which may precipitate a syndrome related to subacute combined degeneration).

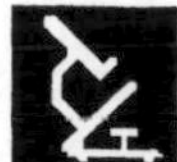

Diagnosis

DIFFERENTIAL DIAGNOSIS

As with acute syndromes, diagnosis depends on combining accurate history, physical and neurologic examinations, and imaging studies. The mnemonic VIBRATED SPASMS (adapted from Wagner and Jagoda, 1997) is useful (see Spinal Cord Syndromes, Acute).

SIGNS AND SYMPTOMS

Symptoms

Paresthesias (numbness, tingling) in limbs and trunk; limb weakness; change in urine or bowel function (either more or less frequent); incontinence; back pain; and root distribution pain, which may encircle the trunk. Patients usually complain most of a progressive gait disorder characterized by leg stiffness, with urgency of urination and constipation. In patients with cervical spine disease, weakness, dysesthetic sensation, and stiffness may be noticed in the hands. Neck or back pain may be present. Symptoms suggesting cranial nerve injury (diplopia, dysarthria, facial numbness, or weakness) are absent.

Signs

Loss of pin sensation below a certain level; "sweat" level; weakness in upper or lower extremities or both sparing the face; increased muscle tone; tenderness over the spine; hyperreflexia; up-going toes; absent abdominal reflexes; loss of anal sphincter tone; and distended bladder. Often patients have a stiff-legged gait and may hyperextend their knees. If there is cervical root injury, a combination of wasting and reflex loss in the arms (due to cervical root injury) and spasticity in the legs may occur. This must be differentiated from ALS, in which there are no sensory signs, but upper and lower motor neuron signs are present. In suspected familial syndromes, search for high arches (present in some spinocerebellar syndromes), and consider examining family members who might be affected subclinically.

LABORATORY PROCEDURES

B_{12} level in suspected combined systems disease; CSF examination for MS: pleocytosis, elevated protein, oligoclonal bands; pleocytosis in myelitis; elevated protein in arachnoiditis. In familial syndromes, more specialized tests may be useful (for example, very long chain fatty acids in adrenomyeloneuropathy).

IMAGING STUDIES

MRI of spinal cord and brain in MS; MRI of the spinal cord for syrinx, epidural, subdural or intramedullary tumor, infarcts, and for evidence of myelitis and arteriovenous malformations (AVMs) x-rays show bony abnormalities in developmental and hereditary disorders and in atlantoaxial dislocations.

SPECIAL TESTS

Rarely spinal cord angiography may be necessary for dural AV fistulas or spinal cord AVMs. This study should be performed in specialized centers due to risk of permanent spinal cord injury.

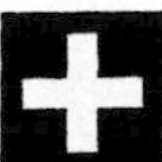

Management

GENERAL MEASURES

Measures that are applicable to all patients with chronic spinal cord conditions include provision of therapy aimed at stretching and strengthening the affected muscles; avoiding decubitus ulcers in severely affected patients; provision of adequate bowel and bladder care; and attention to issues of rehabilitation including assistive devices, wheelchairs, transfer aids, and other appropriate support.

SURGICAL MEASURES

Surgery may be used in cases where there is spinal cord compression and alternative therapies cannot be used. Particularly patients with relatively rapidly progressive syndromes should be considered for surgery early, as accrued spinal cord deficits may not improve even after decompression.

SYMPTOMATIC TREATMENT

Medications for spasticity are useful in this population. Baclofen (Lioresal) or tizanidine (Zanaflex) are commonly used to relieve this symptom. Side effects of Lioresal include fatigue and leg weakness, particularly at higher doses. Side effects of tizanidine include fatigue, hypotension, and occasionally altered liver function tests. Occasionally very spastic muscles may require treatment with botulinum toxin or implantation of an intrathecal pump for Lioresal infusion near the spinal cord.

ADJUNCTIVE TREATMENT

Consider deep vein thrombosis (DVT) prophylaxis as necessary.

Medications

DRUG(S) OF CHOICE

Medical management of chronic spinal cord syndromes depends on the cause. In patients with MS, for example, intravenous steroids are often used to treat individual attacks. To prevent attacks and the progression of disease, subcutaneous or intramuscular immunomodulating therapies (β-interferon 1-a IM, β-interferon 1-a SC, β-interferon 1-b, and glatiramer acetate) and in some cases chemotherapy such as mitoxantrone or methotrexate may be given. For spinal cord compression due to malignancy, decompression, radiation therapy, and/or chemotherapy are used depending on the type of cancer. For compression due to abscess, drainage is done and antibiotics are given. For spondylitic myelopathy, decompression may be performed. Vitamin B_{12}-deficient patients need replacement, orally or IM. For ALS patients, consider riluzole. Unfortunately, some causes, such as radiation-induced myelopathy have no specific treatments.

ALTERNATIVE DRUGS

N/A

Follow-Up

PATIENT MONITORING

Depends on the diagnosis. For example, patients with MS often require routine or frequent follow-up visits.

EXPECTED COURSE AND PROGNOSIS

Depends on the etiology of the spinal cord syndrome.

PATIENT EDUCATION

Patients should be educated generally about the effect of chronic spinal cord injury on sensory and motor function, bowel and bladder activity, and gait. The specific cause and its prognosis should be discussed with the patients. If there are specific societies with information for the etiology, the patient should be made aware of these (for example, the ALS and MS societies).

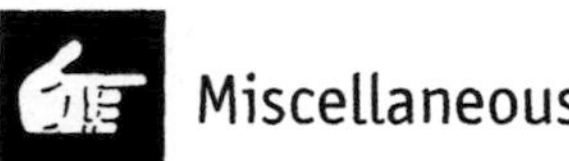

Miscellaneous

SYNONYMS

Chronic myelopathy
Chronic spastic paraparesis

ICD-9-CM: 336.9 Myelopathy, unspecified

SEE ALSO: SPINAL CORD SYNDROMES, ACUTE; MULTIPLE SCLEROSIS; VITAMIN B_{12} DEFICIENCY; SPINAL CORD, NEOPLASTIC CORD COMPRESSION

REFERENCES

- Daw H, Markman M. Epidural spinal cord compression in cancer patients: diagnosis and management. Cleve Clin J Med 2000;67:7–12.
- Mackin G. Optimizing care of patients with ALS. Postgrad Med 1999;105:4–8.
- Rolak L. Multiple sclerosis treatment 2001. Neurol Clin 2001;19:1–19.
- Wagner R, Jagoda A. Spinal cord syndromes. Emerg Med Clin North Am 1997;15:3–15.
- Weiner H, Levitt L, Rae-Grant A. Spinal cord compression. In: Neurology for the house officer. Baltimore: Lippincott Williams & Wilkins, 1999:43–48

Author(s): Lawrence P. Levitt, MD; Stacy Statler, PA-C

Spinal Cord Tumor, Astrocytoma

Basics

DESCRIPTION

Spinal cord astrocytomas (SCAs) are intradural, intramedullary tumors that arise from the gray or white matter of the spinal cord and can affect patients of all ages. They occur most commonly in the cervical and upper thoracic region, but can develop anywhere in the cord. Although most SCAs are low grade, they are all very infiltrative and typically span four to six spinal cord segments at diagnosis.

EPIDEMIOLOGY

Incidence/Prevalence

Spinal cord tumors (SCTs) are relatively uncommon, representing only 0.5% of newly diagnosed tumors in adults. SCAs comprise 6% to 8% of all primary SCTs, approximately 30% of all intramedullary SCTs, and only 3% to 4% of all CNS astrocytomas. They are more common in children, comprising 35% to 60% of all pediatric SCTs, and representing the most common type of intramedullary SCTs.

Race

All races and ethnic groups affected; Caucasians are affected more commonly than blacks, Latinos, and Asians.

Age

Typical presentation is between 25 and 40 years, but can occur at any age. A secondary peak occurs in the pediatric years.

Sex

Males have a higher incidence than females: 4:1.

ETIOLOGY

- The World Health Organization (WHO) classifies astrocytomas of the spinal cord similarly to those of the brain: pilocytic astrocytoma as grade I (50%), fibrillary astrocytoma as grade II (22%), anaplastic astrocytoma (AA; 20%) as grade III, and glioblastoma multiforme (GBM; 8%) as grade IV.
- SCAs are mainly low grade (i.e., grade I, II; LGA). High-grade tumors are less common. The tumors are derived from transformed astrocytes. Pathologic evaluation of LGA reveals mild to moderate cellularity without anaplasia or severe nuclear atypia, minimal mitotic activity and endothelial proliferation, no necrosis, and frequent staining for glial fibrillary acidic protein. High-grade tumors have high cellularity, cellular and nuclear atypia, moderate to high mitotic rate, endothelial proliferation, and necrosis (in GBM).
- Molecular genetic studies of LGA reveal frequent allelic deletions of chromosome 17p, often with loss or mutation of the tumor suppressor gene, *p53*. Amplification of oncogenes (e.g., *MDM2, CDK2, gli*) and deletion of tumor suppressors genes (e.g., *p16*, retinoblastoma) may be present in some tumors.

Genetics

Astrocytomas of the spinal cord are usually sporadic tumors, but can occur in association with neurofibromatosis type 1 (NF-1).

RISK FACTORS

Risk factors for spinal astrocytomas remain unclear, but may be similar to astrocytomas of the intracranial cavity. These include spinal radiation ($\geq$10 Gy), breast cancer, regional trauma, and NF-1.

PREGNANCY

Pregnancy does not affect the clinical behavior of spinal astrocytomas.

ASSOCIATED CONDITIONS

N/A

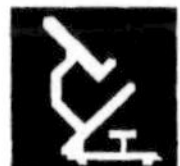

Diagnosis

DIFFERENTIAL DIAGNOSIS

Includes other intramedullary enhancing spinal masses such as ependymoma, metastasis, and abscess. Other disorders that can have a similar neurologic presentation are syringomyelia, multiple sclerosis, transverse myelitis, herniated disc, amyotrophic lateral sclerosis, and vitamin B_{12} deficiency.

SIGNS AND SYMPTOMS

- SCAs are often slow-growing tumors, with an insidious onset of symptoms. The time to diagnosis is typically prolonged (i.e., 6 to 10 months in high-grade SCAs, 5 to 7 years in low-grade SCAs). The presentation varies with tumor location, rate of growth, and amount of edema and compression of regional spinal cord. The most common early symptom (70% to 80%) is slowly progressive localized back and/or radicular pain. Weakness of the lower extremities and gait dysfunction are the next most common symptoms. Sensory symptoms occur next and consist of paresthesias and dysesthesias. Central cord pain syndromes of the legs can develop in some patients. Scoliosis may be noted in children. Dysfunction of bowel and bladder is a late symptom.
- Common neurologic signs include evidence for myelopathy, with weakness and spasticity of the legs and/or arms, reflex asymmetry, loss of abdominal reflexes, Babinski signs, sensory loss, and sphincter dysfunction. Patients with cervical SCA may demonstrate lower motor neuron signs and atrophy of the upper extremities, due to destruction of anterior horn cells.

LABORATORY PROCEDURES

N/A

IMAGING STUDIES

MRI, with and without gadolinium contrast, is the most critical diagnostic test; axial, coronal, and midsagittal enhanced images should be obtained. MRI is more sensitive than CT for intramedullary spinal cord tumors. On T1 images, the tumor is usually hypointense or isointense compared to normal spinal cord and causes diffuse multisegmental enlargement. On T2 images it is hyperintense. Spinal astrocytomas have mild to moderate enhancement after administration of gadolinium. Regions of cyst, peritumoral edema, and areas of hemorrhage may be noted. CT demonstrates a hypodense enlargement of the spinal cord with variable enhancement and edema. Hydrocephalus can be noted in a small percentage of patients.

SPECIAL TESTS

Intraoperative neurophysiologic monitoring with evoked potentials may be helpful during surgical resection to maximize tumor removal and minimize neurologic morbidity. Ultrasound may be helpful for the surgeon to accurately localize the tumor before myelotomy and removal.

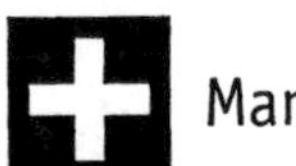

Management

GENERAL MEASURES

Include symptomatic treatment and physical therapy.

SURGICAL MEASURES

Surgical resection is required for biopsy of diagnostic tissue and maximal tumor removal, while minimizing surgical neurologic morbidity. Many low-grade SCAs can be completely resected with modern microneurosurgical techniques if a cleavage plane is discerned. Infiltrative low-grade tumors and most high-grade SCAs will allow only a subtotal resection. Ideal surgical candidates have intact or almost normal gait and neurologic function.

SYMPTOMATIC TREATMENT

Consists of corticosteroids to control symptoms of spinal cord edema and pain control caused by compression of the spinal meninges and other neurovascular structures.

ADJUNCTIVE TREATMENT

- Radiation therapy (RT) should be considered for all adult patients with an SCA, even those of low grade that have undergone an apparently complete resection. All patients with residual tumor or high-grade histology require involved field RT. The recommended doses are 50 to 55 Gy over 6 weeks using 180 to 200 cGy/d fractions. Children with completely resected pilocytic SCAs (WHO grade I) can be followed without RT. Patients with high-grade SCAs that disseminate to the neuraxis may benefit from palliative RT.
- Chemotherapy has a limited role in the treatment of SCAs. It should be considered for patients who cannot undergo surgical resection and for tumors that recur despite surgery and/or RT. Drugs to consider have only modest activity and are the same as those used for astrocytic tumors of the brain; they include nitrosoureas (BCNU, CCNU), PCV (procarbazine, CCNU, vincristine), etoposide, cyclophosphamide, carboplatin, and temozolomide. Intrathecal chemotherapy with methotrexate or cytarabine should be considered for patients with high-grade SCAs that develop leptomeningeal metastases.

ADMISSION/DISCHARGE CRITERIA

Admission is generally reserved for presurgical evaluation and biopsy/resection. Patients can be admitted with progressive spinal neurologic dysfunction from tumor growth or leptomeningeal dissemination. Intravenous dexamethasone may be helpful to reduce spinal cord edema and control pain; new treatment may be necessary (e.g., RT, chemotherapy).

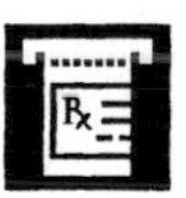

Medications

DRUG(S) OF CHOICE

Dexamethasone (2 to 8 mg/d) may be of benefit to reduce spinal cord edema and often improves pain; it may also relieve transient symptoms of pressure and swelling after RT. Narcotic analgesics may be necessary to control severe pain prior to surgery and/or RT.

Contraindications

None

Precautions

All patients should be on an H2 blocking drug while receiving chronic dexamethasone.

ALTERNATIVE DRUGS

N/A

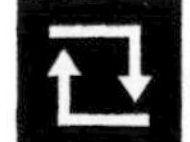

Follow-Up

PATIENT MONITORING

Patients are followed with serial MRI scans and assessment of neurologic function every 3 to 6 months.

EXPECTED COURSE AND PROGNOSIS

- The 5-year survival rate for patients with low-grade SCA after complete resection, with or without RT, is 70% to 80%. After incomplete removal plus RT the survival is lower, with a 5-year rate of 50% to 65%. The prognosis for patients with high-grade SCA is poor, with typical overall survival ranging from 6 to 12 months.
- Factors that improve the prognosis for survival are young age, low-grade histology, relatively intact neurologic function before and after surgery, and complete resection; factors that worsen the prognosis include high-grade histology, older age, significant neurologic dysfunction with poor performance status, and incomplete removal of tumor.

PATIENT EDUCATION

Index—spinal cord astrocytomas:
www.cdickmanmd.com/diseases/inda/inda018.htm
Spinal cord tumor—astrocytoma, benign:
www.medhelp.org/forums/neuro/archive/2276.html
Spine and Nerve Center at MGH/Harvard:
neurosurgery.mgh.harvard.edu/Inkspine.htm

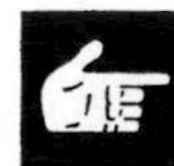

Miscellaneous

SYNONYMS

N/A

ICD-9-CM: 192.2 Malignant neoplasm of spinal cord; 225.3 Benign neoplasm of spinal cord

SEE ALSO: N/A

REFERENCES

- Fehlings MG, Rao SC. Spinal cord and spinal column tumors. In: Bernstein M, Berger MS, eds. Neuro-oncology. The essentials. New York, Thieme Medical Publishers, 2000:445–454.
- Findlay G. Intrinsic spinal cord tumours. In: Vecht CJ, ed. Handbook of clinical neurology, vol 24 (68): neuro-oncology, part II. Amsterdam: Elsevier Science, 1997:497–510.
- Houten JK, Cooper PR. Spinal cord astrocytomas: presentation, management and outcome. J Neuro-Oncol 2000;47: 219–224.
- Jallo GI, Danish S, Velasquez L, et al. Intramedullary low-grade astrocytomas: long-term outcome following radical surgery. J Neuro-Oncol 2001;53:61–66.
- Newton HB, Newton CL, Gatens C, et al. Spinal cord tumors. Review of etiology, diagnosis, and multidisciplinary approach to treatment. Cancer Pract 1995;3: 207–218.
- Sandler HM, Papadopoulos SM, Thornton AF, et al. Spinal cord astrocytomas: results of therapy. Neurosurg 1992;30:490–493.

Author(s): Herbert B. Newton, MD

Spinal Cord Tumor, Ependymoma

Basics

DESCRIPTION

Spinal cord ependymomas (SCEs) are intradural tumors that arise from the ependymal lining cells of the central canal of the spinal cord, affecting patients of all ages. They occur most often in the extramedullary portions of the lumbar spine (60%; cauda equina and filum terminale). In 40% of patients, the tumor is intramedullary and develops within the spinal cord parenchyma. The cervical and upper thoracic cords are the most common (65% to 70%) locations for intramedullary SCEs. Most SCEs are low grade, with less infiltrative capacity than astrocytic tumors. At diagnosis, most SCEs span one to two spinal cord segments.

EPIDEMIOLOGY

Incidence/Prevalence

Spinal cord tumors (SCTs) are relatively uncommon, representing only 0.5% of newly diagnosed tumors in adults. SCEs comprise 12% to 15% of all primary SCTs, approximately 50% to 60% of all intramedullary SCTs, and 30% to 35% of all CNS ependymomas. They are less common in children, comprising 12% to 15% of all pediatric SCT.

Race

All races and ethnic groups affected; Caucasians are affected more commonly than blacks, Latinos, and Asians.

Age

Typical presentation is between 35 and 50 years, but can occur at any age; a secondary peak occurs in the pediatric years.

Sex

Males have a higher incidence than females: 2:1.

ETIOLOGY

- The World Health Organization (WHO) classifies ependymomas of the spinal cord similar to those of the brain. Myxopapillary tumors are classified as WHO grade I and are the most common type of SCEs to arise in the cauda equina and filum terminale. Typical ependymomas are classified as WHO grade II. Anaplastic or malignant ependymomas correspond to WHO grade III.
- SCEs are mainly low grade, and although they are not encapsulated, they are typically well demarcated from surrounding neural tissues. Infiltration of spinal cord or nerve roots is uncommon. Typical histologic features include moderate cellularity, monotonous nuclear morphology, ependymal rosettes, perivascular pseudorosettes, rare or absent mitoses, and very infrequent areas of necrosis; foci of calcification, hemorrhage, and myxoid degeneration may be noted. High-grade tumors are more cellular and have frequent nuclear atypia, mitoses, and regions of necrosis.
- Cytogenetic studies reveal frequent abnormalities of chromosome 22 (30%), including monosomy, deletions, and translocations; less common abnormalities affect chromosomes 9q, 10, 17p, and 13. Molecular studies suggest that amplification of oncogenes (e.g., *MDM2*) and mutation of tumor suppressor genes (e.g., *NF-2*) are involved in transformation of SCEs.

Genetics

SCEs are usually sporadic tumors, but can occur in association with neurofibromatosis type 2 (NF-2).

RISK FACTORS

Risk factors for SCEs remain unclear, but may be similar to ependymomas of the intracranial cavity. These include spinal radiation ($\geq$10 Gy), and NF-2.

PREGNANCY

Pregnancy does not affect the clinical behavior of SCE.

ASSOCIATED CONDITIONS

N/A

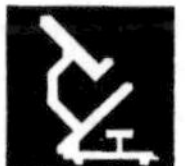

Diagnosis

DIFFERENTIAL DIAGNOSIS

Includes other intramedullary and extramedullary enhancing spinal masses such as astrocytoma, metastasis, and abscess. Other disorders that can have a similar neurologic presentation are syringomyelia, multiple sclerosis, transverse myelitis, herniated disk, and vitamin B_{12} deficiency.

SIGNS AND SYMPTOMS

- SCEs are usually slow-growing tumors, with an insidious onset of symptoms. The time to diagnosis is typically prolonged (i.e., 3 to 5 years). The presentation varies with tumor location, rate of growth, and amount of edema and compression of regional neural structures. Tumors that arise in the lumbar region typically present with low-back pain, with or without sciatica, lower extremity sensory dysfunction (e.g., numbness, paresthesias), bowel and bladder incontinence, and lower extremity weakness. Intramedullary SCEs have a different presentation, with milder, more diffuse back pain, sensory complaints that usually manifest as dysesthesias, and less severe lower extremity weakness and bowel and bladder dysfunction.
- The most common neurologic sign is mild lower extremity weakness. However, it is different between intramedullary and extramedullary SCEs. Intramedullary tumors develop weakness as a late sign and have an upper motor neuron pattern (i.e., spasticity, hyperactive reflexes, Babinski sign). Extramedullary tumors develop weakness earlier and have a lower motor neuron pattern (i.e., flaccidity, hypoactive or absent reflexes, flexor plantar responses). Other frequent signs include sensory loss, sphincter dysfunction, gait disturbance, and loss of abdominal reflexes.

LABORATORY PROCEDURES

CSF analysis and evaluation of cytology are diagnostic (in addition to cranial and/or spinal MRI) for those rare SCEs (high grade, myxopapillary) that disseminate to the leptomeninges.

IMAGING STUDIES

MRI, with and without gadolinium contrast, is the most critical diagnostic test; axial, coronal, and midsagittal enhanced images should be obtained. MRI is more sensitive than CT for intramedullary and extramedullary spinal cord tumors. On T1 images, the tumor is usually hypointense or isointense compared to normal spinal cord and causes a well-demarcated, multisegmental enlargement of the cord or a mass in the cauda equina. On T2 images the mass is hyperintense. SCEs have mild to moderate enhancement after administration of gadolinium. Regions of cyst occur frequently in intramedullary SCEs (50% to 55%; even cranial-caudal distribution). Peritumoral edema may be noted. CT demonstrates a hypodense enlargement of the spinal cord or a mass in the lumbar region with mild enhancement and edema.

SPECIAL TESTS

Intraoperative neurophysiologic monitoring with evoked potentials may be helpful during surgical resection to maximize tumor removal and minimize neurological morbidity. Ultrasound may be helpful for the surgeon to accurately localize the tumor before myelotomy and resection.

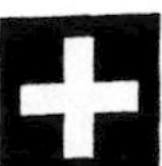

Management

GENERAL MEASURES

Include symptomatic treatment and physical therapy.

SURGICAL MEASURES

Surgical resection with gross-total removal is the treatment of choice for all SCEs. Even intramedullary tumors can be totally removed in most cases, since a clear cleavage plane is often present. Infiltrative low-grade and all high-grade intramedullary tumors will allow only a subtotal resection. Some myxopapillary SCEs of the lumbar region cannot be totally excised due to adherence to, or envelopment of, surrounding nerve roots and vascular structures. Ideal surgical candidates have intact or almost normal gait and neurologic function.

SYMPTOMATIC TREATMENT

Consists of corticosteroids to control symptoms of spinal cord edema and pain control caused by compression of nerve roots, spinal meninges, and other neurovascular structures.

ADJUNCTIVE TREATMENT

- Radiation therapy (RT) should not be considered for SCEs of low grade that have undergone a complete resection. Similarly, RT should be held in patients with extensive subtotal resection until evidence of tumor progression. All patients with high-grade histology require involved field RT. The recommended doses are 45 to 50 Gy over 6 weeks using 180 to 200 cGy/d fractions. Patients with high-grade tumors that disseminate to the neuraxis may benefit from palliative RT.
- Chemotherapy has a limited role in the treatment of SCEs. It should be considered for patients with incompletely resected tumors and tumors that progress despite RT. Drugs to consider only have modest activity and are the same as those used for ependymomas of the brain. They include PCV (procarbazine, CCNU, vincristine), etoposide, cyclophosphamide, cisplatin, carboplatin, and temozolomide.

ADMISSION/DISCHARGE CRITERIA

Admission is generally reserved for presurgical evaluation and resection. Patients can be admitted with progressive spinal neurologic dysfunction from tumor growth. Intravenous dexamethasone may be helpful to reduce spinal cord edema and control pain. New treatments may be necessary (e.g., RT, chemotherapy).

Medications

DRUG(S) OF CHOICE

Dexamethasone (2 to 8 mg/d) may be of benefit to reduce spinal cord edema and often improves pain; it may also relieve transient symptoms of pressure and swelling after surgery or RT; narcotic analgesics may be necessary to control severe pain prior to surgery and/or RT.

Contraindications

None

Precautions

All patients should be on an H2 blocking drug while receiving chronic dexamethasone.

ALTERNATIVE DRUGS

N/A

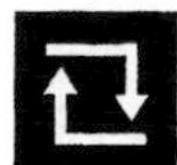

Follow-Up

PATIENT MONITORING

Patients are followed with serial MRI scans and assessment of neurologic function every 6 to 12 months. Patients on chemotherapy may require more frequent assessments.

EXPECTED COURSE AND PROGNOSIS

- The 5- and 10-year survival rates for patients with low-grade SCEs after complete resection (without RT) are 75% to 90% and 65% to 70%, respectively. After incomplete removal plus RT the survival is lower. The prognosis for patients with high-grade SCEs is poor, with typical overall survival ranging from 12 to 18 months.
- The most important prognostic factor is degree of surgical resection. Factors that improve the prognosis for survival and quality of life are complete surgical resection, relatively intact neurologic function before and after surgery, and typical low-grade histology. Factors that worsen the prognosis include incomplete removal of tumor, high-grade histology, significant neurologic dysfunction with poor performance status, and tumor location within the conus medullaris.

PATIENT EDUCATION

Spine and Nerve Center at MGH/Harvard: *neurosurgery.mgh.harvard.edu/Inkspine.htm*
University Southern California Neurosurgery: *www.uscneurosurgery.com/glossary/m/meningioma/htm*

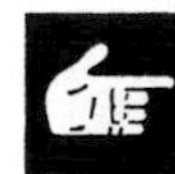

Miscellaneous

SYNONYMS

N/A

ICD-9-CM: 192.2 Malignant neoplasm of spinal cord; 225.3 Benign neoplasm of spinal cord

SEE ALSO: N/A

REFERENCES

- Chang UK, Choe WJ, Chung SK, et al. Surgical outcome and prognostic factors of spinal intramedullary ependymomas in adults. J Neuro-Oncol 2002;57:133–139.
- Epstein FJ, Farmer JP, Freed D. Adult intramedullary spinal cord ependymomas: the result of surgery in 38 patients. J Neurosurg 1993;79:204–209.
- Fehlings MG, Rao SC. Spinal cord and spinal column tumors. In: Bernstein M, Berger MS, eds. Neuro-oncology. The essentials. New York: Thieme Medical Publishers, 2000:445–454.
- Findlay G. Intrinsic spinal cord tumours. In: Vecht CJ, ed. Handbook of clinical neurology, vol 24 (68): neuro-oncology, part II. Amsterdam: Elsevier Science, 1997:497–510.
- Newton HB, Newton CL, Gatens C, et al. Spinal cord tumors. Review of etiology, diagnosis, and multidisciplinary approach to treatment. Cancer Pract 1995;3: 207–218.
- Schwartz TH, McCormick PC. Intramedullary ependymomas: clinical presentation, surgical treatment strategies and prognosis. J Neuro-Oncol 2000;47: 211–218.

Author(s): Herbert B. Newton, MD

Spinal Cord Tumor, Meningioma

Basics

DESCRIPTION

Spinal meningiomas are intradural, extramedullary tumors that arise from the meninges of the spinal neuraxis. They are slow-growing, encapsulated masses that can develop in any location that has continuity with the meninges. The distribution within the spine is as follows: thoracic (75% to 85%), cervical (15% to 20%), and lumbar (2% to 4%); 10% of spinal meningiomas can extend outside of the dura into the paraspinal soft tissues and bone.

EPIDEMIOLOGY

Incidence/Prevalence

Spinal cord tumors are relatively uncommon, representing only 0.5% of newly diagnosed tumors in adults. Meningiomas comprise 20% to 25% of all primary spinal cord tumors in patients over 20 years of age and are extremely rare in children. The estimated incidence of spinal meningiomas is less than 0.18 to 0.23 cases per 100,000 people per year.

Race

All races and ethnic groups are equally affected.

Age

The typical presentation is between 45 to 65 years of age.

Sex

Females have a higher incidence than males: 4:1.

ETIOLOGY

- The World Health Organization (WHO) grades typical low-grade meningiomas (e.g., syncytial, transitional) as WHO grade I, intermediate tumors (e.g., atypical, clear cell) as WHO grade II, and malignant tumors (e.g., anaplastic) as WHO grade III. The vast majority of spinal meningiomas are WHO grade I.
- The cells of origin of meningiomas are transformed arachnoidal cap cells from the outer layer of the spinal arachnoid membrane. Typical meningiomas of the spine are low-grade and demonstrate uniform sheets of spindle-shaped cells, minimal cellular and nuclear atypia, whorl formation, psammoma bodies, and no evidence of mitotic activity or brain infiltration; higher-grade tumors reveal higher cellularity, more prominent nucleoli, high mitotic activity, necrosis, and tissue invasion.
- Molecular genetic studies reveal frequent deletions of chromosomes 22q and 1p. The *NF2* gene (located at 22q12.3) is mutated in up to 60% of meningiomas, with dysfunction of the merlin protein. The majority of meningiomas are positive for estrogen and progesterone receptors. Other receptors of importance include the epidermal growth factor (EGF) and platelet-derived growth factor (PDGF) receptors, both of which stimulate secretion of vascular endothelial growth factor. The ras signaling pathway is activated via stimulation by EGF and PDGF.

Genetics

Meningiomas of the spine are usually sporadic tumors; in rare cases they can be familial.

RISK FACTORS

Risk factors for spinal meningiomas remain unclear, but may be similar to meningiomas of the intracranial cavity; these include spinal radiation ($\geq$10 Gy), breast cancer, regional trauma, and rare familial clusters.

PREGNANCY

In some women, pregnancy can accelerate the growth and increase the clinical symptoms of spinal meningiomas. This is rare compared to cranial meningiomas.

ASSOCIATED CONDITIONS

N/A

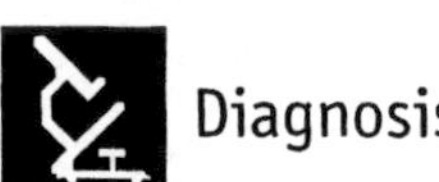

Diagnosis

DIFFERENTIAL DIAGNOSIS

Includes other extraaxial enhancing spinal masses such as schwannoma, metastasis, and abscess. Other disorders that can have a similar neurologic presentation are syringomyelia, multiple sclerosis, transverse myelitis, herniated disc, and vitamin B_{12} deficiency.

SIGNS AND SYMPTOMS

- Meningiomas are slow-growing tumors, with an insidious onset of symptoms. The time to diagnosis is typically prolonged (i.e., 12 to 24 months). The presentation varies with tumor location, rate of growth, and amount of compression of nearby nerve roots and spinal cord. The most common early symptom is pain, which occurs in 42% to 50% of patients. With tumor enlargement pain becomes more prominent, effecting 65% to 85% of patients by the time of initial admission. The pain can be localized and/or radicular (i.e., down an extremity, around the thorax). Leg weakness occurs in 35% to 50% of patients, and is also progressive. Sensory abnormalities develop in 22% to 25% of patients and include paresthesias, numbness, or hot and cold sensations; disturbances of bowel and bladder function can arise in later stages.
- Common neurologic signs include motor weakness (usually of the legs) in 90% to 95% of patients, reflex asymmetry and spasticity of the lower extremities, sensory loss of the extremities (65% to 70%), and sphincter abnormalities (25%). Frank myelopathy can be noted in more advanced patients with spinal cord compression. Up to one third of patients are nonambulatory due to leg weakness and/or pain.

LABORATORY PROCEDURES

Although typically unnecessary with MRI, CSF evaluation usually demonstrates an elevated protein. The WBC is frequently normal; a mild pleocytosis may occur in some cases.

IMAGING STUDIES

MRI, with and without gadolinium contrast, is the most critical diagnostic test. Axial, coronal, and midsagittal enhanced images should be obtained. MRI is more sensitive than CT for tumors of the spinal column. On T1 images, the tumor is usually isointense to spinal cord, while on T2 images it is hyperintense. Spinal meningiomas enhance densely after administration of gadolinium. MRI usually demonstrates a site of dural attachment or a dural tail. The displacement of nerve roots and/or the spinal cord is well delineated by MRI. Meningiomas can cause hyperostotic changes in bones of the spinal column, but less commonly than in the intracranial cavity.

SPECIAL TESTS

Angiography is performed in selected patients to assess vascular anatomy and collateral blood supply prior to surgery. It may also be useful as a prelude to presurgical embolization (to minimize intraoperative bleeding).

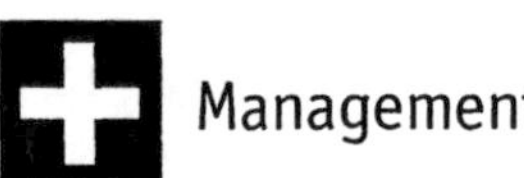

Management

GENERAL MEASURES

In certain patient cohorts, spinal meningiomas are followed conservatively after diagnosis, including those with poor health, elderly patients with small lesions or who are reluctant to proceed to surgery, and patients with small tumors that do not correlate with symptoms. Observation should include an enhanced MRI every 4 to 6 months to monitor for growth. Tumors may remain quiescent if they are stable during the initial observation period. Conservative approaches are unjustified in symptomatic patients and most young patients, especially if growth potential is demonstrated.

SURGICAL MEASURES

Surgical resection is the treatment of choice for most symptomatic patients. The surgical approach varies depending on the location of the tumor. Complete surgical extirpation is the goal whenever possible. Subtotal removal is recommended for tumors intimately associated with spinal nerves and/or vessels. After removal of the tumor, involved bone and dural attachments should also be resected with a wide margin. Dural defects should be repaired with grafts.

SYMPTOMATIC TREATMENT

Consists of corticosteroids to control symptoms of spinal cord compression and pain control due to irritation or compression of nerve roots and other neurovascular structures.

ADJUNCTIVE TREATMENT

- Patients do not require irradiation after complete surgical resection. Conventional external beam radiotherapy (RT) may be of benefit for those infrequent patients with large symptomatic tumors after subtotal removal, for recurrent or progressive tumors that cannot be approached surgically, and for those rare patients with malignant pathology (WHO grade III). It remains unclear whether or not RT provides a survival advantage for patients with spinal meningiomas after subtotal removal or at recurrence, since no clinical trial data have been published. Recommended RT doses are 50 to 55 Gy over 6 weeks, with 180 to 200 cGy per day fractions.
- Chemotherapy has a very limited role in the treatment of spinal meningiomas. It should be considered for patients who cannot undergo surgical resection and for tumors that recur despite surgery and/or RT. Drugs with modest activity in phase II trials against intracranial meningioma could be considered and include mifepristone (RU-486; antagonist to progesterone receptors) and hydroxyurea (induces apoptosis in meningioma cells). Chemotherapy usually induces tumor stabilization; shrinkage is uncommon.

ADMISSION/DISCHARGE CRITERIA

Admission is generally reserved for presurgical evaluation (including angiography in some patients) and surgical resection. Patients with severe spinal cord compression might benefit from admission for intravenous dexamethasone.

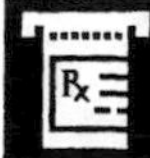

Medications

DRUG(S) OF CHOICE

Dexamethasone (2–8 mg/d) may be of benefit to reduce edema and swelling for patients with spinal cord compression; it may also improve transient symptoms of pressure and swelling after RT; analgesics may be necessary prior to surgery and/or RT.

Contraindications

None

Precautions

All patients should be on an H2 blocking drug while receiving chronic dexamethasone.

ALTERNATIVE DRUGS

N/A

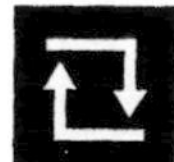

Follow-Up

PATIENT MONITORING

Patients are followed with serial MRI scans and assessment of neurologic function every 6 to 12 months.

EXPECTED COURSE AND PROGNOSIS

- The complete resection rate in most series is 85% to 95%, using preoperative MRI planning and modern microsurgical techniques. Approximately 90% of patients have functional improvement after surgery. Symptomatic patients with neurologic deficits can often improve dramatically after surgery releases pressure on nerve roots and the spinal cord. Tumor recurrence or progression occurs in 3.5% to 7% of patients after complete surgical resection.
- Factors that increase the probability for recurrence include incomplete removal of tumor and all dural attachments, invasion of bone, soft tumor consistency, extradural extension, and malignant histology.

PATIENT EDUCATION

Braintumors.com: *www.braintumors.com*
National Brain Tumor Foundation: *www.braintumor.org*
American Brain Tumor Association: *www.abta.org*
The Brain Tumor Society: *www.tbts.org*
Spine and Nerve Center at MGH/Harvard: *neurosurgery.mgh.harvard.edu/Inkspine.htm*
University Southern California Neurosurgery: *www.uscneurosurgery.com/glossary/m/meningioma/htm*

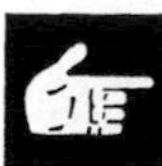

Miscellaneous

SYNONYMS

N/A

ICD-9-CM: 225.4 Benign neoplasm of spinal meninges

SEE ALSO: N/A

REFERENCES

- Fehlings MG, Rao SC. Spinal cord and spinal column tumors. In: Bernstein M, Berger MS, eds. Neuro-oncology. The essentials. New York: Thieme Medical Publishers, 2000:445–454.
- Harkey HL, Crockard HA. Spinal meningiomas: clinical features. In: Al-Mefty O, ed. Meningiomas. New York: Raven Press, 1991:593–601.
- Newton HB, Newton CL, Gatens C, et al. Spinal cord tumors. Review of etiology, diagnosis, and multidisciplinary approach to treatment. Cancer Pract 1995;3: 207–218.
- Sisti MB, Stein BM. Surgery of spinal meningiomas. In: Al-Mefty O, ed. Meningiomas. New York: Raven Press, 1991:615–620.

Author(s): Herbert B. Newton, MD

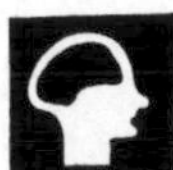

Basics

DESCRIPTION

The spinal muscular atrophies (SMAs) are a group of inherited disorders characterized by lower motor neuron weakness and wasting that is usually symmetrical and slowly progressive. This distinguishes SMA from the progressive muscular atrophy variant of amyotrophic lateral sclerosis (ALS), which is more rapidly progressive and usually fatal. SMA may show a proximal distribution of muscle weakness as in the childhood recessive SMAs due to mutations in the *SMN* gene, or be distal, as is common in dominantly inherited, later-onset forms of SMA. Both upper and lower limb predominant forms of distal dominant SMA are described.

The childhood recessive forms of SMA due to mutations in the *SMN* gene are classified according to severity. Type I (previously known as Werdnig-Hoffmann disease) presents with severe neonatal hypotonia, implying that the loss of motor neurons occurs *in utero*. Infants may require resuscitation and artificial ventilation. Most children with this type of SMA show signs before 6 months of age. By definition they do not achieve the ability to sit unaided and generally succumb to respiratory failure before the age of 2, though patients can survive longer with modern assisted ventilation. Type II SMA (intermediate SMA) is defined by onset in infancy, but affected children achieve the ability to sit but not stand unaided. The long-term outcome is dictated by the degree of respiratory muscle involvement and associated kyphoscoliosis. Approximately 60% of children survive into their 20s. Type III SMA (previously known as Kugelberg-Welander syndrome) is the mildest form, and children in this group achieve the ability to walk unaided. Onset for the majority is in infancy but rare cases of adult onset, even into the 40s and 50s, have been described. Life expectancy is normal and the probability of remaining ambulant in the long term is related to the age of onset. If this occurs before the age of 3 years, only 20% of patients are still ambulant 40 years later compared with 60% of those with an age of onset after 3 years.

EPIDEMIOLOGY

Incidence/Prevalence

Childhood-onset autosomal-recessive SMA is one of the commonest causes of neurologic disability in childhood and has an incidence of 1 in 10,000 live births. Epidemiologic data on other forms of SMA are lacking but taken together they are probably just as common.

Sex

Males and females are affected equally except for Kennedy's disease (spinobulbar muscular atrophy), which is an X-linked form of SMA.

ETIOLOGY

Sporadic cases of SMA in adulthood are not uncommon but most clinically well-characterized forms of the disease are single gene disorders. Inactivating mutations in the survival motor neuron *(SMN1)* gene cause recessive proximal SMA of childhood. Disease severity correlates with the level of residual SMN protein derived from a neighboring gene *(SMN2)*, which varies in copy number. SMN appears to function as a cofactor in ribonucleoprotein metabolism and mRNA splicing. It may have a hitherto unknown function in motor neurons. Another, much rarer, form of infantile SMA with diaphragmatic involvement is due to mutations in another putative RNA interacting protein called IGHMBP2. The X-linked form of bulbar SMA is due to polyglutamine expansion in the first exon of the androgen receptor gene. This leads to partial androgen insensitivity as well as SMA. None of the genes for dominantly inherited forms of SMA has yet been identified. However, scapuloperoneal SMA and distal lower limb SMA have both been linked to different regions of chromosome 12q, while upper limb predominant SMA has been linked to chromosome 7p.

RISK FACTORS

The SMAs are single-gene disorders with no known environmental influence on incidence or progression.

PREGNANCY

There have been occasional reports of women with mild proximal recessive SMA (type III) undergoing significant deterioration during pregnancy. Careful monitoring of respiratory function is advisable.

ASSOCIATED CONDITIONS

N/A

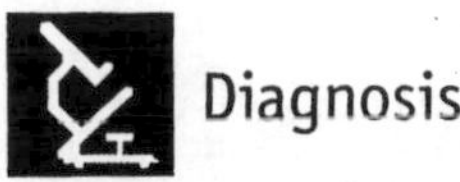

Diagnosis

DIFFERENTIAL DIAGNOSIS

- Childhood recessive SMA: a large number of genetic syndromes lead to neonatal hypotonia, which may be confused with infantile SMA. Rare "SMA-mimic" syndromes occur including cerebellar hypoplasia with anterior horn cell involvement, SMA with congenital contractures, and metabolic disorders due to mitochondrial dysfunction. The key features that distinguish SMA are the normal intellect, sparing of the diaphragm and facial muscles, and the proximal distribution of weakness. The legs are weaker than the arms and are typically held in a "frog-like" posture. SMA with respiratory distress, due to mutations in IGHMBP2, presents with distal muscle weakness and prominent diaphragmatic involvement leading to eventration of abdominal contents into the thorax.
- Other forms of SMA: a detailed description of the many inherited forms of SMA is beyond the scope of this chapter. However, as a general diagnostic point, the appearance of anterior horn cell disease in a patient of any age generally raises fears of ALS. While pure lower motor neuron forms of ALS account for about 10% of cases, these are generally rapidly progressive and many patients ultimately develop upper motor neuron signs. Furthermore, ALS generally has an asymmetrical onset compared with SMA, which is almost always symmetrical. SMA is always a slowly progressive condition, and the majority of patients with later onset, dominantly inherited, SMA have a normal life span and often remain ambulant into old age. There is a degree of confusion among specialists about whether distal SMA should be classified as a pure form of motor neuropathy (the so-called spinal form of Charcot-Marie-Tooth disease) or as an anterior horn cell disease. The identification of the various genes for these disorders will ultimately resolve this argument.
- An important consideration in the differential diagnosis of SMA is multifocal motor neuropathy with conduction block. This presents as slowly progressive asymmetrical wasting and weakness, generally upper in the upper limbs. Nerve conduction studies can be used to demonstrate conduction block (i.e., a reduction in the compound muscle action potential when the nerve is stimulated proximally compared to more distally). This condition responds to treatment with intravenous immunoglobulin.

SIGNS AND SYMPTOMS

See above.

LABORATORY PROCEDURES

Creatine kinase levels may be normal or slightly elevated in different forms of SMA. Levels greater than 1000 IU should always raise the suspicion of a primary myopathy. Neurophysiology is mandatory in cases of suspected SMA at any age as (a) this provides the primary diagnostic confirmation of an anterior horn cell disease, (b) differentiates SMA from a myopathy or peripheral neuropathy, and (c) excludes treatable conduction block neuropathy. Muscle biopsy is often performed in difficult cases where electrophysiology cannot distinguish between a myopathy and denervating disorder.

IMAGING STUDIES

While MRI scanning of muscle is under investigation as a tool for distinguishing neurogenic muscle atrophy from primary myopathies, it is unlikely to replace neurophysiology as the primary diagnostic test.

SPECIAL TESTS

Direct genetic analysis is routinely available for mutations in the *SMN* gene and the trinucleotide expansion associated with Kennedy's disease. For other rarer forms of SMA for which genes have not yet been identified, contact should be made directly with research laboratories undertaking linkage studies.

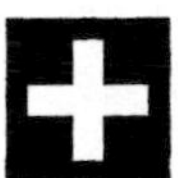

Management

GENERAL MEASURES

The prognosis for infantile SMA presenting with respiratory compromise in the first few months of life is very poor and early and sensitive discussion with the parents is required in deciding when to withdraw ventilation. All children with childhood forms of SMA should be assessed for respiratory compromise on a regular basis. Physiotherapy can limit recurrent infections. A careful assessment for the development of scoliosis is important, as this leads to preventable disability.

SURGICAL MEASURES

Patients who develop painful muscle contractures may benefit from orthopedic intervention. Patients with type II and III SMA may require spinal surgery for scoliosis.

SYMPTOMATIC TREATMENT

Noninvasive ventilation is increasingly being used in type II SMA and prolongs life. A multidisciplinary team in a specialist center is required to support patients on home ventilation.

ADJUNCTIVE TREATMENT

N/A

ADMISSION/DISCHARGE CRITERIA

N/A

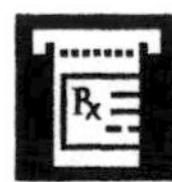

Medications

DRUG(S) OF CHOICE

N/A

ALTERNATIVE DRUGS

N/A

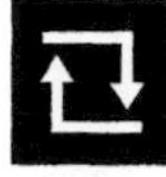

Follow-Up

PATIENT MONITORING

As with other chronic neurologic disorders, SMA is best managed by a dedicated multidisciplinary team (with physiotherapy, occupational therapy, dietetics, and respiratory care specialists) in a specialist setting. The clinical course of the different forms of SMA dictates the pattern of follow-up, but the childhood recessive forms generally require more medical supervision. The role of the neurologist in milder adult-onset forms is primarily diagnostic.

EXPECTED COURSE AND PROGNOSIS

Described above and dependent on the exact type of SMA.

PATIENT EDUCATION

A major issue is that patients are appropriately informed about the pattern of inheritance (dominant versus recessive) of their disorder so that they can make choices about family planning. Referral to a clinical geneticist is usually advisable. For recessive SMA due to mutations in the *SMN* gene, preimplantation genetic diagnosis is available in selected centers.

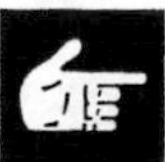

Miscellaneous

SYNONYMS

Kennedy's disease (spinobulbar muscular atrophy)
Werdnig-Hoffmann disease
Kugelberg-Welander syndrome

ICD-9-CM: 335.10 Spinal muscular atrophy, unspecified; 335.0 Werdnig-Hoffmann disease; 335.11 Kugelberg-Welander disease

SEE ALSO: N/A

REFERENCES

- Dubowitz V. Muscle disorders in childhood. Philadelphia: WB Saunders, 1995.
- Munsat T, Davies K. Spinal muscular atrophy. 32nd ENMC International Workshop. Naarden, The Netherlands, March 10–12 1995. Neuromuscul Disord 1996;6(2):125–127.
- Talbot K, Davies K. Spinal muscular atrophy. Semin Neurol 2001;21(2): 189–198.

Author(s): Kevin Talbot, MD, DPhil

Spinocerebellar Ataxias

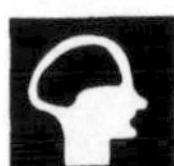

Basics

DESCRIPTION

- The inherited spinocerebellar ataxias (SCAs) represent a group of neurodegenerative diseases characterized by clinical and genetic heterogeneity. This group of disorders encompasses the autosomal dominant cerebellar ataxias (ADCAs) and autosomal recessive Friedreich's ataxia (FRDA); only the ADCAs will be discussed here. Among the ADCAs, new gene loci for mutations are being steadily identified; the corresponding clinical syndromes are labeled as SCA-1, SCA-2, SCA-3 (Machado-Joseph disease), etc. These genetically distinct disorders have overlapping clinical features that make them difficult to diagnose based on clinical features alone.

EPIDEMIOLOGY

Incidence

- 5 per 100,000

ETIOLOGY

- The genetic mutation in five of the ADCA syndromes has been shown to be expansion of an unstable stretch of CAG trinucleotide repeats within the coding region of the respective gene. In the normal population, the CAG repeats are stable; however, when expansion occurs, the number of CAG repeats reaches a threshold at which neurodegeneration occurs and clinical manifestations occur. As a group, the trinucleotide repeat disorders have several common features that are clearly demonstrated in the SCA kindreds with the CAG repeat mutation.
  - —Anticipation: Clinically, it is the occurrence of symptoms at an earlier age along with a more severe disease phenotype or more rapid progression in successive generations. Underlying clinical anticipation is the observed increasing expansion of the trinucleotide repeat sequence in successive generations through parent–child transmissions, i.e., intergenerational instability or meiotic instability.
  - —Inverse correlation between age of onset and repeat number: As repeat number increases, age of onset becomes earlier. There is also a tendency for larger repeat numbers to be associated with more severe disease phenotypes.
  - —Parenteral transmission bias: In a majority of these disorders, intergenerational instability of the repeat is largest in transmission from a father to his offspring.
- The CAG trinucleotide encodes for the amino acid glutamine. Thus, a stretch of CAG repeats results in a polyglutamine tract within the final gene product, i.e., the translated protein. It is thought that this addition to the protein results in a "gain of function" or "change of function" that leads to premature neurodegeneration.

RISK FACTORS

- Family history of ataxia, movement disorder, or gait disturbance

PREGNANCY

N/A

ASSOCIATED CONDITIONS

N/A

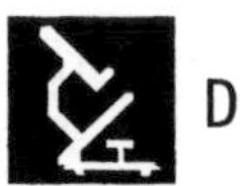

Diagnosis

DIFFERENTIAL DIAGNOSIS

- Other autosomal dominant neurodegenerative diseases:
  - —Huntington's disease; CAG repeat disease
  - —Dentatorubropallidolyusian atrophy; CAG repeat disease
  - —Gerstmann-Straussler-Scheinker disease (prion disease)
  - —Creutzfeldt-Jakob disease, ataxic form (prion disease)
- Autosomal dominant ataxias:
  - —Episodic ataxia type 1
    - -Potassium channel gene mutation chromosome 12p
    - -Associated with interictal myokymia
  - —Episodic ataxia type 2
    - -Point mutation of α subunit of calcium channel gene chromosome 19p
    - -Allelic with familial hemiplegic migraine and SCA-6 (see later)
    - -Responds to acetazolamide
- Autosomal recessive ataxias:
  - —Friedreich's ataxia; GAA repeat expansion
  - —Ataxia telangiectasia
  - —Ataxia with vitamin E deficiency
  - —Bassen-Kornzweig syndrome (abetalipoproteinemia)

SIGNS AND SYMPTOMS

- These disorders demonstrate wide clinical variability, with ataxia the predominant manifestation, in conjunction with other neurologic findings. Clinical variability is evident within a single kindred, between kindreds with the same genotype, and between kindreds with different genotypes. General features among these disorders include a wide range of onset age and anticipation.
- *SCA-1:* SCA-1 is characterized by constant features of gait and limb ataxia, dysarthria, and dysfunction of cranial nerves IX, X, and XII. The disorder will start with ataxia, usually gait ataxia being more severe than limb ataxia, and dysarthria. Pyramidal tract findings (spasticity, hyperreflexia, Babinski signs) and oculomotor findings (e.g., nystagmus, slow saccades, ophthalmoparesis) can be seen early. Only late in the disease course do the cranial nerve palsies occur, leading to dysphagia, recurrent pneumonia, and eventual death. Dystonic posturing or involuntary movements, such as choreoathetosis, also tend to appear late. Mental retardation has been seen only in juvenile-onset cases and tends to appear before any other neurologic manifestations. Anticipation is observed clinically and correlates with larger CAG expansions; larger expansions occur through paternal transmissions.
- *SCA-2:* SCA-2 is characterized by cerebellar ataxia, dysarthria, slow saccades, and peripheral neuropathy. A common initial complaint is muscular cramps at rest. Pyramidal and extrapyramidal features, optic atrophy, and dementia are infrequent features. Anticipation is observed in all kindreds, with larger CAG expansions occurring with paternal transmission.
- *SCA-3/Machado-Joseph disease:* The label of Machado-Joseph disease (MJD) arose in the 1970s in reference to families who exhibited ADCA with wide clinical diversity. However, a disorder with similar phenotypic variability had been described among families of different geographic origin, including Caucasians, the Japanese, and African Americans. It was unclear if these latter families had MJD or another dominant spinocerebellar ataxic syndrome. Subsequent work showed that all of the kindreds had the same genetic mutation, an expansion of CAG trinucleotide repeats in the ataxin-3 gene on chromosome 14. Thus, MJD and SCA-3 are the same disease because they share the same underlying genetic defect. The disorder almost always begins with cerebellar ataxia manifested as an unsteadiness of gait, followed consistently by dysarthria and ophthalmoparesis. Thereafter, a wide range of clinical features may be seen. In early-onset patients (i.e., mid-20s), pyramidal and extrapyramidal features, and facial and lingual fasciculations, are frequently present. In later-onset patients, peripheral neuropathy with weakness and amyotrophy is common. Anticipation has been observed clinically.
- *SCA-4:* This ataxic syndrome is characterized by progressive ataxia, sensory axonal neuropathy, and normal eye movements. Less common features include an extensor plantar response and distal weakness.

- *SCA-5:* Also known as "Lincoln's ataxia," SCA-5 appears to be more benign than the other SCAs, with only the cerebellum affected and brainstem structures being spared. The disease typically begins with a mild disturbance of gait, dysarthria, and incoordination of the upper extremities. Anticipation is seen in successive generations. These manifestations slowly progress over several decades and, in contrast to SCA-1, SCA-2, and SCA-3, pose no threat to shortening the patient's lifespan. This is thought to be due to the lack of brainstem involvement, with a much lower risk of recurrent aspiration pneumonia. SCA-5 is linked to chromosome 11. SCA-5 was described in a large kindred descended from the paternal grandparents of President Abraham Lincoln.
- *SCA-6:* SCA-6 is very unique among the SCAs for three reasons: (i) the function of the gene in which the CAG expansion occurs is known; (ii) the size of the CAG mutation does not change between generations within a kindred; and (iii) SCA-6 is allelic with two other autosomal dominantly inherited conditions: episodic ataxia type 2 (EA-2) and familial hemiplegic migraine (FHM). SCA-6 has been shown to be due to a CAG repeat expansion mutation within the α_{1A} subunit voltage-dependent calcium channel gene on chromosome 19p. This gene is highly expressed in Purkinje cells of the cerebellum, and the α_{1A} subunit is the pore-forming subunit of the calcium channel. The clinical features consist of a slowly progressive gait and limb ataxia, dysarthria, nystagmus, and mild vibration and position sense loss. SCA-6 has a very insidious onset, usually between the ages of 25–70 years, with a slow progression over 20–30 years. The expanded repeat in SCA-6 is stable and does not change in successive generations. Kindreds harboring a larger expansion have earlier onset. In EA-2 and FHM, different missense mutations within the same gene result in truncation of the protein. Thus, these three conditions are considered allelic channelopathies because different mutations within the same gene result in different phenotypes clinically.
- *SCA-7:* This hereditary ataxia is characterized by degeneration of retinal ganglion cells along with cerebellar degeneration and pyramidal signs. Visual complaints including visual loss, progressive photophobia, and difficulty with night vision are the initial symptoms in a majority of patients. Later in the course of the disease, other clinical manifestations appear, including ataxia, dysarthria, ophthalmoplegia, and upper motor neuron signs. Extrapyramidal features are seen occasionally. The gene for SCA-7 is on chromosome 3p and contains a stretch of CAG repeats that are expanded in affected individuals.

LABORATORY PROCEDURES

- Vitamin E level
- Peripheral smear for acanthocytes
- Lipoprotein levels
- Immunoglobulin levels
- α-Fetoprotein

IMAGING STUDIES

- Brain MRI

SPECIAL TESTS

- DNA testing is commercially available for the trinucleotide repeat disorders.

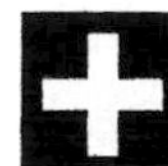

Management

GENERAL MEASURES

- Prevention of falls and aspiration pneumonia are of primary concern.

SURGICAL MEASURES

- Gastric tube placement should be considered when swallowing becomes impaired.

SYMPTOMATIC TREATMENT

- Clonazepam and valproate for associated myoclonus

ADJUNCTIVE TREATMENT

- Mobility aids for ataxia
- Physical therapy

ADMISSION/DISCHARGE CRITERIA

N/A

Medications

DRUG(S) OF CHOICE

- Medications have not proven useful in the treatment of ataxia. Most promising may be the antioxidant *N*-acetylcysteine.

ALTERNATIVE DRUGS

N/A

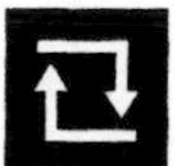

Follow-Up

PATIENT MONITORING

- Patients should be seen routinely for identification of potential complications, such as excessive falls and dysphagia.

EXPECTED COURSE AND PROGNOSIS

- All of the ADCAs are progressive disorders that typically shorten the individual's lifespan; however, variability is the rule, not the exception, in these conditions.

PATIENT EDUCATION

- National Ataxia Foundation. Website: *www.naf@mr.net*

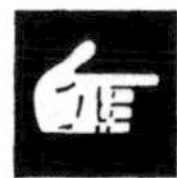

Miscellaneous

SYNONYMS

N/A

ICD-9-CM: 781.3 Ataxia; 334.2 Hereditary ataxia; 334.3 Cerebellar ataxia

SEE ALSO: FRIEDREICH'S ATAXIA

REFERENCES

- Harding AE. Clinical features and classification of inherited ataxias. Adv Neurol 1993;61:1–14.
- Hurd RW, Wilder BJ, Pippenger CE, et al. Treatment of neurodegenerative disease with N-acetylcysteine. Mov Disord 1994; 9[Suppl 1]:60.
- La Spada AR, Paulson H, Fischbeck KH. Trinucleotide repeat expansion in neurologic disease. Ann Neurol 1994;36: 814–822.
- Maciel P, Gaspar C, et al. Correlation between CAG repeat length and clinical features in Machado-Joseph Disease. Am J Hum Genet 1995;57:54–61.
- Zhuchenko O, Bailey J, Bonnen P, et al. Autosomal dominant cerebellar ataxia (SCA6) associated with small polygluta- mine expansions in the alpha 1A voltage- dependent calcium channel. Nat Genet 1997;15:62–69.

Author(s): Paul G. Wasielewski, MD

Stiff Person Syndrome

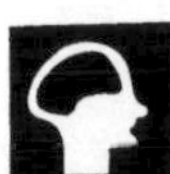

Basics

DESCRIPTION

- Stiff person syndrome (SPS) is a rare disabling disorder of motor function characterized by muscle rigidity and spasms that involve the axial and limb musculature. Continuous contraction of agonist and antagonist muscles caused by involuntary motor unit firing at rest are the hallmark clinical and electrophysiologic signs of the disorder. Except for involuntary global stiffness, the remainder of the neurologic examination is normal.

EPIDEMIOLOGY

Incidence/Prevalence

- The prevalence has not been reported, but it is clear that SPS is rare.

Race

- There is no clear racial or ethnic predisposition.

Age

- The age of onset of symptoms is usually in the fifth decade of life but ranges from the third through the seventh decade. Cases in children are rarely reported.

Sex

- The disease may be more common in women than in men.

ETIOLOGY

- The etiology of SPS is unknown; however, it is believed to be a central nervous system (CNS) disorder. Approximately 10% of patients with SPS have seizures. Drugs that enhance CNS levels of γ-aminobutyric acid (GABA), such as diazepam or valproic acid, improve patient symptoms. One theory proposes that patients with SPS have impaired cortical and spinal inhibitory GABA-nergic intraneurons. The proposed loss of this GABA-nergic input to motor neurons is thought to produce the tonic firing of motor neurons at rest and lead to their hyperactive excitation. Supportive of this theory is that up to 65% of patients with SPS have antibodies against glutamic acid decarboxylase (GAD), which is the rate-limiting enzyme for the synthesis of GABA at the GABA-nergic nerve terminals. The hypothesis is that the anti-GAD antibodies cause a functional impairment in the synthesis of GABA and therefore may play a pathogenic role in the disease. Anti-GAD antibodies have been isolated in both the serum and in the CSF of patients with SPS.
- In a subgroup of patients, SPS is a paraneoplastic disease. In these patients, the stiffness is mostly in the proximal muscles and may predate the detection of the tumor. The most common tumor detected is breast cancer.

ASSOCIATED CONDITIONS

- There are clinical and laboratory associations with autoimmune diseases such as type 1 diabetes, pernicious anemia, thyroiditis, and epilepsy. The autoimmune pathogenesis of SPS is strongly supported by the
  - —Presence of antibodies to glutamic acid decarboxylase (anti-GAD) or anti-islet cell antibodies (anti-ICA) in most patients
  - —Common presence of other autoimmune diseases or autoantibodies in SPS patients and first-degree relatives
  - —Response to immunosuppressive therapy

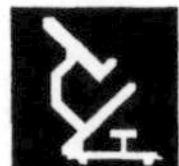

Diagnosis

DIFFERENTIAL DIAGNOSIS

- Diseases that should be differentiated from SPS include chronic tetanus, neuromyotonia, and various types of dystonia and extrapyramidal disease, all of which are easily excluded based on the neurologic examination.

SIGNS AND SYMPTOMS

- SPS is a disabling disorder that begins insidiously and progresses over months to years. Two set of symptoms characterize the disease: stiffness and spasms. Patients first develop a sensation of progressive stiffness that involves the paraspinal musculature. This stiffness manifests over time as paraspinal hypertrophy and lumbar hyperlordosis. To the examiner, the patient's muscles may feel as firm as rocks. Over months the rigidity may extend to involve the extremities. If this occurs, it is not uncommon for the rigidity to be asymmetric. A few cases of extension to the facial musculature have been reported. Superimposed on this set of symptoms, patients experience painful muscle spasms that are triggered by emotional duress, unexpected noise, or tactile stimulation. Collectively these symptoms impair a patient's ability to ambulate effectively. The gait of a patient with SPS often is described as resembling that of Frankenstein's monster. Muscle spasms superimposed on this rigid unsteady gait cause the patient to freeze or fall. The spasms vary in intensity but have been known to be so severe as to cause fractures and to bend the pins used in their repair.

LABORATORY PROCEDURES

- The presence of anti-GAD, anti-ICA, and other autoantibodies helps to support the diagnosis of SPS in a patient with the appropriate clinical presentation but is not necessary for the diagnosis. These antibodies may be isolated from the serum and CSF.

IMAGING STUDIES

- CT and MRI of the brain and spinal cord are normal in patients with SPS. However, neuroimaging is suggested because it can exclude a demyelinating process that could result in some symptoms, such as spasticity, that can mimic SPS.

SPECIAL TESTS

- EMG shows continuous activation of normal-appearing motor unit potentials in affected muscles despite attempts to relax.

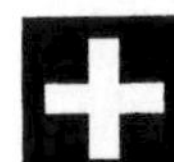

Management

GENERAL MEASURES

- Patients require a significant amount of counseling to educate them on the condition. Attention should be given to how the disorder affects their quality of life. If appropriate, psychological and social services should be offered to support patients as they cope with their disability.

SURGICAL MEASURES

N/A

SYMPTOMATIC TREATMENT

- There is no cure for SPS, but a variety of medications are available to alleviate symptoms. On the basis of the proposed pathogenesis of the disorder, two types of therapy are rationally applied: (i) drugs that enhance CNS GABA-nergic activity, and (ii) immunomodulators.

ADJUNCTIVE TREATMENT

- Behavioral medicine and biofeedback may be helpful in managing the psychological factors that can aggravate symptoms.

ADMISSION/DISCHARGE CRITERIA

- Hospitalization may be indicated for management of severe spasms, spasticity, and pain.

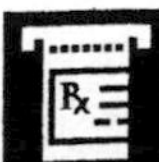

Medications

DRUG(S) OF CHOICE

- *Diazepam* was the first studied and is the most widely used medication. Many patients take 40–60 mg/day; a few take >100 mg/day. Mood changes and sedation are common and should be screened for. Although no controlled trials have been done, most patients with SPS respond to diazepam to some degree and for an extended period of time. The required doses, however, are often so high that diazepam is not easily tolerated and other agents are used as needed.
- *Vigabatrin,* which decreases GABA catabolism, and *tiagabin,* which interferes with GABA uptake, may be helpful.
- *Baclofen* increases GABA activity and thus is efficacious in reducing rigidity and spasms when administered orally/intrathecally. Intrathecal administration has the advantage of minimizing sedation side effects.
- *Corticosteroids* and *azathioprine* have been shown to be effective in treating patient symptoms. Some side effects of corticosteroid use are of particular concern in patients with SPS. IDDM is present in 30% of patients with SPS and complicates therapy, but is not an absolute contraindication. Azathioprine can be effectively used as a steroid sparing agent. Screening for leukopenia and liver dysfunction is important.

ALTERNATIVE DRUGS

- Experience with *intravenous immunoglobulin* and *plasma exchange* is limited but promising.

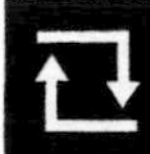

Follow-Up

PATIENT MONITORING

- Regular visits to screen for patient comfort and quality of life are important to the patient, as is routine laboratory work to screen for toxic effects of therapies such as steroids and azathioprine.

EXPECTED COURSE AND PROGNOSIS

- Patients with SPS generally have a progressive course with variable response to treatment.

PATIENT EDUCATION

- Patients can learn more about this disorder through the National Institute of Neurological Disorders and Stroke.
  Website: *www.ninds.nih.gov*

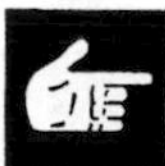

Miscellaneous

SYNONYMS

- Woltman-Moersch syndrome
- Stiff man syndrome

ICD-9-CM: 333.91 Stiff man syndrome

SEE ALSO: NA

REFERENCES

- Gerschlager W, Brown P. Effect of treatment with intravenous immunoglobulin on quality of life in patients with stiff-person syndrome. Mov Disord 2002; 17:590–593.
- Gerschlager W, Schrag A, Brown P. Quality of life in stiff person syndrome. Mov Disord 2002;17:1064–1067.
- Levy LM, Dalakas MC, Floeter MK. The stiff-person syndrome: an autoimmune disorder affecting neurotransmission of gamma-aminobutyric acid. Ann Intern Med 1999;131:522–530.
- McEvoy K. Stiff-man syndrome. In: Samuels MA, Feske SF, eds. Office practice of neurology. New York: Churchill Livingstone, 1996:691–695.

Author(s): Edward A Goldberg, MD

Sturge-Weber Syndrome

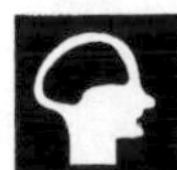

Basics

DESCRIPTION

- Sturge-Weber syndrome (SWS) is a congenital condition affecting the cephalic venous microvasculature.
- The hallmark intracranial vascular anomaly is leptomeningeal angiomatosis, which most often involves the occipital and posterior parietal lobes but can affect both cerebral hemispheres.
- An ipsilateral facial cutaneous capillary vascular malformation usually affects the upper face in a distribution consistent with the first branch of the trigeminal nerve.
- Other findings include glaucoma, buphthalmos, enlargement of the choroid plexus, and seizures.
- Hemiparesis, hemiatrophy, hemianopia, and strokelike events may occur contralateral to the cortical abnormality.
- Calcifications are noted in the external layers of the atrophic cerebral cortex underlying the angiomatosis.
- Nervous, cutaneous, and ophthalmic systems are affected.

EPIDEMIOLOGY

Incidence/Prevalence

- Incidence in the United States is unknown. An estimated 5,000 Americans are affected.

Age

- The typical patient presents at birth with facial capillary vascular malformation.
- Most children have partial seizures by age 3 years.
- Early onset of seizures does not clearly indicate a poor prognosis.

Sex

N/A

Race

N/A

ETIOLOGY

- Congenital. There is a malformation of an embryonic vascular plexus arising within the cephalic mesenchyme between the neuroectoderm and the telencephalic vesicle. Interference with vascular drainage development within these areas between weeks 5 and 8 of gestation subsequently affects the face, eye, leptomeninges, and brain.

Genetics

- Inheritance is sporadic

RISK FACTORS

N/A

PREGNANCY

N/A

ASSOCIATED CONDITIONS

- Glaucoma
- Headache
- Seizure

Diagnosis

DIFFERENTIAL DIAGNOSIS

- Facial capillary vascular malformation
  - —Isolated cutaneous malformation without accompanying glaucoma or CNS disease
- Partial Seizures
  - —Idiopathic
  - —CNS malformation (neuronal migration)
  - —Mesial temporal sclerosis
  - —Hemorrhage
  - —Tumor
  - —Other

SIGNS AND SYMPTOMS

- From 75%–90% of patients with SWS have epilepsy. Seizures probably are caused by hypoxia and microcirculatory stasis.
- From 85%–90% of patients with SWS have facial capillary vascular malformation.
- Other accompanying symptoms are vascular headaches (40%–60%), developmental delay and mental retardation (50%–75%), glaucoma (30%–70%), choroidal hemangioma (40%), hemianopia (40%–45%), and hemiparesis (25%–60%).

LABORATORY PROCEDURES

N/A

IMAGING STUDIES

- Skull x-ray film shows classic "tram-line" or "tram-track" calcifications. These may be a late finding and may not be present initially.
- Angiography demonstrates a lack of superficial cortical veins, nonfilling of the dural sinuses, and a tortuous course of veins toward the vein of Galen. Evidence of venous stasis is characteristic. Arterial distribution is normal.
- CT scan shows calcifications, brain atrophy, and ipsilateral choroid plexus enlargement.
- MRI with gadolinium enhancement shows leptomeningeal angioma.
- SPECT demonstrates decreased cortical perfusion.
- PET demonstrates hypometabolism in areas that correspond to decreased perfusion.
- EEG show electromagnetic abnormalities localized to areas underlying the leptomeningeal angiomatosis. Rarely, affected infants have infantile spasms.

SPECIAL TESTS

Pathology

- Leptomeningeal angiomatosis usually involves the occipital and posterior parietal lobes. It can affect the entire cerebral hemisphere.
- Leptomeninges appear thickened and discolored by the leptomeningeal angiomatosis.
- Enlarged choroid plexus is seen.
- Calcifications are seen in meningeal arteries, cortical and subcortical veins, and cortex underlying the leptomeningeal angiomatosis.
- Laminar cortical necrosis can accompany calcifications, suggesting ischemic damage secondary to venous stasis in leptomeninges and in the cerebral capillary bed.
- Neuronal loss and gliosis can occur.

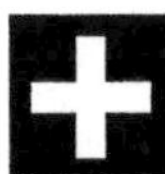

Management

GENERAL MEASURES

- Seizure control
- Symptomatic and prophylactic headache therapy
- Glaucoma treatment to reduce intraocular pressures
- Laser therapy for facial cutaneous vascular malformation
- Management of behavior and learning problems

SURGICAL MEASURES

- For patients with refractory focal seizures, surgery is an option. Procedures include focal cortical resection, hemispherectomy, corpus callosotomy, and vagal nerve stimulation.
- Surgical therapy for intractable epilepsy from SWS uses the same guiding principles as surgical therapy for epilepsy in general.
- There is no conclusive evidence that surgery in infancy is indicated in SWS.
- If glaucoma is poorly controlled by medications, then surgery may be indicated. Trabeculectomy and goniotomy are options.

SYMPTOMATIC TREATMENT

- Seizures: Antiepileptics with focal seizure efficacy and limited side effects
- Strokelike events: Aspirin to inhibit platelet aggregation
- Headaches: Combination analgesics; antimigraine therapy
- Glaucoma: β-Antagonist eye drops and carbonic anhydrase inhibitors decrease production of aqueous fluid. Adrenergic eye drops and miotic eye drops reduce intraocular pressure by promoting drainage.
- Facial cutaneous vascular malformation: Laser therapy started as soon as possible is most successful. Reports show psychological benefits of early removal.

ADJUNCTIVE TREATMENT

N/A

ADMISSION/DISCHARGE CRITERIA

N/A

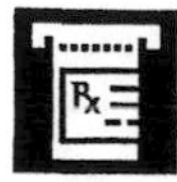

Medications

DRUG(S) OF CHOICE

- Carbamazepine (Tegretol)
- Valproic Acid (Depakote, Depacon)
- Lamotrigine (Lamictal)
- Topiramate (Topamax)
- Tiagabine (Gabitril)
- Oxcarbazepine (Trileptal)
- Aspirin

Contraindications

N/A

Precautions

N/A

ALTERNATIVE DRUGS

N/A

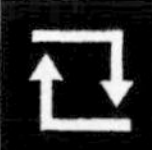

Follow-Up

PATIENT MONITORING

- Child neurologist, ophthalmologist, and dermatologist should follow children with SWS as associated problems dictate.

Possible Complications

- Status epilepticus
- Prolonged strokelike episode
- Hearing disorder
- Behavior problem
- Irretractable headaches

EXPECTED COURSE AND PROGNOSIS

- Some patients are minimally affected, if at all. Others have early-onset seizure, strokelike episodes, and neurologic deterioration. The course is too variable to predict prognosis in any patient.
- Life expectancy is thought to be normal.

PATIENT EDUCATION

- The Sturge-Weber Foundation provides patients with mentors and allows families to network and communicate about emotional and therapeutic management. It is the "first stop" for families of children with SWS. Website: *www.sturge-weber.com*
- Bodensteiner J, Roach FS, eds. Sturge-Weber syndrome. Mount Freedom, NJ: The Sturge-Weber Foundation, 1999:1-95.
- No restrictions to activity except as dictated by associated conditions. Some patients with SWS report severe headache after minor head trauma.
- No special diet is required.

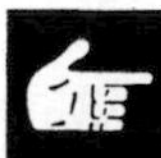

Miscellaneous

SYNONYMS

- Encephalotrigeminal angiomatosis
- Angio-encephalo-cutaneous syndrome

ICD-9-CM: 759.6 Sturge-Weber syndrome

SEE ALSO: N/A

REFERENCES

- Bodensteiner J, Roach FS, eds. Sturge-Weber syndrome. Mount Freedom, NJ: The Sturge-Weber Foundation, 1999:1–95.
- Maria BL. Current management in child neurology. Hamilton, Ontario: BC Decker, 2002.
- Maria BL, Neufeld JA, Rosainz LC, et al. High prevalence of bihemispheric structural and functional defects in Sturge-Weber Syndrome. J Child Neurol 1998;13: 595–605.
- Maria BL, Neufeld JA, Rosainz LC, et al. Central nervous system structure and function in Sturge-Weber syndrome: evidence of neurological and radiological progression. J Child Neurol 1998;13: 606–618.
- Riviello J. Sturge-Weber syndrome. E-medicine Journal, Volume 2, Number 10, October 12, 2001.

Author(s): Bernard Maria, MD, MBA; Kristin Thomas-Sohl, BA

Subclavian Steal Syndrome

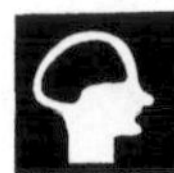

Basics

DESCRIPTION

- Subclavian steal phenomenon describes a state of retrograde vertebral artery flow in the setting of proximal arterial stenosis to the upper limb, causing rerouting of blood from the vertebral circulation. This is a relatively common phenomenon usually recognized by ultrasound. Subclavian steal syndrome refers to the rare situation where neurologic symptoms are caused by this retrograde flow. The treatment of this syndrome is not fully characterized due to its rarity. Subclavian steal phenomenon may be characterized by the territory from which blood is "stolen," or by the severity of hemodynamic disturbances. Territories are classified as vertebro-vertebral, carotid-basilar, external carotid-vertebral, or carotid-subclavian. Severity is classified as stage I: reduced antegrade vertebral flow; stage II: reversal of flow during arm reactive hyperemia testing; or stage III: permanent retrograde vertebral flow. The left vertebral is most commonly affected in this disorder (4:1 ratio).

EPIDEMIOLOGY

- The Joint Study of Extracranial Arterial Occlusion showed angiographic steal occurred in 2.5% (168/6,534) of cases in the study. Of these, only 9/168 (5.3% of angiographic cases) had neurologic symptoms. A European survey showed subclavian steal phenomenon in 324 of 25,000 patients referred for cerebrovascular Doppler ultrasound; of these, only 5% had symptoms suggestive of vertebral dysfunction.
- Males are affected more than females for atherosclerotic subclavian steal phenomenon (approximately 2:1), but females are more likely to suffer from Takayasu's disease. Older patients are more likely to have subclavian steal syndrome of atherosclerotic type; subclavian steal syndrome in Takayasu's disease usually presents in young adults.

ETIOLOGY

- Atherosclerotic vascular disease is the cause of the preponderance of cases of subclavian steal phenomenon and subclavian steal syndrome. In the Far East, there is an increased representation of Takayasu's disease causing subclavian steal syndrome, although the relative frequency is unknown. Nonarteritic causes of subclavian steal phenomenon and subclavian steal syndrome are rare (giant cell arteritis, prior vascular surgery, trauma)

RISK FACTORS

- Usual risk factors for atherosclerotic disease, including smoking, hyperlipidemia, hypertension, diabetes, cardiovascular disease, peripheral vascular disease, family history, and age

PREGNANCY

N/A

ASSOCIATED CONDITIONS

- Most patients with subclavian steal phenomenon have associated carotid circulation stenosis (in the Joint Study of Extracranial Arterial Occlusion, 80% had associated extracranial obstructions). Other atherosclerotic disorders, including cardiac and peripheral vascular diseases, are common in this patient population.

Diagnosis

DIFFERENTIAL DIAGNOSIS

- Differential includes other causes of transient neurologic dysfunction, particularly of the posterior circulation. Intracranial vertebral or basilar stenosis should be considered in this patient population. Embolic lesions from cardiac and other proximal sources may cause similar symptoms. Bickerstaff variant of migraine is characterized by vertebrobasilar symptoms that usually last minutes and are accompanied by headache. Focal seizures occasionally cause vertigo lasting seconds to minutes, representing a simple partial seizure.

SIGNS AND SYMPTOMS

- Subclavian steal syndrome is defined by the presence of vertebrobasilar symptoms in the presence of subclavian steal phenomenon, i.e., retrograde flow in the vertebral arteries precipitated by arm exercise. Symptoms may include vertigo, unsteadiness, visual blurring, and occasionally diplopia and sensory symptoms. Provoking maneuvers for symptoms include ipsilateral arm exercise and neck movement. Hemispheric symptoms have been described in subclavian steal syndrome (aphasia, unilateral field cut, hemi-motor or sensory symptoms.) Whether these symptoms are due to subclavian steal syndrome or concomitant anterior circulation disease is unclear.
- Signs of subclavian steal syndrome include weak or absent radial and ulnar pulses. Blood pressure measured in both arms may show a reduction >20 mm Hg compared to the contralateral arm. A bruit over the subclavian artery may be audible. Unless the patient is symptomatic at the time of neurologic examination, there are no neurologic signs associated with subclavian steal syndrome. Patients should be examined for evidence of peripheral vascular disease and carotid disease.

LABORATORY PROCEDURES

- There are no specific blood tests for subclavian steal syndrome.

IMAGING STUDIES

- There is no specific role for plain radiographs. Magnetic resonance angiography (MRA) may be useful for characterizing the presence of subclavian steal phenomenon. Special techniques, such as phase-contrast MRA and head and neck coils with gadolinium enhancement, may depict the presence of proximal subclavian artery stenosis or occlusion. Angiography can directly show the anatomic features of subclavian stenosis or occlusion, the presence of retrograde vertebral flow, and associated extracranial and intracranial stenoses. Angiography is attended by risks of arterial puncture and reactions associated with contrast medium.

SPECIAL TESTS

- Subclavian steal phenomenon is identified during Doppler ultrasound examination of the carotid and vertebral circulations. Findings may vary from transient decrease in ipsilateral vertebral artery midsystolic velocity (mild) to total vertebral flow (severe). Doppler ultrasound assists in documentation of other vascular lesions (internal and external carotid, contralateral vessels). Transcranial Doppler may further characterize intracranial flow dynamics in the posterior circulation.

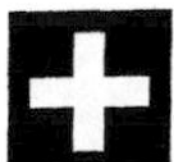

Management

GENERAL MEASURES

- Avoiding specific inciting maneuvers (e.g., arm exercise, neck position changes) may be beneficial.

SURGICAL MEASURES

- Surgical measures may be used when symptoms are severe and well defined by imaging and Doppler ultrasound techniques. Various techniques are used, including carotid-subclavian bypass and axillo-axillary bypass. Published mortality rates for these procedures vary between 0.4% and 2.5%. Transthoracic subclavian and innominate endarterectomies have high mortalities and morbidities and are no longer used.

SYMPTOMATIC TREATMENT

N/A

ADJUNCTIVE TREATMENT

- Percutaneous transluminal angioplasty (PTCA) with or without stent placement is becoming the intervention of choice for subclavian stenosis syndrome. Risks of these procedures include stroke, access site hematoma, and arterial dissection. The decision to intervene is largely dominated by the nature of the symptoms. If the symptoms are mild and not debilitating, avoiding intervention may be the treatment of choice.

ADMISSION/DISCHARGE CRITERIA

- Most patients are evaluated on an outpatient basis unless there are prolonged neurologic symptoms or the differential of TIA is being evaluated. Patients may require admission for surgical procedures or short-stay admission for PTCA with or without stent placement.

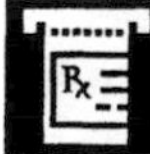

Medications

DRUG(S) OF CHOICE

- There are no specific drug approaches to subclavian steal syndrome. The appropriate use of antiplatelet agents, lipid-lowering medications, and antihypertensives are similar to that for patients with ischemic stroke or transient ischemic attack syndromes.

Contraindications

N/A

Precautions

N/A

ALTERNATIVE DRUGS

N/A

Follow-Up

PATIENT MONITORING

- Patients will require monitoring for their course, as well as progression of concomitant cerebrovascular disease. Repeated Doppler ultrasound is a safe method of monitoring for worsening of vertebral flow reversal.

EXPECTED COURSE AND PROGNOSIS

- The prognosis for subclavian steal syndrome has not been fully characterized due to its rarity. The course varies and depends on the extent of symptoms with exercise and neck movement, as well as the presence of concurrent cerebrovascular disease.

PATIENT EDUCATION

- Patients should be apprised of the pathophysiology of their symptoms, various options for therapy, treatment of risk factors, and proper notification of physicians in case of increasing symptoms.

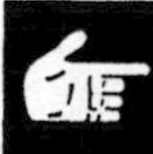

Miscellaneous

SYNONYMS

N/A

ICD-9-CM: 435.2 Subclavian steal syndrome

SEE ALSO: N/A

REFERENCES

- Bornstein NM, Norris JW. Subclavian steal: a harmless haemodynamic phenomenon? Lancet 1986;2:303–305.
- Fields WS, Lemak NA. Joint study of extracranial arterial occlusion VII. Subclavian steal. JAMA 1972;222: 1139–1143.
- Gosselin C, Walker PM. Subclavian steal syndrome: existence, clinical features, diagnosis, and management. Semin Vasc Surg 1996;9:93–97.
- Taylor CL, Selman WR, Ratcheson RA. Steal affecting the central nervous system. Neurosurgery 2002;50:679–688.

Author(s): Alexander D. Rae-Grant, MD

Sydenham's Chorea

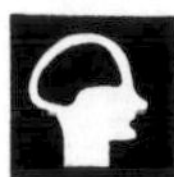

Basics

DESCRIPTION

- First described by Sydenham in 1686, Sydenham's chorea is an immune-mediated acquired chorea that occurs after streptococcal pharyngitis. It may be associated with other features of rheumatic fever (Jones criteria). Chorea refers to involuntary, forceful, random jerks that involve any part of the body. They can include abnormal movements of the respiratory muscles, producing grunts and other sounds. Chorea is present at rest and increases with voluntary movements. Chorea at rest and with posture gives rise to the appearance of a restless child who is unable to sit still. "Piano-playing" movements of fingers, when the hand is held outstretched, and the "milkmaid's grip" when grasping an object, are features of chorea. Volitional movements often are jerky, and the gait often has a lurching quality. Chorea may be accompanied by athetosis, which consists of involuntary movements that have a more writhing, sinusoidal quality.

EPIDEMIOLOGY

Incidence/Prevalence

- Most prevalent acquired chorea in childhood.
- There has been a previous decline in the incidence, with a more recent resurgence of cases.
- Occurs in 10%–20% of patients with rheumatic fever.

Age

- Seen mostly between the ages of 5 to 15 years

Sex

- Female preponderance occurring at a ratio of approximately 2:1 that becomes more evident after age 10 years.

ETIOLOGY

- It is thought that group A β-hemolytic streptococci (GABHS) trigger antistreptococcal antibodies that, by molecular mimicry, cross-react with epitopes on the basal ganglia of susceptible hosts. Genetic susceptibility is suggested by the higher than expected familial incidence of this condition. Although the nature of the relationship between antineuronal antibodies and neuropsychiatric symptoms is not yet known, one hypothesis is that when genetically vulnerable children are exposed to GABHS, antibodies are produced that mistakenly recognize cells within the basal ganglia and cause an inflammatory response. This inflammation is manifest by involuntary movements and psychiatric symptoms. Symptom expression may depend on the epitope recognized by the antineuronal antibody, extent of inflammation, chronicity of the insult, developmental stage of the child's immune system, inherited vulnerability, or a combination of these factors.

RISK FACTORS

- Family history of rheumatic fever, Sydenham's chorea, or post-streptococcal carditis appears to increase the risk of an individual developing Sydenham's chorea.

PREGNANCY

- Women who had Sydenham's chorea in childhood may rarely have a recurrence of symptoms during pregnancy.

ASSOCIATED CONDITIONS

- Rheumatic fever
- Cardiac involvement in 33.7%
- Other neurologic symptoms: Approximately 38.7% had dysarthria. Encephalopathy, with personality changes, emotional lability, disorientation, confusion and, more rarely, delirium, occurred in 10%.
- Other psychiatric symptoms: Obsessive-compulsive symptoms were seen in 82%. Other symptoms included emotional lability, irritability, distractibility, motoric hyperactivity, age-regressed behavior, nightmares, and anxiety. These symptoms may start 2–4 weeks prior to onset of chorea, peak as the motor severity does, and remit shortly after the chorea disappears.

Diagnosis

SIGNS AND SYMPTOMS

- Chorea and emotional lability appear abruptly several months after streptococcal pharyngitis. Although usually fairly abrupt in onset, symptoms may progress in severity over a few weeks and persist for months. In a retrospective study of 240 patients between 1951 and 1976 at the University of Chicago, 81% had generalized chorea and 19% had hemichorea. Duration of chorea ranged from 1–22 weeks (median 12 weeks). Eighty percent had no recurrences.
- Diagnosis is made by establishing a preceding exposure to GABHS, either by history or by elevated antistreptococcal antibody titers (ASO [antistreptolysin-O] or anti-DNAase B). However, in about 20% of cases, no clinical or serologic evidence of a preceding GABHS can be established, because the chorea can lag behind the etiologic infection by 6 months. Without documentation of an antecedent streptococcal infection, the diagnosis of Sydenham's chorea is made by excluding other causes of childhood chorea.

DIFFERENTIAL DIAGNOSIS

- Primary central nervous system vasculitis
- Systemic lupus erythematosus
- Acute encephalitis
- Toxins/drugs
- Wilson's disease
- PANDAS (pediatric autoimmune neuropsychiatric disorders after streptococcal infections)
- G_{M1} and G_{M2} gangliosidoses
- Glutaric aciduria
- Methylmalonic and propionic acidemia
- Antiphospholipid antibody syndrome
- Thyrotoxicosis

LABORATORY PROCEDURES

- Search for evidence of a previous streptococcal infection with ASO titers, anti-DNAase B titers, and a throat swab to determine whether the patient still has streptococcal colonization of the throat. Other tests should include a rheumatological screen with ESR, ANA, RF, and antiphospholipid antibodies. If there is evidence suggesting an acute primary central nervous system infection, cerebrospinal fluid analysis should be performed. When Sydenham's chorea is a consideration, a search should be undertaken for cardiac involvement with electrocardiography and echocardiography.

IMAGING STUDIES

- MRI: Analysis of cerebral MRIs of subjects with Sydenham's chorea and controls in one study demonstrated increased size of the basal ganglia in the Sydenham's chorea group. However, as a diagnostic tool in Sydenham's chorea, cerebral MRI appears to be more helpful in eliminating certain other mimickers than in confirming the diagnosis, as it may often look fairly normal in Sydenham's chorea.

SPECIAL TESTS

- SPECT scan of the brain may show hyperperfusion in the basal ganglia.

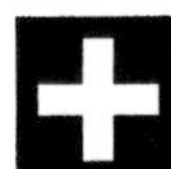

Management

GENERAL MEASURES

- Eradication of streptococcus if still present in the pharynx with antibiotics, and prevention of further infection with antibiotic prophylaxis
- Treatment of cardiac dysfunction if present
- Treatment of chorea
- Treatment of behavior/psychiatric symptoms

SURGICAL MEASURES

N/A

SYMPTOMATIC TREATMENT

- Treatment of chorea (see below). Psychiatric manifestations warrant evaluation and appropriate therapy depending on severity. Cardiac manifestations should be treated and monitored closely.

ADJUNCTIVE TREATMENT

- Measures for physical safety in patients with significant difficulties in ambulation. Difficulties in the realms of behavior, fine motor skills, and cognition should be addressed by a team consisting of the medical provider, psychology/psychiatry, educators, and physical and occupational therapists.

ADMISSION/DISCHARGE CRITERIA

- Admission for rapid evaluation and monitoring if symptoms suggest a primary central nervous system infection or if there are symptoms of cardiac dysfunction. Patients with severe chorea who are unable to ambulate may benefit from initial inpatient rehabilitation.

Medications

DRUG(S) OF CHOICE

- *Prednisone.* In one retrospective study, children treated with prednisone appeared to have a shorter course of chorea that those treated with haloperidol, valproate, or diazepam. Prednisone can cause weight gain, cushingoid appearance, mood lability, psychosis, hypertension, hyperglycemia, electrolyte imbalances, and gastritis. It can suppress the immune system, thereby decreasing the individual's ability to fight off intercurrent infections.
- *Valproate.* In a study of 18 children with Sydenham's chorea, valproate appeared to have a better efficacy than carbamazepine and haloperidol. Side effects can include an allergic skin rash, weight gain, thrombocytopenia, pancytopenia, pancreatitis, hepatic failure, and gastritis.
- *Carbamazepine.* Side effects can include liver dysfunction, an allergic skin rash, leukopenia, pancytopenia, drowsiness, ataxia, and hyponatremia.
- *Haloperidol.* Potential side effects include an acute dystonic reaction, weight gain, hyperthermia, and drug-induced dyskinesias.
- *Pimozide.* Potential side effects include those of haloperidol, with the potential for cardiac dysrhythmias.
- *Benzodiazepines.* Sedation appears to be the main side effect.

ALTERNATIVE DRUGS

N/A

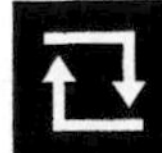

Follow-Up

PATIENT MONITORING

- Monitor response to treatment and for potential side effects of the drug used. Gradually wean medications as symptoms resolve.

EXPECTED COURSE AND PROGNOSIS

- Sydenham's chorea is considered benign and self-limiting. However, on occasion chorea can be so severe as to cause significant impairment in motor function and ambulation. Psychological manifestations may range from minimal to extremely severe. Without treatment the symptoms tend to gradually remit, but may take weeks to a year. Recurrent attacks can occur in up to 20% of cases. Usually there was only one recurrence, on average 1.8 years after the first attack. Recurrences many years after the initial attack are uncommon and suggest that late chorea may be due to reactivation by another mechanism, such as pregnancy or drugs. Patients with Sydenham's chorea may have chorea during pregnancy (chorea gravidarum) and are at higher risk for chorea induced by phenytoin or oral contraceptives.

PATIENT EDUCATION

- Compliance to antibiotic prophylaxis against further streptococcal infection should be stressed.
- Good source for patient information is the website: *www.wemove.org.*

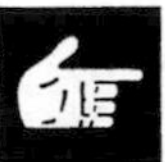

Miscellaneous

SYNONYMS

- Rheumatic chorea
- Chorea minor
- St. Vitus dance
- Encephalitis rheumatica

ICD-9-CM: 392.9 Rheumatic chorea NOS

SEE ALSO: N/A

REFERENCES

- Cardos AF, Eduardo C, Silva AP, et al. Chorea in fifty consecutive patients with rheumatic fever. Mov Disord 1997;12:701.
- Daoud AS, Zaki M, Shakir R, et al. Effectiveness of sodium valproate in the treatment of Sydenham's chorea. Neurology 1990;40:1140.
- Green L. Corticosteroids in the treatment of Sydenham's chorea. Arch Neurol 1978; 35:53.
- Moore DP. Neuropsychiatric aspects of Sydenham's chorea: a comprehensive review. J Clin Psychiatry 1996;57:407.
- Pena J, Mora E, Cardoza J, et al. Comparison of the efficacy of carbamazepine, haloperidol, and valproic acid in the treatment of children with Sydenham's chorea. Arq Neuropsiquiatr 2002;60[2-B]:374.
- Queiroz Campos Araujo AP, Padua PAB, Filho HSM. Management of rheumatic chorea. Arq Neuropsiquiatr 2002; 60[2-A]:231.
- Stollerman GH. Rheumatic fever in the 21st century. CID 2001;33:806.
- Swedo S. Sydenham's chorea. A model for childhood autoimmune neuropsychiatric disorders. JAMA 1994;272:1788.
- Swedo S, et al. Sydenham's chorea: physical and psychological symptoms of St. Vitus dance. Pediatrics 1993;91:706.

Author(s): S. Anne Joseph, MD

Syphilis, Neurologic Complications

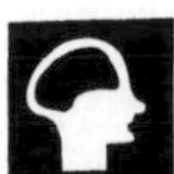

Basics

DESCRIPTION

- Syphilis is a systemic infection that can involve the central nervous system (CNS) during any stage. Neurosyphilis can produce vascular and parenchymatous disease in the cerebrum and spinal cord.

Forms of Neurosyphilis

- *Early and late asymptomatic neurosyphilis:* No clinical neurologic disease. Persistence of CSF abnormalities for >5 years after infection (late asymptomatic neurosyphilis) almost always is followed by clinical neurologic disease.
- *Acute syphilitic meningitis:* Incubation period for meningitis is <1 year. Seen most commonly in HIV-infected individuals.
- *Meningovascular syphilis:* Vascular neurosyphilis is an endarteritis that results in infarction in any vessel territory, but most commonly the middle cerebral artery distribution. Occurs 5–12 years after initial infection. Involvement often occurs with or progresses to parenchymal disease.
- *General paresis:* Meningoencephalitis associated with direct invasion of the cerebrum by *Treponema pallidum.* Develops 15–20 years after initial infection and progresses subacutely over years. Terminal if untreated.
- *Tabes dorsalis:* Parenchymatous form involves the preganglionic portion of the dorsal nerve roots and the spinal cord posterior columns. It is now rare and occurs in untreated patients after 20–25 years of latency. Neurologic damage often irreversible despite therapy.
- *Optic (neuro)syphilis:* Optic involvement takes many forms, including uveitis, retinitis, optic atrophy, perineuritis, and papillitis.
- *Gummas of the CNS:* Gummas, or granulomas, may remain asymptomatic or cause symptoms through compression of CNS meninges and/or parenchyma (extremely rare).
- *HIV and neurosyphilis:* Most common presentations in HIV-infected persons include acute syphilitic meningitis and meningovascular syphilis.

EPIDEMIOLOGY

- True incidence of neurosyphilis is unknown, but 4%–10% of patients with untreated syphilis may progress to neurosyphilis.
- There is no racial, age, or sexual predilection.

ETIOLOGY

- *T. pallidum* subspecies *pallidum* is the causative agent of syphilis. *T. pallidum* invades the CNS very early after initial infection.

RISK FACTORS

- Untreated syphilis at any stage increases the risk of progression to neurosyphilis.
- HIV infection poses a small increased risk, if any, for progression to neurosyphilis.

PREGNANCY

- Neurosyphilis should be treated at the time of diagnosis. Maternal treatment during pregnancy may prevent congenital syphilis.

ASSOCIATED CONDITIONS

N/A

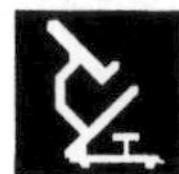

Diagnosis

DIFFERENTIAL DIAGNOSIS

- *Acute syphilitic meningitis:*
  - —Causes of lymphocytic and aseptic meningitis, including viruses
  - —Other spirochetes (e.g., *Borrelia burgdorferi*)
  - —Mycobacteria
  - —Fungi
  - —Autoimmune disease
- *Meningovascular syphilis:*
  - —Other causes of stroke syndromes, including hypertension, cerebral emboli, arteriosclerotic vascular disease, or CNS vasculitis
- *General paresis:*
  - —Tumor
  - —Subdural hematoma
  - —Cerebral arteriosclerosis
  - —Dementia
  - —Multiple sclerosis
  - —Chronic alcoholism
  - —Psychiatric disease
- *Tabes dorsalis:*
  - —Meningovascular syphilis
  - —Adie's syndrome
  - —Diabetic neuropathy (diabetic pseudotabes)
  - —Combined system disease
  - —Peripheral neuropathy
- *Optic (neuro)syphilis:*
  - —Uveitis
  - —Retinitis
  - —Perineuritis
  - —Papillitis
- *Gummas of the CNS:*
  - —Any CNS mass lesion

SIGNS AND SYMPTOMS

- Clinical presentation depends on the particular syndrome. Overlap occurs.
- *Acute syphilitic meningitis:* Symptoms may include stiff neck, confusion, or delirium; fever typically is low grade or absent. Signs may include those of elevated intracranial pressure and cranial nerve palsies. Sensorineural deafness can develops over 1–2 weeks.
- *Meningovascular syphilis:* Most common presentation is hemiparesis, aphasia, or seizures. Symptoms often preceded by premonitory headache, memory loss, or psychiatric disease lasting for weeks to months. Cord involvement may present with paraparesis or paraplegia, sensory abnormalities, urinary or fecal incontinence, or hyperreflexia.
- *General paresis:* Manifestations are variable and can mimic any neuropsychiatric disorder. Onset is insidious, with early manifestations usually psychiatric in nature. Depression is the most common early symptom. Pupillary abnormalities are common and may progress to the Argyll Robertson type (small, fixed pupils that do not react to light and mydriatics, but accommodate normally). Early neurologic features include facial tremors, intention tremors, and impaired speech. Untreated disease may progress to dementia.
- *Tabes dorsalis:* Classic presentation includes lightning pains, paresthesias, diminished deep tendon reflexes, and poor pupillary responses to light. Argyll Robertson pupils are more commonly seen than with paresis. Lightning pains are sudden paroxysms of severe stabbing pain that last for minutes. They may occur anywhere, including viscera (e.g., gastric crisis may mimic appendicitis), but most commonly affect the lower extremities. Loss of vibration sense occurs early and leads to ataxia. Cranial nerve involvement is common.
- *Gummas of the CNS:* Presentation depends on location of the granuloma and mimics a mass lesion.
- *Congenital neurosyphilis:* Presentation is highly variable, but includes optic complications, aseptic meningitis, and cranial nerve palsies.

LABORATORY PROCEDURES

- All patients with suspected neurosyphilis should receive a serum nontreponemal antibody test (i.e., Venereal Disease Research Laboratory [VDRL] or rapid plasma reagin [RPR] tests), a confirmatory treponemal antibody test (i.e., fluorescent treponemal antibody adsorbed [FTA-ABS] or microhemagglutination assay for antibody to *T. pallidum* [MHA-TP] tests), and an HIV test. In neurosyphilis, screening nontreponemal antibody test in most cases will be positive, whereas treponemal antibody test will always be positive.
- Lumbar puncture (LP) recommended when signs or symptoms of neurosyphilis are present, when there is evidence of active tertiary syphilis, with treatment failure during any stage of syphilis, and in HIV infection with latent syphilis or syphilis of unknown duration.

- The VDRL-CSF test is the standard serologic test. When reactive is diagnostic of neurosyphilis, however, negative CSF serology does *not* exclude the diagnosis.
- The CSF FTA-ABS yields more false-positive results, but some experts believe that a negative test excludes neurosyphilis.
- In neurosyphilis, CSF changes may include elevated pressure, mononuclear pleocytosis (up to 2,000 cells per mm^3), elevated protein concentration, reduced glucose, and elevated globulin levels.
- CSF findings are variable and can reflect acute disease or remain completely normal, as in the case of inactive or treated disease.
- In congenital syphilis, CSF findings in neonatal period and infancy are extremely variable.

IMAGING STUDIES

- CNS imaging is nonspecific but has a role in managing complications of syphilitic disease (e.g., hydrocephalus).
- Typical findings of vascular neurosyphilis are seen on cerebral angiography.

SPECIAL TESTS

N/A

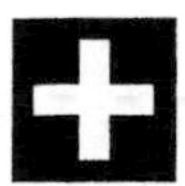

Management

GENERAL MEASURES

- The main focus of treatment for neurosyphilis is administration of appropriate antibiotics.

SURGICAL MEASURES

- Surgical intervention is required for biopsy of a suspected CNS gumma or the management of syphilitic complications (e.g., shunt placement for hydrocephalus).

SYMPTOMATIC TREATMENT

- Antiemetics, hydration, analgesics, and control of fever for those with acute syphilitic meningitis

ADJUNCTIVE TREATMENT

- Physical therapy for gait disorders
- Antiepileptic medications such as gabapentin may be tried for lancinating pains
- Antiepileptic medications if associated with seizures

ADMISSION/DISCHARGE CRITERIA

N/A

Medications

DRUG(S) OF CHOICE

- Penicillin is the only proven therapy for neurosyphilis.
- Current recommended treatment regimen is aqueous crystalline penicillin G 18–24 million units per day, administered as 3–4 million units IV every 4 hours for 10–14 days.
- Alternative regimen is procaine penicillin 2.4 million units IM per day, *plus* probenecid 500 mg PO four times per day, both for 10–14 days.
- For infants and children, recommended regimen is aqueous crystalline penicillin G 200,000–300,000 units/kg/day IV, administered as 50,000 units/kg every 4–6 hours for 10 days.

Contraindications

N/A

Precautions

- In those with confirmed penicillin allergy, skin testing and desensitization are recommended.

ALTERNATIVE DRUGS

- Other antibiotics as an alternative regimen have not been studied and their routine use is not recommended.

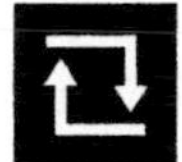

Follow-Up

PATIENT MONITORING

- Patient follow-up is critical to document clinical and serologic improvement/failure, observe for a Jarisch-Herxheimer reaction, and ensure compliance with therapy.
- Serial serum serologic evaluations (with the nontreponemal antibody test, as the treponemal antibody test will remain positive for life) should be performed every 3 months for up to 48 months (or until it normalizes).
- Serial CSF examinations should be repeated 3 months after antibiotic therapy, then every 6 months until the CSF normalizes. Once normal, CSF examination should be repeated annually for the next 2 years.
- Criteria for failure include persistence or development of clinical symptoms, elevation of serum nontreponemal antibody test titer (by two dilutions), failure of serum nontreponemal antibody test to decrease by two dilutions at 24 months, and failure of the CSF to normalize by 6 months (VDRL-CSF test may take up to 2 years to normalize).
- Failure in any form warrants retreatment with penicillin.

EXPECTED COURSE AND PROGNOSIS

- Penicillin is effective in clearing CSF abnormalities and preventing progressive clinical disease in all types of neurosyphilis.
- Antibiotic therapy cannot reverse structural damage that has already occurred.

PATIENT EDUCATION

- Syphilis is a sexually transmitted disease, so patients should be educated regarding safe sexual practices.
- Sexual contacts of patients (over the prior 12 months) should be serologically/clinically evaluated. Epidemiologic treatment is cost effective.

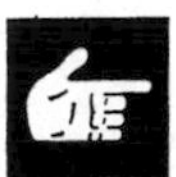

Miscellaneous

SYNONYMS

N/A

ICD-9-CM: 094 Neurosyphilis; 094.0 Tabes dorsalis; 094.1 General paresis; 094.2 Syphilitic meningitis; 094.3 Asymptomatic neurosyphilis; 094.8 Other specified neurosyphilis; 094.81 Syphilitic encephalitis; 094.82 Syphilitic parkinsonism; 094.85 Syphilitic retrobulbar neuritis; 094.87 Syphilitic ruptured cerebral aneurysm; 094.89 Other; 094.9 Neurosyphilis, unspecified

SEE ALSO: N/A

REFERENCES

- Bolan G. Syphilis in HIV infected hosts. In: Cohen PT, et al., eds. The AIDS knowledge base. Philadelphia: Lippincott Williams & Wilkins, 1999:787–799.
- Centers for Disease Control and Prevention. 1998 Guidelines for treatment of sexually transmitted diseases. MMWR 1998;47[No. RR-1]:28–48.
- Hook EW, Marra CM. Acquired syphilis in adults. N Engl J Med 1992;326:1060–1069.
- Marra CA. Neurosyphilis: a guide for clinicians. Infect Dis Clin Pract 1996;5: 33–41.
- Swartz MN, et al. Late syphilis. In: Holmes KK, et al., eds. Sexually transmitted diseases. New York: McGraw-Hill, 1999:487–509.

Author(s): Thomas D. Lamarre, Jr., MD; Julie E. Mangino, MD

Syringomyelia

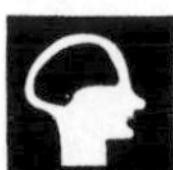

Basics

DESCRIPTION

- *Syringomyelia* refers to an abnormal fluid collection (syrinx) within the spinal cord (myelia). Terminology describing a syrinx (pl. syringes) often is confusing. Expansion of the ependymal lined central canal is termed *hydromyelia.* Expansion of the cavity into the cord and the resultant nonependymal lined cavity is termed *syringohydromyelia.* Often syringomyelia is used as a generic term before an etiology is determined. The accumulation of fluid within the spinal cord is not thought to be the primary manifestation of any disease process. Syringohydromyelia is a secondary process with many etiologies. A useful classification is to divide these accumulations into communicating and noncommunicating varieties. Cavities with cerebrospinal-like that fluid are communicating are usually associated with altered CSF flow at the craniocervical junction (e.g., Chiari malformation) or occult spinal dysraphism (OSD; e.g. diastematomyelia). Highly proteinaceous fluid cavities are generally found in noncommunicating varieties caused by arachnoiditis, vascular anomalies, neoplasm, or trauma to the spinal cord.

EPIDEMIOLOGY

Incidence/Prevalence

- Seen in ~50%–75% of patients with Chiari I malformation and 20%–95% of patients with Chiari II malformation. Reported in approximately 1% of patients following spinal cord injury. Intramedullary spinal cord tumors have a reported incidence of syrinx in 25%–57% of cases.

Age

- Commonly seen in children with the advent of MRI

Sex

N/A

ETIOLOGY

- Precise cause of syrinx formation is still unknown; however, inappropriate CSF flow at the craniocervical junction (Chiari malformation) is associated with syrinx production.

Genetics

- N/A, although up to 2% of syringes have been found in siblings and twins both monozygotic and dizygotic.

Causes

- Chiari malformation (Type 0, I and II)
- Arachnoiditis (Tuberculosis, fungus, syphilis, following subarachnoid hemorrhage, etc.)
- Neoplasm of the spinal cord (usually glial in origin)
- Vascular malformation of the spinal cord
- Trauma of the spinal cord
- Following iatrogenic penetration of the subarachnoid space e.g. lumbar puncture
- Idiopathic

PREGNANCY

Not applicable.

ASSOCIATED CONDITIONS

- Myelomeningocele
- OSD
- Chiari malformation
- Disseminated tumor
- Systemic infection

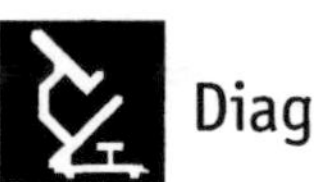

Diagnosis

DIFFERENTIAL DIAGNOSIS

- Chronic demyelinating lesions
- Intramedullary tumors
- Extrinsic compressive lesions of the cord

SIGNS AND SYMPTOMS

Symptoms

- Syringomyelia symptoms tend to be chronic and often are subtle compared to the clinical signs because the patient has years to become accustomed to them. Symptoms include balance disorders, loss of pain/ temperature appreciation in the hands and arms, sphincter disturbance, weakness in the hands, and dysphagia.

Signs

- Decreased pain/temperature appreciation, often in a "shawl" distribution
- Diminished deep tendon reflexes in the arms
- Spasticity in the legs
- Dysesthesia
- Scoliosis
- Muscle atrophy, primarily in the upper extremities
- Motor weakness

LABORATORY PROCEDURES

N/A

IMAGING STUDIES

- MRI
  - —MRI is the test of choice in evaluation of a syrinx. A syrinx will have a CSF signal (black) on T1-weighted images. Contrast may be helpful in discerning tumor or inflammation as a cause of the syrinx. Flow studies (cine mode) of the craniocervical junction often are not useful, yielding many false-negative and false-positive results.
  - —Always evaluate the craniocervical junction in the presence of syrinx (i.e., is a Chiari malformation present?).
  - —Syringes produced by a Chiari malformation often involve the cervicothoracic region, whereas syringes from OSD are found in the distal cord.
  - —If a Chiari I malformation is the cause of the syrinx, hydrocephalus and cervical spine instability should be ruled out first.
- Spine radiographs. Often a syrinx is first appreciated when uncommon curvatures (produced by the underlying syrinx) are found on x-ray films (e.g., a single-curve scoliosis with convexity to the left).

SPECIAL TESTS

- Abdominal reflexes often are diminished or absent in the presence of syrinx, especially in patients with scoliosis

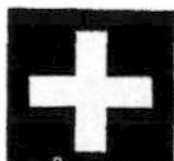

Management

GENERAL MEASURES

- No specific measures; attention to issues such as bladder function, bowel regimen, decubiti in severely disabled patients, and deep vein thrombosis prophylaxis in hospitalized patients

SURGICAL MEASURES

- Communicating syrinx: Consider surgical decompression at hydrostatic sites such as the posterior fossa. Insertion of a tube into the syrinx may provide for chronic decompression. Patients with severe scoliosis may require surgical correction with Harrington rod implantation.
  - —Posttraumatic: Reestablish an open subarachnoid space, usually at the site of a spine fracture. If unsuccessful, then a syringopleural shunt should be placed.
  - —Secondary to Chiari malformation: Craniocervical decompression with or without removal of a cerebellar tonsil
  - —Secondary to neoplasm/vascular malformation: Resection of primary lesion
  - —Secondary to arachnoiditis: Syringopleural shunt
  - —Secondary to OSD: Syringo-subarachnoid stent
  - —Idiopathic: Verify CSF egress from the fourth ventricle. If physiologic result: syringopleural/peritoneal shunt. If no egress and no other cause of syrinx is found: cranio-cervical decompression.
  - —Asymptomatic: If the syrinx is small, consider observation and serial MRI. If the syrinx is large and expanding the spinal cord and no other cause is found, consider craniocervical decompression.

SYMPTOMATIC TREATMENT

- As per general measures, consider measures for spasticity and pain management if applicable.

ADJUNCTIVE TREATMENT

N/A

ADMISSION/DISCHARGE CRITERIA

- If surgery is chosen, patients are brought in electively and observed carefully postoperatively. For both shunt procedures and decompressive procedures, patients normally are discharged in 1–2 days.

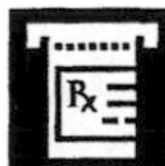

Medications

DRUG(S) OF CHOICE

- There is no medical treatment for syringomyelia.

ALTERNATIVE DRUGS

N/A

Follow-Up

PATIENT MONITORING

- Patients are seen 1 week postoperatively, then in 2 months. At the next follow-up in 6 months, a repeat MRI is obtained to assess the size of the syrinx. If the syrinx is shunted, observe for neurologic deterioration from either shunt malfunction or migration. Shunt infection may occur. Examples of complications of craniocervical decompression are cerebellar ptosis, continued presence of the syrinx, further neurologic compromise, acute hydrocephalus, and ventral compression from a retroflexed dens.

EXPECTED COURSE AND PROGNOSIS

- Approximately 90% of patients in whom hindbrain herniation is the cause of the syrinx have resolution on follow-up imaging.
- Syringopleural shunts and syringo-arachnoid stents do well in combating syringes but require close follow-up and maintenance.
- Syringes of tumor/vascular anomaly origin require that the mass be dealt with efficiently.

PATIENT EDUCATION

- If operative intervention is necessary, patients may resume normal activities once the wound is healed and they are physically back to baseline, usually in a period of weeks. Patients should be educated about the risk of burning their hands due to insensitivity, gait disorders, and bowel and bladder function, if appropriate. Patients should become acquainted with the nature of the illness and the mechanism of neurologic dysfunction.

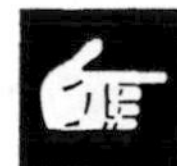

Miscellaneous

SYNONYMS

N/A

ICD-9-CM: 336.0 Syringomyelia/syringobulbia

SEE ALSO: SPINAL CORD SYNDROMES, CHRONIC; CHIARI MALFORMATION

REFERENCES

- Batzdorf U. Syringomyelia: current concepts in diagnosis and treatment. Baltimore: Williams & Wilkins 1991.
- Caplan LR, Norohna AB, Amico LL. Syringomyelia and arachnoiditis. J Neurol Neurosurg Psychiatry 1990;53:106–113.
- Davis CHG, Symon L. Mechanisms and treatment in post-traumatic syringomyelia. Br J Neurosurg 1989;3:669–674.
- Iskandar B, Oakes W. Chiari malformation and syringomyelia. In: Albright L, Pollack I, Adelson P, eds. Principles and practice of pediatric neurosurgery. New York: Thieme, 1999:165–187.
- Johnston I, Jacobson E, Besser M. The acquired Chiari malformation and syringomyelia following spinal CSF drainage: a study of incidence and management. Acta Neurochirurg 1998;140:417–427.
- Logue V, Edwards MR. Syringomyelia and its surgical treatment-an analysis of 75 patients. J Pediatr 1991;118:567–569.
- Oakes WJ. Chiari Malformations and Syringohydromyelia. In: Rengachary S, Wilkins R, eds. Principles of neurosurgery. London, Wolf Publishing, 1994:9.1–9.18
- Oakes WJ, Tubbs RS. Chiari malformations. In: Winn HR, ed. Youman's neurological surgery: a comprehensive guide to the diagnosis and management of neurological problems, 5th ed. Philadelphia: WB Saunders, 2002.
- Tubbs RS, Elton S, Grabb P, et al. Analysis of the posterior fossa in children with the Chiari 0 malformation. Neurosurgery 2001;48:1050–1055.

www.neurosurgery.org

Author(s): R. Shane Tubbs, MS, PA-C, PhD; W. Jerry Oakes, MD

Systemic Lupus Erythematosus, Neurologic Complications

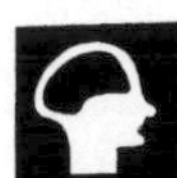

Basics

DESCRIPTION

- Systemic lupus erythematosus (SLE) is a systemic inflammatory disorder that affects almost every organ of the body. Clinical course varies from indolent to fulminant. Neuropsychiatric SLE (NPSLE) includes both the central and peripheral nervous systems

EPIDEMIOLOGY

Incidence/Prevalence

- SLE: 15–50 per 100,000; neurologic involvement: 60%–75% of all SLE patients at some point in disease. Prevalence may be up to 91%, including mood disorder, headache, and cognitive dysfunction.

Race

- All races appear susceptible, although it occurs more frequently in black and Hispanic individuals. Black individuals tend toward increased severity.

Sex

- Women outnumber men 5–10:1. No known gender differences for neurologic involvement.

Age

- Most cases of SLE are diagnosed between 15 and 40 years, although all ages may develop SLE. NPSLE may develop at any time during SLE.

ETIOLOGY

- Although the etiology of SLE is unknown, aberrant regulation of autoreactive antibody production and clearance may be the underlying pathogenesis of SLE. Tissues are damaged by deposition of autoantibodies and immune complexes, which induce antigen-specific immunologic damage or non–antigen-specific complement fixation. The mechanisms of neurologic injury in SLE include direct antibody (antineuronal)-mediated effects, distant effects of systemic inflammation (e.g., cardiac emboli from valvular disease, hemorrhagic stroke from thrombocytopenia), or secondary effects, such as infection, toxicity of medications, or metabolic abnormalities. Although common in other organs (including peripheral nerve), cerebral blood vessel inflammation (vasculitis) is unusual.

Genetics

- Several genes predispose to SLE: HLA classes I and II, including DR2, DR3, and several C4 genes. Ten percent of patients have affected family members.

RISK FACTORS

- Risk factors for NPSLE include antiphospholipid antibody syndrome (positive anticardiolipin IgG in high titer, arterial thrombosis), cutaneous vasculitis lesions, thrombocytopenia, positive anti-SS-B/La, and depressed C3 or C4. Arthralgias/arthritis and discoid rash are protective. Drug-induced lupus rarely involves the nervous system.

PREGNANCY

- SLE does not interfere with conception, and there is no increase in flares during pregnancy. However, there are increased rates of spontaneous abortion, prematurity, and intrauterine death. Differentiating SLE flare from preeclampsia/eclampsia can be difficult, but laboratory abnormalities (anti-DNA antibody titer, decreased complement levels) can assist clinical impression. Prednisone does not cross the placenta and is given safely during pregnancy.

ASSOCIATED CONDITIONS

- CNS autoimmune disorders: multiple sclerosis; primary CNS vasculitis
- Systemic autoimmune disorders: rheumatoid arthritis, polymyositis, scleroderma ("mixed connective tissue diseases"); dermatomyositis; Raynaud's syndrome
- Toxic: drug-induced lupus: procainamide (50%–75% with positive ANA); chlorpromazine, methyldopa, hydralazine, isoniazid, phenytoin, penicillamine. Drug-induced lupus is rarely associated with CNS involvement.
- Anti-phospholipid antibody syndrome (may be separate or a part of SLE)
- Premature atherosclerosis (late-stage SLE)
- Sneddon's syndrome: generalized livedo reticularis and stroke
- Reversible posterior leukoencephalopathy syndrome: associated with SLE nephritis and hypertension

Diagnosis

DIFFERENTIAL DIAGNOSIS

- Autoimmune: multiple sclerosis, primary isolated CNS vasculitis, Behçet's disease, sarcoidosis, mixed connective tissue disease, Susac syndrome
- Psychiatric: depression, schizophrenia
- Epilepsy: partial, partial complex, generalized epilepsy
- Drugs of abuse
- Stroke: cardioembolic, hemorrhagic
- Guillain-Barré syndrome
- Infections: fungal meningitis, bacterial meningitis, herpes simplex virus, Lyme disease, cytomegalovirus, HIV, syphilis, tuberculous meningitis
- Metabolic: hyperuremia, electrolyte imbalances
- Severe hypertension: usually with active nephritis

SIGNS AND SYMPTOMS

- May be seen in isolation or during systemic activity. Non-SLE disorders must be evaluated and ruled out. Generalized disorders are probably from primary CNS involvement of SLE, whereas focal disorders are from distant effects of SLE.

Generalized NPSLE (% Incidence)

- Organic brain syndrome: psychosis (6%), delirium or marked emotional instability. Differentiation between SLE-induced or steroid-induced psychosis is on clinical grounds only. Therapeutic trial of increased or decreased steroids is guided by clinical insight. Infections are very common with acute and subacute altered sensorium.
- Mood disorder: depression (44%), anxiety disorder (13%), personality change
- Cognitive impairment (42%–80%): varies from subclinical impairment to severe dementia
- Headaches (40%–54%): can be migrainous or nonmigrainous; often unresponsive to narcotics
- Chorea: rare; clinically similar to Sydenham's chorea, usually early in disease course; can be associated with antiphospholipid antibodies.
- Retinopathy: usually secondary to vasculitis and accompanies CNS activity
- Vasculopathy: chronic, small-vessel occlusive disorder with cognitive impairment, possibly secondary to chronic immune complex deposition
- CNS vasculitis: rare cause of stroke
- Aseptic meningitis: rare
- Myasthenia gravis: rare

Focal NPSLE

- Seizures (9%–40%): usually secondary to focal ischemia, but must consider infectious and metabolic etiologies
- Peripheral neuropathy (16%–28%): sensory, motor, mixed sensorimotor polyneuropathies, or mononeuritis simplex/multiplex (vasculitic axonal polyradiculopathy). Plexopathy, Guillain-Barré syndrome, autonomic disorder, and transverse myelitis also are seen.
- Cranial neuropathy (6%): visual loss, facial palsy, trigeminal neuralgia, tinnitus, vertigo Stroke (15%)
  - —Stroke usually due to complications from therapy or end-organ damage
  - —Arterial or venous occlusion: related to cardiac emboli, antiphospholipid antibodies
  - —Hemorrhagic: often secondary to thrombocytopenia or hypertension
- Visual disturbances: transient monocular blindness (6%), migraine (10%)
- Myelopathy: due to transverse myelitis, spinal cord infarct, or subdural-epidural hematoma
- Focal demyelinating syndrome: similar to multiple sclerosis, but often has serologic and clinical evidence for antiphospholipid syndrome

LABORATORY PROCEDURES

- CNS involvement of SLE is a clinical diagnosis.
- Serologic evidence for increased disease activity (increased anti-DNA titers, depressed complement levels) can correlate with disease activity. Although studies are conflicting, serum anti-ribosomal-P antibodies appear to correlate with CNS involvement, especially psychosis.
- CSF studies frequently find pleocytosis (usually mononuclear cells, 18%), elevated protein (32%), elevated albumin ratio (24%), oligoclonal bands (28%–70%), and elevated IgG index (70%–90%), although NPSLE did not differ from SLE without neuropsychiatric involvement. Protein and albumin ratio may increase during relapse but is nonspecific.
- CSF studies (including routine and fungal culture, viral studies) are important to exclude infectious complications of immunosuppression. Pleocytosis may be absent despite ongoing fungal infection.

IMAGING STUDIES

- Brain MRI is more useful than CT, reveals distant effects of systemic disease (cardioembolic stroke, hemorrhage), and can show diffuse abnormalities. MR angiography can visualize medium and large vessels.
- Spine MRI can visualize focal lesions (transverse myelitis, infarct) and should be considered when symptoms localize to the spine.
- Conventional angiography is rarely necessary.

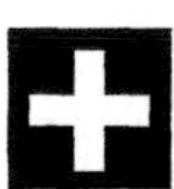

Management

GENERAL MEASURES

- Infections must be considered when new symptoms develop. Postmortem studies in patients with presumed active SLE frequently find active CNS infection (fungal, viral) and quiescent SLE.
- Toxicity/side effects of current medications must be considered.
- Evaluation of seizures includes screening and treatment of active systemic disease, such as uremia, electrolyte abnormalities, metabolic encephalopathy, and hypertension.

SURGICAL MEASURES

- Brain biopsy is rarely needed to confirm diagnosis.
- Sural nerve biopsy can confirm SLE peripheral neuropathy.

SYMPTOMATIC TREATMENT

- See Medications

ADJUNCTIVE TREATMENT

- Counseling is effective for mood disorders and emotional instability.

ADMISSION/DISCHARGE CRITERIA

- Admission may be required for acute confusional state, stroke, infection, or other neurologic complications. Treatment with high-dose corticosteroids or intravenous cyclophosphamide often requires hospitalization.

Medications

DRUG(S) OF CHOICE

- Evidence from controlled clinical trials data is either negative or absent, and most treatment is empiric. Cyclophosphamide is commonly used, but there is little clinical trial evidence supporting its use.
- General: Intravenous cyclophosphamide with high-dose corticosteroids appears to be effective.
- Encephalopathy: Plasmapheresis and cyclophosphamide either 500 mg IV biweekly or 75–100 mg/day PO.
- Seizures: Anticonvulsant usually is sufficient; further immunosuppression usually is not needed.
- Movement disorders: Plasmapheresis with azathioprine or cyclophosphamide is better than corticosteroids.
- Stroke: Treatment is directed by etiology.
  - —Thrombosis: Antiplatelet agents
  - —Emboli: Antibiotics or anticoagulants
  - —Coagulopathy: Plasmapheresis, antiplatelet agents, anticoagulation
  - —Stroke itself is treated according to standard stroke protocols.
  - —If part of antiphospholipid syndrome: warfarin with target INR 3–4
- Transverse myelopathy: High-dose corticosteroids (methylprednisolone >500 mg/day)
- Peripheral neuropathy/plexopathy: Corticosteroids, equivalent of 60–80 mg prednisone daily
- Necrotizing vasculitis: Corticosteroids, immunosuppressive agents, plasmapheresis

Precautions

- It often is difficult to differentiate adverse effects of medications from disease activity. Empiric titration in immunosuppression with careful monitoring is required.
- It is imperative that infectious, metabolic, and hypertensive etiologies be excluded prior to treating neurologic dysfunction as a primary or distant effects of SLE.
- Nonsteroidal antiinflammatory drugs are commonly used in SLE but can cause aseptic meningitis, dizziness, confusion, depression, headache, and worsening of renal dysfunction.

ALTERNATIVE DRUGS

- Autologous stem cell transplant has demonstrated promising preliminary results.
- Azathioprine may be steroid sparing, but efficacy in NPSLE is unknown.
- Plasmapheresis is ineffective in some manifestations of SLE (nephritis).
- Antimalarials (hydroxychloroquine, chloroquine, and quinacrine) are used for cutaneous SLE but can have CNS side effects.
- Methotrexate is used for cutaneous and articular SLE; experience in NPSLE is minimal.

Follow-Up

PATIENT MONITORING

- Clinical monitoring is the best method to follow patients over time. In some patients, serologic studies parallel clinical activity and can be useful for early detection of exacerbations.

EXPECTED COURSE AND PROGNOSIS

- Most CNS events are self-limiting, reversible, and not associated with poor outcome unless multisystem disease activity is present.

PATIENT EDUCATION

- Lupus Foundation of America, 1300 Piccard Drive, Suite 200, Rockville, MD 20850-4303. Phone: 301-670-9292, fax: 800-558-0121, website: *www.lupus.org/lupus/*

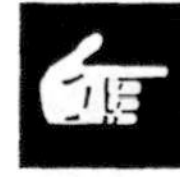

Miscellaneous

SYNONYMS

- Central nervous system systemic lupus erythematosus

ICD-9-CM: 710.0 Systemic lupus erythematosus

SEE ALSO: ANTIPHOSPHOLIPID ANTIBODY SYNDROME, NEUROLOGIC COMPLICATIONS

REFERENCES

- Futrell N, Schultz LR, Millikan C. Central nervous system disease in patients with systemic lupus erythematosus. Neurology 1992;42:1649–1657.
- Karass FB, Ioannidis JPA, Touloumi G, et al. Risk factors for central nervous system involvement in systemic lupus erythematosus. Q J Med 2000;93:169–174.
- West SG, Emlen W, Wener MH, et al. Neuropsychiatric lupus erythematosus: a 10-year prospective study on the value of diagnostic tests. Am J Med 1995;99: 153–163.

Author(s): Robert J. Fox, MD; Lael Stone, MD

Tardive Dyskinesia

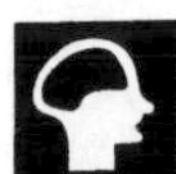

Basics

DESCRIPTION

- Tardive dyskinesia (TD) is a disorder of abnormal involuntary movements most often affecting the orobuccolingual musculature but also truncal and limb musculature. It is associated with antipsychotic drug therapy. TD usually develops after >1 year of treatment, but cases where symptoms of TD appeared within 3-6 months of antipsychotic use have been reported in the literature. Most cases are mild to moderate, but a small percentage can be severely disfiguring and disabling

EPIDEMIOLOGY

Incidence/Prevalence

- The incidence of TD is estimated at 2%–5% per year over the first 5–10 years of treatment with neuroleptic agents.
- Lifetime prevalence is estimated to be approximately 20%, but the range is extremely wide (1%–80%) for those requiring chronic treatment with neuroleptics.

Race

- No information available

Age

- Elderly patients are much more vulnerable.

Sex

- Women are more at risk, with a female-to-male ratio of 1.7:1

ETIOLOGY

- The onset of TD is linked to the use of dopamine receptor-blocking agents, but the exact mechanism is not known.
- There are data suggesting that prolonged receptor blockade by antipsychotic agents may cause hyperactivity of the CNS dopaminergic and noradrenergic systems coupled with reduced activity in the γ-aminobutyric acid (GABA) and cholinergic systems.
- The onset of TD usually has been associated with exposure to antipsychotic agents. Other dopamine receptor-blocking agents, such as the antiemetic agents metoclopramide and prochlorperazine, and the antidepressant amoxapine also can result in TD.
- TD should be distinguished from spontaneous (idiopathic) movement disorders associated with schizophrenia (prevalence of 15%), old age, and brain damage.

Genetics

- No information available

RISK FACTORS

- Higher dose of administered antipsychotic medication
- Longer duration of antipsychotic exposure
- Older age
- Gender
- Psychiatric diagnosis: Patients with mood disorders and/or medical diagnoses receiving antipsychotic medications have a higher incidence than those with schizophrenia.
- Patients who exhibit acute extrapyramidal side effects from neuroleptics may be at greater risk of developing TD.
- Drug holidays: Recent studies have shown that intermittent neuroleptic treatment is *not* helpful and may be detrimental.
- Possibly exposure to anticholinergic use, but the data are controversial.
- Negative symptoms of schizophrenia
- Organic brain damage
- All typical antipsychotics appear to cause TD at a similar rate. No significant difference has been observed among the following factors:
  - —Antipsychotic type: high-potency agents such as haloperidol (Haldol) versus low-potency agents such as chlorpromazine (Thorazine)
  - —Oral agents versus long-acting injectable antipsychotic agents
  - —The newer, atypical antipsychotic agents (risperidone, olanzapine, quetiapine) seem to have a lower incidence of TD. Clozaril has definitely been shown to have a very low incidence of TD.

PREGNANCY

- No information available

ASSOCIATED CONDITIONS

- Tardive dystonia and tardive akathisia

Diagnosis

DIFFERENTIAL DIAGNOSIS

- Tardive dystonia, which consists of
  - —Irregular postures (e.g., Pisa syndrome)
  - —Slow, involuntary twisting movements of face, trunk, or limbs (patients may present with torticollis, blepharospasm, retrocollis, grimacing)
  - —It occurs in 2% of patients treated with antipsychotic agents.
  - —It may coexist with TD and may be even more distressing and disabling.
  - —Use of anticholinergic drugs may lessen symptoms of tardive dystonia.
- Tardive akathisia, which consists of
  - —Motor restlessness
  - —Subjective discomfort
  - —Treatment with benzodiazepines, β blockers, or clozapine may be beneficial
  - —Dopamine depletors, such as reserpine, are effective
- Huntington's disease
- Other basal ganglia disorders

DIAGNOSIS

- Careful clinical assessment is the sole basis for the diagnosis of TD.
- Several quantitative assessment tools have been published, but the most widely used one is the Abnormal Involuntary Movements Scale (AIMS). The AIMS should be assessed for all patients when dopamine receptor-blocking agents are initiated and at least every 3 months while patients continue to be treated with these agents.
- Physicians should not rely solely on patient complaints to make a diagnosis of TD because the early signs and symptoms of this disorder can easily escape notice.
- There are no laboratory procedures, imaging studies, or special tests to diagnose TD.
- TD often becomes evident upon antipsychotic dose reduction or discontinuation.

SIGNS AND SYMPTOMS

- TD is a complex syndrome of irregular, abnormal, repetitive, involuntary movements of the mouth, lips, tongue, limbs, or trunk.
- The buccolinguomasticatory triad of symptoms is most common and consists of
  - —Smacking, puckering movements of the lips
  - —Lateral movements of the jaws
  - —Puffing of the checks with the tongue thrusting and rolling inside the mouth
- Chewing motions (patients frequently bite the inside of their mouths or tongues).
- Athetoid and choreiform movements of the extremities. These movements are involuntary and purposeless.
- Trunk movements: Either anterior-posterior or rhythmical side to side swaying may be present.
- All involuntary movements are exacerbated by stress or anxiety and dramatically subside during sleep.

LABORATORY PROCEDURES

N/A

IMAGING STUDIES

N/A

SPECIAL TESTS

N/A

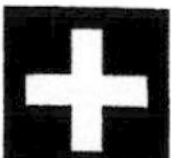

Management

GENERAL MEASURES

- Prevention is the most important aspect of TD management. There is no reliable treatment other than discontinuation of the offending drug.
- Long-term use of antipsychotic agents should be restricted to patients whose chronic illness clearly necessitates it (e.g., schizophrenia). It should be avoided in patients suffering from depression, mania, anxiety, or personality disorders, except in unusual clinical circumstances.
- Ongoing periodic evaluations of the patient's need for long-term antipsychotic agents must be done with an assessment of the risks and benefits of treatment. The dose of medication must be adjusted so that patients receive the lowest antipsychotic dose that is still effective.
  - —There is no reliable treatment of TD other than discontinuation of the offending agent.
  - —Many patients recover spontaneously when antipsychotic agents are discontinued.
  - —TD may improve in some patients even when they continue treatment with antipsychotics.
  - —Anticholinergic medications should be avoided because they may aggravate TD, and it is not known whether long-term use of these agents increases the risk of developing TD.
  - —If an antipsychotic agent is necessary, use clozapine (Clozaril; which has anti-dyskinetic effects) or one of the new atypical antipsychotics (risperidone, olanzapine, quetiapine), which seem to have a much lower incidence of TD.

SURGICAL MEASURES

N/A

SYMPTOMATIC TREATMENT

N/A

ADJUNCTIVE TREATMENT

N/A

ADMISSION/DISCHARGE CRITERIA

- Admission is rarely required unless dyskinesias become so severe that they interfere with breathing or swallowing.

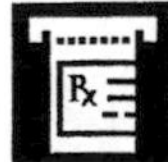

Medications

DRUG(S) OF CHOICE

- Clozapine (an atypical antipsychotic agent) has been found to decrease symptoms of TD in several large studies and may be the treatment of choice, especially for patients who need medications for their psychiatric disorder. Severe TD and particularly tardive dystonia seem to respond best to doses ranging from 300–750 mg/day. The main disadvantages to using clozapine are the potential side effects of agranulocytosis, seizures, and the need for weekly blood monitoring.
- There have been anecdotal reports indicating that risperidone or olanzapine may improve TD, but further controlled studies are necessary to confirm this. One needs to keep in mind that all neuroleptics that have antidyskinetic properties also have been associated with the occurrence of TD.
- Vitamin E (an antioxidant) in doses of 1,600 IU/day has not been consistently shown to be beneficial in all studies. Several case reports have found positive results, but a recent long-term trial found no efficacy of vitamin E in this condition. Patients who have had TD for <5 years appear to have a better response than patients with long-standing TD.
- Clonazepam in doses of 0.5 3 mg/day has been found to reduce movements of TD, but caution must be exercised in chronic use of benzodiazepines.
- Dopamine-depleting medications, such as reserpine in doses of 1-5 mg/day, may alleviate symptoms in up to 50% of patients.
- Calcium channel Blockers may help alleviate TD symptoms. Nifedipine in doses of 20–80 mg/day may be the most effective agent in this class, but further studies are needed to assess its overall place in TD management.

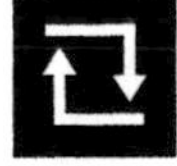

Follow-Up

PATIENT MONITORING

- Patients should be given an AIMS test every 3 months while taking dopamine-blocking agents so that any symptoms of TD can be identified early and discussed at length with the patient.

EXPECTED COURSE AND PROGNOSIS

- We used to believe that the course of TD was progressive and irreversible. More recent data show that in most patients, TD develops to a certain degree and then stabilizes and may even improve. The most frequent pattern is waxing and waning of mild-to-moderate symptoms over many years. Progression to severe TD is not common.

PATIENT EDUCATION

- Each patient should be informed about the long-term risk of developing TD and that the involuntary movements may be irreversible and treatment resistant. At the same time, the patient should be assured that the clinician will make every attempt to minimize the risk of TD and to closely monitor early signs and symptoms.
- Every clinician should obtain informed medical consent from the patient and/or the patient's family. Ongoing education and open communication should occur and should be clearly documented in the patient's record.
- Tardive Dyskinesia/Tardive Dystonia National Association, P.O. Box 4573, Seattle, WA 98145-0732. Phone: 206-522-3166.

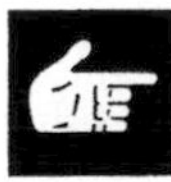

Miscellaneous

SYNONYMS

N/A

ICD-9-CM: 333.82 Orofacial dyskinesia

SEE ALSO: N/A

REFERENCES

- Dauer WT, Fahn S, Burke RE. The diagnosis and treatment of tardive disorders. Med Update Psychiatrists 120–125.
- Egan ME, Apud J, Wyatt RJ. Treatment of tardive dyskinesia. Schizophr Bull 1997; 4:583–609.
- Gardos G. Managing antipsychotic-induced tardive dyskinesia. Drug Saf 1999; 20:187–193.
- Janicak PG, Davis JM, Preskorn S, Ayd FJ Jr. Principles and practice of psycho-pharmacotherapy, 2nd ed. Baltimore: Williams & Wilkins, 1997.
- Kane JM. Tardive dyskinesia in movement disorders. In: Joseh AB, Young RR, eds. Neurology and neuropsychiatry, 2nd ed. Boston: Blackwell Science, 1998:31–39.
- Stanilla JK, Simpson GM. Treatment of extrapyramidal side effects. In: Schatzburg AF, Nemeroff CB, eds. Textbook of psychopharmacology, 2nd ed. American Psychiatric Press, 1998:349–378.

Author(s): Radu Saveanu, MD

Tetanus

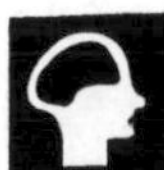

Basics

DESCRIPTION

- Tetanus is a noncommunicable and potentially fatal infection caused by *Clostridium tetani.* Clinically it is characterized by the acute onset of generalized rigidity and reflex spasms.

EPIDEMIOLOGY

Incidence/Prevalence

- The disease is seen worldwide. Tetanus is seen more often in the summer season.

Race

- No information available

Age

- Newborns, because of nonsterile birth conditions, and the elderly have the highest risk for the disease.

Sex

- Male-to-female ratio of 2.5:1

ETIOLOGY

- *C. tetani* is a Gram-positive anaerobic, spore-forming bacteria that is universally found in the environment. The spores enter the body through contaminated wounds. They germinate under anaerobic conditions and produce tetanus toxin (tetanospasmin), which is responsible for the disease. Tetanospasmin inhibits neurotransmitter release presynaptically at the neuromuscular junction, autonomic terminals, and inhibitory neurons of the central nervous system.

Genetics

N/A

RISK FACTORS

- Nonsterile obstetric delivery and contamination of umbilical stump with the organism
- Wounds bearing necrotic tissue, foreign bodies, and associated infection
- Chronic lesions (decubitus ulcers, abscesses)
- Parenteral drug abuse
- Absent or incomplete immunization

PREGNANCY

- Poor obstetric conditions and lack of maternal immunization are risk factors for neonatal tetanus.

ASSOCIATED CONDITIONS

N/A

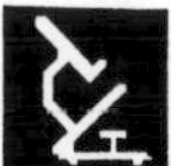

Diagnosis

DIFFERENTIAL DIAGNOSIS

- Other causes of bacterial and viral meningitis
- Rabies
- Hypocalcemic tetany
- Strychnine poisoning
- Tonsillitis
- Peritonsillar abscess
- Dystonic reactions due to phenothiazines

SIGNS AND SYMPTOMS

- The incubation period usually is between 5 and 14 days, although it can be prolonged up to 3 weeks. The distance of injury from the central nervous system determines the length of incubation period. Stiffness of jaw (trismus) usually is the first symptom. A characteristic facial appearance (risus sardonicus) results from sustained contractions of facial muscles. Generalized muscle rigidity involving neck, trunk, and extremity muscles follows. Rigidity of back muscles causes opisthotonus.
- Paroxysmal tonic spasms can occur spontaneously or be precipitated by external stimuli. Pharyngeal muscular spasms cause dysphagia, and spasms of the glottis may lead to death by asphyxiation. Spasms of diaphragmatic, intercostal, and laryngeal muscles are life threatening.
- Autonomic dysfunction (labile hypertension, tachycardia, arrhythmias, hyperhidrosis) can be seen in severe cases.
- Reflexes are increased and sensory examination is normal. Irritability and restlessness are seen, but consciousness is preserved.
- High fever up to 41°C can be seen and signifies poor prognosis.
- Rarely tetanus is localized to an area close to site of injury (local form). Muscles in the region of injury go into intermittent painful spasms. This form is benign and muscular spasms subside spontaneously within weeks. When localized to the head, it is called the cephalic form.
- Manifestations of tetanus increase in severity during the first 3 days after onset, remain stable for 5–7 days, and resolve within 1–2 weeks.
- Neonatal tetanus: Occurs 3–14 days after delivery. Disease is due to nonsterile birth conditions and contamination of the umbilical cord stump. Mothers are unimmunized women. Difficulty in sucking, excessive crying, trismus, opisthotonus, and spasms are clinical signs.

LABORATORY PROCEDURES

- Diagnosis should be made by clinical features and history. There is no single laboratory procedure that gives definite diagnosis in every patient. Routine blood work is nonspecific. Mild leukocytosis is seen.

IMAGING STUDIES

- Imaging studies are not helpful.

SPECIAL TESTS

- Cerebrospinal fluid examination is normal.
- Specimens from the wound may reveal Gram-positive bacilli.
- Anaerobic cultures usually are unsuccessful.
- Neutralization of toxin in mice is the standard method for detection of antitoxin in the serum.

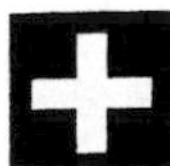

Management

GENERAL MEASURES

- Be sure that the airway is open and ventilation is adequate. Respiratory insufficiency due to laryngospasm or spasms of respiratory muscles is a major problem. Tracheostomy not only facilitates mechanical assistance of ventilation but also reduces the risk of aspiration and protects against suffocation due to laryngospasm. Although some milder cases can be managed without it, every patient should be considered a candidate for tracheostomy.
- Avoid external stimuli and keep the patient in a dim and quiet room.
- All treatments and manipulations should be kept to a minimum to prevent provocation of reflex spasms.
- Stop oral intake to prevent aspiration and start intravenous hyperalimentation because these patients are in an intense catabolic state.
- Monitor fluid and electrolyte balance.
- Position to prevent bedsores, paying attention not to provoke reflex spasms.
- Apply intermittent catheterization if urinary retention develops.
- Prevent deep vein thrombosis with low-dose heparin.

SURGICAL MEASURES

- Surgical debridement of wounds and drainage of abscesses is mandatory because anaerobic conditions are necessary for spore germination. Wounds should be irrigated with 3% hydrogen peroxide three times daily after the procedure.

SYMPTOMATIC TREATMENT

- Muscle relaxation is necessary and mild sedation is desirable.
- Diazepam is very effective. It not only relieves rigidity but also provides sedation. Administer diazepam 0.5–5 mg/kg/day IV in divided doses every 2–8 hours or 5–10 mg whenever spasms occur.
- Phenobarbital 50–100 mg every 3–6 hours or pentobarbital 50–200 mg IV, chlorpromazine 200–300 mg daily, dantrolene, or intrathecal baclofen can be used as muscle relaxants.
- If spasms cannot be controlled by these measures, curarization may be necessary.
- D-Tubocurarine 15 mg/hour IM can be given after ventilatory support. Propofol can be given as sedative.
- Propranolol with phentolamine or labetalol 0.25–1.0 mg/min can be used to decrease sympathetic activity.

ADJUNCTIVE TREATMENT

- Physical therapy can be started 2–6 weeks after the onset of infection, when the spasms disappear. Many patients will also require psychotherapy.

ADMISSION/DISCHARGE CRITERIA

- All patients should be treated in an intensive care unit.

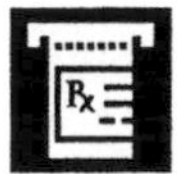

Medications

DRUG(S) OF CHOICE

- Antiserum: Administer human tetanus immune globulin (HTIG) 3,000–6,000 units IM as soon as possible, because antiserum neutralizes only the toxin that has not entered the nervous system.
- Antibiotics: The organism is susceptible to several antibiotics. Metronidazole is first choice: 20–30 mg/kg/day IV over 1 hour in three or four divided doses following a loading dose of 15 mg/kg. Metronidazole should be given for 7–14 days. If metronidazole is not available, penicillin G 100,000 U/kg/day IV in six divided doses can be given.
- Tetanus toxoid: Because tetanus infection does not provide natural immunity against further attacks, active immunization of patients is necessary at the time of diagnosis or during convalescence.

Contraindications

- Known drug allergies

Precautions

- Respiratory function should be monitored during heavy sedation.

Prophylaxis

- Tetanus vaccine (toxoid) is administered with diphtheria and pertussis vaccines at ages 2, 4, 6 months, 12–18 months, and before school (4–6 years). Routine boosters of tetanus with diphtheria (Td) should be given every 10 years.
- Adults who have not been immunized previously should receive two doses of Td 4–8 weeks apart and the third dose 6 months to 1 years after the second dose.
- Nonimmunized female should receive two doses of tetanus toxoid (at least 4 weeks apart) during pregnancy, the last one at least 2 weeks before delivery.
- Management of wound prophylaxis of tetanus depends on current immunization status of the patient. If a patient has received at least three doses of toxoid, there is no need for HTIG. Toxoid booster is required if >5 years (10 years for minor clean wounds) has elapsed.
- For patients who received fewer than three doses, primary immunization series should be started. HTIG 250 units IM should be given prophylactically, except for fresh, clean, minor wounds. Toxoid and antiserum must be given with separate syringes to different sites.

ALTERNATIVE DRUGS

- Pooled human intravenous immunoglobulin may be an alternative to HTIG.

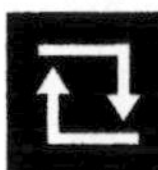

Follow-Up

PATIENT MONITORING

- Sequela are uncommon once the patient heals, although focal deficits such as exotropia and facial muscle paresis have rarely been reported. However, because the infection does not provide natural immunity, primary immunization should be completed.

EXPECTED COURSE AND PROGNOSIS

- Tetanus is self-limited, and patients who recover from the disease have no residual defect. The disease usually subsides within 3–6 weeks. Mortality rate is 50%. For neonatal tetanus, mortality goes up to 60%–80%. Death usually occurs 3–10 days after infection, mostly due to asphyxiation during spasms, cardiovascular insufficiency, or superimposed infections.

PATIENT EDUCATION

- Centers for Disease Control and Prevention. Website: *www.cdc.gov/nip/vaccine/nip-dtp.htm*
- World Health Organization. Website: *www.who.int/gpv-dvacc/diseases/NeonatalTetanus.htm*

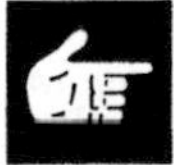

Miscellaneous

SYNONYMS

N/A

ICD-9-CM: 037 Tetanus; 771.3 Tetanus neonatorum; 670 Puerperal tetanus

SEE ALSO: N/A

REFERENCES

- Advisory Committee on Immunization Practices. Diphtheria, tetanus, and pertussis: recommendations for vaccine use and other preventive measures. MMWR 1991;40:1–28.
- Sutter RW, Orenstein WA, Wassilak SG. Tetanus. In: Hoeprich PD, Jordan MC, Ronald AR, eds. Infectious diseases. Philadelphia: JB Lippincott, 1994: 1175–1185.

Author(s): Sevim Erdem, MD

Tics

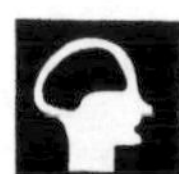

Basics

DESCRIPTION

- Tics are relatively brief involuntary movements (motor tics) or sounds (vocal tics) that usually are intermittent but may be repetitive and stereotypic. They fluctuating or wax and wane in frequency, intensity, and distribution. Typically tics can be volitionally suppressed, although this may require intense mental effort. Motor tics may persist during all stages of sleep. Tics typically are exacerbated by dopaminergic drugs and by CNS stimulants, including methylphenidate and cocaine.
- Premonitory feelings or sensations precede motor and vocal tics in >80% of patients. These premonitory phenomena may be localizable sensations or discomfort, or no localizable, less specific, and poorly described feeling such as an urge, anxiety, and anger.
- The "intentional" component of the movement may be a useful feature differentiating tics from other hyperkinetic movement disorders.

EPIDEMIOLOGY

Incidence/Prevalence

- Reported prevalence rates have varied markedly. The frequency of tics depends on the definition of the phenotype. Transient tic disorders occur relatively commonly in children (3%–15% in different studies), and chronic motor tics occur in approximately 2%–5%, although "chronic" may extend only 2–3 years in many of these individuals.
- Because about one third of patients do not even recognize the tics, it is difficult to derive an accurate prevalence figure.

Age

- Onset is usually in childhood.

Sex

- Boys are much more likely than girls to have chronic tics. The male-to-female ratio in chronic motor tic disorder is approximately 5:1 (between 2:1 and 10:1 in different studies).

ETIOLOGY

- Most of the tic disorders are idiopathic. The pathogenetic mechanisms of tics and Tourette's syndrome are unknown, but evidence supports an organic rather than psychogenic origin.

Genetics

- Probable mixed model of inheritance, rather than simple autosomal mode of transmission.
- Tourette's syndrome is the most common cause of tics, manifested by a broad spectrum of motor and behavioral disturbances.

RISK FACTORS

- Family history of obsessive-compulsive disorder

PREGNANCY

N/A

ASSOCIATED CONDITIONS

- Obsessive-compulsive behavior
- Hyperactivity with attention deficit and impulsive behavior
- Static encephalopathy
- Autistic spectrum disorders
- Neuroacanthocytosis
- Huntington's disease
- Dopamine receptor antagonists
- Cocaine
- Antiepileptic drugs
- Copropraxia (obscene gesture)
- Mannerism
- Stereotypes
- Compulsion

Diagnosis

DIFFERENTIAL DIAGNOSIS

- Abnormal movements that may accompany general medical conditions
- Drugs: stimulants, levodopa, neuroleptics, carbamazepine, phenytoin, phenobarbital, cocaine
- Complex partial seizures
- Neuroacanthocytosis
- Chorea in adults
- Postherpetic chorea in children
- Post stoke
- Frontal lobe syndromes
- Hallervorden-Spatz disease
- Hemifacial spasm
- Huntington's disease
- Inherited metabolic disorders
- Mental retardation
- Movement disorders in individuals with developmental disabilities
- Neurosyphilis
- Periodic limb movement disorder
- Restless legs syndrome
- Tardive dyskinesia
- Tuberous sclerosis
- Wilson's disease

SIGNS AND SYMPTOMS

- Tics may be *simple* or *complex.*

Simple Tics

- Simple tics involve only one group of muscles, causing a brief jerklike movement or a single meaningless sound.
  - —Simple vocal tics: throat clearing, sniffing, animal sounds (e.g., barking), coughing, yelling, hiccuping, belching
  - —Simple motor tics: eye blinking, nose twitching, sticking tongue out, head turning or neck stretching, shoulder jerking, muscle tensing, flexing fingers, blepharospasm, bruxism

Complex Tics

- Complex tics consist of coordinated sequenced movements resembling normal motor acts or gestures that are inappropriately intense and timed. They may be seemingly not purposeful or they may seem purposeful.
  - —Complex vocal tics: parts of words or phrases repeated, talking to oneself in multiple characters, assuming different intonations, *coprolalia* (use of profanity)
  - —Complex motor tics: flapping arms, facial grimaces, picking at clothing, complex touching movements, jumping, shaking feet, pinching, poking, spitting, hair brushing
  - —Also classified as
    - -Transient (duration <12 months)
    - -Chronic (duration >12 consecutive months)
- Neurologic examination in patients with tics usually is normal.

LABORATORY PROCEDURES

- Diagnosis of a tic is generally made during physical examination. If there are no other neurologic findings, tics required no additional diagnostic testing. If other neurologic signs or symptoms are present, further evaluation is guided by that finding.

IMAGING STUDIES

- Imaging studies are not needed routinely in the evaluation of patients with typical history and examination findings and are indicated only to exclude specific illnesses suggested by abnormal historical or examination findings.
- At present, no clinical utility exists for functional imaging studies in the evaluation of tic disorders.

SPECIAL TESTS

- Neuropsychological testing: Patients with difficulties in the school or work setting may benefit from identification of an existing learning disorder so that adaptive strategies can be devised.

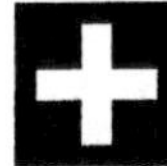

Management

GENERAL MEASURES

- The goal of treatment should not be to completely eliminate all tics but to achieve a tolerable suppression.
- First step is proper education of the patient, relatives, and teachers about the nature of the disorder.
- Counseling and behavioral modification may be sufficient for mild symptoms.
- Medication should be considered when symptoms begin to interfere with activities of daily living.

SURGICAL MEASURES

- There are a few reports of patients with severe motor and phonic tics controlled by high-frequency deep brain stimulation

SYMPTOMATIC TREATMENT

- Symptomatic treatment consists of behavioral management:
  —Positive reinforcement
  —Target behaviors
    -Skill deficiencies
    -Behavior excesses

ADJUNCTIVE TREATMENT

N/A

ADMISSION/DISCHARGE CRITERIA

- Admission for management of tics is rarely necessary.

Medications

DRUG(S) OF CHOICE

- Dopamine D_2 receptor antagonists: Chlorpromazine was reported to dramatically improve tic severity. Since then, several placebo-controlled randomized allocation studies with various neuroleptics (e.g., haloperidol, fluphenazine, pimozide) have confirmed these initial reports. On average, tic severity declines by approximately 50%–80% with neuroleptic treatment.
  —Haloperidol (Haldol): FDA indication for treatment of tics
  —Pimozide (Orap): FDA indication for treatment of tics
  —Fluphenazine (Prolixin): effective anti-tic drug
  —If these three drugs fail to adequately control tics, then risperidone (Risperdal), thioridazine (Mellaril), trifluoperazine (Stelazine), molindone (Moban), or thiothixene (Navane) can be tried.
  —It is not clear whether some of the new atypical neuroleptics, such as clozapine and olanzapine, will be effective in the treatment of tics or other manifestations of Tourette's syndrome.
  —Clonidine: This drug has been used frequently to treat tics. However, no proof exists for anti-tic efficacy after several small trials. A meta-analysis concluded that clonidine has clear efficacy. It may be most appropriate as a first agent in patients with problematic attention deficit hyperactivity disorder (ADHD) and mild tics.
- Mild-to-moderate tic disorder medications
  —Pimozide superior to Haldol in one double-blind study
  —Fluphenazine another good choice
  —Clonidine (Catapres) 0.05 mg PO bid to 0.1 mg PO qid
- Severe tic disorder medications: neuroleptic preparations
  —Haloperidol (Haldol) 0.5–4 mg PO qhs
  —Pimozide (Orap) 1–8 mg PO qhs
  —Risperidone (Risperdal)

Precautions

- Use the lowest dose of medication that achieves acceptable tic suppression.
- Neuroleptics may be associated with various extrapyramidal side effects, including dystonia, akathisia, and tardive dyskinesia in up to 20% of children.
- Sedation, depression, weight gain, school phobia, tardive dyskinesia, hepatotoxicity, prolongation of QT interval with pimozide, akathisia, and acute dystonic reaction

Contraindications

- None of these drugs should be used if there is a known hypersensitivity.
- Pimozide is contraindicated in patients with the long QT syndrome because it may prolong the QT interval. There are a few reports of deaths when pimozide is used in conjunction with macrolide antibiotics, so this drug combination should be avoided.

ALTERNATIVE DRUGS

- Benzodiazepines: Retrospective reports suggest that benzodiazepines, such as clonazepam, reduce tic severity in some patients. The effect is less than that of neuroleptics and is probably nonspecific. Clonazepam (Klonopin) 0.25 mg PO bid to 1 mg PO tid.
- Botulinum toxin injections in motor tics: Botulinum toxin injections may improve urges or sensory tics, as well as observable tics, and may be the treatment of choice for patients with a single, especially problematic, dystonic tic.
- Tetrabenazine: This is a presynaptic dopamine-depleting agent. It has not been reported to cause tardive movement disorders. A retrospective report noted "marked" clinical improvement in 57% of 47 patients with tics. It is not available in United States.
- Guanfacine: This agent was tested in a 2001 randomized controlled trial in children with both ADHD and chronic tic disorders. The drug showed clear superiority to placebo in reduction of both ADHD and tic symptoms, with few adverse effects. It also has been shown to be efficacious in adults with non-tic ADHD.
- An open trial using nicotine patch indicates that nicotine may suppress tics in patients not treated with D_2 receptor-blocking drugs.

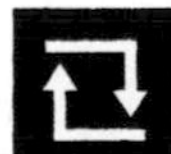

Follow-Up

PATIENT MONITORING

- Because a medication for tics may not have any impact on obsessions or compulsions, and medications for ADHD may worsen tics in some patients, the selection of medications and combination of medications can become quite complex in a situation with associated or comorbid conditions.

EXPECTED COURSE AND PROGNOSIS

- The prognosis for children who develop this disorder between the ages of 6 and 8 is good.
- Symptoms may last 4–6 years and then disappear without treatment in early adolescence.
- When the disorder begins in older children and there is no remission or reduction of symptoms well into the 20s, a chronic, lifelong disorder may be anticipated.

PATIENT EDUCATION

- WeMove. Website: *www.wemove.org*

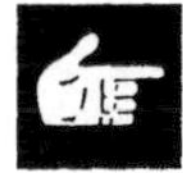

Miscellaneous

SYNONYMS

N/A

ICD-9-CM: 307.20 Tics; 307.21 Tics, transient of childhood; 307.22 Tics and spasms, compulsive

SEE ALSO: TOURETTE'S SYNDROME

REFERENCES

- Kurlan R, Como PG, Miller B, et al. The behavioral spectrum of tic disorders: a community-based study. Neurology 2002;59:414–420.
- Marras C, Andrews D, Sime E, et al. Botulinum toxin for simple motor tics: a randomized, double-blind, controlled clinical trial. Neurology 2001;56:605–610.
- Schlaggar BL, Mink JW. Movement disorders in children. Pediatr Rev 2003;24:39–51.
- The Tourette's Syndrome Study Group. Treatment of ADHD in children with tics: a randomized controlled trial. Neurology 2002;58:527–536.

Author(s): Muhammad I. Akhtar, MD

Torticollis

Basics

DESCRIPTION

- Torticollis is a term used to describe disorders characterized by abnormal postures of the head and neck. Cervical dystonia (CD) is the preferred term for the idiopathic movement disorder that causes involuntary contraction of the cervical muscles, resulting in clonic (spasmodic, tremor) head movements and/or tonic (sustained) head deviation. Head deviation can be described as follows: torticollis, torsion or rotation of the head; anterocollis, flexion of the neck, head forward; retrocollis, extension of the neck, head backward; or laterocollis, tilt of the head to one side.

EPIDEMIOLOGY

Incidence

- CD is the most common form of focal dystonia, onset most commonly in early to mid life with a female predominance. Torticollis and laterocollis are the most common head deviations; retrocollis and anterocollis are more rare. Most patients have combinations of neck deviations depending on the cervical muscles involved. Tremor is common with the tonic head deviation. There may be other dystonias and tremor involving facial, buccal-lingual, mandibular, and other body parts. The clinical course of CD is variable; most patients report some progression of symptoms. Spontaneous remission is rare (10%–20%) Torticollis is a disorder of middle and late life. Torticollis in childhood is more likely to be acquired and nondystonic. In infancy, congenital muscular torticollis is the most common cause of restricted range of motion of the head.

ETIOLOGY

- Torticollis may be dystonic (either idiopathic, cause unknown, or secondary, related to some other process) or nondystonic (due to a mechanical process). The pathologic localization and mechanism underlying idiopathic CD is not well understood. The basal ganglia and vestibular system are implicated. Torticollis has a broad differential diagnosis (see below).

Genetics

- Genetic mechanisms may play a role.

RISK FACTORS

- Torticollis usually occurs spontaneously, and there are no specific risk factors for its development.

PREGNANCY

- Torticollis is not associated with pregnancy. In terms of treatment, botulinum toxin is not approved for use during pregnancy. Other medications should be avoided if possible during pregnancy.

ASSOCIATED CONDITIONS

- Torticollis may be idiopathic or secondary to other conditions (listed below). Head tremor is commonly associated with torticollis and may confuse the examiner.

Diagnosis

DIFFERENTIAL DIAGNOSIS

Dystonic Conditions

- Idiopathic:
  - —Primary focal dystonia (CD)
  - —Associated with more generalized dystonia
- Secondary:
  - —Associated with neurologic degenerative illnesses, e.g., parkinsonism (MSA, PSP, IPD), Huntington's disease, Wilson's disease
  - —Associated with metabolic disorders, e.g., amino acid disorders (such as homocystinuria), lipid storage disorders (such as metachromatic leukodystrophy), Lehigh's disease
  - —Associated with other causes, e.g., perinatal injury (cerebral palsy), infection (encephalitis, Jakob-Creutzfeldt disease, syphilis), head trauma/cervical trauma, multiple sclerosis, stroke
  - —Associated with toxins, e.g., manganese, carbon monoxide, methane
  - —Associated with drugs, e.g., levodopa, dopamine agonists, neuroleptics, dopamine-blocking agents

Nondystonic Head Tilt

- Structural (mechanical):
  - —Cervical spine fracture
  - —Dislocation
  - —Disc herniation
  - —Cervical region abscess
  - —Congenital fibrous bands
- Neurologic:
  - —Vestibulo-visual: fourth nerve palsy, hemianopia
  - —Posterior fossa tumor
  - —Spinal cord tumor
  - —Arnold-Chiari malformation
  - —Focal seizures
  - —Cervical myopathy
  - —Myasthenia gravis
- Psychogenic

SIGNS AND SYMPTOMS

- Head deviation: rotation, tilt, flexion, extension, or some combination
- Tremor: if present, may be essential type involving head ("no direction"), oscillatory, jerky, or spasmodic
- Cervical pain: nonradicular, aching, or radicular
- Palpable spasm and hypertrophy of muscle may be present
- Head deviation can be controlled temporarily by counterpressure and sensory tricks, *geste antagoniste:* touching chin, face, or back of head.
- Exacerbation occurs during periods of fatigue and stress.

LABORATORY PROCEDURES

- With onset in patient <50 years old, obtain serum ceruloplasmin and liver function tests to exclude Wilson's disease.
- Review drug exposure (especially dopamine-blocking agents, i.e., neuroleptics, metoclopramide).
- Consider magnetic resonance imaging of neck to exclude structural etiologies.
- Consider genetic testing if there is a strong family history of dystonia.
- Consider other laboratory studies (ANA, ESR, RPR, CBC, electrolytes, renal, and liver function tests) if history or physical examination suggests the condition.

IMAGING STUDIES

- There is no specific imaging abnormality demonstrable in idiopathic CD. However, appropriate imaging studies may be indicated to identify nondystonic forms of torticollis.

SPECIAL TESTS

N/A

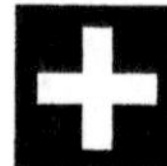

Management

GENERAL MEASURES

- Physical measures such as stretching, heat, and physical therapy may be considered. The role of such measures is limited in idiopathic torticollis.

SURGICAL MEASURES

- Rhizotomy, neurectomy, or myotomy has been advocated for patients who do not respond to chemodenervation and medical pharmacotherapy. Currently the application of basal ganglia ablative surgery (i.e., thalamotomy) and deep brain stimulation is considered only for treatment of more generalized forms of dystonia.

SYMPTOMATIC TREATMENT

- Nonpharmacologic therapies such as biofeedback, hypnosis, relaxation techniques, acupuncture, and other modalities have been used in torticollis but are generally unhelpful. Botulinum therapy has become the standard of care.

ADJUNCTIVE TREATMENT

- There occasionally may be a role for sensory feedback therapy or relaxation techniques in the relief of associative symptoms such as pain.

ADMISSION/DISCHARGE CRITERIA

N/A

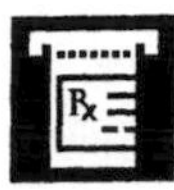

Medications

DRUG(S) OF CHOICE

Chemodenervation, Botulinum Toxin Treatment

- Botulinum injections are the treatment of choice for torticollis (CD), both idiopathic and secondary forms. Botulinum toxin injections block acetylcholine release, causing focal neuromuscular junction blockade. By selectively injecting various doses into affected muscles, the symptoms of CD and other dystonias often are dramatically relieved. Repeated injections often are necessary every few weeks or months, depending on the response.

Contraindications

- Neuromuscular disorders such as Lambert-Eaton syndrome and myasthenia gravis are relative contraindications to botulinum toxin use. It also should be avoided in myopathies and in motor neuron disorders.

Precautions

- Botulinum injections should be administered only by a physician expert in the diagnosis and treatment of dystonias and in the administration of this medication. Side effects are rare when used appropriately. Subcutaneous hematomas and pneumothorax have been reported. Temporary muscle weakness is a predictable response to this therapy. Occasionally temporary dysphagia occurs with higher doses. Secondary resistance to botulinum toxin is becoming an issue in clinical practice.

ALTERNATIVE DRUGS

- Anticholinergic agents (trihexyphenidyl)
  —Often require high doses with significant side effects
  —Dry mouth, urine retention, psychosis
- Tricyclic antidepressants (amitriptyline)
  —Often requires high doses with significant side effects
  —Dry mouth, urine retention, weight gain
- Benzodiazepines (clonazepam, lorazepam)
  —Antispasticity agents (baclofen)
- For tremor component of torticollis
  —Primidone
  —Benzodiazepine
  —β-Blocker

Follow-Up

PATIENT MONITORING

- Patients undergoing botulinum toxin injections should be monitored for response to medication and evaluated at regular appointments, usually every 3 months, for repeated injections. No routine laboratory or imaging studies required.

EXPECTED COURSE AND PROGNOSIS

- Approximately 60%–80% of patients benefit from botulinum toxin injections, usually with reduced but not completely abolished symptoms.

PATIENT EDUCATION

- Patients should be made aware of the risk of muscle weakness, dysphagia, bruising, and rarely pneumothorax with botulinum injections. They should know that treatment is temporary and needs close follow-up. They should understand that torticollis is a treatable condition that usually does not cause major disability.

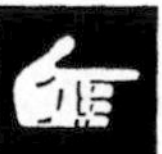

Miscellaneous

SYNONYMS

- Cervical dystonia
- Spasmodic torticollis
- Wry neck
- Stiff neck
- Capitium obstipum
- Rhaebocrania
- See Description

ICD-9-CM: 723.5 Torticollis, unspecified; excludes: 754.1 Congenital; 767.8 Due to birth injury; 300.1 Hysterical; 306.0 Psychogenic; 333.83 Spasmodic; 847.0 Traumatic, current; 333.7 Due to drugs; 333.83 Spasmodic torticollis (idiopathic cervical dystonia)

SEE ALSO: DYSTONIA; DYSTONIC REACTION (BOTULINUM TOXIN, ACUTE CERVICAL DYSTONIA); PARKINSON'S DISEASE

REFERENCES

- Claypool D, Duane D, Ilstrup D, et al. Epidemiology and outcome of cervical dystonia (spasmodic torticollis) in Rochester, Minnesota. Mov Disord 1995;10: 608–614.
- Freidman J, Standaert D. Dystonia and its disorders. Neurol Clin 2001;19:681–705.
- Jankovic J, Leder S, Warner D, et al. Cervical dystonia: clinical findings and associative movement disorders. Neurology 1991;41:1088–1091.
- Jankovic J, Tolosa E. Dystonic disorders, cervical dystonia. In: Jankovic J, Tolosa E, eds. Parkinson's disease and movement disorders, 2nd ed. Baltimore: Williams & Wilkins, 1993.
- Jankovic J, Tolosa E. Dystonic disorders, classification of dystonia. In: Jankovic J, Tolosa E, eds. Parkinson's disease and movement disorders, 2nd ed. Baltimore: Williams & Wilkins, 1993.
- Jankovic J, Tolosa E. Dystonic disorders, surgical treatment. In: Jankovic J, Tolosa E, eds. Parkinson's disease and movement disorders, 2nd ed. Baltimore: Williams & Wilkins, 1993.

Author(s): Peter Barbour, MD

Tourette's Syndrome

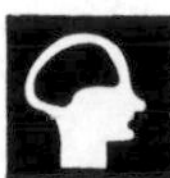

Basics

DESCRIPTION

- Tics are a movement disorder characterized by brief, repetitive, stereotyped movements or sounds. Tic disorders are classified along a spectrum based on severity.
  - —Transient tic disorder: single or multiple motor and/or vocal tics, which have occurred for <1 year
  - —Chronic tic disorder: single or multiple motor or vocal tics, but not both, which have persisted for >1 year
  - —Tourette's syndrome (TS): multiple motor and one or more vocal tics, which have persisted for >1 year

EPIDEMIOLOGY

Prevalence

- The exact prevalence of TS is unknown, but estimates range from 2.9–49.5 per 100,000 children.

Race

- TS has been reported in all races, with no ethnic predominance.

Age

- Tics begin most commonly by age 6–7 years and always before 18 years.

Sex

- Males are more commonly affected than females.

ETIOLOGY

- Penetrance is 70% in females and 99% in males.
- Streptococcal infection may play a triggering role in genetically susceptible individuals.

Genetics

- TS is a genetic disorder with an autosomal dominant pattern of inheritance, although the gene has not yet been identified.

RISK FACTORS

- There are no identified risk factors other than genetic and possibly streptococcal infection.
- In patients with TS, however, stress, fatigue, and excitement may exacerbate tics.

PREGNANCY

N/A

ASSOCIATED CONDITIONS

- 50% of patients with TS have attention deficit hyperactivity disorder (ADHD).
- 50% of patients with TS have obsessive-compulsive disorder (OCD).
- There is a higher incidence of learning disabilities in children with TS.
- Self-injurious behaviors, such as hitting or biting oneself, may occur.

Diagnosis

DIFFERENTIAL DIAGNOSIS

- Chorea
- Myoclonus
- Seizures

SIGNS AND SYMPTOMS

- Tics develop abruptly, with initial tics usually being motor tics. Common motor tics include eye blinking, head jerking, and facial grimacing.
- Vocal tics include throat clearing, sniffing, grunting, and coughing. Coprolalia, which is involuntary swearing, develops in about 10% of patients and is not usually present until 4–7 years after initial symptoms.
- Tics vary in frequency, location, type, and severity. Although initial tics may involve the head, over time the tics often involve the limbs and trunk.
- Tics may spontaneously wax and wane, and there may be periods of days to months when all symptoms disappear. They also change over time, with one tic disappearing and another developing.
- Patients can voluntarily suppress tics for varying periods of time; however, the suppression creates an inner tension and eventually the tics must be released.
- Tics may occur during sleep.

LABORATORY PROCEDURES

- There is no laboratory test that is diagnostic for TS.
- The diagnosis is based on clinical criteria.
- If there is a preceding history of sore throat, tests for streptococcal infection including ASO titer or streptozyme may be indicated.

IMAGING STUDIES

- Neuroimaging studies do not show any structural abnormalities and are not helpful in making the diagnosis

SPECIAL TESTS

- No special tests are indicated.
- EEG and CSF examinations are not helpful.

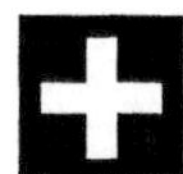

Management

GENERAL MEASURES

- Explaining the nature of TS to the child and family is the most important initial intervention.
- Parents need to know that tics are involuntary and that children should not be punished for symptoms they cannot control.
- They also need to understand that tics are not a sign of psychological disease but that stress can exacerbate the symptoms.
- Any events or conditions that exacerbate tics should be identified and eliminated if possible.
- Parents should be educated to ignore tics as much as possible, because focusing attention on them often increases the frequency of tics.
- Management should focus on educational issues that may result from the tics or associated ADHD or OCD.

SURGICAL MEASURES

- There is no surgical treatment for TS.

SYMPTOMATIC TREATMENT

- Pharmacotherapy is indicated for children whose symptoms impair their psychosocial or educational functioning.

ADJUNCTIVE TREATMENT

- In patients with obsessive-compulsive symptoms, behavioral therapy in conjunction with pharmacotherapy may be helpful.
- Educational intervention may be required to optimize academic success.

ADMISSION/DISCHARGE CRITERIA

- It is very unusual for patients with TS to require admission for their symptoms.

Medications

DRUG(S) OF CHOICE

Tics

- Haloperidol is effective in decreasing tics in about 80% of patients.
- A dose of 0.5 mg qhs is started, with an increase of 0.25–0.5 mg weekly until satisfactory tic control is achieved. Doses >4 mg qd rarely are required. After the tics are controlled for a few months, the medication can be slowly tapered as tolerated.

Contraindications

- None in children with tics other than hypersensitivity to the drug

Precautions

- Patients need to be monitored for lethargy, weight gain, personality changes, cognitive impairment, and school phobia. Tardive dyskinesia is a potential side effect from use of haloperidol, but this rarely occurs in children with tics.
- Clonidine reduces tics in some children and can also be helpful for treatment of ADHD.
- A dose of 0.05 mg qd is started and increased by 0.05 mg q5–7 days to a maximum of 0.2–0.3 mg/day. Clonidine has a short half-life, so tid or qid dosing often is required. The patch form has the advantage of providing a constant level of medication.

Contraindications

- Hypotension

Precautions

- Patients need to be monitored for sedation and hypotension and, in those treated with the transdermal form, skin reaction. It is advisable not to abruptly stop the medication because of the risk of hypertension.

ADHD

- Stimulants such as methylphenidate or dextroamphetamine can improve the attention span and help with impulsive behavior.
- The dose of methylphenidate is 0.3–0.6 mg/kg per dose given 2–3 times qd.

Contraindications

- None

Precautions

- Stimulants may exacerbate tics in some children. Decreased appetite and insomnia may occur.

OCD

- Clomipramine or one of the newer serotonin reuptake inhibitors, such as fluoxetine, sertraline, fluvoxamine, or paroxetine, may help decrease OCD symptoms. These medications usually must be given for 4–6 weeks before improvement is seen.
- The daily dose of clomipramine is 1–3 mg/kg in children and 250 mg in adults. Usual doses of fluoxetine range from 10–40 mg/day, sertraline 50–100 mg/day, fluvoxamine 50–200 mg/day, and paroxetine 20–40 mg/day.

Contraindications

- Clomipramine is contraindicated in patients with hypersensitivity to tricyclic antidepressants. Fluoxetine, fluvoxamine, and paroxetine should not be used in combination with MAO inhibitors. Fluvoxamine also cannot be used with terfenadine, astemizole, and cisapride.

Precautions

- ECG monitoring before and during treatment with clomipramine is recommended.

ALTERNATIVE DRUGS

- Pimozide is as effective as haloperidol for tic suppression; however, because of reported ECG changes at higher doses it is not a first-line drug.
- Fluphenazine is another alternative treatment for tics.
- Guanfacine, which is similar to clonidine, can be used to treat both tics and ADHD.
- Risperidone is an atypical neuroleptic that may improve tics and can be helpful for impulsive and oppositional behavior.

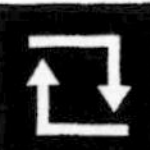

Follow-Up

PATIENT MONITORING

- Patients with mild symptoms who do not need medications can be followed on an as-needed basis. Patients with more severe symptoms will need follow-up every few weeks to months to monitor medication response, school progress, and psychosocial issues.

EXPECTED COURSE AND PROGNOSIS

- Approximately one third of patients have complete remission of tics by late adolescence. An additional third of patients report that their tics significantly lessen in frequency and severity by late adolescence. The remaining third of patients continue to be symptomatic into adulthood, although in some there is continuing gradual improvement throughout life.
- ADHD symptoms tend to improve during the adolescent years, although some patients continue to have symptoms that may affect their occupation.
- OCD symptoms, which tend to begin later than tics, may persist and have a negative impact on the patient's life.

PATIENT EDUCATION

- The Tourette Syndrome Association provides many services for patients, families, physicians, and caregivers. Local chapters throughout the country provide additional services, including support groups. Tourette Syndrome Association, 42-40 Bell Boulevard, Bayside, NY 11361-2820. Phone: 718-224-2999, fax: 718-279-9596, website: *http://tsa.mga.harvard.edu*

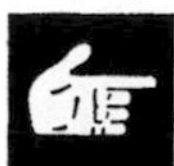

Miscellaneous

SYNONYMS

- Gilles de la Tourette syndrome

ICD-9-CM: 307.21 Transient tic disorder; 307.22 Chronic motor or vocal tic disorder; 307.23 Tourette's disorder; 307.20 Tic disorder not otherwise specified

SEE ALSO: N/A

REFERENCES

- Chase TN, Friedhoff AJ, Cohen DJ, eds. Advances in neurology, Tourette syndrome: genetics, neurobiology, and treatment. New York: Raven Press, 1992.
- Kurlan R, ed. Handbook of Tourette's syndrome and related tic and behavioral disorders. New York: Marcel Dekker, 1993.
- Leckman JF, Cohen DJ. Tourette's syndrome—tics, obsessions, compulsions. New York: John Wiley & Sons, 1999.
- Singer HS, Giuliano JD, Hansen BS, et al. Antibodies against human putamen in children with Tourette syndrome. Neurology 1998;50:1618–1624.

Author(s): Sarah M. Roddy, MD

Transverse Myelitis

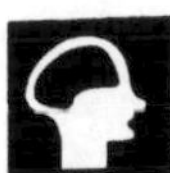

Basics

DESCRIPTION

- Transverse myelitis (TM) is a syndrome of inflammation of the spinal cord, usually involving multiple segments and both gray and white matter, with resultant myelopathy or spinal cord dysfunction.

EPIDEMIOLOGY

Incidence/Prevalence

- TM is uncommon, with an incidence estimated at 1–5 cases per million.

Race

- No study has demonstrated any ethnic predominance.

Age

- All ages affected, with peak incidence in the third and fourth decades.

Sex

- Males and females are equally affected.

ETIOLOGY

- The cause of TM is largely unknown. Approximately one third of cases occur during or shortly after an infectious illness such as mycoplasma, schistosomiasis, cytomegalovirus, Ebstein-Barr virus, mumps, and varicella. Although some infections may attack the spinal cord by direct invasion, it has been hypothesized that other systemic infections may invoke a cell-mediated autoimmune response with sensitization of lymphocytes to spinal cord antigens.
- Another subset of TM is associated with autoimmune disorders including systemic lupus erythematosus (SLE), Sjögren's syndrome, sarcoidosis, and multiple sclerosis.

Genetics

- None identified

RISK FACTORS

- Systemic illness, especially respiratory

PREGNANCY

- Little is known about any relationship of TM to pregnancy.

ASSOCIATED CONDITIONS

- Multiple sclerosis
- SLE
- Devic's disease

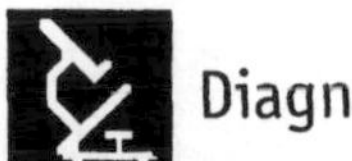

Diagnosis

DIFFERENTIAL DIAGNOSIS

- Extrinsic cord compression
  —Vertebral metastases
  —Benign tumors such as meningioma
  —Disc herniation
  —Spinal canal stenosis
- Spinal arteriovenous malformation
- Epidural abscess
- Spinal cord infarction
- Autoimmune disorders
  —Multiple sclerosis
  —SLE
  —Sjögren's syndrome
  —Sarcoidosis
  —Paraneoplastic
  —Infectious myelitis: bacterial, viral, tuberculous, syphilitic, fungal, parasitic
  —Myelopathy associated with intravenous opiate use

SIGNS AND SYMPTOMS

- TM symptoms develop rapidly over several hours to several weeks. Approximately 45% of patients reach maximal deficit within 24 hours. Most patients develop leg weakness of varying degrees of severity. The arms are involved in a minority of cases. Initial muscle tone is flaccid, with spasticity developing over hours to days. Sensation is diminished below the level of spinal cord involvement. Some patients experience tingling paresthesias or numbness. Bowel and bladder dysfunction occurs in the majority of patients. Many patients with TM complain of a tight banding or girdlelike sensation around the trunk.

LABORATORY PROCEDURES

- Blood work: There are no specific blood tests to diagnose TM, but the following tests should be obtained to identify potential underlying causes: CBC/differential, RPR, ANA, double-stranded DNA, anti-SSA antibody, anti-SSB antibody, serum vitamin B_{12} level, human immunodeficiency virus antibody, human T-cell leukemia virus (HTLV-1) antibody, and serum angiotensin-converting enzyme.

IMAGING STUDIES

- MRI with T2-weighted images and contrast enhancement should be performed of the complete spinal cord urgently. If MRI is contraindicated, myelogram should be performed. The most immediate purpose is to rule out a compressive lesion of the cord requiring surgical decompression. MRI also gives information about inflammation of the spinal cord and may suggest multiple sclerosis, intramedullary tumor, or abscess. Lesions with hyperintense signal on T2-weighted images over several cord segments are often found in TM. Sometimes the cord is swollen. Cranial MRI is helpful to explore the possibility of multiple sclerosis.

SPECIAL TESTS

- Cerebrospinal fluid (CSF) should be sent for cell count, differential, total protein, protein electrophoresis, IgG index, Gram stain, and bacterial culture, cryptococcal antigen, fungal culture, acid-fast bacilli smear and culture, and viral titers or cultures. CSF examination typically shows a lymphocytic pleocytosis with normal or elevated total protein level. Oligoclonal bands are present in 20%–40% of patients with TM.

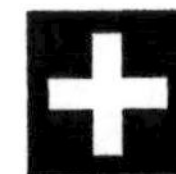

Management

GENERAL MEASURES

- Specific treatment should be given if any underlying cause of TM is detected. Examples include antibiotics for bacterial infections and antiviral agents such as acyclovir for TM associated with varicella-zoster or herpes simplex virus. More aggressive immunosuppression with cyclophosphamide is generally considered if the patient is identified to have SLE. Otherwise, most neurologists would administer high-dose intravenous methylprednisolone for idiopathic or postinfectious TM.
- Respiratory function should be monitored closely with forced vital capacity for hypoventilation in the acute phase for high cervical TM. Patients with high cervical lesions may require intubation for airway protection if they are not handling secretions well.
- Prophylactic treatment should be given for deep vein thrombosis (DVT) in patients who are immobilized with either air compression boots or SQ heparin 5,000 U bid. A high index of suspicion should be maintained for DVT and pulmonary embolism (PE) should suggestive symptoms arise.
- Urinary retention is frequent. Bladder function should be checked frequently in the acute phase to rule out retention. Intermittent catheterization often is required to prevent bladder distention. A bowel program should be taught. Patients with immobilization should have attention to frequent repositioning and padding to prevent decubitus ulceration. Splints and range of motion may be required to prevent joint contractures.

SURGICAL MEASURES

- There are no surgical procedures for TM. Sometimes the cord is shown to be swollen and a spinal cord tumor cannot be excluded. Biopsy of the cord should be cautiously considered in that case.

SYMPTOMATIC TREATMENT

- Spasticity may be a subacute or even long-term problem. It may be ameliorated by
  —Baclofen at a dosage of 10 mg 1–2 times daily titrated up to an effective dose to maximum of 100 mg or even 200 mg daily if severe, divided in 3–4 doses per day.
  —Tizanidine may be used as an alternative agent if baclofen is not tolerated. Start with 2 mg daily and gradually increase by 2 mg every 3–4 days up to a maximum of 32 mg daily in three doses per day. Tizanidine may cause less weakness than baclofen. Liver function tests must be monitored.
  —Diazepam 2–10 mg 3 times a day or clonazepam 0.5–1.0 mg 3 times a day may relieve spasticity but use often is limited to nighttime because of concomitant sedation.
- Bladder dysfunction: Patients may develop several different patterns of bladder dysfunction. Checking postvoid residuals and cystometric studies may help to sort out the problem.
  —Hypertonic bladder: Oxybutynin 2.5–5 mg PO taken 2–3 times per day or propantheline bromide 15-mg PO qhs and 7.5–15 mg tid during the day.
- Constipation
  —Patient's fluid intake should be increased to 2 to 2.5 L daily
  —Bulking agents, stool softeners, rectal stimulation (e.g., with glycerin or Dulcolax suppositories), and Theravac mini-enemas may be helpful.
- Neuropathic pain: Many patients complain of neuropathic pain as a long-term residuum of TM. This should be managed with trials of agents such as gabapentin 100–900 mg PO tid, amitriptyline 25–150 mg PO qhs, or carbamazepine 100–200 mg daily, with gradual increase to 600–1,600 mg daily in 3–4 doses.

ADJUNCTIVE TREATMENTS

- Physical therapy with passive and active range of motion and occupational therapy should be started as soon as possible to prevent contractures and hasten functional recovery.

ADMISSION/DISCHARGE CRITERIA

- Patients are generally admitted for acute evaluation and administration of intravenous steroid therapy. Patients with significant weakness should be evaluated for consideration of inpatient acute rehabilitation.

Medications

DRUG(S) OF CHOICE

- Methylprednisolone 1 g IV qd for 3–5 days followed by an oral taper of prednisone is given for patients with no identifiable infectious. There is no standard taper used in practice, but a typical regimen might be to start with 1 mg/kg prednisone qd and then taper by 10 mg every 3 days.

Contraindications

- Known hypersensitivity to corticosteroids

Precautions

- Diabetes mellitus, hypertension

ALTERNATIVE DRUGS

N/A

Follow-Up

PATIENT MONITORING

- Patients should be monitored to make sure that they are stabilized and followed as outpatients to facilitate rehabilitation during recovery.

EXPECTED COURSE AND PROGNOSIS

- Approximately 45% of patients develop maximal neurologic deficit within 24 hours. In one series, recovery was judged to be good in 33%, fair in 48%, and poor in 25%. Recovery generally begins between 1 and 3 months after onset of symptoms. Back pain or spinal shock at onset is associated with poorer outcome. Recovery is unlikely if no improvement is seen in the first month. TM is generally a monophasic illness, but relapses have been reported in idiopathic or postinfectious TM. Recurrent myelopathic symptoms are frequent in patients with underlying autoimmune illnesses such as SLE or spinal vascular malformations. TM is the first manifestation of multiple sclerosis for some patients. However, most long-term studies record rates of subsequent develop of MS of <25%. The presence of abnormal cerebral white matter lesions on MRI at the time of presentation with TM is associated with a significantly higher risk for subsequent development of MS.

PATIENT EDUCATION

- Transverse Myelitis Association, 3548 Tahoma Place W, Tacoma, WA 98466.
  Phone: 614-766-1806,
  website: *www.myelitis.org*

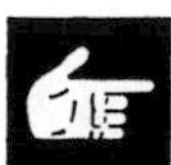

Miscellaneous

SYNONYMS

N/A

ICD-9-CM: 323 Encephalitis, myelitis, encephalomyelitis; 323.9 Unspecified cause of encephalitis. There are other descriptors for viral, postinfectious, and other causes of myelitis.

SEE ALSO: N/A

REFERENCES

- Berman M, Feldman S, Alter M, et al. Acute transverse myelitis: incidence and etiological considerations. Neurology 1981;31:966.
- Ford B, Tampieri D, Francis G. Long-term follow-up of acute partial transverse myelopathy. Neurology 1992:42:250.
- Jeffery DR, Mandler RN, Davis LE. Transverse myelitis: retrospective analysis of 33 cases, with differentiation of cases associated with multiple sclerosis and parainfectious events. Arch Neurol 1993;50:532.
- Ropper AH, Poskanzer DC. The prognosis of acute and subacute transverse myelopathy based on early signs and symptoms. Ann Neurol 1978;4:51.
- Stone LA. Transverse myelitis. In: Rolak LA, Harati Y, eds. Neuroimmunology for the clinician. Boston: Butterworth-Heinemann, 1997:155–165.
- Transverse Myelitis Consortium Working Group. Proposed diagnostic criteria and nosology of acute transverse myelitis. Neurology 2002;59:499–505.

Author(s): D. Joanne Lynn, MD

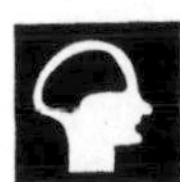

Basics

DESCRIPTION

- Intracranial trauma can be described in terms of mechanism and morphology of injury. Mechanism of injury refers to blunt versus penetrating trauma, whereas morphology describes the presence of focal or diffuse intracranial injury. The initial primary injury results in both global and focal disruption of neural networks. The vulnerable tissue is at high risk for secondary insult.

EPIDEMIOLOGY

Incidence

- Estimate in the United States is 200 per 100,000 (80% mild, 10% moderate, 10% severe)

Race

- Higher incidence in African Americans; appears to be related to increased exposure to firearms and higher rates of homicide.

Age

- Occurs in all ages; majority 15–24

Sex

- Males to females ratio of 3:1.

ETIOLOGY

- Motor vehicle accidents, falls, assaults, and sports-related injuries with resultant
  - —Diffuse axonal injury
  - —Traumatic subarachnoid hemorrhage
  - —Coup-contrecoup injuries
  - —Cortical contusions and lacerations
  - —Subdural, epidural, or intracerebral hematomas

Genetics

N/A

RISK FACTORS

- Alcohol and drug intoxication

PREGNANCY

N/A

ASSOCIATED CONDITIONS

N/A

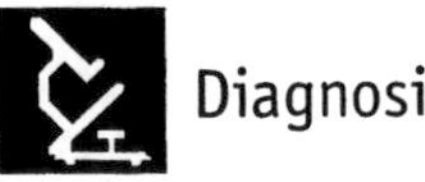

Diagnosis

DIFFERENTIAL DIAGNOSIS

- Other causes of coma

SIGNS AND SYMPTOMS

- Immediate loss or alteration of consciousness
- Period of confusion and posttraumatic amnesia (retrograde and antegrade)
- Signs of trauma
  - —Raccoon's sign
  - —Battle sign
- GCS: defines severity of injury.
  - —Ocular: eyes open spontaneously = 4, to voice = 3, to pain = 2, no opening = 1
  - —Verbal: oriented = 5, disoriented = 4, inappropriate = 3, incomprehensible = 2, no response = 1
  - —Motor: follows commands = 6, localizes = 5, withdraws = 4, flexion posturing = 3, extensors posturing = 2, no response = 1

Definitions

- Severe injury: initial GCS ≤8 or deterioration to this score
- Moderate injury: initial GCS 9–12 without subsequent deterioration
- Mild injury: loss of consciousness or alteration of awareness for <30 minutes; initial GCS 13–15 without neurosurgical pathology or subsequent deterioration

LABORATORY PROCEDURES

- Platelet count, PT, PTT, INR, glucose

IMAGING STUDIES

- Head CT: Initial study assesses for intracranial blood. Perform on anyone with loss of consciousness for >15 minutes.
- Brain MRI is useful for detecting brainstem involvement and diffuse axonal injury.

SPECIAL TESTS

- EEG
  - —Mandatory for induced barbiturate coma. Useful to assess seizure activity. Limited role in predicting outcome.
- Evoked potentials (EPs)
  - —Combination of somatosensory, visual, and brainstem EPs have high correlation with 1-year clinical outcome.

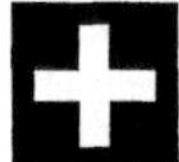

Management

GENERAL MEASURES

- Appropriate emergency department/intensive care unit management is critical. Treatment differs based on severity of injury. Multidisciplinary teams consisting of trauma surgery, neurosurgery, orthopedic surgery, neurology, and rehabilitation services frequently are necessary.

Severe TBI

- Monitor to prevent secondary injury
  - —Intracranial pressure (ICP) monitors: Camino bolts, ventriculostomy; ICP goal: <25 mm Hg.
  - —Cerebral perfusion pressure = MAP − ICP; goal: >70 mm Hg
- ICP control
  - —Hyperosmotic agents (i.e., mannitol, 3% saline); monitor serum osmolality and sodium levels frequently.
  - —Ventricular drainage
  - —Limited use of hyperventilation secondary to risk for ischemia with prolonged use; prophylactic prolonged hyperventilation results in worse outcomes at 6 months
  - —Barbiturate coma
  - —Hypothermia may assist in ICP control, but recent studies found no benefit on outcome
  - —Corticosteroids are not recommended for improving outcome or ICP control
  - —Identify and treat herniation syndromes
- Seizures
  - —Immediate seizures at time of injury do not require anticonvulsant medications; initiate anticonvulsants if seizures are observed after initial resuscitation and stabilization
  - —May contribute to ICP elevations
  - —Routine prophylaxis should not be used beyond 1 week
- Acute hydrocephalus
  - —Usually secondary to intraventricular or subarachnoid hemorrhage
  - —Signs: neurologic deterioration, increased ICP, nausea, vomiting, headache
  - —Ventriculostomy provides acute treatment; ventriculoperitoneal shunting may be necessary
- Agitation
  - —Subtype of delirium occurring during period of amnesia due to increased sympathetic drive; characterized by excessive behaviors
  - —Manage with combination of low-dose anxiolytics and antipsychotics
- Electrolyte abnormalities
  - —Hyponatremia
    - -Syndrome of inappropriate secretion of antidiuretic hormone (SIADH)
      - *Treatment: fluid restriction and avoid hypotonic IV fluids. Refractory cases: demeclocycline (300 mg every 6 hours), fludrocortisone (0.1–0.2 mg/day), hypertonic saline (500 cc over several hours), or oral salt replacement
    - -Cerebral salt wasting
      - *Clinical signs: hyponatremia with hypovolemia, high urine output, normal to increased serum osmolality
      - *Treatment: should focus on hydration and salt supplementation
  - —Hypernatremia
    - -Diabetes insipidus (DI): relatively uncommon
      - *Clinical signs: hypernatremia with polyuria, polydipsia, hypovolemia, increased serum osmolality, low urine osmolality
      - *Treatment: pitressin, vasopressin, fluid supplementation
- General care
  - —Prophylaxis for deep vein thrombosis
  - —Address nutritional needs early
  - —Early initiation of rehabilitation services

Moderate TBI

- Generally ICP is not a concern in this group. Similar management as severe TBI for seizures, agitation, and general care.

Mild TBI

- Treatment should focus on the symptomatic treatment of sequelae. Patients should not engage in activities placing them at risk for recurrent injury until they have been symptom-free for at least 1 week.

SURGICAL MEASURES

- Early surgery warranted for resectable lesion causing a midline shift of >5 mm on CT.
- Decompressive hemicraniectomy with or without tissue resection may be used for refractory increased ICP.

SYMPTOMATIC TREATMENT

- Discussed under General Measures. Sequelae may require treatment of headaches, spasticity, cognitive deficits, and pain.

ADJUNCTIVE TREATMENT

- Rehabilitation services: physical, occupational, and speech therapy; neuropsychological testing and counseling

ADMISSION/DISCHARGE CRITERIA

- All severe and moderate injuries, as well as mild injuries with an abnormal CT, should be admitted. Discharge may be considered when responsive and clinically stable ≥24 hours.

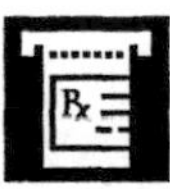

Medications

DRUG(S) OF CHOICE

- Increased ICP
  - -Mannitol at 1 gm/kg loading dose, then repeat boluses of 12.5–50 g
  - -Barbiturates (pentobarbital, thiopental) at 5 mg/kg loading dose, then steady infusion of 1–3 mg/kg/hour to maintain burst-suppression EEG pattern
- Seizures
  - -Acute period: phenytoin at 15–20 mg/kg loading dose, then maintenance dose for a therapeutic level; discontinue after 1 week if there are no witnessed seizures
  - -Long-term: carbamazepine, valproic acid, or levetiracetam are preferred anticonvulsants due to fewer adverse effects on cognition
- Agitation
  - -Agitation in ICU should be treated with short-acting sedatives, analgesics, and soft restraints.
  - -Persistent agitation can be treated with dopamine agonists, anticonvulsants (valproic acid, carbamazepine), β-adrenergic antagonists, antipsychotics, or buspirone.
- Arousal
  - -Arousal, motivation, and responsiveness increase with use of dopamine agonists, psychostimulants, and antidepressants.

Contraindications

- Hypotension and hypoxia worsen clinical outcome. Glucocorticoids have no beneficial role in TBI. Avoid glucose-containing IV fluids.

Precautions

- Rebound increased ICP has been reported with mannitol. IV forms of valproic acid should not be used in the acute phase after TBI. Avoid hyperthermia and hyperglycemia.

ALTERNATIVE DRUGS

N/A

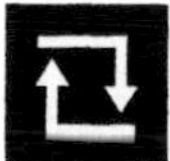

Follow-Up

PATIENT MONITORING

- Monitor through neurology and rehabilitation services for delayed complications

EXPECTED COURSE AND PROGNOSIS

- *Mortality:* Directly related to severity of injury, overall rate = 20/100,000. Higher mortality seen in ages <5 and >65. Severe injury carries a 30% mortality rate.
- *Morbidity:* Some degree of neurologic impairment remains in 10% of patients with mild TBI, 67% with moderate, and 100% with severe. Annual disability rate is 35/100,000.

Posttraumatic Seizures

- Risk is greatest in first year after injury. Recurrent seizures occur in >85% with an unprovoked late posttraumatic seizure.
- Risk factors for posttraumatic seizures:
  - —Intracerebral contusion
  - —Subdural hematoma
  - —Prolonged coma or posttraumatic amnesia
  - —Skull fracture

Delayed Hydrocephalus

- Difficult to distinguish hydrocephalus ex vacuo from symptomatic hydrocephalus. Sequential head CTs are beneficial.
- Presents any time, from >1 month to years after injury. Incidence is 4%.
- Usually a communicating hydrocephalus. May see the classic triad of dementia, gait ataxia, and urinary incontinence.
- Suspect in patients who deteriorate or fail to progress in their rehabilitation.
- Treatment: ventriculoperitoneal or lumboperitoneal shunt.

Postconcussion Syndrome (PCS)

- Diverse symptom constellation: headaches, dizziness, visual blurring, tinnitus, fatigue, sleep disruption, mood changes, impairments in memory, and attention.
- Usually improves over 3 months in >90%.
- Persistence 6 months after injury raises concerns of psychological factors.

Neuropsychological Issues

- Five years after injury, 50% of severe, 14% of moderate, and 3% of mild injuries may still demonstrate neuropsychological impairments.
- Neuropsychological testing can assist with planning of appropriate rehabilitation programs, prediction of functional recovery, and long-term prognosis.

Rehabilitation

- Majority of recovery following any brain injury occurs in first 6 months after injury.
- Specialized postacute rehabilitation programs have been developed to address community reentry and vocational rehabilitation.

PATIENT EDUCATION

- Brain Injury Association, 105 North Alfred Street, Alexandria, VA 22314. Website: *www.biausa.org*

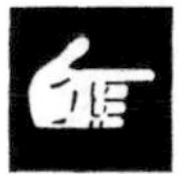

Miscellaneous

SYNONYMS

- Head injury

ICD-9-CM: 854.00 Brain injury NEC

SEE ALSO: CONCUSSION; TRAUMA, SPINAL CORD

REFERENCES

- AANS and Brain Trauma Foundation. Guidelines for the management of severe head injury, 1999.
- Annengers J, Hauser W, Coan S, et al. A population-based study of seizures after traumatic brain injuries. N Engl J Med 1998;338:20–24.
- Kraus J, McArthur D. Epidemiology of brain injury. In: Evans R, ed. Neurology and trauma. Philadelphia: WB Saunders, 1996.

Author(s): Lori Shutter, MD

Basics

DESCRIPTION

- Mild traumatic brain injury (MTBI) or mild head injury is difficult to define compared to moderate or severe injury in which structural damage is evident. Currently, MTBI is considered a traumatically induced physiologic disruption of brain function that may or may not be associated with loss of consciousness.

EPIDEMIOLOGY

Incidence/Prevalence

- It is estimated that two million persons in the United States suffer closed head injuries each year. Approximately 80% of these are due to mild head injury.

Race

- No known differences

Age

- Motor vehicle accidents are the most frequent cause of head injuries. Males between 15 and 24 years old are the group at highest risk.

ETIOLOGY

- Estimates of the relative causes of MTBI in the United States are as follows:
  —Motor vehicle accidents 45%
  —Falls 30%
  —Occupational accidents 10%
  —Recreational accidents 10%
  —Assaults 5%
- Mechanisms of head injury or MTBI include
  —Direct contact injuries
  —Indirect or nonimpact injury (whiplash)
  —Soft tissue injuries
  —Probable cascade of metabolic changes that are known to occur in brain injury
- Most injuries may overlap, i.e., in acceleration/deceleration head movement, forehead collision on the steering wheel, and cervical strain. There is increasing evidence supporting an organic basis in the pathophysiology of MTBI. After both mild and severe head injuries, damage to nerve fibers and nerve fiber degeneration are evident. Cerebral circulation can be slowed and rotational forces may cause shearing of axons. Generally an injury sustained with the head free (such as an automobile accident) is more damaging than an injury sustained with the head fixed (such as sports injuries).

RISK FACTORS

- Motor vehicle accidents are the main cause in the young. Falls are more common in the elderly. Rates of head injury are higher for males at all ages.

PREGNANCY

- No association

ASSOCIATED CONDITIONS

- Alcohol intoxication has been found in almost two thirds of those tested following MTBI due to automobile accidents.

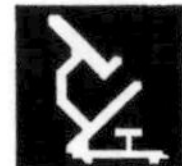

Diagnosis

DIFFERENTIAL DIAGNOSIS

- Usually mild head injury has an apparent source as noted above. Other medical or neurologic conditions may have been responsible for the head injury, such as a seizure disorder or syncope.

SIGNS AND SYMPTOMS

- Headaches are the most common symptom following MTBI. Headache prevalence actually is greater in people with mild head injury than in those with more severe trauma. The onset of headache usually occurs within 2 weeks. There may be more than one type of headache, i.e., they often are mixed with tension and vascular features.
- Neck injuries commonly accompany head injuries and can cause headache. Tension-type headaches may account for 75% of headaches. Recurring attacks of migraine with or without aura can occur. Cluster-type headaches are rare.
- Dizziness is reported by almost half of patients with MTBI. This can have a central origin but probably is more likely from labyrinthine concussion. The dizziness usually is triggered by head movement.
- Other common symptoms include difficulty with attention, concentration, and memory; depression; fatigue; and irritability.

LABORATORY PROCEDURES

- Usually not significant

IMAGING STUDIES

- The most common imaging study is CT scan, although MRI probably is superior in most circumstances. In MTBI, imaging studies usually are normal. Some have recommended CT brain scan for all patients with a Glasgow Coma Score (GCS) <15, an abnormal mental status examination, or any neurologic deficit. Even mild lethargy or memory deficit justifies a CT scan.

SPECIAL TESTS

- EEG evaluation in MTBI remains uncertain. The EEG may be abnormal, usually with slowing, in some patients shortly after a head injury, and this abnormality may decrease or disappear within days to weeks. Some studies have found no EEG abnormalities if there was not a period of amnesia or loss of consciousness.
- Brainstem auditory evoked potentials are useful for assessing the integrity of the auditory pathway. Abnormalities can be found in 10%–20% of patients with posttraumatic syndrome or after MTBI. Approximately 30% of patients with mild MTBI and symptomatic dizziness will have abnormal studies. The degree of abnormality usually increases with the extent of injury.
- Electronystagmography (ENG) has been noted to be abnormal in 40%–50% of patients with MTBI or even "whiplash." ENG may be more sensitive to traumatic abnormalities than the brainstem auditory evoked response.

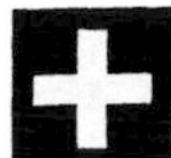

Management

GENERAL MEASURES

- Treatment is individualized for each of the problems diagnosed. Treatment for headaches is similar to treatment of headache in general. If there is a posttraumatic migraine syndrome, the triptan-type medications can be helpful. Education of the patient, family members, other physicians, and, when appropriate, employers and attorneys can be very helpful.

SURGICAL MEASURES

- Generally none for MTBI

SYMPTOMATIC TREATMENT

- Patients with daily posttraumatic headache may need to be placed on some type of preventative medication, usually an antidepressant. Tricyclic antidepressants usually are given first, but selective serotonin reuptake inhibitors also can be tried. Dosing antidepressants for posttraumatic headache is essentially the same as for treatment of depression, although occasionally patients will respond to lower doses. Patients with posttraumatic migraine may benefit from propranolol or a calcium channel blocker (verapamil). Using analgesic medication to decrease pain levels may enable the patient to better concentrate and relax and obtain greater benefits from nondrug therapies. Care must be taken that analgesic rebound headaches do not occur. Antiinflammatory medication and muscle relaxants may be useful for some patients, usually for a limited time frame, i.e., 1–2 weeks.

ADJUNCTIVE TREATMENT

- Headaches associated with myofascial trigger points in the neck or upper back often will respond to trigger point injections of local anesthetic, with or without steroids. These often are helpful but typically last only 2–4 weeks. Other nondrug therapies include biofeedback, physical therapy, massage, and counseling. Psychotherapy may be helpful if there is significant depression, anxiety, frustration, excessive expectations, anger, and unresolved grief and loss. Depression should be treated with antidepressant medication.

ADMISSION/DISCHARGE CRITERIA

- MTBI typically does not require neurosurgical intervention or hospitalization. If there is any uncertainty as to the degree or head injury, a brief hospitalization for observation is perfectly reasonable. Patients with MTBI may be admitted if there are concurrent injuries to other parts of the body. Patients with GCS scores <15, an abnormal mental status, or any neurologic deficit should be considered for admission. The majority of patients with mild head injuries can be sent home and observed.

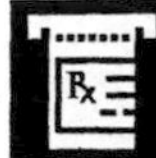

Medications

DRUG(S) OF CHOICE

- Analgesics
- Nonsteroidal inflammatory medications
- Muscle relaxants
- Antidepressants
- Anticonvulsants
- There has been some success with treating chronic daily posttraumatic headache with divalproex sodium. Other anticonvulsant medications currently are being tried for various types of headache.

Contraindications

- Triptan medications are contraindicated in patients with ischemic coronary, cerebrovascular, or peripheral vascular artery disease and pregnancy.
- Propanolol is contraindicated in cardiogenic shock and severe congestive heart failure; sinus bradycardia and greater than first-degree block; and bronchial asthma
- Valproate sodium is contraindicated in patients with significant hepatic disease.

Precautions

- Valproate sodium is associated with hepatotoxicity, pancreatitis, hyperammonemia, and thrombocytopenia. It is known to cause teratogenic effects, such as neural tube defects. Liver function tests and platelet count should be monitored at drug initiation and at regular intervals.

ALTERNATIVE DRUGS

- Not established for MTBI

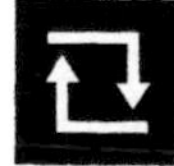

Follow-Up

PATIENT MONITORING

- Outpatient follow-up usually is all that is necessary, but patients may take more time because of multiple symptoms and concerns. Follow-up should be individualized.

EXPECTED COURSE AND PROGNOSIS

- Approximately 80% of patients will recover without significant sequelae. Twenty percent may continue to have symptomatic headache, neck pain, or dizziness. Some will continue to have difficulty with attention, concentration, and memory. Although most patients have a favorable outcome. Some guidelines exist to identify patients at risk for longer periods of incapacity. These include
  —Older patients
  —Patients with previous head injuries
  —Persons who have been high achievers or in demanding occupations
  —Patients who have family or social stressors

PATIENT EDUCATION

- Patients should be educated as to the expected outcome for MTBI. Most MTBI patients do not enroll in support groups or brain injury associations. If patients have symptoms that persist beyond 1 year, they may benefit from contacting the Brain Injury Association.

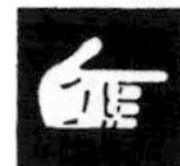

Miscellaneous

SYNONYMS

- Concussion
- Mild head injury
- Mild traumatic brain injury
- Postconcussive syndrome.

ICD-9-CM: 850.0 Concussion; 310.20 Postconcussive syndrome

SEE ALSO: N/A

REFERENCES

- Gean AD. Imaging of head trauma. New York: Raven Press, 1994.
- Kelly KP, Rosenburg JH. Diagnosis and management of concussion in sports. Neurology 1997;48:575–580.
- McCrea M, Kelly J, Kluge J, et al. Standardized assessment of concussion in football players. Neurology 1997;48: 586–588.
- Narayan R, Wilberger J, Povlishock J. Neurotrauma. New York: McGraw-Hill, 1996.
- Packard RC. Seminars in neurology: mild head injury, vol. 14. New York: Thieme Medical Publishers, 1994:1–95.
- Packard RC. Treatment of chronic daily posttraumatic headache with divalproex sodium. Headache 2000;40:736–739.
- Packard RC, Ham LP. Promising techniques in the assessment of mild head injury. Semin Neurol 1994;14:74–83.
- Rizzo M, Tramal D. Head injury and postconcussive syndrome. New York: Churchill-Livingstone, 1996.
- Sturzenegger M, Di Stefano MA. Presenting symptoms and signs after whiplash injury: the influence of accident mechanisms. Neurology 1994;44:688–693.

Author(s): Russell C. Packard, MD

Trauma, Spinal Cord

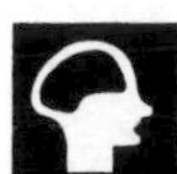

Basics

DESCRIPTION

- Spinal cord injury can be divided into complete or incomplete injuries. Extrication, stabilization, and transport guidelines are followed to prevent exacerbation of current injuries and increase rehabilitation potential.

EPIDEMIOLOGY

Incidence

- Between 30 and 50 per 1,000,000

Injury Levels

- C-spine 55%, T-spine 30%, L-spine 15%

Prevalence

- Approximately 721 per 1,000,000

Age

- All ages; majority 25–44 years; median age at injury is 26 years.

Sex

- Males outnumber females by a ratio of 2.5:1

Race

- Higher incidence in Caucasians

ETIOLOGY

- Motor vehicle accidents 45%
- Falls 17%
- Violence

Genetics

N/A

RISK FACTORS

- Alcohol, drug intoxication, violence

PREGNANCY

N/A

ASSOCIATED CONDITIONS

N/A

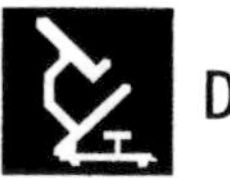

Diagnosis

DIFFERENTIAL DIAGNOSIS

- Transverse myelitis, myelopathy
- Spinal cord ischemia

SIGNS AND SYMPTOMS

- Depend on level of injury, which is defined as the lowest spinal cord segment with intact motor and sensory function.
  —Loss of motor control, tone and reflexes
  —Loss of sensory function within three levels of injury
    -Hand paresthesias should raise concern for cervical injury.
  —Loss of bowel, bladder, and sexual function.
    -Testing involves voluntary motor control, sensory sparing, tone, and reflexes (bulbocavernosus reflex).
- Key levels:
  —Motor:
    -C5: Elbow flexors
    -C6: Wrist extensors
    -C7: Elbow extensors
    -C8: Finger flexors to the middle finger
    -T1: Small finger abductors
    -L2: Hip flexors
    -L3: Knee extensors
    -L4: Ankle dorsiflexors
    -L5: Long toe extensors
    -S1: Ankle plantar flexors
    -S4–5: Rectal tone
  —Sensory: T4- nipple line, T10-umbilicus
- Tetraplegia results from cervical region injury.
- Paraplegia results from injury to the thoracic, lumbar, or sacral segments; conus medullaris; or cauda equina.
- Spinal cord syndromes
  —Complete
    -Loss of all sensory and motor function
    -Reflexes initially flaccid, but hyperreflexia develops over time.
    -Autonomic pathways are disrupted, resulting in urinary, rectal, and sexual dysfunction.
  —Incomplete syndromes
    -Brown-Séquard syndrome (hemisection of cord)
      *Ipsilateral motor weakness and proprioception/vibration loss
      *Contralateral pain and temperature loss
    -Central cord syndrome
      *Weakness of arms greater than legs due to involvement of anterior horn cells
      *Pain/temperature loss at level of injury
      *Reflexes decreased in arms; normal to hyperactive in legs
      *Frequently occurs with hyperextension injuries in the elderly due to cervical spondylosis
    -Anterior cord syndrome
      *Weakness from involvement of corticospinal tracts and anterior horn cells
      *Disruption of spinothalamic pathways results in loss of pain, temperature, and light touch, with sparing of proprioception/vibration
      *Reflexes initially flaccid, but hyperreflexia develops over time.
      *Autonomic pathways are disrupted.
    -Posterior cord syndrome
      *Motor pathways are intact.
      *Dorsal column impairment resulting in proprioception/vibration loss and a sensory ataxia.
    -Cauda equina syndrome
      *Motor involvement results in rectal and bladder paralysis.
      *Sensory loss in area supplied by nerve roots.
      *Reflexes usually are flaccid.
- American Spinal Injury Association (ASIA) Impairment Scale describes the extent of spinal cord injury:
  —A = Complete: No preserved motor or sensory function
  —B = Incomplete: Motor function absent, sensation preserved below the neurologic level
  —C = Incomplete: Motor function below the neurologic level with <50% key muscle grades ≥3/5
  —D = Incomplete: Motor function below the neurologic level with ≥50% key muscle grades ≥3/5
  —E = Normal: Motor and sensory function

LABORATORY PROCEDURES

- CBC, PT, PTT, INR, glucose

IMAGING STUDIES

- Anteroposterior and lateral plain x-ray films of bony spine
- Spinal CT of bony structures if abnormalities present on conventional imaging
- Spinal MRI of spinal cord, and intervertebral and paravertebral soft tissue

SPECIAL TESTS

- Cervical magnetic resonance angiography (MRA) to assess integrity of vertebral arteries with cervical injury.
- Head CT or MRI should be done if traumatic brain injury is suspected.

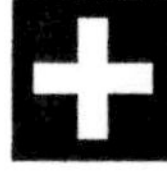

Management

GENERAL MEASURES

- Early immobilization of the spine is mandatory. A detailed neurologic examination, including rectal tone, is necessary to identify level and completeness of injury.
  —Megadose steroids: methylprednisolone, initial bolus 30 mg/kg over 1 hour.
    -Follow with continuous infusion of 5.4 mg/kg/hour for 23 hours if treatment is started within 3 hours of injury. Continue for 48 hours if treatment was started 3–8 hours after injury.
    -No indication for megadose steroids beyond the 8-hour time window.
  —Neurogenic shock
    -Autonomic reflexes lost in high/mid cervical injury disrupting sympathetic tone.
    -Decreased peripheral vascular tone results in expanded vascular space and relative hypovolemia, with hypotension, bradycardia, and warm dry skin.
    -Monitor central venous and pulmonary wedge pressures, with appropriate use of vasopressors.

—Spinal shock
-Loss of tone and spinal reflexes below level of injury. Duration is 2–4 weeks.
—Pulmonary complications
-High tetraplegics require ventilatory support and/or phrenic nerve pacemakers.
—Pain management
-Differentiate between neuropathic and musculoskeletal pain.
-Gabapentin rather than narcotics should be considered for neuropathic pain.
—Autonomic dysreflexia
-Noxious stimuli below the lesion level result in sympathetic discharge with hypertension, reflex bradycardia, sweating, headache, flushing, and piloerection.
-Noted in 45%–85% of injuries at or above T6. Onset $\geq$2 months after injury.
-Common causes:
*Bladder and/or bowel distention
*Pressure ulcers, skin infections
*Urinary tract infections
*Uterine contractions during labor and delivery
-Management:
*Treat underlying inciting factor
*Raise head of bed and treat hypertension pharmacologically
—General care
-Prophylaxis for deep vein thrombosis.
-Gastrointestinal care: Nasogastric tube to manage ileus prior to return of GI motility. Bowel program.
-Monitor for spasticity. Early ranging and medications may prevent contractures.
-Prevent decubitus ulcers.

SURGICAL MEASURES

- Early surgery warranted for locked and dislocated facet joints, or marked spinal instability or deformity that does not respond to closed realignment.
—Decompress and prevent further injury to neural elements to maximize recovery.
—Prevent delayed spinal instability and deformity.
—Allow early mobilization and rehabilitation.

SYMPTOMATIC TREATMENT

- Sequelae of trauma may require treatment of orthopedic, internal, and pulmonary injuries, spasticity, and pain.

ADJUNCTIVE TREATMENT

- Rehabilitation services: physical, occupational, and speech therapy; neuropsychological counseling

ADMISSION/DISCHARGE CRITERIA

- Any evidence of spinal cord injury warrants admission. Transfer to specialized rehabilitation services when the patient is stabilized.

Medications

DRUG(S) OF CHOICE

- Acute injury
—Methylprednisolone
—Vasopressors for shock and hypotension
- Pain
—Neuropathic pain: gabapentin, levetiracetam (Keppra), carbamazepine dilantin
—Musculoskeletal pain: narcotics acutely, nonsteroidal antiinflammatory drugs
- Deep Vein Thrombosis
—Prophylaxis: Enoxaparin (Lovenox) 30–60 mg bid, SQ heparin 5,000 U bid
—Treatment: Anticoagulation with heparin, then coumadin. If contraindicated, IVC Greenfield filter is necessary.
- Spasticity
—Useful drugs: gabapentin, baclofen, tizanidine, diazepam, dantrolene sodium
—Intrathecal baclofen pumps are helpful for excessive spasticity.
- GI issues
—Ileus/gastric motility: metoclopramide 10 mg qid, erythromycin 250 mg bid
—Ulcer prophylaxis: H_2 receptor antagonists or sucralfate
—Bowel program: adequate fluid, diet, and activity level, stool softeners, and glycerin or bisacodyl suppositories

Contraindications

- Hypotension worsens clinical outcome.

Precautions

- Monitor closely for pulmonary complications, DVT, infections, and skin care.

ALTERNATIVE DRUGS

N/A

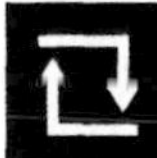

Follow-Up

PATIENT MONITORING

- Long-term monitoring by neurology and rehabilitation for delayed complications

EXPECTED COURSE AND PROGNOSIS

- Clinical course is based on level of injury
—High tetraplegia (C1–C4)
-Requires long-term ventilatory support
—C5: Functional biceps allows greater independence through splinting and orthotics. Generally able to feed self and assist with upper body dressing.
—C6: Presence of wrist extension allows use of tenodesis for greater hand use.
-Generally able to feed self and perform oral-facial hygiene.
—C7: Triceps function significantly increases independence.
-Most are independent with dressing, and bowel and bladder management.
—Thoracic and lumbar paraplegia
-Should achieve full independence with self-care and wheelchair mobility.
- Prognosis for ambulation recovery based on assessment at 1 week:
—ASIA A: 80%–90% remain complete. Only 3%–6% recover functional leg strength.
—ASIA B: 50% become ambulatory.
—ASIA C: 75% become community ambulators. ASIA D: 95% become community ambulators.
- Equipment needs
—Proper wheelchair positioning, cushions
—Bracing may assist with ambulation
- Sexual function
—Education and counseling are essential.
—Adaptive strategies, alternative techniques, mechanical devices, and medications may be useful.
- Psychological
—Depression in 25%–50%.
—Chemical dependency in up to 50%.
—Counseling should be available.

PATIENT EDUCATION

- American Spinal Injury Association, 2020 Peachtree Road, NW, Atlanta, GA 30309. Phone: 404-355-9772; website: *www.asia-spinalinjury.org*

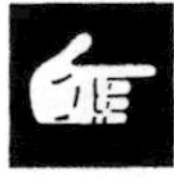

Miscellaneous

SYNONYMS: N/A

ICD-9-CM: 952.00 Spinal cord injury, cervical region; 952.1 Spinal cord injury, dorsal (thoracic); see multiple qualifiers for 952 codes

SEE ALSO: TRANSVERSE MYELITIS

REFERENCES

- American Spinal Injury Association (ASIA). Standards for neurological and functional classification of spinal cord injury. Chicago, IL: ASIA, 1992.
- Bracken MB, Shepard, MJ, Collins EF, et al. A randomized, controlled trial of methylprednisolone or naloxone in the treatment of acute spinal-cord injury. N Engl J Med 1990;322:1405–1411.
- Consortium for Spinal Cord Medicine. Outcomes following traumatic spinal cord injury: clinical practice guidelines for health-care professionals. Paralyzed Veterans of America, Washington, D.C, 1999.
- Yarkony GM. Spinal cord rehabilitation. In: Lazar RB, ed. Principles of neurologic rehabilitation. New York: McGraw-Hill, 1998:121–141.

Author(s): Lori Shutter, MD

Trichinosis

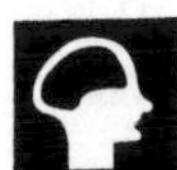

Basics

DESCRIPTION

- Trichinosis is the systemic illness that results from infestation with larvae of the nematode worm *Trichinella spiralis*. It may consist of general, gastrointestinal, neurologic, cardiac, and respiratory manifestations.

EPIDEMIOLOGY

- Incidence in United States has been declining over the past 50 years.
- Currently, cases in United States average <40 years.
- May be acquired by travel in foreign countries.

ETIOLOGY

- Invasion of tissue by worm larvae
- Inflammatory response to infection

Genetics

N/A

RISK FACTORS

- Consumption of undercooked pork or wild game such as deer, bear, horse meat, which contain larvae of *T. spiralis*.
- Recommendations are to cook pork and game meats until well done (not pink), to temperatures of at least 77°C (171°F).

PREGNANCY

- There are reports of trichinosis being transmitted *in utero* from mother to fetus.
- Maternal trichinosis has been associated with spontaneous abortion. Lactation has been reported to be suppressed in postpartum women with trichinosis.

ASSOCIATED CONDITIONS

N/A

Diagnosis

DIFFERENTIAL DIAGNOSIS

- Typhoid fever
- Food poisoning
- Leptospirosis
- Periarteritis nodosa
- Dermatomyositis
- Poliomyelitis
- Meningitis/encephalitis

SIGNS AND SYMPTOMS

- The diagnosis is suggested by the symptom complex of fever, malaise, myalgia, periorbital edema, and eosinophilia.
- The incubation period for appearance of generalized symptoms from time of ingestion varies from approximately 1 day to 7 weeks, with earlier appearance of symptoms generally presaging a more severe course. After the ingested cyst wall is digested in the stomach, the larvae are released and enter the general circulation from the gut. Although they may invade multiple organ systems, they encyst in striated muscle and may persist there for many years. An allergic vasculitis may occur and is responsible for edema and hemorrhage.

General/Abdominal

- Fever, malaise
- Cramping, diarrhea
- Periorbital edema
- Subconjunctival hemorrhages
- Myocarditis
- Maculopapular rash

Neurologic

- Myalgia
- Muscles painful to palpation
- Pain occurring at rest but worse with movement
- Limbs, extraocular muscles, tongue, respiratory, neck muscles
- Weakness and stiffness in affected muscles
- CNS involvement occurs in 10%–20% of cases, and may result from direct invasion of tissue by larvae, obstruction of blood vessels by larvae, toxic vasculitis, or acute host hypersensitivity reaction. In untreated patients with neurologic manifestations, mortality may be as high as 50%.
- Headache
- Seizures
- Meningitis/encephalitis
- Cerebrovascular thrombosis/infarction
- Tinnitus/decreased hearing
- Polyradiculoneuritis

LABORATORY PROCEDURES

Blood Tests

- Eosinophilia
- Elevated muscle enzymes
- Hypoalbuminemia
- Leukocytosis

IMAGING STUDIES

- Neuroimaging may reveal focal areas of infarction, hemorrhage, or thrombosis, in cases where there has been larval invasion of the brain. In some cases, larvae may be found in spun samples of CSF. In cases of pulmonary complications, there may be pneumonia or pleural effusion present on chest x-ray film.

SPECIAL TESTS

- The definitive test for trichinosis is the presence of *T. spiralis* larvae in muscle biopsy of the affected individual. Biopsy may be positive as early as 2 weeks after infection. Serology may be obtained for the presence of *T. spiralis* antibodies. Serologic tests become positive 3–4 weeks after initial infection.
- ECG
  —T wave changes, e.g., inversion
  —Decreased QRS voltage
  —ST-segment depression
  —Premature ventricular contractions
  —Conduction disturbances

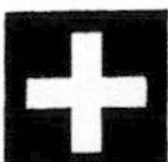

Management

GENERAL MEASURES

- Other than specific treatment of complications, therapy is directed at stopping infection and eradicating the parasite within the host *(vide infra)*. Management of complications is symptom specific, e.g., anticonvulsant therapy for seizures. Corticosteroids may be indicated in moderate-to-severe cases of allergic vasculitis, e.g., prednisone at doses of 60–120 mg/day or higher if needed. Steroids should not be used alone in early cases (<6 weeks after ingestion) because they may prolong the presence of adult worms in the gut.

SURGICAL MEASURES

N/A

SYMPTOMATIC TREATMENT

- Symptomatic therapy is aimed at specific complications. Fluids may be needed for dehydration, or diuretics in cases of severe edema. Antiarrhythmics may be indicated in cases of cardiac complications. Rarely, with severe pulmonary involvement, assisted ventilation may be necessary. Myalgia may respond to conventional doses of salicylates or nonsteroidal antiinflammatory drugs. After the acute phase, physical or occupational therapy may be indicated to restore function in affected muscles.

ADJUNCTIVE TREATMENT

N/A

ADMISSION/DISCHARGE CRITERIA

- Patients with moderate or severe trichinosis will need to be admitted primarily for management of systemic manifestations and complications, e.g., dehydration, or cardiopulmonary or CNS manifestations. The most common cause of death in trichinosis is myocarditis/cardiac failure, which most frequently occurs in weeks 4–8 of infection.

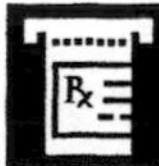

Medications

DRUG(S) OF CHOICE

Intestinal Phase

- Mebendazole 200–400 mg PO tid for 3 days, followed by 400–500 mg PO tid for 10 days
- Albendazole 400 mg bid

Acute Phase

- Corticosteroids 0.5–2.0 mg/kg/day in divided doses for 4–10 days
- Mebendazole 200–400 mg PO tid daily for 3 days, followed by 400–500 mg PO tid for 10 days

Contraindications

- These drugs are contraindicated for use in pregnant women.

Precautions

- Side effects include neutropenia, abnormal liver function tests, myalgia, and fatigue. In patients who develop allergic vasculitis or hypersensitivity reactions, steroids may be combined with antihelminthic treatment.

ALTERNATIVE DRUGS

N/A

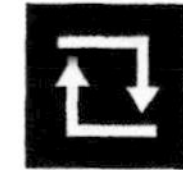

Follow-Up

PATIENT MONITORING

- Patients should be monitored in the first few weeks of the illness for development of neurologic, cardiac, pulmonary, and respiratory complications. Patients may develop hypersensitivity reactions as the result of larval death due to antihelminthic therapy.

EXPECTED COURSE AND PROGNOSIS

- Recovery is complete in a few months in most cases.
- Encysted larvae in muscle may persist for up to decades and be asymptomatic.
- Rarely, there is a chronic syndrome that consists primarily of fatigue.

PATIENT EDUCATION

- Patients should be warned against eating raw or undercooked pork or wild game products, particularly when traveling abroad. They should be instructed in proper cooking and freezing procedures when home processing pork and game products.

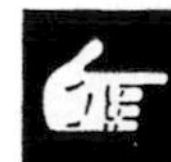

Miscellaneous

SYNONYMS

- Trichinellosis

ICD-9-CM: 124 Trichinosis

REFERENCES

- Clausen MR, Meyer CN, Krantz T, et al. Trichinella infection and clinical disease. QJM 1996;89:631–636.
- Gould SE. Symptomatology and diagnosis. In: Gould SE, ed. Trichinosis in man and animals. Springfield, Illinois: Charles C. Thomas Publisher, 1970:269–307.
- MacLean JD. Trichinosis. In: Hoeprich PD, ed. Infectious diseases: A treatise of infectious processes, 4th ed. Philadelphia: JB Lippincott, 1994:1377–1380.
- Pawlowski ZS. Clinical aspects in man. In: Campbell WC, ed. Trichinella and trichinosis. New York: Plenum Press, 1983:367–398.

Author(s): Barbara S. Giesser, MD

Trigeminal Neuralgia

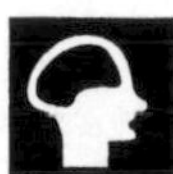

Basics

DESCRIPTION

- Trigeminal neuralgia is a clinical syndrome characterized by recurrent paroxysmal lancinating pain in the trigeminal distribution. The pathogenesis in most cases is idiopathic but may be caused by a local lesion.

EPIDEMIOLOGY

Incidence/Prevalence

- 4–5 per 100,000 population

Age

- Trigeminal neuralgia usually occurs after age 40 years.

Sex

- Slightly greater incidence in females

ETIOLOGY

- The pathogenesis of trigeminal neuralgia is unclear and probably multifactorial.
- Cerebellopontine tumors, schwannoma, multiple sclerosis, or other lesion involving or near the trigeminal nerve or its nucleus may cause trigeminal neuralgia in a minority of cases.
- The proposed theories of pathogenesis for both the idiopathic and symptomatic cases focus on aberrant repetitive discharges that could arise from
  —The vascular compression theory holds that a tortuous artery or vein near the trigeminal nerve compresses the nerve root. The compression increases with age and causes changes in the sensory root entry zone that result in prolongation of electrical impulses in the nerve and reexcitement of the axon leading to repetitive neuronal discharges.
  —Inflammation near or in the trigeminal nerve

RISK FACTORS

N/A

PREGNANCY

- Currently, there is no particular relation of trigeminal neuralgia with pregnancy.

ASSOCIATED CONDITIONS

- Multiple sclerosis
- Brainstem neoplasm
- Vascular compression/vertebrobasilar dolichoectasia
- Trigeminal schwannoma
- Cerebropontine angle tumors: acoustic neuroma, meningioma
- Metastatic infiltration of the base of the skull
- Cavernous sinus lesions: cavernous carotid aneurysm, meningioma, pituitary adenoma, Tolosa-Hunt syndrome, metastasis

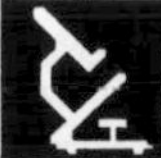

Diagnosis

DIFFERENTIAL DIAGNOSIS

- Need to differentiate from *other causes of pain or cranial pain.*
  —Neuralgia
    -Glossopharyngeal neuralgia
    -Atypical neuralgia
  —Migraine headaches
  —Cluster headache
  —Temporal arteritis
  —Musculoskeletal pain
    -Temporomandibular joint pain
    -Myofascial pain syndrome
  —Local diseases
    -Ocular and periocular diseases, e.g., uveitis, orbital tumor, orbital cellulitis
    -Nasal and paranasal sinus diseases
    -Odontogenic diseases

SIGNS AND SYMPTOMS

- The characteristic pain in trigeminal neuralgia is a paroxysmal, sharp, shooting or lancinating pain in the distribution of one or more divisions of the trigeminal nerve, most commonly in the second and third divisions.
- Pain classically consists of a burst of multiple very brief sharp jabs, each lasting <1 second but adding to 1 to several seconds. The bursts themselves may occur repeatedly for a period of a few seconds to 1 minute. The pain may be excruciating to the point of deep depression or even suicide.
- The pain is triggered by sensory stimuli to the skin, mucosa, or teeth within the area innervated by trigeminal nerve. Pain sometimes can be initiated by chewing, brushing the teeth, or talking.
- In classic idiopathic trigeminal neuralgia, the neurologic examination is normal. There is no sensory or motor impairment in the trigeminal distribution.
- When trigeminal neuralgia results from a lesion involving the trigeminal nerve roots or ganglion, the neurologic examination may show sensory deficits in the trigeminal distribution, weakness or atrophy of the muscles of mastication, or abnormalities in the adjacent cranial nerves, depending on the location.
- Atypical trigeminal neuralgia is characterized by atypical characteristics of pain (e.g., no bursts, continuous pain) or an abnormal neurologic examination that would prompt investigations for an associated structural lesion.

LABORATORY PROCEDURES

- In classic trigeminal neuralgia, there are no accompanying laboratory or radiographic abnormalities. Blink reflexes are normal.
- Additional laboratory tests may be required for other disorders in the differential diagnosis of facial pain, such as ESR for temporal arteritis, or x-ray film of sinus or temporomandibular joint.

IMAGING STUDIES

- Neuroradiologic imaging is recommended in patients undergoing surgical treatment for trigeminal neuralgia, patients with atypical trigeminal neuralgia, or patients with any associated neurologic deficit compatible with an underlying structural lesion.
- In the case of trigeminal neuralgia due to structural lesions such as meningioma, schwannoma of the trigeminal nerve, or infiltration of the base of skull by malignant tumors, CT or MRI with contrast may reveal a lesion along the pathway of trigeminal nerve.
- In idiopathic trigeminal neuralgia, neuroimaging will be normal.

SPECIAL TESTS

N/A

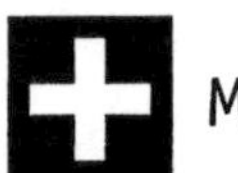

Management

GENERAL MEASURES

- Initial management begins with a trial of carbamazepine, which is the agent of choice. Doses are gradually increased until pain is controlled or side effects become intolerable. Other agents listed in the Medications section can be tried alone or in combination. Approximately 25%–50% of patients eventually will fail to respond to drug therapy and require some sort of surgical intervention.

SURGICAL MEASURES

- Surgical measures are reserved for patients with
  —Surgical lesions
  —Inadequate response to nonsurgical treatment
  —High-dosage medication requirement with intolerable side effects

Extracranial Peripheral Denervation

- Temporary denervation or blocks of the peripheral branches of trigeminal nerve
- Nerve block performed at supraorbital, infraorbital, or mental foramen with alcohol or lidocaine
- Advantages: May be performed in the office. The area of denervation is focal and small. The corneal does not become denervated and permanent dysesthesias are unlikely. Major complications are rare.
- Disadvantages: The procedure is very painful when it is performed without sedation or analgesia in the office. Pain can return in a short period.
- Even with the more permanent peripheral denervations, pain commonly returns within 6–18 months, and repeating the procedure could be more difficult with shorter period of pain relief.

Percutaneous Denervation of Gasserian Ganglion and Retrogasserian Ganglion Rootlets

- Several methods may produce partial denervation of the trigeminal ganglion or its rootlets. A specially designed device is inserted under radiographic control into the cheek, through the foramen ovale, into the gasserian or retrogasserian ganglion. Partial destruction of the trigeminal nerve then is accomplished with radiofrequency thermocoagulation or glycerol.

Percutaneous Radiofrequency Thermocoagulation

- Initial pain relief occurs in >90% of the patients, with recurrence in 22% at 2–6 years and up to 80% with long-term (12 years) follow-up. A smaller area of denervation is associated with a higher recurrence rate.
- Procedure can be repeated, usually with good probability of pain relief.
- Severe dysesthesia follows the procedure in 2%–10% of the patients. Denervation of cornea and keratitis occur in 1%–3% of patients. The incidence of dysesthesias and keratitis tends to increase with more aggressive denervation.

Glycerol Trigeminal Rhizolysis

- Injection of sterile glycerol into the gasserian ganglion and retrogasserian rootlets instead of radiofrequency thermocoagulation.
- Glycerol is a mild denervating agent producing milder denervation with presumably fewer complications such as dysesthesia or keratitis. With mild denervation, the recurrence rate is high (28% after 1 year and 50% after 47 months).

Microvascular Decompression

- Procedure is based on the proposed mechanism that trigeminal neuralgia results from chronic vascular compression of the trigeminal nerve at the root entry zone.
- Procedure is performed through the suboccipital retromastoid craniectomy. The trigeminal nerve then is decompressed by placing a synthetic material, usually a Teflon felt, between the nerve and the vessel.
- One year after the procedure, 75% have pain relief and 9% have partial relief, After 10 years, 64% continue with excellent results and 4% with partial relief of pain.
- Death occurs in 0.2%–2.4% of patients, and other major intracranial complications occur in 1%–2% of patients. Hearing loss occurs in 1%–2% of patients. Facial weakness occurs in approximately 1% of patients, and burning and aching facial pain occur in 3.3%–4.8% of patients.

Choosing the Surgical Procedure

- Due to the invasiveness of microvascular decompression, radiofrequency thermocoagulation or other less invasive procedures are preferred in patients with (i) older age, (ii) significant medical illness, (iii) contralateral hearing loss, (iv) previously good results with radiofrequency thermocoagulation, or (v) multiple sclerosis, because pain recurrence is frequent regardless of procedure type.

SYMPTOMATIC TREATMENT

- See Medications

ADJUNCTIVE TREATMENT

N/A

ADMISSION/DISCHARGE CRITERIA

- Admission may be required when pain is so severe that it has resulted in dehydration.

Medications

DRUG(S) OF CHOICE

- Carbamazepine is the most effective medication with pain relief achieved in 75% of patients.

Dosage

- Medication may be started at a small dose of 50–100 mg twice per day to prevent side effects and increased slowly as tolerated. Usual therapeutic doses range from 600–1,200 mg/day, with the therapeutic drug level of 40–100 g/mL.

Side Effects

- Common side effects include drowsiness, vertigo, nausea, and ataxia.

Contraindications

- History of previous bone marrow depression, hypersensitivity to carbamazepine. Combination with monoamine oxidase (MAO) inhibitors is contraindicated. MAO inhibitors should be discontinued for 14 days before starting carbamazepine.

Precautions

- Hyponatremia can occur. In patients taking carbamazepine, CBC should be taken in the first few months and periodically because of increased risk for aplastic anemia and agranulocytosis. Obtaining these counts may or may not influence risk for these rare but devastating complications. Patients should be advised to contact their physician if they develop symptoms of a hematologic problem, such as prolonged fever, infection, easy bruising, petechial hemorrhage, and symptoms of anemia.

ALTERNATIVE DRUGS

- Alternative medications are phenytoin, baclofen, gabapentin, valproate, mexiletine, and clonazepam, which are generally less effective than carbamazepine but may be better in particular individuals.

Follow-Up

PATIENT MONITORING

- Neurologic examination should be performed periodically. A neurologic deficit suggests an occult structural lesion.

EXPECTED COURSE AND PROGNOSIS

- The clinical course is exacerbating and remitting over many years. Spontaneous remission may occur at any time and last for months or years.
- Medications should be tapered periodically to uncover a remission.

PATIENT EDUCATION

- Trigeminal Neuralgia Association (TNA), P.O. Box 340, Barnegat Light, NJ 08006. Phone: 609-361-1014, fax: 609-361-0982; website: *www.tna-support.org*

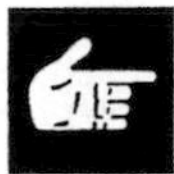

Miscellaneous

SYNONYMS

- Tic douloureux

ICD-9-CM: 350.1 Neuralgia, trigeminal

SEE ALSO: N/A

REFERENCES

- Barker FG, Jannetta PJ, Bissonette DJ, et al. The long term outcome of microvascular decompression for trigeminal neuralgia. N Engl J Med 1996;334:1077–1083.
- Brisman R. Surgical treatment of trigeminal neuralgia. Semin Neurol 1997;367–372.
- Campbell JK, Caselli RJ. Head and other craniofacial pain. In: Bradley WG, Daroff RB, Finichel GM, et al., eds Neurology in clinical practice: principle of diagnosis and management, 2nd ed. Butterworth-Heinemann 1995:1714–1716.
- De Marco JK, Hasselink JR. Trigeminal neuropathy. Neurosurg Clin 1997;8:103–130.
- Fromm GH, Terrence CF, Maroon JC, et al. Trigeminal neuralgia: current concepts regarding etiology and pathogenesis. Arch Neurol 1984;41:1204–1207.
- Gouda JJ, Brown JA. Atypical facial pain and other pain syndromes: differential diagnosis and treatment. Neurosurg Clin 1997;8:87–100.
- Rose CF. Trigeminal neuralgia. Arch Neurol 1999;56:1163–1164.
- Tensor RB. Trigeminal neuralgia: mechanism of treatment. Neurology 1998;51:17–19.

Author(s): Thomas C. Chelimsky, MD

Tuberculosis

Basics

DESCRIPTION

- Tuberculous involvement of the nervous system occurs as meningitis, tuberculoma formation, or spinal arachnoiditis.

EPIDEMIOLOGY

Incidence/Prevalence

- Tuberculous meningitis develops in 1%–2% of tuberculosis cases. Immunodeficiency increases the incidence. From 5%–10% of AIDS patients have tuberculosis, and up to 10% of these patients develop central nervous system (CNS) involvement.

Race

- American Indians have higher rates than African Americans, who in turn have higher rates than Caucasians.

Age

- Seen at any age, but peaks in the pediatric and elderly populations.

Sex

- More common in males than females.

ETIOLOGY

- Mycobacterium tuberculosis is an obligate aerobic bacillus. Transmission of the disease from person to person is through air. Bacilli are expelled as droplet nuclei from patients while they are coughing, sneezing, and talking. Droplet nuclei can stay in the air for hours before they enter the body through the respiratory tract or rarely through the skin and gastrointestinal tract. Bacilli reach the central nervous system by hematogenous dissemination from a primary focus.

Genetics

N/A

RISK FACTORS

- Immunodeficiency
- HIV infection
- Hematologic and reticuloendothelial malignancies
- Immunosuppressive therapy
- Malnutrition
- Chronic renal failure
- Alcohol and drug abuse

PREGNANCY

- A pregnant woman with tuberculosis should be treated because the infection is more hazardous to the patient and fetus than are the drugs. Isoniazid, rifampin, and ethambutol cross the placenta but do not have demonstrated teratogenic effects. Streptomycin can cause congenital deafness. There are no adequate data on pyrazinamide. Tuberculosis during pregnancy is not an indication for therapeutic abortion.

ASSOCIATED CONDITIONS

N/A

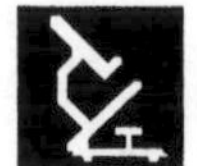

Diagnosis

DIFFERENTIAL DIAGNOSIS

- Fungal or viral meningitis
- Partially treated bacterial meningitis.
- Parasitic infections (cysticercosis, toxoplasmosis)
- Carcinomatous meningitis
- Neurosyphilis
- Sarcoidosis
- Pyogenic brain abscess

SIGNS AND SYMPTOMS

- CNS tuberculosis presents as three different clinical pictures.
  —*Tuberculous meningitis* results from hematogenous dissemination or, more frequently, rupture of granulomas into the subarachnoid space. The cause of the neurologic symptoms is the thick fibrous exudate that especially fills the basal cisterns. Inflammation and compression of blood vessels cause cerebral infarctions. Cranial nerves traversing the exudate are affected. A communicating type of hydrocephalus commonly develops.
    -The onset of symptoms is subacute. Signs of meningeal irritation (headache, vomiting, neck stiffness) are preceded by a prodromal phase lasting 2–3 weeks. Prodromal symptoms are fatigue, night sweats, low-grade fever, anorexia, malaise, and myalgia. Altered consciousness will follow meningeal irritation signs. Cranial nerve palsies, especially involvement of cranial nerves III, IV, and VI, are seen in 20%–30% of patients. Papilledema, seizures, and hemiparesis occur in 10%–15% of patients. Signs of pulmonary or extrapulmonary tuberculosis are often present. If not treated, coma and death will occur within 5–8 weeks.
  —*Tuberculomas* are slow-growing granulomas that can be found in the cerebrum, cerebellum, brainstem, subarachnoid, subdural and epidural spaces, and rarely within the spinal cord. They can occur in isolation or associated with meningitis. They cause headache, seizures, and focal neurologic deficits. Tuberculomas can cause an obstructive type of hydrocephalus.
  —*Spinal arachnoiditis* usually follows intracranial meningitis. Resultant root and cord compression causes pain, paralysis, sensory loss, and sphincter disturbances.

LABORATORY PROCEDURES

- Routine blood tests are nonspecific. Mild anemia, leukocytosis, and increased erythrocyte sedimentation rate are seen. Inappropriate antidiuretic hormone secretion can lead to mild-to-moderate hyponatremia in about half of the patients.
- From 50%–75% of patients with tuberculous meningitis have a positive tuberculin skin test (PPD).

IMAGING STUDIES

- Chest x-ray film shows findings of pulmonary tuberculosis in about 50%–90% of patients with meningitis.
- Cranial CT with contrast and postgadolinium magnetic MRI demonstrate uniform and intense enhancement of basal cisterns and meninges early in the disease. Ischemic infarctions are also detected by either CT or MRI.
- Hydrocephalus is seen as the disease evolves, more commonly in children. Serial CT examinations will help to follow the progression of hydrocephalus.
- Tuberculomas are seen as hypodense, avascular, solid, or ring-enhancing lesions on CT scans. Occasionally they may have central calcification surrounded by a hypodense area with ring enhancement (target sign). On MRI tuberculomas appear isointense to gray matter on T1-weighted images and are either hyperintense (noncaseating lesions) or isointense to hypointense (caseating tuberculomas) on T2-weighted images. They may have surrounding edema. Most often they are located at the corticomedullary junction and periventricular regions. Tuberculomas tend to be infratentorial in children but supratentorial in adults.

SPECIAL TESTS

- CSF examination is the most important investigation. CSF pressure is increased, usually over 300 mm H_2O, and there is pleocytosis. Polymorphonuclear leukocytes predominate in the earlier stages. Lymphocytic pleocytosis is seen within 24–48 hours. White cell count is between 100 and 400 cells/mm^3. CSF protein concentration is high (between 100 and 200 mg/dl) and glucose is decreased (<45 mg/dl). Acid-fast bacilli can be detected by Ziehl-Neelsen stain on CSF examination. The chance of detection of acid-fast bacilli increases with repeated examinations.
- CSF cultures reveal the microorganism in 50%–60% of patients; however, it takes several weeks to obtain the results. Cultures are important for drug sensitivity studies.
- Detection of bacterial DNA with polymerase chain reaction amplification is more sensitive than cultures and provides results within 24–72 hours.
- In tuberculomas without meningitis, CSF is either normal or may show lymphocytic pleocytosis with elevated protein and normal glucose.

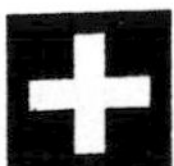

Management

GENERAL MEASURES

- Routine supportive care of the unconscious or paralyzed patient, maintenance of fluid and electrolyte balance and nutrition, and care of urinary bladder are important.

SURGICAL MEASURES

- Ventriculoperitoneal shunt insertion is necessary if hydrocephalus does not respond to medical therapy.
- Surgery for tuberculomas is only indicated in the presence of intolerably high intracranial pressure or in medical failures.

SYMPTOMATIC TREATMENT

- Symptomatic treatment for headaches, vomiting, fever, and seizures is necessary.

ADJUNCTIVE TREATMENT

N/A

ADMISSION/DISCHARGE CRITERIA

- Tuberculosis patients with neurologic involvement must be hospitalized.

Medications

DRUG(S) OF CHOICE

- Multiple-drug therapy is necessary because of the possibility of resistant strains of bacteria. Treatment should include bactericidal drugs that penetrate inflamed and noninflamed meninges. Isoniazid and pyrazinamide always pass the blood-brain barrier, whereas penetration of rifampin, streptomycin, and ethambutol through noninflamed meninges is poor.
- Centers for Disease Control and Prevention recommends a combination of three drugs as initial therapy in adults:
  —Isoniazid (INH) 5 mg/kg/day (maximum 300 mg/day) with pyridoxine 50 mg/day
  —Rifampin 10 mg/kg/day (maximum 600 mg/day)
  —Pyrazinamide 15-30 mg/kg/day (maximum 2 g/day)
- After 8 weeks, stop pyrazinamide and continue INH and rifampin. Short-duration (6 months) treatment is as effective as long-duration (9-18 months) treatment. In persons with delayed response, therapy should continue at least 6 months after the cultures become negative.
- In areas where drug resistance is common or if drug resistance is suspected, either ethambutol 15-25 mg/kg/day (maximum 2.0 g/day) or streptomycin 15 mg/kg/day IM (maximum 1 g/day) should be added as a fourth drug for 2 months.
- For immunosuppressed individuals, streptomycin should be added to the regimen and continued at least 6 months after cultures are negative for a total length of 6-9 months.
- Steroid therapy is controversial but is recommended for patients with focal neurologic signs, increased intracranial pressure, hydrocephalus, spinal block, and altered consciousness. Steroids 1-3 mg/kg/day can be given for 2-3 weeks. The dose should be reduced after 2-3 weeks and stopped at 4-6 weeks.

Contraindications

- Drug allergy

Precautions

- Side effects: Isoniazid causes an axonal sensorimotor polyneuropathy by interfering with pyridoxine metabolism. Supplemental pyridoxine should be administered. Slow acetylators of the drug are more susceptible to neuropathy, whereas fast acetylators are prone to hepatotoxicity. Rifampin causes orange discoloration of body fluids, leukopenia, thrombocytopenia, and hemolytic anemia. Streptomycin is ototoxic, and ethambutol carries a risk of optic neuropathy.

ALTERNATIVE DRUGS

- If resistance or allergy to the standard regimen exists, susceptibility studies should guide treatment.

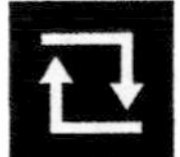

Follow-Up

PATIENT MONITORING

- Repeat lumbar punctures are necessary to monitor response to treatment, and CSF pressure should be measured. Serial CT scans are used to follow hydrocephalus and resolution of tuberculomas. Patients receiving isoniazid should be followed monthly for hepatotoxicity. Color vision and visual acuity should be followed in patients receiving ethambutol, and patients should be asked to report any decrease in acuity.

EXPECTED COURSE AND PROGNOSIS

- Although discovery of antituberculosis agents increased survival, tuberculosis meningitis still carries 20% mortality risk. The prognosis mainly depends on the severity of findings at the initiation of therapy. Therefore, early treatment is the most important factor in the prognosis. Empiric therapy should be started as soon as tuberculosis meningitis is suspected. Other factors that affect the prognosis are
  —Age of the patient (children <years and the elderly have worse prognosis)
  —Nutritional status
  —Presence of miliary tuberculosis
  —Presence of hydrocephalus or cerebral infarction

PATIENT EDUCATION

- Centers for Disease Control and Prevention. Website: *www.cdc.gov/nchstp/tb/faqs/qa.htm*
- American Thoracic Society. Website: *www.thoracic.org/statemnt.html*

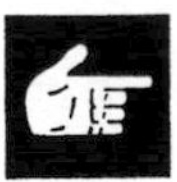

Miscellaneous

SYNONYMS

N/A

ICD-9-CM: 013 Tuberculosis of meninges and central nervous system; 013.0 Tuberculous meningitis; 013.1 Tuberculoma of meninges; 013.2 Tuberculoma of brain; 013.3 Tuberculous abscess of brain; 013.4 Tuberculoma of spinal cord; 013.5 Tuberculous abscess of spinal cord; 013.6 Tuberculous encephalitis or myelitis

SEE ALSO: N/A

REFERENCES

- Centers for Disease Control. Recommended treatment options for persons with human immunodeficiency virus-related tuberculosis infection and disease. MMWR 1988;47:53–58.
- Garcia-Monco JC. Central nervous system tuberculosis. Neurol Clin 1999;17:737–759.
- Glander DA. Tuberculous meningitis. In: Roos KL, ed. Central nervous system infectious diseases and therapy. New York: Marcel Decker, 1997:153–166.
- Jinkins JR, Gupta R, Chank KH, et al. MR imaging of central nervous system tuberculosis. Radial Clin North Am 1995;33:771–786.
- Lin JJ, Harn HJ, Hsu YD, et al. Rapid diagnosis of tuberculous meningitis by polymerase chain reaction assay of cerebrospinal fluid. J Neurol 1995;242:147–152.

Author(s): Ersin Tan, MD

Tuberous Sclerosis

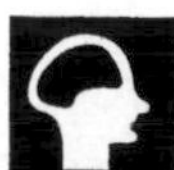

Basics

DESCRIPTION

- The tuberous sclerosis complex is a multisystem autosomal dominant neurocutaneous syndrome that most commonly affects the brain, eye, skin, kidneys, and heart. The clinical manifestations of tuberous sclerosis can be identified in organs derived from all primary stem cell lines, e.g., ectoderm, endoderm, and mesoderm.

EPIDEMIOLOGY

- Tuberous sclerosis occurs in about 1 in 300,000 persons.

ETIOLOGY

Genetics

- Tuberous sclerosis is inherited in an autosomal dominant fashion, with a penetrance of almost 100%. There is considerable variation in the expressivity of tuberous sclerosis. Recent advances in genetic identification have led to the identification of two genes that result in the phenotype of tuberous sclerosis. The first to be identified was TS2, located on chromosome 16p13.3. This gene encodes for the protein tuberin. More recently, TS1 has been identified. This gene, which encodes for the protein hamartin, is found on chromosome 9p34. Tuberin plays a role in cellular growth regulation, and hamartin appears to have an interactive function with tuberin. Approximately 50% of tuberous sclerosis families show genetic linkage to TS2 and 50% to TS1. Approximately 60% of patients have no prior family history and represent new mutations.

RISK FACTORS

N/A

PREGNANCY

N/A

ASSOCIATED CONDITIONS

- Mental retardation. Mental function varies greatly among patients with tuberous sclerosis. Although mental retardation is a characteristic of the disease, approximately 30% of patients have normal intelligence.
- Seizures. Seizures can be refractory and can start in infancy. The following seizure types can be seen in tuberous sclerosis:
  - —Neonatal seizures
  - —Infantile spasms
  - —Lennox-Gastaut syndrome
  - —Simple and complex partial seizures
- Behavioral abnormalities
  - —Hyperactivity
  - —Aggression
- Autism and pervasive developmental disorder
- Malignant transformation
  - —Giant cell astrocytoma
  - —Renal cell carcinoma

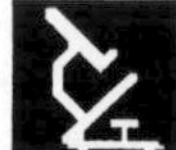

Diagnosis

DIFFERENTIAL DIAGNOSIS

N/A

SIGNS AND SYMPTOMS

- The clinical manifestations in tuberous sclerosis are varied. The following are the revised diagnostic criteria for tuberous sclerosis.
- Major features
  - —Facial angiofibromas or forehead plaque
  - —Nontraumatic ungual or periungual fibroma
  - —Hypomelanotic macules (three or more)
  - —Shagreen patch (connective tissue nevus)
  - —Multiple retinal nodular hamartomas
  - —Cortical tuber
  - —Subependymal nodules
  - —Subependymal giant cell astrocytoma
  - —Cardiac rhabdomyoma, single or multiple
  - —Lymphangiomatosis
  - —Renal angiomyolipoma
- Minor features
  - —Multiple randomly distributed pits in dental enamel
  - —Hamartomatous rectal polyps
  - —Bone cysts
  - —Cerebral white matter radial migrational lines
  - —Gingival fibromas
  - —Nonrenal hamartoma
  - —Retinal achromic patch
  - —"Confetti" skin lesions
  - —Multiple renal cysts
  - —Definite tuberous sclerosis complex: *Either two major or one major and two minor features*
  - —Probable tuberous sclerosis: *One major plus one minor feature*
  - —Possible tuberous sclerosis: *Either one major feature or two minor features*
- The diagnosis is made clinically. Once the diagnosis is suspected, then additional studies should be done to screen the organ systems that usually are affected.
- Neurologic symptoms can include seizures, developmental delay, mental retardation, autism or pervasive developmental disorder, or obstructive hydrocephalus. Renal manifestations can include hypertension or painless hematuria. Cardiac rhabdomyomas tend to be silent unless they cause rhythm or flow problems. They tend to involute with age.

LABORATORY PROCEDURES

- The following diagnostic studies are recommended in the evaluation of a new patient with tuberous sclerosis.
- *Electroencephalogram.* This test is recommended for patients who present with episodes suggestive of seizures but are not particularly useful in the routine evaluation of a patient with tuberous sclerosis.
- *Electrocardiography.* Cardiac arrhythmias sometimes occur even in patients without a cardiac rhabdomyoma. A baseline study is recommended at the time of diagnosis or before surgery.

IMAGING STUDIES

- *MRI/cranial CT.* MRI may be the more sensitive test to determine the presence of cerebral hamartomas, subependymal nodules, radial migrational lines, and giant cell astrocytomas. Larger calcified lesions can be seen on CT scan.
- *Renal ultrasonography* for renal angiomyolipomas.
- *Echocardiography* reveals one or more cardiac rhabdomyomas in more than half the younger individuals with tuberous sclerosis. These tumors tend to involute dramatically and often disappear by adulthood. The most rapid reduction in size occurs in the first 3 years of life.

SPECIAL TESTS

- *Molecular diagnosis.* DNA-based testing is not yet routinely available. Once molecular testing becomes available and there are sufficient data to determine which phenotypes correlate with which gene defects, gene typing at the time of initial diagnosis could be useful.
- *Ophthalmologic evaluation* for retinal hamartomas
- *Dermatologic evaluation*

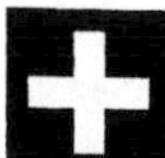

Management

GENERAL MEASURES

- There is no specific treatment for tuberous sclerosis. Care centers for management of symptomatic problems related to tuberous sclerosis, such as epilepsy, mental retardation, and autism, and for monitoring cardiac, renal, and dermatologic manifestations are discussed below.

SURGICAL MEASURES

- Patients with refractory epilepsy may be epilepsy surgery candidates. Large lesions that obstruct cerebrospinal fluid flow should be surgically removed. Occasionally if skin lesions are continually irritated or subjected to trauma, they can be removed surgically or by other dermatologic therapeutic measures.

SYMPTOMATIC TREATMENT

- Associated conditions such as epilepsy should be treated with the appropriate antiepileptic agents

ADJUNCTIVE TREATMENT

N/A

ADMISSION/DISCHARGE CRITERIA

N/A

Medications

DRUG(S) OF CHOICE

N/A

ALTERNATIVE DRUGS

N/A

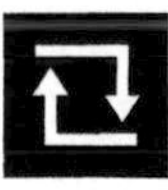

Follow-Up

PATIENT MONITORING

- Once the diagnosis has been established and the extent of organ involvement determined, management includes ongoing monitoring and treatment of associated conditions. Long-term surveillance testing should concentrate on complications that are significant, relatively common, and more easily managed when found early. The following guidelines are designed for long-term clinical management of an asymptomatic patient. Additional studies may be necessary and tailored to clinical symptoms.

Cranial CT and MRI

- Children should undergo neuroimaging once every 1–3 years to monitor for subendymal giant cell astrocytomas and cerebral hamartomas. If cerebral lesions are already present, more frequent neuroimaging may be needed to monitor progression.

Renal Ultrasonography

- By age 10 years, nearly 75% of children with tuberous sclerosis have sonographic evidence of one or more renal angiomyolipomas. During the first decade, the number and size of these lesions tend to increase. The current recommendation is for renal ultrasonography to be done once every 1–3 years. The frequency depends on the results of previous examinations. Patients with large or numerous renal tumors may require referral to a urologist, as well as either CT or MRI of the kidneys to better define the extent of kidney disease.

Echocardiography

- Most patients with tuberous sclerosis who have a cardiac rhabdomyoma remain asymptomatic. It is unusual for patients to become symptomatic after the neonatal period. Occasionally asymptomatic patients may need follow-up echocardiography because the original study raised specific concern about the size and location of a cardiac rhabdomyoma.

Lung Disease

- Pulmonary function tests should be reserved for patients with suspected lung dysfunction.

EXPECTED COURSE AND PROGNOSIS

- Course and prognosis depend on the organ systems involved and the extent of involvement.

PATIENT EDUCATION

- Education with regard to the long-term nature of this disease, as well as the potential for multiple organ involvement, should be outlined in detail.
- Genetic counseling, as well as screening of family members, is an important part of management.
- Seizure care should be explained, and seizure precautions should be followed by patients with seizures.
- Tuberous Sclerosis Alliance offers a comprehensive website for patients and professionals. Website: *www.tsalliance.org/default.asp*

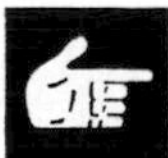

Miscellaneous

SYNONYMS

- Bourneville's cerebral sclerosis

ICD-9-CM: 759.5

SEE ALSO: N/A

REFERENCES

- Arbuckle HA, Morelli JG. Pigmentary disorders: update on neurofibromatosis-1 and tuberous sclerosis. Curr Opin Pediatr 2000;12:354–358.
- Berg BO. Neurocutaneous syndromes: phakomatoses and allied conditions. In: Swaiman KF, Ashwal S, eds. Pediatric neurology principles and practice, vol. 1. St. Louis: Mosby, 1999.
- Cheadle JP, Reeve MP, Sampson JR, et al. Molecular genetic advances in tuberous sclerosis. Hum Genet 2000;107:97–114.
- Crino PB, Henske EP. New developments in the neurobiology of the tuberous sclerosis complex. Neurology 1999;53: 1384–1390.
- Roach ES, DeMario FJ, Kandt RS, et al. Tuberous sclerosis consensus conference: recommendations for diagnostic evaluation. J Child Neurol 1999;14: 401–407.
- Road ES, Gomez MR, Northrup H. Tuberous sclerosis complex consensus conference: revised clinical diagnostic criteria. J Child Neurol 1998;13:624–628.

Author(s): S. Anne Joseph, MD

Vasculitis, Central Nervous System

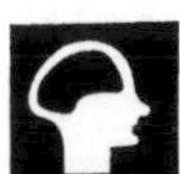

Basics

DESCRIPTION

- Central nervous system (CNS) vasculitis is characterized histologically by inflammation and necrosis of blood vessel walls. Primary (also called isolated) CNS vasculitis is clinically and pathologically limited to the CNS. Secondary vasculitis is associated with widespread systemic vasculitis and at times an identifiable underlying disorder.

EPIDEMIOLOGY

Incidence

- Uncommon with an annual incidence of 30–45 cases per million

Age

- Occurs at all ages, with cases reported as young as 3 years and up to age 78 years.

Sex

- Affects both males and females. Some specific entities show a male preponderance, others a female preponderance.

Race

- No investigations have been done to determine a racial predominance. Some systemic conditions, such as sarcoidosis, may be more common in African Americans.

ETIOLOGY

- CNS vasculitis is a segmental necrotizing vasculitis. The pathogenic events leading to vasculitis are not understood, but several mechanisms have been proposed. Isolated CNS vasculitis usually is granulomatous with infiltrates consisting of monocytes, lymphocytes, and plasma cells. The infiltrate usually is adjacent to a disrupted elastic lamina and involves the intima and adventitia with sparing of the media. It affects mainly small artery and veins, especially in the leptomeninges. Deposition of antigen-antibody immune complexes containing activated complement in blood vessel walls has been implicated in initiating the vascular injury. It leads to endothelial damage, infiltration of neutrophils and monocytes, activation of clotting and kinin pathways, and free radical and proteolytic enzyme release. Other mechanisms include neutrophil and natural killer (NK) cell-mediated vascular damage; a T-cell mediated immune response directed against a specific antigen with secondary macrophage activation and direct damage by cytotoxic T cells; and direct vascular damage by infectious agents and tumor. CNS vasculitis can be associated with a number of systemic conditions. It occurs with systemic vasculitides, autoimmune diseases, infectious diseases, neoplasia, and toxic exposures.

RISK FACTORS

- Risk factors are associated with specific conditions known to cause a secondary vasculitis.

PREGNANCY

- There is no known relationship to pregnancy.

ASSOCIATED CONDITIONS

- *Systemic necrotizing arteritis:* Wegener's granulomatosis, sarcoidosis
- *Autoimmune diseases:* Systemic lupus erythematosus, rheumatoid arthritis, scleroderma, mixed connective tissue disease, dermatomyositis
- *Infectious diseases:* Herpes zoster, cytomegalovirus, syphilis, Lyme disease, fungal infections
- *Neoplasia:* Lymphoma, malignant histiocytosis, meningeal carcinomatosis
- *Toxic:* Radiation, cocaine, heroin, amphetamine
- *Childhood:* Kawasaki disease, Henoch-Schönlein purpura, juvenile rheumatoid arthritis

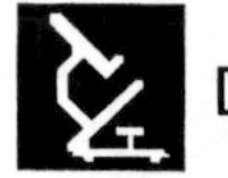

Diagnosis

DIFFERENTIAL DIAGNOSIS

- Primary isolated CNS vasculitis
- Giant cell arteritis
- Takayasu's disease
- Polyarteritis nodosa
- Wegener's granulomatosis
- Behçet's disease
- Systemic lupus erythematosus
- Multiple sclerosis
- Multiinfarct state (atheromatous or hypercoagulable)
- Moyamoya
- Sarcoidosis
- Mixed connective tissue disease
- Infectious (syphilis, tuberculous meningitis, fungal meningitis, bacterial meningitis, herpes simplex virus, cytomegalovirus, Lyme disease)
- Drugs of abuse (cocaine)
- Neoplasia (intravascular lymphoma)

SIGNS AND SYMPTOMS

- CNS vasculitis presents with an acute or subacute onset. Initial symptoms are frequently headache, hemiparesis, confusion, lethargy, and personality change. The disease is progressive, with an accumulation of multifocal symptoms. Among the symptoms are ataxia, aphasia, nausea or vomiting, cranial nerve dysfunction, memory deficits, seizures, and visual changes. CNS vasculitis can cause hemorrhagic and ischemic strokes. Fever and hypertension are sometimes present early in the disease. Funduscopic examination can reveal papilledema or vasculopathy.

LABORATORY PROCEDURES

- Blood tests may be useful for identifying an inflammatory process and possible underlying systemic conditions. These include a CBC with differential, erythrocyte sedimentation rate, serology for syphilis, liver function tests, ANA, anti-ds-DNA, c-ANCA and p-ANCA, lupus anticoagulant, and anticardiolipin antibody. CSF can be normal or have nonspecific abnormalities such as a lymphocytic pleocytosis, mildly elevated protein, and oligoclonal bands. It is critical to rule out CNS infection and examine CSF cytology to rule out a neoplastic meningeal infiltrate.

IMAGING STUDIES

- CT and MRI may identify multiple CNS lesions, but do not evaluate angiitis. An MR angiogram and a cerebral angiography may show sausage-shaped beading appearance of affected vessels, but in many cases they appear normal.

SPECIAL TESTS

- In isolated angiitis of the CNS, a biopsy that includes the leptomeninges and cortical parenchyma is the gold standard for diagnosis and often is necessary to exclude an infectious etiology prior to immunosuppression. Temporal artery biopsy may be necessary to diagnose giant cell arteritis. Skin, muscle, peripheral nerve, conjunctival, and specific organ biopsies may be useful in specific systemic vasculitides, occasionally even when these tissues are not overtly effected.

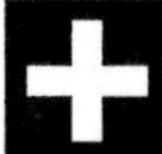

Management

GENERAL MEASURES

- Treatment requires identification of the specific vasculitic syndrome, assessment of organ damage, and treatment of the underlying cause. Medical therapy is primarily immunosuppression with steroids and/or cyclophosphamide. High-dose prednisone 1.5 mg/kg/day or IV methylprednisolone 15 mg/kg/day is the initial treatment. If the response to steroid therapy is poor, oral cyclophosphamide 2 mg/kg/day can be added and often is given with steroids as initial therapy. Long term maintenance therapy consists of prednisone 5–10 mg/day and azathioprine 2 mg/kg/day. IV immunoglobulin has been reported in specific cases to be effective in treating CNS vasculitis.

SURGICAL MEASURES

- There is no surgical treatment, but biopsies may be required for diagnosis.

SYMPTOMATIC TREATMENT

- Aggressive treatment of hypertension, especially if there is renal involvement. Monitor specific organ dysfunction and treat appropriately. Cardiac involvement, such as coronary artery dilatation in Kawasaki disease, may require monitoring with an echocardiogram.

ADJUNCTIVE TREATMENT

- Physical, occupational, speech, and cognitive therapy may be needed, depending on the specific benefits.

ADMISSION/DISCHARGE CRITERIA

- Patients are admitted for the severity of symptoms and deficits, and evaluation for etiology. Certain institutions may require admission for IV methylprednisolone and/or cyclophosphamide therapy. After induction therapy, patients may need subacute inpatient rehabilitation care.

Medications

DRUG(S) OF CHOICE

- *Induction therapy:* Methylprednisolone 15 mg/kg and cyclophosphamide 2 mg/kg
- *Maintenance therapy:* Prednisone 10 mg/kg/day (tapering over 1 year, alternate-day therapy, and azathioprine 2 mg/kg/day)

Contraindications

- Immunosuppression should be avoided or minimized if an infection is identified. Prior history of hypersensitivity or allergic reaction to any of the above drugs may preclude their use.

Precautions

- Steroid therapy can be associated with hypertension and hyperglycemia. Urine should be examined for glucose. Steroids are associated with gastric ulcers, and prophylaxis with H_2 antagonists is recommended. If azathioprine is used, liver enzymes and CBC must be closely monitored. Cyclophosphamide has been associated with hemorrhagic cystitis, infertility, and numerous other toxicities. All of these drugs should be prescribed only by individuals experienced with their potential toxicity.

ALTERNATIVE DRUGS

- Other immunosuppressive drugs may be useful in specific situations (e.g., cyclosporine, methotrexate), but experience is limited.

Follow-Up

PATIENT MONITORING

- Patients are followed to monitor progression of symptoms and efficacy of therapy. This can be done with serial physical examinations. Also, if an abnormality is detected in the CSF, on MRI, or on angiogram, it can be followed serially to evaluate efficacy of therapy. There may be relapses and remissions of the underlying disorder. If an abnormality by angiography was identified, a response to treatment may be seen on serial angiograms.

EXPECTED COURSE AND PROGNOSIS

- Isolated angiitis of the CNS is relatively rare and its clinical course may vary. It may be acute with rapid progression to coma and then death in 3 days to 6 weeks. It also can wax and wane before a spontaneous resolution, followed by a stepwise progression of symptoms. There may be relapses and remissions with long periods of remission or a slow gradual progression over years. Most patients die within 1 year of this diagnosis. A poor outcome is associated with diffuse cerebral dysfunction and altered mental status. Prognosis is better if the symptoms are primarily focal neurologic deficits or perhaps with early treatment. In secondary CNS vasculitis, success depends on treating the underlying autoimmune, collagen/vascular, infectious, or neoplastic disorder.

PATIENT EDUCATION

- There are no support groups or organizations providing information for patients and their families living with CNS vasculitis.
- For Behçet's disease, there is the American Behçet's Disease Association, P.O. Box 280240, Memphis, TN 38168-0240.
- Organizations may exist for the various other systemic conditions.

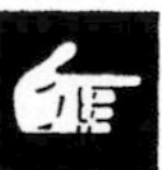

Miscellaneous

SYNONYMS

- Primary angiitis of the central nervous system
- Granulomatous angiitis of the central nervous system
- Isolated angiitis of the central nervous system

ICD-9-CM: 136.1 Behçet's syndrome; 437.4 Cerebral arteritis; 446.0 Polyarteritis nodosa; 446.1 Acute febrile mucocutaneous lymph node syndrome (Kawasaki disease); 446.4 Wegener's granulomatosis; 446.5 Giant cell arteritis; 446.7 Takayasu's disease

REFERENCES

- Alhalabe M, Moore PM. Serial angiography in isolated angiitis of the central nervous system. Neurology 1994;44:1221.
- Ferro JM. Vasculitis of the central nervous system. J Neurol 1998;245:766.
- Hankey JG. Isolated angiitis/angiopathy of the central nervous system. Cerebrovasc Dis 1991;1:2.
- Miller DH, Ormerod EC, Gibson A, et al. MRI brain scanning in patients with vasculitis: differentiation from multiple sclerosis. Neuroradiology 1987;29:226.
- Moore PM. Central nervous system vasculitis. Curr Opin Neurol 1998;3:241-6.
- Moore PM. Neurological manifestation of vasculitis: update on immunopathogenic mechanisms and clinical features. Ann Neurol 1995;37[Suppl 1]:S131–S141.
- Oliveira V, Povoa P, Costa A, et al. Cerebrospinal fluid and therapy of isolated angiitis of the central nervous system. Stroke 1994;25:1693.
- Sigal LH. The neurologic presentation of vasculitic and rheumatologic syndromes. Medicine 1987;66:157.

Author(s): Raymond Ferri, MD; Peter Calabresi, MD

Vertebrobasilar Insufficiency

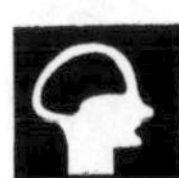

Basics

DESCRIPTION

- Vertebrobasilar insufficiency (VBI) describes a wide spectrum of clinical symptoms caused by compromise of the posterior cerebral circulation. The reduction of blood flow to the brainstem leads to a constellation of brainstem signs and symptoms that are essentially transient ischemic attacks (TIAs) in this vascular territory.

EPIDEMIOLOGY

- Incidence of VBI is about 5–6 per 1,000; vertebrobasilar atherothrombotic disease (VBATD) is about 3 per 1,000; and vertebral artery dissection (VAD) about 1–2 per 1,000.

Sex

- As with atherosclerosis, VBATD affects men twice as often as it does women. For spontaneous VAD, the female-to-male ratio is 3:1.

Age

- VBATD occurs in the late decades of life (70s and 80s). Traumatic causes and vascular anomalies leading to VBI are more common in the younger age group (30s and 40s).

ETIOLOGY

- VBATD is by far the most common cause of VBI, making VBI most common among patients with cardiovascular risk factors such as age, hypertension, diabetes, smoking, and dyslipidemias.
- VBI may result from any disease process that impacts arterial supply to the posterior fossa.
  —Fibromuscular dysplasia
  —Rotational occlusion (Bow hunter's stroke): mechanical occlusion or stenosis of the vertebral artery at the C1-2 level caused by lateral flexion as in traumatic insults
  —Vertebral artery dissection, spontaneous and traumatic
  —Vertebrobasilar aneurysms
  —Dolichoectasia of basilar artery

RISK FACTORS

- As above and hypercoagulable states

PREGNANCY

- The risk of ischemic stroke is not increased during pregnancy but is increased during the first 6 weeks postpartum.

ASSOCIATED CONDITIONS

- Subclavian steal syndrome
- Posterior circulation migraine
- Posterior fossa tumor
- Transtentorial herniation
- CNS vasculitis

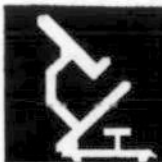

Diagnosis

DIFFERENTIAL DIAGNOSIS

- Benign positional vertigo
- Vestibular neuronitis
- Labyrinthitis
- Multiple sclerosis
- Hemorrhagic stroke
- Ischemic stroke
- Neurosyphilis
- Hypothyroidism/hyperthyroidism
- Meningoencephalitis

SIGNS AND SYMPTOMS

- Vertigo is the hallmark symptom of patients experiencing ischemia in the vertebrobasilar distribution. Many patients describe their vertigo as a nonviolent swaying sensation. Exact incidence is unknown, but up to one third of VBI patients may experience vertigo as the sole manifestation of their illness.
- Visual disturbances (including diplopia)
- Facial numbness or paresthesias
- Dysphagia, dysarthria, hoarseness
- Syncope or presyncope
- Hemisensory or hemimotor extremity symptoms (most commonly contralateral to facial component)

LABORATORY PROCEDURES

- Blood work: There are no specific blood tests to diagnose VBI, but the following blood tests should be obtained to help with differential and treatment options: CBC/differential, electrolyte profile, glucose, coagulation profile, ESR, ANA, RPR, and thyroid function testing.

IMAGING STUDIES

- CT scan helps to rule out CNS hemorrhage or mass effect secondary to cerebellar infarction.
- MRI is far superior to CT scan for brainstem and posterior fossa imaging. MRI is more sensitive to small ischemic areas that characterize branch occlusion of the vertebrobasilar circulation.
- Magnetic resonance angiography (MRA) may be as good as cerebral angiography for detecting occlusions and stenoses of the vertebrobasilar circulation, but because it is a dynamic study it may not be as good for quantifying degree of stenosis.
- Doppler ultrasound and MRA may provide important hemodynamic data on degree of vertebrobasilar stenosis.
- Transcranial Doppler helps assess and monitor vertebrobasilar patency in patients who received intraarterial thrombolysis or/and underwent balloon angioplasty.
- Cerebral angiography is still the gold standard. The characteristic angiographic finding in a dissected vertebral artery is the string or "string and pearl" appearance of the stenotic vessel lumen. Because of the high incidence (up to 40% in some series) of multiple extracranial cervical artery dissections occurring simultaneously in the same patient, four-vessel angiography is the technique of choice in all patients with potential VAD.

SPECIAL TESTS

- Chest x-ray film
- Electrocardiogram
- Consider a lumbar puncture when differential diagnosis is possible meningoencephalitis.

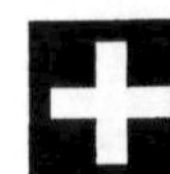

Management

GENERAL MEASURES

- Management is dependent on the underlying etiology, and patient's symptoms and condition
- Airway issues must be addressed for patients with brainstem infarction.
  —Compromise of ninth and tenth cranial nerves can blunt the gag reflex and inhibit even a conscious or awake patient from handling secretions effectively.
  —Secure airway of patient with an unstable course or severe deficits before starting prolonged diagnostic imaging studies.
- Patients with ischemic stroke often are hypertensive, even in the absence of premorbid blood pressure elevations.
  —Given the autoregulatory curve's tendency to shift to the right during hypertension, most experts caution against lowering the blood pressure in the first 24–48 hours after onset of stroke unless extremely elevated.
  —Precipitous drop in blood pressure can significantly impact cerebral perfusion pressure and extend infarction.
  —Consider antihypertensive medication only in cases of concomitant hypertensive emergency (ongoing end-organ damage), mean arterial pressure (MAP) >130 mm Hg, or systolic BP >220 mm Hg.
- Prevent arterial occlusion. If hemorrhagic lesion has been excluded, patients with VBATD and VAD are managed with antiplatelet agents or, in certain circumstances, an anticoagulant such as heparin.

SURGICAL MEASURES

- Endovascular surgery
  - —Intraarterial thrombolysis: High mortality associated with basilar artery occlusion and resulting brainstem infarction has prompted research into reperfusion therapy via intraarterial infusion of thrombolytic agents.
  - —Percutaneous transluminal cerebral angioplasty (PTCA): Increasingly, investigators have described successful dilation of high-grade vertebral artery stenoses in VBATD patients who did not respond to medical therapy.
  - —Balloon angioplasty and stenting: Still experimental in CNS disease. It has been used successfully for cardiovascular diseases. It is now becoming increasingly popular for treatment of VAD and certain cases of VBATD.
- Neurosurgical intervention is indicated for surgical evacuation of cerebellar hemorrhages and to manage cerebellar infarction complicated by hydrocephalus.
- Intravenous thrombolysis (tissue plasminogen activator [tPA]) is now approved for acute stroke within 3 hours. Trials are ongoing for intraarterial urokinase, tPA, and Reteplase for VBI leading to persistent deficits.

SYMPTOMATIC TREATMENT

- Intravenous fluid therapy to provide isotonic hydration and to prevent hyperglycemia, which appears to exacerbate neuronal injury in stroke.
- Treat vomiting with antiemetics. Vomiting may be severe in some brainstem infarctions.

ADJUNCTIVE TREATMENT

- Lipid-lowering statin agents have been shown to be effective in slowing the progression of atherosclerosis.

ADMISSION/DISCHARGE CRITERIA

- Admission is warranted for stuttering VBI symptoms or acute stroke.

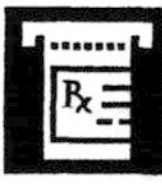

Medications

DRUG(S) OF CHOICE

- Antiplatelet medications constitute first-line treatment for patients with VBATD.
  - —Aspirin 81–650 mg PO qd, not to exceed 1.3 g/day
  - —Clopidogrel (Plavix) 75 mg PO once per day
  - —Aggrenox (combination of extended release dipyridamole 200 mg and aspirin 25 mg) 1 cap PO bid
- Acute heparinization is indicated for stuttering VBI symptoms (crescendo TIAs) or progressive stroke. There is no definite consensus regarding duration of anticoagulation.
  - —Heparin (Hep-Lock) start with 50 U/kg/hour, followed by continuous infusion of 15–25 U/kg/hour. Increase dosage by 5 U/kg/hour q4h PRN using PTT results. If no contraindication, convert heparin to coumadin with INR of 2–3 for 3–6 months.
  - —tPA (Alteplase, Activase) 0.9 mg/kg IV over 60 minutes, with 10% of the dose given as initial IV bolus. Maximum dose: 90 mg. Alternatively, intraarterial therapy 0.6 mg/kg over 30–60 minutes is given. Maximum dose: 60 mg.

Contraindications

- Contraindications for tPA include uncontrolled hypertension, recent surgery or hemorrhage, coagulopathy.

Precautions

N/A

ALTERNATIVE DRUGS

N/A

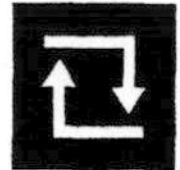

Follow-Up

PATIENT MONITORING

- Patients with VBI warrant admission and close neurologic monitoring until therapy is optimized and patient's clinical condition is stable.

EXPECTED COURSE AND PROGNOSIS

- VBI generally has a more favorable prognosis than carotid territory TIAs because there is less risk of developing a completed stroke. Better collateral circulation may account for improved outcome in these patients.
- Basilar artery occlusion is a rare but devastating complication of VBI. It is associated with a 75%–85% mortality and high rate of neurovegetative states in survivors.
  - —Extracranial dissection: Most patients do remarkably well if they survive the initial crisis. As many as 88% of patients demonstrate complete clinical recovery at follow-up. Severity of neurologic deficits at the time of presentation usually is related directly to the functional outcome.
  - —Patients with intracranial vertebrobasilar dissection constitute a more severely affected subgroup of all patients with VAD and is associated with higher mortality rate.

PATIENT EDUCATION

- *www.stroke.org/supportsearch.cfm*
- Stroke Family "Warn Line." Phone: 1-800-553-6321
- *www.strokeassociation.org/Consumer/support/warmline.html*

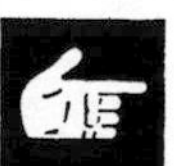

Miscellaneous

SYNONYMS

- Posterior circulation transient cerebral ischemia

ICD-9-CM: 435 Transient cerebral ischemia; 435.0 Basilar artery syndrome; 435.1 Vertebral artery syndrome; 435.2 Subclavian steal syndrome; 435.8 Other specified transient cerebral ischemias; 435.9 Unspecified transient cerebral ischemia

SEE ALSO: N/A

REFERENCES

- Becker KJ, Purcell LL, Hacke W. Vertebrobasilar thrombosis: diagnosis, management, and the use of intra- arterial thrombolytics. Crit Care Med 1996;24: 1729–1742.
- Brandt T, von Kummer R, Muller-Kuppers M. Thrombolytic therapy of acute basilar artery occlusion. Variables affecting recanalization and outcome. Stroke 1996;27:875–881.
- Caplan LR. Vertebrobasilar occlusive disease. In: Barnett HJM, ed. Stroke: pathophysiology, diagnosis and management. New York Churchill Livingston, 1992;1:549–619.
- Culebras A, Kase CS, Masdeu JC. Practice guidelines for the use of imaging in transient ischemic attacks and acute stroke. A report of the Stroke Council, American Heart Association. Stroke 1997;28:1480–1497.
- Lipinski CA, Swanson ER. Vertebrobasilar distribution stroke mimicking transtentorial herniation. Ann Emerg Med 1998;31:640–642.
- Phan TG, Wijdicks EF. Intra-arterial thrombolysis for vertebrobasilar circulation ischemia. Crit Care Clin 1999;15:719–742, vi.
- Sivenius J, Riekkinen PJ, Smets P. The European Stroke Prevention Study (ESPS): results by arterial distribution. Ann Neurol 1991;29:596–600.
- Terada T, Higashida RT, Halbach VV. Transluminal angioplasty for arteriosclerotic disease of the distal vertebral and basilar arteries. J Neurol Neurosurg Psychiatry 1996;60:377–381.
- Whisnant JP, Cartlidge NE, Elveback LR. Carotid and vertebral-basilar transient ischemic attacks: effect of anticoagulants, hypertension, and cardiac disorders on survival and stroke occurrence—a population study. Ann Neurol 1978;3:107–115.

Author(s): Jawad F. Kirmani, MD; Abutaher M. Yahia, MD

Vitamin B_{12} Deficiency

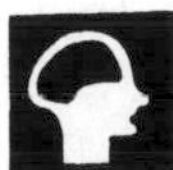

Basics

DESCRIPTION

- Subacute combined degeneration (SCD) is the name given to the spinal cord dysfunction that arises from vitamin B_{12} deficiency. Subacute implies a time course over a few weeks; combined refers to involvement of both the corticospinal tracts (resulting in motor weakness) and the dorsal columns (resulting in vibratory and proprioceptive loss).

EPIDEMIOLOGY

Incidence/Prevalence

- SCD is uncommon.

Race

- No difference

Sex

- No difference

Age

- B_{12} deficiency is more common in the elderly.

ETIOLOGY

- The cause of SCD is vitamin B_{12} deficiency. Rarely the deficiency is not in quantity of B_{12} but rather the precursors of the pathway that processes B_{12} (methylmalonic acid [MMA] and homocysteine [HC]). The classic etiology for B_{12} insufficiency is that of pernicious anemia (PA), wherein the gastric mucosa does not release B_{12} binding factor and patients present with megaloblastic anemia, mental status changes, and evidence of myelopathy. B_{12} is released from bound food in the stomach and bound to intrinsic factor (IF); the B_{12}-IF complex then travels to the distal ilium, where B_{12} is released from IF and absorbed. Pernicious anemia results from antibody formation to IF, reducing the free IF available to bind the vitamin. Pernicious anemia also can result from gastric achlorhydria, most often seen in the elderly, in which increased stomach pH prevents the release of bound B_{12} from food. Also, in today's medical era, malabsorption of B_{12} from the distal ilium may occur from either resection or chronic inflammation of the stomach or ileum, such as sprue or ulcerative colitis. Intestinal bacteria or parasites occasionally may compete for dietary vitamin B_{12}, most notably the fish tapeworm *(Diphyllobothrium latum)*.
- An environmental cause of B_{12} deficiency is that of nitrous oxide abuse; NO_2 interferes with the B_{12} processing pathway and causes an intrinsic deficiency. Patients receiving excess folic acid with B_{12} deficiency may present with spinal cord dysfunction without anemia, as the folate may correct the anemia.
- Gastric carcinomas may be the underlying etiology for pernicious anemia. In patients with clear gastric malabsorption, esophagogastroduodenoscopy (EGD) may be indicated to evaluate for cancerous lesions.

Genetics

N/A

RISK FACTORS

- Infiltrative gastric carcinomas or gastric resection, strict vegetarian diet

PREGNANCY

- Pregnancy may exacerbate an occult B_{12} deficiency, as the needs of the developing fetus may deplete reserves of stored vitamins.

ASSOCIATED CONDITIONS

- Nitrous oxide abuse
- Pernicious anemia
- Terminal ilial resection

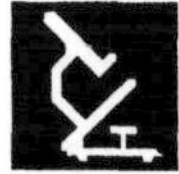

Diagnosis

DIFFERENTIAL DIAGNOSIS

- Myelopathy
- Syringomyelia
- Epidural abscess
- Infectious myelitis, especially tabetic

SIGNS AND SYMPTOMS

- The signs and symptoms of SCD develop subacutely over days to weeks and may vary from overt to insidious in presentation. Patients primarily complain of weakness and imbalance. They may complain of variable degrees of sensory disturbance and even may have a "cord level," i.e., sensory changes ascending to, and ending at, an certain point. Sensory abnormalities vary from numbness to tingling and paresthesias. The imbalance may present as falling, impaired gait, or inability to stand upright without assistance. The weakness may be mild or profound. Reflecting the injury to several ("combined") neurologic pathways, the neurologic examination may reveal a combination of upper and lower motor neuron signs that may be confusing for non-neurologists. Spasticity and positive Babinski signs may coexist with hyporeflexia.
- Signs and symptoms in the upper extremities may or may not be present; this may manifest as the disease progresses. Many patients will have a Lhermitte's sign, which is an electric-like sensation through the spine produced by flexion of the neck, signaling localization to the spinal cord.

LABORATORY PROCEDURES

- Blood work: Vitamin B_{12} and RBC folic acid levels are initially indicated. If they return normal (or low normal) values, then serum MMA and HC levels are checked. MMA and HC both are precursors in the B_{12} metabolic pathway. If B_{12} is deficient, production halts at this point and precursors accumulate; therefore, MMA and HC often will be elevated in B_{12} deficient states.
- If folate is taken to excess in a B_{12} deficient state, HC levels may normalize, whereas MMA levels will remain high.

IMAGING STUDIES

- In any patient with suspected spinal cord dysfunction, MRI of the entire cord, specifically focusing on the region of the presumed level, is indicated. This is done to ensure that abscess or compression is not mimicking SCD. In SCD, high signal on T2-weighted images in the dorsal columns in sagittal views can be seen and is indicative of ongoing degeneration.

SPECIAL TESTS

- The Schilling's test is performed to determine B_{12} malabsorption and to isolate the source. In part I, radiolabeled B_{12} is taken orally and percent absorption is measured. If the absorption is low, the test proceeds until absorption normalizes. In part II, B_{12} and IF are taken together. In part III, B_{12} and IF are given in an acidic milieu to reverse achlorhydria. In part IV, B_{12} and IF are given after 1–2 weeks of antibiotics to treat bacterial overgrowth (bacteria have a propensity for B_{12}).

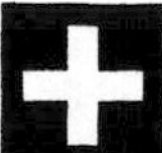

Management

GENERAL MEASURES

- Management of B_{12} deficiency (and SCD) depends upon the underlying etiology. If B_{12} malabsorption is the cause, the vitamin must be replaced.
- Patients should be questioned regarding recreational drug use, specifically abuse of nitrous oxide, or "whippets." Persons with access to NO_2 obviously are at higher risk; this includes those in the dental field and the food industry, where whippets are used in the preparation of whipped cream. NO_2 consumption must be stopped to prevent further CNS injury.
- If a gastric etiology is the cause of B_{12} deficiency, there is a small risk of an underlying gastric carcinoma and consideration should be given for an EGD study.
- The main treatment in the United States is intramuscular (IM) cyanocobalamin. IM replacement should be performed once per week for 2-3 months, then once every 2 weeks for 2-3 months, and then lifelong monthly injections. The level may be checked approximately 2-3 months into treatment to ensure adequacy of therapy. Some resolution of acquired deficits may be observed. The goal of treatment is to prevent further degeneration and dysfunction of the spinal cord.
- Controversy exists as to whether oral vitamin B_{12} is adequate. Oral B_{12} is available in 1,000-μg "nuggets." Currently, some researchers are making a case for large doses of oral B_{12}; oral absorption without IF is 1%–2%, therefore, a 1,000-μg tablet would provide the daily recommended dose of 1–2 μg. However, this is clearly not acceptable as replacement therapy for diminished levels. Oral B_{12} may have a role in maintenance therapy. If the underlying etiology is distal ileal dysfunction, oral treatment may be ineffective.

SURGICAL MEASURES

N/A

ADJUNCTIVE TREATMENT

- Management of gait abnormalities and balance difficulties is best performed by physical therapy.

ADMISSION/DISCHARGE CRITERIA

- Patients are admitted if they are unable to ambulate at presentation. Discharge considerations after evaluation and treatment include ability to perform safely activities of daily living upon discharge. If this is not possible, discharge to inpatient rehabilitation may be necessary.

Medications

DRUG(S) OF CHOICE

- Intramuscular cyanocobalamin

Contraindications

- Anaphylactic reactions

Precautions

- Infections, muscle soreness, focal muscle atrophy from repeated injections

ALTERNATIVE DRUGS

- Oral hydroxycobalamin is sometimes used as a maintenance drug when gastrointestinal absorption of vitamin B_{12} is intact, but careful long-term monitoring of serum B_{12} levels is necessary.
- Cyanocobalamin gel for intranasal administration (500 μg intranasally every week) is indicated for long-term maintenance after a course of replacement with intramuscular cyanocobalamin

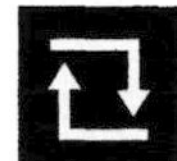

Follow-Up

PATIENT MONITORING

- Once a patient has been diagnosed with B_{12} deficiency, levels should be followed lifelong. Once replacement has occurred and levels have normalized, periodic evaluations (once per year or as needed) is adequate. Patients with a history of nitrous oxide abuse should be offered counseling and periodically assessed for possible relapses.

EXPECTED COURSE AND PROGNOSIS

- Treatment should begin promptly once the diagnosis of B_{12} deficiency is made. Theoretically, degeneration desists as soon as B_{12} levels return to normal. However, acquired abnormalities may not be reversible. Therapy is lifelong.

PATIENT EDUCATION

- Patients should be counseled regarding the necessity of lifelong therapy in case of B_{12} malabsorption. For patients whose underlying etiology is NO_2 abuse, counseling regarding drug abuse is indicated, because some of these patients may relapse.

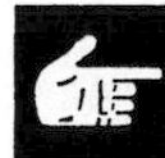

Miscellaneous

SYNONYMS

- Subacute combined degeneration
- B_{12} deficiency
- Pernicious anemia

ICD-9-CM: 336.2 Subacute combined degeneration of spinal cord in diseases classified elsewhere; Deficiency of B complex components: 281.0 Pernicious anemia; 281.1 Other vitamin B_{12} deficiency anemia; 266.2 Vitamin B_{12} deficiency

SEE ALSO: N/A

REFERENCES

- Green R, Kinsella L. Current concepts in the diagnosis of cobalamin deficiency. Neurology 1995;45:1435–1440.
- Layzer R, Fishman R, Schafer J. Neuropathy following abuse of nitrous oxide. Neurology 1978;28:504–506.
- Savage D, et al. Sensitivity of serum methylmalonic acid and total homocysteine determinations for diagnosing cobalamin and folate deficiencies. Am J Med 1994;96: 239–246.
- Stabler S, et al. Vitamin B-12 deficiency in the elderly: current dilemmas. Am J Clin Nutr 1997;66:741–749.
- Stacy C, et al. Methionine in the treatment of nitrous-oxide-induced neuropathy and myeloneuropathy. J Neurol 1992;239: 401–403.

Author(s): Holli A. Horak, MD

Wernicke-Korsakoff Syndrome

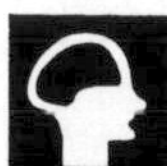

Basics

DESCRIPTION

- Wernicke-Korsakoff syndrome (WKS) is a disorder of the central nervous system in which a lack of thiamine causes an initial acute illness (Wernicke syndrome) followed occasionally by a chronic illness (Korsakoff syndrome). Classic signs of Wernicke syndrome include nystagmus, ataxia, and confusion. Korsakoff syndrome is characterized by a disorder of memory.
- Early replacement of thiamine may abort the acute syndrome, but delay in diagnosis and treatment can cause permanent injury.

EPIDEMIOLOGY

- Wernicke syndrome is frequently underdiagnosed. In one series, only 20% of autopsy cases were suspected in life. Autopsy series frequency for Wernicke syndrome ranges from 0.8%–2.8%. A high level of clinical suspicion is necessary. It is likely that the disease is underreported and underdiagnosed. An estimated 25% of WKS cases were missed when the brains were not examined microscopically.

Incidence/Prevalence

- See Epidemiology

ETIOLOGY

- WKS occurs in the setting of thiamine deficiency. Various states with nutritional deficits may cause this syndrome. Chronic alcoholism with deficient nutritional intake is the most common cause, but other causes include hyperemesis gravidarum, systemic malignancy, chronically ill patients, anorexia nervosa, acquired immunodeficiency syndrome, and postgastroplasty states.
- Thiamine is a vitamin cofactor in many enzymatic reactions important for energy metabolism. Specific areas of the brain susceptible to injury include the paraventricular regions of the thalamus and hypothalamus, the mamillary bodies, the periaqueductal region of the midbrain, the floor of the fourth ventricle, and the superior cerebellar vermis. These areas may show necrosis and gliosis, with vacuolation of the affected brain.

Genetics

- Transketolase in cultured fibroblasts from alcoholics with WKS bind thiamine pyrophosphate less well than control lines. This finding may implicate a hereditary basis for WKS in this population. Recent research suggests that the genetic marker APOE4 is a significant predictor of global intellectual deficits in people with WKS.

RISK FACTORS

- Any condition causing reduced thiamine intake, absorption, or excessive utilization of thiamine can cause WKS.

PREGNANCY

- Hyperemesis gravidarum may precipitate WKS.

ASSOCIATED CONDITIONS

- Alcoholism
- Alcoholic polyneuropathy
- Alcoholic beriberi
- Alcoholic myopathy
- Marchiafava-Bignami disease
- Alcoholic cerebellar degeneration

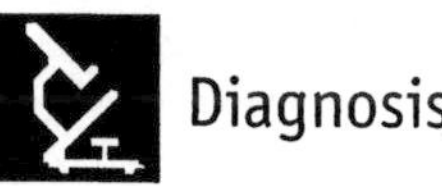

Diagnosis

DIFFERENTIAL DIAGNOSIS

- Diagnosis is based on a high index of suspicion in the appropriate clinical situation. Consider in patients with alcoholism, chronic disease, or poor nutritional intake who show evidence of nystagmus, diplopia, ataxia, confusion, or ophthalmoplegia. Patients with cerebellar or thalamic infarction may have some of the same symptoms. Head injured patients may have unrecognized WKS. Rarely Creutzfeldt-Jacob syndrome may mimic WKS. Paraneoplastic or toxic cerebellar disorders may mimic WKS.

SIGNS AND SYMPTOMS

- The triad of ophthalmoplegia, ataxia, and confusion is classic, but only 19% of patients determined to have Wernicke syndrome show all of these signs. Oculomotor signs: horizontal nystagmus on lateral gaze, bilateral lateral rectus palsies, conjugate gaze palsies, ptosis. Other signs: Paresis of vestibular function may be shown by absent cold water calorics. Confusion with reduced attention, indifference to environment. Unsteady gait due to ataxia. Korsakoff syndrome is diagnosed in the presence of appropriate risk factors, and a defect in learning new material (anterograde amnesia) and a loss of prior memories (retrograde amnesia). Signs of peripheral neuropathy, an associated nutritional disorder, are common. Postural hypotension and syncope are common and related to autonomic insufficiency.

LABORATORY PROCEDURES

- WKS is a clinical diagnosis. Laboratory testing usually is not helpful. Blood pyruvate levels are elevated in untreated cases of Wernicke syndrome. Blood transketolase activity is reduced to as low as one third of normal values, but assays are not readily available.

IMAGING STUDIES

- CT scanning is of no use in WKS. It may help rule out concurrent syndromes causing altered consciousness, such as subdural hematomas, intracerebral hemorrhage, or ischemic disease.
- MRI occasionally can show atrophy of the mamillary bodies or small hemorrhages in affected brain areas. The sensitivity and specificity of this test for WKS are unknown.

SPECIAL TESTS

N/A

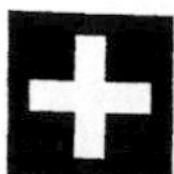

Management

GENERAL MEASURES

- Care must be taken to stabilize the patient medically, particularly noting the presence of hypothermia and treating it if present. Appropriate fluid resuscitation is key, because patients may be dehydrated. Patients should be examined for trauma and assessed for the presence of alcohol intoxication or withdrawal, as well as concurrent drug intoxication or withdrawal. Concurrent pneumonia, subdural hematoma, GI bleeding, pancreatitis, and other sequelae of alcoholism may be present and need to be considered and treated.

SURGICAL MEASURES

N/A

SYMPTOMATIC TREATMENT

- See Medications

ADJUNCTIVE TREATMENT

- Treatment for alcohol withdrawal or delirium tremens may be necessary (see appropriate sections).

ADMISSION/DISCHARGE CRITERIA

- Patients with Wernicke syndrome usually are acutely ill and require admission. Patients with Korsakoff syndrome may require long-term care.

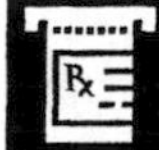

Medications

DRUG(S) OF CHOICE

- Thiamine: 100 mg IV stat, followed by 50–100 mg IM/IV qd until normal intake is reestablished.

Contraindications

- Hypersensitivity to thiamine

Precautions

- Rare cases of angioedema, cyanosis, or anaphylaxis may occur. Common reactions include pruritus, urticaria, and injection site pain.

ALTERNATIVE DRUGS

N/A

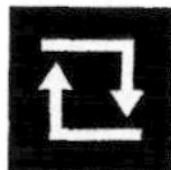

Follow-Up

PATIENT MONITORING

- Patients with WKS are acutely ill and need to be monitored in an ICU or other monitored setting until they are stable.

EXPECTED COURSE AND PROGNOSIS

- Although treatable if caught early enough, the death rate from WKS is relatively high, about 10%–20%. Ataxia improves > nystagmus > cognitive dysfunction.

PATIENT EDUCATION

- When stable, patients should be counseled on avoiding alcohol intake (if appropriate) and maintaining good dietary intake.

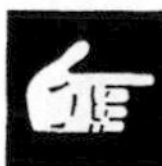

Miscellaneous

SYNONYMS

N/A

ICD-9-CM: 291.1 (alcoholic); 294.0 (non-alcoholic)

SEE ALSO: ALCOHOL, NEUROLOGIC COMPLICATIONS

REFERENCES

- Harper CG, Giles M, Finlay-Jones R. Clinical signs in the Wernicke-Korsakoff complex. J Neurol Neurosurg Psychiatry 1986;49:341–345.
- Zubaran C, Fernandes JG, Rodnight R. Wernicke-Korsakoff syndrome. Postgrad Med J 1997;73:27–31.

Author(s): Alexander D. Rae-Grant, MD

Whipple's Disease

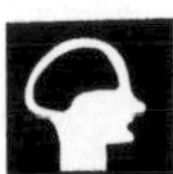

Basics

DESCRIPTION

- Whipple's disease is a rare systemic disorder caused by infection with *Tropheryma whippelii.* It is characterized by diarrhea, migratory arthralgias, lymphadenopathy, fever, dementia, ophthalmoplegia, and myoclonus.
- CNS involvement occurs in 5%–40% of cases and may be present without systemic symptoms.
- Oculomasticatory myorhythmia and oculofacial-skeletal myorhythmia are infrequent but pathognomonic signs of the disease.

EPIDEMIOLOGY

Incidence/Prevalence

- <1,000 cases reported since 1907. Occupational association with farmers, construction workers, and machinists

Race

- Nearly all reported cases are Caucasians.

Age

- Peak in the fifth decade

Sex

- 86% male

ETIOLOGY

- *Tropheryma whippelii,* a Gram-positive bacillus
- Humans are the only known host
- Reservoir unknown
- Infection probably from ingestion
- Pathogenesis unknown
- Spread to CNS is likely hematogenous; several reported cases of endocarditis and embolic strokes

RISK FACTORS

- Exposure to soil or animals

PREGNANCY

- No reported cases

ASSOCIATED CONDITIONS

- Arthritis
- Fever of unknown origin
- Malabsorption
- Diarrhea
- Weight loss
- Pneumonia
- Dementia
- Seizures
- Headache

Diagnosis

DIFFERENTIAL DIAGNOSIS

Systemic

- Celiac sprue
- Rheumatoid arthritis
- Lymphoma
- Inflammatory bowel disease
- Pancreatitis
- Systemic lupus erythematous
- Lyme disease
- Waldenström's macroglobulinemia

Neurologic

- Alzheimer's disease
- Sarcoidosis
- Vasculitis
- Primary or metastatic tumor
- Cerebrovascular accident
- Multiple sclerosis
- Encephalitis
- HIV-related CNS infections
- Tuberculosis
- Creutzfeldt-Jakob Disease

SIGNS AND SYMPTOMS

Systemic

- Arthralgias
- Fever
- Abdominal pain
- Weight loss
- Diarrhea
- Malabsorption
- Uveitis
- Lymphadenopathy
- Increased skin pigmentation

Neurologic

- Dementia
- Ophthalmoplegia, particularly upward gaze palsy
- Myoclonus
- Nystagmus
- Oculomasticatory myorhythmia (OMM): 1-Hz pendular convergent nystagmus with synchronous contraction of muscles of mastication
- Oculofacial-skeletal myorhythmia (OFSM): 1-Hz pendular convergent nystagmus with synchronous contraction of facial and skeletal muscles
  - —OMM and OFSM have not been reported in other diseases.
- Personality changes
- Ataxia
- Cranial nerve deficits
- Hypothalamic symptoms
  - —Insomnia, temperature sensitivity, altered appetite
- Headache
- Seizures
- Focal neurologic deficits

LABORATORY PROCEDURES

- Biopsy: Jejunum is the most common site, but *T. whippelii* has been identified in CNS tissue, lymph nodes, serum, and pleural fluid.
  - —Staining with periodic acid-Schiff (PAS) is strongly suggestive but not diagnostic.
  - —Negative biopsy should be repeated in 1 month if clinical suspicion is high.
- Polymerase chain reaction (PCR) testing provides a sensitive and specific means of diagnosis and monitoring.
- Organisms can be seen by electron microscopy

IMAGING STUDIES

- MRI of brain or spinal cord: Lesions enhance without edema.
  - —May mimic stroke, tumor, demyelinating plaques, or vascular abnormalities.
- CT of brain: Lesions enhance with contrast.
- KUB: Enlarged small intestine, thickened mucosa.

SPECIAL TESTS

- PAS staining
- PCR
- Electron microscopy

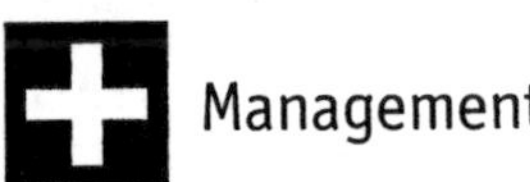

Management

GENERAL MEASURES

- Malabsorption: intravenous hydration and nutritional supplementation

SURGICAL MEASURES

N/A

SYMPTOMATIC TREATMENT

- Antiepileptics for seizures
- Analgesics for headache and arthralgias
- Hydration and symptomatic treatment of diarrhea

ADJUNCTIVE TREATMENT

N/A

ADMISSION/DISCHARGE CRITERIA

- Seizure control
- Facilitate diagnosis
- Parenteral nutrition
- Intravenous antibiotics

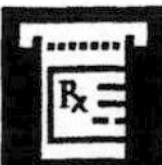

Medications

DRUG(S) OF CHOICE

- Induction treatment for 2–4 weeks
  —Ceftriaxone 2 gm IV bid ± streptomycin 1 gm IV/IM qd *or*
  —Penicillin G 4 million units IV q4h *and* streptomycin 1 g IV/IM qd
- Maintenance treatment for 1 year
  —Trimethoprim-sulfamethoxazole DS PO bid *or*
  —Cefepime 400 mg PO bid
- Recurrence or clinical decline on oral antibiotics requires repeat course of intravenous ceftriaxone for at least 1 month.

Contraindications

- Allergy to cephalosporins or sulfonamides

Precautions

- Folinic acid supplementation should be given with chronic trimethoprim-sulfamethoxazole administration.
- Because of the rare nature of this disease, consultation with an infectious disease specialist is recommended.

ALTERNATIVE DRUGS

- Doxycycline or chloramphenicol may be used for patients allergic to cephalosporins and sulfonamides.

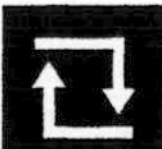

Follow-Up

PATIENT MONITORING

- Repeat jejunal biopsy or CSF PCR at 1 year to verify clearance
- Serial MRI to assess response

EXPECTED COURSE AND PROGNOSIS

- Uniformly fatal prior to advent of antibiotics
- Systemic symptoms routinely respond to antibiotics
- Of CNS manifestations, nystagmus and ophthalmoplegia show the most improvement.
- Recurrence rate is high.

PATIENT EDUCATION

- *www.niddk.nih.gov/health/digest/summary/whipple/whipple.htm*

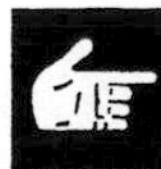

Miscellaneous

SYNONYMS

- Intestinal lipodystrophy

ICD-9-CM: 040.2 Whipple's disease

SEE ALSO: N/A

REFERENCES

- Anderson M. Neurology of Whipple's disease. J Neurol Neurosurg Psychiatry. 2000;68:1–5.
- Dobbins WO III, ed. Whipple's disease. Springfield, IL: Charles C Thomas, 1987.
- Fleming J, Weisner R, Shorter R. Whipple's disease: clinical, biochemical, and histopathologic features and assessment of treatment in 29 patients. Mayo Clinic Proceedings. 1998;63:539–551.
- Fredericks D, Relman D. Localization of Tropheryma whippelii rRNA in tissues from patients with Whipple's disease. The Journal of Infectious Disease. 2001;183: 1229–37.
- Keinath RD, Merrel DE, Vlietstra R, Dobbins WO III. Antibiotic treatment and relapse in Whipple's disease. Gastroenterology. 1985;88:1867–73.
- Louis ED, Lynch T, Kaufman P, Fahn F, Odel J. Diagnostic guidelines in central nervous system Whipple's disease. Ann Neurol. 1996;40:561–68.
- von Herbay A, Ditton HJ, Scuhmacher F, et al. Whipple's disease: staging and monitoring by cytology and polymerase chain reaction analysis of cerebrospinal fluid. Gastroenterology 1997;113:434–41.
- Whipple GH. A hitherto undescribed disease characterized anatomically by deposits of fat and fatty acids in the intestinal and mesenteric lymphatic tissues. Bull Johns Hopkins Hosp. 1907;18:382–391.

Author(s): Todd Czartoski, MD; Christina Marra, MD

Wilson's Disease

Basics

DESCRIPTION

- Wilson's disease (WD) is an inherited disorder of copper metabolism with a wide spectrum of clinical manifestations.

EPIDEMIOLOGY

Incidence/Prevalence

- Estimates of prevalence vary widely (10–30 per million), with a heterozygous carrier rate of 1 in 90.

Race

- No known difference

Age

- Age at diagnosis of WD varies from 3-61 years. Hemolytic anemia presents in early childhood (ages 7-14), chronic liver disease between ages 5 and mid-30s, and neuropsychiatric symptoms between ages 14 and 40.

Sex

- No known difference

ETIOLOGY

- The cause of this illness is a gene mutation causing absence or dysfunction of production of a copper transporting ATPase ATP7B. This ATPase is localized to the hepatocyte trans-Golgi network and transports copper into the secretary pathway for incorporation into ceruloplasmin and excretion into bile. The normal route of excretion of copper in the bile is deficient, and copper accumulates in the liver. When hepatic storage is exceeded, hepatocyte death occurs with copper release into the plasma (where it is bound by ceruloplasmin) and tissue deposition.

Genetics

- WD is inherited as an autosomal recessive disease due to mutation of the ATPase ATP7B gene on chromosome 13. The risk of WD is 40% in a sibling of an index case and 0.5% in a child of an index parent.

RISK FACTORS

N/A

PREGNANCY

- Both penicillamine and trientine have been used successfully for treatment of WD during pregnancy without reports of teratogenicity.

ASSOCIATED CONDITIONS

N/A

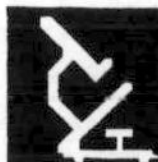

Diagnosis

DIFFERENTIAL DIAGNOSIS

- The differential diagnosis of WD is very large given the wide spectrum of potential presentations and includes the differential diagnosis for each of the conditions listed under Signs and Symptoms.
- Neurologic disorders that are in the differential include
  —Huntington's disease
  —Essential tremor
  —Parkinson's disease
  —Neurologic complications of chronic hepatic encephalopathy
  —Multiple sclerosis

SIGNS AND SYMPTOMS

Hepatic

- Chronic active hepatitis
- Cirrhosis
- Fulminant hepatic failure

Hematologic

- Coombs' negative hemolytic anemia
- Hypersplenism
- Coagulopathy due to liver disease

Renal

- Fanconi's syndrome
- Urolithiasis
- Hematuria
- Proteinuria
- Peptiduria
- Nephrocalcinosis

Neuropsychiatric

- Neurologic symptoms occur at initial presentation in 60% of patients, usually in the third or fourth decade of life.
- Tremor: "wing beating," titubation
- Dystonia of bulbar musculature with resultant dysarthria and dysphagia
- Gait disorder (parkinsonian and/or ataxic)
- Seizures (approximately 6%)
- Personality change: emotional lability, impulsiveness, disinhibition
- Affective symptoms
- Cognitive impairment
- Psychosis

Ophthalmologic

- Kayser-Fleischer (KF) pigmented corneal rings
- Sunflower cataracts
- Night blindness

Other

- Osteopenia
- Arthralgias/arthritis
- Cardiomyopathy/cardiac arrhythmias
- Amenorrhea
- Hypoparathyroidism

LABORATORY PROCEDURES

- Total serum copper levels are of little value.
- Free serum copper is generally elevated.
- Serum ceruloplasmin: Reduced level <20 mg/dL is strongly supportive (normal: 20–40 mg/dL). False-positive low levels may occur in protein deficiency states, heterozygotes for the WD gene who will not develop disease, and hypoceruloplasminemia. False-negative results may be due to elevated levels: ceruloplasmin is an acute phase reactant and levels will increase in response to hepatic inflammation or end-stage hepatic disease, pregnancy, infection, or treatment with estrogens.
- Twenty-four-hour urinary copper excretion often is increased (>100 μg in 24 hours).

IMAGING STUDIES

- Cranial CT scan is abnormal in the majority of patients having neuropsychiatric WD, with generalized atrophy, dilation of the ventricles, and focal areas of low attenuation in the basal ganglia and more diffusely. Brain MRI shows abnormal low signal lesions on T1-weighted images and high signal on T2-weighted images in the putamen, and dorsal and central aspects of the pons.

SPECIAL TESTS

- Slit-lamp ophthalmologic examination for KF rings: Despite a clinical tradition that KF rings must be present once neuropsychiatric signs are present in WD, there are reports of a small percentage of patients with neuropsychiatric signs without KF rings.
- Hepatic copper content via liver biopsy is considered the gold standard for diagnosis by some (normal: 15–55 μg per gram).
- Definitive diagnosis often is based on the presence of two of the following:
  —KF ring
  —Serum ceruloplasmin level <20 mg/dL
  —Typical neuropsychiatric finding

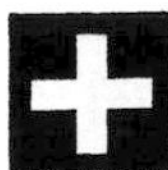

Management

GENERAL MEASURES

- Treatment of WD centers on efforts to restore and maintain normal copper balance within body tissues. Primary treatment is systemic chelation therapy to restore hepatic copper balance.

SURGICAL MEASURES

- Orthoptic hepatic transplantation is recommended for patients with progressive liver failure unresponsive to chelation therapy or acute liver failure due to fulminant hepatitis. Hepatic transplantation results in improvement of neuropsychiatric symptoms.

SYMPTOMATIC TREATMENT

- Physical therapy and treatments that address the many manifestations of WD

ADJUNCTIVE TREATMENT

- Zinc salts should be prescribed in addition to chelation therapy to reduce gastrointestinal copper absorption. Dietary copper should be restricted.

ADMISSION/DISCHARGE CRITERIA

- Admission is required if symptoms are life threatening (e.g., hepatic failure) or if hydration, mobility, and nutrition are compromised.

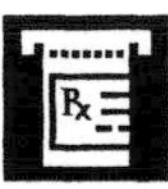

Medications

DRUG(S) OF CHOICE

- Penicillamine (dimethylcysteine), the traditional mainstay for treatment of WD, avidly chelates copper; the complexed copper is excreted in urine. The traditional initial recommended dosage is 1–2 g daily on an empty stomach, but many advocate beginning with a significantly lower dose, such as 250 mg/day with gradual upward titration. Because of the high adverse reaction profile, some authorities recommend induction therapy with less toxic alternatives.
- Zinc acetate or zinc sulfate should be administered at a dose of 50-mg elemental zinc three times per day on an empty stomach.

CONTRAINDICATIONS

- Renal disease and history of penicillamine-induced aplastic anemia or agranulocytosis

Precautions

- Initiation of penicillamine therapy is frequently associated with neurologic deterioration. This has been attributed to mobilization of copper from the liver with redistribution to the brain, although there is evidence against this hypothesis. This problem has led some authorities to recommend induction of therapy with alternative agents such as zinc or ammonium tetrathiomolybdate.
- Penicillamine therapy may cause acute sensitivity reactions, including skin rash, fever, eosinophilia, thrombocytopenia, leukopenia, and lymphadenopathy. Penicillamine should be discontinued until the fever and rash clear. It then can be reinstituted at a reduced dose with concomitant prednisone, or an alternative agent may be considered. Many other adverse reactions are associated with penicillamine, including nephrotic syndrome, Goodpasture's syndrome, a lupus-like syndrome, myasthenic syndrome, polyarthritis, thrombocytopenia, retinal hemorrhages, dysgeusia, and dermatopathy.

ALTERNATIVE DRUGS

- Ammonium tetrathiomolybdate (TM) complexes copper in the gut to prevent absorption and in the bloodstream to reduce tissue deposition. TM is administered in a regimen of 6 doses daily: 3 with meals and 3 between meals, at starting doses of 20 mg at meal time and 20 mg between meals gradually titrated upward (20–60 mg/dose). In initial studies, patients were switched to zinc maintenance therapy after 8 weeks. TM is associated with reversible bone marrow depression and damage to epiphyses in growing bone.
- Triethylene tetramine dihydrochloride (trientine) is a copper chelation therapy. It should be taken on an empty stomach. A typical daily dosage is 750–2,000 mg in three divided doses. Trientine is less toxic than penicillamine, but it has been associated with lupus nephritis and sideroblastic anemia.

Follow-Up

PATIENT MONITORING

- Blood counts and urinalysis should be followed closely during penicillamine therapy because hypersensitivity reactions are not uncommon. Copper concentrations in 24-hour urine collections can be used to guide titration of therapy. A 24-hour cupriuresis >2 g is desirable, and it is recommended that the dose be titrated up until this level is achieved for the first 3 months of therapy if tolerated.

EXPECTED COURSE AND PROGNOSIS

- Most patients will become asymptomatic within 4 months of chelation therapy. After significant improvement occurs, the dose of penicillamine may be reduced by half for lifetime maintenance chelation therapy.

PATIENT EDUCATION

- Compliance with long-term chelation therapy must be encouraged because rapid deterioration has been reported after abrupt discontinuation of penicillamine. Patients should be instructed to follow a low-copper diet.
- Wilson's Disease Association, 4 Navahoe Drive, Brookfield, CT 06804. Phone: 1-800-399-0266, website: *www.medhelp.org/wda/lit.htm*
- Wilson's Disease Association International. Website: *www.wilsonsdisease.org*
- Wilson's Disease Association Copper Content of Various Foods. Website: *www.wilsonsdisease.org/copper.html*

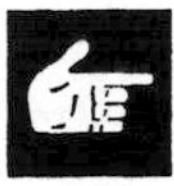

Miscellaneous

SYNONYMS

- Hepatolenticular degeneration

ICD-9-CM: 275.1 Disorders of copper metabolism, Wilson's disease

SEE ALSO: N/A

REFERENCES

- Bax RT, Hassler A. Luck W, et al. Cerebral manifestations of Wilson's disease successfully treated with liver transplantation. Neurology 1998;51:863–865.
- Brewer GJ, Dick RD, Yuzbasiyan-Gurkan V, et al. Treatment of Wilson's disease with ammonium tetrathiomolybdate. I. Initial therapy in 17 neurologically affected patients. Arch Neurol 1994:51:545–554.
- Cuthbert JA. Wilson's disease: update on a systemic disorder with protean manifestations. Gastroenterol Clin North Am 1998;27:655–682.
- Loudianos G, Gitlin JD. Wilson's disease. Semin Liver Dis 2000;20:353–364.

Author(s): D. Joanne Lynn, MD

SECTION IV

Short Topics

Abetalipoproteinemia

Bassen-Kornzweig syndrome; autosomal recessive; disorder of lipid metabolism, develops in first decade of life; symptoms and signs consist of steatorrhea, distal sensorimotor neuropathy, retinitis pigmentosa, ataxia, areflexia, and dysarthria; metabolic defect involves inability to synthesize β-lipoprotein, which reduces concentration of chylomicrons and causes deficiencies of fat-soluble vitamins A, K, and E; neurologic syndrome resembles vitamin E deficiency in other situations; treatment consists of vitamin E supplementation, restricted intake of long-chain fats, substitution with polyunsaturated fats, and rehabilitation.

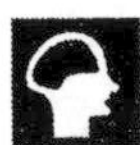

Adie's Syndrome

Tonic pupil syndrome; incidence of 4.7 per 100,000; usually sporadic in origin; female preponderance with typical onset between 20 and 50 years of age; unilateral in 80% of cases; usually develops acutely, with pupillary dilation and poor reaction to light; over time the pupil often becomes miotic; symptoms include difficulty with dark adaptation and reading, photophobia, blurred near vision, and anisocoria; reduced or absent deep tendon reflexes are often noted; cholinergic denervation supersensitivity can be demonstrated with a 0.1% pilocarpine solution; cause of Adie's syndrome remains unclear; symptomatic treatment is not required for most patients.

Adrenoleukodystrophy

X-linked recessive disorder with variable expressivity; adrenoleukodystrophy (ALD) gene encodes an ATP-binding cassette transporter protein; childhood onset most common (between 5 and 10 years of age), may develop in adolescence or adulthood; clinical symptoms are progressive and include withdrawal, dementia, visual loss with optic atrophy, spastic gait, dysphagia, deafness, and seizures; adrenal failure variable; patients enter vegetative state within 1–10 years of onset; MRI shows diffuse demyelination, which predates clinical symptoms; diagnosis requires presence of elevated levels of very-long-chain fatty acids (VLCFA) in plasma and cultured fibroblasts; treatment includes replacement and stress steroids, methods to reduce VLCFA, and bone marrow transplantation.

Adrenomyeloneuropathy

Most common phenotypic variant of ALD; accounts for 25% of phenotypes associated with mutations at ALD locus; onset between 18 and 36 years of age; main clinical features include spastic paraparesis, peripheral neuropathy, and adrenal insufficiency; other commonly noted signs are hypogonadism, impotence, cerebellar dysfunction, and dementia; MRI reveals demyelination, which always predates symptoms; diagnosis requires presence of elevated levels of VLCFA in plasma and cultured fibroblasts; treatment is similar to ALD and includes replacement and stress steroids, methods to reduce VLCFA, such as dietary restriction of VLCFA and Lorenzo's oil (glycerol trierucate oil, glycerol trioleate oil), and bone marrow transplantation.

Adult Polyglucosan Body Disease

Glycogenosis type IV; form of glycogen storage disease with adult onset in the fifth or sixth decade; usually associated with a deficiency of the branching enzyme, but there appear to be other biochemical variants; inheritance is autosomal recessive; characterized by progressive upper and lower motor neuron dysfunction, sensory loss, sphincter abnormalities, neurogenic bladder, and dementia (50% of patients); electrodiagnostic testing demonstrates axonal sensorimotor neuropathy; polyglucosan bodies are periodic acid–Schiff (PAS)-positive, diastase-resistant cellular inclusions; pathology reveals polyglucosan bodies in processes of neurons and astrocytes of gray and white matter, and in the axoplasm of peripheral myelinated fibers; there is no specific therapy.

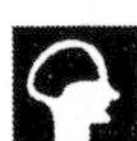

Aicardi's Syndrome

Disorder of cerebral cortical development, with abnormal neuronal migration; only noted in females, probably due to X-linked dominant transmission (lethal to males); presents with severe mental retardation, early seizures (infantile spasms), agenesis or hypoplasia of the corpus callosum, periventricular and subcortical band heterotopias, chorioretinal lacunae, cerebellar abnormalities, fused vertebrae, and hemivertebrae; associated with an increased incidence of choroid plexus papillomas; there is no specific therapy except anticonvulsant treatment; supportive care.

Alexander Disease

Degenerative disease of unknown etiology that affects astrocytes; autosomal inheritance may be noted in some families; usually occurs in childhood; infantile form most common, which presents with severe psychomotor retardation, progressive spasticity, seizures, megalencephaly, and frequent hydrocephalus; juvenile and adult variants are less severe; CT and MRI demonstrate diffuse demyelination with a frontal predominance; pathologic hallmark is diffuse presence of Rosenthal fibers within astrocytic footplates; alpha B-crystallin and HSP27 levels may be elevated in CSF; therapy is nonspecific and consists of seizure medications and other supportive care.

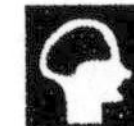

Alpers' Syndrome

Progressive infantile poliodystrophy; grouped into diseases of mitochondrial enzyme defects; exact gene and enzyme defect remains unclear; age of onset before 1 year, with death by age 5; presents with initial psychomotor delay, abrupt onset of seizures, multifocal myoclonus, areflexia, and hypotonia; ataxia, spasticity, and blindness may occur later; 40% incidence of hepatic dysfunction; damage noted in cerebral cortex, cerebellum, basal ganglia, and brainstem; biochemical abnormalities include decreased pyruvate dehydrogenase activity and dysfunction of the citric acid cycle; MRI shows progressive atrophy; diagnosis is by exclusion; no specific treatment, except for anticonvulsants; a trial of pyridoxine may be helpful.

Andersen Syndrome

Type of familial periodic paralysis; autosomal dominant inheritance; linked to mutations of potassium channel Kir2.1 subunit on chromosome 17q23 in some families; attacks may be associated with high, low, or normal potassium levels; administration of potassium may provoke attacks of weakness or arrhythmias; presentation is in childhood or adolescence with dysmorphic features (low-set ears, broad nose, hypertelorism), short stature, periodic paralysis, potassium sensitivity, myotonia, and cardiac disease (prolonged QT interval, ventricular arrhythmias); EMG demonstrates progressive drop in CMAP amplitude during exercise, without myotonic discharges; serum CK shows mild-to-moderate elevation; high incidence of death from arrhythmia and cardiac arrest; acetazolamide may control periodic weakness; antiarrhythmics.

Angelman's Syndrome

Genetic disease that usually is sporadic but may be familial; associated with DNA deletion within chromosome 15q11-13, inherited maternally in most cases; mouse models suggest UBE3A is a strong candidate gene within 15q12; infants are typically normal at birth, with rapid onset of feeding abnormalities and failure to thrive; other features include small head circumference, severely delayed motor development and hypotonia, early onset of seizures, lack of speech development, wide-based and ataxic gait, hyperactivity, rounded facies with a protruding tongue, delayed puberty, and very short adult height; no specific treatment, except anticonvulsants.

Apert Syndrome

Acrocephalosyndactyly; a subtype of craniosynostosis; autosomal dominant; abnormal skull development with coronal suture closure, shortening of the head in the anteroposterior dimension, prominent forehead, and flat occiput; typical facies includes shallow orbits and proptosis of eyes, hypertelorism, maxillary hypoplasia, small nose, low-set ears, and narrow or cleft palate; osseous and cutaneous syndactyly noted often; occasional cardiac, gastrointestinal, and genitourinary malformations are present; mental deficiency often noted; hydrocephalus may develop; maldevelopment of the limbic structures, corpus callosum, and gyri may occur; no specific therapy.

Ataxia-Telangiectasia

Early-onset ataxia syndrome; autosomal recessive inheritance; involves mutations of ATM gene on chromosome 11q22-23, results in dysfunction of DNA repair processes and impaired cell cycle control; clinical features include truncal ataxia, delayed motor development, dysarthria, conjunctival and cutaneous telangiectasias, immune dysfunction with reduced concentrations of IgA and IgG2, recurrent respiratory and cutaneous infections, growth retardation, premature aging, and delayed sexual development; mild mental retardation, oculomotor abnormalities, myoclonus, and peripheral neuropathy may be noted; 15%–20% incidence of malignancies, especially leukemias and lymphomas; serum α-fetoprotein level is elevated; median age at death is 20 years, from respiratory infections and cancer; treatment is supportive (antibiotics).

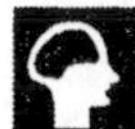

Balint's Syndrome

Symptom complex due to bilateral damage to posterior parietal lobes (e.g., angular gyrus and superior parietal cortex); most commonly caused by watershed infarction; cerebral control of precise eye movements is impaired; clinical features include optic ataxia (defect in reaching under visual guidance), simultanagnosia (inability to recognize a whole picture despite perceiving its parts), and ocular apraxia (defect in voluntary eye movements); inferior altitudinal visual field defects and bilateral hemineglect may be present; patients may deny having any visual dysfunction or deficits.

Behçet's Disease

Inflammatory disorder of unknown etiology, characterized by relapsing/remitting uveitis and recurrent genital and oral ulcers; CNS involvement occurs in 25%–30% of patients; age at onset is the third and fourth decades; men are affected more frequently than women; neurologic signs and symptoms include headache, cranial nerve palsies, seizures, mental confusion, dementia, aphasia, hemiparesis, and papilledema; low-grade fevers are common; laboratory data may include elevated sedimentation rate, anemia, mild leukocytosis, elevated CSF pressure and protein, CSF pleocytosis; CNS involvement may be multifocal (similar to multiple sclerosis); CT/MRI demonstrate focal CNS lesions; immunosuppressive therapy may be of benefit for CNS involvement.

Brill-Zinsser Disease

Recrudescent typhus; flare-up of epidemic louse-borne typhus fever in mild form months to years after the primary attack; infectious agent is obligate intracellular parasite *Rickettsia prowazekii*, which has remained latent in the tissues; symptoms and signs are similar to epidemic typhus fever, lasts 7–12 days, and may include the characteristic rash (often absent), mild fever, headache, malaise, myalgias, photophobia, dizziness, stroke, and mild somnolence or encephalopathy; diagnosis is made by Weil-Felix test (may be negative) or specific rickettsial antibody titers; treatment is with tetracycline antibiotics (doxycycline) or chloramphenicol, and supportive care.

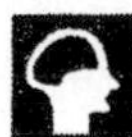

Carnitine Deficiency

Carnitine is an essential cofactor to transport long-chain fatty acids into mitochondria for β-oxidation; muscle carnitine concentration is decreased or absent; primary carnitine deficiency presents in first or second decade as progressive, proximal muscle weakness and hypotonia, reduced or absent reflexes, normal motor milestones, mentation and sensation preserved; atrophy of extremities may be noted; EMG shows diffuse myopathic process; secondary carnitine deficiency occurs with short-chain and medium-chain acyl-coenzyme A dehydrogenase deficiencies, Reye syndrome, and valproate therapy; primary carnitine deficiency is diagnosis of exclusion; treatment consists of oral carnitine, with or without prednisone.

Cerebrotendinous Xanthomatosis

Cholestanol storage disease; caused by mutations in the sterol 27-hydroxylase gene; autosomal inheritance often noted; clinical features become apparent in early adolescence and include cataracts, tendon xanthomas, progressive spasticity and ataxia, dysarthria, mental deterioration (in most cases), sensorimotor neuropathy, distal muscle wasting, and Babinski signs; pseudobulbar palsy, dementia, and myocardial infarction may be noted in late stages; cholestanol levels are increased in plasma, brain, bile, and tendon xanthomas; cholesterol level usually normal in serum; chenodeoxycholic acid level is reduced or absent in bile; treatment with a low cholestanol diet or certain bile acids may be of benefit.

Chagas Disease

South American trypanosomiasis *(Trypanosoma cruzi)*; infection is transmitted by an animal host (e.g., rodents, cats) to humans by blood-sucking reduviid bugs (i.e., "kissing bug"); clinical features include an acute febrile stage with conjunctivitis, facial edema, lymphadenopathy, and hepatosplenomegaly; chronic infection may lead to diffuse (encephalopathy, seizures, chorea) or focal (hemiplegia, ataxia, aphasia) neurologic involvement; disease is slowly progressive without treatment; laboratory abnormalities may include elevated ESR and anemia, and CSF lymphocytic pleocytosis with elevated protein and γ-globulins; diagnosis made by demonstration of organisms in blood, CSF, or biopsy materials, or by serologic and CSF antibody testing; treatment with nifurtimox or benzimidazole usually effective in acute stage.

Chediak-Higashi Syndrome

Autosomal recessive inheritance; characterized by partial oculocutaneous albinism, immunologic defects, hepatosplenomegaly, pancytopenia, and progressive neurologic dysfunction, including psychomotor retardation, seizures, nystagmus, spinocerebellar disorder, and peripheral neuropathy; linked to mutation of CHS1 gene on chromosome 1q42-44; results in defective transport of intracellular proteins, leading to giant peroxidase-positive granules and reduced function of leukocytes and other granule-containing cells (e.g., monocytes, hepatocytes, renal tubular cells); neurons and Schwann cells may have inclusions; predisposition to frequent pyogenic infections; increased risk of lymphoreticular malignancies; therapy consists of anticonvulsants, antibiotics, and other supportive care; no specific therapy exists.

Chorea-Acanthocytosis

Neuroacanthocytosis; Levine-Critchley syndrome; multisystem degenerative disease; characterized by acanthocytes, normal plasma lipids and lipoproteins, and variable neurologic involvement; inheritance usually autosomal dominant, but may be recessive or sporadic; linked to chromosome 9q21; onset in fourth or fifth decade; clinical features include hyperkinetic movement disorder (chorea, orofacial dyskinesias, dystonia), personality changes such as obsessive-compulsive disorder, dementia in late stages, axonal neuropathy with muscle wasting and weakness, reduced deep tendon reflexes, pseudobulbar palsy, and seizures in 40% of patients; MRI shows generalized atrophy and atrophy of caudate nuclei; treatment is symptomatic and supportive.

Cockayne Syndrome

Progressive multisystem disease with autosomal recessive inheritance pattern; clinical features include extreme dwarfism, dysmorphic facies, cachectic habitus, and neurologic deterioration; children are normal at birth, then develop failure to thrive and decreased height, weight, and head circumference by 24 months; cognitive development and speech are rudimentary; gait is limited by progressive spasticity and ataxia; deafness and impaired vision occur frequently; peripheral neuropathy may develop; the brain is small, with atrophic white matter and calcification of the basal ganglia; patchy demyelination is noted in the white matter and peripheral nerves; underlying biochemical abnormality is unknown; no specific treatment.

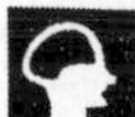

Corticobasal Ganglionic Degeneration

Corticodentatonigral degeneration; degenerative dementia syndrome characterized by diffuse accumulation of pathologic tau proteins within neurons; clinical features reflect dysfunction predominantly of frontal and parietal cortices and include progressive memory loss, dysphasia, psychomotor slowing, apraxia, asymmetric rigidity, dysphagia, postural instability, frontal release signs, oculomotor impairment, asymmetric hyperreflexia, myoclonus, and hypokinetic dysarthria; pathology demonstrates asymmetric frontoparietal atrophy with neuronal loss and gliosis, substantia nigra degeneration, and swollen achromatic neurons; MRI shows asymmetric cortical atrophy most severe in the parietal lobes; PET and SPECT reveal hypoperfusion and hypometabolism in affected areas; treatment involves symptomatic and supportive care; levodopa occasionally may result in modest reduction of rigidity.

Cowden's Syndrome

Gingival multiple hamartoma syndrome; familial cancer syndrome with autosomal dominant inheritance; linked to mutations of PTEN gene on chromosome 10q23; symptoms in young children include progressive macrocephaly, mental retardation, mild-to-moderate delay in motor development, lingua plicata; adults present with facial trichilemmomas, oral papillomas, lingua plicata, and hamartomatous lesions like lipomas, fibromas, and hemangiomas; at young age, increased risk for developing benign and malignant tumors of the thyroid, gastrointestinal tract, breast, retina, and ovary; frequent occurrence of Lhermitte-Duclos disease; management is directed toward surveillance and treatment of the various hamartomatous and neoplastic lesions.

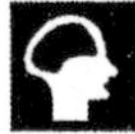

Crouzon's Syndrome

Craniofacial dysostosis; disorder caused by premature fusion of the cranial sutures; autosomal dominant inheritance pattern; linked to mutations in fibroblast growth factor receptor type 2 gene; coronal, sagittal, and lambdoid sutures affected most often; other clinical features include ocular proptosis caused by shallow orbits, visual impairment in 50% of cases, traction and compression in the optic canals can cause optic atrophy and blindness, conductive hearing loss in 55% of patients, headaches, and seizures in up to 12% of patients; mental deficiency is rare; CT with three-dimensional reconstruction is necessary for evaluation and planning of neurosurgical repair.

Crow-Fukase Syndrome

POEMS syndrome (plasma cell dyscrasia with polyneuropathy, organomegaly, endocrinopathy, monoclonal gammopathy, and skin changes); characterized by progressive, symmetric demyelinating sensorimotor neuropathy in association with osteosclerotic and multiple myeloma, Waldenström's macroglobulinemia, plasmacytoma, or angiofollicular lymph node hyperplasia; pathophysiology unknown, probably mediated by immune effectors; mean onset in the fifth decade, often in males; clinical features include moderate-to-severe weakness affecting distal more than proximal muscles, less prominent sensory loss (mostly large fiber), uncommon autonomic symptoms and cranial nerve involvement; common systemic features include hepatomegaly, diabetes mellitus, hypothyroidism, skin hyperpigmentation, and peripheral edema; treatment of underlying disease may stabilize or improve the neuropathy.

Cysticercosis

Most common parasitic disease of the CNS; acquired by ingestion of food contaminated by *Taenia solium* eggs (often undercooked pork); hatched eggs spread via blood to eyes, skeletal muscles, and CNS (brain parenchyma, subarachnoid space, ventricles, spinal cord); parasites may live for years within cysts or die and leave calcified granulomas; cysts in subarachnoid space may incite intense inflammation, causing fibrosis and hydrocephalus; clinical features include new-onset seizures, cognitive impairment, confusion, headache; gait disturbance, focal neurologic deficits, and signs of elevated intracranial pressure; cysts well visualized by CT and MRI; CSF ELISA and complement fixation tests are diagnostic; treatment consists of albendazole and praziquantel, and anticonvulsants.

Dejerine-Sottas Syndrome

Progressive hypertrophic neuropathy; form of hereditary peripheral neuropathy (HSMN type III); autosomal dominant or recessive inheritance patterns can occur; presentation in infancy with progressive generalized muscle weakness, severe sensory loss, limb ataxia, muscular atrophy, and marked hypertrophy of peripheral nerves; appears to be more severe phenotype of Charcot-Marie-Tooth disease; mutations within several different genes involved in peripheral nerve myelination result in a similar phenotype, including PMP22 (17p11.2), myelin P0 (1q22.3), and EGR2 (10q21); treatment is supportive and consists of physical and occupational therapy, orthotic devices, and genetic counseling.

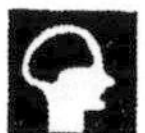

Dandy-Walker Syndrome

Dandy-Walker malformation; 1 in 30,000 births; posterior fossa malformation characterized by complete or partial agenesis of the cerebellar vermis, cystic dilation of the fourth ventricle, enlarged posterior fossa, elevation of the torcula and straight sinus, and hydrocephalus; atresia of the foramina of Luschka and Magendie may be present; patients display delayed motor development, nystagmus, spasticity, titubation, and abnormal cognition; treatment consists of shunting of the ventricles and/or posterior fossa cyst; early shunting and decompression of the cyst may allow more normal development of the cerebellar hemispheres.

Denny-Brown, Foley Syndrome

Benign fasciculation with cramps; disorder characterized by frequent muscle cramping, often accompanied by muscle fasciculations; cramps can occur during sleep or after ordinary physical activity; EMG and nerve conduction testing are benign, without evidence of muscle denervation or peripheral nerve dysfunction; symptoms do not progress to include muscle weakness or atrophy; not accompanied by an increased risk for amyotrophic lateral sclerosis or motor neuron disease; treatment is symptomatic and consists of quinine, phenytoin, or carbamazepine.

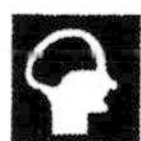

Dentatorubral-Pallidoluysian Atrophy

Degenerative trinucleotide repeat disorder that usually is autosomal dominant, occasionally sporadic; occurs mainly in Japan; caused by unstable expanded CAG repeats within the DRPLA gene, on chromosome 12p12; intergenerational instability occurs; onset at any age, usually in early fourth decade; constant clinical features include cerebellar ataxia, dysarthria, and progressive dementia; less common findings consist of progressive myoclonic epilepsy, opsoclonus, chorea or dystonia, psychiatric abnormalities, and oculomotor disturbances; EEG demonstrates a slow background and frequent epileptiform activity; MRI reveals atrophy of the superior cerebellar peduncles and high-signal abnormalities in the pallidum; no specific therapy available except for anticonvulsants.

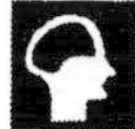

DiMauro Syndrome

Carnitine palmitoyl transferase (CPT1 or CPT2) deficiency; enzymes involved in fatty acid oxidation and energy metabolism within mitochondria; autosomal recessive inheritance pattern; CPT1 deficiency manifests in infancy with nonketotic hypoglycemic coma, hepatomegaly, hypertriglyceridemia, and abnormal liver function, including hyperammonemia (similar to Reye syndrome); condition may improve with medium-chain triglycerides; CPT2 deficiency is lethal in infants but more benign in adults; clinical features include metabolic myopathy with recurrent pain and myoglobinuria; symptoms provoked by fasting, prolonged exercise, cold exposure, infection, or emotional stress; permanent weakness in 10% of cases; no specific treatment.

Dystonia Musculorum Deformans

Idiopathic torsion dystonia; inherited disorder of the basal ganglia with autosomal dominant inheritance; initial onset between 5 and 15 years of age; clinical features include early dystonic involvement of the legs, with rapid progression to involve the arms, neck, head, and trunk; torticollis, lordosis, and scoliosis often develop; pain with movements is unusual; over time, axial musculature may become more impaired than limb muscles; affected muscles often become hypertrophic; MRI usually unremarkable; PET scans may demonstrate reduced glucose metabolism in the basal ganglia; treatment with anticholinergic agents, levodopa, bromocriptine, baclofen, or carbamazepine occasionally improves symptoms.

Emery-Dreifuss Muscular Dystrophy

X-linked muscular dystrophy syndrome characterized by an unusual pattern of weakness: humeroperoneal, which predominantly affects the biceps and triceps in the arms and distal musculature of the legs; severity of myopathic weakness is quite variable; early onset of severe contractures of elbows, knees, ankles, fingers, and spine; a rigid spine typically develops, with limited neck flexion; prominent muscular wasting occurs; heart block is common and often requires a pacemaker; linked to mutation of EDMD gene, localized to the Xq28 locus; expression of the EDMD gene product emerin, which normally is present in the nuclear membrane of muscles and other tissues, is absent; treatment is symptomatic.

Encephalitis Lethargica

von Economo Disease; disease of unknown etiology, presumed to be viral, responsible for worldwide epidemic from 1917 to 1928; epidemic form possibly extinct; now occurs sporadically; affects patients of all ages and sexes; clinical features include acute stage (duration 3–4 weeks) with onset of fever, headache, lethargy, impairment of eye movements and oculomotor control, motor symptoms characteristic of basal ganglia dysfunction, and acute organic psychosis; CSF demonstrates lymphocytic pleocytosis with elevated protein in 50% of patients; parkinsonian syndrome common in postencephalitic phase, unusual features include early age of onset, torticollis, torsion spasms, myoclonus, and facial tics; no specific treatment.

Encephalotrigeminal Angiomatosis

Sturge-Weber-Dimitri syndrome; form of neurocutaneous disorder characterized by a cutaneous vascular port-wine nevus of the face (follows distribution of trigeminal nerve), contralateral hemiparesis and hemiatrophy, glaucoma, seizures, frequent homonymous hemianopsia, and mental retardation; inheritance usually sporadic, may be dominant or recessive; seizures are early onset and difficult to control, they can be focal motor, generalized, or partial complex; occipital lobe most often affected, also involves the temporal and parietal lobes; atrophy noted ipsilateral to facial nevus; calcification involves the cortex and small vessels; skull radiographs reveal trolley-track curvilinear calcifications; treatment includes cosmetic surgery, anticonvulsants, physical and occupational therapy, and supportive care.

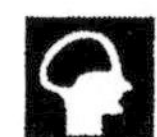

Eosinophilia-Myalgia Syndrome

Interstitial form of eosinophilic myositis and fasciitis; characterized by severe myalgias, muscle cramps, edema and induration of the skin, pulmonary symptoms (e.g., cough, dyspnea), and peripheral blood eosinophilia; in one third of cases, an associated inflammatory polyneuropathy can occur and cause neuropathic symptoms (may be painful); myokymia, myoclonus, and movement disorders occur in some patients; in most cases, related to patients taking certain preparations of L-tryptophan that contained a chemical contaminant (e.g., 1,1′-ethylidenebis); the condition has been most prevalent in the United States; symptoms respond well to glucocorticoids; nonsteroidal antiinflammatory agents and rehabilitation also may be beneficial.

Erb-Duchenne Syndrome

Upper radicular syndrome; weakness of the upper extremity caused by damage to the upper nerve roots (fourth, fifth, sixth cervical roots or upper trunks) of the brachial plexus; weakness affects the deltoid, biceps, brachioradialis, pectoralis major, supraspinatus, infraspinatus, subscapularis, and teres major muscles; flexion of the forearm, abduction and internal and external rotation of the arm, and apposition of the scapula are all severely affected; sensory loss is variable and consists of hypesthesia on the outer surface of the arm and forearm; the biceps reflex is absent; recovery is likely if complete avulsion has not occurred; rehabilitation is of benefit.

Fabry Disease

X-linked disorder of the skin (angiokeratoma corporis diffusum), kidney, blood vessels, neurons, and peripheral and autonomic nervous systems; caused by defective enzyme, α-galactosidase A, with abnormal storage of ceramide trihexoside in affected tissues; incompletely recessive, as some female heterozygotes may be affected; clinical features include paroxysmal burning pains in the limbs, paresthesias, anhydrosis, fever, priapism, hemiplegia, hemianesthesia, dysphasia, and seizures; psychosis and dementia may occur in older patients; cardiac abnormalities may include myocardial ischemia or infarction, congestive heart failure, and aortic stenosis; progressive renal failure is common; no specific treatment; kidney transplant may be lifesaving; phenytoin or carbamazepine may improve neuropathic pain.

Familial Amyloidotic Polyneuropathy

Inherited neuropathy characterized by amyloid deposition into peripheral and autonomic nerves; pathologic evaluation reveals both demyelination and axonal damage; autosomal dominant inheritance pattern; linked to mutations of transthyretin gene, mapped to chromosome 18q11.2-q12.1; onset is between ages 20 and 35 years; initial clinical features include acral sensory loss, chronic diarrhea, and impotence; followed by progressive weakness, sphincter dysfunction, and orthostatic hypotension; cardiomyopathy with heart block may occur, requiring a pacemaker; nephrosis is a late manifestation; the disease is inexorable progressive, no specific therapy exists; liver transplantation and plasma exchange have had little impact on the neuropathy; symptomatic treatment.

Familial Dysautonomia

Riley-Day syndrome; autosomal recessive, slowly progressive condition that affects children, typically of Jewish heritage; clinical features include diminished lacrimation, lack of reflexes, hyperhidrosis, abnormal blood pressure regulation, postural hypotension, intermittent skin blotching, poor temperature control, subnormal growth, and multiple sensory deficits; in addition, children have poor motor coordination, emotional instability, frequent vomiting, and relative insensitivity to pain; seizures, frequent breath-holding episodes, and abnormal EEGs may be noted; overall intelligence is preserved; pathology reveals progressive loss of neurons in sympathetic and parasympathetic ganglia; bethanecol chloride may provide relief from crises, improve gastrointestinal motility, increase tearing, and reduce the incidence of aspiration.

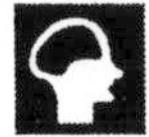

Farber Lipogranulomatosis

Onset in first few weeks to months of life; clinical features include painful swollen joints, hoarseness, vomiting, respiratory difficulties, and limb edema; subcutaneous nodules develop near joints, tendon sheaths, and at pressure points; less common findings include cardiac enlargement, lymphadenopathy, hepatosplenomegaly, macroglossia, and difficulty swallowing; mental development may be impaired; syndrome caused by severe deficiency of acid ceramidase, with accumulation of ceramide and related materials in foam cells within affected tissues; diagnosis is clinical, finding deficiency of acid ceramidase in cultured fibroblasts or leukocytes; no specific treatment.

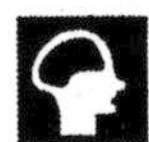

Fatal Familial Insomnia

Prion disease (spongiform encephalopathy) with autosomal dominant inheritance and onset between 18 and 60 years of age; clinical features include progressive insomnia, dysautonomia (hyperhidrosis, tachycardia, tachypnea, hyperthermia, hypertension), dementia, myoclonus, and motor dysfunction (pyramidal tract and cerebellar signs); EEG shows diffuse slowing with infrequent periodicity; pathology reveals prominent neuronal loss and gliosis in the thalamus, with minimal spongiform change; neocortex, basal ganglia, cerebellum, and brainstem are variably affected; syndrome caused by mutation within PrP gene at codon 178, coupled with a methionine at codon 129; no specific treatment; family genetic counseling is indicated.

Fazio-Londe Syndrome

Form of juvenile spinal muscular atrophy, with onset in late childhood or early adolescence; inheritance usually is autosomal recessive, although sporadic cases can occur; clinical features include progressive bulbofacial weakness, dysarthria, dysphagia, and, in some cases, less severe weakness of the arms and legs; wasting of the tongue with visible fasciculations is noted; upper motor neuron signs are absent; respiration may be affected in patients with long-standing disease; symptoms typically remain restricted until end-stage disease; death occurs within 2 years of presentation in most patients, usually from respiratory failure.

Foster Kennedy Syndrome

Defined as ipsilateral optic nerve atrophy and contralateral papilledema; caused by tumors that arise in the retro-orbital region, anterior skull base (e.g., medial sphenoid wing), or inferior frontal lobe and compress the optic nerve; initial tumor growth causes optic nerve damage and atrophy, further growth elevates intracranial pressure and leads to papilledema in the contralateral, intact optic nerve; ipsilateral anosmia may be noted; a central scotoma often is present ipsilateral to the tumor; typically occurs with frontal tumors and meningiomas of the olfactory groove and sphenoid wing.

Friedreich's Ataxia

Autosomal recessive inheritance; prevalence is 2 per 100,000; GAA triplet repeat expansion found in first intron of X25 gene, located on chromosome 9q13-21, codes for conserved protein, frataxin; onset in early teen years; clinical symptoms include progressive gait ataxia, areflexia of lower limbs, impaired vibration and position sense, diffuse weakness, dysarthria, nystagmus, frequent Babinski sign, and hypertrophic cardiomyopathy; MRI usually is normal, may show mild cerebellar atrophy; most patients become nonambulatory within 15 years of symptom onset; treatment is symptomatic (e.g., physical therapy); no specific treatment; death from infection or cardiac disease occurs between 40 and 60 years of age.

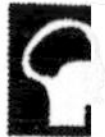

Frontotemporal Dementia

Group of rare progressive dementia syndromes, Pick's disease is the best characterized subtype; clinical features of Pick's disease include initial mild memory impairment, with more pronounced dysphasia (reduced speech output), personality changes, apathy, inattentiveness, and extrapyramidal motor dysfunction; dementia become severe later in the disease; MRI demonstrates focal atrophy of the frontal and temporal lobes; pathology reveals argyrophilic intraneuronal inclusion bodies (Pick bodies) and gliosis in affected areas; associated with mutations in tau gene (involved in microtubule assembly and stabilization) on chromosome 17, with accumulation of abnormal tau proteins in Pick bodies; memory may improve or stabilize with anticholinergic agents.

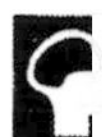

Fucosidosis

Storage disease with onset during the first 2 years of life; clinical features include progressive intellectual and motor deterioration, initial hypotonia that gradually evolves into spastic quadriplegia, decorticate rigidity, anhydrosis, cardiomegaly, failure to thrive, and recurrent respiratory infections; other findings are coarse facies and angiokeratoma corporis diffusum of the skin; caused by mutation of α-L-fucosidase gene on chromosome 1p34.1-36.1; enzyme levels are severely reduced in serum, leukocytes, and cultured fibroblasts; pathology reveals accumulation of fucose-containing oligosaccharides and glycoproteins into vacuoles within affected regions of brain; no specific treatment.

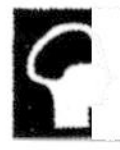

Fukuyama Congenital Muscular Dystrophy

Autosomal recessive disorder linked to chromosome 9q31, the involved gene has not yet been identified; common in Japan but rare elsewhere; infants demonstrate significant muscular weakness and contractures, in combination with moderately severe psychomotor retardation; mild developmental and functional abnormalities of the eyes can be occasionally noted (e.g., myopia and optic atrophy); seizures occur in approximately 50% of patients; MRI demonstrates areas of pachygyria and polymicrogyria, with regions of high-signal abnormality in the white matter; the cerebellum may be mildly affected; no specific treatment; anticonvulsants and physical therapy are of benefit.

Gaucher Disease

Lysosomal storage disease with autosomal recessive inheritance; glucocerebroside accumulates within affected tissues because of a deficiency of β-glucosidase; infantile, juvenile, and adult neuronopathic forms exist, as well as an adult non-neuronopathic form; the infantile form has onset in the first 6–12 months, with poor suck and swallow, dementia, strabismus, opisthotonus, spasticity, organomegaly, and seizures; clinical features of the juvenile and adult forms include dementia with variable onset, seizures, incoordination, splenomegaly, and tics; diagnosis made by demonstration of reduced β-glucosidase in leukocytes or presence of a mutation in the β-glucosidase gene; no specific treatment.

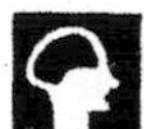

Hallervorden-Spatz Disease

Autosomal recessive disorder with onset in childhood and adolescence; symptoms typically begin with stiffness of gait, distal extremity wasting (hands may become useless), pes cavus, toe walking, risus sardonicus, spasticity and rigidity (painful spasms can develop), speech difficulty with eventual anarthria (comprehension is maintained), hyperactive reflexes, and occasional mild dementia; dystonia, ataxia, and tremor may occur; MRI demonstrates low-signal abnormality in the globus pallidus (eye-of-the-tiger sign); pathology reveals neuronal loss and thinning of myelin in the medial segment of the globus pallidus; underlying biochemical defect unknown, but disease linked to chromosome 20p12.3-p13 in some families; no specific treatment.

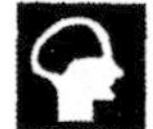

Hand-Schüller-Christian Disease

Multifocal form of Langerhans cell histiocytosis; caused by proliferation of antigen-presenting dendritic cells and antigen-processing phagocytic cells; core features are calvarial lesions, exophthalmus, and diabetes insipidus; short stature; otitis media, constitutional symptoms (fever, weight loss), visual loss, and other endocrine manifestations may occur; symptoms linked to granuloma formation within skull, orbits, and hypothalamic-pituitary axis; MRI reveals multifocal intraparenchymal lesions that may enhance; diagnosis is made by demonstration of Langerhans cells in brain or calvarial biopsy tissue, with a consistent immunohistochemical analysis; treatment consists of corticosteroids and localized radiotherapy; chemotherapy is reserved for refractory disease.

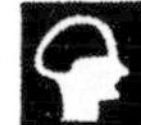

Hepatolenticular Degeneration

Wilson's disease; inborn error of copper metabolism with autosomal recessive inheritance, due to mutations and deletions of P-type ATPase located on chromosome 13q14.3; onset variable in late childhood or adolescence; accumulation of copper in liver leads to cirrhosis; neurologic features are quite variable but can include rigidity, tremor (often "wing beating"), dystonic movements, dysarthria, unsteady gait, reduced dexterity, hypophonic speech, seizures, behavioral abnormalities (affective disorder or psychosis), drooling, and dysphagia; Kayser-Fleischer ring noted in 75% of patients; MRI demonstrates diffuse atrophy, especially of the basal ganglia, and ventricular dilation; initial therapy involves penicillamine, tetrathiomolybdate, triethylene tetramine, or zinc; optimum maintenance treatment is with zinc.

Hereditary Spastic Paraplegia

Genetically diverse group of disorders, usually autosomal dominant, may be recessive, X linked, or sporadic; age of onset variable, symptoms may be mild or severe, all cases are slowly progressive; symptoms of "pure" disorder include spastic gait, with poor coordination, overactive reflexes, Babinski signs, and ankle clonus; sensation usually normal; leg strength may be normal; "complicated" cases present similar to "pure" patients but have additional features, such as amyotrophy, ataxia, myoclonic epilepsy, dementia, optic atrophy, macular degeneration, or choreoathetosis; sphincter dysfunction may occur in late-onset forms; MRI of the spinal cord usually normal; no specific treatment; management is symptomatic.

Hirayama Syndrome

Monomelic muscular atrophy; disorder of unknown origin, often diagnosed in Japan, usually affects young males; onset at approximately 20 years of age in most patients; initial symptoms are progressive weakness and muscular atrophy affecting one limb, typically an arm and hand; patients often are athletes, but the disorder is not clearly related to cervical trauma; symptoms usually stabilize after several years; EMG consistent with a lower motor neuron process; patients must be followed closely even after stabilization of symptoms to rule out other signs of motor neuron disease; no specific treatment; physical therapy may be of benefit.

Hunter Syndrome

X-linked recessive lysosomal storage disease, with accumulation of mucopolysaccharides (dermatan sulfate, heparan sulfate) within affected tissues; caused by deficiency of iduronate-2-sulfatase; two forms, mild and severe; clinical features of the severe form include juvenile onset of joint stiffness, coarse facies, dysostosis multiplex, hepatosplenomegaly, mental deterioration, growth retardation, diarrhea, and occasional pigmentary retinal deterioration; the mild form may be asymptomatic, with short stature, joint stiffness, coarse features, normal intelligence, and hepatosplenomegaly; neither form has corneal clouding; diagnosis via demonstration of excess urinary dermatan sulfate and heparan sulfate, and deficiency of iduronate-2-sulfatase in cultured fibroblasts; no specific treatment.

Hurler Syndrome

Autosomal recessive lysosomal storage disease, with accumulation of mucopolysaccharides (dermatan sulfate, heparan sulfate) within affected tissues; caused by reduced expression of α-L-iduronidase gene (chromosome 4p); most severe form of the mucopolysaccharidoses; onset in infancy with stiff joints, corneal clouding, periarticular swelling, clawhands, chest deformity, dwarfing, coarsening of facial features, hypertelorism, enlarged tongue, mental retardation and deterioration, minimal speech development, and deafness; cardiac disease, abdominal distention, visual loss, and cervical cord compression may occur; zebra bodies containing lipids are noted in the brain; diagnosis via demonstration of excess urinary dermatan sulfate and heparan sulfate, and deficiency of α-L-iduronidase in cultured fibroblasts; no specific treatment.

Hyperekplexia

Form of exaggerated startle response; can result from a brainstem disorder or can be inherited as an autosomal dominant trait with mutations of the α_1 subunit of the glycine receptor (chromosome 5q); clinical features include a sudden motor response to unexpected auditory, tactile, or visual stimuli; the motor response involves a blink, contraction of the face, flexion of the neck and trunk, and abduction and flexion of the arms; the response can be brief or prolonged, falling can occur; in infancy may result in "stiff baby syndrome" due to prolonged tonic spasms; excessive startle syndromes can be regional, such as the "jumping Frenchman of Maine" in Quebec; may respond to clonazepam or valproic acid.

Hyperviscosity Syndrome

Can develop in all forms of leukemia with significant leukocytosis (most severe in myeloid forms), as well as in IgM paraproteinemia; clinical features include headache, blurred vision, tinnitus, vertigo, ataxia, somnolence, severe lethargy and fatigue, and cerebrovascular events (transient ischemic attacks or stroke); encephalopathy, reduced level of consciousness and coma, subarachnoid hemorrhage, spinal cord dysfunction, and seizures may develop; acute treatment consists of leukapheresis or plasmapheresis; definitive treatment of the underlying disease with chemotherapy is beneficial.

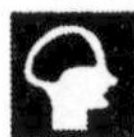

Isaacs Syndrome

Neuromyotonia; slowly progressive myokymia (visible and continuous muscle twitching) that affects children, adolescents, or young adults; clinical features include slowed movements, clawing of the fingers, toe walking, stiffness of muscles, abnormal postures of the limbs (similar to carpal spasm), pseudomyotonia, frequent cramps, and hyperhidrosis; percussion myotonia is not present; oropharyngeal and respiratory muscles may be affected; stiffness and myokymia are present during rest and sleep; rarely occurs as a paraneoplastic syndrome (antibodies to potassium channels); muscle activity abolished by botulinum toxin; disorder may be due to peripheral neuropathy or dysfunction of nerve terminal; phenytoin and carbamazepine usually control symptoms; plasmapheresis and intravenous immunoglobulin may be beneficial.

Jumping Frenchman of Maine

Regional form of hyperekplexia (see above).

Kennedy Disease

Spinobulbar muscular atrophy; X-linked recessive inheritance pattern; onset usually after age 40; clinical features include slowly progressive dysarthria, dysphagia, tongue fasciculations, twitching of limb muscles, and delayed limb weakness, which is more severe proximally; reflexes are lost; upper motor neuron signs and dementia may occur but are extremely rare; gynecomastia is common; disorder caused by CAG expansion mutation within the androgen receptor gene, linked to chromosome Xq11-12; expansion mutation probably causes toxic gain of function of gene product; inverse relationship between the number of repeats and the severity of the disease; no specific therapy.

Kleine-Levin Syndrome

Recurrent hypersomnia; form of sleep disorder that consists of recurrent episodes of hypersomnia and binge eating that last up to several weeks; interval of 2–12 months between episodes; usually affects boys in early adolescence, rare in girls or adults; behavioral and psychological changes can occur, such as disorientation, forgetfulness, depression, depersonalization, hallucinations, irritability, aggression, and sexual hyperactivity accompany episodes of hypersomnia; episodes decrease in frequency and severity with age, uncommon after the fourth decade; patients may have limited improvement with amphetamines, methylphenidate, or lithium; no definitive treatment.

Klippel-Feil Syndrome

Congenital fusion of two or more cervical vertebrae (usually C2–3 or C5–6); embryonic failure of segmentation of chorda-mesoderm that form cervical vertebrae; can be part of other syndromes (i.e., Turner's, Noonan's, Wildervanck's), sporadic, or inherited as autosomal dominant; radiographic evaluation of cervical spine is diagnostic; patients have a short neck, limited head and neck movement; frequent kyphosis, scoliosis, platybasia, and hearing loss; may have weakness and atrophy of arm muscles, mental retardation; craniocervical instability may lead to spinal cord compression and progressive paraplegia; laminectomy is indicated for cord compression.

Klumpke Syndrome

Lower radicular syndrome; weakness of the upper extremity caused by damage to the lower nerve roots (eighth cervical and first thoracic roots or lower trunk) of the brachial plexus; weakness affects the flexor carpi ulnaris, flexor digitorum, interossei, and the thenar and hypothenar muscles; pattern of weakness is similar to a combined lesion of the median and ulnar nerves, with a flattened or simian hand; sensory deficit consists of hypesthesia on the inner side of the arm and forearm, and on the ulnar side of the hand; triceps reflex is absent; Horner syndrome may occur if the inferior cervical ganglion is injured; rehabilitation is of benefit.

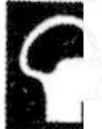

Krabbe Leukodystrophy

Lysosomal storage disease with deficiency of galactocerebrosidase and accumulation of galactocerebroside and psychosine in affected tissues; typical onset in infancy, occasionally can develop in juvenile or adult years; patients are normal at birth, then have progressive irritability, inexplicable crying, fevers, limb stiffness, seizures, feeding difficulty, vomiting, and slowing of mental and motor development; followed by psychomotor deterioration, marked hypertonia, extensor posturing, and optic atrophy; reflexes eventually decrease or disappear, with loss of tone and flaccidity; death by 2 years in most cases; CSF protein is elevated; nerve conduction velocities are reduced; globoid cells are noted in demyelinated regions of affected brain; no specific treatment.

Kugelberg-Welander Syndrome

Spinal muscular atrophy type 3; inheritance can be autosomal recessive or dominant; onset usually is in middle to late childhood, with slow progression into adult middle age; clinical features include proximal weakness of the extremities (most often the legs), with variable amounts of muscle wasting, fasciculations, and occasional elevation of serum creatine kinase activity; bulbar musculature usually is spared; corticospinal tract signs, sensory deficit, autonomic involvement, and mental deterioration do not occur; linked to mutations of SMN gene, located on chromosome 5q11.3-13.1; no specific treatment; multidisciplinary supportive care and genetic counseling are of benefit.

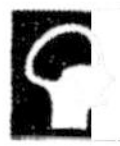

Landau-Kleffner Syndrome

Disorder of childhood characterized by an acquired aphasia, typically in association with a seizure disorder, which occurs in children with previously normal language and motor development, between ages 4 and 7; occasionally the disorder can affect very young children, so speech never develops properly; the disorder can precede or follow the occurrence of seizures and often persists, even though seizures may be well controlled; EEG shows temporal or temporoparietal spikes, or spike-and-wave discharges, which may be almost continuous in some cases; MRI is normal; etiology unknown, possibly a focal encephalitis; valproic acid, ethosuximide, and benzodiazepines may improve the condition.

Laurence-Moon-Biedl Syndrome

Congenital disorder of development with an autosomal recessive inheritance pattern; characterized by early-onset obesity, mental retardation, retinal dystrophy, hypogenitalism and hypogonadism (mostly in males), and coloboma; polydactyly, syndactyly, or both may occur; less common features include renal dysfunction, hypertension, cardiac abnormalities, and liver defects; night vision is impaired early by retinitis pigmentosa, patients often are blind by age 20; lifespan may be normal, although frequently shortened by cardiac and renal disease; no specific neuropathologic changes have been described yet; treatment is symptomatic, with supportive care.

Leber Hereditary Optic Neuropathy

Maternally inherited disorder of the optic nerve, caused by mutations in mitochondrial DNA; mutations have been noted in several genes of complex I of the respiratory chain (e.g., ND1, ND4, ND6); clinical features include onset in adolescence or early adulthood, with progressive, painless cloudiness of central vision (may be asymmetric) that results in bilateral loss of vision (20/200 or finger counting) within several months; optic atrophy is always present; possible associated findings include cardiac preexcitation, postural tremor, dystonia, motor tics, and peripheral neuropathy; treatment remains unclear; corticosteroids, hydroxocobalamin, optic nerve sheath fenestration, and craniotomy with lysis of optic nerve/chiasm adhesions are of unproved value.

Lesch-Nyhan Syndrome

Hypoxanthine-guanine phosphoribosyltransferase (HPRT) deficiency; X-linked recessive; HPRT necessary for recycling of purine bases into nucleotide forms during DNA and RNA synthesis; leads to accelerated synthesis of uric acid and hyperuricemia; onset by 6 months of age with developmental delay, axial hypotonia, appendicular spasticity, mental retardation, choreoathetoid movements, self-mutilation, dysarthria; diagnosis by demonstrating reduced tissue levels of HPRT; allopurinol reduces serum uric acid but does not effect neurologic symptoms; no effective treatment; supportive care.

Letterer-Siwe Disease

Disseminated form of Langerhans cell histiocytosis; caused by proliferation of antigen-presenting dendritic cells and antigen-processing phagocytic cells; affects children <2 years of age; clinical features include a granulomatous rash, lymphadenopathy, hepatomegaly, splenomegaly, fever, and weight loss; pulmonary and bone involvement is common; granulocytosis usually is present; pancytopenia may occur with severe hypersplenism; neurologic involvement usually is absent; course often is fulminant, with poor prognosis; symptoms may improve with corticosteroids; focal lesions may respond to radiotherapy; chemotherapy may be required to achieve clinical remission.

Levine-Critchley Syndrome

Neuroacanthocytosis; familial multisystem neurodegenerative disorder with autosomal dominant or recessive inheritance linked to chromosome 9q21, sporadic cases are rare; onset is usually in the fourth or fifth decade, juvenile onset is uncommon; clinical features include acanthocytosis, hyperkinetic movement disorder (chorea, orofacial dyskinesias, dystonia), psychiatric symptoms (obsessive-compulsive disorder, personality changes), dementia, and axonal neuropathy; neuropathy causes muscle wasting, weakness, and absent reflexes; epileptic seizures occur in 40% of patients; MRI shows atrophy of the caudate nuclei and high signal within the striatum; pathology reveals neuronal degeneration and gliosis within the basal ganglia and substantia nigra; no specific treatment.

Lhermitte-Duclos Disease

Dysplastic gangliocytoma of the cerebellum; rarely noted in hypothalamus and spinal cord; age of onset typically in the third or fourth decade; usually sporadic in origin; clinical features include cerebellar dysfunction (ataxia, dysdiadochokinesia, nystagmus), and symptoms of increased intracranial pressures secondary to hydrocephalus; may be associated with CNS malformations such as hydromyelia, brain heterotopia, and megalencephaly; MRI shows low signal lesion on T1 images, with minimal enhancement; pathology demonstrates altered cerebellar architecture, with pleomorphic ganglion cells replacing the granule cell layer; treatment is surgical resection; role of radiotherapy and chemotherapy is unclear.

Lowe Syndrome

Oculocerebrorenal syndrome; X-linked (long arm) recessive disorder of amino acid metabolism; clinical features include severe mental retardation, delayed physical development, myopathy, and congenital glaucoma or cataracts; general aminoaciduria of the Fanconi type occurs, with renal tubular acidosis and rickets; lysine is the predominant amino acid in the urine; MRI shows various patterns of white matter damage; CNS pathology is inconsistent; the gene encodes a protein similar to inositol polyphosphate-5-phosphatase; no specific treatment.

Lytico-Bodig Disease

Parkinsonism-dementia-amyotrophic lateral sclerosis complex of Guam; syndrome indigenous to the Chamorro natives of Guam; also noted in emigrants from Guam; clinical features include those of Parkinson's disease and dementia, often in combination with amyotrophic lateral sclerosis; supranuclear gaze palsy may be present; pathology reveals the presence of neurofibrillary tangles in degenerating neurons of the substantia nigra and locus ceruleus, loss of anterior horn cells, and scattered granulovascular bodies; Lewy bodies and senile plaques are absent; possibly related to exposure to a neurotoxin, 2-amino-3-(methylamino)-propanoic acid, present in seeds of the plant *Cycas circinalis;* parkinsonian symptoms may respond to levodopa.

Marinesco-Sjögren Syndrome

Early-onset ataxia syndrome; autosomal recessive inheritance pattern; clinical features include ataxia, bilateral cataracts (congenital or can develop in infancy), mental retardation, limited sexual maturation, and short stature; cerebellar dysfunction is manifested by dysarthria, nystagmus, and ataxia of the trunk and limbs; developmental delay always occurs but can vary from mild to severe; other associated features that may be noted are strabismus, hypotonia, pes valgus, and scoliosis; disease progression is slow, with most patients being wheelchair bound by the third or fourth decade; underlying cause is unknown, possibly a lysosomal storage disorder; no specific treatment.

Maroteaux-Lamy Syndrome

Mucopolysaccharidosis type VI; form of lysosomal storage disease, with deficiency of *N*-acetylgalactosamine-4-sulfate sulfatase or arylsulfatase B; accumulation of dermatan sulfate within affected tissues; disease severity can be variable, with mild, intermediate, and severe forms; manifestations of the severe form include growth retardation by 2 or 3 years of age, coarse facial features, corneal clouding, severe skeletal abnormalities, short stature, valvular heart disease, and heart failure; intelligence remains normal; hydrocephalus and cervical cord compression can develop from hypoplasia of the odontoid process; patients may survive into the second or third decade; treatment is supportive and symptomatic.

Meige's Syndrome

Oromandibular dystonia; form of oral-facial dyskinesia; characterized by the combination of blepharospasm and other cranial dystonias; clinical features include forceful blinking and sustained eye closure (with or without spasms of the orbicularis oculi), spasms of the jaw muscles that cause slow forceful involuntary opening of the mouth, deviation of the jaw to one side, protrusion of the tongue, spasms may be forceful enough to dislocate the mandible or fracture teeth; dystonia may spread over time to include the cervical and shoulder musculature; treatment with anticholinergic agents may give partial relief of symptoms.

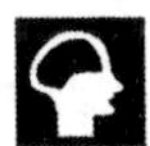

Menkes Syndrome

X linked, localized to gene at Xq13.3, in family of cation-transporting ATPases that transport ions across membranes; lack of gene causes insufficient intestinal absorption of copper and dysfunction of copper-containing enzymes; develops in first few months of life; symptoms and signs consist of male infants with developmental arrest and regression, hypotonia, seizures, failure to thrive, wiry and friable hair, recurrent infections, and hypothermia; very low serum copper levels; no effective treatment; supportive care.

Metachromatic Leukodystrophy

Group of autosomal recessive disorders characterized by degeneration of central and peripheral myelin; several forms are known, late infantile is most common; caused by deficiency of arylsulfatase A, with accumulation of sulfatide in affected tissues; infants between 12 and 30 months develop difficulty with gait, which progresses to flaccid paresis and reduced reflexes (spastic paresis may occur instead); other features include mental deterioration, dysarthria, intermittent pain in the extremities, feeding difficulties, bulbar and pseudobulbar palsies, and optic atrophy; progression to blindness and a vegetative state over 5–10 years; juvenile and adult cases are similar with slower progression; metachromatic lipids are noted on sural nerve biopsy; no treatment available.

Miller-Dieker Syndrome

Associated with abnormal neuronal migration and development of the CNS; distinctive facial dysmorphism occurs, with bitemporal hollowing, short nose with upturned nares, long and thin upper lip, low-set and posteriorly rotated ears, and small chin; other features include lissencephaly and agenesis of the corpus callosum, cardiac anomalies, and severe cerebral dysfunction; death usually occurs in the first decade; linked to abnormality of chromosome 17 in most cases; no specific treatment; supportive care.

Miller-Fisher Syndrome

Miller-Fisher variant of Guillain-Barré syndrome (GBS); consists of the triad of ophthalmoplegia, gait ataxia, and areflexia occurring in isolation; pupillary abnormalities may be noted; limb weakness does not develop; similar to GBS, the disorder often is preceded by a respiratory infection; typically benign course with progression over weeks, followed by improvement; CSF protein usually is elevated; nerve conduction testing is unremarkable; MRI may show high-signal abnormalities within the brainstem; no specific immune therapy is required in most cases.

Möbius Syndrome

Developmental anomaly of the posterior fossa; core features include the combination of congenital facial diplegia and bilateral abducens nerve palsies; associated findings may include other cranial nerve deficits (hearing loss, dysarthria, dysphagia, ptosis, complete ophthalmoplegia), congenital anomalies of the limbs or heart, hypogonadism and anosmia, and mental retardation; facial weakness is more severe in the upper face than below (i.e., more difficulty with eye closure than lip movement); infants have difficulty sucking and lack facial expression when they cry; etiology unclear, may be due to congenital absence of cranial nerve nuclei or vascular damage within the brainstem.

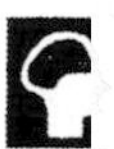

Neuronal Ceroid-Lipofuscinosis (NCL)—Adult Variant

NCL type 4; Kufs disease; form of lysosomal storage disease with adult onset in the third or fourth decade; abnormal autofluorescent lipopigments are present in granular cytosomes within nervous system tissues and other organs; inheritance usually autosomal recessive, may be dominant or sporadic; patients present with either late-onset epilepsy and progressive dementia or progressive motor deficits (ataxia, rigidity), myoclonus may be present; MRI may show cortical and/or cerebellar atrophy; diagnosis is made by light and electron microscopic examination of tissue specimens and by enzyme and mutation testing; no specific treatment; anticonvulsant therapy and supportive care; disease progression is slow over several decades.

Neuronal Ceroid-Lipofuscinosis (NCL)—Juvenile Variant

NCL type 1; Batten's disease; form of lysosomal storage disease with onset between ages 5 and 15 years; abnormal autofluorescent lipopigments are present in fingerprint cytosomes within nervous system tissues and other organs; inheritance usually autosomal recessive; early symptoms include behavioral changes, visual dysfunction, and learning difficulty; symptoms progress to dementia and blindness, with the addition of seizures, myoclonus, and motor dysfunction (pyramidal and extrapyramidal); reduced or absent electroretinogram; MRI may show cortical atrophy; diagnosis is made by light and electron microscopic examination of tissue specimens and by enzyme and mutation testing; no specific treatment; anticonvulsant therapy and supportive care.

Neuronal Ceroid Lipofuscinosis (NCL)—Late-Infantile Variant

NCL type 2; Jansky-Bielschowsky disease; form of lysosomal storage disease with onset between ages 1.5 and 4 years; abnormal autofluorescent lipopigments are present in curvilinear cytosomes within nervous system tissues and other organs; inheritance usually autosomal recessive; clinical features include severe seizures, psychomotor deterioration, and ataxia; seizures often are refractory to anticonvulsant treatment; progressive retinal deterioration, optic atrophy, and visual loss occur, with abolition of the electroretinogram; rapid progression to a vegetative state or death in a matter of months to several years, MRI may show atrophy; diagnosis is made by light and electron microscopic examination of tissue specimens and by enzyme and mutation testing; no specific treatment; anticonvulsant therapy and supportive care.

Opsoclonus-Myoclonus Syndrome

Form of paraneoplastic syndrome, most often noted in children with neuroblastoma and adults with solid tumors (e.g., breast, small cell lung); clinical features consist of constant, arrhythmic motion of the eyes, irregular in direction or tempo, in combination with myoclonus affecting the facial muscles, limbs, or trunk; in adults, may be associated with the presence of anti-Ri antibodies and encephalomyelitis or a cerebellar disorder; eye movement disorder attributed to dysfunction of the paramedian pontine reticular formation; pathology occasionally reveals Purkinje cell loss, neuronal loss in the dentate nucleus, and demyelination of the cerebellar white matter; no specific treatment.

Parinaud Syndrome

Dorsal rostral midbrain syndrome; characterized by supranuclear paralysis of upgaze, defective convergence, convergence-retraction nystagmus, and light-near dissociation; lid retraction (Collier's sign) and skew deviation may be noted; most often caused by compression of the dorsal midbrain and superior colliculi from tumors of the pineal region (e.g., pinealoma, germ cell tumor, glioma); other causes include ischemia and stroke, and demyelinating disease; symptoms are caused by impairment of fiber connections between the oculomotor nuclei; treatment is directed toward the initiating disease process.

Pelizaeus-Merzbacher Disease

X-linked recessive degenerative disease of childhood; linked to defects in the proteolipid gene on Xq22; two forms exist, one that is present at birth (connatal variant) and an infantile variant; both forms present with nystagmus and head tremor; the connatal form also has floppiness, head lag, psychomotor retardation, ataxia, spasticity, and failure to thrive; the classic infantile form shows initial slowing of motor and speech development, in association with ataxia, spasticity, hyperreflexia, optic atrophy, choreoathetotic movements, and eventual regression of psychomotor skills; patients often develop kyphoscoliosis, joint contractures, and incontinence; hearing is preserved; sensory loss does not occur; pathology reveals tigroid changes of the white matter; no specific treatment.

Pick's Disease

Also known as frontotemporal dementia. An uncommon, progressive dementing syndrome that has a prominent language component. Patients present with variable degree of memory impairment, apathy, and personality changes, in association with an early expressive dysphasia. The dysphasia usually begins with reduced verbal output, dysnomia, and non-fluency; patients may become mute. The brain demonstrates focal atrophy of the frontal and anterior temporal lobes (may be "knife-edge"), with neuronal loss, gliosis, Pick bodies (eosinophilic cytoplasmic masses), swollen ballooned neurons (Pick cells), and sparing of the nucleus basalis. Marked caudate and hippocampal atrophy may be noted. Treatment consists of supportive care; there are no specific therapies for Pick's Disease.

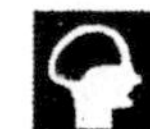

Platybasia

Autosomal dominant congenital malformation, affecting the base of the skull; defined as a skull base in which the angle between the planes of the anterior cranial fossa and the clivus is greater than 140 degrees; foramen magnum is narrowed; patients generally remain asymptomatic; if symptoms occur, the onset is in the second or third decade, related to progressive compression of the cervical spinal cord; clinical features include spasticity, incoordination, nystagmus, and lower cranial nerve palsies; can occur in other syndromes, such as Chiari types I and II, and aqueductal stenosis; treatment requires surgical decompression of the posterior fossa and upper cervical cord.

POEMS Syndrome

Polyneuropathy, organomegaly, endocrinopathy, M protein, and skin changes; associated with osteosclerotic myeloma or plasmacytoma; electrodiagnostic testing of the neuropathy is consistent with demyelination and axonal degeneration, which may be similar to CIDP; see Crow-Fukase syndrome.

Pompe's Disease

Infantile acid maltase deficiency; glycogenosis type 2; lysosomal storage disease with autosomal recessive inheritance; combination of a metabolic myopathy and motor neuron disease; clinical features include initial normal development (for several weeks to months), followed by severe hypotonia, retained mental alertness, generalized weakness, weak cry, dysphagia, areflexia, enlarged tongue, cardiomegaly with congestive failure, and hepatomegaly; respiratory weakness usually will develop, along with an inability to handle oropharyngeal secretions; cardiac failure is the usual cause of death by 12–18 months of age; no specific treatment; supportive care.

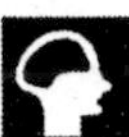

Prader-Willi Syndrome

Sporadic cytogenetic disorder affecting chromosome 15q11-q13, deletions of this region may occur in up to 50% of cases; clinical features include decreased fetal movement *in utero*, infants will have a feeble suck and severe hypotonia; older children have short stature, small hands and feet, narrowed cranial bifrontal diameter, almond-shaped eyes with strabismus, hypopigmentation of the skin, delayed speech development, hypogonadism, hyperphagia, obesity, and mild mental retardation; MRI may show anomalous cortical growth around the sylvian fissure, possibly due to misrouting of long projection axons; may be due to defective hypothalamic function; no specific treatment.

Quadriplegic Myopathy

Syndrome of acute quadriparesis that occurs in critically ill patients; usually develops after administration of high-dose corticosteroids, nondepolarizing neuromuscular blocking agents, or both; most often under treatment for status asthmaticus, organ transplantation, and trauma; clinical features include onset of severe, diffuse extremity weakness, loss of reflexes, and persistent respiratory weakness; ophthalmoparesis and facial weakness may occur; serum creatine kinase levels often are elevated; muscle biopsies reveal myopathic changes with fiber atrophy, fiber necrosis, loss of thick filaments (myosin); treatment consists of discontinuation of offending agents and supportive care.

Raeder Syndrome

Cluster headache; characterized by 1–3 brief attacks of severe periorbital or temporal pain every day for 4–8 weeks, followed by pain-free intervals that may last up to 1 year; chronic form may develop; onset of pain is very rapid, unilateral, and peaks within 5 minutes; pain is constant, excruciating, deep, and nonpulsatile; attacks last from 30 minutes to 2 hours, associated symptoms include ipsilateral scleral injection, lacrimation, nasal stuffiness, ptosis, and nausea; pathognomic feature is instigation of attacks by alcohol in 70% of patients; may be due to abnormal serotonergic activity within the hypothalamus; treatment consists of prednisone, lithium, methysergide, ergotamine, or verapamil.

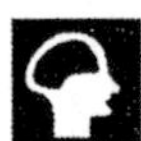

Ramsay Hunt Syndrome

Early-onset ataxia syndrome; etiologically heterogeneous, consists of progressive ataxia in combination with myoclonus (action or intention); in most patients, progressive ataxia develops first, followed by onset of myoclonus; in other patients, myoclonus may be the initial manifestation; the myoclonus may be a manifestation of another disease, such as MERFF (mitochondrial encephalomyopathy with ragged red fibers), Unverricht-Lundborg disease, or progressive myoclonus epilepsy; MERRF, the most common cause, consists of ataxia, myoclonus, seizure activity, myopathy, and hearing loss; no specific treatment; myoclonic activity may respond to valproic acid or clonazepam.

Rasmussen Encephalitis

Disorder of childhood and preadolescence characterized by a unilateral focal seizure disorder, including epilepsia partialis continua, and a progressive hemiplegia induced by focal cortical inflammation and destruction; seizures manifest as repeated clonic or myoclonic jerks that may remain focal or regional; MRI shows focal or hemispheric atrophy; underlying etiology is a chronic focal encephalitis, although an infectious agent is not consistently identified; an autoimmune etiology also has been postulated; treatment with anticonvulsants such as valproic acid or clonazepam often is unsuccessful but may give partial relief; surgical hemispherectomy should be considered for intractable seizures.

Refsum's Disease

Heredopathia atactica polyneuritiformis; autosomal recessive lipidosis with deficiency of phytanoyl-coenzyme A hydroxylase and accumulation of phytanic acid in affected tissues; phytanic acid is exclusively of dietary origin; onset usually in childhood, manifested by progressive night blindness (granular pigmentary retinopathy), limb weakness, gait ataxia, peripheral neuropathy, loss of reflexes, and muscle wasting; less common features include deafness, cataracts, miosis, pes cavus, cardiac arrhythmias, and bone deformities; symptoms are progressive but may have exacerbations with intercurrent illness; treatment with dietary reduction of phytanic acid and phytol may improve symptoms; exacerbations may respond to plasmapheresis.

Rendu-Osler-Weber Syndrome

Presence of telangiectasias within multiple organs, including the brain; telangiectasias are collections of engorged capillaries or cavernous spaces that can originate anywhere in the brain but have a predilection for white matter; brain telangiectasias are associated with similar lesions of the skin, mucous membranes, respiratory system, gastrointestinal tract, and genitourinary system; on occasion the telangiectasias can hemorrhage within the brain or other organs, leading to disability or death; they cannot be identified on angiography or CT; no specific treatment.

Rubella

Infection by rubella, a single-stranded RNA virus, acquired by droplet inhalation; neurologic syndromes include congenital infection, acute encephalitis, postrubella polyradiculoneuritis, and progressive panencephalitis; congenital rubella infection manifests as intrauterine growth retardation, deafness, cataracts, glaucoma, microcephaly, and mental retardation; rubella encephalitis is rare, symptoms include headache, dizziness, lethargy, seizures, behavioral changes, and coma; polyradiculoneuritis presents similar to GBS but has a brief course; rubella panencephalitis presents with dementia, cerebellar syndrome affecting gait and extremity function, spasticity, optic atrophy and retinopathy, lymphocytic CSF pleocytosis, and occasional seizures and myoclonus; no specific treatment.

Scheie's Syndrome

Milder version of Hurler syndrome; autosomal recessive lysosomal storage disease, with accumulation of dermatan sulfate and heparan sulfate within affected tissues; caused by deficiency of α-L-iduronidase; juvenile onset of stiff joints, clawhands, deformed feet, corneal clouding, pigmentary degeneration of the retina, coarse facial features, glaucoma, carpal tunnel syndrome, and deafness; stature and intelligence are normal; psychological disturbances and cardiac dysfunction may be noted; diagnosis via demonstration of excess urinary dermatan sulfate and heparan sulfate, and deficiency of α-L-iduronidase in cultured fibroblasts; no specific treatment.

Schwartz-Jampel Syndrome

Chondrodystrophic myotonia; three forms are recognized; the most common is the late-infantile variant, which is autosomal recessive and mapped to 1p34-p36.1; a neonatal variant, which is more severe and often fatal, is not linked to chromosome 1; and an autosomal dominant variant, which is unmapped; muscles are stiff, especially in the face and thighs; muscle hypertrophy may be noted; EMG demonstrates continuous myotonia, with minimal waxing and waning; other associated features include facial abnormalities (narrow palpebral fissures, pinched nose, micrognathia) and skeletal anomalies (short neck, flexion contractures, kyphosis); treatment is symptomatic; improvement may occur with membrane-stabilizing drugs (phenytoin).

Serotonin Syndrome

Iatrogenic disorder caused most often by the use of serotonin reuptake inhibitor drugs, either alone or in combination with other medications; clinical features include altered mental status and confusion, agitation, myoclonus, hyperreflexia, tremor, incoordination, nausea and diarrhea, low-grade fever, autonomic instability, diaphoresis, and rigidity; occurs after a serotoninergic drug is started or the dosage increased; also may be induced by the use of a selective serotonin reuptake inhibitor (SSRI) in combination with a monoamine oxidase inhibitor or tricyclic antidepressant; other etiologies must be ruled out (i.e., infection, metabolic alteration, substance abuse); treatment consists of drug withdrawal and supportive care.

Sjögren's Syndrome

Vasculitic and inflammatory disorder of unknown etiology, defined by two or more of the following symptoms: xerostomia, xerophthalmia, or keratoconjunctivitis sicca (diagnosed by Shirmer test); most common neurologic complications are sensorimotor peripheral neuropathy and polymyositis; oculomotor and trigeminal sensory neuropathies may occur; CNS involvement can manifest as aseptic meningitis, focal cerebral deficits, seizures, cognitive decline, personality changes, and optic neuropathy; spinal cord may present as myelopathy, transverse myelitis, or intraspinal hemorrhage; CSF may show pleocytosis and elevated protein; MRI can demonstrate high-signal regions of ischemia; symptoms related to vasculitis respond well to corticosteroids; supportive care.

Subacute Sclerosing Panencephalitis (SSPE)

Dawson disease; chronic viral infection caused by a defective measles virus (deficient viral M protein); preadolescent children and young adults are affected (males more often than females); initial clinical features include the gradual onset of forgetfulness, difficulty with homework, and restlessness; followed in weeks to months by incoordination, ataxia, myoclonic jerks of the trunk and extremities, apraxia, loss of speech, and seizures; late-stage disease reveals loss of vision, hearing, dementia, and a rigid quadriplegia; pathology demonstrates neuronal degeneration, perivascular infiltration, demyelination, and gliosis in the cortex, white matter, and deep nuclei; no definitive treatment; stabilization may occur with intrathecal interferon alfa.

Sydenham Chorea

St. Vitus dance; rheumatic chorea; acquired chorea of childhood caused by an autoimmune reaction to infection with group A β-hemolytic streptococcus; clinical features include the onset of rapid, irregular, aimless, involuntary movements of the muscles of the limbs, face, and trunk; patients appear to be very restless; other findings include muscular weakness, hypotonia, emotional lability, irritability, and obsessive-compulsive symptoms; less common manifestations are speech impairment, headache, seizures, and cranial neuropathy; EEG reveals diffuse slowing; CSF often normal, may show pleocytosis; MRI normal or may demonstrate enlargement of the basal ganglia; course benign, with improvement in 4–8 weeks; symptoms may improve with benzodiazepines, valproic acid, or corticosteroids.

Tay-Sachs Disease

G_{M2}-gangliosidosis type I; infantile variant of storage disease with deficiency of hexosaminidase A; autosomal recessive inheritance pattern; normal development until onset of symptoms by 6 months of age; clinical features include irritability and hyperexcitability, exaggerated startle response, delayed cognitive development, motor retardation with hypotonia, hyperactive reflexes, clonus, extensor plantar responses, progressive visual impairment, complete blindness by 1 year in most cases, presence of macular cherry-red spot, and occasional myoclonic seizures; vegetative state occurs by the second year; pathology reveals ballooned neurons in brain, cerebellum, and spinal cord; no specific treatment; supportive care.

Thoracic Outlet Syndrome

Group of disorders that cause compression of the nerves or blood vessels of the brachial plexus; C8 and T1 nerve roots and lower trunk of the plexus can be compressed by cervical ribs, fibrous bands, and hypertrophic scalenus muscles; pain is present in the shoulder, arm, and hand (fourth and fifth digits); use of the limb may exacerbate the pain and induce fatigue; hypesthesia of affected areas may be noted; wasting and weakness of muscles in the hand occurs; EMG is consistent with the appropriate nerve injury; MRI may show distortion or impingement along the pathway of nerves or vessels; surgery and physical therapy are the appropriate treatment.

Tolosa-Hunt Syndrome

Painful ophthalmoplegia syndrome; noncaseating granulomatous disorder of unknown etiology characterized by severe retro-orbital and supra-orbital pain, diplopia, paralysis of cranial nerves III, IV, and VI; less frequent involvement of cranial nerves II, V1, and V2; inflammation involves the superior orbital fissure and cavernous sinus region; visualized clearly on enhanced MRI scans; typical onset in middle to late life; dramatic clinical response to oral prednisone (60–80 mg/day); pain improves rapidly with treatment, ophthalmoplegia may take weeks to months to resolve; differential diagnosis includes syphilis, temporal arteritis, sarcoidosis, and systemic lupus erythematosus.

Trypanosomiasis

See Chagas disease; African form of trypanosomiasis *(Trypanosoma brucei)*; infection usually is transmitted person to person by the tsetse fly, occasionally by other flies or insects; clinical features include an acute febrile stage with rash, lymphadenitis, splenomegaly, arthralgias, asthenia, and myalgias; chronic stage involves the CNS and includes tremor, seizures, confusion, incoordination, headache, paralysis, and eventual coma; laboratory abnormalities may include elevated ESR and anemia, CSF lymphocytic pleocytosis with elevated protein and γ-globulins; diagnosis made by demonstration of organisms in blood, CSF, or biopsy materials, or by serologic and CSF antibody testing; treatment with suramin or eflornithine is effective in the acute stages; melarsoprol for infections of the CNS.

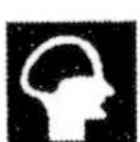

Turner Syndrome

Chromosomal anomaly associated with a 45, X karyotype (X-chromosomal monosomy); major clinical features are female phenotype, short stature, a shieldlike chest, short and sometimes webbed neck, low-set ears, high-arched palate, small mandible, and sexual infantilism; associated findings include cardiac and renal defects, skeletal anomalies, nerve deafness, and congenital lymphedema; psychological testing reveals poor visuospatial and intellectual function, difficulty with attention, and impaired social behaviors; MRI may reveal volumetric loss in the parietal lobes, hippocampus, thalamus, caudate, and lenticular nuclei; treatment consists of hormone replacement therapy to improve growth retardation (recombinant growth hormone) and sexual infantilism.

Vogt-Koyanagi-Harada Syndrome

Characterized by uveitis, retinal hemorrhages and detachment, depigmentation of the skin (i.e., vitiligo) and hair (i.e., poliosis and canities), alopecia, and neurologic symptoms, which are caused by an inflammatory adhesive arachnoiditis; clinical features include headache, dizziness, somnolence, fatigue, ocular palsies, and meningeal signs; sensorineural deafness, hemiplegia, and psychosis are noted less frequently; CSF has elevated pressure and moderate lymphocytic pleocytosis, minimal increase in protein, normal glucose, intermittent elevation of γ-globulin; symptoms last for 6–12 months before improvement; etiology unknown, although a virus is suspected; no specific therapy, although steroids may be beneficial.

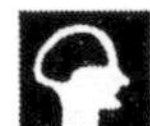

Von Hippel-Lindau Disease

Characterized by coexistence of multiple hemangioblastomas of the CNS, angiomas of the retina, cysts of the kidney and pancreas, capillary nevi of the skin, and systemic neoplasms such as renal cell carcinoma and pheochromocytoma; autosomal dominant inheritance, linked to mutations of tumor suppressor gene on chromosome 3p25.5; onset usually between ages 15 and 50 years; hemangioblastomas are vascular neoplasms that typically develop in the midline cerebellar hemispheres, less often in the medulla and spinal cord; clinical presentation includes headache, ataxia, nausea, emesis, and dizziness; hydrocephalus is common; treatment of choice is surgical resection; radiotherapy may be of benefit.

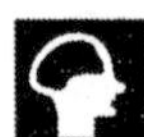

Wegener Granulomatosis

Systemic vasculitis syndrome that primarily attacks the respiratory system and kidneys; diagnostic criteria include oral ulcers, purulent bloody nasal discharge, pulmonary infiltrates or nodules, glomerulonephritis with microhematuria, and biopsy evidence of granulomatous inflammation of arteries or perivascular tissue; neurologic complications include peripheral neuropathy (typically mononeuritis multiplex), stroke, cranial neuropathies, headache, ophthalmoplegia, and ischemic optic neuropathy; most patients have elevated ESR and are cANCA positive; MRI may be normal or reveal ischemic high-signal lesions; angiography usually is normal; brain or lung biopsy may be necessary for diagnosis; treatment consists of prednisone and cyclophosphamide.

Wolman Disease

Storage disease characterized by a deficiency of the enzyme acid lipase, which has been mapped to a gene on chromosome 10q23.2; accumulation of cholesterol esters and triglycerides in affected tissues; infants are normal at birth but have rapid onset of severe vomiting, abdominal distention, malabsorption with diarrhea, poor weight gain, jaundice, fever, diffuse rash, hepatosplenomegaly, and adrenal insufficiency; adrenal calcification is noted on radiographs; neurologic involvement is generally mild and includes delayed intellectual development and mild spasticity; the course is generally quite rapid, death occurs within 3–6 months in most cases; no treatment available.

Xeroderma Pigmentosum (XP)

De Sanctis-Cacchione syndrome; group of autosomal recessive disorders characterized by loss of genes required for excision of damaged DNA and for replication past regions of damaged DNA; mutations can occur in genes mapped to several loci, depending on type of XP (9q34.1, 2q21, 3p25.1, and others); cells are hypersensitive to ultraviolet light and chemical carcinogens; clinical features include early sensitivity to light with blistering and erythema, dwarfism, increased risk of skin cancer, microcephaly, mental retardation, chorea, ataxia, spasticity, peripheral nerve dysfunction (motor neuron disorder, segmental demyelination), hearing loss, and supranuclear ophthalmoplegia; no specific treatment; management includes avoidance of sunlight, reduced exposure to environmental carcinogens, and surveillance for malignancies.

Zellweger Syndrome

Cerebrohepatorenal syndrome; autosomal recessive peroxisomal disorder; symptoms are present at birth, including hypotonia, reduced activity, poor infantile reflexes (Moro, stepping, placing), hypoactive reflexes, characteristic facies (high narrow forehead, round cheeks, wide-set eyes, high-arched palate, small chin); other features include pigmentary retinopathy, optic atrophy, poor suck and swallow, congenital heart disease, cystic renal dysplasia, liver cirrhosis, splenomegaly, genital and skeletal anomalies, and seizures; MRI shows atrophy, poor myelination, pachygyria, and polymicrogyria; caused by dysfunction in multiple enzyme pathways, with increased levels of VLCFAs, bile acid intermediates, pipecolic acid, and phytanic acid; no specific treatment; supportive care.

Index